Textbook of Forensic Medicine and Toxicology

(Revised Third Edition)

Dr. P.C. Dikshit

M.D. (AIIMS), LL.B., FICFMT, FDAME, W.H.O. Fellow
Director Professor and Head (Retd.)
Department of Forensic Medicine and Toxicology
Maulana Azad Medical College and Associated Hospitals, New Delhi, India

Professor and Head (Retd.)
Department of Forensic Medicine and Toxicology
Hamdard Institute of Medical Sciences and Research
and Associated HAHC Hospital, Jamia Hamdard, New Delhi

and

Dr. Chittaranjan Behera

M.D. (AIIMS), MAMS, FIMSA, FICFMT, ICMR International Fellow
Professor
Department of Forensic Medicine and Toxicology
All India Institute of Medical Sciences, New Delhi, India

Peepee Publishers and Distributors Private Limited®

Textbook of Forensic Medicine and Toxicology

Published by:
Pawaninder P. Vij and Anupam Vij

Peepee Publishers and Distributors Private Limited
Head Office: 160, Shakti Vihar, Pitam Pura, Delhi-110 034 (India)

Correspondence Address:
7/31, First Floor, Ansari Road, Daryaganj
New Delhi-110 002 (India)

Ph: 41512412, 9811156083

e-mail: *peepee160@yahoo.co.in*

e-mail: *peepee160@gmail.com*

www.peepeepub.com

join us on facebook.com/pp.publishers

First Edition : 2007

Third Edition : 2022

Revised Edition: 2026

ISBN: 978-81-8445-295-2

Dedicated to

My dear wife Dr. Bharati

and Sons

Kunal and Rahul

who always stood with me during the odds

P.C. Dikshit

Preface to the Third Edition

The book having met with such a large measure of success, we thought it would be desirable to bring out a new edition incorporating the most recent developments in the subject. As we all know that medical science is a rapidly evolving field and one has to be updated in his/her knowledge to keep in pace with these changes. The MCI announced the **"Competency-based Undergraduate Curriculum for the Indian Medical Graduate"** regulation in 2018. This is an outcome driven curriculum that is in line with current global trends. The MCI was replaced by **National Medical Commission (NMC)** in the year 2020. The NMC shall perform the functions as per the National Medical Commission Act, 2019. Recently many amendments have taken place in the law specially in context of sexual offences, artificial reproduction techniques, surrogacy, mental health etc. In this edition, an effort has been made to inform readers about these modifications.

The simple style of writing which was the plus point of the 2nd edition is retained in this edition as well. It will help the undergraduate students to understand the concept of Forensic Medicine in a better way. Extensive use of tables and related colour diagrams provides value addition to the text. We have also rearranged the matter with the object of making the various sections more consecutive than they were previously to make a better sense of them. At the end of each chapters, potential long questions, short notes and multiple choice questions have been added. Besides undergraduates, this book also targets the postgraduates, post-doctoral and students from Forensic Science, Forensic Nursing branches. However, in today's world of rising medical malpractice claims, every physician must be aware of his or her legal obligations, which is why specific devoted chapters such as Legal Procedures and Laws in Relation to Medical Practice are presented with up-to-date information.

We trust that having thoroughly revised, it may prove as useful to the students preparing for examination in the future as it has been in the past. Every effort has been made to ensure that this book is free from any mistake. However, to err is human. Therefore, readers are welcome to post their comments and suggestions to the email: *drchitta75@gmail.com* or *pcdikshit@yahoo.com* to help in improving this book.

P.C. Dikshit

C. Behera

Preface to the First Edition

I feel great pleasure in presenting the book **Textbook of Forensic Medicine and Toxicology**. The book is intended to cater to the needs of medical as well as legal community. The book is student-friendly and written in a simple style covering the whole curriculum of undergraduate students. The book would be beneficial not only for U.G. but for P.G. students and medical officers posted in health care setup. It has been designed in a simpler form with photographs wherever necessary for easy grasp among the students. Moreover, tables, diagrams and salient points have been incorporated for easy understanding and memorization of the subject. To inculcate vast coverage of the subject, quite a number of books and journals have been consulted and advice has been sought from colleagues and teachers. No doubt the book is a departure from the conventional writing.

In the past decade there has been an increase in medical negligence cases. New government laws and regulations have a deep impact on medicine. Biomedical research has created new questions that have not been considered before. There are questions as to whether death has occurred at the moment declared. The spread of AIDS has created new problem for doctors and law enforcement agencies. The criminal law is now involved with prostitutes and homosexuals who can spread the disease. Even malpractice litigation has caused the face of medicine to change. As a result, the field of Forensic Medicine had shown a drastic change.

Keeping this in mind, some of the newer and modern concepts such as DNA fingerprinting, cloning, euthanasia, assisted reproduction technologies have been included with all the details. Older topics such as Sexual Offences, Infanticide, Abortion, Impotence and Sterility, Virginity, Pregnancy, Delivery and Legitimacy have been revised with addition of the related legal amendments. Certain topics like Law in Relation to Medical Men, Road Traffic Accidents, Asphyxial Deaths and Mechanical Injuries can be used as reference chapters. The inclusion of topics such as Moment of Death with different schools of thought, World Scenario in Euthanasia and AIDS and the latest safety measures in vehicles makes the book quite readable. The chapters like Infanticide, Firearms, Forensic Psychiatry have been written thoroughly. In addition, topics like Dysbarism and Barotrauma, Fall From Height, Biological and Chemical Warfare Agents that are usually neglected have been incorporated. The relevant laws and Acts have also been included along with the topics. In addition, chapters on Toxicology have been dealt in Indian context after thoroughly revising and by adding the latest management protocols. Brief index of all the poisonings with their management have been summarized that would fulfil the needs of the undergraduate students during examination. Moreover, the possible questions included in each of the chapter of Part 1 and at the end of Part 2 will help them tremendously.

I feel and sincerely hope that this book will immensely benefit the undergraduate and postgraduate medical students. In addition, the book will help the police officers as well as lawyers while investigating and solving many crime related problems. I trust that this book will be a valuable reference book to all who work in the fields of law and medicine.

Lastly, I feel that the readers are the best judges and their suggestions and healthy criticism will be of immense help in the future for further improvement of this book. The readers can contact me at *e-mail: pcdikshit@yahoo.com*

P.C. Dikshit

Contents

Part 1: Forensic Medicine and Pathology

Part 2: Forensic Toxicology

Competency Based Medical Education in Forensic Medicine and Toxicology for MBBS Students As Per Guidelines of NMC

Number	Competency: The student should be able to:	Page No.
	Introduction and History of Forensic Medicine	
FM 1.1	Demonstrate knowledge of basics of Forensic Medicine like definitions of Forensic Medicine, Clinical Forensic Medicine, Forensic Pathology, State Medicine, Legal Medicine and Medical Jurisprudence	1
FM 1.2	Describe history of Forensic Medicine	2-3
	Legal Procedure	
FM 1.3	Describe legal procedures including Criminal Procedure Code, Indian Penal Code, Indian Evidence Act, Civil and Criminal Cases, Inquest (Police Inquest and Magistrate's Inquest), Cognizable and Non-cognizable offences	5-9
FM 1.4	Describe Courts in India and their powers: Supreme Court, High Court, Sessions Court, Magistrate's Court, Labour Court, Family Court, Executive Magistrate Court and Juvenile Justice Board	7-8
FM 1.5	Describe Court procedures including issue of Summons, conduct money, types of witnesses, recording of evidence oath, affirmation, examination in chief, cross-examination, re-examination and Court questions, recording of evidence and conduct of doctor in witness box	9-12,16
FM 1.6	Describe Offenses in Court including Perjury; Court strictures vis-a-vis Medical Officer	9-10
FM 1.7	Describe Dying Declaration and Dying Deposition	15-16
FM 1.9	Describe the importance of documentation in medical practice in regard to medicolegal examinations, Medical Certificates and medicolegal reports especially • Maintenance of patient case records, discharge summary, prescribed registers to be maintained in Health Centres • Maintenance of medicolegal register like accident register • Documents of issuance of wound certificate • Documents of issuance of drunkenness certificate • Documents of issuance of sickness and fitness certificate • Documents for issuance of death certificate • Documents of Medical Certification of Cause of Death • Form Number 4 and 4A documents for estimation of age by physical, dental and radiological examination and issuance of certificate	12-15, 25, 38-39, 42, 176, 600-604
FM 1.10	Select appropriate cause of death in a particular scenario by referring ICD 10 code	14-15
FM 1.11	Write a correct cause of death certificate as per ICD 10 document	13-14
	Thanatology	
FM 2.1	Define, describe and discuss death and its types including somatic/clinical/cellular, molecular and brain-death, Cortical Death and Brainstem Death	49-51

FM 2.2	Describe and discuss natural and unnatural deaths	6-7
FM 2.3	Describe and discuss issues related to sudden natural deaths	154-161
FM 2.4	Describe salient features of the Organ Transplantation and The Human Organ Transplant (Amendment) Act 2011 and discuss ethical issues regarding organ donation	54-57
FM 2.5	Discuss moment of death, modes of death–coma, asphyxia and syncope	49-58
FM 2.6	Discuss presumption of death and survivorship	61
FM 2.7	Describe and discuss suspended animation	51
FM 2.8	Describe and discuss postmortem changes including signs of death, cooling of body, postmortem lividity, rigor mortis, cadaveric spasm, cold stiffening and heat stiffening	102-111
FM 2.9	Describe putrefaction, mummification, adipocere and maceration	111-119
FM 2.10	Discuss estimation of time since death	119-121
	Autopsy Procedures and Exhumation	
FM 2.11	Describe and discuss autopsy procedures including postmortem examination, different types of autopsies, aims and objectives of postmortem examination	123-132
FM 2.12	Describe the legal requirements to conduct postmortem examination and procedures to conduct medicolegal postmortem examination	123-132
FM 2.13	Describe and discuss obscure autopsy	133-134
FM 2.14	Describe and discuss examination of clothing, preservation of viscera on postmortem examination for chemical analysis and other medicolegal purposes, postmortem artefacts	124-125, 132, 147-150
FM 2.15	Describe special protocols for conduction of medicolegal autopsies in cases of death in custody or following violation of human rights as per National Human Rights Commission Guidelines	276-277
FM 2.16	Describe and discuss examination of mutilated bodies or fragments,charred bones and bundle of bones	135-138
FM 2.17	Describe and discuss exhumation	135
	Crime Scene Investigation	
FM 2.18	Describe and discuss the objectives of crime scene visit, the duties and responsibilities of doctors on crime scene and the reconstruction of sequence of events after crime scene investigation	140-146
	Investigation of Anesthetic, Operative Deaths	
FM 2.19	Describe and discuss special protocols for conduction of autopsy and for collection, preservation and dispatch of related material evidences	151-153
	Asphyxial Deaths	
FM 2.20	Define, classify and describe asphyxia and medicolegal interpretation of postmortem findings in asphyxial deaths	279-282
FM 2.21	Describe and discuss different types of hanging and strangulation including clinical findings, causes of death, postmortem findings and medicolegal aspects of death due to hanging and strangulation including examination, preservation and dispatch of ligature material	282-293
FM 2.22	Describe and discuss pathophysiology, clinical features, postmortem findings and medicolegal aspects of traumatic asphyxia, obstruction of nose and mouth, suffocation and sexual asphyxia	294-299
FM 2.23	Describe and discuss types, pathophysiology, clinical features, postmortem findings and medicolegal aspects of drowning, diatom test and gettler test	299-305
	Thermal Injuries	
FM 2.24	Describe the clinical features, postmortem finding and medicolegal aspects of injuries due to physical agents like heat (heat-hyperpyrexia, heat stroke, sun stroke, heat exhaustion/ prostration, heat cramps [miner's cramp] or cold (systemic and localized hypothermia, frostbite, trench foot, immersion foot)	235-237

FM 2.25	Describe types of injuries, clinical features, pathophysiology, postmortem findings and medico-legal aspects in cases of burns, scalds, lightening, electrocution and radiations	237-249
	Starvation Deaths	
FM 2.26	Describe and discuss clinical features, postmortem findings and medicolegal aspects of death due to starvation and neglect	430-431
	Infanticide	
FM 2.27	Define and discuss infanticide, foeticide and stillbirth	308-310
FM 2.28	Describe and discuss signs of intrauterine death, signs of live birth, viability of foetus, age determination of foetus, DOAP session of ossification centres, Hydrostatic test, Sudden Infants Death syndrome and Munchausen's syndrome by proxy	64-66 310-320
	Identification	
FM 3.1	Define and describe Corpus Delicti, establishment of identity of living persons including race, sex, religion, complexion, stature, age determination using morphology, teeth-eruption, decay, bite marks, bones-ossification centres, medicolegal aspects of age	63-85
FM 3.2	Describe and discuss identification of criminals, unknown persons, dead bodies from the remains–hairs fibers, teeth, anthropometry, dactylography, foot prints, scars, tattoos, poroscopy and superimposition	86-99
	Mechanical Injuries and Wounds	
FM 3.3	Define, describe and classify different types of mechanical injuries, abrasion, bruise, laceration, stab wound, incised wound, chop wound, defense wound, self-inflicted/fabricated wounds and their medicolegal aspects	162-176
FM 3.4	Define injury, assault and hurt. Describe IPC pertaining to injuries	258-261
FM 3.5	Describe accidental, suicidal and homicidal injuries. Describe simple, grievous and dangerous injuries. Describe antemortem and postmortem injuries	176, 258-261
FM 3.6	Describe healing of injury and fracture of bones with its medicolegal importance	267-270
FM 3.7	Describe factors influencing infliction of injuries and healing, examination and certification of wounds and wound as a cause of death: Primary and Secondary	267-270
FM 3.8	Describe and discuss different types of weapons including dangerous weapons and their examination	261
	Firearm Injuries	
FM 3.9	Describe different types of firearms including structure and components. Along with description of ammunition propellant charge and mechanism of firearms, different types of cartridges and bullets and various terminology in relation of firearm–caliber, range, choking	186-191
FM 3.10	Describe and discuss wound ballistics–different types of firearm injuries, blast injuries and their interpretation, preservation and dispatch of trace evidences in cases of firearm and blast injuries, various tests related to confirmation of use of firearms	192-200
	Regional Injuries	
FM 3.11	Describe and discuss regional injuries to head (Scalp wounds, fracture skull, intracranial hemorrhages, coup and contrecoup injuries), neck, chest, abdomen, limbs, genital organs, spinal cord and skeleton	202-219
FM 3.12	Describe and discuss injuries related to fall from height and vehicular injuries–Primary and Secondary impact, Secondary injuries, crush syndrome, railway spine	178-180, 220, 228-231
	Sexual Offences	
FM 3.13	Describe different types of sexual offences. Describe various sections of IPC regarding rape including definition of rape (Section 375 IPC), Punishment for Rape (Section 376 IPC) and recent amendments notified till date	371-379

FM 3.14	Describe and discuss the examination of the victim of an alleged case of rape, and the preparation of report, framing the opinion and preservation and dispatch of trace evidences in such cases	379-388, 591-598
FM 3.15	Describe and discuss examination of accused and victim of sodomy, preparation of report, framing of opinion, preservation and despatch of trace evidences in such cases	393-395, 591-598, 599
FM 3.16	Describe and discuss adultery and unnatural sexual offences–sodomy, incest, lesbianism, buccal coitus, bestiality, indecent assault and preparation of report, framing the opinion and preservation and dispatch of trace evidences in such cases	391, 393-395, 591-598, 599
FM 3.17	Describe and discuss the sexual perversions fetishism, transvestism, voyeurism, sadism, necrophagia, masochism, exhibitionism, frotteurism, Necrophilia	395-398
	Virginity, Pregnancy, Delivery and Legitimacy	
FM 3.18	Describe anatomy of male and female genitalia, hymen and its types. Discuss the medicolegal importance of hymen. Define virginity, defloration, legitimacy and its medicolegal importance	326-329
FM 3.19	Discuss the medicolegal aspects of pregnancy and delivery, signs of pregnancy, precipitate labour superfoetation, superfecundation and signs of recent and remote delivery in living and dead	329-335
FM 3.20	Discuss disputed paternity and maternity	335,360, 401, 415
	Abortion, Impotency and Sterility, Assisted Reproduction Techniques	
FM 3.21	Discuss Pre-conception and Prenatal-Diagnostic Techniques (PC & PNDT)–Prohibition of Sex Selection Act 2003 and Domestic Violence Act 2005	277-278, 345-346
FM 3.22	Define and discuss impotence, sterility, frigidity, sexual dysfunction, premature ejaculation. Discuss the causes of impotence and sterility in male and female	322-324
FM 3.23	Discuss sterilization of male and female, artificial insemination, Test Tube Baby, surrogate mother, hormonal replacement therapy with respect to appropriate national and state laws	348-359, 361
FM 3.24	Discuss the relative importance of surgical methods of contraception (vasectomy and tubectomy) as methods of contraception in the National Family Planning Programme	346
FM 3.25	Discuss the major results of the National Family Health Survey	346-347
FM 3.26	Discuss the national guidelines for accreditation, supervision and regulation of ART Clinics in India	355-358
FM 3.27	Define, classify and discuss abortion, methods of procuring MTP and criminal abortion and complication of abortion. Medical Termination of Pregnancy (Amendment) Act, 2021	337-343
FM 3.28	Describe evidences of abortion–living and dead, duties of doctor in cases of abortion, investigations of death due to criminal abortion	343-344
	Child Abuse	
FM 3.29	Describe and discuss child abuse and battered baby syndrome	317-319
	Torture and Custodial Deaths	
FM 3.30	Describe and discuss issues relating to torture, identification of injuries caused by torture and its sequelae, management of torture survivors	272-275
FM 3.31	Torture and Human Rights Describe and discuss guidelines and Protocols of National Human Rights Commission regarding torture	276-277
	Medical Jurisprudence (Medical Law and Ethics)	
FM 4.1	Describe Medical Ethics and explain its historical emergence	22
FM 4.2	Describe the Code of Medical Ethics 2002 conduct, Etiquette and Ethics in medical practice and unethical practices and the dichotomy	24-28
FM 4.3	Describe the functions and role of National Medical Commission and State Medical Councils	18-22

FM 4.4	Describe the Indian Medical Register	21
FM 4.5	Rights/privileges of a medical practitioner, penal erasure, infamous conduct, disciplinary committee, disciplinary procedures, warning notice and penal erasure	24-25, 28-29
FM 4.6	Describe the Laws in Relation to medical practice and the duties of a medical practitioner towards patients and society	25-28
FM 4.7	Describe and discuss the ethics related to HIV patients	361-367
FM 4.8	Describe the Consumer Protection Act, 2019 (Medical Indemnity Insurance, Civil Litigations and Compensations), Employee's Compensation (Amendment) Act, 2017 and ESI Act (Amendment), 2010	41-43
FM 4.9	Describe the medicolegal issues in relation to family violence, violation of human rights, NHRC and doctors	277-278
FM 4.10	Describe communication between doctors, public and media	29-31
FM 4.11	Describe and discuss euthanasia	58-61
FM 4.12	Discuss legal and ethical issues in relation to stem cell research	46-47
FM 4.13	Describe social aspects of medicolegal cases with respect to victims of assault, rape, attempted suicide, homicide, domestic violence, dowry-related cases	244, 259-260, 277-278, 378,424
FM 4.14	Describe and discuss the challenges in managing medicolegal cases including development of skills in relationship management–Human behaviour, communication skills, conflict resolution techniques	29-32
FM 4.15	Describe the principles of handling pressure–definition, types, causes, sources and skills for managing the pressure while dealing with medicolegal cases by the doctor	31-32
FM 4.16	Describe and discuss Bioethics	22
FM 4.17	Describe and discuss ethical Principles: Respect for autonomy, non-malfeasance, beneficence and justice	22
FM 4.18	Describe and discuss medical negligence including civil and criminal negligence, contributory negligence, corporate negligence, vicarious liability, Res Ipsa Loquitor, prevention of medical negligence and defenses in medical negligence litigations	34-38
FM 4.19	Define Consent. Describe different types of consent and ingredients of informed consent. Describe the rules of consent and importance of consent in relation to age, emergency situation, mental illness and alcohol intoxication	32-33
FM 4.20	Describe therapeutic privilege, Malingering, Therapeutic Misadventure, Professional Secrecy, Human Experimentation	32,37, 33, 43-46, 401
FM 4.21	Describe Products Liability and Medical Indemnity Insurance	38-39, 42
FM 4.22	Explain Oath – Hippocrates, Charaka and Sushruta and procedure for administration of Oath	23-24
FM 4.23	Describe the modified Declaration of Geneva and its relevance	23-24,43
FM 4.24	Enumerate rights, privileges and duties of a Registered Medical Practitioner. Discuss doctor-patient relationship: Professional secrecy and privileged communication	24-26,33-34
FM 4.25	Clinical Research and Ethics Discuss human experimentation including clinical trials	43-47
FM 4.26	Discuss the constitution and functions of ethical committees	45-46
FM 4.27	Describe and discuss Ethical Guidelines for Biomedical Research on Human Subjects and Animals	45-46
	Forensic Psychiatry	
FM 5.1	Classify common mental illnesses including post-traumatic stress disorder (PTSD)	418-419
FM 5.2	Define, classify and describe delusions, hallucinations, illusion, lucid interval and obsessions with exemplification	419-421

FM 5.3	Describe Civil and criminal responsibilities of a mentally ill person	424-428
FM 5.4	Differentiate between true insanity from feigned insanity	425
FM 5.5	Describe and discuss Delirium tremens	418
FM 5.6	Describe the Indian Mental Health Care Act, 2017 with special reference to admission, care and discharge of a mentally ill person	423-424
	Forensic Laboratory Investigation in Medical Legal Practice	
FM 6.1	Describe different types of specimen and tissues to be collected both in the living and dead: Body fluids (blood, urine, semen, faeces, saliva), Skin, Nails, tooth pulp, vaginal smear, viscera, skull, specimen for histopathological examination, blood grouping, HLA Typing and DNA Fingerprinting Describe Locard's Exchange Principle	132, 141 384-385 401-408 410-415 443-444
FM 6.2	Describe the methods of sample collection, preservation, labelling, dispatch and interpretation of reports	132, 384-388, 401-408, 410-415, 443-445
	Emerging Technologies in Forensic Medicine	
FM 7.1	Enumerate the indications and describe the principles and appropriate use for: - DNA profiling - Facial reconstruction - Polygraph (Lie Detector) - Narcoanalysis - Brain mapping - Digital autopsy - Virtual autopsy - Imaging technologies	 410-415 98 390 389 390 134 134 134
	Toxicology: General Toxicology	
FM 8.1	Describe the history of Toxicology	432-433
FM 8.2	Define the terms Toxicology, Forensic Toxicology, Clinical Toxicology and Poison	433-434
FM 8.3	Describe the various types of poisons, Toxicokinetics and Toxicodynamics and diagnosis of poisoning in living and dead	433-435, 441-445
FM 8.4	Describe the Laws in relation to poisons including NDPS Act, Medicolegal aspects of poisons	448-450
FM 8.5	Describe Medicolegal autopsy in cases of poisoning including preservation and dispatch of viscera for chemical analysis	442-445
FM 8.6	Describe the general symptoms, principles of diagnosis and management of common poisons encountered in India	435-441
FM 8.7	Describe simple Bedside clinic tests to detect poison/drug in a patient's body fluids	445
FM 8.8	Describe basic methodologies in treatment of poisoning: Decontamination, supportive therapy, antidote therapy, procedures of enhanced elimination	435-441
FM 8.10	Describe the general principles of Analytical Toxicology and give a brief description of analytical methods available for toxicological analysis: Chromatography–Thin Layer Chromatography, Gas Chromatography, Liquid Chromatography and Atomic Absorption Spectroscopy	445-447
	Toxicology: Chemical Toxicology	
FM 9.1	Describe General Principles and basic methodologies in treatment of poisoning: Decontamination, supportive therapy, antidote therapy, procedures of enhanced elimination with regard to: Caustics Inorganic–Sulphuric, nitric and hydrochloric acids; Organic–Carbolic Acid (phenol), Oxalic and acetylsalicylic acids	452-459
FM 9.2	Describe General Principles and basic methodologies in treatment of poisoning: decontamination, supportive therapy, antidote therapy, procedures of enhanced elimination with regard to Phosphorus, Iodine, Barium	496-500

FM 9.3	Describe General Principles and basic methodologies in treatment of poisoning: Decontamination, supportive therapy, antidote therapy, procedures of enhanced elimination with regard to Arsenic, lead, mercury, copper, iron, cadmium and thallium	460-476
FM 9.4	Describe General Principles and basic methodologies in treatment of poisoning: Decontamination, supportive therapy, antidote therapy, procedures of enhanced elimination with regard to Ethanol, methanol, ethylene glycol	511-522
FM 9.5	Describe General Principles and basic methodologies in treatment of poisoning: Decontamination, supportive therapy, antidote therapy, procedures of enhanced elimination with regard to Organophosphates, Carbamates, Organochlorines, Pyrethroids, Paraquat, Aluminum and Zinc phosphide	561-570
FM 9.6	Describe General Principles and basic methodologies in treatment of poisoning: Decontamination, supportive therapy, antidote therapy, procedures of enhanced elimination with regard to Ammonia, carbon monoxide, hydrogen cyanide and derivatives, methyl isocyanate, tear (riot control) gases	458, 553-556, 541-543, 559
	Toxicology: Pharmaceutical Toxicology	
FM 10.1	Describe General Principles and basic methodologies in treatment of poisoning: Decontamination, supportive therapy, antidote therapy, procedures of enhanced elimination with regard to: i. Antipyretics–Paracetamol, Salicylates ii. Anti-Infectives (Common antibiotics–An overview) iii. Neuropsychotoxicology Barbiturates, benzodiazepine, phenytoin, lithium, haloperidol, neuroleptics, tricyclics iv. Narcotic Analgesics, Anesthetics and Muscle Relaxants v. Cardiovascular Toxicology Cardiotoxic plants–oleander, odollam, aconite, digitalis vi. Gastrointestinal and Endocrinal Drugs – Insulin	 574-575 576 526-529, 551, 576-577, 550 577-578 535-540 575-576
	Toxicology: Biotoxicology	
FM 11.1	Describe features and management of Snake bite, scorpion sting, bee and wasp sting and spider bite	485-496
	Toxicology: Sociomedical Toxicology	
FM 12.1	Describe features and management of abuse/poisoning with following chemicals: Tobacco, cannabis, amphetamines, cocaine, hallucinogens, designer drugs and solvent	377, 504-507, 507-509, 535-536,548-551, 572-573
	Toxicology: Environmental Toxicology	
FM 13.2	Describe medicolegal aspects of poisoning in Workman's Compensation Act	42

Part 1: Forensic Medicine and Pathology

1 CHAPTER

Introduction and History of Forensic Medicine

The origin of medicine is as old as civilization. In the early stages, the mankind used spirituality, herbs, God worship and witchcraft etc. for the cure. Then they felt the need of formulating certain rules and regulations for these practices that led to the origin of Medical Jurisprudence. With advancement of civilization various legal systems came into force and the knowledge of medicine became necessary for the purpose of law and justice and the concept of Legal medicine or Forensic Medicine originated. The term Forensic Medicine, Legal medicine and Medical Jurisprudence are used in different meanings.

Forensic medicine: It is the application of medical knowledge for the purpose of law both civil and criminal, for example in cases of vehicular accidents, the Forensic expert is able to give opinion whether the said injuries are due to vehicular accident or not, duration of injuries, nature of injuries and the cause of death etc. Similarly, in cases of sexual offences, he/she is able to opine whether the sexual act has been committed or not, duration and type of injuries on the person and private parts etc. The Forensic expert not only expertises in his own field but uses the knowledge of other branches of medical science to solve the problems related to forensic medicine, such as while conducting the postmortem in cases of accidental deaths, criminal abortion, anaesthetic deaths and sudden death due to medical and surgical causes.

Medical jurisprudence: It deals with legal aspects of practice of medicine. The concept of doctor-patient relationship, rights and duties of doctors, duties towards the patient and the state in particular the medical negligence etc. are all covered by the term Medical Jurisprudence.

Medical ethics: It deals with the moral principles that guide the members of medical profession when they deal with each other, their patients as well as with the State.

Medical etiquette: It deals with the conventional laws of courtesy observed between the members of the medical profession.

State medicine: It is a term, which was suggested for laws in relation to medical men by Dr. Stanford Emerson Chaille in the year 1949, but now-a-days it stands rejected worldwide. In India few States like West Bengal, Manipur and Assam etc. use the word and the subject is known as Forensic and State Medicine.

Forensic medicine can be divided into a number of sub-branches. **Forensic pathology** deals with morbid anatomy, pathology of injury and different aspects of death with their medicolegal significance. **Forensic psychiatry** is a very interesting branch where legal aspects of mental disorders are studied. **Forensic odontology** where the ability of dentist is undertaken when the question of identification, interpretation of bite marks and age determination arise. A number of factors are found in the teeth that are utilized for identification purposes. **Forensic anthropology** is study of bodily shape and skeletal formation in legal cases and also for the identification purposes.

Forensic science: It is a sister discipline of forensic medicine. Now-a-days this is mainly occupied by the non-medical scientists mainly a biologist or chemist who deals with the criminal aspects of crime investigations. There is a strong link between the forensic experts and forensic scientists as the former collects the evidences during medicolegal autopsy or while examining living persons and the latter carries out the test and gives the opinion. Therefore, both these branches are complementary to each other.

HISTORY OF FORENSIC MEDICINE IN INDIA AND ABROAD

The word forensic medicine came from the Latin word 'forensis' meaning marketplace, as during ancient days the justice used to be dispensed at marketplaces or common meeting places. The total period of forensic medicine can be divided into three phases:

1. Ancient phase: The law and medicine problems were found as written records in China, India, Egypt and Babylon etc. dating back to 5000 BC to 3000 BC. The **Hammurabi code** by King of Babylon is the oldest medicolegal code. Chief justice and Chief physician of the King Zoser of Egypt was the **first medicolegal** expert. Different techniques were developed for the preservation of the dead bodies (mummification). Indian civilization such as excavation remains of the Indus valley civilization (3200-2000 BC) gives the evidence of the use of medicines like *shilajit* and use of weapons made of bronze and copper.

Manu (3102 BC) was the **first lawgiver** in India. His **"Manusmriti"** gives the knowledge about the laws prevalent at that time. Various types of crimes like sexual offences, seduction and adultery have been mentioned. Those who were having mental illness were not allowed to enter into contract. King's permission was required to practice medicine. Definite rules were laid down to learn and practice medicine. It can be presumed that the origin of Medical Jurisprudence can be dated back to 3000 BC. At the same time, a Chinese materia medica provided information about poisons.

The **Vedas** of ancient India were composed between 3000 and1000 BC. The Rig Veda, the oldest one mentions about kings and their administration. Marriage was prohibited in blood relations. The Atharva Veda mentions cure for wounds, snake bite and poisons etc. in the form of mantras or charms while other Vedas mentions crimes like incest, adultery, abortion and drunkenness etc. along with the punishment for them. During this time dead bodies were dissected that can be compared to anatomical dissection as well as pathological autopsy of the present day.

At that time Ayurveda was quite advanced. The first treatise was **Agnivesh Charaka Samhita** supposed to have been composed during 700 BC. Here we find the description of rules of studying ayurveda, duties and rights of the students, privileges they can avail. This can be considered as the origin of medical ethics. In addition, there is a mention of poisons, their symptoms with treatment.

Between third and fourth century BC, the **Arthashashtra** of Kautilya was written. In this book, the penal laws are defined and the rules regarding the application of medical knowledge to legal matters has been mentioned which can be considered as the origin of legal medicine in India. The physicians were allowed to practice only after king's approval, similar to registration with Medical Council today. They were liable to be punished if there was any negligence during treatment. The other crimes like sexual offences, violation in marriage laws etc. were also punishable. There were provisions for the examination of dead bodies like postmortem examination of today. The body used to be kept in oil for examination in cases of sudden deaths. If any dead body that was swollen with eyes protruding out, marks on the neck, was taken granted that he has been killed by strangulation. Signs of death due to hanging, strangulation, drowning etc. have been mentioned. In cases of poisoning the portions of stomach and heart were put in the fire and the nature of flame and sound were noted to determine the nature of poison. Depending on the seriousness of the crimes, different types of punishments like whipping and cutting of body parts were awarded.

Hippocrates the father of western medicine (460 BC to 377 BC) was first to write the code of medical ethics. He practiced in the island of Kos in Greece and discussed the lethality of wounds at large. During 44 BC **Antistius** had **conducted the autopsy** on the body of Julius Caesar who was assassinated.

2. Medieval phase: Justinian court during the 1st to 5th century AD came into existence after the name of **Justinian**, the Roman Emperor who specified the role of medicolegal experts in dealing with medicolegal problems.

During the period of 12th to 15th century AD a Chinese treatise was published named **His-Huan-Lu**. The inquest was made obligatory in all types of unnatural deaths. Different types of injuries were defined and the manner of investigations to be done in these cases was also suggested.

During the period of 1000 AD to 1600 AD India was invaded by several foreign powers like Dutch, the French and East India Company so as to plunder its wealth and establish their colonies. Chaos and uncertainty prevailed in all spheres of life including law and order situation. Lastly, the East India Company conquered and ruled over India in the middle of 18th century until it handed over power to the British crown in 1857.

The **first medicolegal autopsy** was done by **Bartoloneo DE Varignana** in Bologna (Italy) in the year 1302 AD.

The **Constitutio Criminalis Carolina** was published in Germany in 1532 AD which wrote about different types of homicides that were not punishable for example if a criminal who is deprived of his judgment power was not responsible for the act like a murder committed by an insane that is being followed till today.

3. European phase (1600-1947 AD): Paulus Zacchias was the principal physician to Pope Innocent X and Alexander VII and an expert before the court "rota romana", the court of appeal. His works **"medicolegalis"** were published in seven volumes during 1621 to 1635 AD. This work remained an authority in medicolegal matters until the start of 19th century. He was considered as the father of Forensic Psychiatry as well as of legal medicine. An Italian physician **Fortunate Fedele** published the **first book in forensic medicine in 1602**. In 18th century, the post of professorship was created in Germany. **Orphila,** professor of chemistry and legal medicine at Paris is considered as **the father of modern toxicology**.

The British ruled over India till 1947 and introduced their system in every sphere like culture, education, administration, legal system and crime investigation etc. They introduced the allopathic system of medicine. The present legal system in India is a mixture of the English and Roman system, having been modified to suit the Indian conditions. The **first medical school** was established in Calcutta in 1822 that was later on converted into a medical college in the year 1835. Next medical school established in Madras in 1835, which was converted into a college in 1850. In Bombay, first medical college was established in the year 1950.

In 1857, the **first separate chair in medical jurisprudence** was created in Madras Medical College. Governor Lord Harris selected **Dr Urguhart,** a private practitioner and coroner of Madras as the first professor. Among the earlier professors were Dr Mouat, Dr John Moses of Calcutta Medical College, Dr A Porter and Lt. DG Roy of Madras Medical College and Major Collies Barry of Grant Medical College, Bombay. The books that were followed were brought from England. The popular English authors' books were Taylor's Principles and Practice of Medical Jurisprudence and Caspers Medical Jurisprudence.

The **first book for India** was written in 1856 by Dr Norman Chevers. The other books written in 1888 by Dr I B Lyon named Medical Jurisprudence for India, Outlines of Medical Jurisprudence by Lt. Colonel P Henir and J D B Gribel in 1889 and Legal Medicine in India and Toxicology by Major Collies Berry in 1902. Dr Jaising P Modi, lecturer at Agra Medical College and then at Lucknow Medical College since 1918 was a leading medicolegal expert. His first book the Text Book of Medical Jurisprudence and Toxicology was published in 1920. The book became popular not only with medical students but also among the lawyers and judges.

The British rulers subsequently codified the criminal law in India in 1833. The present Indian Penal Code (IPC) came into existence in 1860 and superseded all previous laws. The Criminal Procedure Code (CrPC) came into force from 1973. These laws are being followed till today. The procedure for crime investigation was systematized by the introduction of **Indian Police Act of 1861** and the coroner system by the **Indian Coroners Act 1871**. The coroner system was followed in Calcutta, Bombay and Madras whereas the rest of the country followed the police system.

The practice of modern medicine was first regulated by the formation of Provincial Medical Councils in 1912 according to which the medical practitioners were required to register themselves in the respective State Medical Councils.

In 1916 the **Indian Medical Degrees Act** was passed to recognize the qualifications from recognized institutions and to penalize persons having false certificates to practice medicine.

The **Indian Medical Council Act** was passed in the year 1933 and the Indian Medical Council was established to control the State Medical Councils and to maintain uniformity in medical education throughout the country. Later the Act was amended several times. Recently, the **National Medical Commission Act, 2019** was passed and under this Act, the **National Medical Commission** was established to regulate medical education and practice in India.

One of the greatest contributions India has made to modern criminology is dactylography or fingerprint system for personal identification. Towards the later part of 19th century that is in 1860 AD William Herschel, an Indian Civil Service officer posted at Nadia district of Bengal first used this method for identifying illiterate people while distributing money. After him Edward Richard Henry in 1891 AD developed the method further and published a book entitled **"Classification and use of fingerprints".** By his recommendation the Government of India also adopted this method of identification and established a fingerprint bureau in Bengal in 1897 AD. Subsequently this method was introduced in criminal investigation department of Scotland Yard in July 1901 by Henry himself who was posted there as Assistant Commissioner.

Then the medicolegal work was undertaken and postmortem centers were established at different places. During the time of East India Company, a postmortem was conducted in Madras in August 1693 by Dr Buckley in an alleged case of arsenic poisoning. This was probably the **first medicolegal autopsy of modern India**.

LONG QUESTION

1. Describe history of Forensic Medicine in India and abroad.

MULTIPLE CHOICE QUESTIONS

1. The oldest medicolegal code is:

(a) Hammurabi code (b) Tang code
(c) Code of Neslim (d) Code of Assura

2. The first lawgiver in India is:

(a) Panini (b) Manu
(c) Kautilya (d) Chanakya

3. The Code of Medical Ethics was first written by:

(a) Charaka (b) Manu
(c) Aristotle (d) Hippocrates

4. The first medicolegal autopsy was conducted at:

(a) United Kingdom (b) France
(c) Italy (d) Greece

5. The father of modern toxicology is:

(a) Orphila (b) Paulus Zachias
(c) Fortunate Fedele (d) Norman Chevers

6. The father of Forensic Psychiatry and Legal Medicine is:

(a) Antistius
(b) Bortoloneo DE Varignana
(c) Orphila
(d) Paulus Zachias

7. In British India, the coroner system was followed in all places *except*:

(a) Calcutta (b) Bombay
(c) Madras (d) Delhi

8. In modern India, the first medicolegal autopsy was conducted at:

(a) Calcutta (b) Bombay
(c) Madras (d) Delhi

9. The first book in Forensic Medicine was written by a physician of:

(a) U.S.A. (b) U.K.
(c) Italy (d) Denmark

ANSWER KEY ☞

1. (a)	2. (b)	3. (d)	4. (c)	5. (a)	6. (d)	7. (d)	8. (c)	9. (c)

2 CHAPTER

Legal Procedures

INTRODUCTION

The legal procedures described in this chapter should be followed in the cases where death has resulted from some unnatural cause and under suspicious circumstance. In all these cases, the investigating agency should be informed who conducts further investigations.

Legal procedures in India are based on:

1. The Constitution of India.
2. Code of Criminal Procedure (Cr.P.C.).
3. Indian Penal Code (I.P.C.); and
4. Indian Evidence Act (IEA).

The Constitution of India: It contains 395 chapters and 12 schedules. Sections here are known as articles. Some important contents are described below:

Part III: Fundamental Rights: 5 in number.

1. **Right to Equality (S. 14-18)**

   S. 14: Equality before law.

   S. 15: Prohibition of discrimination on grounds of race, religion, caste, sex, place of birth.

   S. 16: Equality of opportunity in matters of public employment.

   S. 17: Abolition of untouchability.

2. **Right to Freedom (S. 19-22)**

   S. 20: Protection in respect of conviction for certain offences.

   Note: Article 20(2), Constitution of India says that a person shall not be charged and convicted more than once for the same offence. S.300, Cr.P.C., says that person once convicted or acquitted not to be tried for same offence.

   S. 21: Protection of life and personal liberty.

   S. 22: Protection against arrest and detention in certain cases.

3. **Right Against Exploitation (S. 23-24)**

   S. 23: Prohibition of traffic in human beings and forced labour.

   S. 24: Prohibition of employment of children in factories.

4. **Right to Freedom of Religion (S. 25-28)**
5. **Cultural and Educational Rights**

Part IVA: Fundamental Duties (S. 51A)

On 5 August, 2019, the Indian Parliament revoked the Article 370 of the Indian Constitution. The Ranbir Penal Code which was earlier followed in Jammu and Kashmir has thus been dissolved. All central Acts are applicable retrospectively from 31 October 2019 in this region.

The Criminal Procedure Code, 1973 (Cr.P.C.): It deals with the procedure of investigation and trial of offences which is applicable to whole India. However, the provisions of this Code, other than those relating to Chapters VIII, X and XI thereof, shall not apply to the state of Nagaland and some other tribal areas but the concerned state Government may, by notification apply any or all these provisions in these areas. It provides for different classes of Courts and defines their powers. It also formulates duties of police in arresting offenders, dealing with absconders, in the production of documents and investigating offences. It defines offences into two categories: cognizable and non-cognizable. Some cases are triable by both magistrates as well as Courts of Sessions as indicated in S. 2 of Cr.P.C. However, when tried by a magistrate the punishment must be limited to magistrate's powers. The Code also provides for the period of detention undergone by the accused during investigation. The period of inquiry or trial is to be deducted from the sentence of imprisonment awarded by the Court and the balance period of punishment only should be undergone as punishment. A bar of limitation for taking cognizance ranging from 6 months-3 years has been prescribed in certain cases under S. 468.

The Indian Penal Code, 1860 (I.P.C.): It describes various offences and with their punishments in the Courts of law. It defines offences and several categories of the same offence are created such as House Trespass (S. 448-460, I.P.C.) and theft (S. 379-382 and 401 I.P.C.). Besides this, the I.P.C. also provides a chapter on general exceptions in which the right of self defence of person and property, extending to causing deaths in certain circumstances. S. 53, I.P.C. describes various punishments described later on.

The Indian Evidence Act, 1872 (IEA): It relates to evidence on which the Courts could come to some conclusion about the facts of the case.

Criminal law: It relates to the offences that are against the interest of the public namely offences against the person, property, safety of the public as well as security of the state.

Civil law: It deals with disputes between two individuals or parties called the plaintiff and defendant (accused).

INQUEST

An inquest is the investigation into the cause of death in cases of sudden, unnatural and suspicious deaths conducted by the legal authorities such as the police officer, Magistrate or the Coroner etc. The types of inquest are:

Police Inquest [S. 174, Cr.P.C.]

An officer-in-charge of the police station in whose jurisdiction the death has occurred conducts the police inquest. On receipt of information of an unnatural death, the police officer first of all informs the nearest Magistrate and thereby proceeds to the place of death. The police officer then conducts an inquest in the presence of two or more respectable inhabitants of the neighbourhood ***(panchas).*** After the necessary investigation, a report is drawn up on the apparent cause of death as judged by the state of the body, the injuries present on the body, hearsay evidence and circumstantial evidence etc., this document is called inquest report (also known as ***panchnama***). This report is signed by the police officers and the persons present at the inquest. If any foul play or unnatural death is suspected, the police officer forwards the body for postmortem examination to the nearest government hospital along with the written request for conducting the autopsy (postmortem examination) and a copy of inquest report. If the autopsy report confirms that the death is due to an unnatural cause, further inquiry and trial of the case is conducted in the usual manner by the Magistrate concerned to whom the entire records of the case are transferred by the police officer. Police inquest is done in cases where a person: (i) Has committed suicide (ii) Has been killed by another man, or animal, or machinery (iii) Killed in an accident (iv) Died in suspicious circumstances raising reasonable suspicion that some other person has committed an offence.

1. In the above situation when the police officer gets information, he will immediately inform the nearest Executive Magistrate empowered to hold inquest and then proceeds to the place where the body of such person is found. He makes investigation in the presence of two or more respectable persons of the locality, draws up a report regarding the apparent cause of death, describing such wounds, bruises, fractures etc. found on the body and stating the manner and type of weapon that has caused such injuries.
2. The report shall be signed by such police officer and other persons or by so many of them who agree with the same opinion and shall be forwarded to District Magistrate/SDM.
3. When (i) Case involves suicide by a woman within seven years of marriage; or (ii) Case relates the death of woman within seven years of her marriage raising a reasonable suspicion that some other person has committed the offence in relation to such woman; or (iii) Case relates the death of a woman within seven years of marriage and any relative of the woman has made the request in this behalf; or (iv) There is any doubt regarding the cause of death. (v) Police officer for any other reason considers it suitable to do so sends the body to the nearest civil surgeon or medical officer for examination.
4. The following Magistrates will be empowered to hold inquests, namely any District Magistrate or Sub Divisional Magistrate, any other Executive Magistrate empowered by State Government or the District Magistrate.

Magistrates Inquest (S. 176, Cr.P.C.)

- The inquest is done by any District Magistrate, Sub Divisional Magistrate or any other Executive Magistrate or any Magistrate empowered by the State Government.
- Following are the indications of Magistrate's Inquest: (i) Custodial deaths (ii) Deaths due to police firing (iii) Death inside prison (iv) Dowry deaths (v) Clause (i) or (ii) of sub-section (3) of S. 174, Cr.P.C. The case involves suicide by a woman within seven years of marriage or the case relates the death of woman within seven years of her marriage raising a reasonable suspicion that some other person has committed the offence in relation to such woman. In addition, the Magistrate may hold an inquest in the cases done by police. The proceedings of the Magistrate are not judicial

proceedings, they only try to find out the cause of death. After inquest the body is sent for the postmortem examination. The inquest papers must be handed over to the autopsy surgeon for information. During the investigation, the Magistrate shall inform the relatives of the deceased and also allow them to stay during investigation. The differences between police and Magistrate inquest are given under Table 2.1.

Table 2.1: Difference between police and magistrate inquest

Features	Police inquest	Magistrate inquest
Investigating officer	Police officer (above the rank of head constable)	District Magistrate/ SDM
Types of cases	All unnatural deaths	Conducted in cases as specified under S.176 Cr.P.C.
Warrant	Cannot issue	Can issue
Fine/punishment	Cannot impose	Can impose
Exhumation	Cannot allow	Can allow
Value of inquest	Inferior	Superior

Coroner's Inquest

- Coroner's system was introduced in England in 1275 A.D. It used to be followed previously in Bombay (now Mumbai). It was discontinued on 29th July, 1999, when the Coroner's Act, 1871 (vide Sec. 8) was repealed. It no longer exists in India. The Coroner system is prevalent in countries like U.K. and some states of U.S.A.
- The Coroner's Court is a Court of inquiry (not a Court for trial) in which the Coroner conducts the inquest in unnatural, sudden and suspicious deaths. In his Court, the **jurors** are sworn to give a true verdict according to the evidence.
  (a) *Coroner:* He was an officer (a lawyer or a doctor, or both) of the rank of 1st class Judicial Magistrate, appointed by State Government, assisted by a deputy Coroner and had some judicial powers also. He had no power to pass a sentence. He had power to order any medical man to hold postmortem examination and to summon him to give evidence in his Court. Also he had power to order for exhumation for the purpose of identification and for postmortem examination.
  (b) *Jury:* It is a group of (usually 7) responsible, educated persons of good social position called jurors. They helped and assisted the Coroner.

Medical Examiner's System

- It is a newer system. The medical examiner's system for conducting inquest exists in most of the states in the U.S., Canada and Japan.
- Medical examiner is a professional (especially a medical man/forensic pathologist) who is appointed to perform the duties of a Coroner. In this system, the medical examiner visits the scene of crime and conducts further inquest, and conducts autopsy on dead bodies to ascertain the cause of death, so this system is superior to that of police inquest or a Coroner's system.
- The medical examiner neither has judicial functions nor has any authority to order the arrest of any person.

Procurator Fiscal System

A procurator fiscal is a public prosecutor who investigate sudden and suspicious death in Scotland.

COURTS OF LAW IN INDIA

Courts are of 2 Types

1. **Civil Courts:** They try only civil cases.
2. **Criminal Courts:** They try only criminal cases. Classes of criminal courts (S. 6, Cr.P.C.) are:
   (a) Supreme Court (Not given in S. 6, Cr.P.C.).
   (b) High Courts.
   (c) Session Courts.
   (d) Magistrate Courts.

Supreme Court

- It is the highest judicial tribunal (Court) of the country situated in New Delhi. The law declared by it is binding on all Courts (Article 134, Constitution of India).
- **Powers:** It has jurisdiction over all kinds of offences and can pass any sentence including death sentence. It usually considers appeal from lower Courts. The parties dissatisfied with the decisions in High Courts may go for an appeal in the Supreme Court.

High Court

- It is the highest judicial tribunal of the state (Article 214, COI).
- For 28 States and 8 Union Territories of India, there are at present 25 High Courts (Goa, Arunachal Pradesh, Mizoram and Nagaland does not have its own High Courts).
- High Court can pass any sentence authorized by law [S. 28(1), Cr.P.C.] including death sentence.
- The parties dissatisfied with the decision of High Courts can appeal in the Supreme Court.

Session Court

- It is the highest judicial tribunal of the District located at District headquarters. It is established by State Government and presided by a judge appointed by High Court. High Court may also appoint Additional Session Judges and Assistant Session Judges to exercise jurisdiction in a Court of Session.

- **Powers:**
    1. It can carry only those cases which have been committed to it by a Magistrate.
    2. **Session Judge or Additional Session Judge** can pass any sentence authorized by law, but the death sentence must be confirmed by High Court [S. 28(2), Cr.P.C. and S. 366, Cr.P.C.].
- **Assistant Session Judge** may pass any sentence authorized by law except death sentence, or imprisonment for life or imprisonment for more than 10 years [S. 28(3), Cr.P.C.]. It means he may pass sentence of imprisonment of ≤ 10 years.

Magistrate (S.11–23, Cr.P.C.) and Powers of Magistrate

Besides the High Courts and the Courts constituted under any law, there shall be in every state: (i) Courts of Sessions (ii) Judicial Magistrates of the first class and, in any Metropolitan area, Metropolitan Magistrate (iii) Judicial Magistrate of second class; and (iv) Executive Magistrate.

Powers of Magistrates (S. 29, Cr.P.C.)

The Court of Chief Metropolitan Magistrates shall have the powers of the Court of a Chief Judicial Magistrate and that of a Metropolitan Magistrate. The powers of the Court of Magistrate are given in Table 2.2.

Table 2.2: Powers of magistrate

Magistrates	Imprisonment (yrs)	Solitary confinement	Fine (Rs)
Chief judicial	Up to 7	Yes	Unlimited
First class judicial	Up to 3	Yes	10,000
Second class judicial	Up to 1	Yes	5,000

Executive Magistrate

Executive Magistrates namely District Magistrate, Additional District Magistrate, Sub-Divisional Magistrate, Subordinate Executive Magistrate and Special Executive Magistrate (Tahsildar/ Deputy Tahsildar) are the officers of the Executive branch. They are appointed by the state government under section 20 and 21 Cr.P.C. Executive Magistrates are Criminal Courts within the meaning of the Code vide Sec. 6 (iv) Cr.P.C. A Magistrate holding an inquiry under section 176 does not constitute a court. Executive Magistrates are courts inferior to that of the Sessions Judge. Compared to the Judicial Magistrate, functions of an Executive Magistrate are mainly limited to administrative matters, taking preventive measures and issues relating to maintenance of law and order.

Juvenile Justice Board

Children allegedly found to be in conflict with law are not be taken to a regular criminal court for trial. For them, there is provision of **Juvenile Justice Board** (under the Juvenile Justice (Care and Protection of Children) Act 2000 (amended in 2006, 2015, Bill 2021) and provisions of the Criminal Code Procedure) whose role is to hold a child culpable for his/her criminal activity, not through punishment, but counselling the child to understand their actions and persuade them away from criminal activities in the future. At Juvenile Justice Board, all procedures followed are child friendly and the venue is not intimidating. However, juveniles in conflict with law in the age group of 16-18, involved in heinous offences, to be tried as adults (As per 2015 amendment). The Juvenile Justice Board consists of Metropolitan Magistrate or Judicial Magistrate First Class (Principal Magistrate) and two social workers, at least one of whom should be a woman. There can be one or more than one Juvenile Justice Board(s) in each district that are established by the State Government.

Family Courts

As per the provision of The Family Courts Act, 1984, these special courts are designed to deal with legal problems arising out of family relations such as marriage, divorce, alimony, child custody etc. The setup provides a congenial environment away from the intimidating atmosphere of regular courts. These family courts are equipped with counsellors and psychologists. In these courts, special emphasis is put on, settling the disputes by mediation and conciliation.

Labour Courts

As per the provision of Industrial Dispute Act, 1947, these courts are designed to provide high quality, fair and impartial arrangements for the resolution of industrial disputes and the determination of appeals in disputes based on employment law.

OFFENCES

Offence [S. 2(n), Cr.P.C.]: "Any act or omission made punishable by any law for the time being in force and includes any act in respect of which a complaint may be made under S. 20, Cattle Trespass Act, 1871."

Cognizable offences [S. 2(c), Cr.P.C.]: It means an offence for which, (and cognizable case means a case in which), a police officer may, in accordance with the first schedule or any other law for the time being in force, arrest the alleged accused without warrant (Table 2.3).

Non-cognizable offences [S. 2(l), Cr.P.C.]: It means an offence for which, (and non-cognizable case means a case in which), a police officer has no authority to arrest the alleged accused without warrant (Table 2.3).

PUNISHMENTS (S. 53, I.P.C.)

S. 53, I.P.C. describes various punishments such as:

1. Death or Capital punishment.

Table 2.3: Cognizable offences and Non-cognizable offences	
Cognizable offences [S. 2(c), Cr.P.C.]	**Non-cognizable offences [S. 2(l), Cr.P.C.]**
Offences for which a police officer **may arrest** without warrant	Offences for which a police officer **has no authority** to arrest without warrant
Examples	*Examples*
1. Murder (S. 302, I.P.C.)	1. Voluntary causing hurt (S. 319 and 323, I.P.C.)
2. Death due to rash or negligent act	2. Causing miscarriage without a woman's consent (S. 313, I.P.C.)
3. Dowry death (S. 304B and 498A, I.P.C.)	3. Intercourse by a man with his own wife under 15 years of age (S. 375, I.P.C.)
4. Sexual offences (S. 372, 375 and 377, I.P.C.)	4. Bribery (S. 171E, I.P.C.)
5. Theft (S. 379, I.P.C.)	
6. Robbery (S. 392, I.P.C.)	
7. Dacoity (S. 395, I.P.C.)	

2. Imprisonment for life: In 1955, 'transportation for life' was replaced by imprisonment for life.
3. Clause thirdly omitted in 1949.
4. Imprisonment: (1) Rigorous (i.e., with hard labour), (2) Simple imprisonment.
5. Forfeiture of property.
6. Fine.

Summons (Subpoena) (S. 61-69, Cr.P.C.)

- It is a written document compelling the attendance of the witness in the Court to depose evidence, at a particular time and purpose under penalty. The word "summons" is singular, its pleural is "summonses". In many textbooks, the word 'summon' has been used for this document mentioned above, which is incorrect. Although in the textbooks of law, the word "summon" has been used as a verb (e.g., Magistrate can summon any of the relatives of an accused). Summons is also known as "subpoena" (Literally sub = under, poena = penalty).
- The provisions regarding summons are dealt in the S. 61 to 69 Cr.P.C.
- The summons is issued in duplicate signed by presiding officer of the Court and bears the seal of the Court (S. 61, Cr.P.C.). The summons is delivered to the witness through a police officer, an officer from the Court or by any other person. The witness signs the carbon copy and returns it to the Court. According to S. 66, Cr.P.C., if the witness is a government servant the summons can be sent to the head of the office in duplicate and the head in turn serves it to the concerned person. When summons are issued to produce a document or any other article required for investigation or trial (S. 91, Cr.P.C.) the person in possession of the said document or article may send it instead of attending personally. If the witness fails to attend the Court without any valid reason, he will be penalized in the form of paying damages in civil cases, but in criminal cases notice will be served under **S. 350, Cr.P.C.** After hearing from the witness if the Court thinks that there was no proper reason for not attending the Court, a bailable/non-bailable warrant may be issued to procure his attendance in the Court **(S. 172-174, I.P.C.** and **S. 87, Cr.P.C.).**
- If a witness receives two summons on the same date from the same type of Court he will attend the Court from which he received the summons first and will inform the other Court. If he receives two summonses, one from Criminal Court and the other from Civil Court, he will attend the criminal Court first with intimation to the Civil Court because Criminal Courts have priority over Civil Courts and also the higher Courts have priority over lower Courts. The witness would not leave the Court without the permission of the presiding officer.
- In civil cases certain amount of money is paid to the witness towards his expenses for attending the Court, which is called **conduct money.** This amount is paid to the witness while serving the summons. At times the money is paid in the Court itself. If the witness thinks that the amount paid is less and not according to his status and expenses he can pray to the presiding officer in the Court for additional amount. Even he can ignore the summon if no amount is paid in civil cases.
- However, in criminal cases no conduct money is paid but the witness must attend the Court in the interest of the state or in the interest of justice. The government usually pays TA and DA to attend such Courts. If the witness does not attend the Court he will be charged for contempt of Court.
- After getting the summons the witness appears before the Court on the specified date and time with the records called for. Before deposing the evidence, the witness has to take the oath.

Warrant Cases *Vs.* Summons Cases (Table 2.4)

Warrant case [defined in S. 2(x), Cr.P.C.] means a case relating to an offence punishable with death, imprisonment for life or imprisonment for a term exceeding 2 years.

Summons case [defined in S. 2(w), Cr.P.C.] means a case relating to an offence and not being a warrant case. So a summons case means a case relating to an offence punishable with imprisonment of a term ≤ 2 years.

Table 2.4: Cr.P.C.

Chapter 19 (XIX) (S. 238-250, Cr.P.C.)	Chapter 20 (XX) (S. 251-259, Cr.P.C.)	Chapter 21 (XXI) (S. 260-265, Cr.P.C.)
Trial of **"Warrant cases"** by Magistrate	Trial of **"Summons cases"** by Magistrate	**"Summary trial"**

COURT PROCEDURES

Include:

1. Oath (S. 51, I.P.C.).
2. Examination of witness:

   S. 137, IEA defines the Examination-in-Chief, Cross-examination and Re-examination.

   S. 138, IEA describes the Order of examination in the following sequence:

   Examination-in-Chief → Cross Examination → Re-examination.
3. Questions put by the Court: According to S. 165, IEA, the Judge has power to ask any question at any time.

Oath (S. 51, I.P.C.)

- The witness stands in the witness box and takes the oath. The main aim of taking oath is affirmation that the witness will tell the truth during the evidence. He takes oath (Vide **S. 4 and 6, Indian Oath Act 44 of 1969)** as follows: "I do (swear in the name of God)/(Solemnly affirm), that what I shall tell, be the truth, the whole truth and nothing but the truth." Affirmation is a secular form of oath where the witness does not have to mention a deity or holy book. The oath is to be taken while appearing as witness in all the Courts other than High Courts and Supreme Court, which is administered by the presiding officer himself. In cases where the witness appears before a bench of judges or magistrates, one of the judges or the magistrate can administer the oath (S. 2, Indian Oath Act 44 of 1969). **Oath taking is not required for a child witness (<12 years).**
- **Perjury (S.191, I.P.C.)** means willfully giving false evidence under oath or unable to tell what he knows or believes to be the truth. Punishment for perjury is incorporated under **S. 193, I.P.C.** with imprisonment up to 7 years and fine. **S. 344, Cr.P.C.** describes the summary procedure for trial for giving false evidence.

Examination-in-Chief (S. 137, IEA)

- After the oath, the witness will be examined by the lawyer of the party that has called him. It is also known as **direct examination.** In criminal cases, the state becomes a party so the burden of proof is always on the prosecution. It is always presumed that the accused is innocent unless otherwise proved. Before giving the evidence, the doctor should always go through the previously prepared report. If needed he can meet the public prosecutor and go through the files and other records. The doctor should help the public prosecutor to frame the questions so that proper facts are elicited. The medical witness is usually asked questions as to when he first saw the body and time of conduction of the postmortem examination etc. The question pertaining to description of the injuries, duration of injuries and possibly about the weapon of offence are also asked during examination-in-chief.
- Normally **leading questions** are **not allowed** but where the Court is satisfied that the witness is a hostile one **(S. 142, IEA)** then only leading questions can be asked. A **leading question** as defined under **S. 141, IEA,** is any question that suggests the answer which the person putting it wishes or expects to receive. For example, "Did you carry out the postmortem examination?", "Did you find a five cm laceration on the forehead?" To an ordinary witness, question such as "Did you see the accused inside the restaurant?" or "Have you seen him beating A?" are asked. The answer to the question must be in a conclusive manner as "Yes" or "No". In civil cases also, the same procedure is followed.

Cross-Examination (S.137, IEA)

- During the cross-examination, the lawyer of the opposite party, i.e., the lawyer of the accused (defence lawyer) examines the witness.
- The main objectives of cross-examination are: (i) To elicit facts favorable to his client (ii) to find out the weak points in the case (iii) to verify the accuracy of the facts already told. The defence lawyer always tries to discredit the witness and tries to prove that the report given is not correct and biased one. It is not necessary that the question should be confined to the facts told in examination-in-chief. The defence lawyer may even ask questions pertaining to the qualifications, experience etc., especially in the type of the case in question. During this time the Court observes whether a particular question should be answered or not. The Court has power to disallow a question if it is intended to insult or harass the witness but if it is relevant to the case the Court cannot disallow.
- The witness can be compelled and has to answer the question that relates to the case even if it is harmful to the witness or it exposes his fault or negligence **(S. 147, IEA).** If a witness is forced to answer a question that goes against him, he cannot be arrested or prosecuted or cannot be taken as proof against him for any criminal proceedings. When a question is not audible, the witness can request to repeat the same and when the question is not understood properly he can again ask to explain. The witness should be clear, direct and precise in his answer.

- When a witness is harassed and humiliated he may become angry, hostile and tense. His intellectual faculties are blunted so as to loose the power of giving proper evidence. He may ask the Court for some time to be in proper shape for further evidence. He may volunteer certain facts that are relevant to the case even if not asked by the lawyer.
- In cross-examination, the **leading questions are allowed (S. 143, IEA).**
- There is no time limit for cross-examination.

Re-Examination (S. 137, IEA)

This is done by the lawyer who has called the witness. The main aim of re-examination is to clarify the points raised in cross-examination and correct the mistakes done. However, the lawyer should not bring any new points during the examination that has not been raised in the examination-in-chief. If any new point arises, the witness should be cross-examined again. Raising a new point should be done after taking permission from the Court. Leading questions cannot be asked except with permission of the court.

Questions Put by the Court

- According to **S. 165, IEA,** the judge has power to ask any question at any time. The judge may ask any question to clarify doubts in the evidences.
- According to **S. 311, Cr.P.C.,** the Court is also empowered to examine any person in attendance (though not summoned as a witness), or to re-examine any witness already examined, if the Court thinks that it is essential to arrive at a decision.

The deposition is handed over to the witness. After reading carefully and thoroughly the witness signs at the end of each page with date. Any mistakes in the deposition should be brought to the notice of the Court and then he can correct it with his initials. He should not leave the Court without prior permission. The TA and DA are usually paid in the Court.

CODE OF CONDUCT OF A DOCTOR INSIDE THE WITNESS BOX

The doctor is an expert witness to the Court, not belonging to any party even though one party has called him. The Court and the society want him to be impartial and assist the Court to reach a proper conclusion for the sake of justice. This has been well put by the famous French medicolegal authority in 19th century **Brovardel.** He said, "Where the law has made a physician a witness, he should remain a man of science. He should remember that he has no victim to avenge, no guilty person to convict and no innocent person to save."

The doctor in the witness box should appear as a man of professional competence and integrity. He should be well dressed and look sober, prepare the facts of the case and take all relevant records or articles in his custody to the Court. The doctor should never be nervous inside the Court and speak loudly and clearly so that the presiding officer can record the deposition.

It is essential that he should use no medical jargon and if medical terms are to be used a short explanation can be added. An expert may refresh his memory **(S. 159, IEA)** by reference to the professional treatise. The writing that is used to refresh the memory can be cross-examined by the opposite party.

The doctor should never be over confident or arrogant. He should always use "Sir" or "Your honour" while addressing the Court. He should never use adjectives or exaggerations like very large bruise, severe pain etc. and never loose the temper even if provoked by the opposite lawyer.

The doctor should not avoid any question. If the answer is not known, always say, "I don't know." Nobody expects the doctor to know everything. Do not alter your findings to what is said in the statement. The answers should always be brief and to the point.

If the lawyer limits the answer to "yes" or "no" which is not possible at times, the doctor can tell the judge that it requires explanation because you have taken the oath not only to speak truth but the whole truth. Always answer "in my opinion but not as I think or imagine or I am not sure etc". When the answer demands quantity or number, the doctor should not tell the number unless he knows the exact number or quantity such as in cases of age estimation, the answer should be given within certain limits. The doctor should always answer within his own speciality. He should never comment on the points where he has little or no experience at all.

When the lawyer reads a paragraph from the book and asks to comment the doctor should always be careful. He must read the paragraph carefully including even the paragraphs before and after it to come to the conclusion. He must see that the book is a recent edition and the views expressed must be latest. He may or may not agree on these views. It is not necessary to agree upon everything written in the book. It should be remembered that views expressed in the book by reputed authors are taken as evidence even if the witness doesn't agree to it.

When attempts are made to influence the witness by one party or the other, he must report to the senior police officer or to the Court so that the corrupt person can be penalized and at the same time he and his family members are given protection.

A medical witness cannot claim professional privilege. He has to answer each and every question asked after obtaining the permission of the Court. A witness whether medical or otherwise is completely immune from actions for defamation (libel or slander) for anything he says in the witness box. This is quite important otherwise the witness will not disclose the actual facts because of fear of legal action later on.

Volunteering of statements: At times the public prosecutor leaves certain ambiguities in the evidence and the defence lawyer also puts ambiguous questions. As a result the witness gives incomplete answers. The defence lawyer takes the advantage of these during an argument. When certain ambiguity is left or a general statement given by him is not applicable to the facts of the case in hand, the medical witness should come forward and volunteer for a statement making the position clear. When such statements are volunteered, the Court writes "As statements volunteered. The statement has the same value as other statements given by the witness in response to questions put to him. The advocates of both the parties have a right to cross-examine such volunteered statements.

MEDICAL EVIDENCE

According to S. 3, IEA, evidence means all statements, which the Court permits or requires to be made before it by the witness, in relation to matters of fact under inquiry, and such statements are called oral evidence.

All documents produced for the inspection of the Court are called documentary evidence. Before accepting the documents the Court must be satisfied regarding the identification and the place of seizure of such documents. Ordinarily the value of medical evidence is only corroborative. It proves that the injuries could have been caused in the manner alleged and nothing more. The defence makes use of the medical evidence to prove that the injuries could not possibly have been caused in the manner alleged and thereby discredit the eyewitness.

Types of Evidence

A. **Oral evidence (S. 59, IEA): S. 159, IEA** states that all facts, except the contents of documents or electronic records may be proved by oral evidence.

   Direct evidence: The oral evidence must be direct **(S. 60, IEA),** for example when it refers to a fact that could be seen, heard or perceived, it must be the evidence of that person who saw/heard/perceived it. It must be direct if it refers to an opinion or to the grounds on which that opinion is held. The evidence must confirm to the matters in question, e.g., a knife that has caused stab injury or a medical prescription that resulted in the ill effects to the patient.

   Indirect evidence (Circumstantial): At times the other surrounding facts are taken into consideration that are consistent with the direct evidence for example 'A' committed murder of 'B' with knife at a particular place, date and time. Here 'C' will depose that he saw 'A' on that day, date and time with a knife in hand just before the murder. This evidence of 'C' has a bearing to the fact.

   Hearsay evidence: Here the persons other than the witness give the statement. For example during the trial 'A' told that 'B' had told him that he has seen 'C' while committing the crime. Here 'B' can give the direct evidence as he has seen 'C' committing the crime. However, the evidence of 'A' will be hearsay evidence.

B. **Documentary evidence (S. 61-90, IEA):** It includes all documents including electronic records produced before Court during trial. **S. 29, I.P.C.,** defines the word "document" as "Any matter expressed or described upon any substance by means of letters, figures, marks or by more than one of these means intended to be used or which may be used as evidence of that matter." According to **S. 29A, I.P.C.,** the word **"electronic record"** shall have the meaning assigned in Information Technology Act, 2000.

Proof of contents of the documents (S. 61, IEA): The contents of documents may be proved either by primary or secondary evidences.

Primary evidence (S. 62, IEA): It means the document itself produced for inspection of the Court.

Secondary evidence (S. 63, IEA): It means and includes the certified copies, copies made from the original by mechanical process, copies made from or compared with the original and oral accounts of the contents of a document given by a person who has himself seen it. Electronic evidence/Digital evidence is a secondary evidence admissible in court subject to certain conditions, under **S. 65 IEA.** Tape-recorded statements are admissible as evidence *(K.S. Mohan vs. Sandhya Mohan AIR 1993 Mad 59)*. Evidence must confirm to the matters in issue and is admitted on the basis of relevance and admissibility.

Varieties of documentary evidence: Documentary evidence is of the following types:

1. ***Medical certificates:*** Medical certificates are regarded as the simplest form of documentary evidence. They are issued by a registered medical practitioner (RMP) in respect of ill health, age and mental condition. The certificates are also issued in cases of death. It is a vital document that may be needed during cremation, transportation outside state and in certain insurance claims etc. It is accepted in the Court of law as a piece of evidence as to the facts stated in the medical certificate. Even the doctor who has issued it may be summoned to the Court of law to testify the contents of the certificate on oath and if needed cross-examination can be done. Thus the medical practitioner must exercise due care and skill in issuing such certificate. The certificate must state the exact nature of illness and should contain doctor's opinion in clear language. In case of ill health the doctor should write the exact nature of illness, the duration of illness and probable period of absence in cases of employed persons. The signature of the patient

should be at the bottom with the date indicating that he has attended the clinic and the doctor has examined him while issuing the certificate. The signature of the patient is to be verified by the doctor.

2. ***Death certificate:*** It is essential that identification and cause of death is to be determined for the lawful disposal of the dead body. **The Registration of Birth and Death (RBD) Act, 1969** came into force from 1st April 1970. According to this Act all the births and deaths are to be registered throughout India. Before issuing death certificate the doctor must inspect the body and satisfy that the person is dead. He is legally bound to issue the certificate indicating the cause of death if he has attended the patient during his last illness. According to the recommendation of **Brodrick Committee** a doctor should not be allowed to issue a death certificate unless he has attended the deceased at least once during seven days preceding death. He cannot charge any fee for issuing a death certificate. He cannot delay or refuse to issue a certificate. He may subsequently sue the legal heirs for his pending dues. He must refuse to give a certificate on the following grounds: (A) If he is not sure about the cause of death. (B) Any suspicion of foul play. (C) Death by violent and unnatural cause, drugs, poisoning etc. If he is not sure regarding the cause of death and suspects some foul play he should not issue the certificate, instead he should inform the police. Issuing a false certificate **(S. 197, I.P.C.)** is punishable under **S. 193, I.P.C.** with imprisonment that may extend to 7 years and also fine. It is a general belief that physician can write anything on death certificate for monetary games. Due to this people try to lure the doctor to produce false certificates for various purposes.

   Death certificate is a predicament in any doctor's practice. The relatives of the deceased may plead, persuade, pressurize, offer a price and at times even threaten the doctor. He may be tempted at times on humanitarian grounds to issue a certificate. The doctor may certify death in doubtful cases but must not give a cause of death and should inform the police. Failure to do so may result in the doctor being prosecuted under **S. 39, Cr.P.C.** Under **S. 17(1)(b) of RBD Act, 1969,** any person may obtain an extract from the registrar relating to any death after paying the requisite fee, though it will not disclose particulars regarding the cause of death as entered in the register. This confidentiality can be overridden in public interest.

   International format of death certificate: The death certificate recommended by WHO for international use is in two parts: Part I (Disease or condition directly leading to death) and Part II (Other significant conditions contributing to the death but not related to disease or condition causing it). *Part I:* It is categorized into 3 subsections that are inter-related to each other: (a) *Immediate/recent cause:* The disease or condition directly leading to death; and (b) *Intermediate/Intermediary causes* viz, the morbid conditions, if any, giving rise to the cause mentioned in (a). (c) is the *underlying cause* to (a) and/or (b). Thus (a) must be due to (b) which must be due to (c), etc. When many conditions are involved, the doctor should write the full sequence–one condition per line, with the most recent condition (immediate cause) at the top (in line a) and the other intermediate conditions are listed in line b to then sequentially and in the last line, the underlying cause should be mentioned. As per the recommendations of 43rd World Health Assembly 1990, an additional line (d) has been added below (c). The basic pathological condition is the one, which is mentioned on the lower most line, and this is the one that is used for statistical and epidemiological purposes. The approximate interval between the onset of each events and the time of death should be mentioned in hours, days, weeks, or months. *Part II:* Any condition that is not related to Part I (disease or condition causing it) and contributing to death. In this certificate, the doctor should specify in Part I the underlying pathological condition that lead to death. No clinical manifestations or mode of death should be included in Part I. Part II of the form should preferably be left blank unless there is any contributory factor in the death. The cause of death should be coded with reference to International Statistical Classification of Diseases and Related Health Problems code (ICD-10) for mortality statistics purpose. International forms are used by various municipal authorities in our country and are available for doctors. Doctors should necessarily affix their rubber stamp after putting signature on death certificate with date.

Examples of Completing a Death Certificate As Per ICD-10 Document

Case 1

A 53-year-old male was admitted to hospital with history of fever and cough. He was tested Covid-19 positive on the same day. He was a diabetic since last 20 years. He developed pneumonia after 2 days of admission and was under oxygen support. His condition remained critical for last two days as he developed acute respiratory distress syndrome. He died on 14th day of admission on to the hospital.

Part I				
		Cause of death	**Time interval from onset to death**	**ICD-10 Code**
• Report disease or condition directly leading to death on line a	**a**	Acute respiratory distress syndrome	2 days	J80
• Report chain of events in due to order (if applicable)	**b**	Due to: Pneumonia	12 days	J18.9
• State the underlying cause on the lowest used on line c	**c**	Due to: COVID-19	14 days	U07.1
Part II Other significant conditions contributing to death but not related to the disease or condition causing it (time intervals can be included in brackets after the condition)		Diabetes (20 years)		E 11.9
Manner of death 1. **Natural** 2. Accident 3. Suicide 4. Homicide 5. Pending investigation **Autopsy:** Yes/**No**				

Case 2

A 60-year-old female while crossing the road, hit by a car accidentally. She was immediately admitted to the hospital for open fracture of lower end right tibia. She was known diabetic since last 10 years and hypertensive since last 20 years. She received screw fixed operation for his right tibia and had been in the hospital for one month. On 30th day patient deteriorated becoming severe breathless and had sudden collapse showing signs of pulmonary embolism. Patient died after 2 hours.

Part I				
		Cause of death	**Time interval from onset to death**	**ICD-10 Code**
• Report disease or condition directly leading to death on line a	**a**	Pulmonary embolism	2 hours	I26.0
• Report chain of events in due to order (if applicable)	**b**	Due to: Fracture of right tibia	30 days	S82.31
• State the underlying cause on the lowest used on line c	**c**	Due to: Victim was a pedestrian and hit by a car	30 days	V03
Part II Other significant conditions contributing to death but not related to the disease or condition causing it (time intervals can be included in brackets after the condition)		Diabetes (10 years), Hypertension (20yrs)		E 11.9, I10
Manner of death 1. Natural 2. **Accident** 3. Suicide 4. Homicide 5. Pending investigation **Autopsy: Yes**/No				

International Classification of Diseases and Related Health Problems (ICD)

The ICD is designed collaboratively by World Health Organization (WHO) and other international centers to promote international comparability in collection, processing, classification, and presentation of mortality statistics. It also provides a format for reporting causes of death on the death certificate.

The ICD-10 is the 10th revision of ICD, which has 3 volumes, out of these first contains main classification of diseases and related health problems. The core classification of ICD-10 is the three-character code, which is the mandatory level of coding for international reporting to the WHO mortality database and for general international comparisons. These unique codes provide a common language that allows health professionals to share health information across the globe. It contains around 55000 unique codes for injuries, diseases and causes of death (Examples are cited in Table 2.5). The classification is also divided into 21 chapters. The first character of the ICD code is a letter, and each letter is associated with a particular chapter with few exceptions.

On 18 June, 2018, the WHO released the new International Classification of Diseases (ICD-11) which will be come into effect on 1 January 2022. The new ICD-11 also includes new chapters, on traditional medicine and sexual health. Gaming disorder has been added to the section on addictive disorders.

Table 2.5: Examples of use of ICD-10 code for causes of death		
Chapter	**Code range**	**Description with ICD-10 code**
XX	V01-Y98	**External causes of morbidity and mortality** • Accidents (V01-X59) – Transport Accidents(V01-V99) ° Pedestrian injured in collision with car, pick-up truck or van (V03) • Intentional self-harm (X60-X84) – Hanging, strangulation and suffocation (X70) – Drowning and submersion (X71) • Assault (X85-Y09) – Assault by sharp object (X99) – Assault by blunt object (Y00) • Event of undetermined intent (Y10-Y34) – Falling, jumping or pushed from a high place, undetermined intent (Y31)

3. ***Medicolegal report:*** These are the legal documents prepared by the doctor at the request of investigating officers usually in criminal cases like injury cases, sexual offences, murder and poisoning cases. These reports are made in both living and dead individuals. The request usually comes from police officer or magistrate. Medicolegal report is usually prepared in two parts. The first part consists of observations and findings of the cases while the second part consists of the opinion and conclusion. The doctor starting the examination of the individual should write in detail his name, date, time and place of examination. The identification marks should be noted and the consent has to be taken because any examination without consent is regarded an assault in law. The victim should be explained the purpose and outcome of such examination before taking the consent. A lady RMP should examine the female patient **[S. 53(2) Cr.P.C.]**. Where the lady doctor is not available a female attendant should be present at the time of examination whose signature should be taken in the report. All the findings are observed in detail and a report is prepared. The opinion or conclusion drawn should not be biased one as it is subjected to cross-examination in the Court of law. The opinion must be kept pending till the reports are available in cases where necessary investigations are required. The negative findings should also to be pointed out in the report. These reports are produced in the Court of law. The doctor who has made the report should attend the Court to testify under oath, and then only they are admissible as evidence. If the doctor is not available someone else can attend the Court to testify his signature and handwriting as evidences.
4. ***Dying declaration:*** The major purpose of dying declaration is to render it admissible. Dying declaration is any evidence from a person who dies before the case is heard. Such a declaration must have corroborative evidence to support it before it can be accepted **(S. 157, IEA)** in courts of law. The dying declaration has been incorporated in **S. 32 of IEA** that reads as "a statement written or verbal of relevant facts made by a person who is dead or who cannot be found, or who has become incapable of giving evidence or whose attendance cannot be procured, without an amount of delay or expenses which under the circumstances of the case appears to the Court unreasonable" are themselves relevant facts in the following: (i) When it relates to the cause of death. (ii) When a statement made by a person as to the cause of his death or as to any of the circumstances of the transaction which resulted in his death. Such a statement are relevant whether the person who made them was or was not at the time when they were made under expectation of death and whatever may be the nature of proceeding where his cause of death comes in question. The above provisions were made on mainly two grounds: (i) At times the victim being the only eyewitness to the incident, exclusion of his or her statement will not be justified to meet the justice. (ii) Impending sense of death is taken as equal to oath and it is believed that the person will speak truth at the time of impending death. In United States under the Federal Rules of evidence, a dying declaration is admissible if: (i) It constituted the last words of a person who was dying or thought he was dying; and (ii) That person was aware that he or she was dying; and (iii) That person made a statement, based on their actual knowledge, that relates in some way to the cause or circumstances of his or her death.

Recording the dying declaration: Depending of the availability of time, the magistrate should be called to record the declaration. In the absence of magistrate, the doctor should record it. The police officer can also record it either at the site of accident or when the patient is being taken to the hospital. Even any lay person like the panchayat head or the relatives can record the declaration depending upon the situation. However, the weightage of dying declaration becomes less and less in the descending order of recording by above mentioned individuals.

Procedure: In the hospital admitted cases; the treating physician first tries to stabilize the patient's and then informs the police. If the doctor thinks that the patient life is in danger he will arrange for the dying declaration. The police will inform the area magistrate for the purpose. The doctor first has to certify that the patient is in perfect mental condition to make a declaration, i.e., the patient is in **"compos mentis"**. If the magistrate is not available or there is much delay of his arrival then the doctor will write the declaration. The police should be discouraged to be near the patient so as to avoid the undue influence. The doctor should be there throughout the declaration to check the mental condition. If during declaration the patient becomes unconscious or unfit for a declaration the recordings will be stopped at that time putting the signature of the person who is recording it along with date and time. The declaration is recorded again when the doctor declares the patient fit. If the dying person is unable to speak but able to make sign in answer to questions this can be recorded and regarded as verbal statement. It can also be recorded in the form of questions and answers. If at any stage a particular point is not clear he can be asked to make it clear. At the end the declaration is read before the patient who puts his signature or thumb impression. It is also signed by the recording magistrate, the doctor and the witness mentioning the date and time. The declaration may take in the form of first information report of a statement before the police **(S. 162, Cr.P.C.)** during investigation. There is no prescribed form to record a dying declaration and no rigid rule can be followed. When a deceased person makes more than one dying declaration then they should be taken as one for the purpose of conviction. If the subject matter differs in these two declarations efforts should be made to reconcile. If at all the differences exist about the facts that should be covered by the explanation to the **S. 161, Cr.P.C.** and to be considered as a matter of fact in each case. If the person survives after making a declaration then he is called to the Court and his evidence is taken. Therefore, the dying declaration recorded earlier acts as corroborative evidence. The value of declaration given in the court of law is more compared to the one recorded before.

5. ***Dying deposition:*** There is no provision of dying deposition in the Indian Evidence Act therefore it is not followed in India. Here the Magistrate records the evidence after administering oath. The accused or his lawyer is present and they are allowed to cross-examine the victim. The difference between dying declaration and deposition mentioned in Table 2.6.

WITNESS

S. 118, IEA states about the person who may testify as witness in Courts of Law and reads as "All persons shall be competent to testify unless the Court considers that they are prevented from understanding the questions put to them, or from giving rational answers to those questions as a result of tender age, extreme old age, disease of mind or body or any other cause of the same kind." Even a mentally ill person, lunatic is not incompetent to testify unless he is prevented by his lunacy from understanding the questions put to him. Various types of witnesses are:

Common witness (Ordinary witness): Common witness is a person who has seen or observed the facts. It has to be proved that he/she was capable of perceiving the facts or has actually seen the facts. This principle is known as "first hand knowledge rule". For e.g. 'A' told in the Court that he had seen 'X' and 'Y' fighting in a garden on a particular date and time.

Expert witness: S. 45, IEA deals with opinion of experts. They are not only medical experts, but also experts in other subjects. It states that when a Court has to form an opinion upon a point of foreign law or of science or art or identifying the handwritings and fingerprints that are relevant facts. Such persons because of their professional training and experience are capable of drawing a conclusion on the facts observed by them or by others and are called experts. They also give expert opinion on hypothetical questions as well as on matters of common knowledge. The answer should be given by an expert witness after understanding the questions clearly and whenever possible in a guarded manner, the examples like the findings are consistent with the alleged history, does not mean that another mechanism cannot produce the same findings. Conclusions must be based on the facts because it is more important than the opinions.

Hostile witness: Hostile witness is one who purposefully makes statements contrary to the fact or has some interest or motive for concealing truth. **S. 191, I.P.C.** states that whoever, being legally bound by an oath or by an express provision of law to state the truth, or being bound by a law to make a declaration upon any subject, makes any statement which is false, and which

Table 2.6: Difference between Dying declaration and Dying deposition

S. No.	Dying declaration	Dying deposition
1.	Followed in India	Followed in Western countries
2.	It is merely the recording of a statement of a dying person	It is a full-fledged court procedure, so also known as "court by the bedside"
3.	Recorded by the Magistrate, doctor, police officer, panchayat head or relative	Recorded always by Magistrate
4.	The accused and his lawyer need not be present	They have to be present
5.	Oath: Not administered	Has to be administered
6.	Cross examination: Not allowed	Allowed
7.	Leading question: Not allowed	Allowed
8.	It loses its value if the victim survives, but it acts as corroborative evidence	It retains its value if the victim survives
9.	Less value	More value

he either knows or believes to be false or does not belong to be true, is said to give false evidence. The common as well as expert witnesses can be hostile.

LONG QUESTIONS

1. What is inquest? Discuss different types of inquest prevalent in India and which is the best?
2. Discuss various types of documentary evidences in medicolegal practices.
3. Discuss various types of evidences.

SHORT QUESTIONS

1. Cross-examination.
2. Dying declaration.
3. Powers of magistrates.
4. Types of witness.
5. Magistrate's inquest.
6. Subpoena.
7. Difference between police and magistrate inquest.
8. Expert witness.
9. Hostile witness.

MULTIPLE CHOICE QUESTIONS

1. The present criminal procedure code has been enacted in the year:

(a) 1947 (b) 1963
(c) 1973 (d) 1985

2. Section 174 I.P.C. deals with:

(a) Inquest (b) Murder
(c) Exhumation (d) Inquiry

3. Death sentence can be given by which court?

(a) Central administrative tribunal
(b) Sessions court
(c) Magistrate court
(d) Chief judicial magistrate court

4. Summons is a written document of the court:

(a) Compelling attendance of a witness
(b) Guarantee money to witness
(c) Providing legal immunity to a witness
(d) That can be attended at will

5. Conduct money is paid to a witness if he/she comes from a distance of more than:

(a) 5 kms (b) 7 kms
(c) 10 kms (d) Any distance

6. Conduct money is the expenses paid to a witness for attending court in:

(a) All criminal case
(b) Civil case
(c) Both civil and criminal case
(d) Only murder case

7. The court may permit for leading questions during Examination-in-Chief, if the witness is a:

(a) Hostile witness (b) Expert witness
(c) Common witness (d) Character witness

8. During recording of evidence in court, leading questions are usually allowed during:

(a) Examination-in-Chief (b) Cross-examination
(c) Re-examination (d) Questions put by the Court

9. Dying declaration ideally is to be recorded by:

(a) Police (b) Medical officer
(c) Magistrate (d) Session's Judge

10. The witness is liable to be prosecuted for 'perjury' is defined in I.P.C. section:

(a) 82 (b) 83
(c) 191 (d) 193

ANSWER KEY ☞

1. (c)	2. (a)	3. (b)	4. (a)	5. (d)	6. (b)	7. (a)	8. (b)	9. (c)	10. (d)

3 CHAPTER

Laws and Ethics in Medical Practice

INTRODUCTION

The medical profession is guided by a code of ethics which are formulated by the National Medical Commission and State Medical Council along with World Medical Association (WMA). The ethics are nothing but the moral principles that guide the members of medical profession. The enforcement is done by the National Medical Commission (NMC) and State Medical Council.

Indian Medical Degrees Act, 1916

The Act was passed to grant the title in respect of the qualification of Western medical science.

MEDICAL COUNCIL OF INDIA (MCI)

In 1934, First **Medical Council of India (MCI)** was established by the **Indian Medical Council (IMC) Act, 1933**. Its primary function was to standardize both training in medicine and the accreditation of medical and surgical proficiency. In 1956, the IMC Act was repealed and a redesigned Act came into force which was called **Indian Medical Council (IMC) Act, 1956.** The purpose of MCI established under this Act was to maintain a medical register for India and for the matters concerned with it. Subsequently amendments of this Act were done in year 1964, 1993 and 2001 for face-lifting of MCI.

Following allegation of irregularities and corruption in MCI, on 15th May 2010, the Central Government brought an ordinance which superseded the MCI. The Government constituted a **Board of Governor (BoG)** to perform its functions. There was a plan by the Central Government to reform the MCI for which Indian Medical Council (Amendment) bill brought in the Parliament. However, the Government was unable to pass the bill and the autonomy of the MCI was again restored in year 2013 as per old IMC Act, 1956. In July 2017, the Supreme Court allowed the Central Government again to replace the MCI with the Board of Governors (BoG) consists of five specialized doctors to monitor the medical education system in India.

The **Niti Ayayog** has recommended the replacement of Medical Council of India (MCI) with National Medical Commission (NMC). In year 2019; the Central Government passed the National Medical Commission Bill, 2019 in both houses of the Parliament. The National Medical Commission Act, 2019, was notified vide the Gazette Notification dated 8th August, 2019.

The National Medical Commission (NMC) Act, 2019

The aims of the Act are to repeal the Indian Medical Council Act, 1956 (**IMC Act**) and constitute the National Medical Commission (**NMC**), which shall supersede the Medical Council of India (**MCI**).

NATIONAL MEDICAL COMMISSION (NMC)

S. 3, Central Government shall constitute the NMC. The NMC became functional on 25th September, 2020 replacing the Board of Governor (BoG). The head office of the commission is at New Delhi.

A. **Constitution and Composition of the NMC: S. 4,** NMC consists of 33 members and they are as follows:

1. **One chairperson:** Shall be a medical professional of outstanding ability, proven administrative capacity and integrity, possessing a postgraduate degree in any discipline of medical sciences from any university and having experience of not less than twenty years in the field of medical sciences, out of which at least ten years shall be as a leader in the area of medical education.

2. **Ten *ex officio* members:** The following persons shall be the *ex officio* members of the Commission,

   (a) The President of the Under-Graduate Medical Education Board.

   (b) The President of the Post-Graduate Medical Education Board.

   (c) The President of the Medical Assessment and Rating Board.

   (d) The President of the Ethics and Medical Registration Board.

   (e) The Director General of Health Services, New Delhi.

   (f) The Director General, Indian Council of Medical Research.

   (g) One Director of any of the All India Institutes of Medical Sciences, to be nominated by the Central Government.

   (h) Two persons from amongst the Directors of Postgraduate Institute of Medical Education and Research, Chandigarh; Jawaharlal Institute of Postgraduate Medical Education and Research, Puducherry; Tata Memorial Hospital, Mumbai; North Eastern Indira Gandhi Regional Institute of Health and Medical Sciences, Shillong; and All India Institute of Hygiene and Public Health, Kolkata to be nominated by the Central Government.

   (i) One person to represent the Ministry of Health and Family Welfare, Government of India, not below the rank of Additional Secretary, to be nominated by the same Ministry.

3. **Twenty-two part-time members:** The following persons shall be appointed as part-time members of the Commission:

   (a) Three members to be appointed from amongst persons of ability, integrity and standing, who have special knowledge and professional experience in such areas including management, law, medical ethics, health research, consumer or patient rights advocacy, science and technology and economics.

   (b) Ten members to be appointed on rotational basis from amongst the nominees of the States and Union territories, under clauses (c) and (d) of sub-section (2) of section 11, in the Medical Advisory Council for a term of two years in such manner as may be prescribed.

   (c) Nine members to be appointed from amongst the nominees of the States and Union territories, under clause (e) of sub-section (2) of section 11, in the Medical Advisory Council for a term of two years in such manner as may be prescribed.

S. 5, the Central Government shall appoint the Chairperson and part-time members on the recommendation of a search committee headed by Cabinet Secretary.

S. 6, they shall hold office for a term not exceeding 4 years and shall not be eligible for extension or reappointment further. Also, such person shall cease to hold office after attaining the age of 70 years. However, the term of office of an *ex officio* member shall continue as long as he holds the office by virtue of which he is such member.

S. 7, Central Government may remove the Chairperson and other members who (a) has been adjudged an insolvent (b) has been convicted of an offence (c) has become physically or mentally incapable of acting as member (d) is of unsound mind and stands so declared by a competent court (e) has acquired such financial or other interest as is likely to affect prejudicially his functions as a member (f) has so abused his position as to render his continuance in office prejudicial to public interest. However, no member shall not be removed for the reason described under clauses (e) and (f), unless the member has been given a reasonable opportunity of being heard in the matter.

S. 8, there shall be a **Secretariat for the Commission,** headed by a **Secretary**. The Secretary to be appointed by the Central Government in accordance with provisions of S. 5. The Secretary shall be appointed for a term of four years and shall not be eligible for any extension or re-appointment. The Secretary shall discharge such functions of the Commission as are assigned to him by the Commission. All orders and decisions of the Commission shall be authenticated by the signature of the Secretary. The Commission may delegate such of its powers of administrative and financial matters, as it deems fit, to the Secretary.

S. 9, Chairperson shall be the administrative head of the Commission and shall preside the meeting of Commission. If the Chairperson is unable to attend a meeting, any other member, being the President of an Autonomous Board, nominated by the Chairperson, shall preside at the meeting. The Commission meets at least once every quarter and all acts of the Commission are decided by a majority of the members present and voting. In the event of equality of votes, the Chairperson, or in his absence, the President of the Autonomous Board nominated under sub-section (2), shall have the casting vote. No act done by the Commission shall be questioned on the ground of the existence of a vacancy in, or a defect in the constitution of the Commission. A person who is aggrieved by any decision of the Commission except the decision by Ethics and Medical Registration Board (sub-section (4) of section 30) may prefer an appeal to the Central Government against such decision within thirty days of the communication of such decision.

B. **Main Functions of the NMC are as follows: S. 10.**

(a) Laying down policies for maintaining a high quality and high standard medical education and make necessary regulations.

(b) Laying down policies for regulating medical institutions, medical research and medical professionals and make necessary regulations.

(c) Assessing the requirements of human resources and infrastructure in health care.

(d) Ensuring compliance by the State Medical Councils with the regulations made under this Act for effective functioning.

(e) Laying down policies and codes to ensure observance of professional ethics in medical profession and to promote ethical conduct during the provision of care by medical practitioners.

(f) Exercising appellate jurisdiction with respect to the decisions of the Autonomous Boards and ensuring co-ordination among the Autonomous Boards.

(g) Framing guidelines for determination of fees and all other charges in respect of 50% of seats in private medical institutions and deemed to be universities.

C. **The Medical Advisory Council: S. 11,** Central Government shall constitute an advisory body to be known as the Medical Advisory Council. The members are as follows:

(a) The Chairperson of the Commission shall be the *ex officio* Chairperson of the Council.

(b) Every member of the Commission shall be the *ex officio* member of the Council.

(c) One member to represent each State, who is the Vice-Chancellor of a Health University in that State, to be nominated by that State Government.

(d) One member to represent each Union territory, who is the Vice-Chancellor of a Health University in that Union territory, to be nominated by the Ministry of Home Affairs in the Government of India.

(e) One member to represent each State and each Union territory from amongst elected members of the State Medical Council, to be nominated by that State Medical Council.

(f) The Chairman, University Grants Commission.

(g) The Director, National Assessment and Accreditation Council.

(h) Four members to be nominated by the Central Government from amongst persons holding the post of Director in the Indian Institutes of Technology, Indian Institutes of Management and the Indian Institute of Science.

If there is no Health University in any State or Union territory, the Vice-Chancellor of a University within that State or Union territory having the largest number of medical colleges affiliated to it shall be nominated by the State Government or by the Ministry of Home Affairs in the Government of India. If there is no University in any Union territory, the Ministry of Home Affairs shall nominate a member who possesses such medical qualification and experience as may be prescribed.

Role of Medical Advisory Council: It shall advise the NMC on measures to enhance equitable access to medical education. The states and Union territories may put forth their views and concerns before the Commission through Medical Advisory Council. The Council shall meet at least twice a year and all acts of the Council are decided by a majority of the members present and voting **(S. 13).**

D. **National Examination:**

1. ***National Eligibility-cum-Entrance Test:*** **S. 14,** there shall be a uniform National Eligibility-cum-Entrance Test for admission to the undergraduate and postgraduate super-specialty medical education in all medical institutions. The NMC shall conduct the test in English and in other languages, through designated authority. For all India seats, the designated authority of Central Government shall conduct the common counselling for admission; whereas the designated authority of the State Government shall conduct the common counselling for the seats at the State level.

2. ***National Exit Test (NEXT):*** **S. 15,** a common final year undergraduate medical examination, to be known as the National Exit Test shall be held for granting licence to practice medicine as medical practitioners and for enrolment in the State Register or the National Register. Any person with a foreign medical qualification shall have to qualify National Exit Test for the purpose of obtaining licence to practice medicine as medical practitioner and for enrolment in the State Register or the National Register. The National Exit Test shall be the basis for admission to the postgraduate broad-specialty medical education in medical institutions which are governed under the provisions of this Act.

The NMC shall conduct the test through designated authority and shall become operational within three years from the date of commencement of Act. The designated authority of the Central Government shall conduct the common counselling for All India seats and the designated authority of the State Government shall conduct the common counselling for the seats at the State level.

E. **Autonomous Boards: S. 16,** the Central Government shall constitute four **Autonomous Boards** under the supervision of the NMC. They are as follows: (a) The Undergraduate Medical Education Board (b) The Postgraduate Medical Education Board (c) The Medical Assessment and Rating Board (d) The Ethics and Medical Registration Board.

S. 17, each Autonomous Board consists of a President and four members (two whole-time and two part-time). The president and the members of the autonomous board are appointed by the Central Government except a part-time member who shall be chosen from amongst the elected members of the State Medical Council. Each Autonomous Board, except the Ethics and Medical Registration Board, shall be assisted by advisory committees for the efficient discharge of the functions. The Ethics and Medical Registration Board shall be assisted by ethics committees of experts. Every Autonomous Board shall meet at least once a month. All decisions of the Autonomous Boards shall be made by majority of votes of the President and members.

Main Functions of Autonomous Board

(a) **The Undergraduate Medical Education Board: S. 24,** the board shall (i) Determine standards of medical education at undergraduate level. (ii) Develop competency based dynamic curriculum at UG level. (iii) Develop competency based dynamic curriculum for addressing the needs of primary health services, community medicine and family medicine to ensure health care in such areas. (iv) Framing guidelines for setting up of medical institutions for imparting undergraduate courses. (v) Determining the minimum requirements and standards for conducting courses and examinations for undergraduates in medical institutions. (vi) Determine standards and norms for infrastructure, faculty and quality of education in medical institutions providing undergraduate medical education. (vii) Facilitating development and training of faculty members teaching undergraduate courses. (viii) Granting medical qualification at the undergraduate level.

(b) **The Postgraduate Medical Education Board: S. 25,** the board shall (i) Determine standards of medical education at postgraduate level. (ii) Develop competency based dynamic curriculum at PG and super-specialty level. (iii) Frame guidelines for setting up of medical institutions for imparting PG and super-specialty courses as per global norms and needs of the country. (iv) Determine standards and norms for infrastructure, faculty and quality of education in medical institutions conducting PG and super-specialty medical education. (v) Facilitate development and training of the faculty members teaching PG and super-specialty courses. (vi) Facilitate research and the international student and faculty exchange programmes relating to PG and super-specialty medical education. (vii) Specify norms for compulsory annual disclosure, electronically or otherwise, by medical institutions in respect of their functions that has a bearing on the interest of all stakeholders including faculty, the Commission and the Central Government. (viii) Grant of recognition to the medical qualifications at the PG and super-specialty level. (ix) Promote and facilitate PG course in Family medicine.

(c) **The Medical Assessment and Rating Board: S. 26,** the board shall (i) Determine the procedure for assessing and rating the medical institutions for their compliance with the standards laid down by the Undergraduate Medical Education Board or the Postgraduate Medical Education Board. (ii) Grant permission for establishment of a new medical institution, or to start any postgraduate course or to increase number of seats. (iii) Carry out inspections of medical institutions for assessing and rating such institutions. (iv) Take such measures, including issuing warning, imposition of monetary penalty, reducing intake or stoppage of admissions and recommending to the Commission for withdrawal of recognition, against a medical institution for failure to maintain the minimum essential standards specified by the Undergraduate Medical Education Board or the Postgraduate Medical Education Board.

(d) **The Ethics and Medical Registration Board: S. 27,** the Ethics and Medical Registration Board shall perform: (i) Maintains a register called **National Register** where the names, address, recognized qualifications possessed by all licensed medical practitioner either enrolled directly with NMC or with any State Medical Council. The State Medical Council which maintains the State Register shall supply copy of the same to Ethics and Medical Registration Board, so that the doctor's name is automatically registered in the National Register. The Ethics and Medical Registration Board maintains a separate National Register for Community Health Providers (S. 32). (ii) Regulate professional conduct and promote medical ethics. (iii) A medical practitioner or professional who is aggrieved by the decision of the Ethics and Medical Registration Board may prefer an appeal to the Commission within sixty days of communication of such decision.

Community Health Provider: S. 14, shall grant limited licence to practice medicine at mid-level as Community Health Provider to such person connected with modern scientific medical profession who qualify such criteria as may be specified by the regulations. The number of licenses shall not exceed one-third of the total number of licensed medical practitioners registered under sub-section (1). They may prescribe specified medicine independently, only in primary and preventive health care.

All medical qualifications which have been recognized before the date of commencement of this Act and are included in the Second Schedule and Part II of the Third Schedule to the Indian Medical Council Act, 1956, shall also be recognized medical qualifications for the purposes of this Act, and shall be listed and maintained by the Commission in such manner as may be specified by the regulations.

STATE MEDICAL COUNCIL (SMC)

Introduction

The State Medical Councils are autonomous bodies established under the State Medical Council Act. It consists of a set of members of the profession from the State by election, as well as by direct nomination by State Government.

- Members from RMPs at the State (elected).
- Members directly nominated by the State Government.
- **President and Vice-President:** They are elected by the members from among themselves.
- **Registrar:** He is the in-charge of the day-to-day administration.

Duration of members is for a maximum period of 5 years, or till new office is formed.

Functions

1. **Maintenance of state medical register (SMR):** The SMR contains the name, address, qualifications and date of qualification of every person who is registered under this Act. On registration, a number is allotted with a certificate and then the registered person is considered as "Registered Medical Practitioner" (RMP).
2. **Disciplinary control:** The SMC has power to erase the name of any doctor from the register when the RMP has been convicted of criminal offence or professional misconduct.
3. **Warning notice:** In case of first offence, doctor may be warned not to repeat the same.
4. **Penal erasure (Professional death sentence):** It means erasure of the name of the doctor from the register permanently when the offence is confirmed beyond doubt allowing not to practice the profession. The doctor then may apply for restoration at various fixed intervals. If the doctor is dissatisfied from the decision of SMC, he can appeal to the Central Health Ministry.

Under NMC Act 2019, states shall establish their respective State Medical Councils within three years of functioning of NMC. These Councils shall have a role similar to the NMC, at the State level.

MEDICAL ETHICS AND BIOETHICS

Ethics: It is concerned with moral principles, values and standard of conduct. The word ethics is derived from the Greek word 'ethos' which means 'character'.

Medical ethics: It is concerned with the moral principles that guide the members of medical profession when they deal with each other, their patients as well as with the state. It is closely related to law.

Ethics in medical practice is necessary as the doctors are dealing with the life of the patients. They have the power to cure as well as the power to kill a patient. It is required to ensure highest care to the community.

Bioethics: It is derived from Greek 'bio-life' and 'ethicos-moral'. It is the study of the ethical issues emerging from advances in biology and medicine.

Historical Emergence of Medical Ethics: (i) In 18th Century BC, the codes of conduct were laid by **Hammurabi,** well-acclaimed ruler of Babylon. These rules are testimony to the fact that the concept of medical ethics was well formulated early in the history of mankind. (ii) In 5th Century BC, **Hippocratic ethical code** attributed to the ancient Greek physician Hippocrates. (iii)In 9th century AD, the first book dedicated to medical ethics **"Adab al-Talib" (Conduct of a physician)** was written by Muslim physician Ishaq bin Ali. He described physicians as "guardians of soul". (iv) In 15th century AD, the concept of written consent and patient-physician contract was adopted and enforced by an Ottoman Empire court. (v) In 17th century AD, German philosopher "Immanuel Kant" laid the foundation of a secular-based theory of freedom and autonomy. (vi) In 1803, **Thomas Percival,** an English physician first used the term 'medical ethics. (vii) In 1847, The American Medical Association adopted its first code of ethics, largely based on Percival's work. (viii) In 1948, **Nuremberg Code:** The principles in this code were articulated in the context of the Nuremberg trials in 1947 at the end of World war II. As per this code, the voluntary consent of the human subject is absolutely essential. It is considered as the most important document in the history of clinical research ethics. (ix) In 1964, **Declaration of Helsinki:** The World Medical Association (WMA) General Assembly at Helsinki, Finland, developed a set of guidelines to safeguard the rights and well-being of subjects participating in clinical research. (x) In 1979, the US government to set up **'International Ethical Guidelines for Biomedical Research Involving Human Subjects'** that submitted the report (Belmont report), which stressed on three basic ethical principles: autonomy, beneficence and justice. These guidelines were made in view of unethical research conducted by the United States Public Health Service (Tuskegee Syphilis Study) was surfaced in 1979. (xi) In 1980, the **Indian Council of Medical Research (ICMR)** first released a policy statement on ethical considerations involved in research on human subjects. (xii) In 2000, ICMR revised the guidelines in the face of controversies and introduced "Ethical Guidelines for Biomedical Research on Human Subjects" and latest amendments was done in 2017.

Principles of Medical Ethics and Bioethics: (i) **Autonomy:** It is the rights of the individual to make decisions regarding health care procedures. (ii) **Justice:** Patient should share (more or less) equally in the costs and benefits of the health care system. (iii) **Beneficence:** Health care providers must strive to benefit their patient. Patient's welfare is the first consideration. (iv) **Non-maleficence/Do not harm:** Health care providers must not hurt their patient. (v) **Confidentiality:** Health care providers to maintain the confidentiality of all personal, medical and treatment information of the patient.

Oaths, Codes and Declarations

(i) **Hippocratic Oath (5th Century BC):** It is written in ionic Greek by Hippocrates, the 'Father of Western Medicine'. It is the oldest code of medical ethics which is being followed till date. However, the original version of the oath has been modified and numerous translations and variations have emerged for medical students to take, usually at graduation time.

It reads as follows:

"I swear by Apollo the physician, by Aesculapius, Hygeia and panacea and I take to witness all the Gods, all the Goddesses to keep according to my ability and judgment the following oath":

"To consider dear to me as my parents him who taught me this art; to live in common with him and if necessary to share my goods with him; to look upon his children as my own brothers, to teach them this art if they so desire without fee or written promise; to impart to my sons and the sons of the master who taught me and the disciples who have enrolled themselves and have agreed to the rules of the profession, but to these alone, the precepts and the instruction. I will prescribe regimen for the good of my patients according to my ability and my judgment and never do harm to anyone. To please no one will I prescribe a deadly drug, nor give advice which may cause his death. Nor, will I give a woman a pessary to procure abortion. But I will preserve the purity of my life and my art. I will not cut for stone, even for patients in whom the disease is manifested. I will leave this operation to be performed by practitioners (specialists in this art). In every house where I come I will enter only for the good of my patients, keeping myself far from all intentional ill-doing and all seduction, and especially from the pleasures of love with women or with men, be they free or slaves. All that may come to my knowledge in the exercise or my profession or outside or any profession or in daily commerce with men, which ought not to be spread abroad. I will keep secret and will never reveal. If I keep this oath faithfully, may I enjoy my life and practice my art, respected by all men and in all times; but if I swerve from it or violate it, may the reverse be my lot."

(ii) **Charaka's Oath (150-200AD):** It is an ancient Indian oath mentioned in 'Charaka Samhita' written by Charaka. It contains several uniquely Hindu elements, including the requirements to lead the life of a celibate, eat no meat and carry no arms.

It reads as follows *"I shall be free from envy, not cause another death, and pray for the welfare of all creatures. Day and night, I shall not desert a patient, not commit adultery, be modest in my attire and appearance, not be drunkard or sinful, while entering a patient's house, be accompanied by a person known to the patient."*

(iii) **Sushruta Oath (888-700 BC):** He was a physician and surgeon in ancient India and is known as the 'Father of Indian Medicine', 'Father of Plastic Surgery' and 'Father of Brain Surgery'. His works are compiled as Sushruta Samhita or Compendium of Sushrut which is considered as a foundational text of Ayurveda.

The new student was expected to study for at least 6 years and before starting his training, he had to take a solemn oath. The oath can be compared to that of Hippocrates.

"Thou shalt renounce all evil desires, anger, greed, passion, pride, egotism, envy, harshness, meanness, untruth, indolence and other qualities that bring infamy upon oneself."

"Thou shalt clip thy nails and hair close, observe cleanliness . . . and dedicate thyself to the observance of truth, celibacy and the salutation of elders..."

"The preceptor, the poor, the friendly, the travellers, the lowly, the good and the destitute – those thou shalt treat when they come to thee like thy own kith and kin and relieve their ailments..."

(iv) **Declaration of the World Medical Association (WMA):** The World Medical Association is an international organization representing medical organizations and physicians across world. It is advisory body for medical profession which was established in the year 1947 at Paris. The WMA council meets bi-annually. It issues policy statements on a range of ethical issues related to medical professionalism, patient care, research on human subjects and public health.

(a) ***The Declaration of Geneva (1948):*** It is one of the oldest policies by the 2nd General Assembly in Geneva in 1948. It builds on the principles of the Hippocratic Oath, and is now known as **'The Modern Hippocratic Oath'.** It has been amended several times. Most recently, on October 13, 2017, at Chicago, USA, the WMA adopted a revised version of the substance to the Hippocratic Oath.

At the time of being admitted a member of the medical profession, the physician shall pledge: (i) I solemnly pledge to dedicate my life to the service of humanity. (ii) I will give to my teachers the respect and gratitude which is their due. (iii) I will practice my profession with conscience and dignity. (iv) The health of my patient will be my first consideration. (v) I will respect the secrets which are confided in me, even after the patient has died. (vi) I will maintain by all means in my power the honour and the noble traditions of the medical profession. (vii) My colleagues will be my brothers. (viii) I will not permit considerations of religion, nationality, race, party politics or social standing to intervene between my duty and my patient. (ix) I will maintain the utmost respect for human life from the time of conception; even under threat, I will not use my medical knowledge contrary to the laws of humanity. (x) I make these promises solemnly, freely and upon my honour.

(b) ***International Code of Medical Ethics (1949):*** It was adopted by the *3rd General Assembly of the World Medical Association, London, England in 1949. Subsequently it was amended at 22nd World Medical Assembly, Sydney, Australia (1968), 35th World Medical Assembly, Venice, Italy (1983), 57th WMA General Assembly, Pilanesberg, South Africa (2006). It is a code based on the declaration of Geneva* to establish the ethical principles of the physicians worldwide, based on his duties in general, to his patients and to his colleagues.

(c) ***Declaration of Helsinki (1964):*** Statement of ethical principles of medical research involving human subjects (amendment 2013) (Please refer 'Human Experimentation' below).

(d) ***Declaration of Sydney (1968):*** Declaration on determination of death and the recovery of organs *Adopted by the 22nd WMA, Sydney, Australia, 1968 (amendment in 1983, 2006, 2016).*

(e) ***Declaration of Oslo (1970):*** Statement on therapeutic abortion was adopted by the *24th World Medical Assembly, Oslo, Norway, 1970 (amended in 1983, 2006).*

(f) ***Declaration of Tokyo (1975):*** Guidelines for the physicians concerning torture and other cruel, inhuman or degrading treatment or punishment in relation to detention and imprisonment was adopted in *29th WMA, Tokyo, Japan, 1975 (amended in 2006).*

(g) ***Declaration of Lisbon (1981):*** Declaration on the right of a patient was adopted *34th WMA, Lisbon, Portugal, 1981(amended in 2005, 2015).*

(h) ***Declaration of Malta (1991):*** Declaration on hunger strike was adopted by the 43rd WMA, Malta (amended 1992).

(i) ***Declaration of Taipei (2016):*** Declaration of Taipei on Ethical Considerations regarding Health Databases and Biobanks was adopted in *67th WMA General Assembly, Taipei, Taiwan, 2016.*

(j) **Declaration Chicago (2017):** Statement of quality assurance in medical education *was adopted by the 68th WMA General Assembly, Chicago, USA, 2017.*

INDIAN MEDICAL COUNCIL (PROFESSIONAL CONDUCT, ETIQUETTE AND ETHICS REGULATIONS, 2002)

The Medical Council of India brought into force the ethical regulations in year 2002 called the Indian Medical Council Regulations, 2002 (recent amendment 2009, 2019 and 2020). They are binding on all doctors in India. There are 8 chapters in the regulation describing (i) Code of medical ethics. (ii) Duties of physicians to their patients. (iii) Duties of physicians in consultation. (iv) Responsibilities of physicians to each other. (v) Duties of physicians to the public and to the paramedical profession. (vi) Unethical acts. (vii) Misconduct. (viii) Punishment and disciplinary action.

As per the regulation, at the time of making an application for registration, the applicant shall submit a duly signed Declaration (see Appendix 1). The applicant shall also certify that he/she had read and agreed to abide by the same.

Appendix-1

A. DECLARATION

At the time of registration, each applicant shall be given a copy of the following declaration by the Registrar concerned and the applicant shall read and agree to abide by the same:

1. I solemnly pledge myself to consecrate my life to service of humanity.
2. Even under threat, I will not use my medical knowledge contrary to the laws of humanity.
3. I will maintain the utmost respect for human life from the time of conception.
4. I will not permit considerations of religion, nationality, race, party politics or social standing to intervene between my duty and my patient.
5. I will practice my profession with conscience and dignity.
6. The health of my patient will be my first consideration.
7. I will respect the secrets which are confined in me.
8. I will give to my teachers the respect and gratitude which is their due.
9. I will maintain by all means in my power, the honour and noble traditions of medical profession.
10. I will treat my colleagues with all respect and dignity.
11. I shall abide by the code of medical ethics as enunciated in the Indian Medical Council (Professional Conduct, Etiquette and Ethics) Regulations 2002.

I make these promises solemnly, freely and upon my honour.

Signature ....

Name ....

Place ....

Address ....

Date ....

Rights and Privileges of Registered Medical Practitioner (RMP)

(i) Right to practice medicine (ii) Right to choose a patient, except in emergency (iii) Right to issue a certificate (iv) Right to add title to his name (v) Right to recover his fees (vi) Right of appointment to public hospitals (vii) Right to give expert evidence in the court of law (viii) Right to dispense medicine.

The use of Red Cross Emblem by the doctors is prohibited. **S. 12 of Geneva Convention Act 1960** prohibits its use and allied emblem without the approval of Central Government. The medical as well as paramedical staffs using it can be penalized under S. 13 of the above Act with fine upto Rs.500 and forfeiture of the property on which it has been used. It can be used by the armed forces medical services, their personnel units, installations and means of transport.

Duties of A Medical Practitioner

The RMP has multiform duties towards the patient, colleagues and State. Some of these are as follows:

A. Duties and Responsibilities in General

(i) **Character of physicians:** A physician shall uphold the dignity and honour of his profession. He should be modest, sober, patient, prompt in discharging his duty without anxiety. He should render service to humanity and reward or financial gain should be a subordinate consideration for him.

(ii) **Maintaining good medical practice:** Physician should practice methods of healing founded on scientific basis and should not associate professionally with anyone who violates this principle. He/she should try continuously to improve medical knowledge and skills. Physician should participate in professional meetings as part of Continuing Medical Education (CME) programmes, for **at least 30 hours every 5 years.** He/she should affiliate with associations and societies of allopathic medical professions and involve actively in the functioning of such bodies.

(iii) **Maintaining of medical records:** Physician shall maintain the medical records pertaining to his/her indoor patients **for a period of 3 years** from the date of commencement of the treatment. On the request of by the patients/authorised attendant or legal authorities, the medical records should be issued within the period of 72 hours. Efforts shall be made to computerize medical records for quick retrieval.

(iv) **Display of registration number:** Physician shall display the registration number accorded to him/her by NMC/SMC in his/her clinic and in all his prescriptions, certificates, money receipts given to patients. The physician shall display as suffix to their names only recognized medical degrees or such certificates/diplomas and memberships/honours which confer professional knowledge or recognizes any exemplary qualification/achievements.

(v) **Use of generic names of drugs:** Physician should prescribe drugs with generic names (not in brand name) preferably in capital letters. The physician shall ensure that there is a rational prescription and use of drugs.

(vi) **High quality assurance in patient care:** Physician should not employ in connection with his/her professional practice any attendant who is neither registered nor enlisted under the Medical Acts in force and shall not permit such persons to attend, treat or perform operations upon patients wherever professional discretion or skill is required.

(vii) **Exposure of unethical conduct:** A physician should expose, without fear or favour, incompetent or corrupt, dishonest or unethical conduct on the part of members of the profession.

(viii) **Payment of professional fees:** A physician should announce his fees before rendering service and not after the operation or treatment is under way. Physician rendering service on behalf of the state shall refrain from anticipating or accepting any consideration.

(ix) **Evasion of legal restrictions:** The physician shall observe the laws of the country in regulating the practice of medicine and shall also not assist others to evade such laws.

B. Duties Towards Patients

(i) **Duty to exercise necessary care and skill:** When a patient comes to a doctor, the doctor has right to refuse him but once he starts treating the patient his duty towards the patient starts. For patients coming to the hospital for treatment, the duty towards the patient arises when the patient gets treatment. However, in cases of emergency the doctor cannot refuse the patient and only after giving the first aid and other life saving measures, if available with due precautions he can refer the patient to the nearest hospital where advanced facilities are available. The doctor should use reasonable skill and care according to his knowledge and qualification for treating the patient. In addition, in case of minors, the doctor has the duty to exercise such care and skill even though the fee is being paid by the guardian.

(ii) **To examine the patient properly:** It is the duty of the doctor to examine the patient thoroughly after obtaining proper history from him or from his attendant.

(iii) **To prescribe proper medicines:** The doctor should prescribe proper medicines after carefully evaluating the patient. In patients getting treatment from government hospitals, if the medicines are not available, the doctor should advice the patient to purchase them from the market. When the doctor prescribes a wrong medicine or does not provide proper instructions that causes harm to the patient, he will be liable to the damages.

(iv) **Duty to inform the risks:** The doctor should inform the patient about the disease and possible risks involved with the treatment. If the patient is not of sound mind the guardian should be informed about them. Only after obtaining the consent the doctor should start the treatment. In circumstances where the doctor feels that there are chances of psychological upset once he discloses all the risks to the patient, he can withhold some of the risks.

(v) **Duty to give proper instructions:** The doctor should give full instructions to the patient or to the attendants regarding the proper administration of medicines and type of diet to be taken. He should also mention the dose and frequency of the medicines to be used. In addition, in cases of any untoward reaction the patient should be advised to report immediately.

(vi) **Instructions to those patients who cannot take care of themselves:** In cases of mentally ill or comatose patients, their attendants or guardians should be properly instructed about the use of medicine.

(vii) **Duty in relation to operations:** After careful diagnosis when the surgeon thinks that it is necessary to operate the patient, he should explain the nature and extent of operation to the patient. The possible risks involved in these cases and any alternative method available should also be explained. He must obtain consent before performing operation. He must not experiment on the patient. He should be sure that no swabs or any instrument are left inside the body after operation. He must take postoperative care properly to avoid any complication.

(viii) **Inform third parties:** In cases of patient suffering from infectious diseases, the doctor should not only warn the patient but also the third party, i.e., relatives, friends and co-workers, thus proper precautions can be taken by them. He also has duty to inform the health authorities about the infectious diseases.

(ix) **Poisoning cases:** When the doctor attends a suspected poisoning case, he has to do the stomach wash with plain water so that the sample can be sent for chemical analysis. He has to preserve vomitus, blood and urine for chemical analysis. After that he should treat the patient with suitable antidote and then carry out further management. The doctor should inform the police in case of suspected homicidal poisoning.

C. Duties Towards Colleagues

(i) **Conduct in consultation:** When a patient comes to him after leaving another doctor, he must not criticize that doctor in front of the patient. Also, he should not criticize the medicines prescribed by that doctor earlier in order to gain cheap popularity. He/she not be indulged in any rivalry or enmity and insincerity in consultations.

(ii) **Consultant not to take charge of the case:** When any specialist examines or treats another doctor, he should not demand any fees from him. It is the professional courtesy he has to extend to his colleagues.

(iii) **Dependence of physicians on each other:** A physician should consider it as a pleasure and privilege to render gratuitous service to all physicians and their immediate family dependents.

(iv) **Appointment of substitute:** It is a professional courtesy of a physician to accept the request of a colleague to attend his patients during his temporary absence from his practice, only when he has the capacity to discharge the additional responsibility.

D. Duties Towards State

(i) **Notifiable diseases:** A doctor is bound to inform the communicable diseases like cholera, plague etc. to the Health authorities.

(ii) He is also bound to **inform the birth and death** to proper authorities. If a doctor fails to inform, a civil suit can be brought against him, but not a criminal suit.

(iii) **Geneva Convention (1949):** A medical practitioner is bound to treat or provide medical aid in cases of person wounded or sick of the armed forces (I Convention), ship wrecked persons (II Convention); prisoner of war (III Convention) and civilians of enemy nationalist (IV Convention). All the above categories of persons should be treated without any discrimination based on race, religion or political grounds.

(iv) It is a duty of doctor to **inform police or magistrate** of medicolegal cases brought to him during his medical practice.

E. Duties of Physician in Consultation

(i) **Unnecessary consultation should be avoided:** The physician should request for consultation for justifiable reasons in the interest of the patient only and not for any other consideration. It should be done judiciously and not in a routine manner while consulting pathologists/radiologists or asking for any other diagnostic lab investigation.

(ii) **Consultation for patient's benefit:** In every consultation, the benefit to the patient is of foremost importance.

(iii) **Punctuality in consultation:** The physician should observe utmost punctuality in attending a consultation referred to him/her.

(iv) **Statement to patient after consultation:** All statements to the patient or his representatives should take place in the presence of the consulting physicians, except as otherwise agreed. Differences of opinion should not be divulged unnecessarily.

(v) **Treatment after consultation:** The attending physician can make subsequent variations in the treatment if any unexpected change occurs, but at the next consultation, reasons for the variations should be discussed/explained. The attending physician may prescribe medicine at any time for the patient, whereas the consultant may prescribe only in case of emergency or as an expert when called for.

(vi) **Patients referred to specialists:** An attending physician should send a case summary of the patient while referring the patient to a specialist. The specialist shall communicate his opinion in writing to the attending physician.

(vii) **Fees and other charges:** A physician shall clearly display his fees and other charges on the board of his chamber and/or the hospitals he is visiting.

Recent Amendment in Indian Medical Council (Professional Conduct, Etiquette and Ethics) Regulations, 2002

A. 2009 Amendment

Gift to doctors run **afoul** of MCI Ethics regulation:

1. Medical practitioner shall not receive any gift, travel facility or hospitality from any pharmaceutical or allied health care industry and their sales people or representatives.
2. He shall not receive any cash or any monetary grant.
3. But it permits funding for medical research, study etc. provided the money is received through the approved institutions.
4. It also permits the doctors to work for pharmaceutical and allied health care companies in advisory capacity, as consultants, researchers and treating doctors.

B. 2019 Amendment

Submission of false or wrong information by a Medical Faculty in the Declaration Form submitted at the time of assessment by Council, will be treated as misconduct both by the Medical Faculty and the Dean/Head of Department countersigning the Declaration Form.

C. 2020 Amendment

Consultation Through Telemedicine

In view of COVID-19 pandemic, on 25 March, 2020, the Board of Governors (BOG) instituted by the Central Government for regulating medical education and the medical profession in India, issued the Telemedicine Practice Guidelines in partnership with the NITI Aayog. The Guidelines are included in the Indian Medical Council (Professional Conduct, Etiquette and Ethics) Regulations, 2002 (Amendment 2020) and violation thereof, would constitute 'Misconduct' under the regulations.

1. **Definition of Telemedicine (As per WHO):** The delivery of health care services, where distance is a critical factor, by all health care professionals using information and communication technologies for the exchange of valid information for diagnosis, treatment and prevention of disease and injuries, research and evaluation, and for the continuing education of health care providers, all in the interests of advancing the health of individuals and their communities.
2. **Definition of Telehealth (As per NEJM Catalyst):** The delivery and facilitation of health and health-related services including medical care, provider and patient education, health information services, and self-care via telecommunications and digital communication technologies.

   Scope: (i) The guidelines are meant for registered medical practitioner (RMP). (ii) The guidelines cover norms and standards of the RMP to consult patients via telemedicine. (iii) Telemedicine includes all channels of communication with the patient that leverage Information Technology platforms, including Voice, Audio, Text and Digital Data exchange.
3. **The guidelines specifically explicitly exclude the following:** (i) Specifications for hardware or software, infrastructure building and maintenance. (ii) Data management systems involved; standards and interoperability. (iii) Use of digital technology to conduct surgical or invasive procedures remotely. (iv) Other aspects of telehealth such as research and evaluation and continuing education of health care workers. (v) Does not provide for consultations outside the jurisdiction of India.

Guidelines for Telemedicine in India: (a) ***Decision for Telemedicine consultation:*** The RMP should exercise his/her professional judgment to decide whether a telemedicine consultation is appropriate in a given situation or an in-person consultation is needed in the interest of the patient. (b) ***Identification:*** Both patient and the RMP need to know each other's identity through proper mechanism. Where the patient is a minor, after confirming the age, tele consultation would be allowed only if the minor is consulting alongwith an adult whose identity needs to be ascertained. (c) ***Mode of telemedicine:*** Primarily there are 3 modes of consultation: Video, Audio or Text (chat, images, messaging, email, fax etc.). (d) ***Consent of patient:*** If, the patient initiates the telemedicine consultation, then the consent is implied. If a health worker, RMP or a caregiver initiates a telemedicine consultation, an explicit consent is required which can be sent by the patient via an email, text or audio/video message. The RMP must record this in his patient records. (e) ***Exchange of information for patient evaluation:*** RMP would use his/her professional discretion to gather the type and extent of patient information (history/examination findings/Investigation reports/past records etc.) required to be able to exercise proper clinical judgement. If he/she feels the information received is inadequate, then he/she can request for additional information from the patient. If a physical examination is critical information for consultation, RMP should not proceed until a physical examination can be arranged through an in-person consult. (f) ***In emergency:*** In all cases of emergency, the patient must be advised for in-person interaction with an RMP at the earliest. However, if this is not possible emergency consult for immediate assistance or first aid etc., may be offered. (g) ***Prescription of medicines:*** RMP may prescribe medicines via telemedicine only when RMP is satisfied that he/she has gathered adequate and relevant information about the patient's medical condition and prescribed medicines are in the best interest of the patient. RMP must prescribe medicines as per Indian

Medical Council (Professional Conduct, Etiquette and Ethics Regulation, 2002 and not in contravention with Drugs and Cosmetics Act and Rules. RMP cannot prescribe Schedule X of Drug and Cosmetic Act and Rules. (h) ***Misconduct:*** In telemedicine practice, some examples of misconduct by RMP are: (i) Insisting on telemedicine, when the patient is willing to travel to a facility and/or requests an in-person consultation. (ii) Misusing patient images and data, especially private and sensitive in nature (e.g., RMP uploads an explicit picture of patient on social media etc.). (iii) Prescribe medicines from the specific restricted list of drugs. (iv) Solicit patients for telemedicine through any advertisements or inducements. (i) ***Fees:*** Teleconsultation fees can be charged in the same way as in-person consultations from the patient and RMP should give a receipt/invoice for the same. (j) ***Rights to discontinue teleconsultation:*** The RMP can choose not to proceed with the consultation at any time. At any step, he /she may refer or request for an in-person consultation. The patient has the right to choose to discontinue the teleconsultation at any stage.

Unethical Acts

According this regulation, unethical acts in medical practice includes the following:

(i) **Advertisement:** Soliciting of patients directly or indirectly, by a group of physicians or by institutions or organization shall be constructed as unethical acts. A physician should not exhibit publicly the scale of fees except in the waiting hall of the patients or in his chamber. The doctor can publish any change in address in newspapers or journals. He can even publish about his timings, interruption or restarting of the practice after a long interval in the press. The doctor can write to the lay press in his name on matters of public interest and even can deliver public lectures and can give talks on the radio. He should not use an unusually large signboard in front of his clinic/nursing home and should not write on it anything other than his name, qualification and the name of his specialty. The same should be contents of his prescription letter or letter head, which may in addition contain his address, registration number and telephone number. Printing of self-photograph in letterhead or signboard is unethical. It is unethical to fix a signboard on a chemist shop or in places where he does not reside or work. He should not advertise himself through manufacturing firms directly or indirectly. (ii) **Patent and copyrights:** Physician may patent surgical instruments, appliances and medicine or copyright applications, methods and procedures. However, it shall be unethical if the benefits of such patents or copyrights are not made available in situations where the interest of large population is involved. (iii) **Running an open shop (Dispensing of drugs and appliances by physician):** A physician should not run an open shop for sale of medicine for dispensing prescriptions prescribed by doctors other than himself or for sale of medical or surgical appliances. (iv) **Rebates and commission (cut practice/fee splitting/dichotomy):** A physician shall not give, solicit, or receive nor shall he offer to give solicit or receive, any gift, gratuity, commission or bonus in consideration of or return for the referring, recommending or procuring of any patient for medical, surgical or other treatment. A physician shall not directly or indirectly, participate in or be a party to act of division, transference, assignment, subordination, rebating, splitting or refunding of any fee for medical, surgical or other treatment. (v) **Secret remedies:** The physician should not prescribe or dispense secret remedial agents of which he does not know the composition. The physician should not manufacture or promote the use of such secret remedial agents. (vi) **Human Rights:** The physician shall not aid or abet torture nor shall he be a party to either infliction of mental or physical trauma or concealment of torture inflicted by some other person or agency in clear violation of human rights. (vii) **Euthanasia:** Practicing euthanasia by a physician shall constitute unethical conduct. Passive euthanasia is now legal in India. However, it cannot be practiced by the treating physician alone. For passive euthanasia a medical board takes decision. (viii) **Pharmaceutical and allied health sector industry:** A medical practitioner shall not receive any **gift, cash, monetary grants, travel facilities** or **hospitality** like hotel accommodation from any pharmaceutical or allied health care industry and their sales people or representatives for self and family members for vacation or for attending conferences, seminars, workshops, CME programme etc. as a delegate or under any pretext. Receipt of funding for medical research or study should be through approved institutions and should be fully disclosed. As per section 6.8.1, action shall be taken in case of violation and the quantum of punishment is as per the cost of the bribe: (a) More than Rs. 1000 and upto Rs. 5000-Warning/ Censure (b) More than Rs. 5000 and upto Rs. 10000-Removal from Indian or State Medical Register for 3 months (c) More than Rs.10000 and upto Rs. 50000-Removal from Indian or State Medical Register for 6 months (d) More than Rs.50000 and upto Rs. 100000-Removal from Indian or State Medical Register for 1 year (e) More than Rs.100000-Removal from Indian or State Medical Register for more than 1 year. (ix) **Endorsement of any drug or product:** A medical practitioner should not endorse any drug or product of the industry publically.

Professional Misconduct

It is also known as **infamous conduct or disgraceful act.** It is the improper conduct of the doctors in the professional aspect. What really constitutes misconduct is controversial. However, as per Indian Medical Council (Professional Conduct, Etiquette and Ethics) Regulation, the NMC has enlisted the acts or behaviour that constitutes the professional misconduct. If the doctor's act falls in any of the enlisted acts, he is liable for disciplinary action. The conduct of the doctor is judged by the professional men of good repute and competence. The NMC or SMC is also empowered to act against an act done by the doctor even if it is not included in the list. The following are the few examples of professional misconduct for which action can be taken.

(i) ***Any unethical acts mentioned above.*** (ii) ***Adultery or improper conduct:*** Adultery is no longer criminal offence in India. However, improper conduct or association of a male or female doctor with a patient (both male or female) or their attendants is punishable, so far as professional misconduct is concerned. (iii) ***Association with unqualified persons:*** He should not use touts and agents for fetching patients. (iv) ***Addiction:*** He should not use any drugs of addiction that can hamper the practice. (v) ***Alcohol:*** He should not practice medicine under the influence of alcohol, which interfere with the skilled performances. (vi) ***Abortion:*** The doctor should not perform an abortion that is not under the provisions of MTP Act and he should not assist any unqualified person while performing criminal abortion. (vii) ***Advertisement:*** (a) A physician should not contribute to the lay press articles and give interviews regarding diseases and treatments which may have the effect of advertising himself or soliciting practices; but is open to write to the lay press under his own name on matters of public health, hygienic living or to deliver public lectures, give talks on the radio/TV/internet chat for the same purpose and send announcement of the same to lay press. (b) He should not use an unusually large signboard and write on it anything other than his name, qualifications obtained from a University or a statutory body, titles and name of his specialty, registration number including the name of the State Medical Council under which registered. The same should be the contents of his prescription papers. (c) He should not affix a signboard on a chemist's shop or in places where he does not reside or work. (viii) ***Disclosing the patient's secrets,*** except the situations where he/she is bound by the law to reveal, e.g., in case of notifiable diseases. (ix) ***Refusal to treat*** a patient on religious grounds. (x) ***Running a chemist shop*** for the sale of medicine or for dispensing prescriptions of other doctors. (xi) ***Issuing false certificates*** in connection with sick benefit insurance or passport etc. (xii) ***Assisting*** a person who has no qualification to attend or treat a patient. (xiii) ***Not maintaining medical records*** of his/her indoor patients for 3 years and refuses to provide the same within 72 hours, ***when the patient requests for it.*** (xiv) ***Conducting sex determination tests*** with intent to terminate the life of a female fetus, unless indicated in the MTP Act. (xv) ***Not displaying registration number*** in his/her clinic and prescription. (xvi) ***Publishing photographs or reports*** of his/her patient without consent in medical or other journal or social media in a manner by which the patient's identity could be made out. (xvii) ***Convicted by court of law.*** (xviii) ***Contravening drugs and cosmetics Act,*** especially prescribing steroids/psychotropic drugs when there is no absolute medical indication and selling "H' and 'L' drugs and poisons to the public except to his patient. (xix) ***Violating the existing ICMR guidelines*** while doing drug trials and other research involving volunteers and patients. (xx) ***Claiming as specialist when the physician does not have special qualification.*** (xxi) ***In vitro fertilization or artificial insemination without informed consent*** of female patient and her spouse as well as the donor. (xxii) ***Submission of false or wrong information*** by a Medical Faculty in the Declaration Form submitted at the time of assessment by Council, will be treated as misconduct both by the Medical Faculty and the Dean/Head of Department countersigning the Declaration Form (amendment 2019). (xxiii) ***Misconduct in telemedicine practice:*** (Please refer details–Consultation through telemedicine).

Punishment and Disciplinary Action for Professional Misconduct

The list of professional misconduct given under regulation is not a complete one, the doctor can be penalized for a conduct even though it is not on the list depending on the nature.

Disciplinary Committee: The Ethics and Medical Registration Board of NMC shall ensure compliance of the code of professional and ethical conduct through the State Medical Council in a case where such State Medical Council has been conferred power to take disciplinary actions in respect of professional or ethical misconduct by medical practitioners under respective State Act.

Disciplinary Procedures: After receipt of any complaint of professional misconduct, the appropriate medical council (state medical council) would hold an inquiry. During the inquiry, the medical practitioner will be given an opportunity to be heard in person or by pleader. A decision on the complaint has to be taken within 6 months from filing the complaint. During the pendency of the complaint, the council may restrain the physician from performing the procedure or practice under scrutiny. If State Medical Council does not take a decision within 6 months of filing the complaint, the Ethics and Medical Registration Board of NMC can impress upon the concerned State Council to decide the complaint in a time-bound manner. It can also withdraw the complaint to itself for expeditious disposal. Professional incompetence shall be judged by the peer group prescribed by the NMC.

Punishment: If a doctor found guilty of professional misconduct, he/she may be issued **warning notice** or his/her name may be erased from the medical register **(Penal erasure)** for a specified period or permanently. If the name is permanently removed, it is termed as **Professional death sentence.** The erasure from the register is widely publicized through the local press as well as publications of different Medical Associations/Bodies/Societies.

Appeal and Limitation: A person aggrieved by the decision of State Medical Council can file an appeal to the National Medical Commission, India within 60 days from the date of receipt of the order passed by State Medical Council. Further extension may be granted by the MCI if it is satisfied that the appellant was prevented by sufficient cause from filing the appeal within 60 days.

Communication Skills

Communication skills are the abilities a person use when giving and receiving different kinds of information. The ability to communicate effectively is a core competency for doctors. Communication skills of the doctors could be enhanced by training and experience. The National Medical Commission of India reaffirms the need to include training in communication skills in the MBBS curriculum.

Benefits of good communications skill in medical practice: It builds an optimal doctor-patient relationship, that leads to better compliance, better health outcomes, decreased litigation, and higher satisfaction both for doctors and patients.

Components of communication skills: There are 3 basic components of effective communication (i) **Verbal:** It includes the written and spoken word. (ii) **Non-verbal:** It includes attentive posture, eye contact, facial expression, and encouraging the patient to talk using cues such as nodding etc. (iii) **Paraverbal:** It includes tone, pitch and pacing of the voice.

Common barriers to effective communication: Common barriers to good communication between doctor and patient include: (i) **Use of medical jargon** (language understand by the doctor). (ii) **Language barrier:** Language difference and inability to communicate in a simple language by the doctor. (iii) **Cultural and social barriers:** Social values, belief and cultural perceptions of health, sickness, and medical care of patients and families may differ with that of the physicians. (iv) **Low health literacy** among patients. (v) **Arrogance** among physicians. (vi) **Time management:** Lack of enough time dedicated to the doctor-patient encounter, and frequent interruptions while the patient is narrating his problems. (vii) The **physical setup** of the clinic etc.

Essential skills of effective communication are: (i) **Active listening:** The physician should actively listen to the patient the using nonverbal (e.g., eye contact) and verbal (e.g., words of encouragement) techniques and spend time with patient. The physician needs to listen to his/her patients' stories and how the illness affected his/her patients' life. The doctor should not interrupt the patient while he/she is talking. It creates trust in doctor-patient relationship which is a prerequisite for therapeutic success. (ii) **Empathy:** It is the capacity to understand and relate to the patient's illness experience and emotions. It is a skill that promotes professional satisfaction for the doctor and allows for more effective care, as patients are more likely to be open with an empathetic doctor. (iii) **Other essential skills** are like **patience, calm and confident, being honest and open minded, giving and receiving feedback** etc.

Communicating with the patient: There are 3 main goals for doctor-patient communication (a) **A good interpersonal relationship** (b) **Facilitating exchange of information** (c) **Inclusion of patient in decision making.**

The doctor should (i) Put the patient at ease and comfort. (ii) Introduce himself/herself to the patient and explain his/her role in the patient's care. (iii) Greet the patient with smile and cheerful voice, can shake hands with the patient, but not to force physical contact if the patient is uncomfortable. (iv) Sit at patient's level and make eye contact when appropriate. (v) Maintain privacy of the patient, acknowledge and greet others in the room. (vi) Maintain a professional appearance (proper dress with neat and clean appearance). (vii) Show respect to the patient. (viii) Review the medical record of the patient and ask basic get-to-know-you questions to the patient. (ix) Elicit the patient's full set of concerns. (x) Acknowledge and respond to the patient's ideas, feelings, and values. (xi) Summarize and affirm agreement with the plan of action with the patient etc.

Communicating with the attendant: The doctor should (i) Discuss with patient attendants frequently and explain them dynamic nature of the disease. (ii) Expresses support and build partnership with them. (iii) Alleviate patient attendant's concern, respect their experience and praise their efforts. The doctor should (iv) Never express shock and should try to convince attendant that all efforts are being made to bring situation under control or will be controlled. (v) Always explain about the necessity and yield of expensive investigations and risks/benefits involved in invasive procedures to the patient's attendants. (vi) Extremely cautious while managing difficult encounters and breaking bad news.

Communicating with the colleagues: These skills also extend to a doctor's ability to collaborate and work as part of a larger team of medical professionals. **The doctor should** (i) Not talk low about his/her colleagues or scold residents, fellows or other students in front of patients or attendants. (ii) Show greatest courtesy to all staffs including nurses, paramedical staffs and other supporting staffs. (iii) Explain the role and responsibility of his/her colleagues/staffs and make them realise that they are a part of the team. (iv) Lead the team by setting examples. (v) Teach the juniors/medical staffs about basics and the principles of management of commonly encountered diseases in his/her ward which will keep them motivated. (vi) Do audit and get feedback about his/her work which will improve professional practice. (vii) Appreciate work of his/her colleagues. (viii) Give positive criticism only, whenever required.

Doctors and Media

Role of media: (a) Media is a very effective medium for the dissemination of timely health care and wellness information (b) The social media can be used for professional networking (c) It is also being used to improve professional education (d) It can be used for organizational promotion (e) It can quickly spread information and mobilize large numbers of people to facilitate greater progress toward public health goals.

Nowadays, doctors have been portrayed by media in very different ways. Sometimes, stories about doctors in the media have reinforced positive impressions of medical practitioners. However, occasionally, the media has sown seeds of distrust in a profession that is committed above all else to doing no harm.

The doctor should: (a) Follow the guidelines about advertisement and sharing of information in lay press by doctor mentioned in Indian Medical Council (Professional Conduct, Etiquette and Ethics) Regulations, 2002. (b) Follow institutional policies, especially for those low in their institutional hierarchy, from medical students to entry-level employees. (c) Should continue to operate under the professional principle of first doing no harm. (d) Obtain informed consent from the patient before posting information and images online. (e) Protect patient information by deidentifying the information and or image while posting online (f) Declare conflict of interest and any financial interest linked to their posts in social media. (g) Respect the colleagues and profession in their social media interaction.

The doctor should not: (a) Offer medical advice to individuals on social media. (b) Involved in sensationalist social media posts. (c) Allow bias to influence their reporting and must be sure that all statements that they make are well thought-out, measured, and free from ambiguity. (d) Breach the confidentiality of the doctor-patient relationship when working with any media outlet. (e) Violate institutional policy. (f) Accept sponsorship on personal social media accounts and or supporting products for financial gain. (g) Comment negatively about medical profession or colleague.

Challenges in Managing Medicolegal (MLC) Cases

A medicolegal case (MLC) can be defined as "a case of injury or ailment, etc., in which investigations by the law-enforcing agencies are essential to fix the responsibility regarding the causation of the injury or ailment". MLC examination and reporting is one of the legal responsibilities of all doctors. MLC cases *have to be dealt with due care and proficiency.* MLC to be made by the doctor who has examined the patient first. In case it has not been made in the casualty, it can be made in the ward also. Police has no say in making the case as medicolegal or not. The decision to label a case as MLC should be based detailed history, thorough clinical examination and sound professional judgement. However, it has been *seen with avoidance, anxiousness and even fear by doctors due to many challenges they faced.*

The challenges while dealing with MLC cases are: (i) Difficulty in making decision a case as MLC or not (ii) Unavailability of proper, or complete history while examining a patient and preparing MLC (iii) Absence of attendants/relatives for history (iv) Absconding of patient in fear of intimation to police (v) Unwillingness of the patient party for MLC (vi) Patient or their relatives request or any external pressure to label a case as MLC (vii) Patient or relatives wish to be referred to higher or preferred center (viii) Referred case from another hospital (ix) Delayed treatment in emergency/critical cases due to confusion (x) Difficulty in dealing with violent public and managing crowds (xi) Uncooperative and careless attitude of the police (xii) Inadequate support from hospital staff (xiii) Problems related to preservation of evidence material, documentation (xiv) Giving opinion for 'fit for statement' (xv) Mortuary and autopsy related issues (xvi) Attending court as witness etc.

Conflict

Conflict can be defined as a disagreement within oneself or between people that causes harm or has the potential to cause harm (Saltman *et al.* 2006). It should not be confused with disagreement which is a situation where people have a different opinion about something and often also argue. However, it can lead to conflict. There are many factors that precipitate the transition from a disagreement to a conflict like difference in ideas, perspectives, priorities, preferences, beliefs, values and goals etc.

In medical practice, conflicts can occur between physicians, between physicians and staff, and between the staff or the health care team and the patient or patient's family. It can arise due to diversity of values, skills, priorities, prohibitive environments and organizational structures. Many factors can accelerate the conflict which includes differing goals and individual differences, problems with communication and feedback, power and rivalry, lack of support and collegiality, and the absence of role modelling and expertise.

Types of conflict: The conflicts could be (i) **Intrapersonal:** Conflict experienced by a single individual, when his or her own goals, values or roles diverge. (ii) **Interpersonal:** Conflict between two or more persons due to differences in goals, value, and styles. (iii) **Intragroup:** Conflict within a group or team, where members conflict over goals or procedures; and (iv) **Intergroup:** Conflict between groups inside and outside an organization disagree on various issues.

The negative outcomes of the conflicts in medical practice are: (i) It may lead to litigation. (ii) It can lead violent confrontation. (iii) It can adversely affect productivity, morale, and efficient patient care. (iv) It can lead to poor mental health among medical professionals etc.

Conflict management: It is the process of planning to avoid conflict where possible and organizing to resolve conflict where it does happen, as rapidly and smoothly as possible. It is important that the parties involved in conflict do not unnecessarily end up being in any kind of emotional stress during the resolution process of the conflict. Striking a balance between resolving the conflict to find the decision and maintaining the emotional wellbeing of people involved will be critical to successful conflict management.

Conflict Resolution techniques: In conflict situation, the **Thomas-Kilmann model** identifies an individual's behaviour along two dimensions: assertiveness and cooperativeness. Assertiveness involves taking action to satisfy your own needs, while cooperativeness involves taking action to satisfy the other's needs.

In this model, there are 5 modes to deal with conflict:

(i) **Forcing/competing:** In this technique, the goal is to win and often interpreted as a "male" way of doing things. A person with authority and power can force his/her opinion and resolves the conflict without giving any chance to the other party/person. It is characterized by high assertiveness and little cooperativeness. It can be used if the conflicts are unnecessary and mostly destructive for the team. It is effective when quick decisive action is needed, however, it is likely to be unpopular with others.

(ii) **Accommodating:** In this technique, the goal is to yield and often interpreted as a "female" way of doing things. One of the parties gives into the wishes or demands of another. It is characterized by low assertiveness and high cooperativeness. It is effective to resolve a small conflict quickly and easily. However, a larger or more important issue may not be solved in a meaningful way and should absolutely be avoided.

(iii) **Avoiding:** In this technique, the goal is to delay or walk away. It works when the issue is relatively trivial. It is useful for calming down the conflict when there is a lot of "heat" in the situation. It as a short-term strategy and rarely works to achieve long-term change. It is characterized by low assertiveness and low cooperativeness. In this technique, neither party's concerns are met.

(iv) **Compromising/Negotiating:** In this technique, the goal is to find middle ground by negotiating or splitting any differences of opinion and both parties "win some and lose some". It is characterized by moderate assertiveness and cooperativeness. It is a quick way to achieve an expedient solution and may be helpful in settling complex issues temporarily. It may be used as a backup style when collaboration and competition fail.

(v) **Collaborating:** In this technique, the goal is multiple participation and a "win-win" negotiations for both sides. It is the most time-consuming and most complex style of conflict management strategy. The components for this style of conflict management are digging into the issues, exploring them in depth, and confronting differences. It is characterized by high assertiveness and high cooperativeness. It is the method of choice to be adopted for resolution of a conflict when possible.

CONSENT

It is defined as voluntary agreement, compliance and permission. **S. 13 of Indian Contract Act** defines that "two or more persons are said to consent when they agree upon the same thing in the same sense". According to **S. 14 of Indian Contract Act**, consent is said to be free, when it is not caused by: (i) Coercion, as defined in section 15; or (ii) Undue influence, as defined in S. 16; or (iii) Fraud, as defined in S. 17; or (iv) Misrepresentation, as defined in S. 18; (v) Mistake subject to the provisions of S. 20, 21, 22.

Reasons for obtaining the consent: To examine, treat or operate upon a patient without consent is regarded as assault in law, even if it does not cause any harm and beneficial and done in good faith, for which the patient may sue the doctor for damages. If the doctor fails to give the requisite information to a patient before asking for his consent for a particular operation or treatment he may be charged for negligence.

Types of Consent

1. Implied.
2. Express (i) Oral (ii) Written (Informed).

Implied Consent: This type of consent is specifically stated by the patient and is seen in routine medical practice and is quite adequate. In these situations, consent is implied in the sense that patient has come to physician with a physical condition or ailment for examination and treatment. When a patient holds out his arm for an injection. It is also an implied consent.

If the procedure of diagnosis is simple and straightforward, the risk is negligible and uncommon and the conduct of the patient implies willingness to undergo treatment. In spite of all the precautions, if there is the slightest fear of complication, the doctor should seek express consent.

Express Consent: May be written or verbal, and should be obtained for any procedure beyond the routine physical examination, like operation, collection of blood, blood transfusion etc. The nature and consequences of the procedure should be explained before obtaining consent. Oral consent in the presence of a disinterested third party is as good as written one.

Doctrine of Informed Consent: In informed consent, the doctor informs the patient about his/her condition or disease, nature of the proposed treatment, i.e., whether surgical or medicinal methods to be used, availability of any alternative procedure, the possible risks and benefits of the procedure and the percentage of chances of success and failure.

The patient should be explained in a simple language that he can understand fully and give consent in the presence of third party who acts as a witness. Once the consent is obtained any untoward reaction or harm cause to the patient cannot lead to charge of negligence for the doctor.

Exceptions to the Informed Consent

1. **Emergency:** In an emergency condition it is usually assumed that the patient will give consent. In these cases, the consent is taken as implied **(S. 92, IPC)**.
2. **Incompetence:** The incompetent patients may be treated without their permission as generally it is regarded that incompetent patients are unable to make rational decisions. In this category the patients of unconscious, delirious, senile or grossly psychotic nature are included. When patients are in intensive care unit they are treated without informed consent.
3. **Therapeutic privilege:** In this category the physician can be excused of obtaining informed consent when disclosure of information could have a detrimental effect on the patient.
4. **Waiver:** The last exception allows a patient to waive his right to informed consent. In these cases, the patient may delegate the right to the physician or to a third party especially the close relatives to make the decision for him.

If one of the exceptions to the informed consent applies, the physician should document the exception. Under these circumstances full disclosure and consent should occur. However, in emergency situations time may not permit such disclosure and consent. If patient is incompetent or therapeutic waiver is used, a surrogate should give informed consent for the patient.

Informed Refusal: The doctor has a duty to inform the patient that he has a right to refuse the treatment or investigations to be undertaken. After listening to the doctor, the patient can refuse to consent for the proposed investigation/treatment.

Rules of Consent: Consent should be obtained necessarily before every medical examination. In routine medical practice, formal consent to medical examination is not required as the patient presents himself in a manner that implies consent.

Written consent is not necessary in each and every case that comes to the doctor for examination and treatment. However, it should be obtained to prevent litigations in the court of law if necessity arises. In medicolegal cases written consent must be taken.

Any procedure beyond routine physical examination such as operation, blood transfusion, collection of blood etc. requires express consent. In these cases, it must be obtained before the act and not at the time of admission into the hospital.

The consent should be full, free, voluntary, clear, informed, direct and personal. There should be no undue influence, fraud, and misrepresentation of the facts, compulsion and threat of physical injury, death or other consequences. The doctor should inform the patient that he has the right to refuse to submit himself to the examination and that the results may go against him/her. If he/she refuses to consent it is an absolute bar for examination except under **S. 53, CrPC.** Written consent is taken for specific procedure individually. It is not same as blanket permission obtained for general procedure where the surgeon can decide in the operation theatre itself about the type and extent of operation. The doctor should explain the object of the examination to the patient and he should be informed that the findings would be embodied in a medical report.

In criminal cases, the victim cannot be examined without consent. The court also cannot compel a person to get himself medically examined against his will. In cases where, the person is arrested on the charge of committing some offence and the examination of his body can provide some evidences toward the commission of the crime, he can be examined by a Registered Medical Practitioner even without his consent and if necessary by using reasonable force **(S. 53(1), CrPC). S. 53(2), CrPC** mentions that when the case relates to a female examination should only be conducted by a female Registered Medical Practitioner or in the presence of female assistant such as Nurse.

Under **S. 54, CrPC** an arrested person can also request to be examined by a doctor to detect any evidences in his favour. Under **S. 87, IPC** a person above 18 years of age can give consent to suffer any harm if the act is not intended and not known to cause death or grievous hurt. Under **S. 88, IPC** a person can give consent to suffer any harm if the act is not intended and not known to cause death or grievous hurt when the act is done in good faith and for the benefit of the person.

Under **S. 89, IPC** a child under 12 years of age or a person of unsound mind cannot give consent to suffer any harm for an act which may cause grievous hurt or death even if done in good faith, but the consent has to be obtained from the guardian of the child or insane person. Under **S. 90, IPC** consent given by an insane person or given under fear of injury, death etc. or due to misconception of a fact is invalid. Under **S. 92, IPC** any harm caused to a person in good faith even without the person's consent is not an offence if the circumstances were such that it was impossible to obtain consent of the person or his lawful guardian at that material time for that thing to be done for the benefit of the person. However, the act should not extend to intentionally causing hurt other than for preventing death, grievous hurt or curing of disease or infirmity.

Professional Secrecy

In the Hippocratic Oath there is an affirmation by the doctor that whatever in connection with my professional practice or not in connection with what I see or hear in the life of men, which ought not be spoken of abroad, I will not divulge, as reckoning that all such be kept secret.

Even the places where oath is not formally given in qualifying convocation ceremony, there is an implied acceptance of its spirit and intentions as the ideal standard of his professional behaviour. Therefore, both on ethical grounds and also because it may be used in the civil courts for breach of confidence, the doctor should respect this professional secrecy to the utmost of his ability. The following examples may be kept in mind: (i) Doctor should not discuss any point with others relating to the patient's illness that he came to know in his professional practice except with the consent of the patient. (ii) If the patient is a major a doctor should not disclose anything learnt about his illness even to his parents without obtaining his consent. (iii) In case of husband and wife the facts relating to the nature of illness of one should not be disclosed to the other without the consent. (iv) If the doctor examines a domestic servant at the request of the master who is paying the fees still he should not disclose the nature of his illness even to the master without the consent of the servant. (v) Doctors in government service are bound by code of professional secrecy even if they are treating the patients free of cost. (vi) Criminals in police custody has right not to allow the treating doctor to disclose the nature of illness to any person. However, once the person is convicted he has lost this right and the doctor can disclose to the proper authorities for the sake of justice. (vii) While reporting any case report in a medical journal care should be taken not to disclose the identity of the person. (viii) When a person submits himself for medical examination before taking life insurance policies, the doctor can disclose the result to the proper authorities because here the concept of implied consent will apply. (ix) A doctor should not disclose any information about the illness of his patient without his consent even when requested by a statutory body except the notifiable diseases. (x) Examination of the dead body at times may reveal certain facts that affect the reputation of the deceased as well as the family members. Thus, the doctor should not disclose the fact to the relatives, e.g., pregnancy discovered in an unmarried girl during autopsy examination.

Exceptions to professional secrecy: The rules of professional secrecy can be broken in certain situations that are known as **privileged communication.**

Privileged Communication

It is a statement made bona fide upon by the doctor to the concerned authority to protect the interest of the community or state. To be privileged it must be disclosed only to the concerned person or authority. If the plea of privileged facts is communicated to more than one person then the doctor must obtain the consent from the patient. If he fails to give consent, then the doctor can communicate to concerned authority to protect the interest of the community. **Following are some of the examples of privileged communications:**

Infectious diseases: If anybody having infectious diseases gets an employment, the doctor should persuade not to undertake the job till he is completely cured. If somebody is found to be suffering from infectious diseases during his employment, he/she should also be asked to go on leave till he/she is cured. If the patient refuses, the doctor can inform his employer about his illness, e.g., a school teacher who is suffering from tuberculosis or cook of the hostel suffering from typhoid.

Notifiable diseases: Medical person has statutory duties to notify births, deaths and notifiable diseases to the Public Health Authority.

Suspected crimes: The doctor must inform the police of commission of crimes such as homicides, suspected suicides (**S. 39, CrPC**: Public to inform police of certain offences).

Servants and employees: When an employee is suffering from a serious diseases such as colour blindness in drivers, epilepsy in cooks, they should be persuaded to change their profession, otherwise the employer should be informed about the illness.

Sexually transmitted diseases: Person having a sexually transmitted disease intending to join in swimming pool or going for marriage, should be persuaded not to join the swimming pool or go for marriage. If he does not comply, then the doctor should inform concerned person or authority.

In patient's interest: If the patient is having suicidal tendency, the parents/guardians may be informed about so that they can take proper care and provide proper treatment.

Court of law: In the court of law, the doctor cannot claim the privilege about the illness of his patient. When asked to communicate regarding the illness of his patient, he should appeal to the court of providing information in writing in order to avoid disclosing secrets learnt during the treatment of the patient. However, if the court rejects his application he has to communicate before the court of law. Nevertheless, under **S. 126 and 129, IEA**, a lawyer can claim the privilege in a court of law about any communication made to him by his client.

Negligent suits: When a patient files any suit of negligence against a doctor and he employs another doctor to examine the patient, the information thus acquired is not privileged and he can divulge it in the court of law.

Self-interest: When a patient files a civil or criminal suit, the doctor can disclose information learnt during his professional practice.

MEDICAL NEGLIGENCE (MALPRAXIS)

Introduction

The law of negligence is applicable to the conduct of all individuals whether layman or professional. In addition, certain ethical standards are applied to the professionals. Whenever a privilege is bestowed upon an individual, concomitant duties and obligations are attached and the physician is no exception.

In present times doctors cannot be sure that they will never be threatened with an action for negligence. Patients are ready to sue even though they had received excellent treatment with complete cure and without cost. There are three reasons for this: (i) Transfer of hospitals to the State or Central Government (ii) Cost are met out of national funds (iii) There is a provision of free legal aid for the patient.

It is difficult to appreciate that severe disability resulting from an accident during the course of treatment is not necessarily negligence but unfortunately patient may allege negligence and seek compensation.

In **Hatcher Vs. Black and others** (1954) Lord Denning compared negligence with a dagger. The doctors' professional reputation is as much dear to him as his body, perhaps more so, and an action for negligence could wound his reputation as severely as a dagger to his body.

Professional negligence: It is defined as "Want of reasonable care and skill or willful negligence on the part of the medical practitioner while treating a patient resulting in bodily injury, ill health or death".

Negligence was first defined by **Justice Baron Alderson** in 1856 "The omission to do something which a reasonable man could do or doing something which a prudent and a reasonable man would not do". It could be defined as a failure to perform the duty to exercise a reasonable degree of skill and care in the treatment of patient.

In 1934 **Lord Wright** defined it as: (i) There must be a duty owed (ii) Breach of that duty either by omission or commission (iii) Direct causation (iv) Damage.

To summarize the doctor owes a duty towards the patient, the doctor was in breach of that duty as a result of which the patient suffered damage. There is a direct relationship between the dereliction of duty and the damage.

Medical negligence is no different in law from any other type of negligence. Negligence medical or otherwise is a civil wrong than as a "tort". Rarely the medical negligence may be renewed from a civil action between doctor and patient to the criminal courts, where the state prosecutes the doctor for a severe degree of reckless and dangerous *action, amounting to criminal negligence.*

Duty of the doctor to choose a patient: The doctor has right to refuse any patient. Thus, any patient who comes to a doctor, he can either refuse or accept for the treatment. Once the doctor accepts the patient, his duty towards the patient starts. The doctor can refuse to accept the patient in the following circumstances: (i) When patient does not belong to his/her specialty (ii) Facilities of treatment are not available at his place (iii) Doctor is not well or any member of the family is sick (iv) When he is busy in important family functions.

Duty of the doctor during an emergency: During emergency he is morally and ethically bound to provide the best of help he can do to save the life of the patient and see that the patient if not accepted by him, can reach the nearest hospital. Here no patient-doctor relationship is established. So, if some damage occurs, the patient cannot sue the doctor.

Absence of reasonable care and skill: The duty to exercise reasonable care and skill exists when a doctor-patient relationship is established. This may be true even if the patient is unconscious and quite unaware of the doctor's presence.

A doctor who deals with a patient with the intent to act as a healer establishes a doctor-patient relationship immediately and from that moment he has a legal obligation to exercise due care and skill. Any breach of that duty is a ground for the negligent action.

When a doctor examines a patient for some other purpose than providing advice and treatment, i.e., he is not present as a healer, no doctor-patient relationship is established and there is no duty of care. When a doctor examines a medicolegal case like sexual assault, alcoholics and insurance etc., he is there not as a healer and thus no relationship exists, but there is a duty not to damage. Thus, if he breaks the needle while taking blood sample, he is liable to pay damages. On the other hand, if he reports the findings to the employer and insurance company, no action for damages arises.

Degree of competence: A doctor must possess reasonable degree of proficiency and he must apply it while treating the patient. A highly qualified doctor will be held negligent if he fails to apply his greater knowledge with sufficient degree of care. Conversely an inexperienced doctor may be negligent if he attempts to do some procedure, which is beyond his capability except in an emergency. The degree of competence is not a fixed quality but varies according to the qualification and experience of the doctor.

There is a minimum level of competence for all doctors who have qualified in the examinations and registered in the State Medical Councils or the National Medical Commission. This minimum level is set to protect the public from insufficiently qualified doctors. Beyond this minimum point there is a whole spectrum of proficiency from a newly graduated doctor to a senior specialist. No doctor is expected to possess all up-to-date knowledge nor he can apply all known diagnostic and therapeutic techniques. However, a doctor of a particular status as regards his grading and experience is expected to have a standard of knowledge and capability corresponding to his status in the profession for example a house surgeon is not expected to possess the same skills as that of a consultant surgeon. A house surgeon volunteering to perform a major surgical operation (not an emergency) might be held guilty of negligence if he causes damage to his patient. This applies to all other specialties such as anesthesia, medicine and so on. On the other hand, if a junior doctor performs any operation or treats a patient in an emergency and there is no other medical facility available even if there is damage to the patient he will not be held negligent provided that he has acted in good faith.

Breach of duty of care: It will not be incorrect to say that categories of negligence are never close which means that it is impossible to draw a complete list of things that can cause negligence in action because of the advancement of medical technology day by day. Any action of the doctor can be a ground for negligence provided the patient is not satisfied and damage occurs to him.

A doctor is not liable for errors of judgment either in diagnosis or treatment as long as he applied a reasonable standard of skill. Negligence is not a matter of a doctor making a mistake but it is not trying hard enough to prevent complications, lack of care and attention for the consequences. A doctor can misdiagnose and

Table 3.1: Differences between civil and criminal negligence

Features	Civil negligence	Criminal negligence
Offence	No specific and clear violation of law	There is specific violation of a particular criminal law in question
Negligence	Simple absence of care and skill	Gross negligence, inattention or lack of competency
Conduct of physician	Compared to a generally accepted standard of professional conduct	Not compared to a any single test
Consent for act	Good defence in court of law cannot recover damages	Not a defence; can be prosecuted
Trial	Civil court	Criminal court
Evidence	Strong evidence is sufficient	Guilt should be proved beyond reasonable doubt
Punishment	Damages to be paid	Imprisonment

mistreat a patient without being negligent in spite of the fact that another practitioner of greater skill and ability would have had more success in the same situation. A doctor is not an insurer of as one famous judge said and he doesn't guarantee to provide the best possible care but only care which is reasonably adequate and consistent with his professional status.

Who sets the standard? The court will rely upon the evidence of competent practitioner in the relevant field of medical practice. Approved practice is a criterion for reasonable care. In almost all defence cases it is argued that what was done, was done in accordance with general approved practice. Court gives much importance to the expert evidence in the relevant field. A doctor is not negligent if he acts in accordance with general accepted practice. The court pronounces the practice negligent if there are some inherent defects in it. It is not enough to repute negligence by saying that he did it what everybody does. A risky practice may well be held negligent not withstanding that it is widely followed.

The court pronounces the practice negligent if this is not a usual and normal practice. The practice adopted is one which no professional man of ordinary skill would adopt.

A medical practitioner when deviates from normal practice it must be established that he is free to exercise his judgment, discretion and the new procedure was done with the consent of the patient for his benefit. Anyone who adopts a noble course of treatment or omits to use some form of diagnosis or treatment, which has gained general approval, must be able to justify his actions if something goes wrong. In these cases, success is the best justification.

Duty to inform the risks: In a hospital, no matter what care is taken there is always a risk. Always there is some risk in every operation under general anesthesia. It is an important question as to what extent the doctor is obliged to inform his patient or relatives about these risks? When there is some known risk they should be informed before obtaining the consent, then there is no room for negligence. For example, in an electroconvulsive therapy there is risk of fracture of dorsal vertebrae thus the written consent of the patient must be taken. The doctor is not expected to inform all possible treatment and risks. He is not negligent if he has not informed about remote risks.

Retention of swabs, packs, instruments and drainage tube etc.: Responsibility of recovery of swabs used in operation theatre lies with the surgeon. During an operation the surgeon puts the swabs inside the cavity and it is his duty to remove them after the operation. He must use reasonable degree of care in the circumstances and this depends upon the evidences. He cannot say, "I relied upon the nurse." He must ask the nurse if everything is all right. The circumstances when the nurse's count will be of immense value are that the emergency situation was such that the surgeon was not able to carry out the count without endangering the patient's life.

To avoid negligence, the surgeon must satisfy the following: (i) Counting system is efficient and the person working is familiar with it (ii) System was followed during the operation and the count showed that the number is all right (iii) He must take all reasonable precaution that swabs used were recovered (iv) He must do a visual and manual search of the field (v) In these cases the plaintiff has only to prove that he has suffered damage and the onus is upon the surgeon to prove that he is not negligent.

Precautions Against Medical Negligence

The doctor should take following precautions: (i) Never guarantee a cure. (ii) Obtain informed consent from the patient. (iii) Diagnosis to be confirmed by proper investigation depending upon the nature of case. (iv) Reasonable skill and care to be taken. (v) Proper, accurate and legible records to be maintained. (vi) Immunization to be done specially tetanus in cases of injuries. (vii) Sensitivity test to be performed before injecting the drugs known to cause hypersensitivity reactions specially in cases of penicillin, streptomycin and antivenins. (viii) Patient or his attendant should be advised that the medicine should be given in the proper dosage and in time and no telephonic consultation should be done. (ix) Consultation to be undertaken with appropriate specialist in case of need. (x) Never criticise your colleagues regarding his professional ability. (xi) During labour, the patient should not be left unattended when she is undergoing labour. (xii) In case of absence from practice the patient should be informed or qualified substitute should be arranged. (xiii) A written informed consent should be obtained before carrying out surgery and anaesthesia and the detailed surgical procedures and possible risks should be explained to the patient. (xiv) Anesthesia should be given by an expert in the field. (xv) Before a surgical operation, the surgeon should make sure that all the instruments are in good working condition and proper count of the instruments should be done by the nurse before and after completing the operation. (xvi) Whenever a death occurs from anaesthesia or during surgical operation the doctor should report to the police. (xvii) For carrying out any research work on the patient his consent should be taken. (xviii) No female patient to be examined without the presence of a third person preferably a female or by a female Registered Medical Practitioner. (xix) The doctor should be well versed with the advanced medical knowledge in the field. (xx) **Defensive medicine** is one where the doctor advises each and every test or radiological examination of the patient before starting the treatment. This is done to avoid charge of negligence in future. However, this becomes quite costly for the patient. (xxi) Physician must not practice **defence by denial** and claim that patient is not his which becomes abandonment.

Contributory Negligence

Contributory negligence is the absence of reasonable care on the part of the patient or his attendant that combines with the negligent action of the doctor resulting in the damage completed off directly and without which damage should not have occurred. The examples are: (i) Not to provide proper history to the doctor (ii) Failure to follow the line of treatment (iii) Refusal to take up the suggested advice (iv) Leaving the hospital against the doctor's advice (v) Failure to seek further medical treatment if the signs or symptoms persists.

If the doctor and the patient are negligent simultaneously, the doctor can take a good defence, otherwise the contributory negligence is a partial defence in civil suit only and has no place in criminal negligence. When the patient consents to take the risk of the injuries and its effects, then he cannot claim damages. When the doctor is not negligent and it is the patient alone who is negligent, it is called **"negligence of the patient"**.

Limitations of Contributory Negligence

1. **Last clear chance doctrine:** In this rule the person who is negligent may recover the damages if the doctor discovered the injury while there was still time to avoid the injury but he failed to do so.
2. **Avoidable consequences rule:** In these cases, the doctor was found to be negligent and he was sued for the same and after that the negligence of the injured person occurs. In these situations, the patient is not guilty of contributory negligence since his actions were not the cause of the injury.
3. **Error of judgment:** It is a well established fact that a doctor is not expected to do a miracle. The courts do not condemn an honest exercise of judgment even though other doctors may disagree. To cover up an error of judgment is held to be negligent conduct.

Therapeutic Misadventure

A misadventure is an accident or unexpected damage to the patient when the doctor is attending the patient during the treatment is called therapeutic misadventure. It can occur during diagnosis or during experimentation.

Since almost every therapeutic drug has side effects, the doctor should explain the possible side effects while prescribing any drug to the patient. When there are more than one drugs that can be prescribed for a particular disease, then the doctor should prescribe the drug having lesser side effects. As hypersensitivity reactions to some of the drugs are quite common thus when a doctor prescribes a particular drug, he should obtain very particularly the history of hypersensitivity reactions before starting treatment and at the same time should be equipped with life saving measures if required. The doctor is not liable for the damages caused by administration of a drug unless the element of negligence exists.

Examples of some of therapeutic misadventures: (i) A hot water bottle or heating pads causing burns. (ii) Foetal and neonatal deaths occurring inside uterus while the mother is given some drugs for treatment during pregnancy. (iii) Hypersensitivity reaction caused by administration of penicillin, streptomycin, tetracycline etc. (iv) Radiological procedures during diagnostic methods can prove fatal. (v) During barium enema, rupture of rectum causing peritonitis.

Respondent Superior (Vicarious Liability)

The employer is responsible not only for the wrongful deeds committed by him, but also the wrongful deeds of his employees. The doctor usually employs or supervises other members of staff who are less qualified. He distributes the work amongst and supervises them. If one of the members does any negligence, then the principal doctor is held responsible for the act of that member, known as respondent superior. It is also referred to as liability for the act of another. For the acts of general practice, the consultant or the principal doctor is responsible for the act of his assistants such as interns, house surgeons or residents. All of these may be sued along with the head consultant by the patient. When two doctors are working as partners both are liable for negligence for the other even if one has no role to play in the management of the patient.

Doctrine of Res Ipsa Loquitur

Usually the professional negligence of a doctor must be proved in the Court of law by the experts in the field and the patient has to prove the negligence of the doctor. Nevertheless, in cases of res ipsa loquitur which means **"the facts or things speaks for itself"** the patient need not prove the negligence. The rule will be applicable if the following conditions are satisfied: (i) That in the absence of negligence the injury would not have occurred. (ii) Doctor had exclusive control over the injury producing instrument or treatment. (iii) There is no contributory negligence by the patient.

Following are the **few examples** of res ipsa loquitur: (i) Breaking of a needle during injection (ii) Failure to remove swabs from the abdomen during operation (iii) Prescribing overdose of medicine (iv) Burns resulting from application of hot water bottle (v) Failure to give tetanus toxoid in cases of injury resulting tetanus.

This doctrine is applied to both civil and criminal negligence. It cannot be applied against several defendants.

Doctrine of Common Knowledge

This doctrine is based on the assumption that the issue of negligence in a particular case is not related to the technical matters which are within the knowledge of medical profession. It is different from res ipsa loquitur where the patient need not produce evidences regarding the standard of care by the doctor. However, in doctrine of common knowledge the patient must prove the causative factors that had resulted in negligence but he need not produce the evidences to establish the standard of care.

Novus Actus Interveniens

Novus actus interveniens is a Latin term which means a new intervening act. It is an act or event that breaks the causal connection between a wrong or crime committed by the defendant and subsequent happenings. The new event relieves the defendant from responsibility for the happenings. A Latin term for an intervening unforeseeable event that occurs after the defendant's negligent act and operates to precipitate or worsen the plaintiff's loss. The defendant is not liable for the loss precipitated or aggravated by such an event. A break in the chain of causation arises where there is a new intervening act or 'novus actus interveniens'. The term is different from nova causa interveniens, which means a new intervening cause.

A break in the chain of causation means that when this occurs the courts interpret this to mean that the accused's conduct was not the cause of the harm or injury. This is unusual but when it does occur it will result in the accused being acquitted. A break in the chain of causation arises where there is a new intervening act or **'novus actus interveniens'**.

There are two cases which probably best illustrate the principles of causation. These are the cases of **R v Jordan (1956)** and **R v Smith (1959)**.

1. In **R v Jordan (1956)** the defendant stabbed the victim who was admitted to hospital where he died 8 days later. In hospital the victim had been given antibiotics to which he was allergic and he had also been given large amounts of intravenous fluid. At the time of his death the stab wounds were starting to heal. In the Court of Appeal, it was stated that the direct and immediate cause of death was pneumonia. Two doctors expressed the opinion that death had not been caused by the stab wound, which was mainly healed at the time of the death, but by the medical treatment the victim received. The court held that the defendant was not liable for the death.
2. In **R v Smith** the defendant had been involved in a fight with another soldier at their army barracks. During the fight the defendant stabbed the other soldier twice with his bayonet, medics were called and took the injured man to the medical station. On the way, the man was dropped two times and on arrival at the medical centre he did not receive the appropriate treatment and the medical officer did not diagnose the seriousness of his injuries and that his lung had been punctured in the attack. The soldier died and the defendant was convicted of murder. He appealed claiming that if the victim had received the appropriate medical treatment he would have survived. The conviction was upheld as the stab wound was the "operating and substantial cause" of death.

This principle means an 'unrelated action intervening' and it is accepted rarely as a plea in the courts when an element of negligence is there. It is applied to cases of injuries resulting from assault and accidents and implies that the person is responsible for his actions as well as for their logical consequences. When a doctor is negligent resulting in deviation from logical sequence of events, the responsibility for subsequent disability and death in such a case may pass from the original incident to the later negligent action.

Defences Available in Cases of Negligence

(i) No duty owed to the plaintiff (ii) The duty was discharged according to the prevailing standard (iii) It was a therapeutic misadventure (iv) It was error of judgment (v) *Contributory negligence:* It can be taken as defence in cases of civil negligence only (vi) *Res judicata:* Once the case has been decided it cannot be taken to another court. Only appeal can be made. (vi) *Limitations*: The case should be filed within two years from the date of alleged negligence. If it is alleged that there was a breach of duty to take care under some particular contract between doctor and patient, then the period is three years from the date of breach of contract.

The following points are not good defences: (i) There was no contractual relationship between the doctor and the patient (ii) Service was rendered free of charge (iii) The medical man had no bad motive.

Products Liability

In medical practice, many medical products, e.g., pacemakers, stents, defibrillators, IUDS, kidney dialysis filters, drugs etc. are used for a variety of health issues, ranging from heart problems, kidney failure, joint replacements and contraception etc. Sometimes, the patient can get damages (injury/death) as a result of defective medical products/drugs. If a doctor correctly installs a defective medical device and damages occurred to the patient, the liability of negligence would lie on the manufacturing company.

The plaintiff must demonstrate that the product was defective at the time the damage occurred and the defect was the proximate cause of injury or death. If it is proved, the manufacturer is liable for negligence. The manufacturer has to prove that it did not breach its duty of care, i.e., it must prove that its product was free of defects at the time it was placed on the market.

A medical products liability claim differs from a medical malpractice claim in that a medical products liability claim is a lawsuit against a manufacturer, not a doctor. However, doctors also have a duty to inform patients about alternatives in treatment and side effects and to properly install a medical device. Hence, a patient injured by a defective medical product can have both a medical products liability claims against a manufacturer and a medical malpractice claim against the doctor. If the hospital has not taken adequate steps for repair/maintenance of a medical device, then the hospital can also be held responsible.

Clinical Establishments (Registration and Regulation) Act, 2010

Clinical Establishments (Registration and Regulation) Act, 2010 was introduced by Government of India in order to achieve the mandate of Article 47 of the Constitution for improvement in public health. This law, after enactment by Parliament, came into effect in 11 states (Arunachal Pradesh, Himachal Pradesh, Mizoram, Sikkim, Uttar Pradesh, Bihar, Jharkhand, Rajasthan,

Uttarakhand, Assam and Haryana) and all Union Territories except Delhi. The Delhi government proposed 'The Delhi Health Bill, 2019' for implementation clinical establishment Act. It is expected that other states would also adopt this legislation.

The main purpose of the law is to provide a legislative framework for the registration and regulation of clinical establishments in the country and also seeks to improve the quality of health services through the National Council for Standards by prescribing minimum standards of facilities and services which may be provided by them. Salient features of this Act are:

- This Act will apply to a clinical establishment owned, controlled or managed by—(a) The Government or a department of the Government; (b) A trust, whether public or private; (c) A corporation (including a society) registered under a Central, Provincial or State Act, whether or not owned by the Government; (d) A local authority; and (e) A single doctor, but does not include the clinical establishments owned, controlled or managed by the Armed Forces.
- Central Government to establish a Council to be called the National Council for clinical establishments that will be inclusive of DGHS, Medical Council (now NMC), Dental Council, Pharmacy Council and Nursing Council of India and other members as described in Act (S. 3) and States to constitute State Medical Councils consisting of State Medical Council, State Dental Council, State Pharmacy Council and State Nursing Council and other members (S. 8).
- State Government to establish District Registration Authority for each district headed by District Collector (S. 10).
- No person shall run a clinical establishment unless it has been duly registered in accordance with the provisions of this Act (S. 11) and establishment should fulfill the conditions of the minimum requirement of personnel and provisions for maintenance of records and reporting (S. 12).
- After application for registration of clinical establishment, a provisional registration will be issued which will be valid for 12 months (S. 15 to S. 17) before expiry of which, application for permanent registration should be made (S. 24 to S. 27) which will be granted when a clinical establishment fulfills the prescribed standards for registration by the Central Government (S. 28).
- Permanent registration will be valid for a period of 5 years.
- Cancellation of registration: If, at any time after any clinical establishment has been registered, the authority is satisfied that: (a) The conditions of the registration are not being complied with; or (b) The person entrusted with the management of the clinical establishment has been convicted of an offence punishable under this Act (S. 32).
- **S. 40:** Whoever contravenes any provision of this Act shall, if no penalty is provided elsewhere, be punishable for the first offence with fine which may extend to ten thousand rupees, for any second offence with fine which may extend to fifty thousand rupees and for any subsequent offence with fine which may extend to five lakh rupees.
- **S. 41:** Monetary penalty for non-registration.–(1) Whoever carries on a clinical establishment without registration shall, on first contravention, be liable to a monetary penalty up to fifty thousand rupees, for second contravention with a monetary penalty which may extend to two lakh rupees and for any subsequent contravention with a monetary penalty which may extend to five lakh rupees. (2) Whoever knowingly serves in a clinical establishment which is not duly registered under this Act, shall be liable to a monetary penalty which may extend to twenty-five thousand rupees.
- **S. 42:** Disobedience of direction, obstruction and refusal of information-monetary penalty which may extend to five lakh rupees.
- **S. 43:** Penalty for minor deficiencies: Deficiencies that do not pose any imminent danger to the health and safety of any patient and can be rectified within a reasonable time, shall be punishable with fine which may extend to ten thousand rupees.
- **Clinical Establishments (Central Government) Amendment Rules, 2018:** It is effective from 18 May, 2018. **S. 8A,** which prescribes minimum standards for Medical Diagnostic Laboratories (or Pathological Laboratories). However, in this amendment there is not mention of the qualification of authorized signatory at basic composite laboratories
- **Clinical Establishments (Central Government) Amendment Rules, 2019 (amendment in part IIIa).** Prescribes the "minimum standards for different categories of clinical establishments of Allopathy and AYUSH" by adding **S. 8B.**
- **Clinical Establishments (Central Government) Amendment Rules, 2020:** According to the notification, M.Sc. Pathology / Medical Biochemistry / Medical Microbiology candidates with at least 3 years of experience or training in the laboratory can generate and sign test reports. They can also perform medical tests. The test must be of their respective specialty. The candidate need not record any opinion or interpretation of laboratory results. The test report generated must have a disclaimer that the reports are strictly for the use of medical practitioners and are not a medical diagnosis.

CONSUMER PROTECTION ACT, 1986 ('OLD ACT')

The Consumer Protection Act, 1986 [Syn, CPA, COPRA] came into force on 15 April, 1987 is a welfare legislation mainly tilting towards the consumer similar to Industrial Dispute Act that favors the workers.

The Act envisages a three-tier quasi-judicial machinery, i.e., District Consumer Disputes Redressal Forum at the District level,

State Consumer Disputes Redressal Commission at the State level and National Consumer Disputes Redressal Commission at the National level. The **District Forum** consists of three members presided by a retired or serving district judge. It entertains claims up to rupees twenty lakhs. The **State Commission** consists of three members presided by a serving or retired High Court Judge. It entertains claims between rupees twenty lakhs and one crore. The **National Commission** consists of five members presided by a retired Supreme Court judge, which entertains claims above rupees one crore.

Procedure: The complaint can be lodged at any of the places with or without engaging a lawyer by paying a nominal fee. The complaint may be filed with the district forum by: (i) Consumer to whom the service has been provided or had been agreed to be provided (ii) Any recognized consumer association (iii) One or more consumers where numerous consumers have the same interest (iv) State or Central Government.

If the complaint relates to any service the district forum shall refer the copy of the complaint to the opposite party directing him to submit a reply within thirty days. Here it is not necessary for the parties to be represented by the lawyers so the disputes are settled on the basis of evidences put before him. The district forum has the same powers as that of a civil court under the Code of Civil Procedure 1908. Every proceeding before the district forum shall be deemed to be a judicial proceeding within the meaning of section 193 and 228 of the IPC 1860.

If the district forum is satisfied that the goods supplied were having some defects specified in the complaints and that any of the allegations contained in the complaint about the services are proved, it will issue an order to the opposite party either to remove the defect, replace the goods or provide adequate compensation. However, if the complaint is not proved it will be dismissed and the court directs to pay the costs of the opposite party not exceeding more than rupees ten thousand. But there is a provision that the aggrieved party if not satisfied can appeal in the State Commission within thirty days from the date of order. Here also if the party is not satisfied they can appeal to the National Commission and finally to Supreme Court within thirty days of the date of order.

Limitation period: The complaint should be filed in all the above forums within two years from the date on which the cause of action has arisen.

Penalties: For the non-compliance of the order made by district forum, State Commission or National Commission the trader or the person shall be punished with imprisonment ranging from one month to three years and fine from rupees two thousand to ten thousand.

Interpretation of the Act by the Supreme Court

1. Since the enactment of the Act there was a controversy whether the provisions of the Act are applicable to the persons who are rendering medical service to the patients. In this regard there was a difference of opinion between the State Commissions, National Commission and various high courts. The said controversy came to an end by the landmark judgment delivered by the Supreme Court in the case of **Indian Medical Association Council vs V.P. Shantha and others**.
2. The Apex Court arrived at the conclusions that service rendered to patient by medical practitioner except where the doctor renders service free of charge to every patient or under a contract of personal service, by way of consultation diagnosis and treatment both medical and surgical would fall within the ambit of service as defined in section 2(1)(0) of the Act.
3. The fact that the medical practitioners belong to the medical profession and subject to the disciplinary actions of Medical Council of India (now NMC) or State Medical Council constituted under the provisions of the Indian Medical Council Act would not exclude the services rendered by them from the ambit of the Act.
4. A 'contract of personal service' has to be distinguished from 'contract for personal service'. In the absence of relationships of master and servant between the patient and the medical practitioner the service rendered by a medical practitioner to the patient cannot be regarded as service rendered under 'contract of personal service' but such services are regarded as being rendered under a 'contract for personal service' and is not covered by exclusionary clause of definition of service contained in S. 2(1)(0) of the Act.
5. The expression 'contract of personal service' in S. 2(1)(0) of the Act cannot be confined to contracts for employment of domestic servants only and the said expression would include the employment of a medical officer for the purpose of rendering medical service to the employer. The service rendered by a medical officer to his employer is outside the purview of 'service' as defined in S. 2(1)(0) of the Act.
6. Service rendered free of charge by a medical practitioner attached to a hospital/nursing home or a medical officer employed in a hospital/nursing home where such services are rendered free of charge to everybody, would not be 'service' as defined in S. 2(1)(0) of the Act. The payment of a token amount for registration purpose only at the hospital/nursing home would not alter the position.
7. Service rendered at a non-government hospital/nursing home where no charge whatsoever is made from any person availing the service and all patients (rich and poor) are given free-service is outside the purview of the expression 'service' as defined in S. 2(1)(0) of the Act. The payment of a token amount for registration purpose only at the hospital/nursing home would not alter the position.
8. Service rendered at a non-government hospital/nursing home where charges are required to be paid by the persons availing

such services fall within the purview of the expression 'service' as defined in S. 2(1)(0) of the Act.

9. Service rendered at a non-government hospital/nursing home where charges are required to be paid by persons who are in a position to pay, and persons who cannot afford to pay are rendered service free of charge, would fall within the ambit of expression 'service' as defined in S. 2(1)(0) of the Act irrespective of the fact that the service is rendered free of charge to persons who are not in a position to pay for such services. Free service, would also be 'service' and the recipient a 'consumer' under the Act.
10. Service rendered at a government hospital/health center/ dispensary where no charge whatsoever is made from any person availing the services and all patients (rich and poor) are given free service, is outside the purview of the expression 'service' as defined in S. 2(1)(0) of the Act. The payment of a token amount for registration purpose only at the hospital/ nursing home would not alter the position.
11. Service rendered at a government hospital/health center/ dispensary where services are rendered on payment of charges and also rendered free of charge to other persons availing such services would fall within the ambit of the expression 'service' as defined in S. 2(1)(0) of the Act irrespective of the fact that the service was rendered free of charge to persons who do not pay for such service. Free service would also be 'service' and the recipient a 'consumer' under the Act.
12. Service rendered by a medical practitioner or hospital/nursing home cannot be regarded as service rendered free of charge, if the persons availing service has taken an insurance policy for medical care where under the charges for consultation, diagnosis and medical treatment are borne by the insurance company and such service would fall within the ambit of 'service' as defined in S. 2(1)(0) of the Act.
13. Similarly, where, as a part of the conditions of service, the employer bears the expenses of medical treatment of an employee and his family members dependent on him, the service rendered to such an employee and his family members by a medical practitioner or a hospital/nursing home would not be free of charge and would constitute 'service' under the S. 2(1)(0) of the Act.

THE CONSUMER PROTECTION ACT, 2019

This new Act was notified on 15th July 2020 and brought into effect on 20th July 2020. The Act was enacted for **faster disposal** of consumer complaints in Consumer Forums and Courts across the country.

The features of the new Act are as follows:

1. **S. 2(7),** the definition of '**consumer**' now includes any person who 'buys any goods' or 'hires any services' whether through offline or online transactions, electronic means, teleshopping, direct selling or multi-level marketing.
2. The Act has inserted the definition of "**e-commerce**" which means buying or selling of goods or services including digital products over digital or electronic network.
3. **S. 2(17),** the Act has inserted the definition "**electronic service provider**" which is defined as a person who provides technologies or processes to enable a product seller to engage in advertising or selling goods or services to a consumer and includes any online market place or online auction sites.
4. **S. 2(34),** the concept of "**product liability**" has been newly introduced and is defined as the responsibility of a product manufacturer or product seller of any product or service to compensate for any harm caused to a consumer due to defective product manufactured, sold or deficiency in services relating thereto.
5. **S. 10, Establishment of Central Consumer Protection Authority:** The Act introduces the establishment of a Central Consumer Protection Authority (CCPA) by the Central Government. The CCPA is a regulatory authority and shall be empowered to impose penalties, recall goods, cause withdrawal of services, provide refunds and investigate into matters.
6. **E-Filing of Complaints:** Consumer can file complaint online.
7. The proceedings and Evidence can be done through **video-conferencing**.
8. **S. 88, Penalty for Noncompliance of Central Authority** shall be punished with imprisonment for a term which may extend to 6 months or with fine which may extend to 20 lakh rupees or with both.
9. **S. 89, Penalties for Misleading Advertisement:** The CCPA can impose penalty on a manufacturer or an endorser up to 10 lakh rupees and imprisonment for up to 2 years for false or misleading advertisement. For every subsequent offence, the fine may be extended to 50 lakh rupees and imprisonment up to 5 years. The CCPA can also prohibit the endorser for misleading advertisement from endorsing of a particular product or service for a period up to 1 year. For every subsequent offence the period of prohibition may extend to 3 years. However, there are certain exceptions when an endorser shall not be held liable for such penalty.
10. **S. 90, Punishment for Manufacturer for Sale of Adulterated/ Spurious Goods:** In case of the first conviction, a competent court may suspend any licence issued to the person for a period of up to two years and in case of second or subsequent conviction, may cancel the licence permanently.
11. **S. 74,** the new Act provides early disposal of cases through **mediation.**
12. **Enhancement of Pecuniary Jurisdiction:** The different level of commission has been given a higher pecuniary limit to entertain consumer complaints. The District Commission can now entertain consumer complaints where the value of goods or services paid does not exceed 1 crore rupees. The State Commission can entertain disputes where such value

between 1 and 10 crore rupees and the National Commission can exercise jurisdiction where such value exceeds 10 crore rupees.

Medical Indemnity Insurance

Medical indemnity insurance is also known and referred to as medical malpractice insurance or cover. It is contract under which the insurance company agrees in exchange for the payment of premiums, to indemnify (cover) the insured doctor as a result of his claimed professional negligence.

The purposes of medical indemnity insurance are: (i) To fund legal costs (including hiring lawyer and court fees) to defend such claims in the court of law (iii) To pay compensation to a patient or third party arising from a claim made against a doctor on ground of professional misconduct or negligence.

EMPLOYEES' COMPENSATION (AMENDMENT) ACT, 2017

Previously, the act was known as **'Workmen's Compensation Act 1923'** (The Principal Act). This amended act received the Presidential assent on April 12, 2017. The act extends to whole of India, except for employees covered under the provisions of the Employees' State Insurance Act 1988 and for the members serving in the Armed Forces of India. The purpose of the act is to compensate the employees for the injury or death caused by industrial accidents including occupational disease during their employment subject to certain exceptions as laid down in the Act.

Salient features of the act are:

1. **Duty to inform the employee (S.17A):** At the time of appointment, the employer needs to inform an employee of his rights to compensation in writing as well as through electronic means.
2. **Change in penalties (S.18A):** If the employer fails to inform the employee of his rights to compensation, the employer is liable for penalty. The minimum penalty payable has been enhanced to Rs. 50,000 and may be extended upto Rs. 1,00,000.
3. **Personal injury:** To claim compensation following conditions must be satisfied (a) Personal injury must have been caused to the workmen (b) Such injury must have been caused by an accident (c) The accident must have arisen out of and in the course of employment (d) The injury must have resulted either in death of the employee or in his/her **total or partial disablement** for a period exceeding three days.
4. **Occupational disease:** (a) An **occupational disease** is any chronic ailment that occurs as a result of work or occupational activity. (b) The list of occupation diseases is listed in Part A, B and C of Schedule III contract. (c) Examples of few occupation disease are like infections due to contamination, infrared radiations, chemicals, lung cancer by asbestos dust etc. (d) *Length of service required:* For diseases specified in (i) Part A: No specific period, (ii) Part B: 6 months (iii) Part C: As specified by the Central Government.
5. **Poisoning cases:** (a) As per this act, the following poisons/ toxins are implicated as causative agents among the list of occupational diseases (Schedule III): Arsenic, lead (except tetraethyl lead), phosphorous, mercury, manganese, cadmium, benzene, halogenated hydrocarbons, nitrous fume, carbon disulphide, chromic acid or bichromate of ammonium, potassium, sodium and organophosphates. (b) During employment, if the workman contracts any of the mentioned occupational disease peculiar to that employment, he/she becomes eligible for payment of compensation under the Act.
6. **Employer is not liable when:** (a) Disablement not exceeding 3 days (b) Accident due influence of drugs, disobeyed orders, disregards of safeguards (c) *Doctrine of added peril:* If injury occurred at the time of doing any other work which is not assigned to the employee by the employer.
7. **Role of doctor:** (a) Medical examination of injured workmen for assessment of part of body injured, nature of injury (simple/grievous) and for issuing sickness certificate and fitness certificate. (b) The doctor needs to examine the workmen for degree of disablement whether partial or total. Also needs to certify the percentage in case of permanent partial disablement. (c) Establishment of causal relationship between injury and malignancy as per Ewing's postulates. (d) Assessment of loss of earning capacity and issue of certificate. (e) Maintenance of injury report register. (f) In case dispute between administration and employee, the doctor may have to appear before commission to give evidence. (g) Pre-placement medical examination of the workmen. (h) Periodical medical examination for important occupational disease. (i) Supervision of working environment. (j) Heath education.
8. **Amount of compensation:** (a) *In case of death:* 50% of the monthly wage of the deceased workman, multiplied by the relevant factor or Rs. 1,20,000; whichever is more. (b) *In case of total permanent disablement:* 60% of the monthly wage, multiplied by the relevant factor; or Rs. 1,20,000; whichever is more. (c) *In case of (total or partial) temporary disablement:* Half-monthly payment of the sum equivalent to 25% of "monthly wages". (d) As per the new rule (2020) notified by the government, Rs 15,000 will be considered as wage for calculating compensation under the Act.
9. **Appeal:** Appeals can be made against orders related to compensation, distribution of compensation, award of penalty or interest, only if the amount in dispute is at least Rs. 10,000.

THE EMPLOYEES' STATE INSURANCE ACT, 1948

The Employees' State Insurance Act came into force from 19th April 1948. The act was amended in 2010.

Salient Features of the Act

1. **The purpose of the act** is to protect the employees against financial distress arising out of events of sickness, disablement or death due to employment injuries and to provide medical care to insured persons and their families.
2. **ESIC and ESI Scheme:** Under this act, a statutory corporate body set up called Employees' State Insurance Corporation ("ESIC") which is responsible for the administration of the ESI Scheme, a self-financed comprehensive social security scheme.
3. **Applicability:** The ESI Scheme applies to factories and other establishments, viz. Road Transport, Hotels, Restaurants, Cinemas, Newspaper, Shops and Educational/Medical Institutions wherein ≥10 persons are employed (in some states it is still 20). From 1st August, 2015, ESI Corporation has extended the benefits of the ESI Scheme to the workers deployed on the construction sites.
4. **Eligibility:** Employees with a monthly maximum salary of Rs. 21,000 (wage limit) are entitled to get the benefits of the scheme.
5. **Areas covered:** ESI scheme covers more than 34 States and Union Territories of India
6. **Contribution Rates:** The ESI Scheme is financed by contributions from employers and employees. As per latest revision w. e. f. 01.07.2019, the rate of contribution by employer is 3.25% of the wages payable to employees. The employees' contribution is at the rate of 0.75% of the wages payable to an employee. Employees, earning less than Rs. 137 a day as daily wages, are exempted from payment of their share of contribution. Only the employer's contribution is paid for such people.
7. **Benefits:** (a) *Medical Benefit:* The insured's medical expenses are covered through affordable and reasonable health care facilities. (b) *Maternity benefit:* The beneficiary can avail 100% of the daily wages for upto 26 weeks which can be extended to a further one month based on the medical advice. In the case of miscarriage, the benefit is 6 weeks, while in the case of adoption it is 12 weeks. (c) *Sickness benefit:* During medical leave, the worker can avail 70% of the daily wage for a maximum of 91 days which can be availed in two consecutive periods. (d) *Disablement benefit:* For temporary disablement of the worker is eligible for a monthly wage of 90% until he/she recovers. In the case of permanent disability, 90% of the monthly wage can be availed for the entire life. (e) *Unemployment benefit:* A maximum of 50% of the average monthly wage in the case of involuntary loss of non-employment or due to permanent invalidity due to injury for a period of 24 months. (f) *Dependents benefit:* The dependents of the insured receive financial assistance in case of illnesses or injuries while at work. (g) *Funeral expenses:* An amount of Rs.15,000 towards funeral costs shall be paid to the dependents or to the individual who does the last rites of the insured. (h) *Other benefits:* The insurer is also eligible for other benefits like old age medical care, physical and vocational rehabilitation etc. (i) The ESIC also runs many medical and nursing colleges across the country.

HUMAN EXPERIMENTATION

All research involving human subjects should be conducted in accordance with basic ethical principles, which have equal moral force and guide the conscientious preparation of proposals for scientific studies. These are: (i) ***Respect for persons:*** This incorporates at least two fundamental ethical considerations. (ii) ***Respect for autonomy***: This requires that those who are capable of deliberation about their personal choices should be treated with respect for their capacity for self determination. (iii) ***Protection of persons with impaired or diminished autonomy:*** This requires that those who are dependent or vulnerable be afforded security against harm or abuse. (iv) ***Beneficence:*** This refers to ethical obligation to maximize benefit and minimize harms and wrongs. This principle gives rise to norms requiring that the risks of research be reasonable in the light of the expected benefits and that the research design be sound enough to safeguard the welfare of the research project. (v) ***Justice:*** This refers to the ethical obligation to treat each person in accordance with what is morally right and proper to him/her.

Human experimentation may be: (i) ***Therapeutic experimentation***: It is concerned primarily with improving the condition of a particular patient under treatment. (ii) ***Research experimentation:*** It is concerned primarily with using a human subject as a means of expanding scientific knowledge for the benefit of humanity. (iii) ***Innovative experimentation:*** These are therapeutic procedures that have not yet earned a place in medical practice.

The Declaration of Geneva: The Declaration of Geneva of the World Medical Association binds the doctor with the words, "The health of my patient will be my first consideration."

International Code of Medical Ethics: It declares, "Any act or advice which could weaken physical or mental resistance of a human being may be used only in his interest."

The purpose of biomedical research involving human subjects must be to improve the diagnostic, therapeutic and prophylactic procedures and understanding of the etiology and the pathogenesis of the disease. In current medical practices, most of these procedures involve hazards. Medical progress is based on research that ultimately rests in past on human subjects.

Special caution must be exercised in the conduct of research, which may affect the environment, and the welfare of animals used for research must be respected. The results of the laboratory experiments must be applied essentially to human beings to further scientific knowledge and to help the suffering humanity.

World Medical Association (WMA) has prepared the following recommendations as a guide to every doctor in biomedical research involving human subjects. It must be stressed that the standards as drafted are only a guide to physicians all over the world. Doctors are not relieved from the civil, criminal and ethical responsibility under the laws of their own countries.

Helsinki Declaration

The code of ethics known as Declaration of Helsinki was drawn in 1964 and revised many times including latest in 2008 as follows:

Basic principles: (i) Biomedical research involving human subjects must conform to the generally accepted scientific principles and should be based on adequately performed laboratory and animal experimentation. (ii) It should be based on a thorough knowledge of scientific literature. (iii) Design and the performance of each experimental procedure involving human subjects should be clearly formulated in an experimental protocol which should be transmitted to a specially appointed independent committee for consideration, comment and guidance. (iv) Biomedical research involving human subjects should be conducted only by scientifically qualified person and under the supervision of a clinically competent medical person. (v) Responsibility for the human subject must always be with medically qualified person and never rest on the subject of the research, even though the subject has given his/her consent. (vi) Biomedical research involving human subjects cannot legitimately be carried out unless the importance of the objective is in proportion to the inherent risk to the subject. (vii) Every biomedical research project involving human subjects should be preceded by careful assessment of predictable risks in comparison with foreseeable benefits to the subject or to the others. (viii) Concern for the interest of the subject must always prevail over the interest of science and society. (ix) Right of the research subject to safeguard his/her integrity must always be respected. (x) Every precaution should be taken to respect the privacy of the subject, to minimize the impact of the study on the subject's physical and mental integrity and on the personality of subjects. (xi) Doctors should abstain from engaging in research projects involving human subjects unless they are satisfied that the hazards involved are believed to be predictable. (xii) Doctor should cease any investigation if the hazards outweigh the potential benefits. (xiii) In publication of results of his/her research, the doctor is obliged to preserve the accuracy of his results. (xiv) Reports of experimentation that are not in accordance with the principles laid down in this declaration should not be accepted for publication. (xv) In any research on human beings, the subject must be adequately informed of the aims, methods, anticipated benefits, potential hazards of the study and discomfort it may entail and that he/she is at liberty to abstain from participation in the study and is also free to withdraw consent to participation at any time. (xvi) Doctor should then obtain the subject's freely given informed consent in writing. (xvii) Doctor should be particularly cautious if the subject is in a dependent relationship to him/her or may consent under duress. In that case, an independent doctor who is not engaged in the investigation and is completely independent of his official relationship should take informed consent. (xviii) In case of legal incompetence, informed consent should be obtained from a legal guardian in accordance with national legislation. (xix) If the person is physically or mentally incapacitated and cannot give informed consent or when the subject is minor, permission from the responsible relative replaces that of the subject in accordance with national legislation. (xx) Research protocol should always contain a statement of ethical considerations involved and should indicate that the principles enunciated in the present declaration are complied with.

Medical research combined with professional care (clinical research): (i) In the treatment of the sick person, the doctor must be free to use a new diagnostic and therapeutic measure, if in his/her judgment it offers hope of saving life, reestablishing health or alleviate suffering. (ii) Potential benefits, hazards and discomfort of a new method should be weighed against the advantages of the best current diagnostic and therapeutic methods. (iii) In any medical study, every patient including those of a control group, if any should be assured of the best-proven diagnostic and therapeutic methods. (iv) Refusal of the patient to participate in a study must never interfere with the doctor-patient relationship. (v) If the doctor considers it essential not to obtain informed consent, the specific reasons for this proposal should be stated in the experimental protocol for transmission to the independent committee. (vi) Doctor can combine medical research with professional care, the objective being the acquisition of new medical knowledge only to the extent that medical research is justified by its potential diagnostic or therapeutic value for the patient.

Non-therapeutic biomedical research involving human subjects (Non-clinical biomedical research): (i) In the purely scientific application of medical research carried out on a human being, it is the duty of the doctor to remain protector of the life and health of that person on whom biomedical research is being carried out. (ii) Subjects should be volunteers, either healthy persons or patients for whom the experimental design is not related to the patient's illness. (iii) Investigator and the investigating team should discontinue the research if in his/her or their judgment it may, if continued be harmful to the individual. (iv) In research on man, the interest of science and society should never take precedence over consideration related to the well being of the subjects.

Salient features of Helsinki Declaration: (i) Extensive animal research is an absolute prerequisite to the use of an innovative technique in the treatment of human beings. (ii) Most difficult innovative cases will be those in which prior animal research is impossible or would be uninformative. (iii) Treatment should be given cautiously and its after effects noted and appreciated. (iv) Experiment on volunteers can only be justified if they do no significant harm to the subject and the results are likely to be beneficial. (v) It would be unethical to do something merely by way of experimentation that is which is not strictly related to cure patient's illness. (vi) There must also be no great risk in proposed experimentation even if the patient consents to run the great risk. (vii) In considering whether a new treatment is as efficacious as an old one, side effects of the two treatments and their costs should be considered.

ICMR-National Ethical Guidelines for Biomedical and Health Research Involving Human Participants, 2017

In India, the first ethical guidelines for biomedical and health research called "Policy Statement on Ethical Considerations Involved in Research on Human Subjects" was prepared in year 1980 by Indian Council of Medical Research. Subsequently, it was revised in year 2000, 2006 and the latest revised guideline was released on 12 October, 2017. **New sections have been added on informed consent process, vulnerability, biological materials, biobanking and datasets, responsible conduct of research, sociobehavioral research, research in emergencies or disasters**. The guidelines have 12 sections focusing on different areas of research and the corresponding ethical requirements.

The guideline states that medical and related research using human beings should necessarily ensure that: (i) **Purpose of such research** is directed towards the increase of knowledge about human conditions in relation to its social, cultural and natural environment. (ii) **Research is conducted** under such conditions that the subjects are dealt with in a manner conducive to and consistent with their dignity and well being. (iii) Research must be subjected to a regimen of **evaluation** at all stages.

General Principles: (i) *Principle of essentiality:* Whereby the research is considered absolutely essential after a due consideration of all factors and options involved. (ii) *Principle of voluntariness, informed consent and community agreement:* Whereby, the subjects are fully apprised of the research and the impact and risks on him and others; and he retains the right to abstain from further participation in the research irrespective of any obligation they may have entered, subject to only minimal restitutive obligations of any advance consideration received. (iii) *Principle of non-exploitation:* Whereby as a general rule the research subjects are remunerated for their involvement in the research or experiment. (iv) *Principle of privacy and confidentiality:* Whereby, the identity and records of the subjects are kept confidential as far as possible. (v) *Principle of precaution and risk minimization:* Whereby, due care and caution is taken at all stages of a research to ensure that the subjects are put to minimum risk and generally benefit from the experiment. (vi) *Principle of professional competence:* Whereby, the research is conducted at all times by competent and qualified persons who act with total integrity and impartiality and who have been made aware of the ethical considerations. (vii) *Principle of accountability and transparency:* Whereby, the research experiment will be conducted in a fair, honest, impartial and transparent manner after full disclosure of all aspects of their interest. (viii) *Principle of maximization of public interest and of distributive justice:* Whereby, the research or experiment and its subsequent applicative use are conducted and used to benefit all human kind. (ix) *Principle of institutional arrangement:* Whereby, there shall be a duty on all persons connected with the research to ensure that all the procedures required to be complied with and all institutional arrangements required to be made in respect of the research and its subsequent use or application are duly made in a transparent manner. (x) *Principle of public domain:* Whereby, the research is brought into public domain so that its results are generally made known through scientific and other publications. (xi) *Principle of totality of responsibility:* Whereby, the professional and moral responsibility, for the due observance of all the principles, guidelines and prescriptions rests with all those involved in conducting the experiment. (xii) *Principle of compliance:* Whereby, there is a general and positive duty on all persons, conducting with any research entailing the use of a human subject to ensure that these guidelines are adhered in letter and spirit.

Ethics Committee (EC)

All research proposals on biomedical, social and behavioral science research for health involving human participants, their biological material and data to be reviewed and approved by an appropriately constituted EC to safeguard the dignity, rights, safety and well-being of all research participants.

The institution is responsible for establishing an EC and shall provide logistic support, such as infrastructure, staff, space, funds, adequate support and protected time for the Member Secretary to run the EC functions. An institution can have one or more than one EC, e.g., EC for postgraduate research, EC stem cell research and therapy and EC for animal research etc. for to review large numbers of research proposals. An institution that does not have its own EC (user institution) may utilize the services of the EC of another institution (host institution). Every EC should have written SOP (standard operating procedure) according to which the committee should function. The SOP should be prepared based on the ICMR and CDSCO guidelines.

Composition: (i) The head of institution shall appoint all EC members including Chairperson and member secretary. (ii) ECs should be multi-disciplinary and multi-sectoral. (iii) There should be adequate representation of age and gender. (iv) Preferably 50% of the members should be non-affiliated or from outside the institution. (v) The number of members in an EC should preferably be between 7 and 15 and a minimum of 5 members should be present to meet the quorum requirements. (vi) The EC should have a balance between medical and non-medical members/technical and non-technical members, depending upon the needs of the institution. (vii) The EC should have legal expert/s, social scientist/philosopher/ethicist/theologian and lay person(s).

Functions: (i) To provide competent review of scientific, medical, social and ethical aspects of the research proposals. (ii) Undertake review free from bias and influence. (iii) Provide advice to the researchers on all aspects of welfare and safety of research participants. (iv) To protect dignity, rights and wellbeing of potential research participants. (v) To ensure universal ethical values and international scientific standards in terms of local community values and customs. (vi) To assist in the development and education of research community responsive to local health care requirements. (vii) To recommend appropriate compensation for research related injury, whenever required. (viii) To carry out monitoring visits at study sites as and when needed.

STEM CELL RESEARCH (SCR)

Stem cells are undifferentiated cells characterized by the ability to extensively proliferate, usually arise from a single cell (clonal), and differentiate into different types of cells and tissue (potent). There are several sources of human stem cells including embryonic stem (ES) cells, embryonic germ (EG) cells, and adult stem cells. Research in human stem cells provides hope for new treatments for degenerative, incurable and irreversible diseases such as diabetes, spinal cord injury, Parkinson's disease, Alzheimer's disease and myocardial infarction. Stem cells and their derivatives fall under definition of "drug" as per the Drugs and Cosmetics Act 1940, and are categorized as "IND" or "INE" when used for clinical application.

Human SCR both in basic and clinical research raises many ethical and political issues. In India, there is no legal provision to regulate the SCR, but guidelines were made to tackle scientific, technical, as well as perceived challenges. These guidelines seek to facilitate safe, ethical, and regulated translational and clinical SCR by engaging all stakeholders proactively. Recently, an updated new guideline "the National Guidelines for Stem Cell Research 2017" was made on stem cell research (SCR). It was drafted under a collaborative effort from the Indian Council of Medical Research (ICMR) and Department of Biotechnology (DBT). The guidelines reiterate that any stem cell use in patients, other than that for hematopoietic stem cell reconstitution for approved indications, is investigational at present. The guidelines do not apply to research using (a) Nonhuman stem cells and their derivatives; (b) Hematopoietic stem cells (where standard of medical care has been established); and (c) PRP (platelet-rich plasma) and autologous chondrocyte/osteocytes implantation (categorized as "other cell-based applications").

Salient Features of National Guidelines for Stem Cell Research 2017

1. The Institutional Committee for SCR (IC-SCR) and the Institutional Ethics Committee (IEC) need to be mandatorily registered with National Apex Committee for Stem Cell Research and Therapy (NAC-SCRT) and Central Drugs Standard Control Organisation (CDSCO), respectively.
2. The clinical trials only to be undertaken at institutes with registered IC-SCR and IEC, conducting studies only at Good Manufacturing Practice (GMP) and Good Laboratory Practice (GLP) and have certified facilities for processing of stem cell products and derivatives (SCP&D). Institutes must obtain mandatory accreditation from National Accreditation Board for Testing and Calibration Laboratories (NABL), when processing stem cell products and derivatives (SCP&D) for human use.
3. The clinical research undertaken by medical professionals registered with the Medical Council of India (MCI) (Now NMC) having an MCI-approved postgraduate qualification in the domain area of the specific trial.
4. **Categorization of Research (S. 8):** 3 categories (a) *Permissible:* Research involving establishment of ESCs (embryonic stem cells) and iPSCs (induced pluripotent stem cells) (b) *Restrictive:* Research involving human preimplantation embryos processed by in IVF (*In vitro* fertilization)/LCSI (intracytoplasmic sperm injection)/ SCNT (somatic cell nuclear transfer) to derive ESC lines (c) *Prohibited:* Research involving human germline gene therapy and reproductive cloning.
5. **Basic Research (S. 10):** *In vitro* studies largely fall in under permissible category require prior approval of IEC and IC-SCR, except studies involving established human stem-cell lines registered with the IC-SCR. *In vitro* studies on preimplantation human embryos must be carried out within 14 days of fertilization or formation of primitive streak, whichever is earlier. Derivation of new ESC or iPSC lines from human embryonic or somatic cells, respectively, must have prior approval of IC-SCR and IEC. Uterine implantation (human/animal) of manipulated cells with the intent of developing a whole organism is prohibited.
6. **Translational Research Including Clinical Trials (S. 11):** (a) *Preclinical studies:* Require approval from IEC (humans), IAEC (small animals) and CPCSEA (large/ nonhuman primates). Product testing must include safety, biodistribution, immune rejection studies, single-.and repeated-dose toxicity studies, tumorigenicity, genotoxicity, developmental toxicity studies and biodistribution studies. (b) *Clinical studies:* Require clearances from IC-SCR, IEC and CDSCO, and must be registered with CTRI. Follow-up period of minimum 2 years is mandatory. Establishing DSMB is mandatory for each study. All adverse events must be reported to IEC, CDSCO, NAC-SCRT through IC-SCR. Trial records must be maintained for minimum of 15 years. Patient confidentiality is to be maintained by all means.
7. **Banking (S. 14):** Umbilical cord banking (UCB) or ESC/iPSC lines are permitted only in institutions licensed by CDSCO. Commercial banking of all other biological materials is not permitted yet. Such banks, if involved in stem cell research,

should constitute an IC-SCR (NAC-SCRT registered), and have an SOP for banking and release. Biological materials can only be released to institutes with registered IC-SCR and IEC, must constitute IC-SCR (NAC-SCRT registered), and have an SOP for banking and release. Biological materials can only be released to institutes with registered IC-SCR and IEC.

8. **Procurement (S. 15):** Biological material can be procured only from the institutions that have IEC. Only IEC and IC-SCR shall review and approve the process of procurement. If cells/tissues have been developed utilizing IVF method, clearance from the NAC-SCR mandatory. Archival period for stem cell lines and related information is 10 years. For procurement of fetal or placental tissue, processes must comply with all obligations under the MTP Act, 1971. The medical person responsible for care of the pregnant woman and the investigator using the fetal material shall not be the same. Informed consent for fetal tissue donation should be obtained in advance and not just before or at the time of the procedure. If there is disagreement between parents, the mother's wish shall prevail. Consent for donation of blastocysts for establishment of human ESC lines should be obtained from the donor at least 24 hours in advance. Donors retain the right to withdraw consent until the blastocysts are actually used in cell line derivation.
9. **Exchange (S. 17):** Import of stem cell lines for basic research does not require no objection certificate or prior approval from any government agencies, but those required for clinical trials and originating oversees require import clearance from CDSCO. For export of indigenously developed cell lines, IEC and IC-SCR clearances must be obtained and submitted along with the MTA during the review of such research proposals.
10. **Levels of Manipulation (S. 4.2):** Stem cells whether autologous or allogenic, require variable degree of *in vitro* or *ex vivo* processing before their use for clinical application/transplantation/translational research. They are at 3 levels. (a) *Minimal:* Processing period must be within 72 hours; approvals from CDSCO, IC-SCR and IEC (b) *Substantial:* CDSCO approval only after IC-SCR and IEC clearances (c) *Major:* CDSCO approval after clearances from NAC-SCRT through IC-SCR and IEC.
11. Human participants enrolled for clinical trials are not liable to pay any charges toward procedures, investigations, and/or hospitalization related to the trial.
12. **Ethical Aspects (S. 4.1)** (a) *Video consenting* is mandatory, i.e., as per CDSCO guidelines for audio-visual recording. (b) *Screening of six communicable diseases* (human immunodeficiency virus 1 and 2, hepatitis B virus, hepatitis C virus Treponema pallidum, human T lymphotropic virus, and cytomegalovirus) or any other risk factors for genetic diseases) is mandatory. (c) *Intellectual property rights* of donated material will not vest with donor, but may be shared (to be mentioned in informed consent form). If commercialization brings any financial benefit, may be passed on to donor/community.
13. Investigators should demonstrate respect for *autonomy and privacy* of those who donate gametes, blastocysts, embryos or somatic cells for stem cell research.
14. **Publicity (S. 19):** Advertising and publicity of any kind through any mode by the clinicians are not permitted and is prosecutable offence as per Indian Medical Council (Professional Conduct, Etiquette and Ethics) Act.

LONG QUESTIONS

1. What are the functions of National Medical Commission?
2. What are duties of a Registered Medical Practitioner?
3. What is infamous conduct in professional respect? When is the warning notice issued to Registered Medical Practitioner?
4. Define negligence and how will you prove it?
5. Describe the precautions one can take to prevent negligence.
6. What is consent? Describe the "Doctrine of informed consent".
7. Discussed the salient features of Consumer Protection Act.
8. Define consent, the various types of consent, laws in relation to consent and the general rules to be followed for taking consent.
9. Discuss the professional and ethical duties and conduct of a medical practitioner.
10. Discuss medical negligence in detail. Enumerate various types of negligence.

SHORT QUESTIONS

1. Informed consent.
2. Vicarious liability.
3. Professional secrecy.
4. Privileged communication.
5. Contributory negligence.
6. Human experimentation.
7. Consent.
8. Consumer Protection Act.
9. National Medical Commission Act.
10. State Medical Councils.
11. Functions of Medical Council of India.
12. Differentiate between Civil and Criminal Negligence.

13. Res ipsa loquitor.
14. Conflict resolution techniques.
15. Challenges in medicolegal cases.
16. Communication skills.
17. Different types of oath.

MULTIPLE CHOICE QUESTIONS

1. Indian Medical Degrees Act was passed in the year:

(a) 1916 (b) 1920
(c) 1925 (d) 1930

2. The National Medical Commission Act was passed in the year:

(a) 2017 (b) 2018
(c) 2019 (d) 2020

3. All are true for National Medical Commission, *except*:

(a) It consists of 43 members
(b) It maintains the standards of medical education in India
(c) It recognizes the foreign medical education
(d) It shall grant limited license to community health provider

4. Warning Notice is issued to a doctor in cases of:

(a) Prescribing medicine under influence of alcohol
(b) Conviction by a court of law for offences involving moral turpitude
(c) Dichotomy
(d) All of the above

5. In case of an unconscious patient with head injury requiring emergency surgery with no relative to give consent, the doctor should:

(a) Wait for relative for the consent to operate
(b) Operate only with consent of police
(c) Operate only with medical superintendent's consent
(d) Operate without consent

6. When the doctor is not negligent and it is the patient alone who is negligent, it is called:

(a) Negligence of the patient
(b) Contributory negligence
(c) Defences of negligence
(d) Contributory negligence by the plaintiff

7. The law does not consider the following doctrine in a charge of criminal negligence:

(a) Vicarious liability
(b) Novus-actus interveniens
(c) Contributary negligence
(d) Res ipsa loquitur

8. The guideline for clinical drug trial or other research involving patient is issued by:

(a) National Medical Commission
(b) Indian Medical Association
(c) Drug control of India
(d) Indian Council of Medical Research

9. The doctor should keep records of in-patients for a minimum period of:

(a) 3 years (b) 5 years
(c) 7 years (d) 10 years

10. The time limit for filing complaint in consumer court is:

(a) 6 months (b) 1 year
(c) 2 years (d) 3 years

ANSWER KEY

1. (a)	2. (c)	3. (a)	4. (d)	5. (d)	6. (a)	7. (c)	8. (d)	9. (a)	10. (c)

4 CHAPTER

Moment of Death

THANATOLOGY

Thanatology is the branch of science that deals with death in all its aspects.

Death

The definition of death created little or no problem for centuries until 1960 when organ transplantation caused minute scrutiny to be director at the phenomenon of death itself.

Section 46 I.P.C. states that death denotes the death of a human being unless the contrary appears from the context.

Section 2(b) of the Registration of Births and Deaths Act defines death as 'permanent disappearance of all evidence of life at any time after live birth has taken place.

Black's Law Dictionary (Black 1951) in United States defines death as "The cessation of life, the ceasing to exist", defined by physicians as total stoppage of circulation and cessation of vital functions, thereupon such as respiration and pulsation.

Shapiro (1969) defined death as "the irreversible loss of the properties of living matter". However, it is difficult to appreciate his claim that this definition satisfies the practical requirements for death certification.

Calne (1970) gave a more practical definition that states "when destruction of the brain has been established, the individual has died no matter what the state of the rest of his body", giving four signs for such a diagnosis: (i) Deep, irreversible coma with fixed, dilated pupils and absent cranial nerve reflexes (ii) No spontaneous respiration (iii) Absence of electrical brain activity (iv) Cessation of circulation in the retinal vessels.

Rentoul and Smith (1973) defined death as "complete and persistent cessation of respiration and circulation".

In a case of **Smith v/s Smith** in a fatal automobile accident both husband and wife sustained injury. Husband died on the spot and the wife was taken to the hospital where she remained unconscious for 17 days and then died. The petitioner argued that the deaths were simultaneous, since there was no evidence of brain activity after accident and the physicians were unsuccessful to revive her by resuscitation. The inference was that resuscitative efforts were maintaining the body in a state of animation although it could not be shown that life existed. The Court did not accept the contention. They quoted Black's definition of death and stated that breathing though unconscious is not dead.

The living body depends upon the integrity of three principal interdependent systems circulation, respiration and enervation. Failure of one of them will cause failure of the other two. This leads to the death of the individual. There are two phases of death: (i) *Extinction of the personality is immediate sign of vital process:* This is somatic death. (ii) *Progressive disintegration of the body tissue:* This is molecular death or cellular death that occurs sometimes later.

Somatic Death

This is the form of death referred to in common parlance. The issue of its occurrence might have considerable legal implications, but the decision when death has occurred is always a medical one. Its onset is usually not difficult to detect even by lay people if the dying person is under observation during the last minute of life. It is said to have occurred when a final expiration is followed by continuous immobility of the chest, loss of pulse and alteration of the features. These changes indicate that respiration and circulation have been stopped and the brain will stop functioning if it has not been so. Residual heart movement is not of practical importance as they are insufficient to maintain the circulation. Somatic death can be detected by ECG that will show flat line within minutes.

The recent development in medical techniques has posed a number of problems, whereas for so many years it was accepted that death has occurred if respiration and circulation have ceased for more than 10 minutes. Now it is possible for methods such as cooling the whole body to 15ºC or 59°F or less to stop the heart and respiration for an hour or longer and restart them again at will. During this period, ECG and EEG shows no electrical activity and body looks like a corpse. This leads to the view that it is not the cessation of the respiration or circulation but it is their failure to return that indicates death. Thus, we are driven from a positive to negative approach. Therefore, the doctor while taking decision must satisfy himself that not only respiration and circulation has stopped, but their failure has persisted to such a period that under no circumstances it is possible for the person to come to life again.

Finally, death can be defined as "Permanent and irreversible stoppage of respiration, circulation and brain function so called, **tripod of life**".

The diagnosis of death by auscultation of the chest can be difficult in cases of excessive fat, emphysema, apex beat below the rib, poorly beating heart and shallow diaphragmatic respiration. All these conditions damp the conduction of heart sound with body wall.

Diagnosis of recent death is also very difficult whenever the death of the person has not been observed. Whenever a doctor is called to certify a patient as dead that is brought by ambulance, he must insist that the body must be removed to a well-lit room where he can carry out his examination. Even though the condition is satisfactory, the error can occur in the examination.

The signs of life can be detected by special methods like Oscilloscope, ECG and EEG etc. It can never be assumed that attempted resuscitation is pointless. On the other hand, resuscitative measures should always be continued for half an hour. In cases of electric shock and drug overdose, treatment should continue until death. In a case of a young woman 23 years old found lying on a beach at 8:10 AM near Liverpool apparently dead, police was informed. The doctor failed to see any movement for 15 minutes and certified her dead. A pathologist came later, examined her and agreed with the diagnosis. About two hours later when the postmortem was to start, one of the persons noticed flickering of eyelids and formation of tear. She was immediately taken to intensive care unit where she was survived. On investigation, it was found to be a case of overdose of barbiturate.

This case emphasizes the importance of examination of the body by the doctor before certifying it. If the doctor fails to detect heart sound or respiration after adequate auscultation, he must measure rectal temperature. When the rectal temperature is below 75ºF (23.9ºC) it is to be diagnosed as dead. On Ophthalmoscopic examination, there is segmentation of blood in retinal blood vessels. If still there is any doubt, the patient should be taken to intensive care unit for further investigation of heart and brain function.

Major N.C. Kapoor reports a case of resuscitation after cessation of vital functions for 15 min. A Hindu 80 years old male was brought to medical college, Calcutta at 10 PM on July 13, 1925 suffering from severe dyspnea resulting from laryngeal obstruction due to malignant growth. Tracheostomy was done immediately when he suddenly stopped breathing. No heart sounds were audible on auscultation, pupils were dilated and eyes were fixed. Artificial respiration was started and tracheostomy was performed when he was apparently dead, the chest was being flickered by wet towel, there was no pulse at the wrist. After 15 minutes when every body had given up the hope, patient's chest was flicked in a forcible manner and the patient took a shallow breath. The heart sounds were audible and pulse was palpable.

Molecular Death

The occurrence of clinical death implies the failure of the body as an integrated system. For some time afterwards, life continues in the separate tissues, which constitute the body. These only die after varying periods depending upon the ability of the tissue to function without blood supply. This is called molecular or cellular death. The nervous tissue dies rapidly and the vital centers die in about 5 minutes. The muscles live longer and they will constrict to direct electrical stimuli up to 3 hours. The corneal reflex and pupillary reflex disappear at the time of death. The pupil reacts to the drugs like atropine that causes dilatation up to 4 hours and eserine/physostigmine that causes contraction up to 1 hour. The cornea can be removed for transplantation up to 6 hours and blood can be transfused for up to 6 hours of death. Therefore, we die in bits and pieces.

The legal definition of death depends upon the diagnosis of somatic death. The distinction between somatic and molecular death becomes important because in order to remove essential tissues and organs for transplantation there is a relatively short time for the biological properties of living matter to persist after somatic death. With somatic death, there is complete generalized anoxia of the tissue and consequently stoppage of metabolic process carried out by the tissue cells. The metabolic process of the ganglionic cells stops in minutes, which are most sensitive whereas that of connective tissue stops in hours, which are the least sensitive.

Errors in Diagnosis of Death

Generally, there is no difficulty in the diagnosis of somatic deaths. However, in some cases the heart sounds and breath sounds diminish greatly. Errors occur if proper clinical examination is not done or hurriedly done in patients with kidney failure and Cheyne-Stokes respiration etc. Nevertheless, there are occasions when the distinction between death and suspended animation poses a real difficulty.

Suspended animation: This is a death like state in which vital functions of the body are at such a low pitch that they cannot be determined by ordinary methods of clinical examination. Practitioners of yoga can induce this death like state voluntarily. In addition it can be involuntarily due to: (i) Severe shock following accident (ii) Electrical shock (iii) Poisoning (barbiturate) (iv) Drowning (v) Epilepsy (vi) Sunstroke (vii) Cholera; and (viii) Hysteria.

Suspended animation lasts for seconds to hours and by ordinary clinical methods, distinction is not possible. However, methods like ECG and EEG can be used to reach a diagnosis.

Moment of Death

1. The classical concept of so-called **tripod of life** does not hold good now as lungs and heart could be maintained on artificial support system. Any attempt to determine the moment of death in such patients by the help of classical criteria results in a stalemate. Dr Christian Bernard did the first heart transplant on 3rd December, 1967 in Capetown.
2. The second major factor responsible for a fresh appraisal of moment of death is the growing practice of organ transplantation. A **beating heart**, which is the ideal specimen for transplantation cannot be taken out of an individual because of: (i) If we were to apply to classical criteria, because the heart is beating in the prospective donor, he is obviously not dead. (ii) On the contrary, if we wait for his heart to stop to resolve the ethical dilemma, the heart becomes useless for transplantation and chances of such a heart surviving in the recipient are very dim.

Therefore, the people all over the world were trying to find out the legal definition of death, as most of the countries had no such definition. In 1968 **Bruce Tucker**, a labourer fell down from a multistory building. His heart was taken out by the transplantation team while it was beating being declared brain dead on the ground of extensive Craniocerebral damage. His brother William Tucker appealed in the Court in the State of Virginia, USA. The Court verdict was that doctor had not acted lawfully. The jury as directed by the Court decided on the facts of the case and opined that a person having suffered irreparable brain damage and whose bodily function cannot be sustained without continuous artificial assistance is dead. Therefore, the loss of brain function was taken into account for declaring a person dead. Before coming to the modern concept of moment of death, we consider two questions:

(i) What is it that is so central to your humanity, that when you loose it you are dead? (ii) Whether death is an event or process?

If we consider death to be an event then the end point of existence is very clear and sharp. Nevertheless, the 50 trillion cells of the body do not die at a time. Probably they die turn by turn. Therefore, how many cells whether 10%, 20% or 90% will die to declare an individual dead? Is there any point of no return after which no artificial means will be able to revive the person and will be called dead? Let us clarify the fact with an example:

What we call a person who has just been decapitated but whose heart is still beating. If we go by the concept of point of no return, we would pronounce him dead but if we go by old method, he is not dead. It is absurd to wait for asystole in a decapitated man who has reached the "point of no return". Therefore, the modern concept of brain death is now taken into account.

Brain Death

Philadelphia Protocol (1969): It determined death on the basis of: (i) Lack of responsiveness to internal and external environment (ii) Absence of spontaneous breathing movements for 3 minutes, in the absence of hypocarbia and while breathing room air (iii) No muscular movements with generalized flaccidity and no evidence of postural activity or shivering (iv) Reflexes and responses: (a) Pupils fixed, dilated, and nonreactive to strong stimuli (b) Absence of corneal reflexes (c) Supraorbital or other pressure response absent (both pain response and decerebrate posturing) (d) Absence of snouting and sucking responses (e) No reflex response to upper and lower airway stimulation (f) No ocular response to ice water stimulation of inner ear (g) No superficial and deep tendon reflexes (h) No planter responses (v) Falling arterial pressure without support by drugs or other means (vi) Isoelectric EEG (in the absence of hypothermia, anaesthetic deaths and drug intoxication) recorded spontaneously and during auditory and tactile stimulation.

Further, it was added that these criteria shall have been present for at least 2 hours and two physicians other than the physician of a potential organ recipient should certify that death. As the protocol insists on a two-hour delay, this precludes the use of any organs for transplantation.

The concept of brain death goes back as far as 1959 when two French physicians **Mollret and Loudon** described a condition "*Coma depasse*" that is literally a state beyond coma. Again, the adhoc committee of Harvard Medical School revived it. The committee was constituted mainly after Bruce Tucker's case and incorporates surgeons, anaesthetists, forensic expert, legal personnel, philosophers etc. It was declared that it is futile to cling to the older concept, as heart and lungs could be maintained indefinitely. It was declared in fact that the brain was synonymous with the individual, and the death of the brain should be equated with the death of the individual.

Brain was considered superior to heart and lungs because: (i) Brain is the seat of consciousness and hence of the individuality of the person (ii) Brain cannot be kept on artificial support, making stoppage of its functioning irreversible (iii) Brain controls, integrates and coordinates the whole body system, making it master of the orchestra, so to say. Then it was necessary to formulate criteria, which would indicate brain death known as Harvard Report (1968).

Harvard Criteria

1. **Unreceptivity and unresponsivity:** Total unawareness to externally applied stimuli and inner need and complete unresponsiveness to even the most intense painful stimuli.
2. **No movements:** No spontaneous muscular movements in response to stimuli such as pain, touch, sound or light for a period of at least one hour.
3. **Apnoea:** Absence of spontaneous breathing for at least one hour and when patient is on ventilator, the total absence of spontaneous breathing may be established by turning off the respirator for 3 minutes and observing whether there is any effort on the part of the subject to breath spontaneously.
4. **Absence of elicitable reflexes:** Irreversible coma with abolition of central nervous system activity is evidenced in part by the absence of elicitable reflexes. The pupils are fixed and dilated and does not respond to a direct source of bright light. Ocular movement and blinking are absent. There is no evidence of postural activity. Corneal and pharyngeal reflexes are also absent. Stretch tendon reflexes also cannot be elicited.
5. **Isoelectric EEG:** Has confirmatory value.

All these tests should be repeated after 24 hours with no change. Further it is stressed that the patient be declared dead before any effort is made to take him off the ventilator if he is then on a ventilator. This declaration should not be delayed until he has been taken off the respirator and all artificially stimulated signs have ceased. By this time all over the world, it was agreed that brain death was indeed equivalent to individual death. However, they did not agree regarding the criteria fixed by Harvard school. There are three distinct school of diagnosing death: (i) French school that is similar to Harvard (ii) English school that is similar to Harvard (iii) Austro-German school that includes Harvard criteria and bilateral serial angiography of internal carotid and vertebral artery criteria. A negative angiogram for more than 15 minutes proves death.

Critical issues involving brainstem death: Since the brain contains 14 billion neurons, how many neurons should be dead to declare a person dead and should one wait until the last neuron is dead? It was argued that even if one neuron is alive that shows electrical activity you cannot pronounce a person dead. However, the argument that remained was that how much human one remains after loosing 90% of the brain's tissue. In addition, it was argued that since we do not know where the seat of consciousness lies, it is only reasonable to assume that some consciousness does remain even if a single neuron is left.

Then a new school emerged known as American school, led by Mohan Dass and Chou in 1971 that summarized the criteria of brain death at the University of Minnesota Health Services Center.

Minnesota Criteria (1971)

The criteria for brainstem death was formulated by **Mohan Dass and Chou** as follows: (i) Known but irreparable intracranial lesion (ii) No spontaneous movement (iii) Apnea when tested for a period of 4 minutes at a time (iv) Absence of brainstem reflexes: (a) Dilated and fixed pupil (b) Absent corneal reflexes (c) Absent Doll's head phenomenon (d) Absent ciliospinal reflexes (e) Absent gag reflex (f) Absent vestibular response to caloric stimulation (g) Absent tonic neck reflex (v) EEG not mandatory (vi) Spinal reflex not important (vii) All the findings above remain unchanged for at least 12 hours.

Brainstem death can be pronounced only if the pathological processes responsible for states (i) to (iv) above are deemed irreparable with presently available means.

The basic teaching of the American school was not the brain, but the brainstem death, after which there is the point of no return that should be equated as death. There were several reasons for this equation: (i) Medullary neurons are most resistant to anoxia, if they are dead then higher centers are also dead (ii) Brainstem is responsible for the vital functions because it is the seat of respiratory and circulatory center (iii) Brainstem is necessary for proper functioning of the cortex as all sensory and motor nerves pass through this gateway.

Immediately after an individual is put on respirator and other life support system, a systemic examination is done to exclude the possibility of brainstem death. If Minnesota criteria is fulfilled, life support systems should be withdrawn and the person is to be declared dead.

Brainstem Death and Organ Transplantation

For centuries, there has been a dread of being declared dead while still alive. However, it is only since 1959 that there have been conceptual and practical problems with the diagnosis of death following the description of "brain death". The ability to ventilate bodies who are brain dead in intensive therapy units preceded the developments of transplant surgery. The concept of brain death is not simply a convenience invented to satisfy the demands of transplant surgeons.

The diagnosis of death is traditionally made using the **triad of Bichat** that states that death is "the failure of the body as an integrated system associated with the irreversible loss of circulation; respiration and enervation". This is also known as somatic death or clinical death. Death is now accepted as synonymous with brainstem death. The brainstem is a small area of the brain that controls respiration and circulation. If this area is dead, the person will never be able to breathe spontaneously or regain consciousness.

Molecular death may be defined as "the death of individual organs and tissues of the body consequent upon the cessation of circulation". Different tissues die at different rates depending on their oxygen requirement. Thus, within four minutes ceasing of the blood supply to the brain, the central nervous system is irreversibly damaged.

Some authorities recognize a third concept of apparent death that is also known as a suspended animation. It may occur under certain specialised conditions for example drowning or hypothermia. Severe brain damage which does not involve the brainstem may result in a persistent vegetative state. These patients breathe spontaneously, open and close their eyes, swallow and make facial grimaces. However, they show no behavioural evidence of awareness. It is in these cases that the moral dilemma of "allowing some one to die" arises.

The above dilemma does not apply to those who are brainstem dead. These patients are dead irrefutably and unequivocally. Switching off a ventilator under these circumstances would not kill the patient but would discontinue ventilating a corpse.

In 1976 the Conference of the **Medical Royal Colleges and Faculties of the United Kingdom** issued guidelines on the subject of brainstem death. These guidelines are regularly updated and used by doctors in intensive care units throughout the UK.

Diagnosis of Brainstem Death

Exclusions: (i) Where the patient may be under the effects of drugs, e.g., therapeutic drugs or overdoses. (ii) Where the core temperature of the body is below 35°C (iii) Where the patient is suffering from severe metabolic or endocrine disturbances which may lead to severe but reversible coma, e.g., diabetes.

Preconditions of diagnosis: (i) Patient must be deeply comatose (ii) Patient must be maintained on a ventilator (iii) Cause of the coma must be known.

Personnel who should perform the tests: (i) Brainstem death tests must be performed by two medical practitioners (ii) Doctors involved should be experts in this field. Under no circumstances are brainstem death tests performed by transplant surgeons (iii) At least one of the doctors should be of consultant status. Junior doctors are not permitted to perform these tests (iv) Each doctor should perform the tests twice.

Tests to be performed: Before the tests are performed the core temperature of the body is taken to ensure that it is above 35°C. The diagnosis of brainstem death is established by testing the function of the cranial nerves which pass through the brainstem. If there is no response to these tests the brainstem is considered to be irreversibly dead: (i) Pupils are fixed in diameter and do not respond to changes in the intensity of light (ii) There is no corneal reflex (iii) Vestibulo-ocular reflexes are absent, i.e., no eye movement occurs after the instillation of cold water into the outer ears (iv) No motor responses within the cranial nerve distribution can be elicited by painful or other sensory stimuli, that is the patient does not grimace in response to a painful stimulus (v) There is no gag reflex to bronchial stimulation by a suction catheter passed down the trachea (vi) No respiratory movements occur when the patient is disconnected from the ventilator for long enough to ensure that the carbon dioxide concentration in the blood rises above the threshold for stimulating respiration, i.e., after giving the patient 100% oxygen for 5 minutes the ventilator is disconnected for up to 10 minutes. If no spontaneous breathing of any sort occurs within that 10 minutes the brainstem is incapable of reacting to the presence of the carbon dioxide and is thus dead.

When two doctors have performed these tests twice with negative results, the patient is pronounced dead and a death certificate can be issued. It is at this stage that a decision concerning the use of organs for transplantation purposes may be raised and the decision made as to the whether the corpse should be maintained on the ventilator until the organs may be harvested.

Organ Transplantation

Advances in medicine have enabled the use of several organs for transplant purposes. It is now possible to harvest from a cadaver the eyes, kidneys, liver, pancreas, small intestine, lungs and heart. From the living donor it is possible to transplant one kidney. The cornea of the eye may still be suitable for transplant up to 24 hours after death, other organs such as the heart, are very sensitive to low oxygen levels and deteriorate very quickly following the cessation of circulation. It is this, which has led to the controversy regarding the ventilation of corpses prior to harvesting of organs. To prevent premature declaration of death by the physician eager to obtain organs for his patients, due precautions have been incorporated in UK Human Tissue Act 1961 and in India, Anatomy Act 1984 and Human Organ Transplantation Act 1994 (Amendment in 2011, rules 2014) that covers transplantation of human organs and tissues.

The UK Human Tissue Act, 2004

The Key Points of this Act are:

- It regulates the removal, storage and use of human tissue. This is defined as material that has come from a human body and consists of, or includes, human cells.
- It creates a new offence of DNA 'theft'. It is unlawful to have human tissue with the intention of its DNA being analysed, without the consent of the person from whom the tissue came.
- It makes it lawful to take minimum steps to preserve the organs of a deceased person for use in transplantation while steps are taken to determine the wishes of the deceased, or, in the absence of their known wishes, obtaining consent from someone in a qualifying relationship.

Offences Under the Human Tissue Act, 2004

- Removing, storing or using human tissue for Scheduled Purposes without appropriate consent.
- Storing or using human tissue donated for a Scheduled Purpose for another purpose.
- Trafficking in human tissue for transplantation purposes.
- Carrying out licensable activities without holding a licence from the HTA (with lower penalties for related lesser offences such as failing to produce records or obstructing the HTA in carrying out its power or responsibilities).
- Having human tissue, including hair, nail and gametes (i.e., cells connected with sexual reproduction), with the intention

of its DNA being analysed without the consent of the person from whom the tissue came or of those close to them if they have died. (Medical diagnosis and treatment, criminal investigations, etc., are excluded).

The first four offences only apply in England, Wales and Northern Ireland, although the Human Tissue (Scotland) Act 2006 has similar offences and penalties. The offence of DNA theft applies UK-wide.

It also states that if a person, either in writing at any time or orally in the presence of two or more witnesses during his lifetime has expressed a request that his body or any specified part of his body might be used after his death for therapeutic purposes or for purposes of medical education or research, the person lawfully in possession of his body after his death may unless he has reason to believe that the request was subsequently withdrawn, authorize the removal from the body of any part or, as the case may be, the specified part; for use in accordance with the request. British Department of Health has issued cards for donors to carry, indicating their wish to donate organs, if they died.

This Act also provides for obtaining permission for postmortem examination when no medicolegal investigation is being carried out. The person who is legally in charge of the body such as hospital authorities may give permission for autopsy if they are satisfied after reasonable enquiry that there are no surviving close relatives and that the deceased had not objected to such an examination during his lifetime.

Memorandum of British Transplantation Society: British transplantation society has issued a memorandum that states that Human Tissues Act should be amended to clarify the legal aspects. The society has proposed 'Codes of Practice' for organ transplantation with salient features as: (i) Two doctors who are not members of the transplantation team should do the certification of the death of the donor and of the two one should be qualified for at least five years. (ii) As far as decision of switching off the respirator is concerned, it should entirely base on the decision of the treating physicians. This decision should have no connection with the requirements for transplantation. (iii) When it is decided to switch off the ventilator, the willingness for organ donation should be discussed with the relatives. (iv) Surgeon of the transplantation team should ensure that the death has already occurred and the deceased had requested for the donation during his lifetime and that the relatives now has no objection in removal of the organs for the purpose of transplantation. (v) In situations where relatives object to the decision of the deceased for removal of his organs for transplantation, their decision should be respected. (vi) In a medicolegal case, the coroner's permission should be obtained before removing the organs and the surgeon should report any matter of medicolegal significance to the authorities.

The Transplantation of Human Organs Act, 1994 India

An Act to provide for the regulation of removal, storage and transplantation of human organs and tissues for therapeutic purposes and for the prevention of commercial dealings in human organs and for matters connected there with or incidental thereto. This Act came into force on February 4, 1995. **The Amendment of the Act was done on September 2011 and rules were notified in 2014.** The Act amended to include tissues with the exception of blood. The principal Act renamed as **"The Transplantation of Human Organs and Tissues Act, 1994" (TOHOTA)**. It gave a legal recognition to brainstem death.

A. Important Definitions Mentioned in the Act

1. *Section 2 (d):* "**Brainstem death**" means the stage at which all functions of the brainstem have permanently and irreversibly ceased and is so certified under sub-section (6) of section 3.
2. *Section 2 (e):* "**Deceased person**" means a person in whom permanent disappearance of all evidence of life occurs, by reason of brainstem death or in a cardiopulmonary sense, at any time after live birth has taken place.
3. *Section 2 (f):* "**Donor**" means any person, not less than eighteen years of age, who voluntarily authorizes the removal of any of his human organs and tissues or both for therapeutic purposes under sub-section (1) or sub-section (2) of section 3.
4. *Section 2 (g):* "**Hospital**" includes a nursing home, clinic, medical centre, medical or teaching institution for therapeutic purposes and other like institution.
5. *Section 2 (h):* "**Human organ**" means any part of a human body consisting of a structured arrangement of tissues which, if wholly removed, cannot be replicated by the body.
6. *Section 2 (ha):* "**Human Organ Retrieval Centre**" means a hospital – (i) which has adequate facilities for treating seriously ill patients who can be potential donors of organs in the event of death; and (ii) which is registered under sub-section (1) of section 14 for retrieval of human organs.
7. *Section 2(hb):* "**Minor**" means a person who has not completed the age of eighteen years.
8. *Section 2 (i):* "**Near relative**" means spouse, son, daughter, father, mother, brother, sister, grandfather, grandmother, grandson or granddaughter. *The later four relationships were added in the 2011 amendment.*
9. *Section 2 (k):* "**Payment**" means payment in money or moneys worth but does not include any payment for defraying or reimbursing:
   (i) The cost of removing, transporting or preserving the human organ and tissue or both to be supplied; or
   (ii) Any expenses or loss of earnings incurred by a

person so far as reasonably and directly attributable to his supplying any human organ and tissue or both from his body.

10. *Section 2 (m):* "**Recipient**" means a person into whom any human organ and tissue or both is, or is proposed to be transplanted.
11. *Section 2 (o):* "**Therapeutic purposes**" means systematic treatment of any disease or the measures to improve health according to any particular method or modality.
12. *Section 2 (oa):* "**Tissue**" means a group of cells, except blood, performing a particular function in the human body. *Bone marrow as a tissue has been added in 2011 amendment.*
13. *Section 2(ob):* "**Tissue Bank**" means a facility registered under section 14A for carrying out any activity relating to the recovery, screening, testing, processing, storage and distribution of tissues, but does not include a Blood Bank.
14. *Section 2 (p):* "**Transplantation**" means the grafting of any human organ and tissue or both from any living person or deceased person to some other living person for therapeutic purposes.
15. *Section 2 (q):* "**Transplant co-ordinator**" means a person appointed by the hospital for coordinating all matters relating to removal or transplantation of human organs or tissues or both and for assisting the authority for removal of human organs in accordance with the provisions of section 3. The transplant coordinator shall be a doctor or senior nursing staff member having a good communication and independent of transplant team.

B. Regulatory Bodies

1. **Authorization Committee (Sec. 9(4)** shall be constituted at state level or hospital level and approval of this committee is required before removing or transplanting human organ or tissue or both. The members of the committee at state level are (i) Chairperson–Medical practitioner officiating as Chief Medical Officer or any other equivalent post in the major government hospital of the district. (ii) Two senior registered medical practitioners chosen from such medical practitioners who are residing in the concerned state/district and who are not part of any transplant team. (iii) Secretary of health or director health or nominee. (iv) Two senior persons of high integrity, credibility and social standing (preferably one female) who may be doctors, lawyers, chartered accountants, judges, police personnel, etc.

   A hospital authorization committee can be constituted at a hospital which do >25 transplants per year (*As per amendment in 2011*).

2. **Appropriate Authority (Sec. 13):** The Centre and State shall appoint this committee whose functions are as follows: (i) To grant registration of hospitals for transplantation (ii) To inspect hospitals periodically for examination of the quality of transplantation (iii) To investigate if any complaint and take appropriate action. It has the powers of a civil court to summon any person, request documents, and issue search warrants.
3. **Advisory Committees (Sec. 13A, 2011 amendment):** The Central Government and the State Governments, shall constitute an Advisory Committee for a period of two years to aid and advise the Appropriate Authority to discharge its functions. The advisory committee shall consist of: (i) One administrative expert not below the rank of Secretary to the State Government, to be nominated as Chairperson of the Advisory Committee. (ii) Two medical experts having such qualifications as may be prescribed. (iii) One officer not below the rank of a Joint Director to represent the Ministry or Department of Health and Family Welfare, to be designated as Member-Secretary. (iv) Two eminent social workers of high social standing and integrity, one of whom shall be from amongst representatives of women's organisation. (v) One legal expert who has held the position of an Additional District Judge or equivalent. (vi) One person to represent non-governmental organisations or associations which are working in the field of organ or tissue donations or human rights. (vii) One specialist in the field of human organ transplantation, provided he is not a member of the transplantation team.

C. Process of Organ/Tissue Donation for Transplantation

1. **Process for Living Donor Transplants**

   (a) *A living donor wants to donate organs or tissues after death*

   (i) A person above 18 years can authorize to donate his/her body organs or tissues for therapeutic purpose at any stage of life but parental consent is required in case of a minor. However, consent of next to kin is required after death to remove any organ or tissues for the purpose of transplantation.

   (ii) Such an authorisation must be made in writing, and in the presence of two or more witnesses (at least one of whom is a near relative of the donor). If this authorisation has been made, and has not been revoked at any point of time before the death of the potential donor, the person in possession of the body of the person is duty-bound to facilitate such donation (Sec. 3(2)). However, the consent of the near relative, or person in lawful possession of the body, is required before donation irrespective of whether the donor has authorised the donation of his/her organs or tissues.

(iii) If a potential donor is admitted to the Intensive Care Unit of any hospital, the registered medical practitioner (RMP) is under a duty, in consultation with transplantation coordinator, if available to ascertain whether the person has authorised the donation for organs or tissues (Sec.3(1A). The hospital shall proceed to obtain the documentation for such authorisation. If the potential donor has not authorised donation, the RMP must make the aware that person or near relative that there is an option to donate organs after death. If the person consents to donation, **Certification of brainstem death** shall be done by a board of medical experts upon his/her death. The Human Organ Retrieval Centre is then informed by the hospital (in writing) about the authorised donation for necessary action.

(iv) No human organ is to be removed from the body of a person in the event of his brainstem death unless such death is certified by **board of medical experts** (Sec. 3(6)) consisting of the following: (i) Registered medical practitioner/ in-charge of hospital. (ii) Independent registered medical practitioner, being a specialist, to be nominated by registered medical practitioner incharge of the hospital from the panel of names approved by appropriate authority. (iii) Registered medical practitioner treating the person whose brainstem death has occurred. (iv) A neurologist or a neurosurgeon to be nominated by the registered medical practitioner (i), from the panel of names approved by the appropriate authority.

In the event of the non-availability of a neurosurgeon/neurologist, a surgeon/physician and an anaesthetist/intensivist could be nominated from a panel already approved by the appropriate authority. Such surgeons/ physicians Anaesthetist/Intensivist shall, however, not associate with the removal of the organs from the donors or its transplantation into the recipients in any time before the members of the transplant team arrive (*amendment in 2011*).

(b) *Living donor wants to donate organs or tissues before death*

(i) **To a near relative:** The Act permits the transplantation of human organs and tissues if the donor and recipient are near relatives. Near relatives must seek approval from an Authorisation Committee before the organ can be transplanted.

(ii) **To a near relative who is a foreign national: (Section 9(1A)):** Where the donor or the recipient being near relative is a foreign national, prior approval of the Authorization Committee shall be required, before retrieving or transplanting the human organ or tissue or both. In case of foreign donors donating to their relatives in India, the transplantation is permitted only in near-related donors. Indian living donors wanting to donate to a foreigner other than near relative shall not be permitted.

(iii) **To a person who is not a near relative:** The person may donate their organs or tissues to any person who is not a near relative, only for reasons of affection or attachment towards the recipient or for any other 'special reasons'. This affection, attachment or 'special reason' must be demonstrated to an Authorization Committee, which will grant approval to the transplant if it is satisfied about the altruistic nature of the donation.

2. Process of Cadaver Transplants

(a) *The potential donor consented to donation before her death*

The RMP is duty-bound, in consultation with the transplant co-ordinator (if available) to find out from the near relatives of the donor whether he/she had at any time before her death authorised the removal of any of her organs or tissues after death.

D. **Special Circumstances**

(i) When any dead body is lying in the hospital or prison for more than 48 hours and not claimed by any of the near relatives (**Unclaimed body**), the management in-charge of the hospital or prison or any authorized employee of that hospital or prison in this behalf can permit for removal organ or tissues.

(ii) When **a postmortem examination is mandatory either for medicolegal or pathological purposes**, the doctor conducting such an examination can authorize for the removal of organs after satisfying himself that the organs to be removed are not required for such examination. The authorization for removal of organs is subject to no objection from the deceased before his death.

(iii) **Section 9(1C):** Human organs or tissues or both **shall not be removed from the body of mentally challenged person** before his death for the purpose of transplantation.

(iv) **Swap donations:** In near relatives**, organ donation by swapping** of donors between pairs of unmatched donor and recipient is permitted. It needs approval from authorization committee.

(v) **Special provision for removal of corneas:** Enucleation of corneas has been permitted by a trained technician.

E. **National, Regional, and State Registries and Networking (Sec. 13-C, D)**

The Central Government may establish a National Human Organs and Tissues Removal and Storage Network at one or more places and Regional Network. The Central Government shall maintain a national registry of the donors and recipients of human organs and tissues.

India now has transplantation and tissue organizations at a three-tier level. (i) **National Organ and Tissue Transplant Organization (NOTTO), located at Safdarjung Hospital at New Delhi** is the main central body for overall supervision. The website for NOTTO is www.notto.nic.in. (ii) Regional Organ and Tissue Transplant Organization (**ROTTO**) at regional level (at Chennai, Mumbai, Kolkata, Chandigarh and Guwahati) which coordinates transplantation related activities. (iii) State Organ and Tissue Transplantation Organization (**SOTTO)** which is responsible for coordinating activities at the state level.

F. **Registration of Hospitals and Tissue Banks (Sec. 14A)**

Registration is mandatory for the hospitals that are engaged in removal, storage and transplantation of human organs and tissue banks. For a hospital wanting to register for transplantation, an application for registration should be made to the appropriate authority as specified in Form 12 or Form 13 or Form 14 or Form 15, depending on organ, tissue, or eye bank, and the application is accompanied by fee as specified. Permission is valid for 5 years. In case, they violate any of the conditions specified in this Act, their registration is liable to be cancelled after proper inquiry.

G. **Penalties for Violations**

(i) Any person or hospital who are associated in the removal of any human organ without authority shall be liable to punishment with imprisonment for a term of 10 years and with fine which may extend to 20 lakh rupees but may extend to one crore rupees. (ii) If a registered medical practitioner is convicted for violating the conditions of this Act, his name would be removed from the medical register for a period of three years for first offence and permanently for subsequent offences.

ETHICAL ISSUES IN ORGAN DONATION

Both living organ donation and cadaveric donation raises several ethical concerns. The ethical issues related to organ and tissue procurement and transplantation are often discussed in light of such principles as autonomy, benevolence, non-maleficence, free and informed consent, respecting the dignity, integrity and equality of human beings, fairness and the common good.

(i) **Donor autonomy and consent:** *Autonomy* of a donor must be preserved, and the donor must be fully informed of potential short-term and long-term risks. The decision of organ donation should be made in an environment that is conducive to thoughtful decision making without undue influence or coercion.

From a living donor, a free and *informed consent* must be taken which is an ethical and legal requirement. Consent from relatives/legal guardian is required for the deceased donation. As per WHO, *explicit consent* is defined as a system in which cells, tissues or organs may be removed from a deceased person if the person had expressly consented to such removal during his or her lifetime. In some European countries, the practice of *presumed* (rather than expressed) *consent* is followed for organ procurement. Individuals are presumed to want to donate their organs upon brain death unless they have expressly objected to doing so.

(ii) **Religious, cultural and personal values:** Actually, no religion formally obliges one to donate or refuse organs. Most religion believes the human body is always a personal body, the body of a person, hence, the decision is left upto an individual's conscience and/or to their family. However, due to advancements of medical technology, many religious and moral dilemmas have impacted biomedical ethics.

(iii) **Risks and benefits:** Removal of an organ from a living donor is the only operation that is done specifically to help another person. The donor becomes a patient to benefit another person who is already a patient. So, living organ donation would seem to violate traditional first rule of medicine–*primer non nocere* (First, do no harm). Transplants between living persons raise the question whether it can ever be ethical to mutilate one living person to benefit another. This principle of non-maleficence is the most serious ethical problem in living donor transplants. Before deciding to donate organs, the living donor needs to have an accurate understanding of the risks and the potential benefits associated with the donation.

(iv) **Distributive justice:** The allocation of organs, cells and tissues should be guided by clinical criteria and ethical norms, not financial or other considerations. Priority should be given to those who have great need and who are expected to benefit greatly. Time on waiting list is also an important criterion and should be considered. While formulating policy of distribution of organs, social aspects such as social worth, social status, occupation, race, and so forth should not be considered. It should be equitable, justified and transparent.

(v) **Commercialization in organ donation:** As long as a shortage of organs remains, ethical issues are likely to persist. To fill the gap between the supply and demand organ, many a times, organ trafficking, transplant tourism, and commercialization occurs. There is a need to prevent commercialization of organs.

Certification of Death

The terms such as syncope, heart failure or cardiac failure should not be used on part 1 of the certificate. Most commonly, the physicians use the term cardio respiratory arrest that should not be used as everyone dies of stoppage of circulation and respiration. It is important to specify the underlying pathological cause of the cardiac or respiratory arrest. Similarly, the term 'coma' is quite unacceptable as it a clinical symptom and not underlying pathological entity. Also, the term 'asphyxia' should be avoided especially when it is not qualified by the underlying cause of death.

Some of the older textbooks give account of the various modes of death but these are irrelevant in legal medicine. These are:

Bishop's Classification of Modes of Death

Death occurs due to the stoppage of the functions of any of the three main organs (Bishop's tripod of life) namely heart, brain and lungs. Depending on the functions of these organs, the mode of death comprises: (i) *Syncope*: Failure of functions of heart with its circulatory system (ii) *Asphyxia*: It comprises failure of the respiratory system (iii) *Coma*: Failure of nervous system signifies mode of death as coma.

Bishop laid emphasis on the mode of death or the three proximate causes of death. This classification is useful to the law enforcing agencies and non-professionals for interpretation of medical evidence as to cause of death.

EUTHANASIA

The word euthanasia is derived from the Greek word '*Eu*' meaning good and '*thanatos*' meaning death. It means **'good death'** or to **'die well'**, with the basic theme of 'mercy killing'.

Euthanasia is the intentional killing by act or omission of a dependent human being for his or her alleged benefit. The key word here is "intentional". If death is not intended, it is not an act of euthanasia.

It may be defined as the doctrine or theory that in certain circumstances when owing to disease, senility or the like, a person's life has permanently ceased to be either agreeable or useful, the sufferer should be painlessly killed either by himself or by another. In the last decade, the use of **advanced directives or living wills** has become increasingly common. However, with these also problems can arise. All over the world and especially in North American continent, there is increasing support for euthanasia and its consequences. The medical profession finds itself caught in a conflict between the Hippocratic Oath and the question "whose life is it anyway?"

Euthanasia evolves the strong feelings in every one including doctors. It can be classified based on the acts of induction as active and passive and based on the will of the patient as voluntary, involuntary and non-voluntary euthanasia.

Active Euthanasia (Positive Euthanasia)

It is a positive merciful act, to end useless suffering or a meaningless existence. It is an **act of commission** that is when a doctor takes steps to end patient's life, e.g., giving large doses of drugs or giving a lethal injection to hasten death. It is also called **euthanasia by action.**

Passive Euthanasia (Negative Euthanasia)

It means discontinuing or not using extraordinary life sustaining measures to prolong life. It includes **acts of omission** such as failure to resuscitate terminally ill or hopelessly incapacitated patient or a severely defective infant. It is intentionally causing death by not providing necessary and ordinary (usual and customary) care or food and water. It implies not using measures that would probably delay death and permits natural death to occur. It is also called **euthanasia by omission.**

Voluntary euthanasia: When the person who is killed has requested to be killed with his consent.

Non-voluntary: When the person who is killed made no request to be killed such as in persons incapable of making their wishes like persons in irreversible coma.

Involuntary euthanasia: When the person who is killed made an expressed wish to the contrary.

Assisted suicide: Someone provides an individual with the information, guidance and means to take his or her own life with the intention that they will be used for this purpose. When it is a doctor, who helps another person to kill himself or herself it is called "physician assisted suicide".

What is not Euthanasia?

There is no euthanasia unless the death is intentionally caused by what was done or not done. Thus, some medical actions that are often labelled "passive euthanasia" are not a form of euthanasia, since the intention to take life is lacking. These acts include not commencing treatment that would not provide a benefit to the patient, withdrawing treatment that has been shown to be ineffective, too burdensome or is unwanted, and the giving of high doses of painkillers that may endanger life, when they have been shown to be necessary. All those are part of good medical practice, endorsed by law, when they are properly carried out.

Views on Euthanasia

There are both protagonist and antagonist views on euthanasia:

1. **Protagonist views:** It advocated euthanasia on the ground that the patient, if willing should be allowed to die a dignified death instead of prolonging the same through the torture of pain and disease. The protagonist plead that it is a tremendous economic and psychological burden on the patient's relatives to support an incurable patient and have often expressed death wishes for such a patient. They also argue that medical sciences too have its limitations and it cannot cure all the diseases.

2. **Antagonists views:** They claim that medical science has made such a rapid progress and its capabilities are so great that the disease, which seems incurable today, will become curable tomorrow. They remind the doctor of the Code of Medical Ethics and Hippocratic Oath by which the doctor swears to preserve the life and prevent further damage. They remind that euthanasia is against religion and that the crimes against society would increase and would amount to legalizing murder and suicide. If legalized euthanasia could be misused by doctors coming with hand in hand with relatives for material gains or otherwise. It may also encourage people to commit suicides.

History of Euthanasia

(i) About 400 B.C., Hippocratic Oath was given as "I will give no deadly medicine to any one if asked, nor suggest any such counsel". (ii) Swift, in his early 19th century treatise on the laws of Connecticut, stated, "If one counsels another to commit suicide, and the other by reason of the advice kills himself, the advisor is guilty of murder as principal." This was the well-established common law view, as was the similar principle that the consent of a homicide victim is wholly immaterial to the guilt of the person who caused his death. The right to life and to personal security is not only sacred in the estimation of the common law, but it is inalienable. Moreover, the prohibitions against assisting suicide never contained exceptions for those who were near death. Rather, the life of those to whom life had become a burden, of those who were hopelessly diseased or fatally wounded and even the lives of criminals condemned to death, were under the protection of law, equally as the lives of those who were in the full tide of life's enjoyment, and anxious to continue to live. Even the prisoner who persuaded another to commit suicide could be tried for murder, even though victim was scheduled shortly to be executed. (iii) The earliest American statute explicitly to outlaw assisting suicide was enacted in New York in 1828. (iv) Between 1857 and 1865, a New York commission led by Dudley Field drafted a criminal code that prohibited aiding a suicide and, specifically, furnishing another person with any deadly weapon or poisonous drug, knowing that such person intends to use such weapon or drug in taking his own life. (v) In 1920, the book "Permitting the Destruction of Life not Worthy of Life" was published. In this book, authors argued that patients who ask for "death assistance" should, under very carefully controlled conditions, be able to obtain it from a physician. This book helped support involuntary euthanasia by Nazi Germany. (vi) In 1935 the Euthanasia Society of England was formed to promote euthanasia. (vii) In October of 1939 amid the turmoil of the outbreak of war Hitler ordered widespread "mercy killing" of the sick and disabled. The Code named "Aktion T 4", was the Nazi euthanasia program to eliminate "life unworthy of life" and it at first focused on newborns and very young children. (viii) The Nazi euthanasia program quickly expanded to include older disabled children and adults. (ix) In 1973 in America, the Patient Bill of Rights was created that includes informed consent and the right to refuse treatment. (x) In Netherlands, Dr Gertrida Postma received life sentence for giving her dying mother a lethal injection. (xi) In 1980, Pope John Paul II issued declaration in euthanasia opposing mercy killing but permitted the use of painkillers to ease pain and the right to refuse life sustaining means. (xii) In California, the Hemlock Society founded by Derek Humphery advocated legal change and also distributed how to die information. Also, the campaign for assisted dying was launched in America. Right to die societies was also formed in Germany and Canada. (xiii) In 1984, the Netherlands Supreme Court approved voluntary euthanasia under certain conditions. (xiv) In 1990, in America, the Medical Association adopted the position that with informed consent, physician can withhold or withdraw treatment from a patient near death. The Hemlock of Oregon introduced the Death with Dignity Act. (xv) In 1995 Australia's Northern Territory approved a euthanasia bill. (xvi) The euthanasia bill went into effect in 1996 and was overturned by the Australian Parliament in 1997. (xvii) In 1997, the U.S. Supreme Court ruling in the **Washington vs. Glucksberg** was that "More specifically, for over 700 years, the Anglo American common law tradition has punished or otherwise disapproved of both suicide and assisting suicide". (xviii) In 1998 the U.S. State of Oregon legalized assisted suicide. In Switzerland the firm Dignitas was established to offer physician-aided suicide. (xix) In 1999 Dr. Jack Kevorkian **(Known as 'doctor death')** sentenced to a 10-25 years prison term for giving a lethal injection to Thomas Youk. (xx) In the year 2000 the Netherlands legalized euthanasia. (xxi) In 2002 Belgium legalized euthanasia.

Current Legal Scenario Around the World

Euthanasia is illegal in most countries. A few countries like Netherlands, Belgium and Luxembourg legalized active euthanasia. Physician-assisted dying is legalized in Canada. Physician-assisted suicide is legal in the state of Western Australia and state of Victoria, Australia. Similarly, countries like Switzerland, and Germany legalized assisted suicide with some conditions. In USA, practice of active euthanasia is illegal in all states. However, in USA state like Oregon, Washington, Vermont, Colorado, Montana, New Jersey, California, Hawaii and district of Columbia legalized assisted suicide.

Legal Status in India

Article 21 of the Constitution of India says that every individual has a right to live, as a natural right embodied in it. Recent Supreme Court judgment (*Gian Kaur v. State of Punjab*) has clarified further on that. It says that article 21 guarantees 'right to live' but doesn't in any way imply 'right to die' and hence extinction of natural life is illegal. As per this verdict suicide, assisted suicide or euthanasia are not permissible.

However, section 92 I.P.C. prevents euthanasia. Section 92 I.P.C. provides immunity to doctors for any act done in good faith for the benefit of a person without his consent. But under the first and second sub clause of this section, which states that this exception doesn't extend to the intentional causing of death, or attempting to cause death or for an act which is known to cause death. In effect it prohibits euthanasia.

Ms. Aruna Ramchandra Shanbaug Case

On 27 November, 1973, **Ms. Aruna Shanbaug** while working as Nurse in King Edward Memorial (KEM) Hospital, Mumbai, sexually assaulted and strangulated with a dog chain by a sweeper. Ligature strangulation caused hypoxic ischemic brain damage for which she remained in a persistent vegetative state. Her family abandoned her, however, the nurses at the KEM hospital continued to take care of her.

On 17 December, 2010, Pinki Virani, a social activist-cum-journalist made a plea in Supreme Court for permitting euthanasia of the victim. The Supreme Court sought a medical report of her health condition from the Government of Maharashtra. A three-member medical expert committee examined her and opined that she was in Permanent Vegetative state. **On 7th March 2011, the Supreme Court rejected the plea for active euthanasia, however permitted passive euthanasia under proper guidelines**. However, in its judgment, the Supreme Court declined to recognise Pinki Virani as the "next friend" of the victim instead treated the staff of KEM hospital as the "next Friend". The court laid down following guidelines for passive euthanasia. (i) A decision for discontinuation of life support has to be taken by the parents or spouse or other close relatives and in absence of any of them, a next friend or the doctor attending the patient. (ii) The decision should be taken in the best interest of the patient. (iii) The decision requires approval from High Court bench consists of at least two judges. (iv) Regarding the medical condition of the patient, a committee of three of doctors appointed by the High Court bench shall submit report. (v) At the time of decision, two witness shall be present and the document must be counter signed by a first-class judicial magistrate.

On 25 February 2014, a three-judge bench of Supreme Court observed that the 2011 judgment in Aruna Shanbaug case is flawed and based on a wrong interpretation of the Constitution bench judgment in *Gian Kaur v. State of Punjab case of 1996*. The court observed that euthanasia can be allowed only by legislature and referred the issue to a constitution bench. Aruna Shanbaug died on May 18, 2015 due to pneumonia after being in a coma for period of 42 years.

On 9 March, 2018, a five-member consituition bench of **Supreme Court** in the case of *Common Cause v. Union of India* (referred as Common *Cause* judgment) **legalized passive euthanasia also called Physician Assisted Suicide (PAS).** The petition was filed in Supreme Court in year 2005 by an NGO 'Common cause' seeking a direction for recognition of 'living will'. The Supreme Court also legalized a **'living will'** made by terminally-ill patients for passive euthanasia.

A **living will (synonym to advance directive)** also known as advance care directive or advance medical directive is a document prescribing a person's wishes regarding the medical treatment the person would want if he/she was unable to share his/her wishes with the health care provider. The Black's Law Dictionary defines an Advance Medical Directive as, a legal document explaining one's wishes about medical treatment if one becomes incompetent or unable to communicate.

The Supreme Court also laid down guidelines on who would execute the living will and how a nod for passive euthanasia would be granted by a medical board set up to determine and carry out any advance directive.

(a) **Procedure for Execution of the Advance Directive**

(i) The person must be an adult of sound mind and has complete understanding of the directive. (ii) The advance directive should also specify the name of a person who will be the authorised agent of the executor and will be responsible for medical decision in case the executor becomes incapable or incompetent of the same. (iii) The executor is required to sign the advance directive in presence of two, preferably independent, attesting witnesses. (iv) It must be countersigned by the jurisdictional Judicial Magistrate of First Class (JMFC). (v) The jurisdictional JMFC and both the witnesses shall then record their satisfaction regarding the fact of voluntary execution and absence of any form of coercion or inducement or compulsion and that the document was executed with complete understanding of all the relevant information and consequences. (vi) There shall be multiple copies of the advance directive including a digital copy and each of the hardcopy of the document will be kept in custody of JMFC. (vii) The JMFC shall inform regarding the advance directive to the immediate family members and a copy will also be entrusted to the treating physician.

(b) **Procedure for Implementation of the Advance Directive**

(i) The treating physician shall ascertain the genuineness and authenticity of the advance directive with the jurisdictional JMFC. (ii) The physician shall thereafter apprise the guardian/close relative or the executor about the nature and gravity of illness, forms of treatment available and the consequences of not seeking medical treatment. (iii) A Medical Board assembled by the hospital comprising the Head of the treating Department and three other experts from particular specialities shall visit the patient and in presence of close relative/guardian deliberate on whether to certify or not to certify enforcement of withdrawal or refusal of further medical treatment. (iv) This decision of the Board shall be referred to as a preliminary opinion which will be informed to the jurisdictional collector. (v) The collector thereafter will constitute another Medical Board comprising the Chief District Medical Officer of the district as the Chairman and three other expert doctors from the specialities specified in the judgment with practice of over 20 years. The doctors of this board should not have been members of the earlier Medical Board assembled by the hospital. This medical board shall then, depending on their opinion endorse the certificate to carry out the directions given in the living will. (vi) Before effectuating the advance directive, the Chairman of the Medical Board shall mandatorily communicate the jurisdictional JFMC. (vii) Then the JMFC shall also visit the patient and examine all relevant aspects, and after being satisfied he/she may authorise the implementation of the decision. (viii) **In case where the hospital medical board takes a decision not to follow an advance directive while treating a person**, then it shall make an application to the medical board constituted by the jurisdictional collector for consideration and appropriate action on the advance directive. (ix) **If permission to withdraw medical treatment is refused by the Medical Board constituted by the jurisdictional collector**, it would be open to the executor of the Advance Directive or his family members or even the treating doctor or the hospital staff to approach the High Court by way of writ petition under Article 226 of the Constitution.

In cases where there is no advance directive, the hospital medical board shall discuss with the family physician and the family members and record the minutes of the discussion in writing. During the discussion, the family members shall be apprised of the pros and cons of withdrawal or refusal of further medical treatment to the patient and if they give consent in writing, then the Hospital Medical Board may certify the course of action to be taken.

Revocation of advance directive: It can be revoked by the executor at any stage before it is acted upon and implemented. It is mandatory that the withdrawal or revocation of an advance directive must be in writing and the same procedure as provided for recording of advance directive shall be followed for revocation as well.

Difference Between Active and Passive Euthanasia

S. No.	Feature	Active Euthanasia	Passive Euthanasia
1.	Definition	Positive merciful act, to end useless suffering or a meaningless existence	Discontinuing or not using extraordinary life sustaining measures to prolong life
2.	Nature of Act	Act of commission	Act of omission
3.	Procedure	Giving large doses of drugs or giving a lethal injection to hasten death	Permitting to die by not resuscitating terminally ill or hopelessly incapacitated patient or a severely defective infant
4.	Legalized in countries	Netherlands, Belgium, Luxemburg	India, some USA states, Germany, Spain

Presumption of Survivorship

The presumption of survivorship is a legal concept that deals with legal rights following the deaths of two people where the evidence of the sequence of their deaths is unknown.

Assume that a husband and wife are killed in a single car accident. The beneficiaries of their wills are different. The order in which they died is crucial in determining who will be the eventual beneficiary. Since both died within short period of time, the postmortem examination cannot determine who died earlier and who later.

A general presumption that, when it is uncertain in what order two or more individuals have died, the order of death is to be determined by their age (the younger individual withstand better than the older, hence the younger shall be deemed to have survived the elder), gender (males are more resilient than females), physical status (strong and robust person can withstand better than weak, debilitated and diseased person), nature and severity of injuries (extent of haemorrhage and involvement of vital organs) etc.

Presumption of Death

An individual is presumed to be alive until they are announced dead. When there is absence of direct proof of death, such as the discovery of remains (e.g., a body or skeleton) attributable to that person, the death of that person can only be presumed. The issue of presumption of death arises in case of inheritance of property or succession of property of a person, insurance claim etc. when the individual is alleged to be dead and the body is not found.

In India, presumption of death is governed by sections 107 and 108 of the Indian Evidence Act, which allows for presumption of death for a person **missing for 7 years** to be raised in appropriate proceedings before the court.

Section 107 IEA. Burden of proving death of person known to have been alive within 30 years,–When the question is whether a man is alive or dead, and it is shown that he was alive within **30 years**, the burden of proving that he is dead is on the person who affirms it.

Section 108 IEA. Burden of proving that person is alive who has not been heard of for 7 years–the question is whether a man is alive or dead, and it is proved that he has not been heard of for **7 years** by those who would naturally have heard of him if he had been alive, the burden of proving that he is alive is the person who affirms it.

LONG QUESTIONS

1. Discuss the medicolegal aspects of thanatology.
2. Discuss in detail the moment of death with special reference to organ transplantation.
3. Define euthanasia. What are the various types? Discuss the legal status in India.

SHORT QUESTIONS

1. Brain death.
2. Brainstem death.
3. Suspended animation.
4. Harvard criteria.
5. The Human Organ Transplant Act 1994.
6. Euthanasia.

MULTIPLE CHOICE QUESTIONS

1. Thanatology is a science that deals with:

(a) Death in all its aspects
(b) Effects of electricity on body
(c) Hypothermia
(d) Identification

2. The pupils react to eserine after death for about:

(a) 30 minutes (b) 1 hour
(c) 2 hours (d) 3 hours

3. Suspended animation can be seen in following conditions *except:*

(a) During practice of yoga (b) Barbiturate poisoning
(c) Drowning (d) Brain haemorrhage

4. As per Transplantation of Human Organs (Amendment) Act 2011 following can be signatory of the brainstem death certificate *except:*

(a) Registered medical practitioner in-charge of hospital
(b) Neurologist
(c) Treating registered medical practitioner
(d) Pathologist

5. As per the provisions in Transplantation of Human Organs and Tissues (Amendment) Act 2011, Rules 2014, following are true *except:*

(a) Blood is not included as tissue
(b) Bone marrow as a tissue has been added
(c) In near relatives, swapping donation is permitted
(d) Retrieval of eyes/cornea only in hospital settings

6. Active euthanasia is legalized in all countries *except:*

(a) Netherland (b) Luxembourg
(c) Belgium (d) France

7. Which is legalized in India?

(a) Passive euthanasia
(b) Active euthanasia
(c) Involuntary euthanasia
(d) Non-voluntary euthanasia

ANSWER KEY ☞

1. (a)	2. (b)	3. (d)	4. (d)	5. (d)	6. (d)	7. (a)

5 CHAPTER

Identification

Identification means to determine the individuality of a person. Identity can be established by recognizing the physical characteristics. When the person is known by his name with complete address, it is known as **complete identification.** However, in certain circumstances only other details like age, sex etc. can be established that is known as **partial identification.**

The question of identification in living persons arises in criminal cases like assault, murder, rape etc. and even in new-born cases when babies get interchanged in hospitals. In civil cases like marriage, inheritance, insurance and disputed sex etc. identification plays an important role. In the dead especially unknown medicolegal cases, police play an important role in the matter of identification. Police official has to investigate the case and advertise the details including identifying features of the unknown person in the newspapers and media etc. For this purpose, he has to take photographs and fingerprints. He has to find out the relatives who identify the person before conduction of medicolegal postmortem. Sometimes, the identification becomes very difficult if the body is destroyed or mutilated in fires, explosions and other mass disasters. In such cases various other parameters of identification can be established from the fragmentary or mutilated remains.

CORPUS DELICTI

Corpus delicti refers to the body of the criminal offence, which is an essential part of the crime. It not only includes the body of the victim but also the weapon of offence, clothing, drawings and photographs of the deceased. The main purpose of corpus delicti is to establish the identity of the person. However, the Court has passed death penalty even though the body has not been recovered and identification not being established.

The following points are taken into consideration for the purpose of identification in a dead person: (i) Age (ii) Sex (iii) Religion (iv) Complexion (v) General development including stature (vi) Anthropometric measurements (vii) Fingerprints and footprints (viii) Superimposition (ix) Teeth (x) DNA fingerprinting; and (xi) Personal belongings. Features to be examined for identification known as biometric profiling are given in Figure 5.1.

In cases of living person in addition to the above features the following criteria are taken into consideration: (i) Speech and voice (ii) Handwriting (iii) Gait (iv) Habits (v) Memory (vi) Education.

While establishing identification, it is advisable to use maximum number of criteria.

There are methods available by which to establish positive undeniable identification that are: (i) Fingerprints, footprints, handprints and lip prints (ii) Dental patterns (iii) Frontal sinus pattern (iv) Skull suture patterns and vascular grooves (v) Normal and abnormal bone comparisons (vi) Other fortuitous comparisons.

AGE

To establish the identity of an individual, estimation of age is to be done. It depends on:

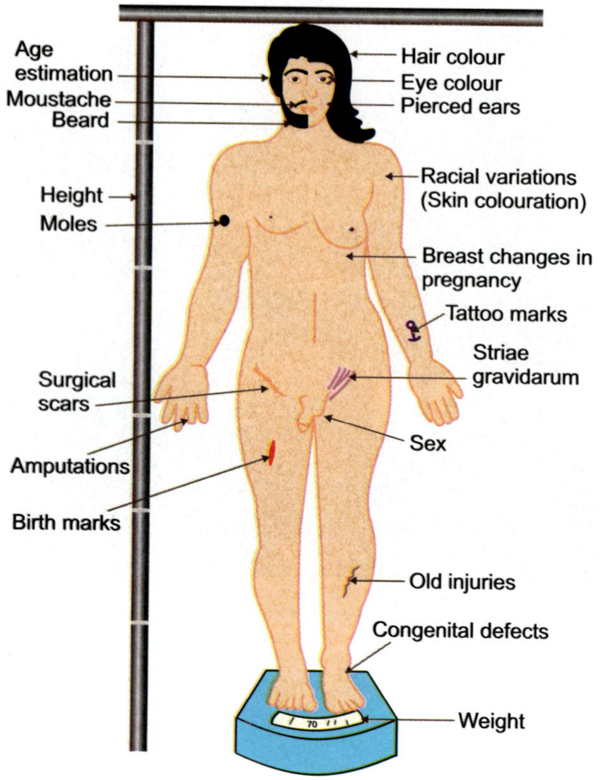

Figure 5.1: Biometric profiling: Features to be examined for identification

Physical or Morphological Features

Physical feature includes height and weight of the person. Starting from the intrauterine life up to certain periods of extrauterine life, height and weight of the individual has some relationship with the age.

Determination of intrauterine age: Intrauterine age of the foetus can be calculated using the Hasse's rule and Morrison's rule.

Rule of Hasse (1895): According to this rule the age of the foetus is calculated by the square root of the crown heel length in centimeters. For example, if the crown heel length is 16 cm, the age of the foetus is about 4 weeks intrauterine life.

Rule of Morrison (1964): This rule states that the crown heel length of the foetus in centimeters, divided by five gives the age in months. For example, if the length is 40 cm, the age is 8 months. It is applicable after 5 months of intrauterine life.

Intrauterine age is that period starting from time of conception till delivery. The various terms used for describing products of conception are: (i) *Ovum:* From fertilization till second week of gestation. (ii) *Embryo:* From second week of gestation till third month of intrauterine life. (iii) *Fetus:* From third month of gestation till full term.

The age of the fetus can be determined by some of the features as given in Table 5.1 and Figures 5.3 to 5.6.

Ossification centers: (i) *Lower end of femur (Figure 5.2) and upper end of tibia:* The knee joint is flexed and a transverse incision is made into the joint starting from lower end of femur till upper end of tibia. The incisions are given parallelly and continued until the largest part of ossification center. The center appears as brownish red surrounded by bluish white cartilage. The sections can be continued till the diaphyseal center. The diameter of center is 2-5 mm at 37-38 weeks, increasing to 6-8 mm in full term fetus. (ii) *Centers of foot:* These can be shown by making an incision between the web of third and fourth toes, when the foot is grasped behind the heel. The incisions are extended backwards through the sole of foot and heel.

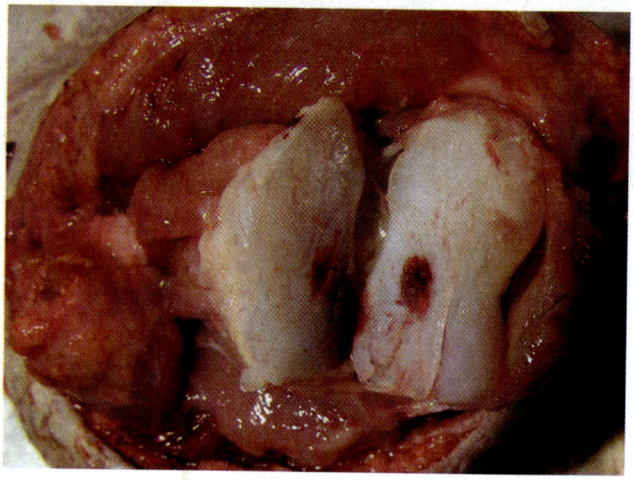

Figure 5.2: Ossification center lower end of femur

Determination of extrauterine age: A full term foetus is 19-20 inches (50 cm) in length and 6-7 pounds by weight. At six months of age, it is 24 inches (60 cm) and by one year of life it is 27 inches (68 cm) in length. At the age of four years, the child becomes 40 inches (100 cm) in length. Weight has little relation with the age of the person. The weight of the infant increases one pound every month until five months of age when it doubles and **trebles by a year**.

Development of Secondary Sexual Characteristics

1. **Growth of hair:** The appearance and growth of hair in males and females vary with the attainment of maturity.

Appearance/graying of hair	Males (Years)	Female (Years)
Pubic hair	14-15	13-14
Axillary hair	15-16	14-15
Beard and moustache	16-17	Absent
Other body parts	17-20	Absent
Graying of scalp hair	40	40
Graying of pubic hair	55	55
Balding	45	Less common

Table 5.1: Intrauterine feature of foetus				
Age (Months)	**Length (cms)**	**Weight**	**Ossification Centers**	**Features**
1	1	2.5 gms	Clavicle	Eyes as two dark spots, Mouth as cleft; beginning of formation of limbs
2	4	10 gms	Long bone shafts	Anus as dark spots; Placenta forms, human appearance demarcated from the limbs, mouth and nose; Feet and hands webbed
3	9	30 gms	1st, 2nd, 3rd sacral vertebras	Pupillary membrane appears; neck and palate forms; placenta fully developed, heart 4 chambered. Alimentary canal is situated in the abdominal cavity; sex bud appears. Limbs, finger and toes well developed but nails remain as membranes
4	16	120 gms	Lower segments of sacrum	Sex can be differentiated; skin covered with fine downy lanugo hair; Ear ossicles are ossified; Skull bones are partly ossified; Brain convolutions begin to develop. Gall-bladder is formed and meconium is found in duodenum
5	25	400 gms	Calcaneum and ischium	Light hairs over scalp, downy hair whole body; Meconium beginning of large intestine. Nails distinct and soft. Skin covered with vernix caseosa. The germs of permanent teeth are present in jaw
6	30	800 gms	Manubrium sterni	Eyelashes and eyebrows appear; Testes close to kidneys. Skin red and wrinkled. Gall-bladder contains bile and meconium present in upper part of large intestine which starts showing sacculation. Cerebral hemispheres cover the cerebellum
7	35	0.9-1.2 kg	Talus	Nails thick; Pupillary membrane disappears; Eyelids open; Meconium in whole of large intestine; Testis at external inguinal ring. Placenta 350-400 gms; Bile in gallbladder; Caecum in right iliac fossa
8	40	1.5-2 kg	–	Left testis in scrotum. Scalp hair thick, skin rosy red and covered with soft lanugo hair except for the face. Nails reach tips of fingers, but not tips of toes. Meconium reaches the rectum. Cerebral convolutions well developed
9	45	2.5-3 kg	Lower end of femur	Posterior fontanelle is closed; Scalp hair are 4 cm long, thick and dark both testis in scrotum. Downy hairs disappear on the body except on the shoulders. Vernix caseosa found in the joint flexures. Scrotum shows wrinkling. Nails grow beyond tips of fingers but only tip of toes
10	50-53 (CR length 30-33 cm)	2.5-5 kg	Upper end of tibia, cuboid	Scalp hair 3-5 cm long, dark. Male 100 gms more than female. Head circumference 33 cms; Anterior fontanelle 4 × 2.5 cm wide. Posterior fontanelle closed. Face not wrinkled; lanugo hairs absent except on the shoulders. Cartilages formed in nose and ear. Umbilicus situated between pubis and xiphisternum. Scrotum contains testicles; vulva closed and labia majora cover labia minora and clitoris. Meconium in rectum

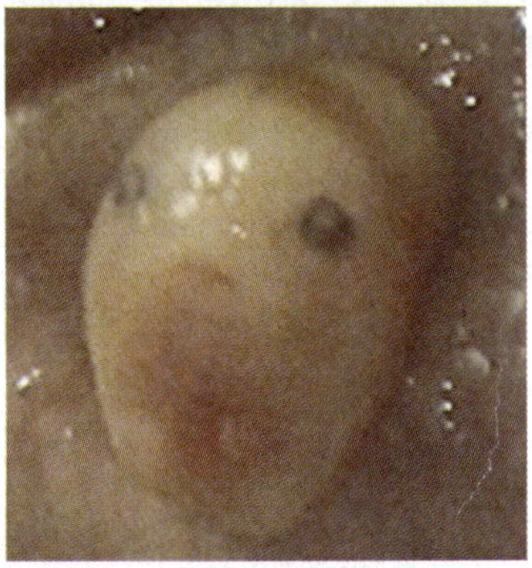

Figure 5.3: Foetus with formation of eyes, mouth as cleft (Age one month I.U.L.)

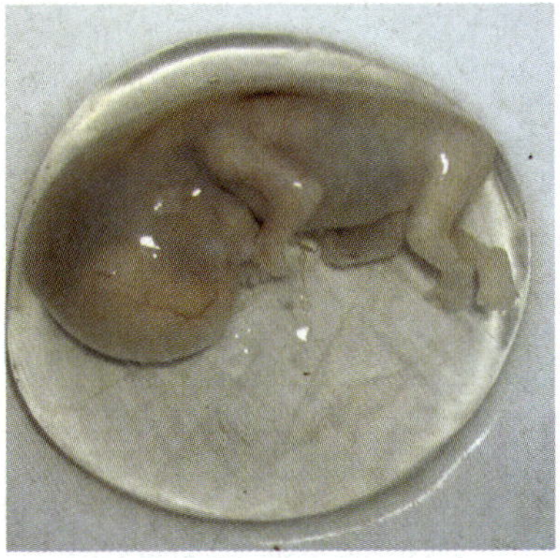

Figure 5.4: Foetus 2-3 months I.U.L. inside the amniotic sac with neck formation

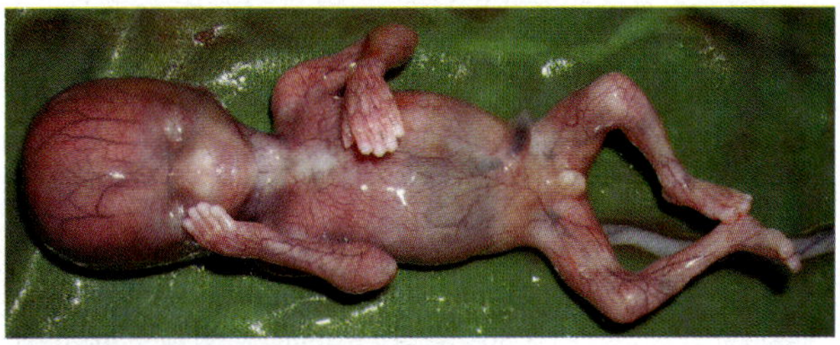

Figure 5.5: Foetus of age 4 months I.U.L. showing appearance of sex

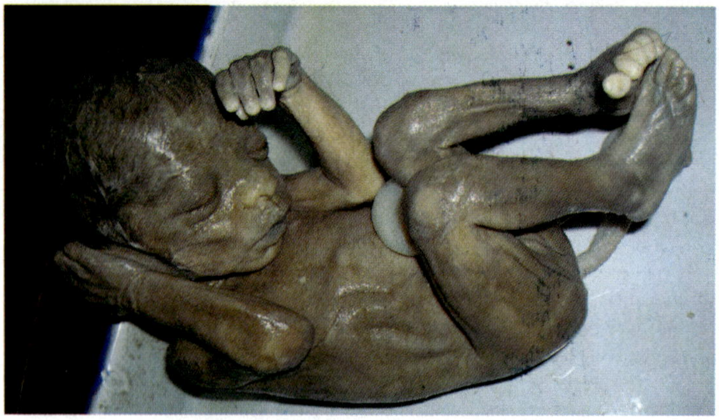

Figure 5.6: Foetus 7-8 months I.U.L.

Hair start developing in the following stages in males and females over genitalia (after Tanner) (Table 5.2).

2. **Development of breasts in girls:** Stages of growth of breast depending on the nutrition and sexual practices at an early age are depicted as under:

Development of breast	Age (years)
• Breast and papillae are elevated as a small mound and there is enlargement of areolar diameter	11-12
• More elevation of breast and papillae and enlargement of areolar diameter	13
• Areola and papillae project over the level of breast	14
• Only papillae project over the level of breast	15
• Only papillae projects over the surface and areola merges with the breast	15-16

Other Physical Features

(i) Hoarseness (deepening) of voice occurs in males by 15-17 years (ii) Adam's apple is more prominent in males by 16-18 years (iii) Stature starts decreasing after 25 years of age at the rate of 1 mm per year (iv) Arcus senilis is the circular opacity at the limbus of cornea that develops by 40 years (v) Females achieve menopause by 40-45 years (vi) Cataract never occurs in the eyes before 55 years except when the precipitating factors cause it early (vii) Creased or wrinkled appearance of skin develops after 55 years (viii) Partial deafness could develop after 65 years of age.

Laboratory Tests

(i) Absence of nucleated RBCs in the peripheral blood occurs by 24 hours after birth.

(ii) Fall of reticulocyte count (2%) in the peripheral blood by 10 days after birth.

(iii) Replacement of foetal hemoglobin by adult hemoglobin is completed by 6 months to two years of age.

(iv) **Molecular Methods:**

A. ***DNA-based methods:*** It includes telomere shortening, mitochondrial DNA deletions, circular excision of T cell receptors or signal-joint-T cell receptor excision circles (sjTRECs) and DNA methylation. However, the use of these techniques in real cases has been limited for several reasons, including the role of environmental effects and disease effects, the low methodological accuracy, and tissue and gender specific variations.

(a) *Telomere shortening:* The end parts of the chromosomes are called telomeres with repetitive (TTAGGG) n sequences. It plays an important role in protecting the DNA and keeping it stable. Human telomeres shorten in an age-dependent manner. **Ren *et al.*** (2009) studied telomere length in peripheral blood leukocytes (PBLs) of Tibetan population. The formula for age estimation according to telomere shortening was Y = -16.539X + 236.287 (Y: age, year; X: mean TRF length in kb). However, the mean telomeric restriction fragment (TRF) length in males shorter than females.

(b) *Mitochondrial DNA deletions (mtDNA deletions):* Oxidative stress causes damage to mitochondrial DNA (mtDNA) so that mtDNA deletions accumulate. The rationale for this method is that increasing number of mtDNA deletions observed with age. The most frequently reported mtDNA deletion associated with ageing is a 4977-bp deletion (mtDNA-4977) which is used for predicting age. However, age range that can be estimated is very wide, which is accurate for ages under 20 years and above 70 years. There is also heterogeneity of mitochondrial deletions in different tissues.

(c) *Circular excision of T-cell receptors or signal-joint-T-cell receptor circles (sjTRECs):* T-lymphocytes carry specific receptors called T-cell receptors (TCR). During the process of growth in human, the TCR experiences intervention and it can be lost or circulated again to become episomal DNA. The missing or circulating TCR is then referred to as the signal-joint-T-cell receptor excision circles or sjTRECs. The sjTRECs levels decline with age, and negative correlations between sjTREC levels and age have been demonstrated which is the basis of age estimation.

Table 5.2: Tanner's stages of growth of pubic hair

Stages	Growth of hair	Age
Stage 1	Prepubertal no pubic hair, fine brown vellus hair	Less than 12 years
Stage 2	Sparse not extending on to mons pubis, light pigmented at the base of penis	12-13 years
Stage 3	Darker, coarse extending on to mons pubis, pigmented and start curling and spreading	13-14 years
Stage 4	Covering most parts but not going up to thighs	14-15 years
Stage 5	Dense hair extending to the inner thighs and dark mature pubic hair	More than 15 years

(d) *DNA methylation:* Aging leads to epigenetic alterations, including changes in DNA methylation, through both multiple distinct and intersecting age-related mechanisms. Many age estimation methods based on DNA methylation biomarkers, using several biological fluids, such as blood, blood stains, saliva, semen stains, etc. are developed. **Maulani *et al.*** (2020) revealed The MAD (mean absolute deviation) of the estimated age from DNA methylation was about 3 to 5 years, which was better than other methods such as those based on telomere length or signal-joint T-cell receptor excision circles. The ELOVL2 gene was a commonly used DNA methylation marker in age estimation.

B. ***Protein-based methods:*** It includes advanced glycation end products (AGEs) and aspartic acid racemization (AAR).

(a) *Advanced glycation end products (AGEs):* AGEs (e.g., pentosidine, N-carboxymethyllysine (CML), pyralline and furosine) are collection of heterogeneous end products that produced from the protein glycation process. With increasing age, these products are accumulated in various body tissues. AGEs can be analysed using calorimeters or spectrophotometers which changes from yellow to brown. This colour change is used as a marker of age estimation, however, there is no standard procedure for testing AGEs. This method has limited use for predicting age and only accurate for identification of age above 45 years.

(b) *Aspartic acid racemization (AAR):* This method was first described in 1975 by Helfman and Bada. Aspartic acid exists both in D and L forms. During ageing process, L-amino acid are transformed into D-amino acid by racemization, which gradually accumulates in tissues. D-aspartic acid increases correspondingly with age in dentin of human teeth. For prediction of age, the aspartic acid-based technique is quite accurate within an error rate of ± 3 years.

(v) **Radiocarbon Analysis:**

The ^{14}C content in the human body reflects the ^{14}C content of atmospheric CO_2 at the time. The rationale of the method is to determine the year of tooth formation based on levels of radiocarbon present in tooth enamel.

Dental Study

The approximate age of the individual can be determined from the examination of teeth in both the jaws. After birth and during developing years, the close estimation of age can be made by the presence of deciduous dentition and its stages of eruption, the period of mixed dentition, stages of eruption of permanent teeth and loss of deciduous teeth. There are twenty temporary teeth and thirty-two permanent teeth in human jaw. The deciduous and permanent teeth erupt earlier in the lower jaw except the lateral incisors that erupt earlier in the upper jaw. The teeth erupt about a year earlier in the females.

The permanent molar erupts first in the lower and on the left side and then on the right side. The eruption of tooth depends on the hereditary, environmental, nutritional and endocrinal factors. There are 32 permanent teeth comprising four incisors, two canines, four premolars and six molars in each of the jaw. The temporary teeth are twenty in number comprising four incisors, two canines, and four molars in each jaw. At 6-7 years of life, first permanent molars erupt behind the second temporary molars. The premolars replace the temporary molars. The amount of wearing in the premolars and molars gives some indication of age after complete dentition. Root formation occurs after completion of the crown and as the root becomes longer, the crown erupts through the bone and finally comes out of the jaws. The tooth calcifies from crown to neck to roots. When permanent tooth erupts, the overlying root of its deciduous predecessor undergoes resorption until only the crown remains that falls off. By assessing the stage of eruption of teeth and extent of completion of calcification of root fairly accurate estimate of age of the individual can be made. In old age, either the tooth falls off decayed or the crown is worn away to the sockets.

Dental Anatomy (Figure 5.7): The development of tooth begins with the formation of cellular tooth germ within the alveolar bone in the shape of the crown. The tooth has a crown, neck and root that are embedded in the jaw. There are certain differences in the appearance of deciduous and permanent teeth (Table 5.3).

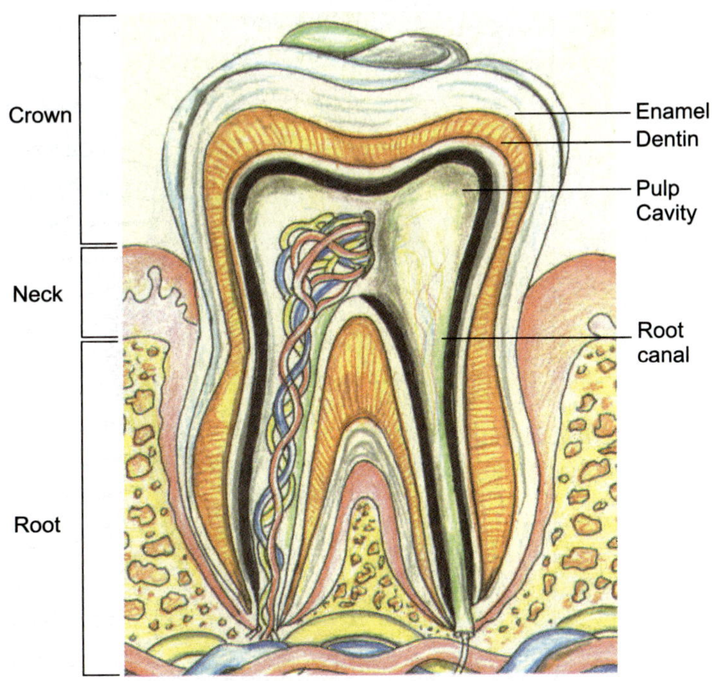

Figure 5.7: Different parts of tooth

Table 5.3: Differences between primary and secondary dentition		
Features	**Temporary teeth**	**Permanent teeth**
Size and weight	Smaller and lighter	Larger and heavier
Colour	China white	Ivory white
Incisors	Vertical	Projected forwards
Neck	More constricted	Less constricted
Presence of ridge	Between neck and body	No ridge
Root of molars	Smaller and more divergent	Longer and less divergent
Replacement by	Permanent teeth	Not replaced
Total number	Twenty	Thirty two
Types	No premolars, 8 molars	8 premolars and 12 molars

Incisors: The incisors have chisel shaped crown that is convex on labial surface and concave on lingual surface, with a constricted neck and has single root. They have chewing surface and cutting edge.

Canines: The canines are larger compared to the incisors, the crown is conical shaped that is concave on its labial surface but slightly concave on its lingual surface. The masticatory edges tapers and projects beyond the level of other teeth. It has a single root and have single cusp.

Premolars: The premolars are also known as bicuspids. They are smaller and shorter than the canines and the crown is circular. The chewing surface is bicuspid with a groove between them. They have a single root but may have double root in some of the races.

Molars: The molars are the largest of the entire tooth, the crown is cubical that is convex on its lingual and labial surface. In upper jaw, first molar has stable configuration with 4 cusps, second molar is very different individually with 3 cusps and third molar is less mineralized than others and may have chalky spots. Also, upper molar has three roots. In lower jaw, first molar has got 5 cusps, 3 buccally and 2 lingually whereas second and third molars have 4 cusps each.

Determination of Age from Dentition in Children

At birth, the rudiments of all temporary teeth and first permanent molars are there. In children and young persons, the chronological calcification and eruption of teeth gives their ages.

The age of appearance of the permanent and secondary dentition is as given in Table 5.4 and Figure 5.8.

Table 5.4: Age of appearance of deciduous and permanent teeth		
Type of teeth	**Age of eruption of temporary teeth**	**Age of appearance of permanent teeth**
Lower central incisor	5-6 months	7-8 years
Upper central incisor	6-7 months	7-8 years
Upper lateral incisor	7-8 months	8-9 years
Lower lateral incisor	8-9 months	8-9 months
Canines	1½ years	11-12 years
First premolar	Absent	9-10 years
Second premolar	Absent	10-11 years
First molar	1 year	6-7 years
Second molar	20-30 months	12-14 years
Third molar	Absent	17-25 years

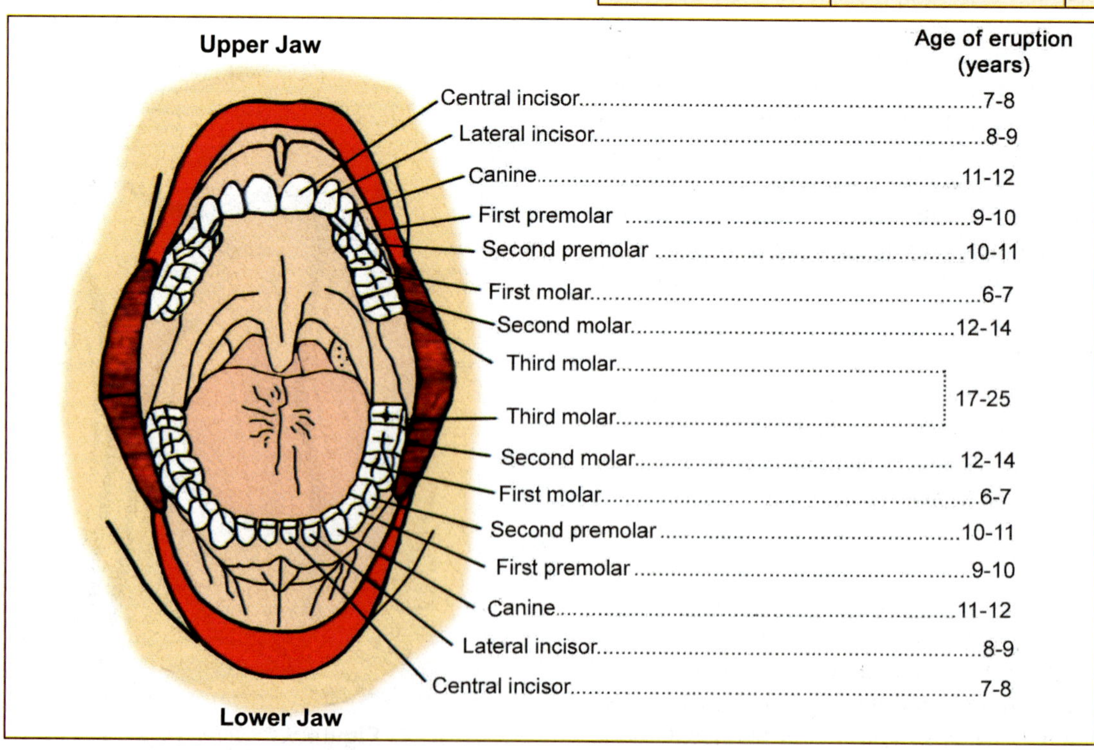

Figure 5.8: Age of eruption of permanent teeth

Wisdom tooth: The third molar is also known as the wisdom tooth. During the age of 14-25 years, the stage of development of third molar is of particular importance to determine the age. The lateral oblique X-ray of maxilla and mandible will show the development of third molar and root completion of second molar. Orthopantomogram also helps to know the status of eruption of third molar. The body of jaw grows posteriorly and the ramus is elongated after eruption of second molar and a space is created for third molar. The third molar erupts between 17-25 years of age.

Spacing of the jaw: When the second molar erupts, the ramus of the mandible grows behind and the body of the jaw also increases in length for the eruption of third molar teeth. The eruption of third molar is quite irregular as it can erupt within 17-25 years. The space for third molar should be examined for its hardness, if present whenever dental examination is being carried out. It is to be noted whether the space is half formed or fully formed by inserting the finger beyond the second molar.

Mixed dentition: Mixed dentition is the period when both the temporary and permanent teeth are present in the jaw. It is the period starting from 6th year of life when the first molar erupts and till the canine falls that is up to 11 years.

Successional teeth: These are ten in each jaw. The permanent teeth replace the temporary ones except the permanent premolars that erupt in place of deciduous molars.

Superadded teeth: These do not have deciduous predecessors and erupt behind the temporary teeth. All permanent molars are superadded as the first permanent molar erupts while other deciduous teeth are present.

Impacted teeth: In some individual, third molar never erupts in oral cavity as the jaw space is inadequate. This is seen particularly in mandibular third molar that remains trapped and are called impacted teeth.

There are a particular number of teeth in different ages in children (Table 5.5).

Table 5.5: Number of teeth in different ages

No. of teeth	Type of teeth	Age (Years)
20	Temporary	5
21-24*	Mixed	6
24**	Mixed	7-11
24-28***	Permanent	12-14
28****	Permanent	14-17
32*****	Permanent	17-25
32	Permanent	> 17

* Due to eruption of first permanent molar.
** Due to eruption of other permanent teeth replacing the temporary ones.
*** Due to eruption of second molar.
**** There is no eruption of third molar but space may be present.
***** Due to eruption of last permanent molar or wisdom tooth.

Boyde's formula: Boyde in 1963 suggested a method for determining the age up to a few months after birth from structural features of the enamel. The so-called cross striations of the enamel prism are thought to be daily increments of growth. In this formula, the numbers of cross striations formed from birth when a particularly prominent incremental line, the **neonatal line** is formed until death is counted.

Stacks' method: It is a method of age determination in fetuses and infants between 5 months in utero and postnatal age of 7 months which is based on the weight of the erupting teeth.

Determination of Age from Dentition in Adults and Older Age

Age changes in mandible: In the mandible the center of ossification of jaw appears at second month of intrauterine life and symphysis menti fuses by 18-20 years. The changes in mandible with age are given in Table 5.6 and Figure 5.9.

Table 5.6: Age changes in mandible

Features	Infancy	Adult	Old age
Angle formed by ramus with body	Obtuse	Right angle	Obtuse
Body	Shallow and small	Thin and elongated	Shallow and big
Ramus	Short and oblique	Stunted	Long and oblique
Condylar process	At lower level than coronoid process	Above the level of coronoid process	Neck of condylar process is bent backwards
Mental foramen	Placed near to the lower border of ramus and mandible	Midway between upper and lower border	Near the alveolar margin

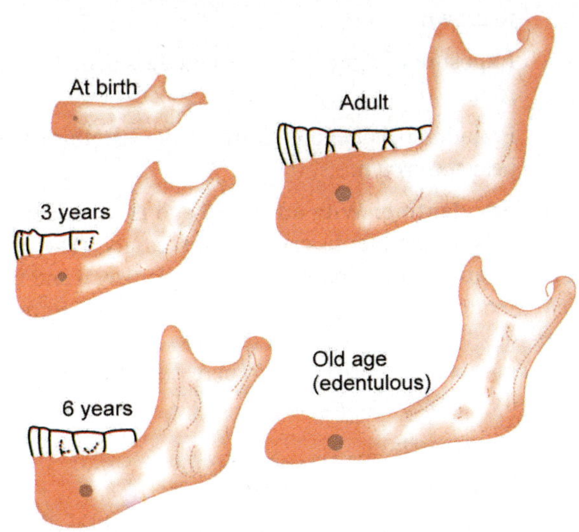

Figure 5.9: Appearance of mandible at different ages

When eruption has ended and the person has achieved adult dentition, it is necessary to apply other methods that occur due to the normal wear and tear and age of the person.

Gustafson's method: This method is used for estimation of age in the adults by studying the progressive changes in an individual tooth. Pathological conditions can alter each of the factors separately (Figure 5.10).

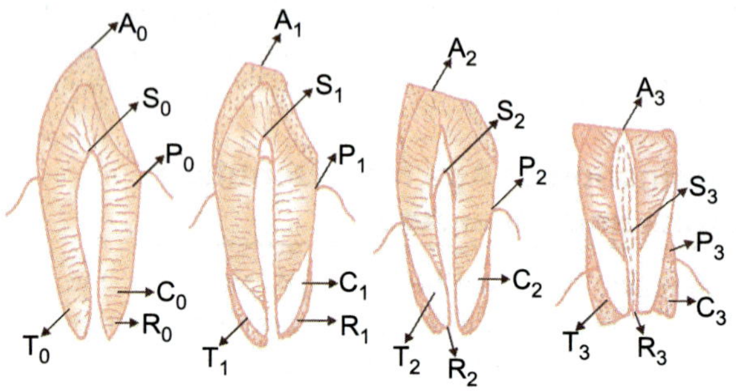

Figure 5.10: Gustafson's method

i. **Attrition:** It is wearing and tearing on the opposing mastication surface of the teeth of the upper and lower gums due to continuous friction. The four degrees of attrition are:

   A_0— No attrition.

   A_1— Attrition within enamel.

   A_2— Attrition within dentine.

   A_3— Attrition exposes to soft pulp.

ii. **Periodontosis:** When the maintenance of teeth and gums is bad, there is regression of gums and periodontal tissue. There is loosening of the teeth, exposure of length of root and deposition of stony hard debris over a long period. According to the length of exposure of root, the periodontosis is of following degrees:

   P_0— No Periodontosis or no root exposure.

   P_1— Exposure of less than 1/3rd of the part of the root next to crown.

   P_2— Exposure of more than 1/3rd but less than 2/3rd of the root.

   P_3— Periodontosis beyond 2/3rd of the length of the root near the crown.

iii. **Secondary dentine:** With advanced age there is deposition of secondary dentine tissue in pulp cavity. The process progress until whole of pulp cavity is replenished and the size of cavity decreases. In mandibular teeth, it starts from above and in maxillary from below. It is due to ageing, pathological conditions, dental caries etc. There are four degrees of secondary dentine formation:

   S_0— No deposition.

   S_1— Deposition in the upper part.

   S_2— Deposition in the half of the pulp cavity from above.

   S_3— Almost whole of the pulp cavity is involved.

iv. **Root resorption:** It is another decaying change involving both cementum and dentine that shows grooves. First apex is involved and then it extends upwards.

   R_0— No root resorption.

   R_1— Seen only in some parts.

   R_2— Seen over a large area.

   R_3— Involves both cementum and dentine.

v. **Cementum apposition:** Cementum deposition increases due to change in the surface of tooth near the end of roof and forms incremental lines. It occurs on the surface of the root in four degrees:

   C_0— Only normal layer of cementum is noticed.

   C_1— Slightly greater than normal.

   C_2— Thick layer has occurred.

   C_3— When a heavy layer is present.

vi. **Root transparency:** It occurs in the root from below upwards in the lower jaw and above downwards in the upper jaw due to rarefaction of dentine tissue:

   R_0— No transparency noticed anywhere.

   R_1— Transparency noticeable mostly over apical region.

   R_2— Transparency upto 1/3rd from the apical region.

   R_3— Transparency noticeable up to 2/3rd of the length of the root from apex.

Out of the six criteria, transparency of the root is the most reliable one for age estimation. The **anterior teeth are most suitable** as they erupt earlier and the changes are also present earlier than others. This method is **applicable only in dead bodies**.

The tooth is first examined by naked eye and then sectioned. Before the teeth is extracted, the degree of periodontosis is noted. The tooth is then ground down on a glass slab to about 1 mm size and transparency is noted. Then it is grounded to 1/4 mm for microscopical examination.

The preceding factors are assessed and given a point value according to the degree of departure from the normal. The average is ascertained from an erupted tooth, which has not exhibited any of these factors. When the total points have been allotted for particular teeth, then these values are compared with the points obtained from a series of teeth of accurately known age. This comparison is carried out on a graph by drawing regression lines showing the relation of the point values of teeth of known age. The estimated age is usually found within an error of ± 3.5 years.

Point formula as given by Gustafson is An+Pn+Rn+Cn+Tn +Sn = Total points that indicates the age in years.

Estimation of age from transparency of root: In 1963, **Miles** stated that transparency of root is a good marker for age and for this purpose anterior tooth are mostly used. The tooth is grounded up to thickness of 1mm and placed on a dotted paper and outline of tooth is made, then the dots visible through transparent root are counted. All dots lying in the area of tooth are counted and the percentage of the two is used to know the age.

Estimation of Age from the Bones

Skeletal age can be determined from the ossification of bones that is helpful in the determination of age. The human bones develop from a number of ossification centers. At 11-12th week of intrauterine life there are 806 ossification centers that at birth are reduced to 450. Adult human is made up of 206 bones. The time of appearance of center of ossification and the process of union of the epiphysis with the diaphysis at the metaphysis have a sequence and time that is utilized towards determination of age (Figure 5.11 and Tables 5.7 and 5.8).

Ossification centers are studied up to the age of 20-22 years, thereafter the skull vault sutures, union and activity of sternum, changes in shape of mandible and changes in pubic symphysis are taken in to account.

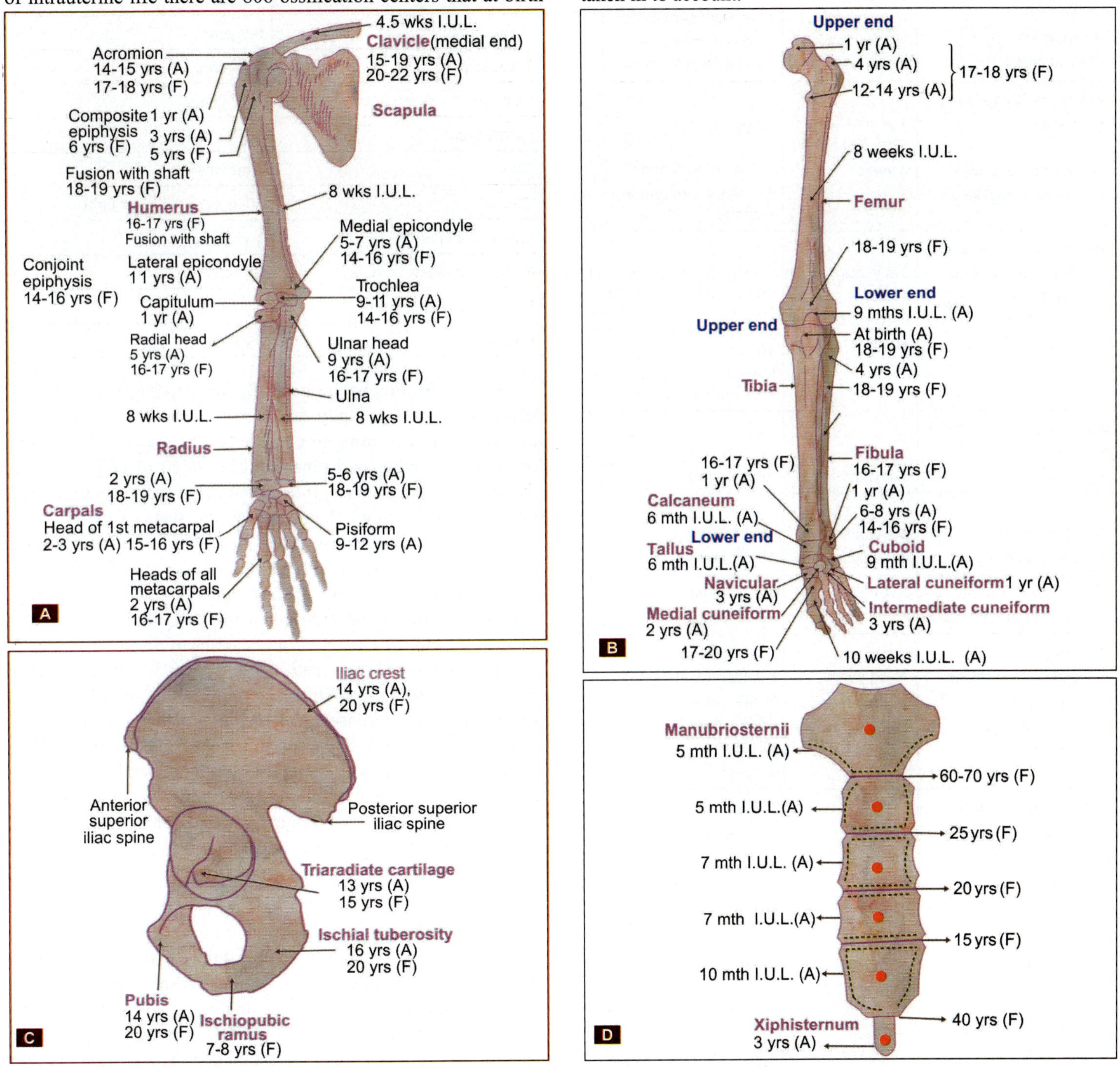

Figure 5.11: Appearance and fusion of ossification centers (A) Upper limb (B) Lower limb (C) Hip bone (D) Sternum (A = appearance, F = Fusion, I.U.L. = Intrauterine life, Yrs = Years)

Table 5.7: Ossification centers and their fusion

Centers of bones	Appearance	Fusion
Clavicle medial end	15-19 years	20-22 years
Sternum Manubrium: Body -1st segment -2nd segment -3rd segment -4th segment Xiphoid process:	 -5 months IUL -5 months IUL -7 months IUL -7 months IUL -10 months IUL 3 years	 60-70 years 14-25 years from below upwards; 3rd and 4th–15 years 2nd and 3rd–20 years 1st and 2nd–25 years >40 years with the body
Humerus (Upper end) • Head • Greater tubercle • Lesser tubercle	 1 year (All three unite at 6 years) 3 years 5 years	 18 years 4-5 years with head 5-7 years with greater tubercle
Humerus (Lower end) • Medial epicondyle • Capitulum • Trochlea • Lateral epicondyle	 5-6 years 1 year 9-10 years 10-12 (11) years	Capitulum, trochlea and lateral epicondyle form conjoint epiphysis at 14 years, unites with shaft at 15 years Medial epicondyle unites with shaft at 16 years
Radius • Upper end • Lower end	 5-6 years 1-2 years	 15-16 years 18-19 years
Ulna • Upper end • Lower end	 8-9 years 5-6 years	 16-17 years 18-19 years
Head 1st metacarpal Head other metacarpals	2 years 1½ to 2½ years	15-16 years 16-17 years
Hip bone • Triradiate cartilage • Iliac crest • Ischial tuberosity • Sacrum	 11-13 years 14-15 years 15-16 years 8 months IUL	 Disappears at 14-15 years 18-20 years 20-22 years 25 years
Femur (Upper end) • Head • Greater trochanter • Lesser trochanter ***Femur (Lower end)***	 1 year 4 years 14 years 9 months IUL	 17-18 years 17 years 15-17 years 17-18 years
Tibia • Upper end • Lower end	 10 months IUL 1 year	 16-17 years 16 years
Scapula • Coracoid base • Acromion process	 10-11 years 14-15 years	 14-15 years 17-18 years

Table 5.8: Age of ossification of hand and foot bones

Type of bone	Age of ossification
Capitate	2 months
Hamate	3 months
Triquetral	2-3 years
Lunate	3-4 years
Scaphoid	5-6 years
Trapezium	5-6 years
Trapezoid	5-6 years
Pisiform	9-12 years
Calcaneum	5 months IUL
Talus	7 months IUL
Cuboid	10 months IUL or at birth
Lateral cuneiform	1 year
Medial cuneiform	2 years
Intermediate cuneiform	3 years
Navicular	3 years

The ossification begins centrally in an epiphysis that spreads peripherally and gradually takes up the osteological details of the bony part, it is going to constitute, e.g., upper end of femur, lower end of radius and ulna etc. The union of epiphysis with diaphysis in long bones is interpreted as united, recently united, uniting and non-united, depending on the stage of union. When the epiphyseal lines persist, it will be called as **recently united**. The anatomical evidence of bony union differs from radiological union by about three years and radiographs give an earlier time of union. In the living subjects while determining the age of subjects to help the Courts of law in cases of disputes relating to age, the radiological examination of the bones is to be undertaken (Figures 5.12 to 5.20). While determining the age of a subject for medicolegal purposes, the standard value obtained from examination of the number of subjects should be the guiding criteria, as individual variations for bony union tend to occur. The degree of growth and development of bones to some extent is affected by the dietary, environmental, hereditary and endocrinal factors in different individuals belonging to different regions and culture. Ossification occurs earlier in tropical climates compared to temperate zones. In females, epiphyseal union occurs 1-2 years earlier than males.

Maturation score for estimation of skeletal age: To minimize the errors of epiphyseal union, **Mckern and Stewart** in 1957 suggested a scheme of scoring involving seven combinations of various segments. The total score is applied to prediction equation for more accurate age estimation. The scoring is given based on the degree of epiphyseal union that is:

Degree of union	Scoring
No union	1
1/4th union	2
1/2 union	3
3/4th union	4
Complete union	5

The various segments considered for the purpose of scoring are: (i) Humerus (proximal end and medial epicondyle) (ii) Radius (distal end) (iii) Femur (head and distal end) (iv) Iliac crest (v) Sacrum (lateral portion and 3/4th segments).

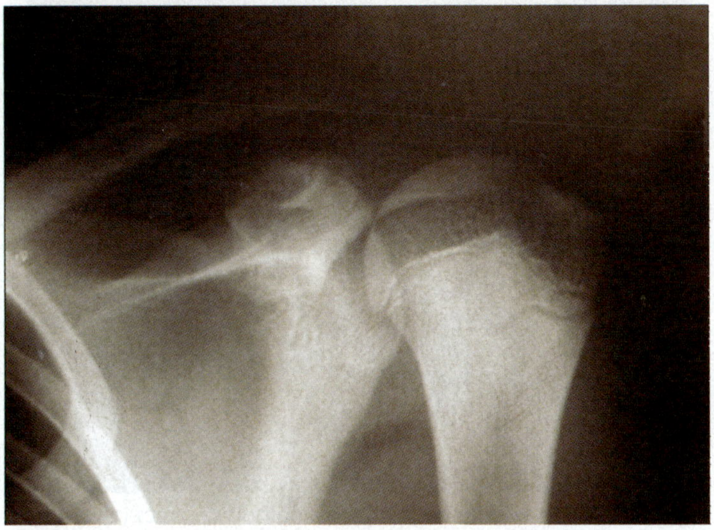

Figure 5.12: X-ray of shoulder joint. Note the nonunion of head and appearance and union of coracoid process (Age = 14-18 years)

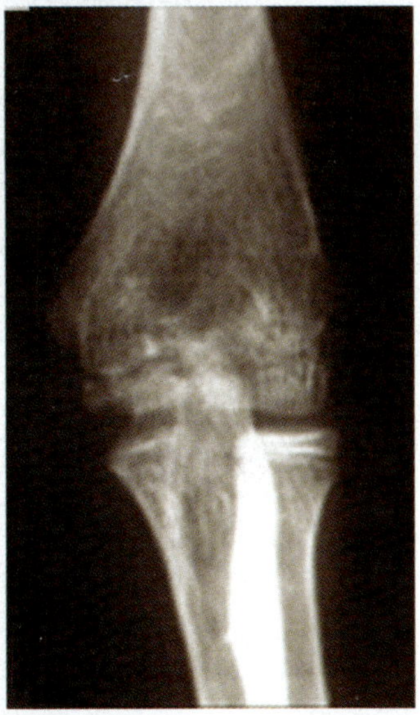

Figure 5.13: X-ray of elbow joint. Note the appearance of medial epicondyle, capitulum, trochlea, heads of radius and ulna and non union of medial epicondyle, conjoint epiphysis and non appearance of lateral epicondyle (Age = 9-11 years)

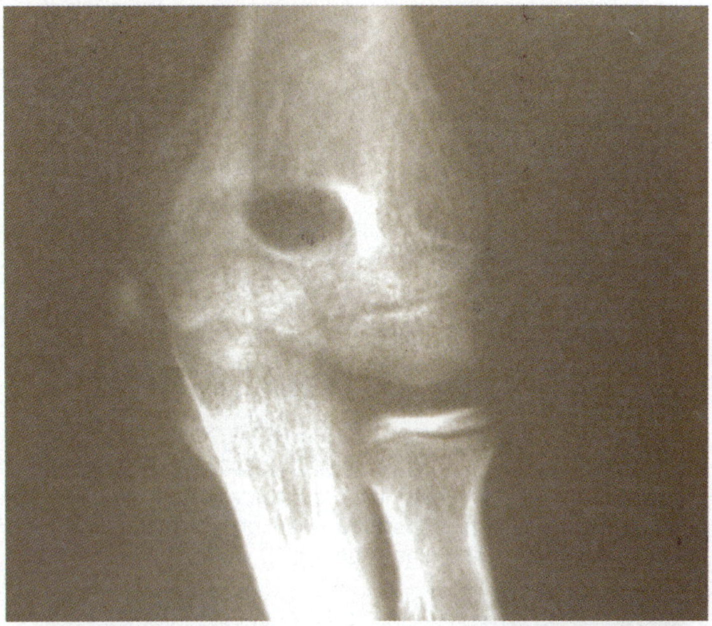

Figure 5.14: X-ray of elbow joint. Note the appearance of medial epicondyle, lateral epicondyle that are united and ununited heads of radius and ulna (Age = 11-14 years)

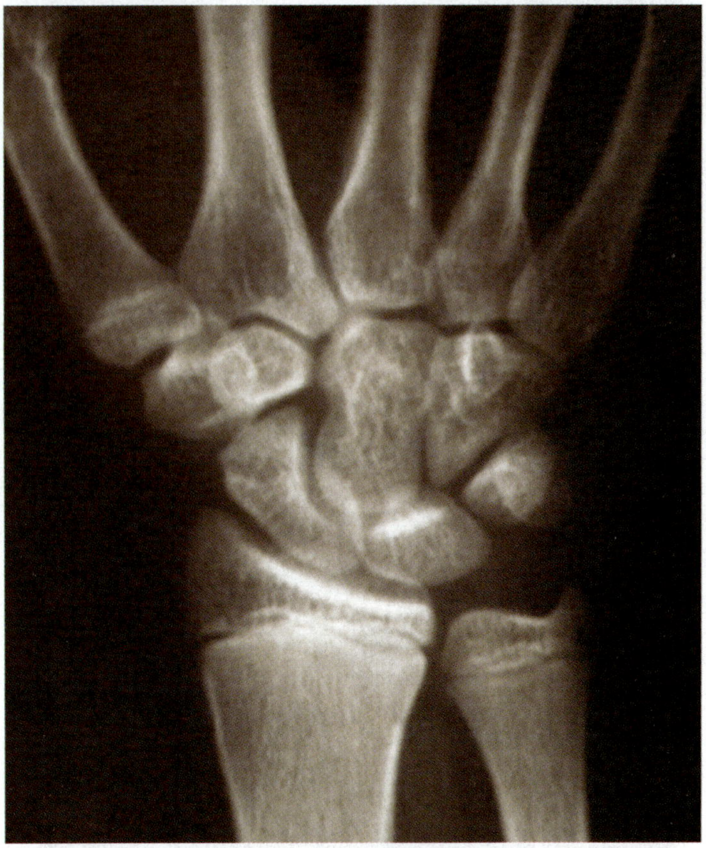

Figure 5.15: X-ray of wrist joint. Note the appearance of carpal bones and unossified head of first metacarpal (Age = 12-17 years)

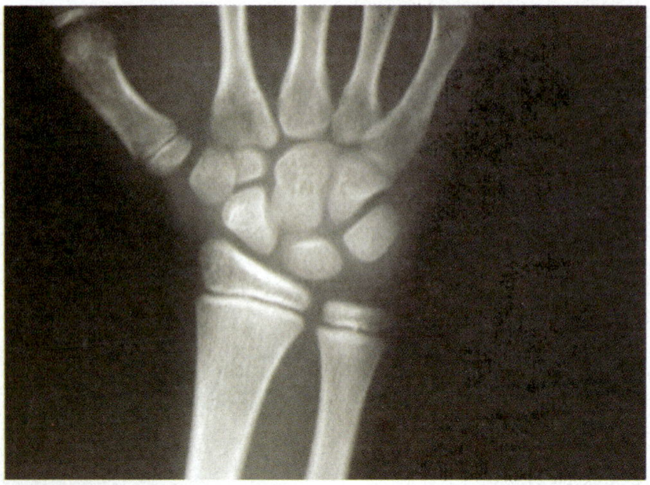

Figure 5.16: X-ray of wrist joint. Note the appearance of carpal bones except pisiform, unossified head of first metacarpal and lower ends of radius and ulna (Age = < 12 years)

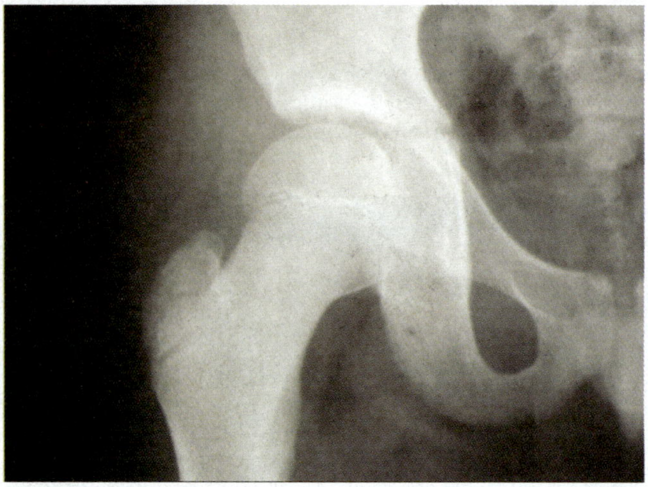

Figure 5.17: X-ray of pelvis. Note unobliterated triradiate cartilage, non union of head and greater trochanter of femur and non appearance of lesser trochanter (Age = 11-14 years)

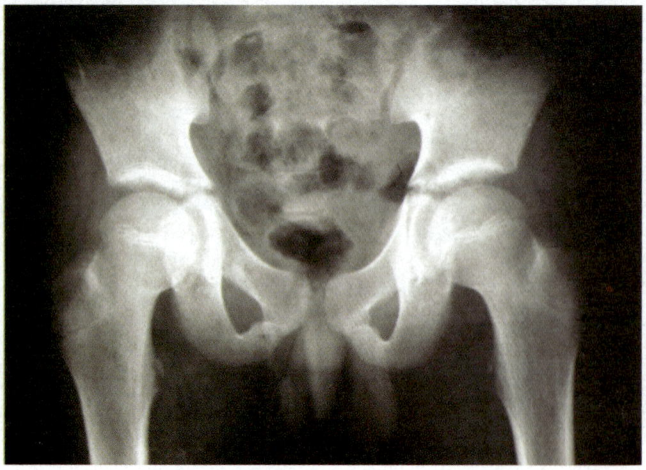

Figure 5.18: X-ray of pelvis. Note the unobliterated triradiate cartilage and non union of head, greater and lesser trochanter (Age = 14-15 years)

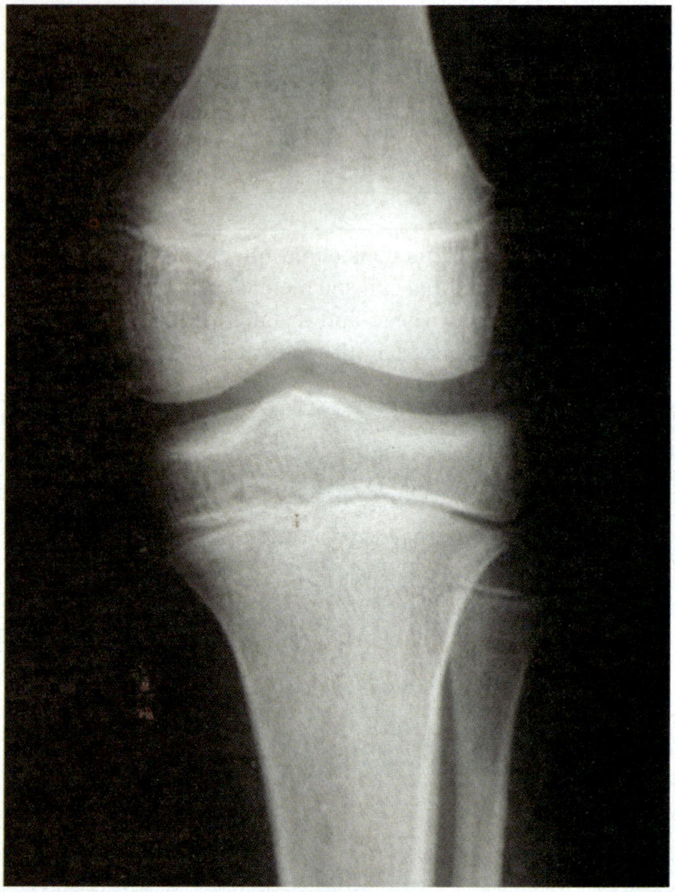

Figure 5.19: X-ray of knee joint showing non union of lower end of femur and upper ends of tibia and fibula (Age = < 17 years)

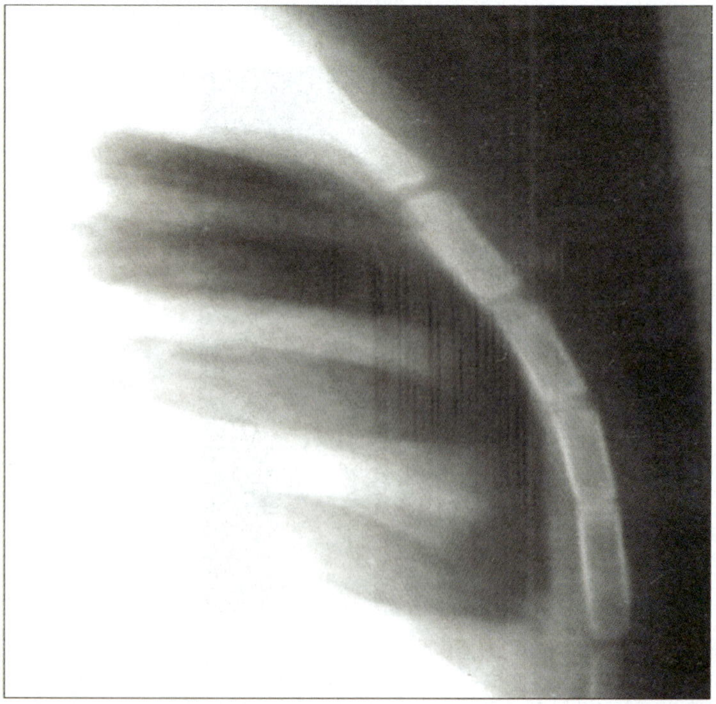

Figure 5.20: X-ray of sternum lateral view. Note the non union of 1st, 2nd and 3rd parts of sternum (Age = 15-20 years)

Sutural Closure of Skull (Figures 5.21 and 5.22)

Closure of sutures of skull has some bearing with the milestones of life. Absence of any signs of closure of any sutures of the skull, points to the strong possibility of the age having not exceeded thirty years. Evidence of commencing union of the sutures is always noticed first in the endocranial surface, then on the ectocranial one (Figures 5.21 and 5.22). As a rule, inner surface closes 5-10 years before the outer. The closure of ectocranial suture is quite variable and it may not close at all **(lapsed union)**. Lapsed union is seen more commonly in sagittal suture. The sutural closure occurs earlier in males than females. Estimation of age from closure of sutures of skull can be given within the range of 10 years between 30 and 60 years and even more in higher age groups. The chronological ages for sutural closure are as follows: (i) Lateral and occipital fontanelle closes at 2 months after birth. (ii) Posterior fontanelle closes at 6-8 months of birth. (iii) Anterior fontanelle closes at 1½-2 years of birth. (iv) Metopic suture closes at 2-4 years but may extend upto six years. (v) Basiocciput and basisphenoid fuses at 18-20 years. (vi) Sagittal suture is the first to start closing endocranially at about 25 years at its back portion close to parietal eminence. The fusion is complete both ectocranially and endocranially by 35-40 years. (vii) Coronal suture starts closing endocranially by 25-30 years in its lowest part, close to the junction with the sphenoid. It is completely closed at 40 years. (viii) Lambdoid suture starts closing endocranially at 25-35 years and terminal closure occurs by 45-50 years. (ix) Pterion starts closing at 40 years and completely closes by 65 years. (x) Mastoido-occipital suture starts closing at 45 years of age and complete closure occurs by 80 years. (xi) Asterion also closes by 80 years. (xii) Parieto-temporal suture closes by 70 years.

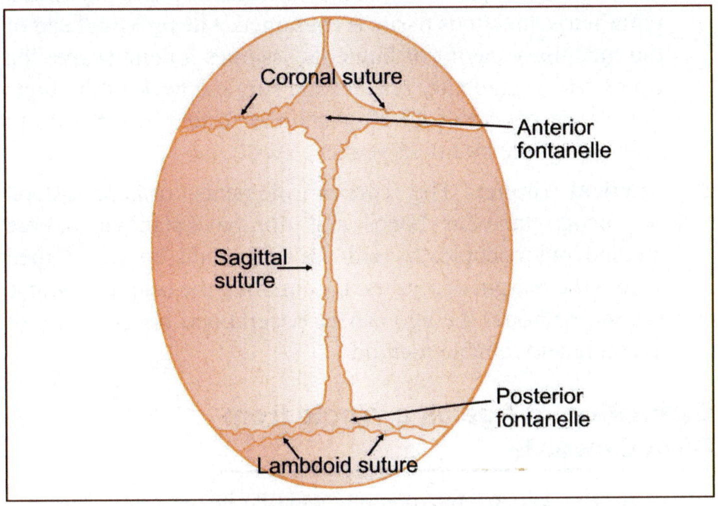

Figure 5.21: Sutures of skull

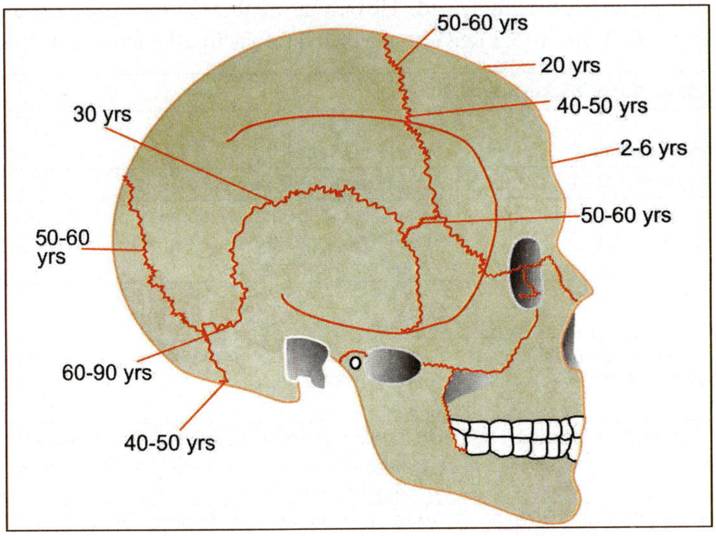

Figure 5.22: Ages of sutural closure of skull

Age Changes in Bones in Adults and Old Age

Changes in scapula: Scapula is a delicate bone and is often too damaged to be helpful. It requires experience to interpret and also the changes do not seem to be constant. The changes are not as closely identified with age as desired. The changes in the scapula are divided into two categories:

1. **Changes due to ossification after maturity:** (i) Lipping of glenoid fossa begins at 30-35 years. (ii) Lipping of clavicular facet begins at 35-40 years. (iii) Appearance of 'plaque; or 'facet' on the underside of acromial process thus prolonging the acromial tip from 2-8 mm at 35-40 years. (iv) Increasing demarcation of the triangular area at the base of scapular spine begins at 45-50 years. (v) Appearance of crista scapularis that tend to become more broader at the base and prominent at the apices with advancing age.

2. **Changes due to atrophic process after maturity:** (i) *Surface vascularity*: This is seen as number of fine lines in less than 25 years old. This visibility is slowly diminished and finally disappears with advancing age. (ii) *Deep vascularity:* Deep vascularity is seen as fine lines but only by transillumination by the age of 25-30 years and they tend to diminish with advancing age. (iii) Atrophic spots are areas of bone atrophy that starts appearing around 45 years and usually start in infraspinous area. (iv) *'Buckling' and 'pleating'* of infraspinous area is due to irregular atrophy of bone and is the result of diminished vascularity. It begins around the age of 40 years and there is absorption of cancellous tissue.

Changes in pubic symphyseal surface: Ageing is responsible for the fundamental contribution and provides a better guide than skull sutures for age estimation. Todd's system (Figure 5.23) states estimation of age from 10 stages of metamorphosis. Mckern and Stewart that is a more reliable method have replaced Todd's system. In this method symphysis pubis is divided into three components of which, six stages (0-5) are studied of metamorphic changes. A total score of three components is obtained which in turn is translated into age provided the individual is male. Various changes in the three components are given under Table 5.9. Joint lipping begins along the vertebral edge during the last two stage of component 3 at about 35-40 years.

Rough estimate of age from pubic symphysis	
Pubic symphyseal changes	**Age (Years)**
Symphyseal surface is even	≤ 20
Surface is markedly ridged and irregular called billowing, the ridges running transversely across the articular surface	20-25
Billowing gradually disappears and the articular surface becomes granular with sharp anterior and posterior margins	25-35
Articular surface is smooth and oval	35-45
Narrow and beaded rims develop in and around the margins of articular surface and some erosion of the surface starts	45-50
Varying degree of erosion with breaking down of ventral margin	≥ 50-60
Surface becomes irregularly eroded	60

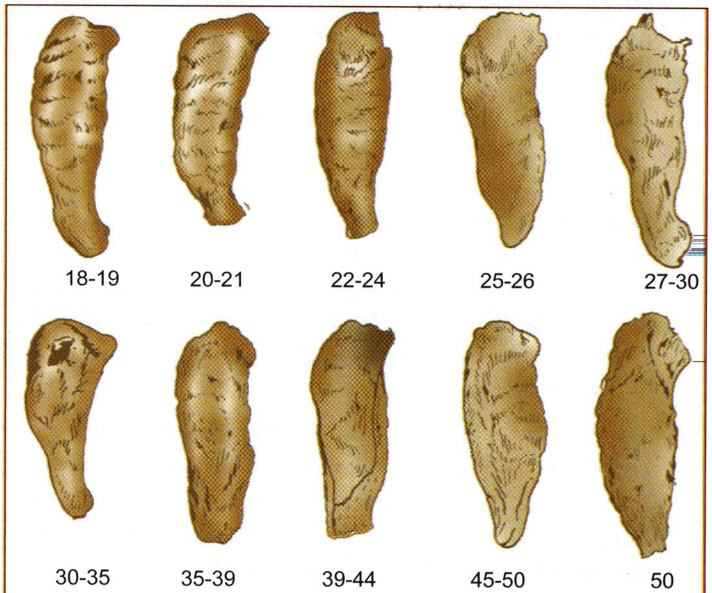

Figure 5.23: Age changes (in years) in pubic symphysis (After Todd's)

Age changes in the vertebra: (i) By the time the deciduous dentition is completed, the vertebral arch unites posteriorly and at the same time the arches and bodies of lowest lumbar vertebra begins to fuse. (ii) Posterior parts begin to fuse by 6 years and at the same time the arches of the first cervical vertebra unite posteriorly. (iii) Upper and lower surfaces of immature vertebra show a series of radial furrows up to 10 years. (iv) Furrows gradually fades on the upper and lower surfaces between 21-25 years. (v) Lipping of vertebra is seen usually after 45 years. (vi) Osteophytic outgrowth from anterior and lateral margins become visible by 40-45 years. The second cervical vertebra up to the age of about three years consists of three pieces that is two lateral portions that constitute the arch, the body and the dens.

Age changes in internal bone structure: Two structural components are studied that is:

1. **Cancellous tissue:** For studying this, humerus and femur are mainly considered and out of the two, humerus is used on priority basis. The methods used are radiological examination of bones and longitudinal section of bones in which resorption pattern of cancellous tissue is examined. The proximal end of the medullary cavity of humerus assumes a cone shape, the tip of which gradually reaches the surgical neck of the bone during the period of 40-50 years and further ascends up to epiphyseal line by 60-75 years.
2. **Cortical tissue:** The cortical elements osteon, osteon fragments, lamellar bones and non-haversian canals are studied microscopically and the age could be ascertained within the margin of 5 years. By counting the osteons in cross section of bone, the age can be ascertained but it is not an accurate and reliable method.

Estimation of Age as a Whole from Birth Onwards

To know the age of the person, usually horoscopes, hospital birth certificates, school admission certificates and matriculation certificates are being used. However, in the Courts horoscopes and affidavits about age are not relied upon. In all such cases, the

Table 5.9: Changes in pubic symphyseal surface (Mckern and Stewart)			
Stages	**Component 1 (Dorsal half of joint surface)**	**Component 2 (Ventral half of joint surface)**	**Component 3 (Whole surface)**
0	Dorsal margin absent	Ventral beveling absent	Symphyseal rim is absent
1	Slight margin formation starts in middle 3rd	Ventral beveling present at the superior extremity and ventral border	Dorsal rim appears at superior end of the dorsal margin, it is smooth and raised above the symphyseal surface
2	Dorsal margin extends over the entire border	Beveling extending downwards	Dorsal rim is complete and ventral rim starts forming
3	Formation of plateau (filling of grooves and resorption of ridges) begins in middle third of the dorsal surface	Bony extension (ventral rampart) begins from either or both extremities	Symphyseal rim is complete and the surface is finely granular
4	Visible billowing still present and plateau extends over most of the dorsal surface	Ventral rampart extends still further but gaps are still visible	Rim begins to break down, is sharply defined. The surface becomes smooth and flat with no lipping of ventral edge
5	Billowing disappears completely and the surface becomes flat and slightly granular	Ventral rampart is complete	There is further breakdown of rim and rarefaction of symphyseal surface

age of the individual is to be determined from certain parameters that are used as a whole. These are:

1. **First 15 days after birth:** The changes that occur in the umbilical cord, umbilical vessels and the skin of the newborn helps in determining the age within first 15 days after birth.
2. **First 6 months after birth:** In the first 6 months after birth the age of the infant can be estimated from the following parameters: (i) Posterior fontanelle closes within 6 weeks of birth (ii) Pterion and asterion closes (iii) Temporary teeth start erupting (iv) Foetal hemoglobin is changed to adult type.
3. **Between 6 months and 2 years:** (i) All temporary teeth erupt (ii) Ossification centers for heads of humerus, femur, all tarsal and carpal bones appear (iii) Anterior fontanelle closes at 1½ years.
4. **Between 2 and 6 years:** (i) Two halves of mandible fuse by second year (ii) Metopic suture close by 2-6 years (iii) Greater and lesser tubercles of head of humerus appear at 3 and 5 years respectively (iv) Condylar part of occipital bone fuse with the squamous part and basi-occiput (v) Medial epicondyle and upper end of radius appear by 5-6 years (vi) Head of first metacarpal appear (vii) Greater trochanter of femur appear at 4 years (viii) Center for xiphisternum appears at 3 years.
5. **Between 6 and 12 years:** (i) Ischio-pubic ramus fuses by 6-7 years (ii) Pisiform bone appear between 9 and 12 years (iii) Coracoid process of scapula appear at 10-11 years (iv) Upper end of ulna appear by 8-9 years (v) Trochlea appear at 9-10 years (vi) Lateral epicondyle appear between 10 and 12 years (vii) All temporary teeth are shed and permanent teeth erupt except third molars (viii) Secondary sexual characters appear on the body.
6. **Between 12 and 18 years:** The secondary sexual characters are well developed at this age. The bones around elbow joint, shoulder joint, hip joint, ankle and knee joint ossify during this period of life. The various changes are: (i) Upper end of radius fuses with the shaft. (ii) Olecranon fuses with the shaft. (iii) Third molar teeth erupt between 17 and 25 years and roots of other erupted teeth calcify. (iv) Head, greater and lesser trochanter of femur fuse with the shaft and lower end of femur, upper and lower end of tibia and fibula unite with their respective shafts. (v) Coracoid process fuses with scapular body at 16 years and acromion unites by 18 years. (vi) Bony replacement of the cartilage between basi-occiput and basi-sphenoid commences at about 17 years. (vii) Third and fourth part of sternum fuses by 15 years.
7. **Between 18 and 25 years:** By this age long bone epiphysis unites with their shaft: (i) Lower end of radius and ulna unite with their respective shafts at 18-19 years. (ii) Iliac crest unites with the ilium and ischial tuberosity unites with the ischium of hip bone by 20 years. (iii) Sternal end of clavicle unites with the sternum by 21 years. (iv) Secondary centers in articular facet of the rib is complete by 20-25 years. (v) Bony replacement of cartilage between basi-occiput and basi-sphenoid is complete by 20-25 years. (vi) Second and third part of sternum fuses by 20 years and first and second part unite by 25 years. (vii) All parts of sacral vertebra unite with each other.
8. **Between 25 and 35 years:** (i) Coronal, sagittal and lambdoid sutures of the skull start closing endocranially by 25-35 years and sagittal sutures close usually by 30-35 years. (ii) Age changes on symphysis pubis are characteristic after 25 years.
9. **Between 35 and 50 years:** The following changes are seen: (i) Coronal and sagittal suture closes by 35-40 years. (ii) Lambdoid suture closes by 50 years. (iii) Xiphoid process unites with the body at about 40 years. (iv) Age changes in symphysial surface of pubis are seen in this age group. (v) Articular surfaces of some bones may show changes such as lipping and loss of joint space. (vi) Glenoid cavity of scapula first shows such changes whereas bodies of lumbar vertebra and inner border of ischial tuberosities usually show lipping by 40 years and other joints of the body shows lipping by 45-50 years. (vii) Hyoid and thyroid cartilage ossify.
10. **Above 50 years:** (i) Mastoid, occipital, squamous and parieto-mastoid sutures close in very old age. (ii) Parietal suture may not close throughout the life. (iii) Manubrio-sternal joint fuse by 60 years. (iv) Laryngeal and costal cartilages calcify. (v) Long bones become lighter and brittle whereas skull bones become thinner and lighter as the diploe is absorbed. The fractures are common in old age owing to these changes. (vi) Degenerative changes like formation of arcus senilis in the eyes, wrinkling of the skin, silvery white deposition of atheromatous plaque in the arteries is common in old age. The chances of development of osteoporosis in the bone are more with advanced years of life.

Various Ages of Medicolegal Importance

1. **Criminal Responsibility:**
   i. *Under S. 82 I.P.C.,* the child of less than 7 years is not held responsible for the crime.
   ii. *Under S. 168* of the Indian Railways Act 1989, if the person under 12 years is guilty of offence under (a) S. 150 (maliciously wrecking or attempting to wreck a train; punished with death/imprisonment for life/10 years) (b) S. 151 (damage to or destruction of certain railway property; punishment with imprisonment for 5 years or fine or both) (c) S. 152 (maliciously hurting or attempting to hurt persons travelling by railway; punishment with imprisonment for life/10 years) (d) S. 153 (endangering safety of persons travelling by railway by willful act or omission; punished with imprisonment for 5 years) and (e) S. 154 (endangering safety of persons travelling by railway by rash or negligent act or omission; punished with imprisonment for one year or with fine or both), the court may require father/guardian

of such person to execute a bond for such amount and for such period for good conduct of the aforesaid person.

iii. *S. 83 I.P.C.:* The child of 7-12 years is presumed to be capable of committing an offence if he has attained sufficient maturity of understanding the nature and consequences of his conduct.

iv. *S. 89 I.P.C.:* The child of less than 12 years cannot give valid consent to suffer any harm that may occur for an act done in good faith for its benefit.

v. *S. 87 I.P.C.:* The adult of more than 18 years can give valid consent to suffer any harm that may result from an act not intended and not known to cause death.

2. **Judicial Punishment:** According to the Juvenile Justice (care and protection of children) Act 2000 (amendment 2015, bill 2021), *juvenile* means a boy or a girl who is less than 18 years of age. Delinquent juvenile when commits an offence, no death sentence and no life imprisonment is awarded. The juveniles are sent to juvenile homes by the Juvenile Justice Board when they commit an offence. Juveniles who are between the age of 16 and 18, if committed heinous crime, shall be tried like adults.
3. **Infanticide:** If the baby is of less than 6 months of intrauterine life, the charge of infanticide cannot be supported.
4. **Criminal Abortion:** A woman who has passed the childbearing age cannot be charged of procuring criminal abortion.
5. **Identification:** To identify a person, age is important.
6. **Impotence and Sterility:** Woman is sterile after menopause and the boy is sterile before puberty though not impotent. In India there is no legal limit on age of persons who can be declared impotent. There have even been allegations of rape against people more than 80-year-old.
7. **Rape:** Sexual intercourse with his own wife below 15 years and other girl below 18 years even with her consent is rape (S. 375 I.P.C.).
8. **Majority:** A child is major on completion of 18 years but attains majority on completion of 21 years when under guardianship of Courts or wards (S. 3, Indian Majority Act).
9. **Evidence (Witness):** A child of any age can give evidence if the Court is satisfied about his truthfulness (S.118 I.E. A).
10. **Employment:** A child of less than 14 years cannot be employed in a factory, mines or other hazardous employment. A person who has completed 15 years of age is allowed to work in a factory like an adult if certified by a doctor.
11. **Kidnapping:** It is removing a person from lawful guardianship. Consent of the person and intention of kidnapper is immaterial. It is an offence to: (i) Kidnap a child with the intention of taking any movable property of a child less than 10 years (S. 369 I.P.C.). (ii) Kidnap a minor from lawful guardianship of less than 16 years boy and less than 18 years girl (S. 361 I.P.C.). (iii) Kidnapping or maiming a minor for purpose of begging. (iv) To procure a girl for prostitution, if she is less than 18 years (S. 366A I.P.C.). (v) To import a girl to India from a foreign country for illicit intercourse, if she is less than 21 years (S. 366 I.P.C.).
12. **Abduction:** S. 362 I.P.C. defines abduction as compelling by force or inducing by any deceitful means any person to go from any place. Abduction is not punishable but when combined with some other intent as under sections 364 to 369 I.P.C. that prescribes punishments for aggravated forms of kidnapping or abduction. Abduction can occur against person of any age.

SEX

Criteria for determination:

(i) Likely indicators of sex are outline of face, figure, clothing, habits etc.

(ii) Highly probable indicators are external sexual characteristics, breast, buttock etc.

(iii) Certain or stronger evidence are penis, testis, prostate etc. in males and vagina, uterus, ovaries etc. in females.

(iv) **Nuclear Sexing:** It is technique for genetic sex determination. It can be determined by demonstration of Barr body in female somatic cells, Davidson body in female neutrophils, fluorescent body (Y chromatin) in male somatic cells, karyotyping and polymerase chain reaction (PCR).

A. ***Cytogenetics***

(a) *Barr Body or Sex Chromatin Bodies:* 1940's two Canadian scientists Murray L. Barr and E. G. Bertram noticed a dark staining mass in the nuclei of cat brain cells. They found these spots in female but not in males and thought the spot was a tightly condensed X chromosome. In 1961, Lyon studied the condensation of X chromosome mechanism for inactivating the genes on the chromosome which is called the Lyon hypothesis/Lyonization. It is present in the nucleus only during interphase and disappears during mitosis. It called sex chromatin bodies and later named as Barr Body which is used a vital tool for determination of sex of the individual. It is present in different somatic cells (seen in all nucleated cells not in RBC) of buccal mucosal cells, pulp tissue, vaginal smears, and hair follicle etc. of a female. The buccal mucosa smear method is the most popular because of minimal inconvenience to the person. It is present in 30 to 40% of female cells. It is mostly seen adjacent to the nuclear membrane, basophilic, measuring about 0.8 to 1.1 μm in diameter (Figure 5.24A, B, C). In some cells like neurons, barr body can be observed adjacent to the nucleolus or even free in the nucleoplasm. The shape can be plano-convex,

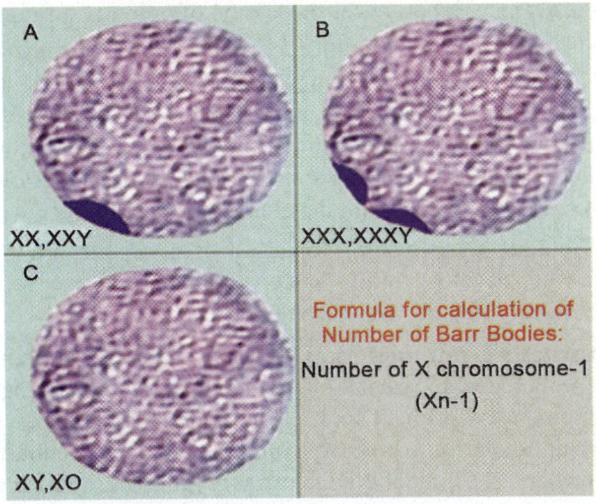

Figure 5.24 A, B, C: Barr body in different karyotypes

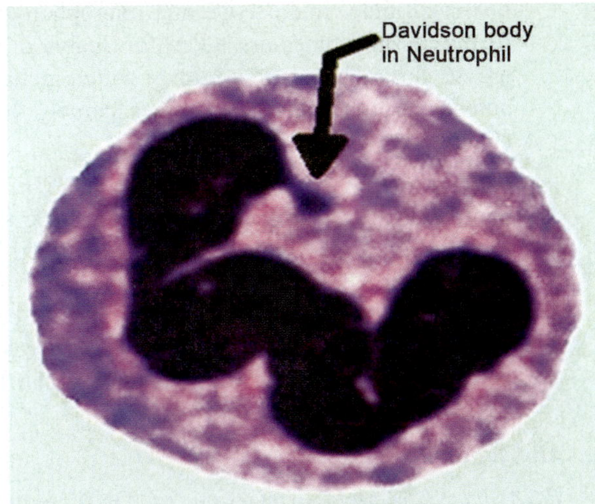

Figure 5.25: Davidson body (Drumstick appearance)

biconvex, triangular, spherical, or rectangular when observed under ordinary microscope in oil immersion or high power. Occasionally, they resemble the letter V, W, S, or X under electron microscope. For calculation of number of Barr bodies, the formula: number of X chromosome -1 (Xn-1) can be used. **Chromatin positive**–XX individuals have one barr body and XXY individuals (Klinefelter syndrome) are male, but have a Barr body. XXX (Trisomy X) or XXXY individuals have two barr bodies. **Chromatin negative**–XY individuals (male) have no barr body and XO individuals (Turner's syndrome) are female but have no barr bodies. Hence, the criteria to identify the gender using Barr body is ambiguous. In putrefied bodies sex chromatin cannot be made out. The frequency of Barr body is decreased during pregnancy, women on oral contraceptives, in newborn females and their mothers on the 1st postpartum day. The study of Barr bodies is advantageous in that it can be studied with simple staining techniques like Giemsa, Methylene blue etc. under an ordinary compound microscope. Special stains such as PAP stain, feulgen and guard stain, orcein, hematoxylin and eosin, cresyl violet, carbol fuchsin, and fluorescent stains are also used to visualize them.

(b) *Davidson's Body:* **Davidson and Smith in 1954** described the presence of drumstick appendage in the neutrophil of the peripheral blood smear. He observed that six drumstick appendages were present in 300 neutrophils examined in case of females but in males no drumstick appendages were found even in 500 neutrophils examined. Actually, neutrophils nuclei have five forms appendages namely drumsticks, racquet forms, sessile nodules, small clubs and minor lobes but only drumstick appendage is sex-specific (found in female) which is called Davidson's body (Figure 5.25). Like Barr body, it is also an inactive X chromosome but present in neutrophils of female. The size of drumstick is about 1.5 μ in diameter, which is attached to the body of the nucleus by means of a thin stalk. The incidence of drumsticks varies between 1% to 17% with an average of 2.9%. These variations could be under different circumstances like during the menstrual cycle, after the administration of adrenocorticotropic hormone and insulin, with senility and with cachexia.

(c) *Chromosome-Specific Fluorescence: Y-Chromosome Specific:* Fluorescent dye such as quinacrine dihydrochloride, binds with the distal portion of the long arms of the Y chromosome produces bright fluorescent in the nuclei of cells in metaphase under fluorescence microscope. The **quinacrine positive bodies** in males range from 45-80% and 0-4% in females. It is commonly referred as **f-body.** The Y-chromosomes can be detected in dental pulp tissue by using fluorescent dyes for about a year. In non-dividing cells (cells in interphase), a similar staining Y chromosome produces a brightly fluorescing pin-point spot which is called the "**Y-body**".

X-Chromosome Specific: Fluorescent Feulgen reaction using Acriflavin Schiff reagent for X-chromosomes that is seen as a bright yellow spot in the nuclei. The fluorescent bodies are seen in 50-70% cells in females and 0-20% cells in males.

(d) *Karyotyping:* It is a technique to determine the size, shape and number of chromosomes in a sample of body cells. The cells are subjected to grow in laboratory, the chromosomes are isolated and special staining is done. The chromosomes are observed under microscope and microphotographs of the chromosomes are taken for analysis. There are 46 chromosomes in a human which include 44 autosomes and 2 sex chromosomes, namely, 46, XX (female) or 46, XY (male).

(e) *Fluorescent in situ Hybridization (FISH):* The complementary sequences on interphase X and Y chromosomes are labeled with multi-colored DNA probes (e.g., FITC, Cy3). This procedure allows visual confirmation of not only the presence but the number of X and Y chromosomes. It can provide a more complete identification of gender than PCR-based techniques.

B. ***Molecular Genetics***

DNA based Method: Detection of DNA sequences specific to X and Y chromosomes through the use of PCR has been employed frequently as a method of gender determination. Amelogenin, SRY, and DYS14 genes are reliable indicators for sex determination.

Amelogenin Gene: It is most widely used as a marker of sex typing. The Amelogenin gene is located on both chromosomes X and Y, showing dimorphism in length.

Method:

(i) First isolation of DNA from available tissue.

(ii) Amplification of AMEL gene by polymerase chain reaction (PCR) by using specific primer: presence of X-specific bands at 330 base pair (bp) and Y-specific bands at 236 bp. Male (XY) is distinguished from female (XX) by the presence of two bands whereas female sample showed only one, i.e., X-specific bands on the agarose gel or SDS page.

(v) **Biopsy:** In intersex cases having unpredictable sexual morphological features, biopsy from the primary gonads namely testicles or ovaries can determine definitely as to whether the person is sexually active male or female or neither.

(vi) **Hormone hormonal measurement:** Gonadal hormones, especially estrogens and androgens, have long been found to account for some sex differences.

Concealed Sex

The person dresses himself/herself similar to that of the opposite sex. The treatment to concealed sex lies in simply undressing the person.

Intersex

Intersex means intermingling of features of both sexes in varying degree in one individual. Though these cases are not presently seen in forensic practice, still one can diagnose them in life. They are intimately connected with sports, service, admission to school, medical science, inheritance, succession of property, of marriage, rape etc. Types of intersex are:

Gonadal Agenesis: There is lack of development of gonads or secondary sexual characters and nuclear sexing is negative. The chromosomes can be demonstrated by microscopic examination but there is no sex chromosome. In addition, morphological features of either sex are not developed during puberty.

Gonadal dysgenesis: Gonads or sex organs are present but fail to develop during puberty. There are two types of medicolegally important syndromes:

Turner's syndrome: Morphology is that a female, but there is no proper development of feminine features during puberty. Development of primary and secondary sexual features is not observed. Short stature (most common feature), webbed neck amenorrhea, sterility and high urinary gonadotropin, etc. are seen. Ovaries do not contain sufficient follicles. Nuclear sexing is positive. Sex chromosome is XO and the total number of chromosomes is 45 instead of 46 (45, XO). The cause is usually defective polarization during cell division in the process of development of spermatozoa. It is also referred as to as congenital ovarian hypoplasia syndrome and is the most common sex chromosomal abnormality found in females.

Klinefelter's syndrome: In this condition, the anatomical structure is male but the nuclear sexing is female. The sex chromosomal pattern is XXY due to an extra chromosome. It is usually diagnosed when secondary sexual characters fail to develop during puberty. Testicles are small and firm and nonfunctional. Azoospermia with a normal or small penis and gynaecomastia are seen. There is scanty pubic hair, moustache and beard. Nuclear sexing is positive for a female.

Sex chromosome pattern is XXY and the total is 47 instead of 46 due to non-polarization of sex during cell division. Sperms contain XY or XX chromosomes and only one of these goes to each sperm but in case of Klinefelter's syndrome both the sex chromosomes remain in the same sperm and leads to the XXY pattern.

True hermaphroditism or bisexuality: The individual possesses two testicles or two ovaries or one testicle or one ovary neither of which functions fully and properly. Hence contradictory secondary sexual features are present in the individual. Nuclear sexing is either positive XX type or negative XY (male type).

Pseudohermaphroditism: Individual has contradictory features of both the sexes. Both groups are either of a male type or female type. In **male pseudohermaphroditism**, the nuclear sex is XY but sex organs and features are that of a female due to testicle feminization. In **female pseudohermaphroditism**, the nuclear sex is XX but sex organs and features are of a male due to adrenal hyperplasia.

Determination of Sex from Bones

General features of bones: The female bones are usually smaller, thinner and lighter than bones of the males in adults whose bones are bigger thicker and massive. The bones in case of males have more prominent ridges and the processes are more marked compared to females. Also, in males the shaft of bones have coarser surface and articular surfaces are wider compared to females where the shaft of long bones are smooth and articular surfaces are smooth and round. As an average, the weight of the skeleton of a 73 kg adult male might be about 10.5 kg and of a 60 kg adult female might be about 7.8 kg (International Commission on Radiological Protection). While determining the sex from the bones the percentage of accuracy from independent skeletal part (as given by **Krogman 1964)** is: (i) Whole skeleton (100%) (ii) Pelvis and skull (98%) (iii) Pelvis alone (95%) (iv) Skull alone (92%) (v) Skull and long bones (96%) (vi) Pelvis and long bones (98%) (vii) Long bones alone (80-85%).

Pelvis alone is sufficient for determination of sex especially in adults in more than 90% of cases. In case of children and fetus even from the examination of the pelvis sex can be determined with fair accuracy. Even in adolescents' greater sciatic notch is the single most important criteria from which sex can be determined. The sex differences in pelvis, skull, mandible, sacrum, clavicle, femur, humerus, radius, ulna and sternum are given in Figures 5.26 to 5.33 and Tables 5.10 to 5.18.

Medicolegal aspects: The question of determination of sex arises in cases of (i) Marriage (ii) Divorce (iii) Legitimacy (iv) Impotence (v) Rape (vi) Heirship.

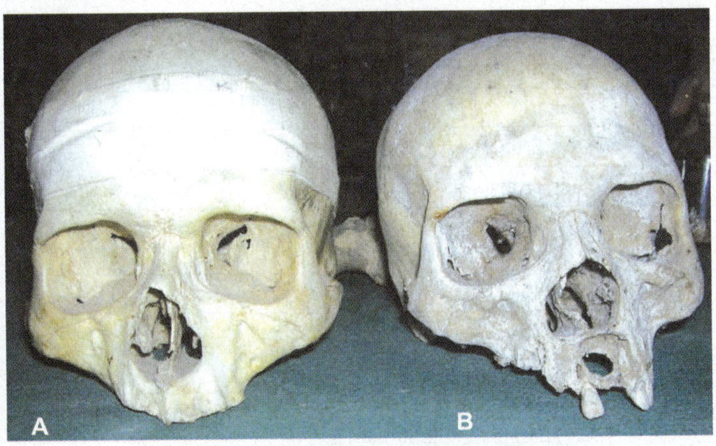

Figure 5.26: (A) Male and (B) Female skull

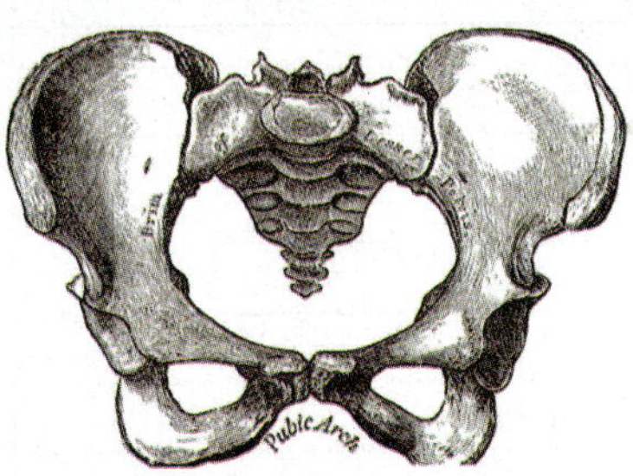

Figure 5.27: Female pelvis (bowl shaped, widely separated ant. sup. iliac spines, subpubic arch U-shaped)

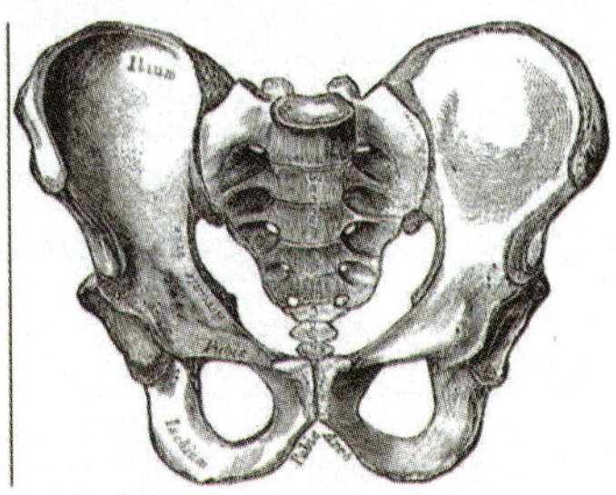

Figure 5.28: Male pelvis (deep funnel shaped, ant. sup. iliac spines not widely separated, subpubic arch V-shaped)

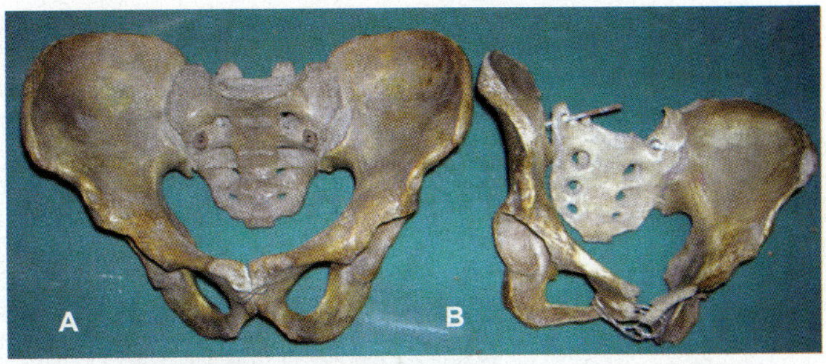

Figure 5.29: (A) Male pelvis and (B) Female pelvis

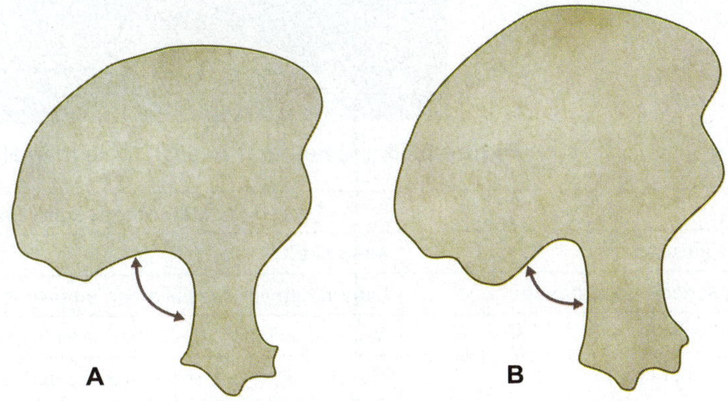

Figure 5.30: Greater sciatic notch (A) Large, wide and shallow in females (B) Small, narrow and deep in males

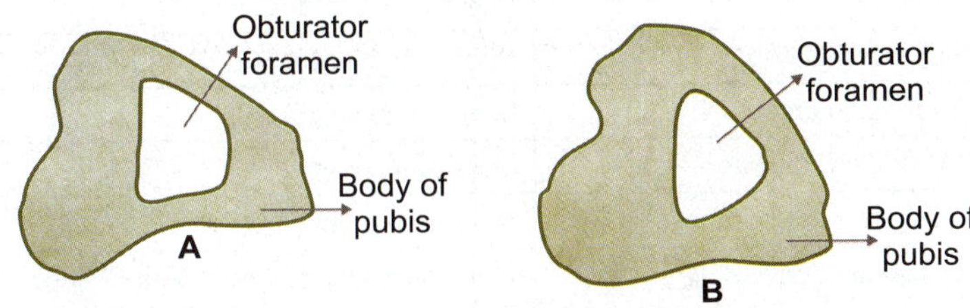

Figure 5.31: (A) In female pelvis body of pubis is broad, square and obturator foramen is small, triangular with apex forwards. (B) In males, body of pubis is narrow and triangular and obturator foramen is large, oval with base upwards

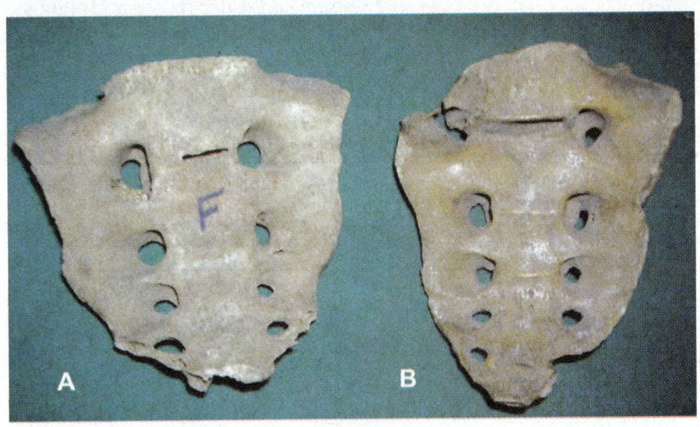

Figure 5.32: (A) Female and (B) Male sacrum (short and wide in females and long and narrow in males)

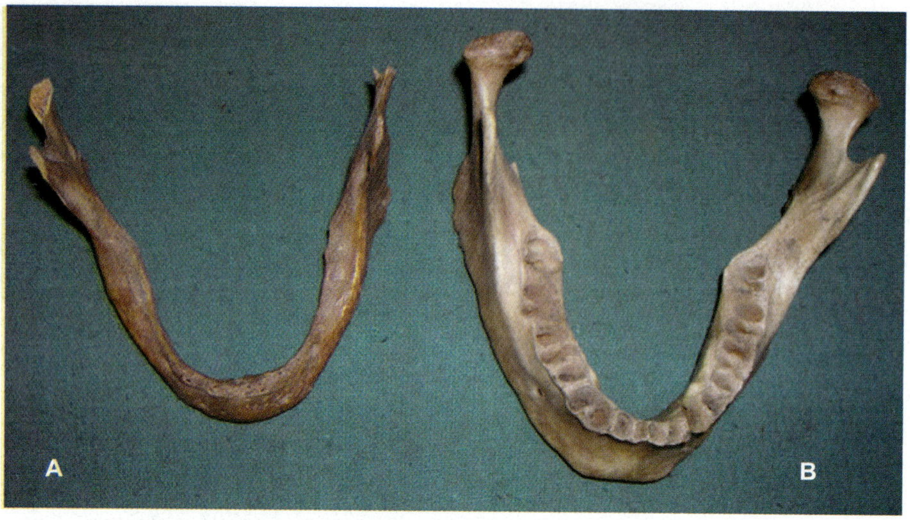

Figure 5.33: (A) Females and (B) Male mandible (square chin in males and rounded in females)

Table 5.10: Differences between male and female skull (Fig. 5.27)

Features	Male skull	Female skull
General appearance	Larger, heavier, massive and surface is rough	Lighter, smaller and surface is smooth
Capacity	More capacious (10% > than females/1500-1550 cc)	Less capacious (10% < than males/1300-1400 cc)
Architecture	Muscle ridges are more marked and prominent over occipital and temporal areas	Less marked
Frontal and parietal eminences	Small, less prominent	Large, more prominent
Frontal surface	Irregular	Smooth
Glabella	Well marked and prominent	Less marked and less prominent
Supraorbital ridges	More prominent	Less prominent
Zygomatic arches	More prominent	Less prominent
Mastoid processes	More prominent	Less prominent
Occipital protuberances	More prominent	Less prominent
Occipital condyles	Well marked and prominent. Facets are long and large	Less marked and prominent. Facets are small and broad
Digastric groove	More deep	Less deep
Fronto-nasal junction	Distinctly angulated	Smoothly curved
Cheek bones	Laterally arched, rough and large	Compressed, smooth and small
Palate	Larger and wider (U shaped) due to relative length of cheek, tooth and jaw	Smaller and narrower (parabola shaped) due to relative length of cheek, tooth and jaw
Orbits	Smaller and square placed low down with round edges	Larger and rounded placed higher up with sharp margins
Forehead	Steeper and less rounded	More rounded and full
Nasal apertures	Narrow and placed higher up	Broad and placed lower down
Teeth	Larger, lower first molars may have five cusps	Smaller, lower first molars have four cusps

Table 5.11: Differences between male and female humerus

Features	Male humerus	Female humerus
Average length	32.5 cm	30 cm
Vertical diameter of head	48.7 mm	41.5 mm
Transverse diameter	44.6 mm	38.9 mm

Table 5.12: Differences between male and female mandible		
Features	**Male mandible**	**Female mandible**
Size	Larger, thicker and heavier	Smaller, thinner and lighter
Chin	U or square and more prominent	V shaped and less prominent
Anatomical angle (between body and ramus)	Less than 125° more prominent and everted	More obtuse, less prominent and inverted
Height of symphysis menti	Greater and higher up	Smaller and shorter
Condyles	Larger	Smaller
Muscular impressions	More prominent	Less prominent

Table 5.13: Differences between male and female pelvis		
Features	**Male pelvis**	**Female pelvis**
General framework	Deep, funnel shaped. Massive and rough	Shallow, bowl shaped. Less massive and smooth
True pelvis	Narrow and deep	Wide and shallow
Pelvic brim	Heart shaped	Circular
Pelvic outlet	Smaller	Larger
Ilium	Curve is more prominent, more sloped with less rounded margins	Curve is less prominent, less sloped with more rounded margins
Iliac crest	More prominent	Less prominent
Anterior superior iliac spine	Not widely separated	Widely separated
Pre auricular sulcus	Not prominent, narrow and shallow	Prominent, broad and deep
Acetabulum	Wide and deep, diameter about 52 mm	Small and narrow, diameter about 46 mm
Symphysis pubis	Higher and bigger in depth and narrow in width. Margins of pubic arch are everted and no parturition pits on the dorsal border	Lower, wider and rounded. Margins of pubic arch not everted and parturition pits on the dorsal border of bone of parous woman
Subpubic angle	70°-75° (acute) and subpubic arch is V-shaped	90° (acute) and subpubic arch is U-shaped
Greater sciatic notch	Smaller, deeper and narrower and less than right angle	Wider, larger and shallower and forming a right angle
Sciatic notch index = $\frac{\text{Width of sciatic notch}}{\text{Depth of sciatic notch}} \times 100$	4-5	5-6
Obturator foramen	Large, oval shaped with base upwards	Small, triangular with the apex directed forwards
Ischial tuberosity	More or less inverted	Everted
Pubis (body)	Narrow and triangular	Broad and square
Pubis (ramus)	In continuation of body	Narrow appearance
Pelvic index = $\frac{\text{Anteroposterior diameter}}{\text{Maximum transverse diameter}} \times 100$	>95	<95
Keil index = $\frac{\text{Surface area of acetabulum}}{\text{Surface area of ilium}} \times 100$	13.57 (Range 12.17-15.05)	12.57 (Range 10.42-14.01)

Table 5.14: Differences between male and female sacrum		
Features	**Male sacrum**	**Female sacrum**
General	Long and narrow, sacral promontory is well marked and anterior curvature is equally distributed along its length	Shorter and wide with less prominent sacral promontory. Anterior curvature is straight in upper half and sharply curved in lower half
Sacroiliac articular surface	Large and extends upto 2.5-3 vertebral bodies	Small and extends upto 2-2.5 vertebral bodies
Coccyx	Less movable	More movable
Sacral index = $\frac{\text{Inter iliac breadth}}{\text{Pelvic breadth}} \times 100$	112	116
Ischiopubic index= $\frac{\text{Pubic length (in mm)}}{\text{Ischial length (in mm)}} \times 100$	73-94	91-115
Corporobasal index of sacrum = $\frac{\text{Breadth of 1st sacral vertebra}}{\text{Breadth of base of sacrum}} \times 100$	45	40.5

Table 5.15: Differences between male and female femur		
Features	**Male femur**	**Female femur**
Head	Larger and forms about 2/3rd or a sphere	Small and forms less than 2/3rd of a sphere
Neck	Forms obtuse angle (125° with the shaft)	Almost right angle with the shaft
Vertical diameter of femoral head	47-49 mm	43-45 mm
Bicondylar width	74-89 mm	67-76 mm
Trochanteric oblique length	450 mm	390 mm

Table 5.16: Differences between male and female sternum		
Features	**Male sternum**	**Female sternum**
Body	Bigger, longer and more than twice the length of manubrium	Shorter and less than twice the length of manubrium
Level of upper border	At the level of lower part of body of second thoracic vertebrae	At the level of lower part of body of third thoracic vertebrae
Ashley's rule of 149	Combined midline length of manubrium and body > 149 mm	Combined midline length of manubrium and body < 149 mm
Manubrium	Smaller	Bigger
Sternal index = $\frac{\text{Length of manubrium}}{\text{Mesosternal length}} \times 100$	46.2	54.3

Table 5.17: Differences between male and female clavicle		
Features	**Male clavicle**	**Female clavicle**
Length	> 175 mm	< 103 mm
Circumference	More	Less

Table 5.18: Differences between male and female radius and ulna		
Features	**Male**	**Female**
General features	Larger, thicker and heavier	Smaller, thinner and lighter
Curvature of radius	Less curved	More curved

STATURE

There is a progressive diminution in stature as age advances, the annual diminution being 0.06 cm. The stature diminishes during afternoon and evening by **1½-2 cm**. Body is said to increase in stature after death by about **2 cm** due to loss of muscle tone, relaxation of joints and tensions of interventricular discs. To calculate stature of an individual, to the total length of entire skeleton 2½-4 cm are added for the thickness of soft parts. In calculating the stature from bones, more than one bone should be taken into consideration and the long bones of lower limbs give a closer estimate than that of upper limbs. The highest correlation with stature is given by femur (r = 0.8) and tibia (r = 0.8) followed by humerus (r = 0.7) and radius (r = 0.7). A combination of bones is more reliable than a single bone in calculation of stature. For measuring the length of bones, sliding calipers can be used but Osteometric board (Figure 5.34) measures the length of the bone more accurately.

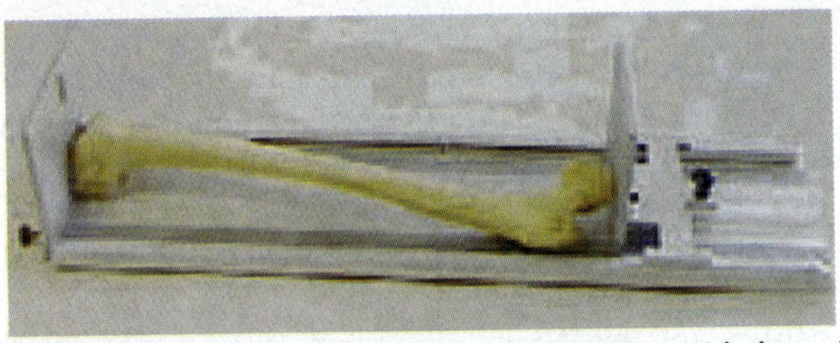

Figure 5.34: Measuring femur with osteometric board

After measuring the length, to calculate the stature it is multiplied by **multiplication factors** as given by **Pan (1924)** for East Indians (Hindus). The multiplication factors are as follows: (i) Humerus 5.30 (ii) Radius 6.90 (iii) Ulna 6.30 (iv) Femur 3.70; and (v) Tibia and fibula 4.48.

In case of dismembered or fragmented body, the stature can be calculated as: (i) Stature is equal to the length between the tip of one middle finger to that of the opposite when the arms are fully extended. (ii) Length of one arm is taken and twice this length + 30 cm for two clavicle + 4 cm for sternum is equal to the total stature. (iii) Length from vertex to symphysis pubis is roughly half of stature. (iv) Length from sternal notch to symphysis pubis is measured and multiplied by 3.3, which gives the stature. (v) Length of forearm from tip of olecranon process to tip of middle finger equals 5/19 of the stature. (vi) Height of head from top of head to tip of chin (as vertical length) = 1/7th of the total stature. (vii) Length of vertebral column is measured that equals 35/100 of the total height. (viii) Maximum length of foot is taken and divided by 0.15 that gives stature.

The regression equations given by Trotter and Gleser, Dupurtuis and Hadden can also be used for calculating the stature.

RACE

Race can be determined by:

1. **Complexion:** It has limited value as complexion varies from person to person even in the same race. Skin colour is brown in Indians, fair in European while Negroes are black. It is determined by melanin granules and melanocytes. Also skin colour changes during decomposition and burns etc.
2. **Eyes:** Eyes are dark in Indians though brown eyes are also found. Europeans have blue or gray coloured eyes.
3. **Hair:** Hair are black and thin in Indians, light brown to reddish in Europeans and straight or weary and thick in Mongolians, Indians and Europeans. They are frizzy or wooly (arranged in tight spirals) in Negroes. On histological examination, Mongoloid hairs are coarse and dark and circular on cross-section. In addition, dense uniform pigmentation is seen with a dark medulla. Negroes have hair that are elongated and oval in cross-section with irregular distribution of dense pigment. Caucasian hair are oval or cuneiform with fine or coarse pigment.
4. **Skeleton:** The race can be devised from several indices such as:
   i. ***Cephalic index or index of breadth:*** It is calculated as maximum breadth of the skull divided by maximum length of the skull multiplied by 100. The length and breadth of skull are best measured by sliding calipers. In the absence of sliding calipers, the osteometric board can be used. The index varies in different races as shown in the Table 5.19.

Table 5.19: Variations in cephalic index in different races

Types of skull	Cephalic index	Race
Dolichocephalic (long headed)	70-75	Aryans, Negroes
Mesati cephalic (medium headed)	75-80	Europeans, Chinese
Brachycephalic (short headed)	80-85	Mongolians

   ii. ***Brachial index*** (Radio-humeral) $= \frac{\text{Length of radius}}{\text{Length of humerus}} \times 100$
   (In Europeans, brachial index is 74.5 and 78.5 in Negroes)

   iii. ***Crural index*** (Tibio-femoral) $= \frac{\text{Length of tibia}}{\text{Length of femur}} \times 100$
   (It is 83.3 in Europeans and 86.2 in Negroes)

   iv. ***Humero-femoral index*** $= \frac{\text{Length of humerus}}{\text{Length of femur}} \times 100$
   (This index is 69 in Europeans and 72.4 in Negroes).

   v. ***Dental peculiarities:*** The race can be devised from several dental peculiarities as described later in this chapter.

FORENSIC ODONTOLOGY

It is the application of dentistry to forensic problems. It is important for: (i) Interpretation of bite marks. (ii) Personal identification for establishing the individuality of the person especially in mass disasters.

Bite Marks

Interpretation of bite marks: Police may sometimes bring objects for examination like apple or piece of cheese. The unusual bite mark on the objects may be due to some dental abnormality. 'Plastic' marks on objects such as butter, cheese, lard, wax or chocolates should be interpreted and for this they are to be stored in refrigerator to prevent them from melting or flowing; they are not deep frozen as they may brittle and crack.

Fruits especially Apples are preserved in Campden solution (Meta bisulphate fluid) used for fruit bottling. Photographs are taken with film plane at right angles to the bite. Salivary traces should be swabbed. Bites are commonly seen in cases of: (i) *Child abuse:* In child abuse, the marks are seen anywhere on the body such as arms, hands, shoulders, cheeks, buttocks and trunk. Bites are examined whether the size of the mark is same as of adult dentition; if it is of small size, could be due to bite by the sibling and when it is of different size it could be an animal bite. (ii) *Sexual assault:* Sexually oriented bites can be caused at any parts of the body namely breasts, neck, shoulders, thighs, abdomen, pubis or vulva. (iii) Police officers by the resisting offenders. (iv) In sporting events like football and wrestling. (v) In assaults anywhere on the body.

Medicolegal aspects of bite marks: (i) Self inflicted bite marks seen at accessible parts of the body such as shoulders or arms etc., usually seen in psychiatric patients, teenage girls and old children. (ii) Can be accidental at times resulting from falls on to the face and during fits; biting of tongue and lips will also be there.

Nature of bite marks: Bite mark comprise a crop of punctate haemorrhages varying from small petechiae to large ecchymoses merging into a confluent central bruise. Front teeth cause bite marks from canine to canine with an invariable gap at either side representing the separation of upper and lower jaw. A circular or shallow oval is human bite and deep parabolic arch or U-shaped is characteristic of an animal bite. Teeth may cause clear separate marks that run into each other as continuous, intermittently broken lines. There may be abrasions, bruises and lacerations or a combination of all these. Suction petechiae without teeth marks in sexual assault are caused by human bites, have a sucking effect and due to the rupture of small venules petechial haemorrhages result. Identification from bite marks is possible if incisors and canines has some characteristic features.

Bite Mark Investigation

1. **Photographing bite mark:** Bite mark is photographed from different angles; from a directly perpendicular viewpoint with a plane of film at right angles to that of the lesion, with an accurate scale.
2. **Swabbing of saliva:** To identify or exclude assailant as 80% of the people are 'secretors' who exude blood group substances in the saliva. Plain cotton wool swabs are rubbed on to the bite after moistening with water or saliva. These are then deep frozen and sent to serology laboratory.
3. **Impression of bite mark:** Plastic substance is laid over the bite mark that hardens and produces permanent negative cast of the lesion. Plastic substance is made with a rubber or silicone based medium containing a catalytic hardener or Plaster of Paris (water based plaster).
4. Skin carrying the bite is removed and preserved in formalin for future examination; formalin causes shrinkage and distortion and makes tooth matching difficult.

Matching the bite mark with the suspect's dentition: (i) Full informed consent before examination of the suspect in writing to be taken. (ii) Oral consent with at least one witness, if not written to be taken. (iii) Dentition examined and points determined and recorded by diagram and writing. (iv) Photographs can be taken.

The points to be noted in bite marks are: (i) Presence of full or partial denture and were they worn at the time of incidence. (ii) Number of teeth in the upper and lower jaw. (iii) Charting of missing teeth. (iv) Estimate of bite overhang; whether there is an edge-to-edge occlusion or an undershoot projection of lower teeth. (v) Recording of any broken teeth or teeth with significant individual abnormalities are charted and described. (vi) Any irregularity or marked variation in cutting edge profile of any front teeth. (vii) Evaluation of size and prominence of any teeth especially canines and incisors. (viii) Any developmental abnormalities are to be noted. (ix) Recording of any abnormality in orientation of any tooth such as twisting (rotation), anteroposterior tilting, double row of teeth or any gap or irregular spacing. For this: (a) Six upper and six lower front teeth give the most information. (b) Canines may provide particular help. (c) Premolars and molars are rarely useful due to being posteriorly positioned in the jaw.

Identification from Dentition

Identification of the dead from dentition: The teeth helps in identification of the individual as no two sets of teeth are identical. This is particularly important in: (i) Disasters such as aviation accidents, marine accidents and air crashes in cases of mutilated or burned bodies. (ii) To identify the unknown in accidents, suicides or homicides.

Identification in mass disasters includes the: (i) *General or reconstructive identity:* This includes classification of the unknown by age, sex and race. (ii) *Comparative method*: To confirm or exclude personal identity against antemortem dental records.

General/Reconstructive identity: In fragmented bodies or skeletonized remains from jaw remnants and teeth, the following features are easily recognized.

Sex of the person: There are certain differences in male and female dentition (Table 5.20).

Table 5.20: Differences in male and female dentition

Findings	Males	Females
Size of upper central and lateral incisors	Different	Same
Size and shape of the teeth	Mandibular teeth are less pointed and bigger	Mandibular teeth are more pointed and smaller
Mandibular first molar	Has a fifth cusp	Fifth cusp is absent
Pulp tissue from tooth (Fluorescent staining for intra nuclear F body)	Absent	Present

Race of the person: In civilized societies, first molar is the longest and third molar is smallest whereas in primitive races, first molar was smallest and third molar was longest in size.

1. **'Shovel'** shaped upper central incisor is seen in Mongoloids. Posterior surface have a depression centrally with two marginal bars, causing the back of tooth to appear like a coal shovel with turned up edges. This is found in 91% of Chinese, Japanese and Tibetans; 84% Eskimos; 46% Palestinian Arabs, 90% Finns and rarely in Negroes and Australians aborigines. In White races, lateral incisors in upper jaw are smaller than the central especially in females; is less marked or absent in Negroid and Mongoloids.
2. **Long pointed canine roots** are not seen in the Mongoloids.
3. **Enamel pearls:** Are small nodules of enamel on the tooth surface, are frequent in Mongoloids.
4. **Carabelli's cusp:** Small nodules on lingual surface of maxillary molar is common in white races and is rare in others.
5. **Taurodontism (Bull tooth):** These are common in Mongoloids; the pulp cavity of molars is wide and deep and the roots are fused and bent.
6. **Congenital lack of third upper molar** is common in Mongoloids.
7. **Large teeth with more cusps** in their molars even up to eight with two lingual cusps on mandibular first premolars are common in Negroid races.

Age of the person: (i) By eruption of deciduous and permanent teeth. (ii) Gustafson's criteria that was later modified by Johanson. (iii) Comparative identification from the teeth by charting.

Charting the Teeth

On the charts following peculiarities are recorded: (i) Any extractions, recent or old from the condition of the socket (ii) Any fillings, number, position and composition (iii) Artificial teeth whether of gold, porcelain or stainless stain (iv) Prosthetic work in mouth such as bridge work or braces (v) Any crowned teeth (vi) Any broken teeth (vii) Pathological conditions in teeth, jaws or gums (viii) Congenital defects such as enamel pearls, carabelli's cusps or ectopic teeth (ix) Malpositioned teeth that are rotated or tilted (x) General state of care and hygiene like caries, plaque, tobacco staining, gingivitis etc. (xi) Racial pointers such as shovel shaped upper central incisors and multi-cusped molars.

Chart designation of teeth: In the middle of nineteenth century, the designation of teeth was based upon anatomical names such as upper and lower jaws and left and right in relation to midline. Latin names were used depending on the function of the teeth. There are various systems for charting of the teeth such as:

1. **Zigmondy system:** First system was given by Zigmondy in 1861. He numbered the permanent teeth with arabic numerals 1 to 8 from midline backwards. The quadrants were denoted by a line drawn between the central incisors bisected by a line separating the upper and lower teeth. The deciduous teeth were given Roman numerals I to V and individual teeth were denoted by the quadrant sign.

8 7 6 5 4 3 2 1	1 2 3 4 5 6 7 8	**Permanent**
8 7 6 5 4 3 2 1	1 2 3 4 5 6 7 8	
V IV III II I	I II III IV V	**Deciduous**
V IV III II I	I II III IV V	

Every type of tooth has same designation so the angle of mandible was used to differentiate and the following numbers were given such as:

6 = upper right first molar; 3 = upper left canine and 2 = lower right lateral incisor etc.

Disadvantages: This method could not be easily adopted in the typewriters. As far as hand written system is concerned this system is very simple to use.

2. **Palmar's notation:** This method was devised by dentist Palmar in 1870 and 1891 as:

Right	8 7 6 5 4 3 2 1	1 2 3 4 5 6 7 8	**Left**
	8 7 6 5 4 3 2 1	1 2 3 4 5 6 7 8	

3. **Universal (Cunningham) system:** Cunningham in 1883 proposed that it would be simpler to avoid the quadrant symbols by using a straightforward numbering notation. Cunningham's notation involved numbering the teeth 1 to 32 and lettering the deciduous teeth A to T, starting at the posterior upper right and continuing in a clockwise direction. In this system, the teeth are numbered from 1-16 from right to left in the upper jaw and 17-32 from left to right in lower jaw. The Universal system was followed by the International Society of Forensic Odontology. However, it underwent a number of modifications in USA.

Right	1 2 3 4 5 6 7 8	9 10 11 12 13 14 15 16	**Left**
	32 31 30 29 28 27 26 25	24 23 22 21 20 19 18 17	

It is the best method of charting but the disadvantages are that it is difficult to learn and the risk of selecting the wrong number is great.

4. **Haderup system:** Haderup devised a notation published in 1902 which made use of the plus and minus sign and retaining the anatomical classification of single teeth as

devised by Zsigmondy. To differentiate between the left and right sides the '+' for the maxilla and '–' for the mandible were placed in front of the number for the left side and behind for the right side, the sign thus being towards the midline. For the deciduous teeth a zero was additionally placed in front of the number. This notation was adopted by the Scandinavian countries.

Permanent teeth,

8+	7+	6+	5+	4+	3+	2+	1+	+1	+2	+3	+4	+5	+6	+7	+8
8–	7–	6–	5–	4–	3–	2–	1–	–1	–2	–3	–4	–5	–6	–7	–8

Deciduous teeth,

05+	04+	03+	02+	01+	+01	+02	+03	+04	+05
05–	04–	03–	02–	01–	–01	–02	–03	–04	–05

5. **FDI notation:** A two digit notation capable of indicating tooth and quadrant was developed. Each permanent and deciduous quadrant was designated by a separate number in a clockwise direction followed by Zsigmondy's number at a meeting of the *Federation Dentaire Internationale* in Bucharest in 1971. This was adopted as the International Standard and was adopted subsequently by the American Dental Association, International Standard Organizations, the International Association for Dental Research and the World Health Organization. From the Forensic Odontologist's point of view the acceptance of this notation by Interpole for identification purposes was a significant step in international communication. The system is known as the FDI notation.

Permanent teeth,

18	17	16	15	14	13	12	11	21	22	23	24	25	26	27	28
48	47	46	45	44	43	42	41	31	32	33	34	35	36	37	38

Deciduous teeth,

55	54	53	52	51	61	62	63	64	65
85	84	83	82	81	71	72	73	74	75

The disadvantage of this method is that teeth could be confused in the change over from one 2-digit notation to another.

6. **Modified FDI system:** In this method, the tooth and quadrant are designated by a separate number. Right quadrant was designated by 2 and 3 and left was designated by 1 and 4 in permanent teeth. In deciduous teeth right quadrant was designated by 6 and 7 and left quadrant by 5 and 8.

Advantages of dental charting: The dental charting is better for forensic purposes involving telegrams or telephones. However, in such cases, good photography is also necessary and in no case should telegrams or telephone calls alone be relied upon.

Medicolegal aspects of Dental study: (i) *Identification of the individual:* From the dental study, age, sex and race of the person can be identified as described before. Other factors for identification include: (a) Habits such as chewing tobacco (b) Peculiarity in setting of the teeth may be familial and may help in identification (c) Teeth resist decomposition so they are important for identification even for a long time after death as peculiarity of setting of teeth, evidence of any missing tooth or any artificial dentures help in proving the identity of the person (d) Occupation can be known if there is a notch under tooth as in case of tailors. (ii) *Grievous hurt:* Fracture dislocation of tooth amounts to grievous hurt according to section 320 (7) I.P.C. (iii) *Cause of death:* The teeth resist putrefaction and the amount of deposition of heavy metals can be detected for a considerable period after death, that is especially helpful in poisoning cases as well as in mass disaster. (iv) *In chronic phosphorus poisoning*: Evidence of phossy jaw and affection of teeth and gums are characteristic. (v) *Bite mark:* Over the articles or food help towards detection of the criminal. Bite mark on private parts, breasts, cheeks, neck of a girl are suggestive of some sexual instinct. (vi) *Artificial dentures:* When dislodged can sometimes cause choking in the elderly. (vii) *Pink teeth:* In putrefied bodies, near gum line, teeth are of pink colour. It is due to dentine being stained by haemoglobin products.

SCARS (Figure 5.35)

Identification from scars: The scar develops whenever there is injury to the dermis. It is a mass of fibrous tissue that is covered by epithelium. Incised, lacerated, penetrating and crushing injuries can cause the scars. The scars can be formed in burns, scalds, corrosive acid injuries, electricity and radiation injuries.

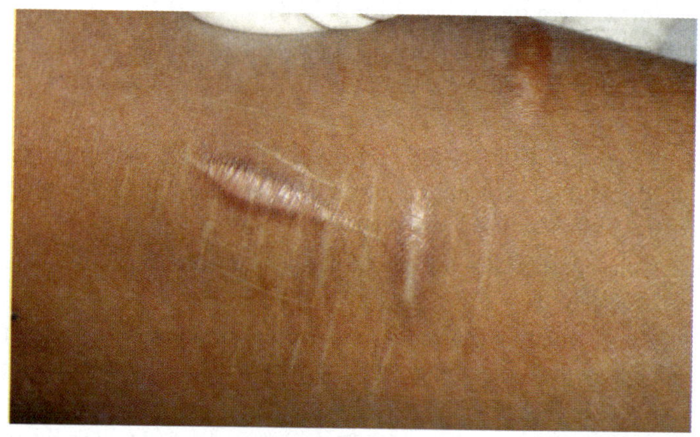

Figure 5.35: Scar

All these result in disfiguration of the part. The scars are used to identify the person. The formation of scar and time required for its formation depends on the size, site, and nature of injury, whether the wound was infected and mode of healing whether by first or second intention. In an incised wound with healing by first intention the reddish linear scar forms within 10-14 days. The scar may form within 7-8 days when the wound heals with the formation of scab in superficial cuts. In a moderately infected area, the scar formation occurs in 2-3 weeks times. When the healing is by secondary intention, and when there is chronic suppuration with infection, the scar may take 4-6 weeks to form. In cases of thermal, chemicals and electricity burns, the scar may form in several weeks to months even after grafting.

Age of scars: To ascertain the time elapsed since injury, the assessment of the age of scar is important. The time taken for the scar to develop depends upon the nature, site and size of the injury, supervening infection of the wound, vascularity of the area and the age and sex of the individual. The scars at an early stage are red and sensitive due to blood supply from small capillaries and as blood supply gets obliterated the scar becomes shrunken, depressed, irregular and smaller in size with irregular and insensitive surface. The various stages of scar formation with the passage of time since the infliction of the injury are:

Time since infliction of injury	Characters of scar
5-6 days	Reddish, soft, tender and sensitive scar with firm union of wound edges
End of 14 days	Scar is soft, pale and sensitive
2-6 months	Soft, brownish or coppery reddish scar with no corrugation
After 6 months	Scar is white, firm, tough, glistening and corrugated

The age of scar can be determined to be fresh, recent, old or late from the following features:

- *Fresh scar* (Within first few weeks): Soft and sensitive or pale yellow ecchymosis around contusion or scab formation.
- *Recent* (Few weeks to 2-3 months): Brownish or copperish red, soft and not irregular.
- *Late* (About 3-6 months): Similar to the scar of 2-3 months and usually shows no corrugation.
- *Old* (More than 6 months): White, glistening, contracted and tough in consistency.

Examination of scar: While examining the scar, following points are to be noted: (i) Shape, size, direction of the scar (ii) Site of the scar (iii) Colour of the scar, whether reddish, brownish, copperish (iv) Surface whether it is irregular, thick, tough or firm in consistency and whether it is glistening or dull (v) Whether it is tender or sensitive (vi) Whether is it freely mobile or fixed (vii) Evidence of marks of surgical interference from marks of stitches and incisions.

Disappearance and erasing of the scar: Superficial linear scars may disappear within a few years but scars resulting from large wounds, ulcers, skin diseases that involve whole thickness of skin are permanent. The scar if faint can be made prominent by rubbing or applying heat locally. The scar can be examined with a hand lens or under UV light. In the dead, the scar tissue can be examined microscopically by staining for reticuli and elastic tissue. The scar can be erased by excision and skin grafting. This may result in the formation of less obvious scar. If a person wants to efface the scar, he may get the part tattooed or may burn it but that in itself result in further scarring.

Medicolegal importance of scar: (i) Scar helps in identification of an individual. (ii) Age of the scar will tell us the time of infliction of injury. (iii) Shape of the scar will give an idea about the nature of weapon or other causative agent: (a) Scars from stab or punctured wounds are usually triangular and smaller than the causative weapon (b) In incised wounds and surgical incisions that have healed by first intention, the scar is linear and straight but if the wounds are infected, the scar is thick and wide (c) Scars from infected lacerated wounds healing by second intention are irregular, thicker, broader and firmer (d) Scars from severe burns are prominent, irregular, thick and adherent (e) Vaccination scars are usually circular or oval, and slightly depressed (f) Scars resulting from corrosives, radiation burns are irregular and thickened. (iv) Striae gravidarum, linea albicantes and old tears in the cervix and posterior commissure indicates previous pregnancy. (v) Disfiguration caused on the face by scars resulting from assault, accident or vitriolage amounts to grievous hurt.

EXAMINATION OF HAIR (TRICOLOGY)

The hair can be examined by naked eye and hand lens as well as by simple microscopy with adequate photomicrography. Certain features like spatial configuration (curl, wave) and physical features such as softness, brittleness etc. are apparent only by naked eye and with hand lens examination. The examination of hair can provide information relating to the purpose of identification and also it has evidentiary value.

Anatomy of Hair

Hair consists of a bulb or root and a shaft with distal termination of tip (Figure 5.36).

During the period of growth, the hair follicle lengthens and during its resting phase, the hair follicle shrinks, the hair ceases to grow and the hair bulb alters. This type of hair is readily shed and has shriveled, distorted bulb whereas the bulb of forcibly plucked

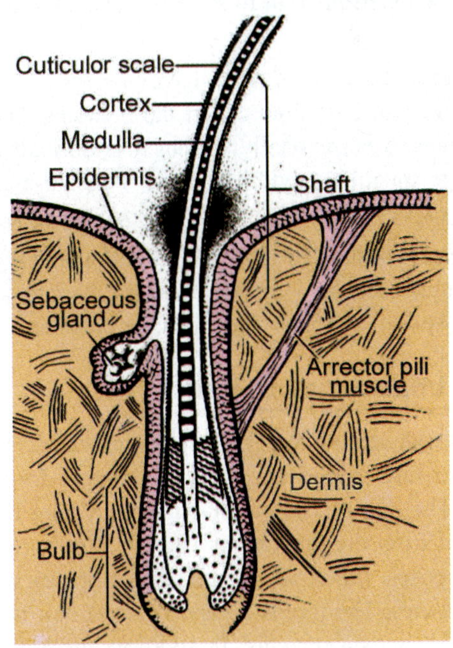

Figure 5.36: Different parts of hair

actively growing hair is rounder and much of the follicle is pulled out of the skin with the bulb.

Hair bulb: The bulb is formed within the follicle in the skin. To pluck a lock of healthily growing hair, considerable force is required.

Hair shaft: The hair shaft is composed of keratinized mass of cortex that forms the bulk of the hair, which has an outer scaly covering or cuticle and a central core, medulla.

Cuticle: The cuticle is a layer of thin, microscopic, nonpigmented scale like plates, each attached at its lower end to the hair cortex. The thickness of cuticle layer depends upon the thickness of individual scales and the degree of overlapping occurs. Cuticle is usually thin and sometimes thick consisting of ten to twenty layers of scales.

Cortex: The cortex forms most of the substance of a hair. It has abundant keratin that is responsible for the charring and acrid odour when the hair is burnt. The cortex is responsible for the strength, the elasticity and the shape of the hair. The cortex is made up of closely set, longitudinally arranged, elongated cells with pointed ends and without nuclei. The fibrils within these cells may have granules on their surface. The cells are held together by cement. The hair when stretched is narrowed and pigment granules are separated in longitudinal direction. Continued stretching causes hair to break and untreated hair is resistant to deforming stresses. The cortex is pigmented, the degree of pigmentation varies from complete absence and sometimes quite intense. A large range of natural colours is present in natural hair of humans. Animal hair may show alternate bands of pigment. Granular pigment of hair is easily seen in hair mounted in an isorefractile medium. Transverse sections of hair enable the distribution of the granules to be determined in relation to the center and periphery of the cortex.

Medulla: Many hairs also have a central, occasionally eccentric core that is hollow called the medulla. The hair is so darkly pigmented occasionally so that it is difficult to visualize medulla. The medullary width is quite variable along the hair shaft and is expressed in relation to the diameter of the shaft.

Tip: The tip of the hair is at its termination that is pointed and non-medullated. Repeated injuries cause the damage to the cuticle so that the exposed and unprotected cortex splits and frays.

Forensic Importance of Hair

Hair resists the destructive tendencies of adverse conditions such as exposure to gastric juice, prolonged drying, soaking and burial. The hair resists putrefaction for a long time and can be recovered from the graves many years after burial. For most forensic purposes, the durability of hair compares with most of the elastic tissues. The forensic importance of hair is to establish the identity of human remains. In addition, the hair is a source of establishing the association between a suspected person and a particular crime, or between a victim and a weapon or vehicle. From medicolegal point of view hair is important as: (i) Important clue is provided when the similar hair may be detected on the alleged weapon and on the body of alleged assailant. (ii) Victim's hair remains identifiable long after the commission of crime and provides valuable physical evidence. (iii) In rape and sodomy, the hair detected on the body of the victim and underclothing of the suspect will provide valuable corroboration. (iv) In bestiality, the presence of animal hair in and around the genitalia, body and clothing of the accused is important evidence. (v) In road traffic accidents, presence of hair of the victim adhering to the car will provide valuable evidentiary proof. (vi) Stains of mud on the hair are suggestive of road traffic accident in some muddy area or struggle in an open field. (vii) Pubic hair matted with seminal discharge may be suggestive of sexual offence. (viii) In asphyxial deaths, salivary stains are present sticking to beard and moustache. (ix) Blood stains on the body hair suggest assault. (x) Many poisonings such as arsenic, thallium and lead can be detected from hairs. (xi) In burns and close range firearm injuries, hair shows singeing. (xii) Age, sex, race and certain individual characters like bleaching, dyeing and waving of the hair can be deduced from examination that would help in individualization. (xiii) Nature of weapon whether sharp or blunt can be estimated from examination of hair. (xiv) Approximate time of death can be calculated from the growth of hair on the face. The growth rate is 0.4 mm per day. (xv) Colour of the hair along with evidence of dirt, grease sticking to the hair may give an idea about the occupation of the person.

The hair can be collected and fixed for transportation and storage by touching them with a sticky surface of transparent adhesive tape, and then pressing gently this tape to the glass slide. Isolated hair must be kept and labeled separately. When a sample of hair is submitted for examination, the following questions need to be answered from medicolegal point of view:

1. **Is the sample hair or some other fiber?** Few of the fibers can be burnt to note the source. Vegetable fibers burn readily without producing a disagreeable odour and leave sharply bent ends. Animal hair burn with difficulty, with odour of burnt feathers and show curved and rounded bead like ends. Human hair gets curled, blackish, brittle, shriveled, distorted and twisted. Human and animal hair consists of a root, cuticle, cortex and the medulla. Certain chemical tests with sulphuric acid and caustic soda can help in differentiating hair from the fiber. The appearance of cotton fibres may be mistaken for hair that appears microscopically as shown in Figure 5.37.

2. **Whether the hair of human or animal origin?** Certain gross and microscopic findings help to differentiate the human and animal hair that are summarized in the Table 5.21. The microscopical appearance of human and animal hair is shown in Figures 5.38 and 5.39.

Table 5.21: Differences between human and animal hair

Features	Human hair	Animal hair
General appearance	Thin, fine and usually brown or black coloured	Thick, coarse and may be different
Cuticle and cuticular scales	Short, broad and irregular margins are placed transversely. The pattern of cuticle is type VII of Moritz	Large with marked step like or wavy projections. The cuticle is other than type VII of Mortiz
Cortex	Well striated and broad; 4-10 times broader than medulla	Narrow, rarely more than twice or as broad as medulla
Medulla	Continuous, narrow, fragmented or absent sometimes	Continuous, broader and always present
Medullary index = $\frac{\text{Diameter of the medulla}}{\text{Diameter of hair shaft}}$	Less than 0.3	More than 0.5 (3.5)
Deposition of pigment granules	Concentrated towards periphery of the cortex and is usually light in the medulla and may not be continuous	Heavy deposition in the medulla may be uniform, central or peripheral
Precipitin test	Specific to humans	Specific to animals

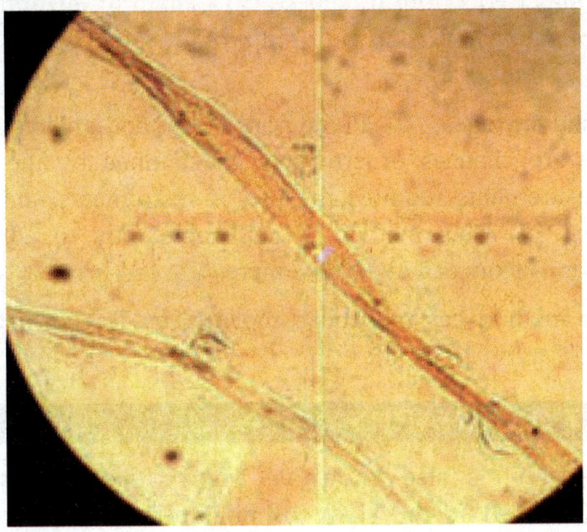

Figure 5.37: Microscopical appearance of cotton fibre

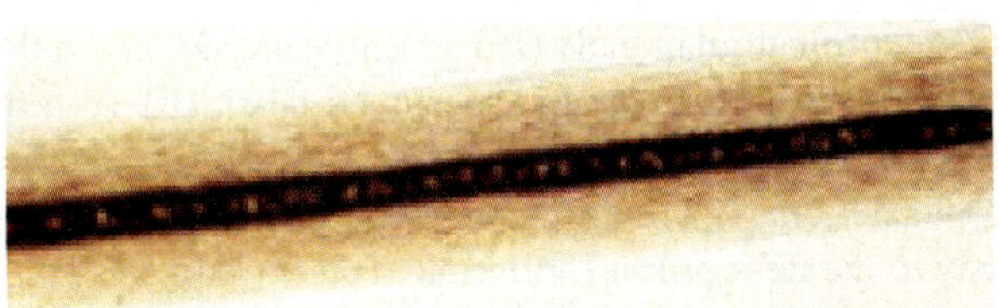

Figure 5.38: Microscopical appearance of animal hair

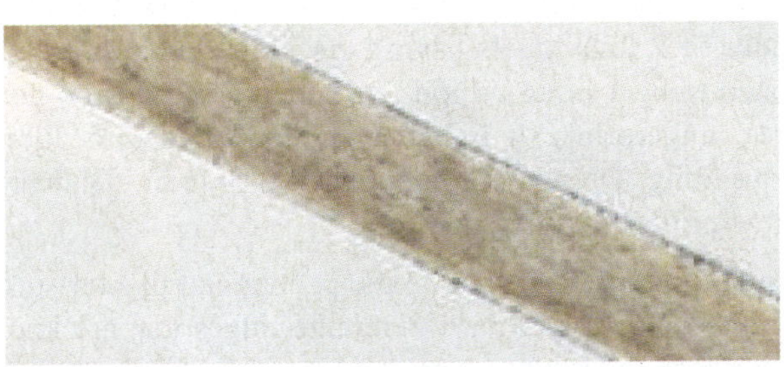

Figure 5.39: Microscopical appearance of human hair

3. **If the hair is human, part of body from where it is derived?** The length of the hair and colour etc. are noted to determine that to which part of the body does it belong. The characteristic features of hair derived from various body parts are: (i) Scalp hairs are long, soft and taper towards the tip. They are circular on cross-section. (ii) Beard and moustache hair are straight, thick and triangular on cross-section. (iii) Axillary and pubic hairs are short, wavy and curly with split ends. They are oval on cross-section. (iv) Eyebrow, eyelashes and nostril hair are thick, straight, bristly, stiff and tapering. They are triangular and kidney shaped on cross-section. (v) Body hairs are soft, fine and flexible. They do not show pigment cells in cortex and the medulla is thin. (vi) Downy hair of foetus or newborn lack medulla and have no pigment cells.

4. **Is the hair of male or female?** The hair in male are thick, coarse and dark compared to that in case of females. Beard and moustache are specific to males. Upper boarder of pubic hair is classically almost horizontal in the female and rises towards the umbilicus in the males. Some physiological and pathological conditions cause gross alterations of hair growth such as hirsutism particularly in females. The **Barr bodies** can be detected in the hair bulb in about 70% of females and only about 7% of the males.

5. **The race of the person to whom hair belongs?** Indians have dark and fine hair; of Japanese and Chinese are dark, coarse and straight whereas those of Negroes are curly and wooly.

6. **What is the age of the person to whom the hair belongs?** The age of the person can be deduced from the hair but within certain limits. The lanugo hairs of the newborn are fine, downy, soft and nonpigmented. These hairs are non-medullated and cuticular scales have smooth and free edges. The hairs of an adult are coarser, pigmented and medullated

having a complex cuticular pattern. Grey hairs are apparent after the third decade of life and are devoid of any pigment. Balding in man may begin in the second or third decade. In females, there is often loss of axillary hair and increase of facial hair at menopause.

7. **Has the hair been dyed, bleached or is there any evidence of disease?** The hair colour can be changed artificially by dyeing or bleaching. To bleach dark hair, hydrogen peroxide is used and to render grey hair dark natural colourants such as *henna*, plant juices or hair dyes are used. People working in certain industries have their hair dyed automatically. Those in copper factories may have greenish hue in the hair, miners working with cobalt exhibit bluish tint. Bleached or coloured hairs are dry, brittle, lusterless and rough. The scalp is also coloured with the hair and the colouring is not uniform. The newly growing hair will be of the original colour. The hair colour is lighter in diseases such as kwashiorkor, malnutrition, and certain vitamin deficiencies. The use of hair dyes produces local dermatitis.
8. **Was the hair pulled or did it fall naturally?** If the hair has fallen naturally, the hair root is distorted and atrophied and the hair sheath is absent whereas when it is forcibly extracted, the hair sheath is ruptured. In case of forcible extraction, the hair bulb is swollen, larger and irregular but when the hair has fallen naturally, the hair bulb has smooth, rounded end.
9. **If there is presence of any injury to the hair and the nature of injury?** Repeated injury to the tip of the hair damages the cuticle and the exposed cortex splits and frays. Blunt force injury and cutting hair by blunt scissors result in flattening and splitting of hair shaft. The hairs cut by a sharp weapon have a clean uniform cut surface. Hair when singed are swollen, fragile, curled and twisted. They emit a peculiar odour and from them the carbon deposits can be detected.
10. **Is there any relation with sexual assault?** In rape and sodomy, the hair detected on the victim or undergarments of accused are important corroborative proof.

ANTHROPOMETRY (BERTILLION'S SYSTEM)

In 1883, **Alphonse Bertillon** a French Law enforcement officer and biometric researcher created anthropometry, an identification system based on unchanging physical measurements that was the first scientific system police used to identify criminals. He found that several physical features and the dimensions of certain bones or bony structures in the body remain practically constant throughout adult life. He concluded that these measurements can be used to distinguish a person from the other. **This system is based on fourteen identical measurements**, a standardised photographic portrait (frontal and profile), the classification of facial and body characteristics, and the notation of scars and tattoos. These were recorded on cards that were filed according to a complex method, so that they could be matched and retrieved. Bertillon's system (called anthropometry, *bertillonage*, or *signaletics*) was adopted by police departments and correction systems in many jurisdictions in Europe and America.

Principle: As the body measurements are not expected to change after 21-22 years (except stature), this method is only applicable to adults after 21 years.

Data to be recorded: (i) Descriptive data such as hair, eyes, complexion, shape of nose, ears, chin, iris colour etc. (ii) Bodily marks like moles, scar, tattoo etc. (iii) Bodily measurements such as: (a) Height (b) Stretch that is length of body from left shoulder to right middle finger when arm is raised (c) Bust that is length of torso from head to seat, taken when seated (d) Length of head from crown to forehead (e) Width of head from temple to temple (f) Length of right ear (g) Length of left foot (h) Length of left middle finger (i) Length of left cubit from elbow to tip of middle finger (j) Width of cheeks (k) Length of left little finger (iv) Photographs of front and right profile views of the head and face are also taken.

Disadvantages: (i) Photographs are not always reliable as there are chances of error when examined by the experts (ii) Measurements requires the use of instruments and trained operators (iii) This method is applicable only to adults (iv) Calculation errors can always be there.

The method has now been replaced by fingerprint system (Dactylography).

DACTYLOGRAPHY

Dactylography is also known as **Henry Galton System** of identification. It is the study of fingerprints as a method of identification. The ultimate positive identification of the dead body presented in an unidentified state is a major goal of the medicolegal expert. There are many reasons to establish effective positive identification namely (i) To resolve the anxiety of the next of kin of a person missing and presumed dead. (ii) To settle the estate of the person missing and assumed dead. (iii) To establish the corpus delicti. (iv) To allow the medicolegal official to release the body to the next of kin for burial.

Since the turn of the century, fingerprints have been used as a very effective means of establishing identity of the individual. It is a most accurate and unfailing method of positive identification. The odds of 2 individuals having the same fingerprint had been estimated to be 1 in 64 billion, even identical twins do not have identical fingerprints. It is better method of identification than DNA profiling. DNA profiling would be same in identical twins but fingerprints are different.

Introduction: The skin on the palmar and planter surface is certainly wrinkled with narrow minute ridges that are known as friction ridges and is also completely free from hair and sebaceous glands. However, there is profusion of sweat glands. **The dermal carvings or fingerprints appear for the first time from the 12-16 weeks of intrauterine life and their formation gets completed by 24th week, i.e., 6th month I.U. life**. The ridge thus formed during the foetal period does not change the course of alignment throughout the life of the individual until destroyed by mutilation.

Fundamental Principles of Fingerprinting

First principle: Fingerprinting is an individual characteristic; no two fingers have been observed to possess identical ridge characteristic.

Second principle: A fingerprint will remain unchanged during an individual's lifetime. Though it is not possible to change one's fingerprint, there has been no lack of effort on the part of criminals to obliterate them. If an injury reaches deeply enough into the skin and damages dermal papillae, a permanent scar will form. For this to happen such a wound would have to penetrate 1-2 mm beneath the skin's surface. Presence of such permanent scars would serve as a new and additional characteristic for the purpose of identification.

Third principle: Fingerprinting has general ridge characteristics that permit them to be systemically classified.

Absence of fingerprint: **Adermatoglyphyia** (immigration delay disease) is a rare genetic disorder in which there is absence of ridges on fingers and toes as well as on the palms and soles. It is an autosomal dominant condition associated with mutated SMARCARD1 gene. **Naegeli syndrome** is a rare autosomal dominant form of ectodermal dysplasia associated with mutated KRT14 gene in which there is also absence of fingerprints. The fingerprint-based identification is not possible in these cases.

Loss of fingerprint: It is associated with **Hand-foot syndrome**, which is developed due to adverse of various chemotherapeutic agents used for cancer treatment like **capecitabine**. There are many **dermatological conditions** which causes temporary loss of fingerprint like lepromatous leprosy, lichen planus, secondary syphilis etc.

History of fingerprinting: In the B.C. era, fingerprints were used on pottery to indicate the make and brand. Clay slabs with fingerprints nearly 3000 years old have been found in Intan khanan and tomb in Egypt. Thumbprints were used as official seals or documents by Chinese emperors since 240 B.C. The work of **Grew (1684) and Biloo (1685)** are among the earliest scientific descriptions of dermatoglyphics.

Purkinje's contribution in **1823** is an important landmark because he classified the varieties of finger patterns systematically for the first time. He pursued a treatise commenting upon diversity of ridge pattern on the tips of fingers and distinguished a variety of patterns of fingerprints.

W.J. Herschel in 1858 began the first known official use of fingerprints in India on a large scale. He used it to prevent fraudulent collection of army pay accounts and for purposes of identity on other documents. **Henry Faulds in 1880** wrote a comment on practical use of fingerprints for identification of criminals.

Francis Galton began his observations around 1890 and published his book on fingerprints in 1892. He established the individuality and permanence of fingerprints and devised the first scientific method of classifying fingerprints.

Juan Vucetich in 1891 installed fingerprint files as an official means of criminal identification. He based his system on the patterns identified by Galton.

The first fingerprint bureau in the world was officially established in Calcutta in June 1897. In 1901, fingerprinting for criminal identification was officially introduced in England and Wales. Edward Richard Henry, IG of police in Lower Bengal did extensive study on fingerprints to develop a register for classification of fingerprints. The system of **Henry and Vucetich** forms the basis of modern ten digit fingerprint identification.

Importance of Fingerprinting

(i) Identification of criminals whose fingerprints are found at the scene of crime (ii) Identification of fugitive through fingerprinting comparisons (iii) Assistance to prosecutors in presenting their cases in the light of defendants' previous records (iv) Exchange of criminal identifying information with identification bureau of foreign countries in cases of mutual interest (v) Assistance to probation or parole officers and to parole board for their enlightenment in decision making (vi) Imposition of more equitable sentences by the Courts (vii) Identification of persons and maintenance of identity records (service or criminal) (viii) Identification of unknown deceased persons (ix) Identification of persons suffering from amnesia (x) Recognition by the government of honored dead (xi) Identification of disaster work (xii) Prevention of hospital mistakes in the identification of infants (xiii) Identification of missing persons (xiv) Identification of licensing procedures for automobiles, firearms (xv) Identification of unconscious person (xvi) Problems of mistaken identity (xvii) Establishing correct identity in cases of kidnapping (xviii) Detection of bank forgeries (xix) This uniqueness makes fingerprints a good modality for biometric identification including national registration, immigration, building and door access, and other settings.

Classes of Fingerprints

All fingerprints are divided into three major classes on the basis of their general pattern (Figure 5.40). These are:

- ***Loops 60-70% (67%):*** Ridges start on one side then run parallely and end on the same side. May be medial (ulnar) loop or lateral (radial) loop.

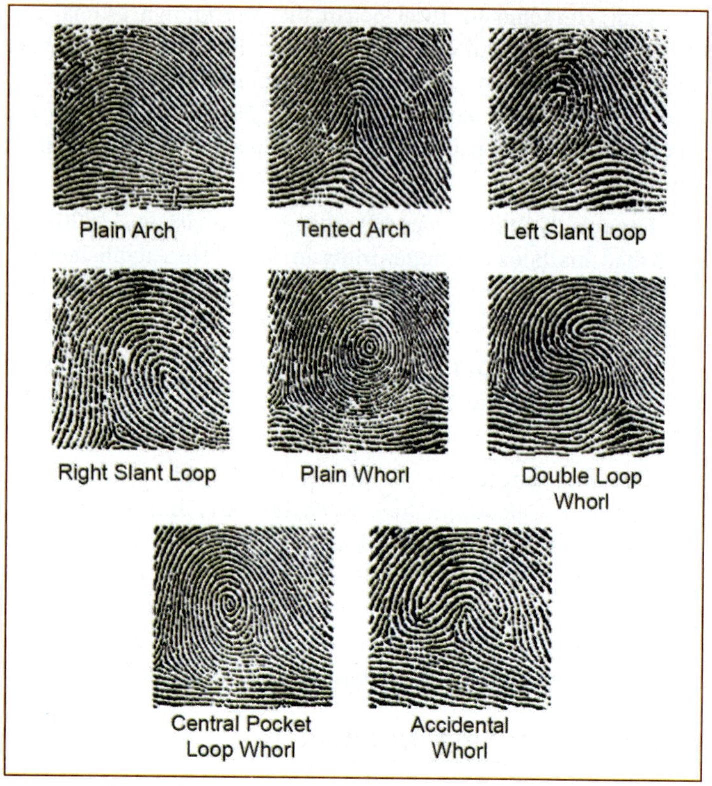

Figure 5.40: Various classes of fingerprints

- ***Arches 5-10% (6-7%):*** Ridges start on one side and after a backward course end on the opposite side.
- ***Whorls 30-35% (25%):*** Multiple circular or oval ridges one around another.
- ***Composite 1-2%:*** Combination of more than one pattern.
- ***Accidental:*** No specific ridge pattern.

Characteristics of fingerprints: Each fingerprint being different from the other but all fingerprints have common characteristics among themselves (Figure 5.41), which are:

1. **Pattern area:** It is that part of a loop or whorl in which appears the core, deltas and ridges with which we are concerned in identifying.
2. **Type line:** Are ridges that determine the pattern area of loops and whorls. Arches lack presence of type line.
3. **Delta or triradius:** It is formed when a ridge bifurcates and the two arms of the bifurcating ridge diverge or when two adjacent ridges running side by side diverge causing an interspace within which the pattern lies.
4. **Core:** Core is the central portion of the pattern and the type of core varies with the type of pattern.

The three basic pattern types arch, loop and whorl are subdivided into nine subtypes for the purpose of classification.

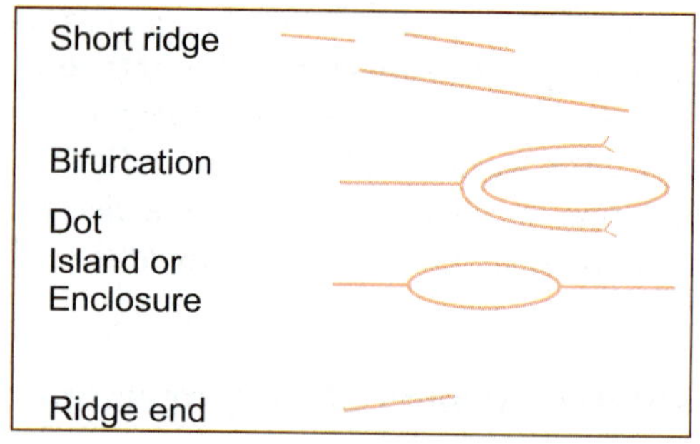

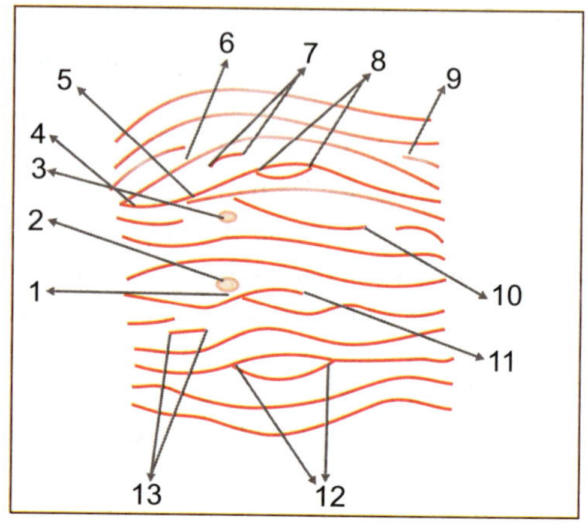

Figure 5.41: Characteristics of fingerprints: (1) Bifurcation (2) Dot (3) Dot (4) Bifurcation (5) Bifurcation (6) Ridge end (7) Short ridge (8) Island (9) Ridge end (10) Ridge end (11) Ridge end (12) Island (13) Short ridge

Basic pattern	Pattern type	Symbol	No. of deltas present
Arch	i. Plain	A	Nil
	ii. Tented	T	Nil
Loop	i. Radial	R	One
	ii. Ulnar	U	One
Whorl	i. Plain	W	Two
	ii. Central pocketed loop	C	Two
	iii. Double loop		
	–Lateral pocket loop	S	Two
	–Twinned loop	S	Two
	iv. Accidentals	X	Two or more than two

Types of fingerprints obtained at the scene: The form of fingerprints obtained at a scene of crime may be classified under the following categories:

1. **Visible prints:** These are visible to the naked eye, they may be formed when a visible or coloured contaminants are present on the fingers of the perpetrator, it will leave a visible print, for example a blood print, an inked print, a colour print, a paint print, a dirt print. These visible prints are photographed directly for the purpose of comparison and maintenance of records.
2. **Plastic prints:** Formed when the fingers or the palm comes in contact with soft surface such as soap, butter, wax, soft

putty, tar, grease or freshly painted surface. Plastic prints should not be dusted with fingerprint powder and should not be photographed with the help of direct or side lighting.

3. **Latent prints:** These are such impressions that are not visible to the naked eye. Whenever the fingers or palm come in contact with any polished or smooth surface, they leave an invisible image on that surface of contact due to perspiration. This invisible image of fingers or palm is known as latent fingerprint. Sweat glands become more active when a person is nervous or excited and the hands perspire more than normal during this state of mind. Thus, a perpetrator of crime leaves behind invisible print impressions on whatever surface he touches during the act. The latent finger impressions then detected are converted to visible prints through fingerprint powders and chemical sprayer solutions so that they may be photographed, preserved and used for identification.

Printing of fingerprints: Fingerprint impressions thus obtained are a reverse of actual pattern on the skin surface. The essential material needed to obtain fingerprints include Printer's ink, paper or card, inking slab, inking rubber or cotton pad, benzene, alcohol, kerosene or gasoline and soap. Fingerprint impressions can be obtained as:

1. **Rolled impressions:** By nail to nail rolling of fingers.
2. **Plain or dab prints:** These are unrolled impressions obtained by direct contact.

For rolled prints, following precautions should be taken: (i) Hands should be properly wiped. (ii) Arm should be kept relaxed and not try to help in rolling the fingers. (iii) Rolling of the fingers and thumb should be in the following manner, the thumb should be rolled towards the subject's body and the fingers are rolled away from the body that is thumb in and fingers out. (iv) Not too much ink should be used or excessive pressure applied on the fingers. (v) Unglazed papers are better for fingerprints. (vi) If a particular finger is missing or is so defective or deformed that it is not possible to obtain an impression, this fact should be specified in ink on the space allotted for that. (vii) Deformities on fingers like cut marks, scars shall be fully described and it should be noted whether they are temporary or permanent in nature.

Fingerprints Classification System

There are over fifty classification systems in use in different countries that are based on Galton, Henry and Vucetish systems. The famous ten digit classification systems and the single digit classification involve less famous features. Of these systems the best known is the **Battley system.** The classification of fingerprint is a method through which the fingerprint impressions are transformed into a formula to facilitate the recording and searching of the fingerprints. In the ten-digit system, it is analyzed under the following seven systems:

1. **Primary classification system (Henry system):** Scores are allotted for presence of whorl pattern in different fingers of each hand.

Whorl in right thumb or right index finger	16 scores
Whorl in right middle or ring finger	8 scores for each place
Whorl in right little finger or left thumb	4 scores
Whorl in left index or middle finger	2 scores
Whorl in left ring or left little finger	1 score
Fingers where no whorls	No scores

Scores are then arranged as $\frac{\text{R.T.+R.R.+L.T.+L.M.+L.L.+1}}{\text{R.T.+R.M.+R.L.+L.I.+L.R.+1}}$

1 is added for the purpose of calculation. The total score of numerator is multiplied by denominator. (2) Major division system (3) Secondary classification system (4) Sub-secondary classification system (5) Second sub-secondary classification system (6) Final classification system (7) Key classification system (For the right thumb only).

After the complete analysis of the seven systems, the complete Ten digit formula may be represented in the following manner for fingerprint for maintenance of records at each step (i) Key (ii) Major (iii) Primary (iv) Secondary (v) Sub-secondary (vi) Second sub-secondary (vii) Final.

Latent Fingerprints

Powdering and lifting latent impressions: A black or grey fingerprint powder is adequate in most places. Black powder should be used for light coloured and white objects and grey powder for black or dark coloured backgrounds. Among other powders, aluminium powder is used as a substitute for grey powder. The Dragon's blood (a natural powder) may be employed on both dark and light coloured surfaces. A fluorescent type of powder is used for developing latent prints on multicoloured surfaces.

Magnetic brush and powders are used to increase the efficiency in development of latent prints. The magnetic brush marks with magnetic powders only, which are available in many colours grey, black, red, yellow etc. The two types of lifting medium employed in latent fingerprint work are: (i) Transparent cellulose tape in 1.5 or 2.0-inch width rolls (ii) Opaque rubber lifter.

Chemical methods of developing latent prints: Perspiration consists of about 98% water with traces of salts like sodium, chloride, sulphates, phosphates, carbamates, lactic acid, fatty acid, glucose and urea. Chemical methods make use of the presence of chlorides, which will react with chemicals to produce visible prints. The following methods are used:

- **The Iodine method:** Made visible by the absorption of iodine fumes that react with fatty acids. The ridges of the print appear yellowish brown or brownish against the background. It is used for old prints.
- **Silver nitrate method:** Sodium chloride reacts with silver nitrate to form silver chloride, which is an unstable white substance that darkens when exposed to light breaking in

to silver and chlorine that appear reddish brown against background.

- **Ninhydrin method:** Reacts to amino acids and gives purple reddish brown stains.
- **Osmium tetraoxide method:** It is used for recent prints. In the presence of fatty substance, osmium tetraoxide is reduced to free osmium that is dark in colour.
- **Chemical print method:** Trade name in aerosol type container used as spray.
- **Hydrofluoric method:** On glass, waxy substance of the print itself repels the liquid.
- **Tannic acid method:** Sets the albumin making the latent prints visible.
- **Osmic acid method:** Osmic acid spray when exposed to light turns black.
- **Mercuric iodide method:** Fumes of mercuric iodide are used.
- **Bromine method:** Bromine vapours are used.
- **Reducing agents:** Organic reducing agents like amidol, pyrogallol or hydroquinone is used.
- **Fleming's reagent method:** Mixture of osmic acid, chromic acid and glacial acetic acid is exposed to diazine fast yellow dye that fluoresces in UV light.

Factors making satisfactory fingerprinting of dead body difficult: Wrinkled skin of the finger pads resulting from immersion of the body in water and injection of air or various liquids into fingerpads has been advocated.

If immersion is prolonged or decomposition is advanced or in some instances of radiant burns, the skin of the hands and fingers can be peeled away from the underlying tissue. Fingerprints can be made by inserting the technicians finger into the 'skin glove' inking the area to be printed and rolling. Where the epidermis is absent, skin can be used for producing useful fingerprints.

In dead bodies with contractures and with decomposing tissues, removal of the fingers from hands may permit more satisfactory printing.

Points of comparison between two fingerprints: (i) Ridge pattern (ii) Ridge endings (iii) Missing ridge (iv) Gap in two ridges (v) Ridge breaking (vi) Ridge bifurcation (vii) Ridge reunion (viii) A dot in ridge gap (ix) A stud in ridge (x) An island formation (xi) A lake formation (xii) A dot in the lake (xiii) Union of two ridges (xiv) Starting of a new ridge in between two ridges (xv) Presence of a scar (xvi) Distance between delta and core (xvii) Number of ridges between delta and core (xviii) Direction of any particular ridge.

Points necessary for establishing complete identity: Different countries have developed their **minimum number of points** for establishing complete identity of the fingerprints based on their personal practical experience for presentation before the Court. These are:

France 16, Australia 12, Japan 12-14, Canada 10-16, Interpol 12, US 7-12, Spain 10-12, New Zealand 8-12, Israel 10-12.

In India, Maharashtra 12, Assam 7-12, Kerala 7, West Bengal 6, Madras 8-10, Bihar 7, Orissa 5-7, Central Fingerprints Bureau (Calcutta) 9.

In 1973, the first All India Forensic Science Congress held at Srinagar adopted a resolution stating that the minimum number of points for establishing the identity beyond doubt in case of fingerprint examination should be fixed at 8. However, if there are 6 or 7 points of identity a qualified opinion can be offered by the expert on his responsibility.

The fingerprint experts of **New Scotland Yard**, London however recommended that at least **16 identical points** should be established. Certain American experts are of the opinion that at least 12 identical points should be established. **US, FBI** is of the opinion that if there are **12 points** of similarities in the two impressions, the identity is absolute.

Certain Indian experts are of the view that in partially blurred or smudged impressions, 3 identical points are sufficient to establish the identity. Supreme Court in 1978 upheld the opinion on 8 points. Under **section 293 Cr.P.C.**, the report of the director of a fingerprint bureau is admissible as evidence without his physical presence in the Court.

Maintenance of fingerprint records: Federal Bureau of Investigation (F.B.I.) USA maintains more than two crores of fingerprints. There is systemic maintenance of separate files for different types of prints. In 60% of the world population there is no whorl in any finger, so according to primary classification, the score is one. On the basis of this scoring, 1,024 divisions are made called **pigeon holes.**

Poroscopy

Poroscopy was described by **Locard.** The ridges on the fingers and hands are studded with microscopic pores, formed by mouths of ducts of subepidermal sweat glands. Each millimeter of a ridge contains 9-18 pores. These are permanent and immutable during life and vary in size, shape, position, extent and number over a given length of ridge in each individual. This method of examining pores is called poroscopy and is useful when only fragments of fingerprints are available.

Electronography

X-rays propagate themselves by a waveform motion just as does visible light. It was discovered by German physicist Plank that in some instances X-rays behave more as bullets or bundles called quanta. This means that X-rays are able to cause the ejection of electrons from their orbits round the nucleus of the atom and impart to these electrons a velocity which carries them away from the parent atom to become photoelectrons. This particular characteristic of X-rays can be used for a technique known as electronography. Electronography is a method whereby metallic elements can be made to produce a recordable emission when irradiated by a high kilovoltage monochromatic X-ray beam. For the proper functioning of electronographic technique, primary beam should be capable of causing the ejection of electrons and it must be so homogenous and of such a short wavelength that it does not itself have a photographic effect.

Emission electronography: Here X-ray beam is first passed through a copper filter of 1 cm thickness. This was found to be the optimum thickness of copper necessary to remove all the soft wavelength components and render the beam practically homogenous. The use of the emission electronographic method for the visualization of routine fingerprints is more advantageous. This method substitutes for the multiplicity of factors involved in the other techniques such as lights, lenses, focusing, positioning, black and grey powders, fluorescent substances, UV light etc. This is a routine procedure, which results in a well-defined print against a clear background.

The pure metallic powders are admittedly, not so adherent to the fingerprint deposit as are the grey and black powders. They can, if necessary be brushed off and the normal police powders reapplied to the fingerprint deposit. The demonstration then carried out by the present methods. Thus, there is never any danger or detriment to the fingerprint deposit by trying the electronographic method. If the normal police practice fails to satisfy in a particular case, the metallic element can be sieved over the already treated print. It will adhere to it and the electronographic method can be used.

Method: To the fingerprint deposit, metallic powder is to be applied by sieving it through a 400-mesh sieve so that it drops in a free fall on to the suspected area. The excess powder is removed by blowing or tapping leaving the fingerprinting visualized against its background. Recording film should be mounted on the fingerprint and in intimate contact with it. If the object can be enclosed in a cassette, it is placed in the cassette containing a layer of clear film.

The recording film is then placed with its emulsion surface in contact with the treated print. This is again covered with a layer of clear film. The cassette is then closed with cardboard packing to ensure intimate film object contact. The cassette with suitably selected filters on top is placed under the X-ray tube. An X-ray exposure is given and backgrounds are eliminated entirely and the palm prints stand out quite clearly.

This technique can be applied to metallic objects also. In case of metallic objects, extremely differential results can be obtained. This is because finely powdered lead dust emits much more readily under the action of the primary beam than does the lead sheet.

Grenz Rays

Grenz ray unit is also extremely useful in many fingerprint investigations, especially when used in conjunction with Polaroid papers. It is simpler to use than electronography and provides an immediate result. Its only application is to objects that can be penetrated by the beam and are of a fairly homogenous structure.

FOOTPRINTS

The offender at the scene of crime may also leave footprints. It can be of barefooted person or of the shoes. Small portion of footprint or shoe is sufficient for comparison. In case of shoe print, primary markings are caused by the make of shoes, soles and secondary markings are caused by changes due to usage. The footprints are used for identification of offenders and as well as of newborn children in hospitals.

LIP PRINTS (CHEILOSCOPY)

Lip prints can be found over wine glass, love letters, on private parts etc. **Le Moyne Sunder** (1950) pointed out that wrinkles and cracks of lips have certain individualistic characteristics like fingerprints. Japanese authors **Kazuo Suzuki and Yasuo Tsuchihashi** 1970 classified lipprints in the following ways (Figure 5.42): (i) *Type I or long vertical grooves:* Clear cut lines or grooves running vertically across the lip. (ii) *Type II or short vertical grooves:* Vertical or straight grooves that disappear half way into the lip instead of covering entire breadth of lip but incomplete length. (iii) *Type II or branching grooves:* These are grooves that branch or fork. (iv) *Type III or diamond grooves:* These are grooves that intersect. (v) *Type IV or reticular grooves:* Reticular or net like. (vi) *Type V or other types:* These include the rectangular or other non-classifiable irregular lip prints.

NAIL STRIATIONS

Striations over nails are said to be permanent but diseases destroying the nails can affect them.

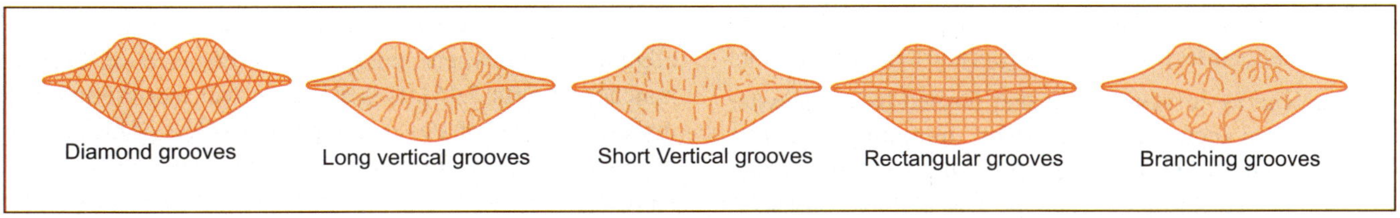

Figure 5.42: Different types of lip prints

PALATOPRINTS

Rugae present over the anterior third of palate are also considered permanent and can be used for identification.

FRONTAL SINUSES

Frontal sinuses can be found in over 95% of the population and they can be compared with fingerprints. Like fingerprints, sinus patterns are unique for the person, the structure is permanent and fixed. Unlike fingerprints the bony sinuses can very rarely be altered by infection or injury. The frontal sinuses are classified based on: (i) Size of each frontal sinus (ii) Comparison between right and left frontal sinuses (iii) Polar coordinate dimensions from frontal sinus prints.

X-ray of the skull is taken in occipitomental plane and the comparison is made to the line of frontal septum, upper border of the sinuses, partial septa and supraorbital ridges.

TATTOO MARKS

Tattoo marks are fairly good for identification of both living and dead. It gives wide range of identification information about the persons. The identity, mental makeup, social status, desires and inclinations of the person can be known from tatoo marks.

They provide information about identification, nationality, religion, God, Goddess (Figure 5.43), occupation, name of person/relative/lover, language, habits such as drug addiction etc. Tattoo of flower, obscene figure or God of worship describes information about mental makeup of the person.

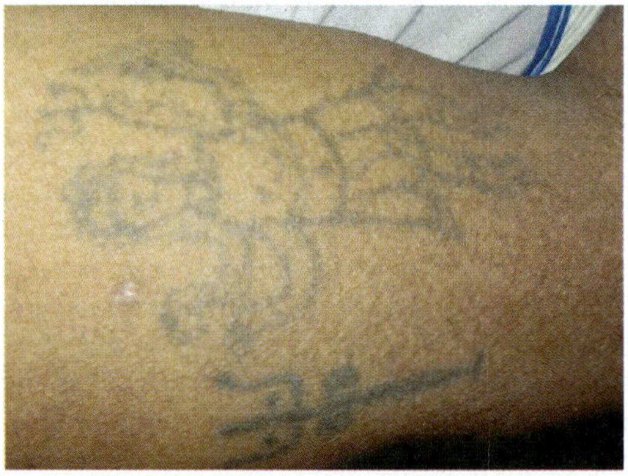

Figure 5.43: Tattoo mark of Goddess

Faded tattoo marks can be made visible by rubbing, by UV light or by burning. In dead bodies tattoo pigment may be found in regional lymph glands at autopsy. Artificial obliteration strongly suggests that the person is trying to conceal his identity. Tattoo in few cases may cause infection, sepsis, ulcers and keloid formation.

Tattooing can be involuntary as that formed by gunpowder or voluntary when they are produced by imprinting pigments of different colours in the dermis, by multiple puncture method mechanically or by electrical device. The pigment used in tattooing are carbon dust, Indian ink, Prussian blue, vermillion or lead tetroxide etc. The duration of tattoo is fairly permanent and can even stay for life if the pigment is introduced in the dermis or on covered parts of the body. They may fade if the pigments are placed in the subepithelial level or exposed parts of the body due to sunlight or on those parts which undergo constant friction for 8-10 years. They can be removed by surgical operation, local use of corrosive agents, electrolysis, by dissolving the pigments and washing them away, by applying carbon dioxide snow and by inflicting deep burns over the area.

SUPERIMPOSITION

It is the technique by which a particular skull recovered can be matched with the photograph. It is very helpful for identification. **Professor Brash** in 1935 first suggested that the photographs of the missing person and the skull could be superimposed as an identification technique. Since then various scientists have utilized this technique in many criminal cases. Mr. G. Webster gives a detailed description of the superimposition technique adopted in the Plumbago Pit case. Recently in the Corn field crime case of Peru, Dr. Basauri P also used superimposed photographs, besides forensic odontology, for identification purposes. In all these cases the technique generally adopted has been described as follows:

More recent photograph is better (Figure 5.44). Even photograph of lateral view can be used.

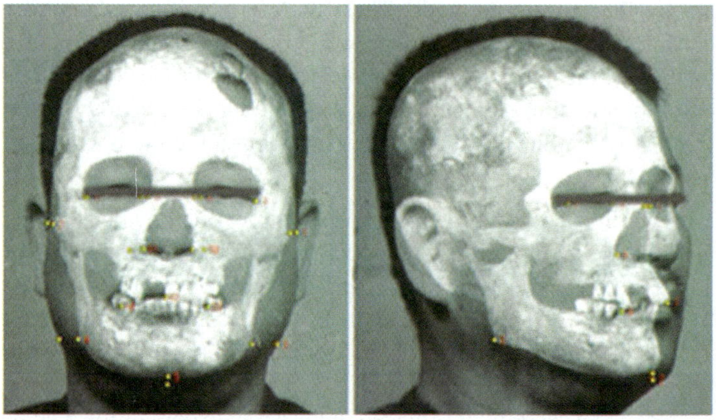

Figure 5.44: Superimposition image of a skull and facial photo

From the original photograph a negative retake is made. Two negatives are prepared one of the persons and the other of the skull. The original photograph may be a bust, a full length photo of the individual or a group photograph. In any case only the face is reproduced on the negative of definite format.

Appropriate magnification is done to achieve maximum alignment and where interpupillary distance of both exactly matches (Figure 5.45). It is a known fact that the interpupillary distance of a person never changes regardless of his age. The two negatives are then superimposed by keeping over each other and various points are compared. The contours, soft tissue thickness and anatomical relationship on the superimposition image are

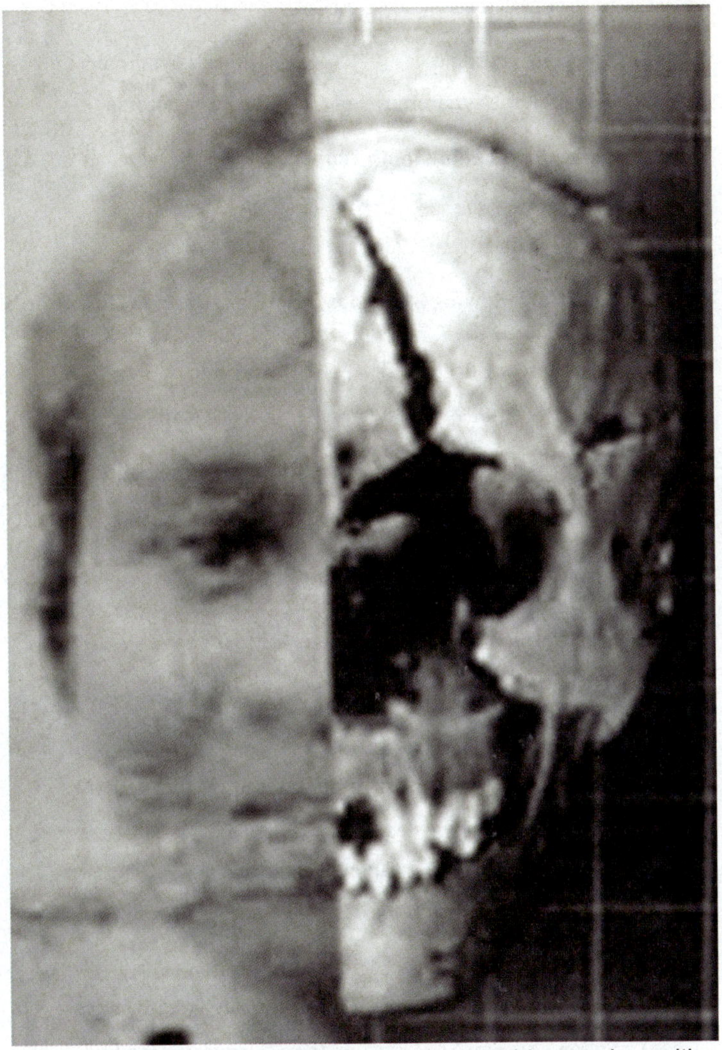

Figure 5.45: Comparison involved in photographic superimposition

examined to judge whether or not the unknown skull is of the presumed person. A computer assisted superimposition system for improving the accuracy and rapidity for identity has been developed.

The canthus, nasion, nasal spine and lower border of nose and upper jaw, supraorbital ridges, angle of jaw, external auditory meatus and teeth etc. are compared and a photograph is taken which is analysed for similarities and dissimilarities to arrive at a conclusion.

In this technique there is often criticism that there is nothing scientific in adjusting the size of the negative image of the skull to fit in with the image of the face. In fact, it is possible to fit a skull with photographs of different persons. Also the real size of the face has not been brought about in the above technique. To be more scientific, the two negatives should be enlarged to the life size, independently, and they should then be superimposed.

This test has more of negative value as it can definitely rule out a combination of a photo and a skull though only a possibility of a match can be established.

LONG QUESTIONS

1. What is identification? Discuss various points to establish the identity of a person.
2. Define and describe Corpus Delicti. Enumerate the points to identify a living person.
3. How you will proceed to determine the age of a person of 16 years? What is its medicolegal significance?
4. Discuss the medicolegal aspects of age.
5. Discuss the role of dentition in age determination.
6. Discuss in detail the various aspects of forensic odontology and its application in identification of a person.
7. Discuss in detail the medicolegal significance of dactylography.
8. What is the medicolegal significance of hair?

SHORT QUESTIONS

1. Intersex.
2. Tattoo marks.
3. Superimposition.
4. Scar.
5. Sutures of skull.
6. Dactylography.
7. Latent fingerprints.
8. Poroscopy.
9. Electronography.
10. Klinefelter's syndrome.
11. Turner's syndrome.
12. Difference between temporary and permanent teeth.
13. Difference between male and female skull.
14. Difference between male and female mandible.
15. Difference between male and female sacrum.
16. Differentiate between animal and human hair.
17. Difference between male and female pelvis.
18. Lip prints.

MULTIPLE CHOICE QUESTIONS

1. In Turner's syndrome the chromosomal pattern is:

(a) 46 XY (b) 45 XO
(c) 47 XXY (d) 48 XXY

2. The chin in cases of male looks:

(a) Triangular (b) Square
(c) Rounded (d) Flattened

3. **The degree of accuracy in sexing adult skeleton remains for pelvis alone is:**
   (a) 80 percent (b) 85 percent
   (c) 95 percent (d) 98 percent

4. **Hair usually starts appearing as in pubic region in females at the age of:**
   (a) 11 years (b) 13 years
   (c) 15 years (d) 16 years

5. **For the contract marriage the age of in female should be:**
   (a) 15 years (b) 16 years
   (c) 17 years (d) 18 years

6. **Rule of Haase was formulated to calculate the:**
   (a) Age (b) Sex
   (c) Stature (d) None of the above

7. **Cheiloscopy is used to identify a person from:**
   (a) Palato prints (b) Lip prints
   (c) Foot prints (d) Fingerprints

8. **Total number of teeth at the age of 8 years in females is:**
   (a) 12 (b) 16
   (c) 20 (d) 24

9. **The appearance of centre of ossification in case of olecranon is:**
   (a) 5 years (b) 7 years
   (c) 9 years (d) 11 years

10. **The most common pattern of fingerprint is:**
    (a) Loop (b) Whirl
    (c) Arch (d) Composite

11. **The different pieces of sternal body become a single one at the age of:**
    (a) 16 years (b) 20 years
    (c) 25 years (d) 30 years

12. **The anterior fontanelle usually closes between:**
    (a) 6-9 months (b) 9-12 months
    (c) 12-18 months (d) 18-24 months

13. **For an offence of kidnapping of a female from lawful guardianship, the age of the female must be below:**
    (a) 16 years (b) 18 years
    (c) 21 years (d) 25 years

14. **Absence of fingerprints found in:**
    (a) Naegeli syndrome (b) Turner's syndrome
    (c) Klinefelter's syndrome (d) Swyer syndrome

15. **The permanent canine tooth erupts at:**
    (a) 9-11 years (b) 10-12 years
    (c) 11-12 years (d) 12-14 years

16. **Which of the following is the most reliable criteria in Gustafson's method?**
    (a) Transparency of the root (b) Attrition
    (c) Cementum apposition (d) Root resorption

17. **For the employment in the factory, the age of the child must not be below:**
    (a) 10 years (b) 12 years
    (c) 14 years (d) No age bars

18. **Cephalic index is calculated to determine the:**
    (a) Age of the person (b) Sex of the person
    (c) Race of the person (d) None of the above

19. **Which of the following is the main part of corpus delicti?**
    (a) Identification of the dead body
    (b) Identification of the weapon of offence
    (c) Identification of clothing
    (d) All of the above

20. **Identification of the face using a skull X-ray is known as:**
    (a) Salton's system (b) Gustafson's method
    (c) Superimposition (d) Locord's principle

21. **The surest method of identification is by:**
    (a) Cephalic index (b) Fingerprints
    (c) Handwriting (d) DNA fingerprinting

22. **The difference between a female pelvis and a male pelvis are all *except:***
    (a) Subpubic angle 90° or more
    (b) Wider greater sciatic notch
    (c) Large obturator foramen
    (d) Well-marked preauricular sulcus

23. **The characteristic feature of male sternum:**
    (a) Body is longer and more than twice in length of the manubrium
    (b) Breadth is less compared to the female
    (c) Body of the sternum is shorter and one and half times the length of manubrium
    (d) Body after sternum is less than twice in length of manubrium

24. According to which Section of Indian Penal Code, a child under seven years of age is not liable for offence?

(a) Sec. 82 IPC (b) Sec. 83 IPC
(c) Sec. 84 IPC (d) Sec. 85 IPC

25. Medial end of clavicle fuses at:

(a) 18 years (b) 22 years
(c) 24 years (d) 26 years

26. Palato-print is commonly taken from which part of palate?

(a) Anterior part (b) Posterior part
(c) Lateral wall (d) Medial wall

27. Ischial tuberosity fused at the age of:

(a) 16-17 years (b) 18-19 years
(c) 20-22 years (d) 23-25 years

28. Pure Mongolians are:

(a) Brachycephalic (b) Dolicocephalic
(c) Mesaticephalic (d) Mesocephalic

29. Fingerprint impression made on soft substrate are called:

(a) Visible print (b) Chance print
(c) Plastic print (d) Latent print

30. To estimate the age of 16 years, following X-rays are advised:

(a) Elbow, hand, oblique view of jaw
(b) Wrist, pelvis, oblique view of jaw
(c) Knee, pelvis, skull
(d) Ankle, shoulder, pelvis

31. Method to know the age of infants from the weight and height of the erupting teeth:

(a) Stack's Method (b) Boyde's Method
(c) Gustafson's Method (d) Ashely's Method

32. The system of identification on the basis of fingerprints is known as:

(a) Anthropology (b) Thanatology
(c) Galton system (d) Bertillon system

33. The chance of two persons having identical fingerprints:

(a) One in thirty-six thousand million
(b) One in sixty-four thousand million
(c) One in fifty-four thousand million
(d) One in sixty-six thousand million

34. Ashley's rule is used for the determination of:

(a) Stature (b) Age
(c) Sex (d) Race

35. All are features of Klinefelter syndrome *except:*

(a) Barr body absent
(b) XXY chromosomal pattern
(c) Male phenotype
(d) Azoospermia

ANSWER KEY

1. (b)	2. (b)	3. (c)	4. (b)	5. (d)	6. (a)	7. (b)	8. (d)	9. (c)	10. (a)
11. (c)	12. (d)	13. (b)	14. (a)	15. (c)	16. (a)	17. (c)	18. (c)	19. (a)	20. (c)
21. (b)	22. (c)	23. (a)	24. (a)	25. (b)	26. (a)	27. (c)	28. (a)	29. (c)	30. (a)
31. (a)	32. (c)	33. (b)	34. (c)	35. (a)					

6 CHAPTER

Changes After Death

The various changes produced in the body after death help in finding out the time since death that has a great value in medicolegal parlance. These are:

1. **Immediate changes:** (i) Unconsciousness and loss of reflexes (ii) Permanent cessation of circulation (iii) Permanent cessation of respiration.
2. **Early changes:** (i) Eye changes (ii) Skin changes (iii) Muscular flaccidity (iv) Contact flattening and pallor (v) Cooling of the body (vi) Cadaveric lividity (vii) Rigor mortis.
3. **Late changes:** (i) Putrefaction (ii) Adipocere (iii) Mummification.

Unconsciousness and Loss of Reflexes

After death, there is loss of consciousness and spinal reflexes with no response to painful stimuli. Rarely after death, coordinated muscle group activity remains, that could be due to surviving cells in the spinal cord.

Permanent Cessation of Circulation and Respiration

This is ascertained by the careful examination of heart and lungs by stethoscope for 5 minutes that is repeated at short intervals. At times heart sounds may not be audible as in case of suspended animation, in an obese and in conditions when apex of heart lies behind a rib etc. In cases of doubt, supplementary tests as given below have to be carried out.

Tests for circulation: (i) ***Magnus test:*** This is done by tying a ligature lightly at the base of the finger, sufficient to cut off venous channels, without occluding arteries. The finger remains white if circulation has stopped. Otherwise, at the site of ligature a bloodless zone appears and the area beyond it gradually becomes blue and swollen. (ii) ***Diaphanous test (Transillumination test):*** The hand with closed fingers is to be held against a strong source of light. During life it is scarlet, red and translucent. (This colour is also seen in CO poisoning). However, after death it is opaque and yellow (yellowish colour is also seen in anemia and syncope). (iii) ***I card's test*:** Hypodermic injection of 20% alkaline fluorescein is given. There is no discolouration of skin if circulation has stopped. The skin is yellowish green if circulation is going on. (iv) ***Finger nail test:*** When the pressure is applied on nail bed, it turns pale if circulation is going on but when the pressure is withdrawn it becomes red. (v) During life on the application of heat to the skin, true blister appears alongwith the line of redness. (vi) When a small artery is cut there is no jerky flow of blood after death. (vii) EEG shows an Isoelectric line after death.

Tests for respiration: (i) ***Mirror test:*** When a mirror is held in front of mouth and nostrils, it becomes dim due to condensation of warm moist air that comes from lungs indicating life. This test is quite useful in a cold weather. (ii) ***Feather test*:** There is no movement of cotton fiber or feather that is held in front of mouth and nostrils, if the respiration has stopped. (iii) ***Winslow test*:** A glass of water is placed on the chest, its surface will be seen to move if respiratory movements are continuing. Likewise, if a mirror is placed on the chest the reflection of a beam of light focused on it will move, if the respiration is continuing.

Changes in the Eyes

1. **Changes in cornea:** After death the eyeballs become softened, cornea looses its luster and the corneal reflex is lost. The cornea becomes hazy and opaque like a dimmed glass. The rise in temperature and humidity hastens the process whereas closed eye delays it. In some conditions haziness of cornea can also be present before death like in uraemia, narcotic poisoning and cholera etc. The transparency is retained longer in cases of apoplexy, CO poisoning and HCN poisoning.
2. **Tache noire de la sclerotique:** The formation of Tache noire de la sclerotique is also seen after death. It is an early and important sign of death. It appears after the passage of few hours to 2 days after death. It is believed to form due to the desiccation of tissues as it is formed only when the eyelids remain open after death. *Tache noire* is triangular in shape and is present over cornea, often outside the globe. It also undergoes colour changes from yellowish to brown to black (Figure 6.1).

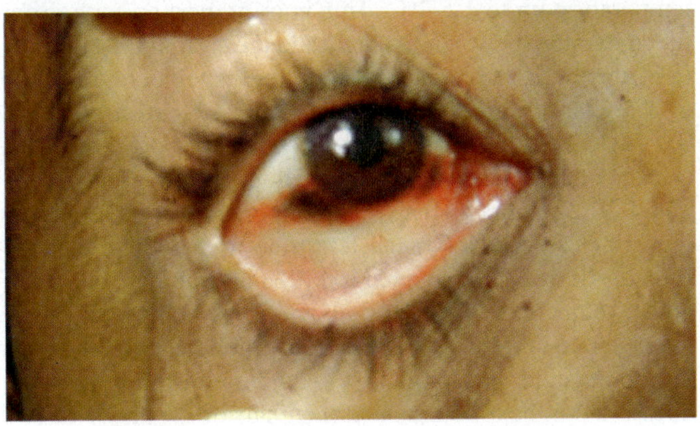

Figure 6.1: Tache noire de la sclerotique

3. **Changes in pupil:** The pupils usually assume a mid-dilated position that is the relaxed neutral position of the pupillary muscle, though they may alter in position later on due to rigor. Although the pupil reacts to atropine and eserine resulting in dilatation and constriction of pupil after somatic death. There may be marked difference in the degree of dilatation of each pupil, but this has no significance as a diagnostic sign either of a brain lesion or of drug intoxication. **The pupil responds to atropine for up to 4 hours and to eserine up to 1 hour**. The shape of the pupil changes as a result of uneven relaxation from circular to oval, polygonal or triangular. When pressure is applied by fingers on two or more sides of the eye balls, it retains the round form in the living persons or in those who are apparently dead.
4. **Intraocular tension:** Intraocular tension becomes 14 g immediately after death from the normal value of 14-25 g and by the end of 2 hours it becomes zero. Intraocular tension is measured by tonometer.
5. **Ophthalmoscopic examination of retinal vessels:** The blood columns of the retinal vessels show fragmentation after death. This change is observed by an Ophthalmoscopic examination within a few minutes after death. It lasts for about an hour. This is the well known **'trucking'** of blood in the retinal vessels (Kevorkian sign), when loss of blood pressure allows blood to break up into segments, similar to trucks in a railway train. On Ophthalmoscopic examination, the retina appears pale for first two hours and then the optic disc outline becomes hazy in about 6 hours and finally blurred in about 8 to 10 hours after death.
6. **Biochemical changes:** There are certain biochemical changes after death that are seen in various body fluids such as blood, CSF, bile, pericardial fluid, urine, synovial fluid and vitreous humor. The vitreous humour is considered the best fluid as it is unaffected by contaminants and is easy to obtain without distorting any body part. The eyelids are retracted and the needle is introduced near the outer canthus and the fluid is withdrawn gradually. There is a marked and progressive rise in the potassium concentration up to 100 hours after death. Besides potassium, the levels of vitreous sodium, vitamin C, etc are helpful in estimating the time since death. The levels of enzymes like lactic dehydrogenase (LDH) and glutamic oxalic transaminase also increases after death.

Changes in the Skin

The skin becomes pale due to drainage of blood from small vessels and appears ashy white after death. It looses its elasticity due to which an incised wound will not gape. However, edges of ulcers and wounds caused during life retain blue or red colour after death. Even the icteric hue produced by jaundice and phosphorous poisoning is not affected. In deaths due to drowning, the skin retains its normal appearance. The pallor of the skin is hardly a reliable sign of death as in deaths due to CO poisoning, some colour remains on the face. Postmortem staining is of pinkish or cherry red appearance in carbon monoxide poisoning and in dead bodies left in cold storage.

Muscular (Primary) Flaccidity

This is also a sign of somatic death and lasts for one to two hours. At about the time of death all the muscles of the body relax and loose their natural tone. As a result the jaw drops, the thorax collapses and the limbs fall quite loose. There is relaxation of facial musculature and ironing out of skin creases resulting in a younger looking person. The smooth muscles of iris relax and the pupil assumes a mid position. The sphincters of the body relax and the wounds do not gape. This is known as primary flaccidity. This relaxation of the muscles is due to high ATP content that permits splitting of the actin-myosin cross bridges.

Postmortem Cooling of the Body (Algor Mortis)

The normal body temperature taken orally is 96.7-99°F (36-37.2°C) whereas the normal rectal temperature is 0.5-0.75°F higher than the oral temperature that is 36.5-37.5°C. During sleep, the temperature of the body is lowered by 1°F and while exercising it is higher by 2-3°F. This temperature range is maintained in health and the balance of heat production and heat loss is also maintained. When the rectal temperature falls below 75° F, it is indicative of death and when it falls below 70°F, it is an evidence of certain death. During life, the body looses heat due to radiation, convection and vaporization and heat loss by conduction is not an important feature. After death, the production of heat ceases but loss of heat continues and the body keeps on cooling until the temperature of body is same as that of the environment. This fall of body temperature after death is due to radiation and convection. When body lies in a cool atmosphere, conduction also plays a role. The surface of the body cools more rapidly than the interior. Within few hours, the body feels cold which is quite unreliable sign for estimating the time since death.

The ideal method to note the body temperature is by recording the visceral temperature. The visceral temperature is recorded by making a small midline incision in the peritoneal cavity and placing the bulb of thermometer in contact with the inferior surface of liver and taking the temperature *in situ*. In calculating the fall of temperature after death, it is assumed that body temperature was normal at the time of death. Nevertheless, in certain cases temperature may be raised or low at the time of death. As in case of a sphere the periphery will cool rapidly than the center, similarly in human body the peripheries cool rapidly and the temperature in the center of the body remains unchanged up to 4 hours after death. The metabolic process like glycogenolysis provides some heat to the core of the body. The fall in body temperature is not uniform at the beginning and at the end, when the body temperature remains within 7°F of the atmospheric temperature. Due to this drawback, postmortem cooling is not an ideal method of estimating time since death.

The disappearance of body warmth is one of the earliest sign of deaths. Today progressive fall of body temperature is accepted as a suggestive sign of death but its main value lies in the estimation of time since death.

The use of a thermometer for measuring body temperature was first proposed by **Dowler (1849-50).** The temperature of the corpse is nowadays measured by inserting a chemical, 10 inches long thermometer with reading from 70-110°F (21-44°C), about 4 inches in to the rectum. The thermometer is inserted this much deep in the rectum enabling recording the temperature of the inner core of the body. The outer layer of the body that is 50% of the total body mass have low temperature and can easily be influenced by environmental conditions. In addition, the temperature of inner core varies from place to place. This drawback can be overcome if the thermometer is left *in situ* for 3 minutes. Nowadays, electronic thermocouple with digital reading is a better way of recording the temperature.

The Newton's law "rate of loss of heat at any instance is directly proportional to the temperature difference between the surface of the object and its surrounding" applies well to bodies after death. The loss of heat cannot be considered as a sure sign of death until the body has lost 15-20 degree of normal body temperature.

Variations of Rectal Temperature

Low rectal temperature: Rectal temperature of 90°-94°F (32°-34.5°C) may be observed in (i) Cholera (ii) Long periods of exposure to cold (iii) Congestive cardiac failure and (iv) Cases of severe collapse.

High rectal temperature: Rectal temperature is elevated in (i) CO poisoning (ii) Coronary thrombosis (iii) Ruptured aortic aneurysm (iv) Heat stroke (v) Pontine haemorrhage (vi) Infections (vii) Asphyxial deaths.

Exercise or struggle prior to death may raise the rectal temperature up to 1.5-2°C. This is in proportion with difference in temperature between the body and the surroundings. According to **Simpson**, in temperate the body looses temperature at the rate of 1.5°C/hour during the first six hours after death followed by 0.9-1.2°C/hour in the next six hours when the body is clothed. The surface of body takes about twelve hours and internal organs take about 20-24 hours to reach the temperature of the environment. Nevertheless, it takes much less time in a tropical country like India. A study was conducted in 1902 in Bombay Famine Hospital where temperature is seldom above 37°C. During this study, the average rate of fall was 1½ times the difference between body and air temperature during the first two hours followed by half of the above rate in next 2 hours and then half of the above rate during next two hours assuming that the body temperature is normal at time of death. It took about 12-15 hours after death for body temperature to equalize with that of the surrounding.

In fact, the cooling of the inner core depends upon the loss of heat through the surface layers, which are about one inch in thickness and have heat insulating properties better than core. During the first 1-3 hours after death or until a significant flow of heat commences through these layers, very little cooling takes place. At this time, cooling is retarded by chemical changes like glycogenolysis, which can produce 140 calories, sufficient to raise a 70 kg body temperature by 2°C (3.6°F). Then during next 6-9 hours, cooling is rapid. After 12 hours, the body temperature reaches that of surrounding resulting in a slow fall again. Overall, the fall of body temperature assumes the form of "sigmoid" curve (Figure 6.2). This sigmoid curve is divided into: (i) An initial plateau (ii) A practically straight line during the period of quickest cooling and (iii) Slow falling. There are certain variations from "standard cooling curves" in conditions of person dying with high or low temperature, obese, heavily clothed and in thin or unclothed person (Figure 6.3).

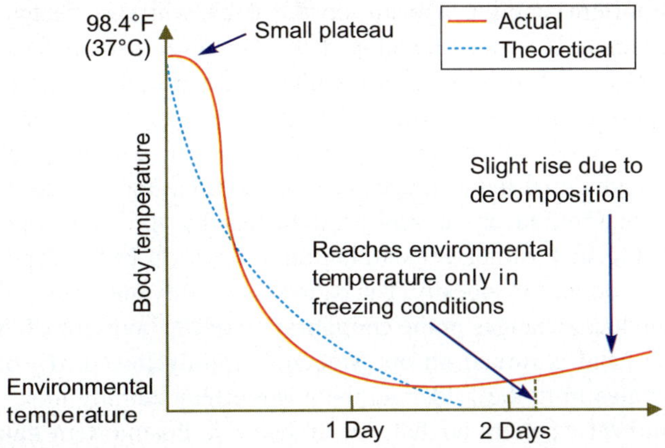

Figure 6.2: Standard cooling curves of the body *(From Legal Aspects of Medical Practice Churchill Livingstone London)*

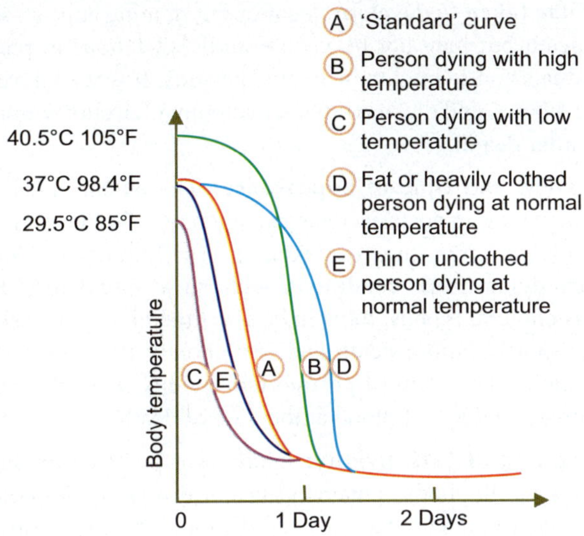

Figure 6.3: Variations from standard cooling curves

Glaister and Rantoul in 1966 calculated the time interval after death in hours as:

$$\text{Time interval after death} = \frac{37.2\ °\text{C–Rectal temperature}}{\text{Rate of fall of temp./hour}}$$

Time since death can also be calculated as:

1. Normal body temp. – Rectal temp. × 0.67 (in °F) = Time since death or 37.2 °C – Rectal temperature × 2 (in °C).
2. Rate of fall of temp. is 1.5 °F/hour (or 0.5 °C/hour).
3. Normal body temp. – rectal temp. (°F)/0.5.

Factors Influencing the Rate of Cooling

1. **Environment temperature:** In a body of 70 kg and 5.9" height lying in supine position facing air temperature between 40-75 ºF, the curve is of usual **sigmoid shape**. As the environmental temperature decreases, cooling quickens and at the temperature of 40 ºF, it is 2½ times more rapid than when it was kept at 75 ºF.
2. **Body size:** Body size is expressed as:

$$\text{Size factor} = \frac{\text{The surface area exposed to cooling}}{\text{Body mass}}$$

Total surface area of the body is not radiating heat to the surroundings. For example, the inner aspects of arms and legs lie opposed to other skin surface, so heat radiated is again reabsorbed into the body. When body is in "mummy" position or supine position with arms by the sides, about 80% of the body surface looses heat and in crouched position only 60% loose heat. Therefore, in the former position cooling is rapid (because 80% is greater surface than 60%).

3. **Presence or absence of clothing or other covering on the body:** In a clothed or covered body, the cooling is slow due to insulation.
4. **Movement and humidity of the atmospheric air:** When air movement occurs, there is increased cooling due to the increased convection of heat. A body cools rapidly in the open than a closed room. In moist air there is increased cooling which is better conductor of heat. On the other hand, dry air retards cooling.
5. **State of nutrition and development of body:** The rate of cooling of an obese or heavy body is slower than cooling of small body, because body fat retards cooling. Cooling of the large body as compared to small body depends not only on absolute body mass, but also on size or the surface area of the body relative to its mass. Therefore, cooling of infants is rapid than that of adults. They are not only smaller but the surface area of the body of a child relative to its mass is larger than adults.
6. **Manner of death:** In cases where death precedes with lot of muscular activity and the glycogen is exhausted resulting in minimal heat production by glycogenolysis, the cooling is rapid. There is also rapid cooling in case of deaths due to hemorrhage, wasting and chronic diseases. On the other hand, body remains warm for longer time in asphyxial deaths. Bodies immersed in water will cool rapidly than air, because water is a better conductor of heat than air. Bodies cool more slowly in water containing sewage or other putrefying organic material than fresh or sea water. Bodies cool more rapidly in running fluids than in the stagnant fluid.

Medicolegal aspects: (i) Postmortem cooling of the body is a sure sign of death (ii) It is one of the parameters for estimating time since death.

Postmortem Caloricity

Postmortem caloricity is the rise of the body temperature for the first two hours or so after death. This rise in body temperature occurs due to various reasons: (i) Heat regulating center has been disturbed before death such as in cases of **heat stroke** (ii) Increased heat production in muscles due to convulsions in cases of **tetanus** and **strychnine poisoning** (iii) Deaths due to excessive bacterial activity like **septicemia**, **cholera** and **fever** (iv) Increased heat production due to **glycogenolysis**.

Postmortem Lividity

Postmortem lividity is also known as hypostasis, livor mortis, subcutaneous hypostasis, postmortem staining, cadaveric lividity, suggilations, vibices etc. Postmortem lividity is the bluish purple discolouration, which appears under the skin of the dependent parts of the body after death due to capillovenous distention (Figure 6.4). The intensity of colour of hypostasis depends upon the amount of reduced haemoglobin in the blood. Large amount of reduced haemoglobin produces deep purplish blue colouration of the stain. It is quite difficult to distinguish between cyanosis and P.M. staining. Postmortem lividity is produced because of: (i) Stoppage of circulation (ii) Stagnation of blood in blood vessels (iii) Tendency of the blood to sink by force of gravity.

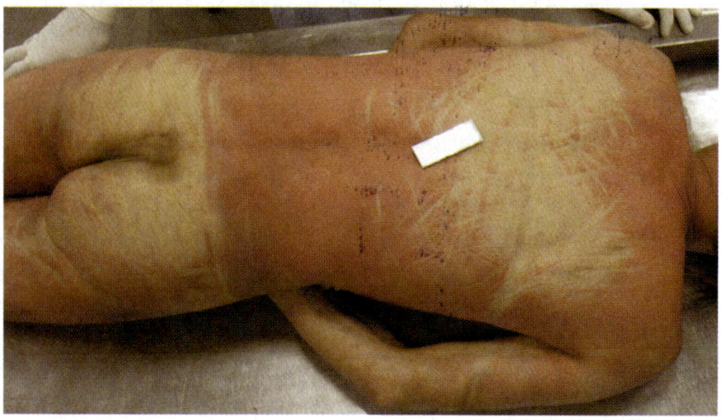

Figure 6.4: Hypostasis with contact flattening over the back

The dependent parts of the body attain a purplish blue hue while the pressure areas become pale due to drainage of blood from these areas. The colour of hypostasis is purplish blue due to the following reasons: (i) In recently dead or dying tissue oxygen dissociation takes place and this continues until equilibrium is reached between oxygen tension in the capillaries and the surrounding tissue. (ii) Reflux of venous blood from the venular end of the capillaries, which adds to the blueness.

Distribution and location: The distribution of postmortem lividity is patchy to start but with passage of time, it gradually enlarges to cover all the dependent areas of the body. The colour of hypostasis blanches out on pressure. The purplish blue colour of hypostasis is more marked in fair coloured skin than the dark. The colour fades in persons suffering from anaemia, wasting diseases like lobar pneumonia, TB, cancer etc. In addition, postmortem staining may not develop in a body that has been in a constant motion after death. Hypostasis appears on dependent parts of body except pressure areas and its location and distribution depends upon the position of the body after death. In supine position, the postmortem staining appears on the back while in deaths due to hanging, it is well developed on the lower part of legs and forearms. In deaths due to drowning, one can find the formation of hypostasis over the front of head, neck, upper part of chest and abdomen. When the body is recovered in a prone position, subconjunctival hemorrhages can be seen that may be confused with that produced in asphyxial deaths by the inexperienced pathologist. Postmortem staining does not form in the depths of folds produced by obesity. The pattern of lividity may be modified by the local changes in the configuration of the body for example if the head is turned on one side and slightly flexed, the blood gravitates in to the folds and the postmortem staining looks like linear bruise pattern on that side of the neck. Postmortem staining does not form at the areas of tight bands such as collar bands, belt, waistband etc.

Time taken to develop: Postmortem staining appears shortly after death but may not be visible until 1/2-1 hour in plethoric individuals and 1-4 hours in anemic persons. It is well developed within 4 hours and the maximum development occurs within 6-12 hours after death.

Extent and time of appearance: The extent and time of appearance of hypostasis depends upon: (i) Volume of blood in circulation at the time of death; and (ii) Fluidity of blood. In persons dying from conditions with slow circulatory failure such as cholera, typhus, tuberculosis or uraemia, hypostasis may appear shortly before death and is markedly developed shortly after death. The extent of postmortem lividity depends upon the amount and fluidity of blood at the time of death.

Fixation of P.M. lividity: Fixation of postmortem staining occurs when the body remains static for 6-8 hours at one place. This is due to the fact that the coagulation in the capillaries takes place in 6-8 hours making the staining permanent. Nevertheless, there will be no fixation if the blood remains persistently fluid due to fibrinolysis.

Shifting of P.M. lividity: Postmortem staining can shift from one part of the body to another due to the movement of the body after death. This is due to the fact that it takes about 6-8 hours for the stain to fix and prior to that period, the staining can keep on shifting as the blood remain fluid. In addition, the shifting also occurs during decomposition as the clotting blood liquefies again. When the body is moved, areas of old staining will disappear and new ones appear on the dependent part. However, lividity to a lighter degree remains due to staining of tissues by haemolysis. As vessel walls become permeable, the blood leaks through and stains the tissues. At this stage, pressure does not blanch the hypostatic area. Postmortem staining at different areas of body indicates the different position of the body after death.

Cause of death: It can be ascertained to some extent by examination of the colour of the P.M. staining, as certain poisons impart distinctive colour to the P.M. staining (Table 6.1).

Table 6.1: Various conditions and causes of death ascertained by the colour of hypostasis	
Colour of hypostasis	**Cause of death**
• Cherry red	Carbon monoxide poisoning
• Bright red	Hydrocyanic acid poisoning
• Reddish brown, brown or deep blue	Nitrates, potassium chlorate, aniline poisoning
• Dark brown	Phosphates poisoning
• Bright red	Burns
• Pink	Cold and refrigerated bodies
• Grayish brown	Septic abortion due to Cl. welchii

Internal hypostasis: It also occurs on the dependent parts of internal organs like lungs, liver, kidney etc. In heart, it simulates coronary occlusion and in lungs it simulates pneumonia. Hypostasis on coils of intestine gives them a strangulated appearance. When putrefaction sets in, haemolysis of red blood cells and diffusion of blood pigments in to the surrounding tissues occurs, where it undergoes secondary changes and formation of sulphmethaemoglobin occurs. Microscopically, the capillary endothelium and the surrounding cells show lytic changes. Only the cellular outline is visible and not the capillaries. Similar changes are seen in a contusion microscopically. It is not possible to know whether the pigment in a stained putrefied area is from the contusion (extravascular) or congestion (intravascular). As decomposition sets in the colour of the hypostasis changes from dusky colour to brown to green and finally it disappears. In mummification the colour changes to brown to blackish with the desiccation of the body (Tables 6.2 and 6.3).

Table 6.2: Differences between P.M. lividity and contusion		
Features	**P.M. Lividity**	**Contusion**
Cause	Engorged vessel	Rupture of vessels
Cuticle	Not injured	May be injured
Site	Dependent parts	Any where
Appearance	Not elevated	Elevated, swollen
Colour	Uniform	Different colour changes with time
Edges	Clear	Not clear
Cut section	Blood in the vessels	Blood outside vessels
Pressure	Not seen in pressure areas	Little lighter over the area of pressure or support

Table 6.3: Differences between P.M. staining and congestion		
Features	**P.M. Lividity**	**Congestion**
Redness	Dependent part	All over the organ, uniform
Mucous membrane	Dull and lusterless	Normal
Exudate	Not inflammatory	Inflammatory exudate may be seen
Hollow viscus	When stretched alternate stained and unstained areas	Uniformly congested

Medicolegal aspects of P.M. lividity: (i) P.M. lividity is a sign of death (ii) It is suggestive of the time passed since death (iii) It can signify cause of death (iv) Distribution of hypostasis helps in elucidating the position of body after death.

Contact Flattening and Pallor

In supine position the muscles of calf and buttocks remain flat due to loss of muscle tone. Once hypostasis has appeared these areas are more easily delineated because they are pale. The areas that are not subjected to pressure are coloured by hypostasis. Contact pallor also occurs internally. In supine position, the larynx sinks downwards on the spine and presses on the oesophagus, mucosa of which is found to have transverse bands of pallor at the level of cricoid cartilage.

Rigor Mortis

Rigor mortis is postmortem stiffening of voluntary and involuntary muscles of the body that develops at variable periods after death and succeeds the state of primary muscular flaccidity. Its physical characteristics have been investigated and it is found to have two physical properties; plasticity and elasticity. There is no measurable shortening of the muscles during rigor mortis unless they are subjected to tension. Muscular shortening only occurs when they are stretched. Therefore, it is equal to the last stretch reflex in a muscle. Rigor mortis represents the last systole. When rigor mortis is developed fully in the joints, they become fixed, extended or flexed depending on the position of the body at the time of death. The flexion attitude is due to shortening of the muscles of forearm and legs. Once rigor mortis is broken down by force, it does not reappear. However, when it is not broken it passes off spontaneously and is followed by a phase of secondary muscular relaxation.

Rigor mortis first appears in involuntary muscles like heart and causes contraction of heart muscle that may rarely be mistaken for cardiac hypertrophy. During the secondary muscular relaxation, dilatation of the heart occurs that should not be mistaken for dilatation of chambers of heart or myocardial degeneration. In view of the above postmortem changes, it is not possible to determine at autopsy whether heart stopped in systole or diastole.

Due to rigor mortis contraction of erector pilorus muscle occurs resulting in cutis anserina or goose skin. In deaths due to drowning goose skin develops due to agonal contraction of the muscles. The cause of goose skin cannot be differentiated in drowning deaths. Development of rigor mortis in muscles of iris results in inequality of pupils. Therefore, the state of pupil after death is not indicative of their antemortem appearance. Due to onset of rigor mortis in seminal vesicles emission of seminal fluid occurs.

Mechanism of development of rigor mortis: The chemical changes which occur in muscles immediately after death are similar to those which occur in living muscle. **Baldwin** has described the mechanism of changes in living muscles of the body. The initial muscle contraction requires immediate energy being supplied by ATP, which is converted to ADP. Terminal phosphate radical in ATP is very rich in energy. Phosphogen (creatine phosphate) donates phosphate to ADP and ATP is restored. Phosphate freed from ATP is utilized in a complete phosphorylation process, which is necessary for conversion of glycogen to lactic acid. The new energy rich phosphate bonds formed by this process are initially used to resynthesize ATP from ADP. The energy for muscle contraction is therefore ultimately obtained from breakdown of glycogen and the formation of lactic acid, which is transferred by the blood to liver for resynthesis of glycogen. All the above processes are anaerobic in nature and that is why specific enzymes are involved during these metabolic processes.

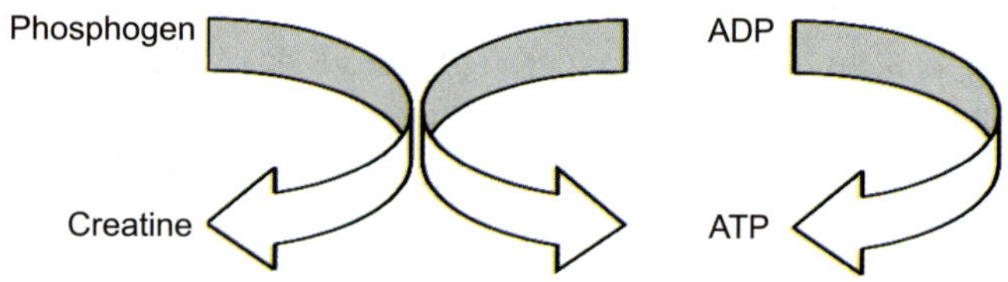

Chemical basis of rigor mortis: It has been noted that there is a gradual loss of ATP in the muscles after death. In addition, it is considered that the development of rigor mortis also depends upon breakdown of this compound. When an animal is narcotized and suddenly killed, the ATP reduction is gradual and rigor mortis is delayed. Whereas when there is struggle before death, the ATP is reduced quickly and the onset of rigor mortis is also quick. Therefore, the fall of level of ATP is directly related to the onset of rigor mortis.

Loves suggested that the destruction of ATP after death is balanced for a variable period by resynthesis from ADP. As long as this equilibrium is maintained, rigor mortis will not develop. Synthesis of ATP from glycogenolysis can only continue as long as glycogen is available in the dying muscles. However, after death the muscles cannot replenish their glycogen stores via the blood. The time of onset of rigor mortis is directly proportional to the glycogen content of the muscle at the time of death. It depends upon whether the muscle was in a state of rest or activity before death. If the person is taking insulin injections, rigor mortis develops rapidly.

A study has been conducted to know the nature of myosin macromolecule. These molecules occur as long linear polypeptide chains possessing polar and nonpolar side chains, which follow each other alternately on both the sides of main chain. Voluntary muscles of the body consist of muscle fibres and each of these muscle fibres consists of densely packed myofibrils extending throughout its whole length. Myofibrils are contractile elements and are made up of two types of protein filaments; myosin and actin.

These filaments are arranged in interdigitating arrays with short lateral projections extending from myosin filament towards the actin filaments. In relaxed state actin filament interdigitate with myosin only to a small extent. However, under the influence of nervous stimulation actin filaments are drawn into myosin filament resulting in contraction of muscles (Figure 6.5). The mechanism by which the sliding movement takes place is not known. Fall in ATP concentration allows the overlapping actin and myosin filament to combine as rigid links of inextensible actomyosin and accounts for the hardness and rigidity. After death the muscle passes in two phases: (i) A delay period during which the elasticity does not change appreciably. (ii) A terminal phase of rigor in which ATP disappears from the muscle and muscle rapidly becomes inelastic. The extensibility of the muscle begins to fall when ATP drops to 85% (is at its lowest) of its original value.

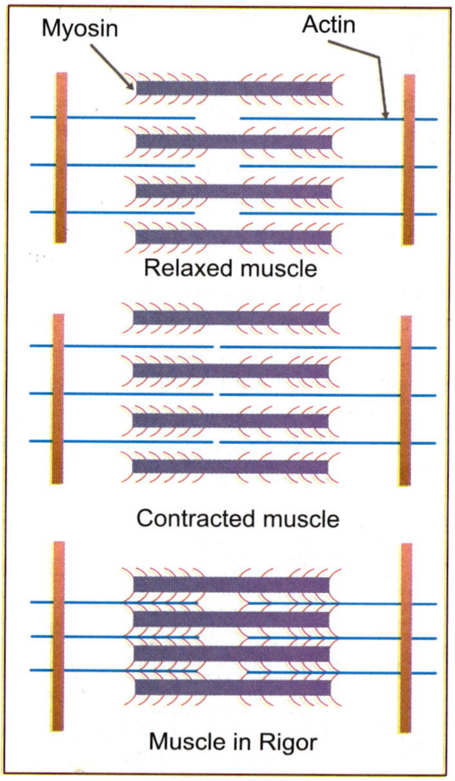

Figure 6.5: Schematic arrangement of the myosin and actin filaments in the muscle fibre

Order of appearance of rigor mortis: Rigor mortis appears first in involuntary muscle like heart. In voluntary muscles, it is commonly described as commencing in eyelids then in the neck muscles and lower jaw and then spreading to upper limbs, thorax, abdomen and the pelvis and lastly to the lower limbs (**Nysten's Law**), as shown in Figure 6.6.

It is generally accepted that rigor mortis passes off in the same order as it appears. **Shapiro** states that rigor mortis does not follow any anatomical sequence. Rigor mortis develops sufficiently at the ankle or wrist joint but elbow or knee allows 5-10 degrees of movement and hip or shoulder joints have even greater degrees of movement. He suggests that since rigor mortis is a

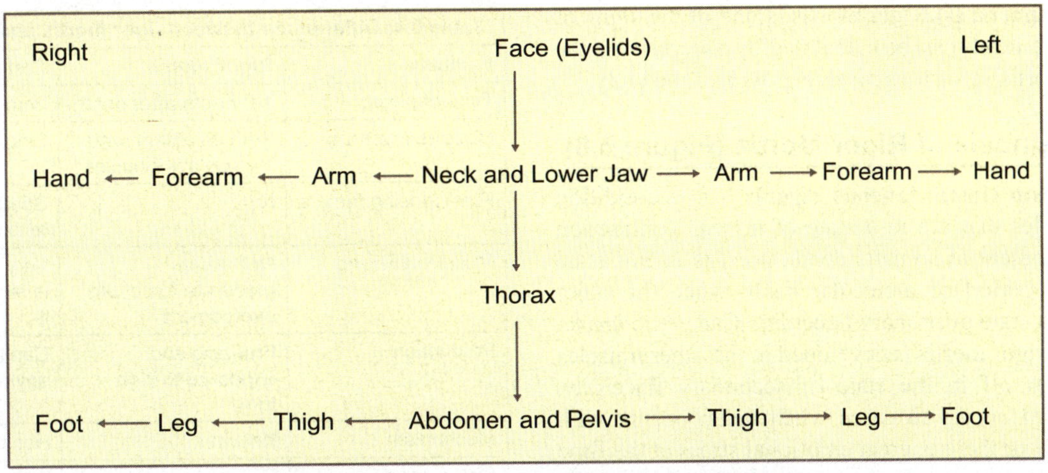

Figure 6.6: Order of appearance of rigor mortis

physiochemical process, it is most likely to develop simultaneously in all the muscles. It develops quickly in small masses of muscles than larger muscles. Therefore, variation in different sizes of joints and muscles controls its development. It appears from proximal (bigger joint) to distal (smaller joint). This hypothesis of Shapiro is important from medicolegal point of view as it emphasizes the difficulty of estimating postmortem interval from distribution of rigor mortis.

Rate of onset and duration of rigor mortis: There is great variation in the onset and duration of rigor mortis and as a general rule, when onset is rapid, duration is short and vice versa. In tropical climate, rigor mortis begins after 1-2 hours of death and takes next 1-2 hours to develop completely in all the muscle groups. In summers, it may last only for 18-36 hours. In temperate climates, rigor mortis begins to develop in 3-5 hours and takes further 2-3 hours for complete development and the total duration being 24-48 hours during winters. To summarize, rigor mortis takes 12 hours to develop, remains for further 12 hours and takes next 12 hours to pass off.

Demonstration of rigor mortis at autopsy: The body is kept in supine position on the autopsy table and the pathologist tries to lift the leg by putting the hand above the knee joint under the thigh. The knee joint will not flex due to stiffness once rigor has developed (Figure 6.7). In the same way, there will not be any flexion movements at the elbow joint. Other muscle groups such as jaw etc. should also be examined for the development of rigor mortis by trying to flex them.

Conditions that Influence Rigor Mortis

1. **Environmental temperature:** When the environmental temperature is high, onset of rigor is rapid and the duration is short. When body is lying at a temperature below 10°C, it is unusual for rigor mortis to develop. When environmental temperature is raised, rigor mortis appears in the usual manner. Air movement and clothing worn by the person at the time of death also indirectly influences the development of rigor mortis by regulating the temperature of the body.

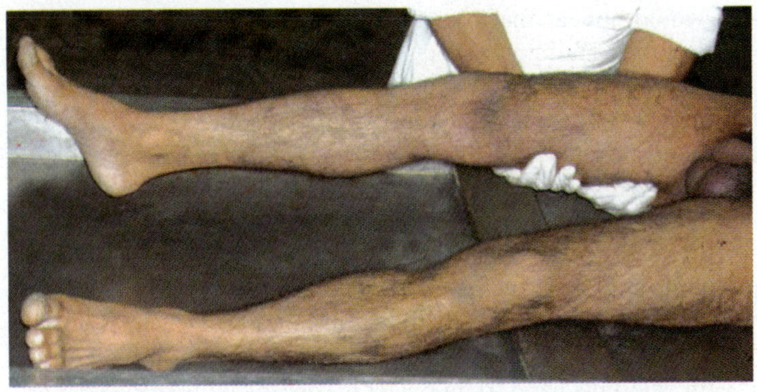

Figure 6.7: Demonstration of rigor mortis at autopsy

2. **Degree of muscular activity before death:** After prolonged muscle activity and in certain disorders, there is rapid onset of rigor mortis and the duration is short. This occurs in soldiers dying in a battlefield and persons dying from convulsive disorders like tetanus, strychnine poisoning.
3. **Age:** There is no scientific data available to support the hypothesis that rigor mortis does not develop in a fetus of less than 7 months of intrauterine life. It appears in stillborn fetus equally as in liveborn. In healthy adults, it appears slowly, is well marked and stays for longer period. In children and old, it is feeble and rapid in onset.
4. **Nature of death:** The development of rigor mortis varies with the nature of death such as: (i) During exhaustion, in wasting disease like TB, cancer and cholera and in violent deaths such as deaths due to firearm, electrocution and lightning, it is of rapid onset and of short duration. (ii) In conditions such as apoplexy, severe hemorrhage, pneumonia and nervous disease the onset of rigor is delayed. (iii) In strychnine poisoning, the onset is rapid and duration is short. In organophosphorous poisoning, it appears early whereas it is delayed in CO poisoning. (iv) In gas gangrene and other bacterial infections, it appears as well as disappears quickly. (v) It may not appear at all in deaths due to septicemia.

Medicolegal aspects: (i) Rigor mortis is one of the signs of death (ii) Time since death can be calculated by ascertaining the presence of rigor mortis in various muscle groups of the body.

Differential Diagnosis of Rigor Mortis (Figure 6.8)

1. **Cadaveric spasm (instantaneous rigor):** It is a condition when the muscles that are in a state of normal contraction at the actual moment of somatic death, persists in this state throughout the period of molecular death when the other muscles are in a state of primary flaccidity. Cadaveric spasm continues until rigor mortis is developed in the other muscles and only passes off in the state of secondary flaccidity. Cadaveric spasm occurs in cases when death occurs with extreme rapidity or there is great emotional stress at the time of death. The spasm is primarily a vital phenomenon and is originated by normal nervous stimulation of the muscles. It would appear that persistence of contraction after death is due to the failure (reason not known) of the chemical process required for active muscular relaxation to occur during molecular death. Cadaveric spasm may affect the whole body but usually a group of muscles is involved. In suicidal deaths, the weapon of offence is firmly grasped in hand and similarly grass or weeds may be held firmly in the hands of the victim in deaths due to drowning. In deaths occurring in mountains and jungles, branches of shrubs and trees are found firmly clenched in the fist. At times, in homicidal deaths buttons, clothes, hair of the assailant are firmly caught in the hold of the victim's hand. If an object is kept in hand during primary flaccidity and then rigor mortis develops, this grasp is not so firm as that of cadaveric spasm. It has been seen that cadaveric spasm can develop in the whole body in poisoning due to Dinitro-orthocresol. The differences between rigor mortis and cadaveric spasm are enumerated under Table 6.4.

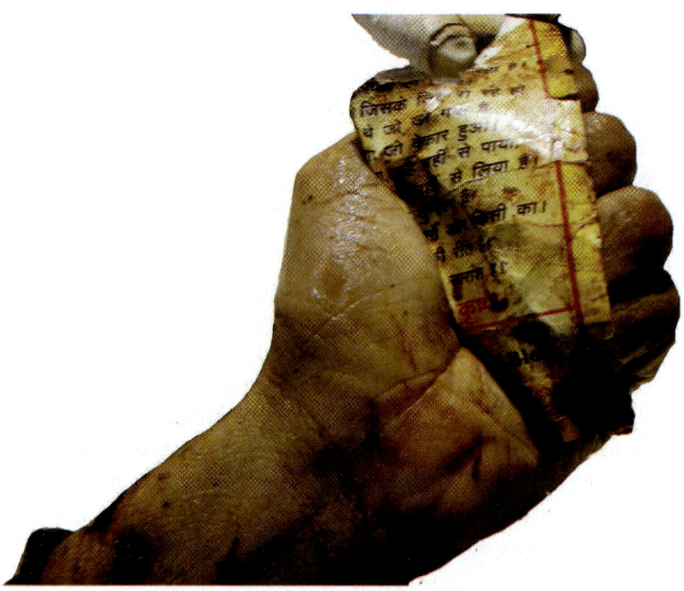

Figure 6.8: Cadaveric spasm

Table 6.4: Differences between rigor mortis and cadaveric spasm

Features	Rigor mortis	Cadaveric spasm
Time of onset	1-2 hours after death	Immediate
Muscles involved	Both voluntary and involuntary muscles	Single group of muscles
Predisposing factors	Nil	Sudden death, extreme tension and exhaustion
Muscle stiffening	Not marked, moderate force can overcome it	Very marked, great force is required to overcome it
Production	Freezing and exposure to high temp	Can't be produced by any method
Mechanism	Known	Not known
Molecular death	Occurs	Does not occur
Electrical stimuli	No response	Positive response
Medicolegal significance	In calculating time since death	Mode of death can be known

2. **Heat rigor (heat stiffening):** Heat rigor is a condition of postmortem stiffening or rigidity of the muscles caused by coagulation of muscle proteins, when body is exposed to high temperatures of 65° C and above. Heat rigor occurs in circumstances when death has resulted due to fire in multistory buildings, aircraft accidents, motor car accidents, burning etc. Rigor mortis does not develop in the muscles that have undergone heat stiffening but heat stiffening can occur after rigor mortis. Heat rigor persists until the muscles undergo softening or putrefaction sets in. In heat rigor, shortening of the muscles occurs resulting in flexion of the joints of the upper and lower limbs called **pugilistic attitude**. The contraction of muscles by heat stiffening may be sufficiently forceful to cause tearing of the tissues called **heat rupture**, that should be differentiated from a lacerated wound (Table 6.5).

Table 6.5: Difference between heat rupture and lacerated wound

Features	Heat rupture	Lacerated wound
Production	Exposure to heat	Blunt force trauma
Site	Fatty areas	Anywhere
Effect on vessels	Bridging of veins, vessels and nerves remain intact	Tearing of the vessels and nerves

3. **Cold stiffening:** In cold climate, tissues of the body are frozen at sub-zero temperature after death and muscles become rigid and hard and this condition simulates rigor mortis and called cold stiffening. There is extreme coldness of the body and when the joints are forcefully flexed, crackling of the ice of the synovial fluid in the joints occurs. Freezing usually occurs before the onset of rigor mortis and if thawing takes place, the initial rigidity passes off and rigor mortis develops.

4. **Gas stiffening:** Gas stiffening occurs in bodies with advanced state of decomposition when a false rigidity is produced due to accumulation of gases in the tissues. The face is swollen, eyes bulge out, abdomen is distended and the scrotum is

swollen. This occurs in bodies with advanced decomposition. As a result, it is best seen in dead bodies recovered from water because of rapid decomposition that have imbibed much fluid.

5. **Rigor mortis in a live person:** Symptoms similar to rigor mortis is reported in a live patient after cardiac surgery (Chakravarthy, 2010). The probable reason for this premortem stiffening of muscle is due to decrease or absence of blood supply to the muscles. The likely factors that may have predisposed are intense low cardiac output status, use of unusually high dose of inotropic and vasopressor agents and sepsis. In such case, before declaration of death and while calculating time since death, careful examination and interpretation should be done.

Secondary Relaxation

Muscles become soft and flaccid due to breaking down of actomyosin and the reaction to various juices becomes alkaline. There is no response to electrical stimuli during the phase of secondary relaxation.

Putrefaction

Putrefaction is a final stage in the changes following death and is a sure sign of death. It usually follows disappearance of rigor mortis. It results from breakdown of complex organic compounds into simpler forms (inorganic compounds) by the action of bacteria, fungi and protozoa etc. In the process, various enzyme systems of the body are involved. Whereas autolysis is a aseptic process where organic compounds are broken by the enzymes of the body. Putrefaction is brought about mainly by the action of anaerobic bacterial enzymes, fungi and insects. The agent commonly responsible is **Cl. welchii** that causes hemolysis, liquefaction of postmortem clot, emboli, thrombi, breakdown of tissues and gas formation. Immediately after death, there is breakdown of cell membranes and they also become permeable. The cytoplasm containing lytic enzymes is released causing autodigestion of the cells and tissues. This autodigestion occurs without any bacterial influence. At times, this autodigestion may start even before death as in intracranial lesions. Maceration of dead fetus inside the uterus results from autolytic fermentation. Also, there is early softening and liquefaction of brain and other internal organs. In newborns and infants, the autodigestion by acid gastric juice is a common finding. As a result, there is softening and rupture of stomach and esophagus. Following changes are brought about after death due to putrefaction: (i) Colour changes (ii) Evolution of foul smelling gases (iii) Effects produced by pressure of the gases (iv) Appearance of maggots (v) Conversion of soft parts in to thick semifluid black mass which separates from the bones and fall off leaving the skeleton exposed **(colliquative putrefaction)**.

Constituents of Putrefying Mass

1. **Acids:** (i) Formic acid (ii) Acetic acid (iii) Butyric acid (iv) Lactic acid (v) Palmitic acid (vi) Oxalic acid and (vii) Succinic acid.
2. **Imino and Amino acids:** (i) Leucine (ii) Tyrosine.
3. **Aromatic compounds:** (i) Indol (ii) Skatol.
4. **Mercaptans in anaerobic putrefaction:** (i) Cl. welchii (ii) B. proteus (iii) B. coli (iv) Streptococcus and staphylococcus.

Mechanism of putrefaction: Putrefaction is brought about mainly due to the action of: (i) Anaerobic bacterial enzymes that originate from the bowel (ii) Anaerobic fungi (iii) Insect larvae (proteolytic enzyme system) (iv) Protozoa (v) Adult insects.

Shortly after death bacterial and coliform organisms make their way to the tissues from the gastrointestinal tract through the blood vessel, respiratory tract and open skin wounds. Blood acts as a good media for distribution of these organisms and it also provides nutrition to them. The fall in oxygen concentration and rise of hydrogen favours bacterial growth and their spread. Bacteria liberate a number of enzymes, one such enzyme is **lecithinase** liberated by Cl. welchii that hydrolyses the lecithin, which is present in all cell membranes including the red blood cells. This enzyme is responsible for postmortem haemolysis of blood. During the process of putrefaction, the soft parts of the body are affected first and the bones are affected much later.

Colour changes: It is the first external sign of putrefaction in a dead body. The greenish discolouration of the abdomen over right iliac fossa is due to the presence of caecum that lies superficially and close to the abdominal wall (Figure 6.9). As the contents of the caecum are more fluid and full of bacteria that is why it develops putrefaction at the earliest. Even internally the undersurface of liver shows the discolouration which is in contact with the caecum. The putrefaction then spreads to other parts of the body (Figure 6.10). The greenish discolouration is due to the change in the blood pigment and as a result of formation

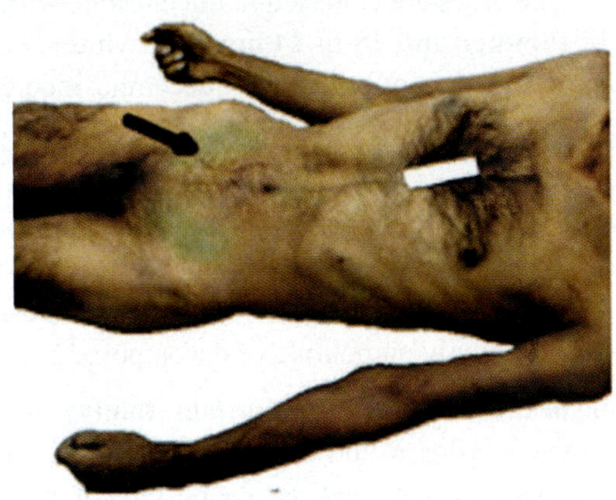

Figure 6.9: Decomposition changes with greenish discolouration of abdomen

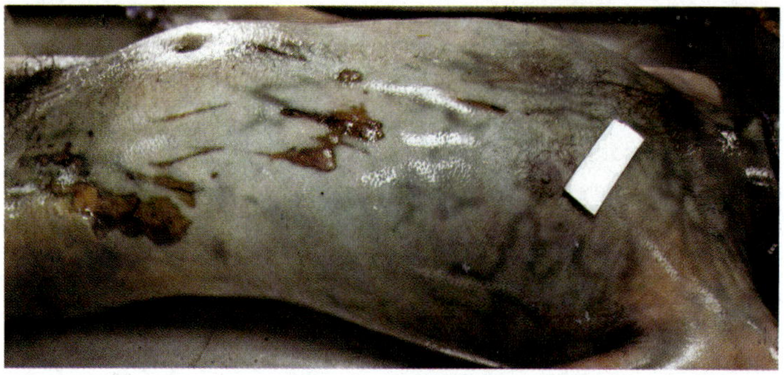

Figure 6.10: Chest and abdomen showing greenish discolouration

of sulphmethhaemoglobin which is formed by the action of hydrogen sulphide on methaemoglobin. The colour appears in **12 to 18 hours in summer** and **18 to 24 hours in winter**. The green colour changes to dark green and later purple or dark blue with the passage of time. In floating bodies with head downwards, greenish discolouration is seen first over face and neck then over other parts of the body. The colour change is more marked in a fair complexioned body.

Marbling of the skin: The marbling of skin occurs due to haemolysis and decomposition of blood in the superficial veins of neck and chest that stains the vessel walls. It appears as purplish red, bluish or greenish streaks against background of black or green skin. The marbling of skin occurs in **24 to 36 hours in summer** and **36 to 48 hours in winter** (Figure 6.11A and B).

Evolution of gases in the tissues: During this stage, the proteins and carbohydrates are split into simpler compounds. As a result, a number of gases such as hydrogen sulphide, phosphonetted hydrogen, methane, carbon dioxide, ammonia and hydrogen are formed during the process.

The offensive odor emitting out of a dead is due to formation of **hydrogen sulphide gas** and **Mercaptans**. In the early stages the gases are noninflammable but as putrefaction progresses lots of hydrogen sulphide is formed which can be ignited to burn with a blue flame. The gases are collected in the intestine **within 12 to 18 hours in summer and 18 to 24 hours in winter**. Following effects are produced due to formation of decomposition gases.

1. **Postmortem bleeding:** Wounds caused during life and after death bleed due to pressure of gases inside the vessels. Therefore, their nature whether antemortem and postmortem cannot be made out. There is no trace of coagulation but this has no effect on meningeal hemorrhages. Postmortem bleeding is just only outpouring of decomposed blood.
2. **Shifting of the position of postmortem staining:** It may shift in any direction due to the pressure of the gas in the blood vessels. Thus, it does not indicate the position of the body.
3. **Displacement of blood:** Occurs from the cavities of the heart.

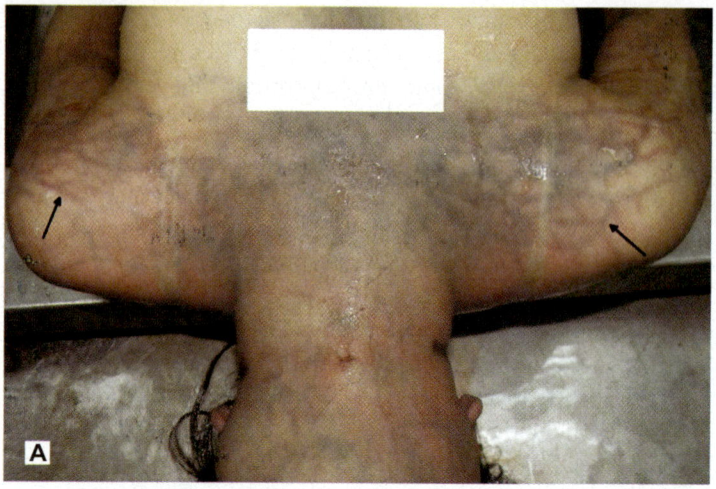

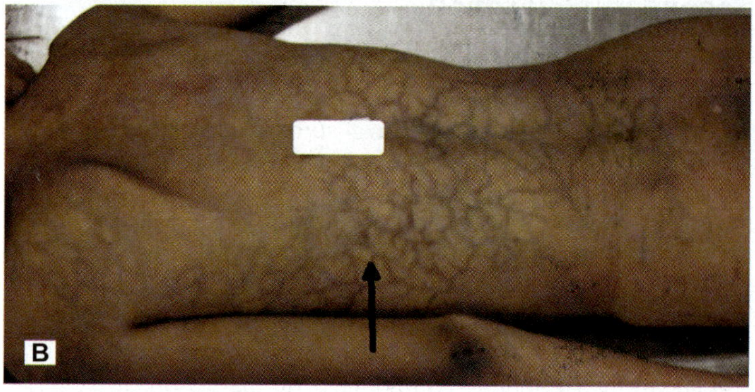

Figure 6.11A and B: Decomposition changes with marbling over upper limbs and chest

4. **Bloating of the features:** The gases at different places render the features bloated and distorted appearance. In the advanced stages, identification becomes impossible, the face is swollen and discoloured, eyes bulge out and tongue protrudes out caught between the teeth. The lips are swollen and the tissues of the neck become swollen. There is accentuation of the natural grooves and bulging of the eyes that may simulate facial features of strangulation (Figures 6.13, 6.14, 6.15 and 6.16).
5. **Distension of abdomen:** The abdomen becomes distended (Figure 6.15) and on opening a loud voice is heard due to release of gases. The female breasts are distended and scrotum and penis are swollen (Figure 6.12). Whole body is swollen leading to distortion of the facial features causing difficulty in identification.
6. **Formation of vesicles:** There is blister formation at different parts of the body that contains reddish fluid and blood and there is slippage of skin at different places. This is caused by the gas pressure forcing the blood stained fluid, air or liquid fat between the epidermis and dermis (Figures 6.13, 6.15 and 6.16).

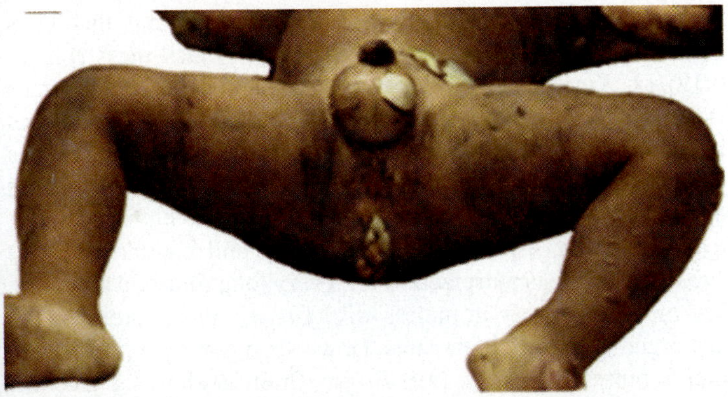

Figure 6.12: Decomposition changes with swelling of penis, scrotum and prolapse of rectum

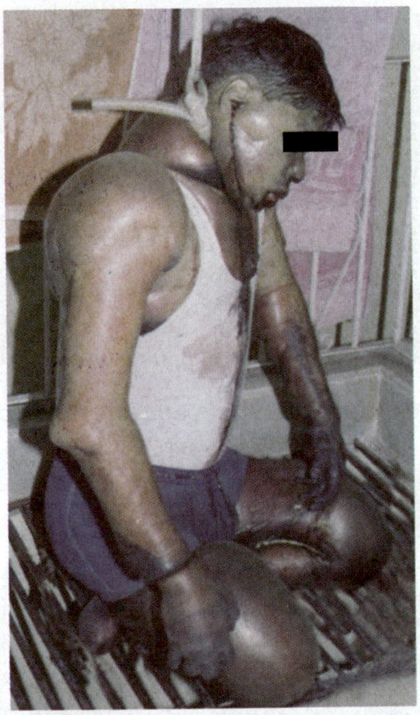

Figure 6.13: Decomposition changes with formation of postmortem blisters

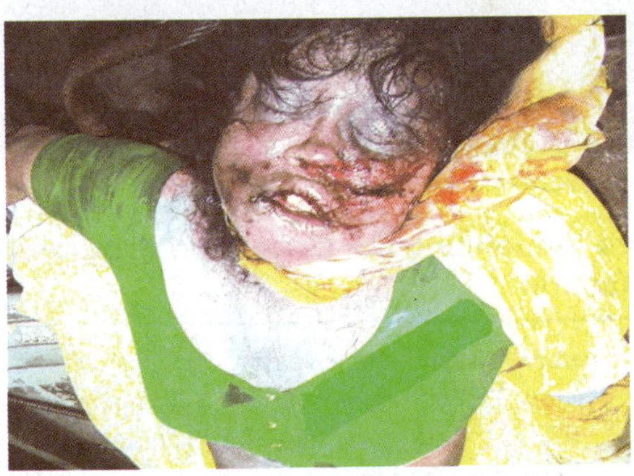

Figure 6.14: Decomposition changes with blotting of features and purging of fluid

7. **Postmortem purge:** Extrusion of fluid from mouth and nostrils along with stomach contents is known as postmortem purge (Figures 6.14 and 6.16).
8. There is **escape of urine and faeces** and prolapse of the rectum as the sphincters relax (Figure 6.12).
9. In advanced stage of putrefaction, **expulsion of fetus** occurs from the uterus because of the pressure of the gases it contains.

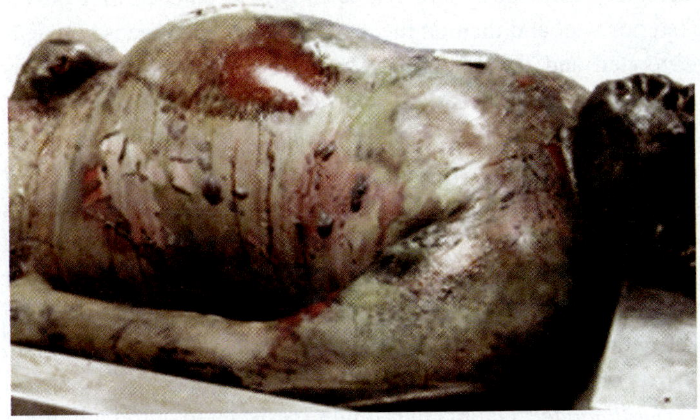

Figure 6.15: Decomposition changes with formation of postmortem blisters, slippage of skin, purging of fluid and distended abdomen

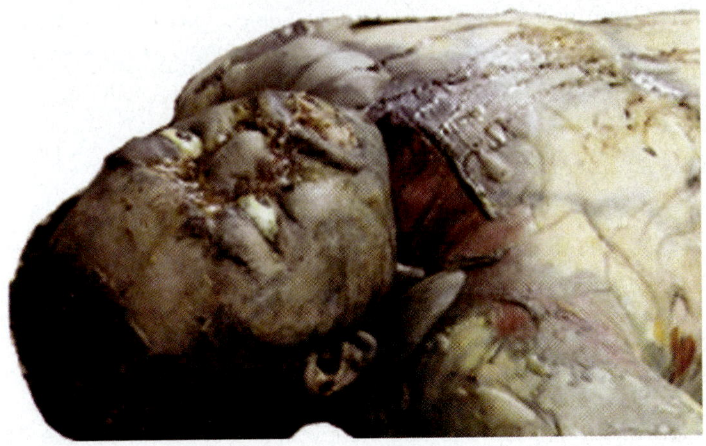

Figure 6.16: Decomposition changes with formation of blisters, purging of fluid and bulging out of eyes

10. **Floating of body:** In deaths due to drowning, the body first sinks in water and after formation of sufficient gases, the body floats. It may occur in about 24 hours in summer and 2-3 days in winter.

Colliquative putrefaction: Colliquative putrefaction is conversion of soft parts into a thick semifluid black mass. Walls of abdomen becomes soft and burst open as a result the stomach and intestine comes out. In the final stage of putrefaction, cartilage and ligaments are softened and ultimately the bones are destroyed.

Putrefaction of internal organs: Internally, decomposition proceeds at the same rate as is seen externally. Putrefaction of internal organs depends upon firmness, moisture content, density and quantity of blood. The blood decomposes and the colouring matter transudes into tissues colouring them. The viscera becomes softened and greasy. The changes seen are: (i) *Larynx and trachea*: Their mucous membrane becomes softened and colour changes to brownish red and later on greenish. (ii) *Stomach and intestine*: They show dark red to brownish patches first on the posterior wall and then on the anterior wall. The mucosa appears macerated and the whole intestine becomes a dark soft pulpy mass. (iii) *Spleen*: It softens and liquefies in two to three days. (iv) *Omentum and mesentery:* Depending on the amount of fat present they become grayish green and dry out. (v) *Liver:* Liver softens and becomes flabby in 12 to 24 hours in summer. Blisters appear on its surface in 24 to 36 hours. The liver assumes a **"honeycoomb" or "foamy" appearance** due to formation of air bubbles (Figure 6.17). The liver develops greenish discolouration that later changes to coal-black and extends to the whole organ. The organism responsible for the gas production is Cl. welchii. (vi) *Gallbladder*: Gallbladder is quite resistant to putrefaction but the bile pigments diffuse through its walls to the adjacent tissues quite early. (vii) *Pancreas*: It softens and becomes hemorrhagic. (viii) *Heart*: It dilates and becomes flabby, soft and shows blisters filled with gases (Figure 6.18). (ix) *Lungs:* Gaseous bullae are formed under the pleura which later coalesce and the lungs soften, collapse and are reduced to a small black mass (Figure 6.19). (x) *Kidneys:* Kidneys become soft and flabby. The surface looses its luster and becomes dull. The cortex becomes dark and later turns greenish. (xi) *Adrenal glands*: The medulla liquefies and the cortex softens from within outwards and the gland appears like a cyst. (xii) *Bladder*: Bladder is also highly resistant to putrefaction, especially if it is empty and contracted. (xiii) *Prostate:* It resists putrefaction for a very long time and this is the last organ to putrefy in males. (xiv) *Uterus*: Virgin uterus is the last organ to putrefy in females. However, a gravid or postpartum uterus putrefies rapidly. (xv) *Brain:* Brain is showing greenish discolouration as putrefaction initiates and then converted to semi-fluid mass that is soft and flabby and finally turns to pasty liquid due to liquefaction (Figure 6.20).

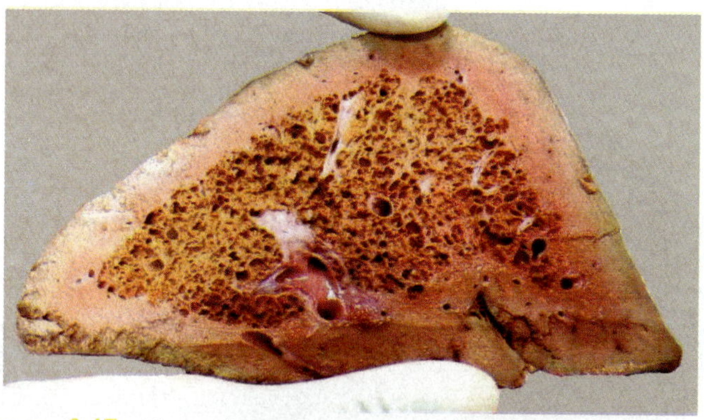

Figure 6.17: Liver showing honeycoomb appearance due to decomposition (*Courtesy:* Dr Venkatesh J, SR, AIIMS, Delhi)

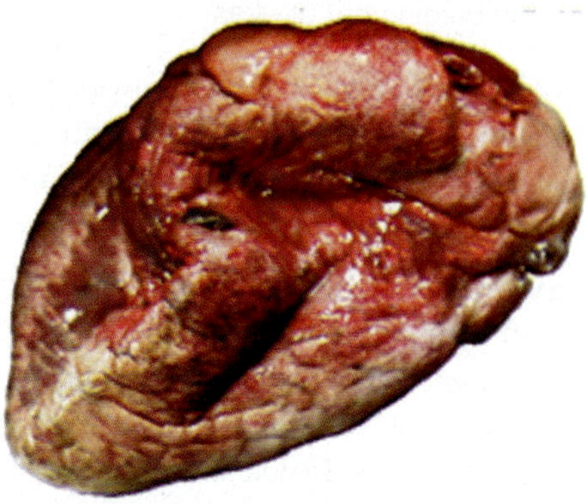

Figure 6.18: Heart showing the decomposition changes

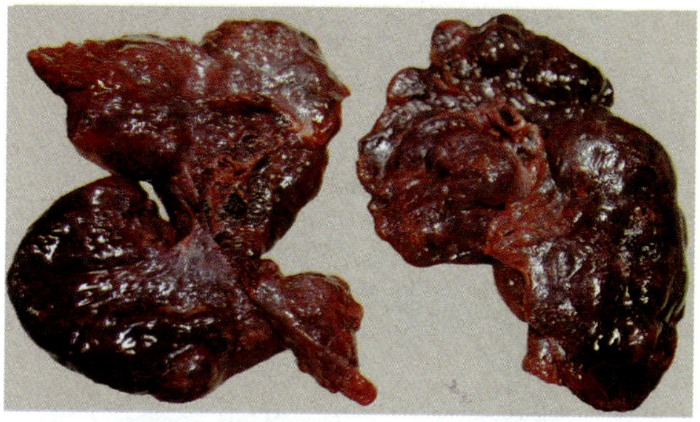

Figure 6.19: Lung showing decomposition changes

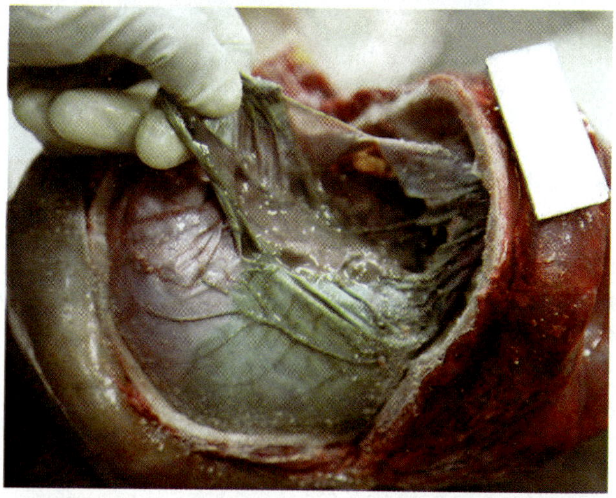

Figure 6.20: Brain showing liquefaction due to decomposition

Factors Influencing the Onset and Progression of Putrefaction

(i) ***Temperature:*** At temperature below 50°F putrefaction slows down and below 32°F, it is almost arrested. Temperature between 50°F and 70°F (21°C-38°C) is ideal for bacterial growth and at more than 70°F putrefaction is accelerated. (ii) ***Moisture:*** It is necessary for bacterial growth. Organs containing water putrefy rapidly and dry organs putrefy slowly like hair, teeth and bones.

(iii) ***Influence of air and light*:** Air influences putrefaction by its temperature and moisture content. Flies and insects avoid decomposed body parts. (iv) ***Clothes:*** Initially clothes hasten putrefaction by maintaining body temperature. The areas underneath the tight clothing develop putrefaction slowly due to bloodlessness in these area. Also, clothes protect against flies and insects. (v) ***Condition of the body:*** In fat and flabby bodies putrefaction is accelerated due to retention of heat. (vi) ***Age of the deceased*:** Dead bodies of newborn and stillborn are sterile. Thus, putrefaction occurs very slowly with the invasion of external bacteria. In old people putrefaction is delayed due to less moisture content. (vii) ***Cause of death:*** (a) Acute diseases lead to rapid decomposition due to increased temperature and increased bacteria. (b) In septic diseases due to increased bacterial activity rapid decomposition occurs. (c) ***Chronic diseases:*** In diseases with general oedema, rapid decomposition occurs. In emaciated and anemic individuals, putrefaction is delayed due to less amount of blood, atrophy and dryness of tissues. (viii) ***Poisons:*** In poisoning due to arsenic, antimony and zinc putrefaction is retarded due to inhibitory effect of poisons on organisms. In chronic arsenic and antimony poisoning due to their preservative action on the body tissues, putrefaction is retarded. In chronic alcoholism and strychnine poisoning putrefaction is rapid.

Medicolegal aspects: (i) Putrefaction is a sign of death (ii) It helps in calculating time since death (iii) It helps in identification of individual as hair, teeth and bones resist putrefaction (iv) Sex can be determined in putrefied bodies as prostate and nulliparous uterus resist putrefaction.

Casper's dictum: The body putrefies twice as rapidly when taken out of water and eight times faster when taken out of grave and placed in air. These differences in rate of putrefaction are given by Casper as: Air : Water : Grave = 1 : 2 : 8.

APPEARANCE OF MAGGOTS (ENTOMOLOGY)

Crimes or sudden deaths may expose the human bodies to the natural effect of the environment including invasion by the sarcosaprophagous insects. These insects have sense organs highly adapted to the detection of corpses.

Forensic entomology: Forensic Entomology is the application of insect biology to the investigation of crime. It is mainly concerned with the determination of time since death, place of death and occasionally manner of death. Forensic Entomology is based on the arrival of different species of these insects that is: (i) On the sequence with which they make their appearance on the carrion. (ii) On the recognition of the development stage of the offspring of the different species thus helping estimating the time elapsed since death.

Application of Entomology is restricted most effectively to the first six months after death. After death, invasion of an unprotected body by sarcosaprophagous insects and other small fauna comes in successive waves.

Historical Perspectives of Forensic Entomology

(i) The earliest known reference is in 13th century Chinese manuscript '**The Washing Away of Wrongs'.** (ii) In 1850, the first application of entomology to forensic science happened when **Dr Bergeret d' Arboris** determined the date of death of a child. (iii) In late 19th century, the following workers, **Megnin** in 1887, **Yovanitch** in 1888 and **Glaister and Brash** in 1937 in Britain in the notorious Buxton case determined time since death from the appearance of maggots. (iv) In the second half of 20th century, **Nuorteva** (1977), **Smith** (1986) and **Greenberg** (1991) studied Forensic Entomology.

Entomotoxicology: The study of the usefulness of insects as alternative toxicological samples is known as entomotoxicology. In cases where conventional tissues and fluids samples have degraded or are no longer available for toxicological analysis, insects, larvae, and other arthropods that did feed on corpse can be used. The drugs or poisons that can be detected are mercury, malathion, barbiturates, benzodiazepines, amphetamines, opiates, acetaminophen and salicylates etc.

Current Perspectives

1. (A) **Time of death (Larval development):** The first approach is the estimation of maggots developing in the body (Figures 6.21 to 6.23). For this purpose, the knowledge of life histories of flies of families **Calliphoridae (blowflies), Sarcophagidae (fruit flies) and Muscidae (Houseflies)** has an important application in forensic medicine.

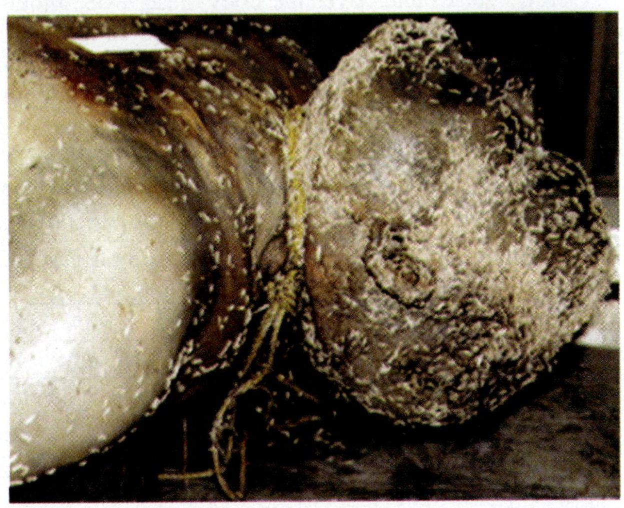

Figure 6.21: Body showing advanced decomposition with appearance of maggots

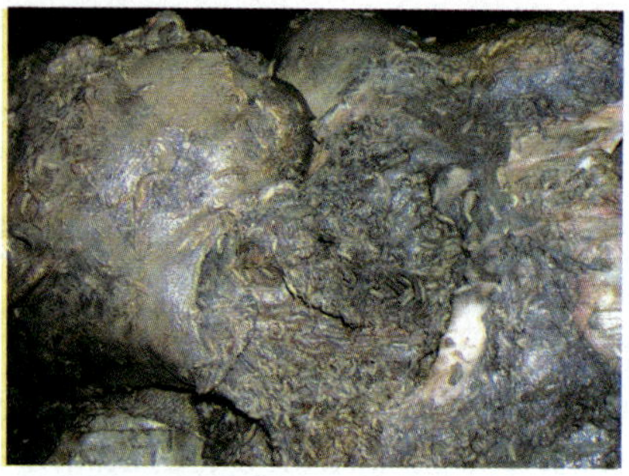

Figure 6.22: Body showing advanced decomposition of maggots and partly eaten up soft tissues

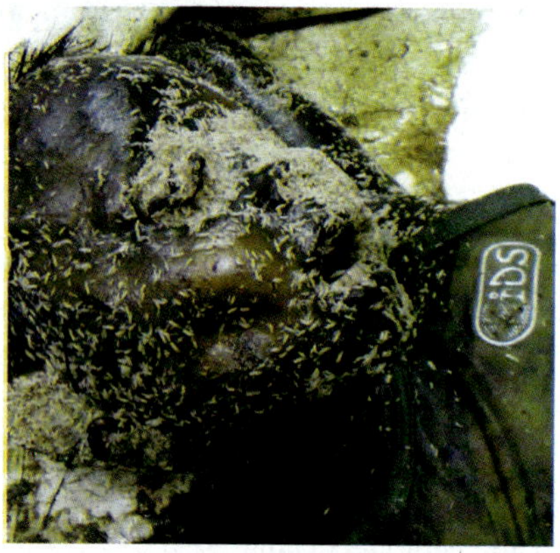

Figure 6.23: Body showing decomposition changes with formation of maggots

Adult flies lay eggs in the shadowed crevices of the corpse. After 4-5 days of emergence as an adult fly, the eggs are laid. The hatching of the eggs takes 1-2 days in cold and a few hours in warm atmosphere. The eggs of the fly are destroyed by heat, desiccation and any change in the position of the corpse since flies place eggs in microclimatically protected areas in the corpse. The young larvae on hatching start to erode the wounds over the body, nose, eyes, mouth or the anus and other soft tissues and moult three times to develop into third instars larvae. It starts to eat carrion. The larvae causes mechanical destruction of tissues by mouth hooks, secrete proteinases, lipases and collagenases and cause extraintestinal digestion of the feeding substrate. Fully grown larvae stops eating **(Post feeding larvae)** and then migrate away from the carcass and settle under the turf and then it evolves into white puparia **(White prepupa)**. The skin becomes tanned that is hard and changes to brownish colour. The hardened larval skin functions as an outer covering within which true pupation takes place. After pupal rest and metamorphosis, adult flies break the anterior end of the puparium and emerges and finally its wings grows. The adult flies at first eat the carbohydrates and then the proteins. **Oviposition** that is the laying of eggs occurs after 4-5 days.

The most common insect found in relatively fresh corpse is the Blow fly (Diptera) that comprises Blue bottle fly (Calliphora), Green bottle fly (Lucilla) and the common house fly (Musca domestica). The differences between the blue bottle and the common house flies are (Table 6.6).

(B) **Time of death (Faunal succession):** Insect fauna on the body will change with the time and as decomposition progresses. The nature of fauna that is the composition of the species will change with the passage of time. Knowledge of appearance of new species and decrease in numbers of other species which were previously present will unable the entomologist to arrive at an estimate of how long the body has been lying in that location. The invasion of corpse by insects depends upon whether the remains are found in open air, buried in ground or immersed in water.

In the open, there are eight successive waves of insect invasions:

Wave 1: This is the immediate wave after death. The larvae of various species of genera Calliphora and Musca are commonly found. **Calliphora** include mostly blow flies commonly observed in meat and milk products that spend summer and winter in the human environment. The genus **Musca** of the Muscidae contains house flies that inhabit in the human settlement areas all year around.

Wave 2: This wave of insects arrive upon the formation of odour in the corpse. Most commonly observed genera of flies are **Sarcophagidae, Lucila and Cynomyia**. Sarcophga (the

Table 6.6: Differences in general features and life cycle of Blue bottle and Common housefly

Features	*Blue bottle (Calliphora)*	*Common housefly (Musca domestica)*
• Invades	Dead flesh, preferably fresh	Decomposed flesh but mostly attracted to garbage and manure
• Size of flies	Large, 6-14 mm long, iridescent blue abdomen	Small
• Eggs	Yellow, banana shaped, 17 mm long	White and smaller
• Optimum temperature for egg hatching	6-7°C and no hatching occurs if the temperature is <4° C	4-16°C
• Hatching time	8-14 hours	8-12 hours
• Total cycle duration	8-10 days	32 (4°C) to 9 (16°C) days
• First maggot stage	8-14 hours	36 hours
• Second maggot stage	2-3 days	1-2 days
• Third maggot stage	4-5 days	3-4 days

flesh flies) are very similar to blow flies. They are viviparous and females give birth to about 150-200 larvae in groups of 10 to 20 at a time.

Wave 3: The most common genera of this wave include **Dermestes** (skin beetles) and **Aglossa** (butterflies and moths). Colonization occurs after the body fat becomes rancid. At this time the odour resulting from butyric acid is usually at its most overwhelming. This occurs in about 3 to 6 months in Northern Europe or places with similar temperature variations. Length of time can be much shorter in warmer places. Dermestids could start coming a day after death instead of 3-6 months.

Wave 4: Following butyric fermentation of fat, the second process is the caseic fermentation of the protein matter. This fermentation attracts mostly cheese or ham eating flies that is the genus of **Piophilia** (Skipper fly or ham and cheese fly). Furthermore, these flies would be more abundant and exclusively colonize a corpse of the large flies so that the previous wave cannot penetrate the body. Insects of this wave include Fannia and other small Coleoptera with metallic colours. Flies of Drosophilidae, Sepiridae and Sphaeroderidae may also found in this wave, if putrid liquids exude present on the body.

Wave 5: This wave coincides with ammoniacal fermentation and includes insects of the genus **Ophyra**. Upon the evaporation of sanious fluid, the so called 'humpbacked' flies of family Phoridae appear. Occasionally some flies of family Thyreophoridae may also be seen in this stage. They are primarily however flies of desiccated remains.

Wave 6: This is the stage of **mites** that absorb the remaining fluids and therefore the remains are desiccated. The flies are no longer seen. This stage takes about a year after death to reach in Europe.

Wave 7: This wave includes those flies that live on furs, hairs, fabrics and similar natural materials in museum. The major insects of this group are members of the **Coleoptera** order.

Wave 8: This occurs about three years after death. Various species of **Coleoptera** genera invade the area where the remains are found primarily to consume the debris left by earlier members of beetle order.

In buried remains the sequence of appearance is as follows: (i) Calliphora and Muscina (ii) Ophyra (iii) Phoridae (Diptera) invade the body a year after the death (iv) Coleoptera, are seen in second year after death.

2. **Place of death:** Since some of the species appear in a particular geographic area or a particular locality, from the examination of the insects, the particular geographic and ecologic place can be known.
3. **Cause and manner of death:** Actual event that lead of death is especially important in advanced putrefied bodies. Under normal conditions, when no wounds are present, flies lay eggs in natural orifices to avoid desiccation of eggs. If body has wounds, these blowflies would lay eggs in these wounded areas of the body that act as sheltered and moist spots for the developing eggs. In case of murder or suicide, the tissues may be entirely consumed by maggots when body is discovered, they accumulate and store in their tissues the toxic substances. From their toxicological analysis, presence and concentration of toxins can be known. Even if the human tissues are not completely consumed by maggots, it is better to test the maggots than the decomposing human remains since living tissues are easier to analyze than dead and decomposing ones. Hence, it is helpful in determining the cause of death in poisoning deaths, drug abuse deaths etc.
4. **Identification of unidentified corpse:** Extraction and characterization of human DNA from gut content of maggots/pupae recovered from unidentified copses can be used for identification of those unidentified bodies.

Areas of Controversy in Entomology

(i) ***Role of temperature in larval development:*** Temperature affects the rate of maggot development. Higher the temperature, more is the rate of development. Fluctuating temperature affect maggot development and there are different effects in different species and the effect on one specie is different than on the other. Acquiring a sequence of data from weather station, together with temperature measurements at the scene, enable the calculation of sequence of temperatures over the relevant periods. (ii) ***Variations in larval development:*** Insects from the same species but different localities develop at different rates. (iii) ***Myiasis:*** Invasion of living tissues by maggots is myiasis. Some species lay eggs on the living person or an animal and may lead to incorrect estimation of minimum time of death. It is common in the US, Southern Europe and Middle East. (iv) ***Role of temperature in fly activity:*** Flies lay eggs at a particular temperature and in the dark also. (v) ***Problems with the faunal succession:*** The differences in weather, location, season and the extent of interference by other animals means that it is very difficult to predict what species will arrive and when. A faunal succession will always occur on a dead body if it lies in nature for any length of time.

Practical guidelines: Insects can be collected from a corpse or its surroundings in three groups, namely, maggots, insects from soil and other insects. (i) ***Maggots:*** Maggots are immersed and killed in a very hot (almost boiling) water and transferred to a solution of acetic alcohol that is 3 parts 70% alcohol and 1 part glacial acetic acid. Killing in hot water over immediate immersion in preservative has two advantages: (a) Death of maggots is instantaneous so exact moment of death can be known and the estimation of age of maggots will help in determining the time since death. (b) Hot water kills maggots in a "relaxed state" in which they are fully stretched. Measurements of maggots can then be compared with measurements from experimental work. (c) If maggots are immersed in preservative to kill them, they will shrink and any measurements will be difficult to interpret.

Rearing of maggots can be done that is they can be kept alive on some meat or liver and reared to adult stage. Any puparia either empty or with the pupae inside them should be preserved in a specimen tube. All the containers carrying live specimens must be perforated for gaseous exchange. A large number of maggots should be collected. (ii) ***Soil insects:*** The soil samples should be collected in specimen bags from which insects can later be extracted in the laboratory. Each soil sample should be as much as would fit into a 'pint' bottle. Soil should not be compacted.

Skeletonization

The skeletonization is the reduction of the dead body to skeleton after removal of soft parts and tissues. The time required depends on variable factors such as: (i) Duration of body in water (ii) Seasonal and climatic variations (iii) Amount of water in soil (iv) Access of air (v) Acid content of soil. Depending on the duration of the body in water, fish and other aquatic animals eat away flesh in a few days. In hot climate when body is lying on ground the decay process may take about 5-10 years. If the body is lying exposed vultures, jackals and rats eat away the flesh within a short period. In an uncoffined buried body, it takes about one year for skeletonization. In air tight coffins the decaying of body is delayed for several decades. In a deeply buried body due to lower temperature, exclusion of air and absence of animals, skeletonization is markedly delayed. Acidic soil causes disintegration of body in about 25 to 100 years whereas neutral soil is quite protective.

Adipocere

Usually putrefaction is the final change occurring in a dead body. Adipocere formation or saponification replaces the putrefaction changes when the body remains submerged in water for appreciable time, buried in moist graves or waterlogged soil. The substance so formed is called adipocere and its properties are between *adipo* (fat) and *cere* (wax) (Figure 6.24).

Properties: (i) Soft, waxy looking substance (ii) Greasy to touch (iii) Dull white to dark brown in colour (iv) Disagreeable rancid odour (v) Specific gravity is less than water (vi) It is inflammable and burns with faint yellow flame (vii) Soluble in ether and alcohol (viii) When fresh, it is soft and moist and when old it is dry and brittle (ix) On fracture, it exhibits traces of fiber and blood vessels.

Composition: Gradual hydrolysis and hydrogenation of preexisting fat like olein that is converted to higher fatty acids like palmitic acid, stearic acid, hydroxystearic acid, glycerides etc. Hard waxy character is due to hydroxystearic acid, calcium soaps and proteins that occur as incidental components.

Certain bacterial enzymes liberated from decomposing protein are necessary for the hydrogenation of unsaturated body fats into saturated firmer fats. In early stages, there is formation

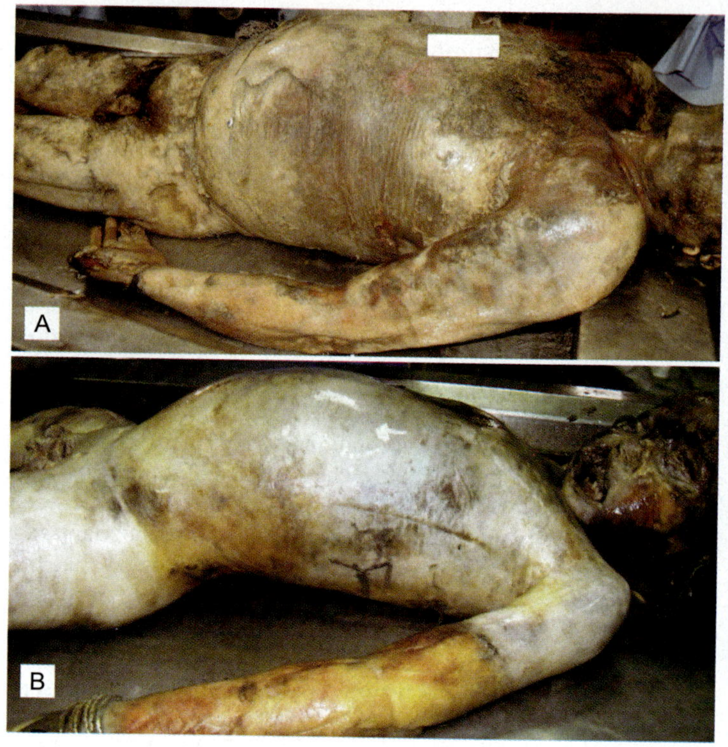

Figure 6.24: Adipocere formation

of ammoniacal soap. Water is essential for the change as it takes part in the synthesis and removes glycerine formed during hydrolysis of fat. Moist conditions are necessary during which adipocere formation takes place but at times it has been seen in dry conditions. Enzymes are also essential. At times it occurs inside the sealed coffins also. Common sites of formation are female breasts, cheeks, face, buttocks and the limbs. It is patchy in distribution and is quite unusually extensive. Since the facial features are preserved, it helps in identification. Nature of wounds remains unchanged and type of weapon can be known from the appearance of wounds. Slight amount of adipocere formation may occur in the muscles whereas internal organs are never affected.

Time: It occurs rapidly in bodies submerged in water than damp soil. In obese persons and mature newborn it is formed quickly. The adipocere formation is accelerated by heat and retarded by cold. In India, it has been reported varying from **3-35 days**. The time taken to develop has been given by Modi (7-35 days) and Mackenjie (3-15 days).

Medicolegal aspects: (i) Adipocere formation is a sign of death (ii) Identification is possible (iii) Nature of wounds and cause of wounds can be found out (iv) Time since death can be calculated.

Mummification

It is a modified form of putrefaction and is characterized by drying or shriveling of the tissue due to dehydration of the body constituents. The body assumes a dried, shrivelled, dark and leathery appearance (Figure 6.25). When climate is dry and warm with a free circulation of air around the dead body, the putrefaction is inhibited. Due to high temperature and moving air the body fluids evaporate rapidly, organism cannot thrive due to lack of moisture and mummification sets in. It begins in the exposed parts of the body like face, hands etc. and then spreads to other parts. The skin hardens, becomes leathery and adheres to the bones. It emits cheese like odor. The external appearance in a mummified body is preserved thus helping in identification. As the wounds remain intact, the cause of death can be determined. Internal organ thickens and becomes dark brown.

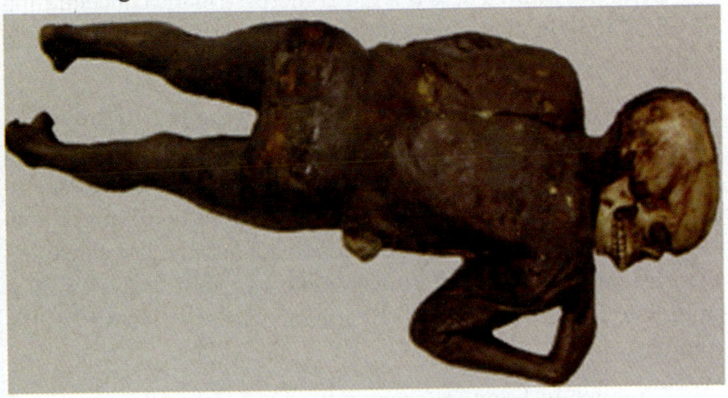

Figure 6.25: Mummified body

It is observed in Rajasthan when the bodies are buried in shallow graves of dry sandy soil. Bodies of newborn infants mummify when concealed in or kept on top of trees, rafters of roof or in steel trunk and left open. At times few parts of a dead body are mummified and other parts show adipocere formation. Time varies greatly for its formation. The average time it takes is from **few months to 1 year** and even at times upto 2 years. The time is also influenced by temperature, place of disposal and size of the body.

Medicolegal aspects: (i) Mummification is a sign of death (ii) Identification is possible (iii) Nature of wounds and cause of wounds can be found out (iv) Time since death can be calculated.

Estimation of Postmortem Interval (Figure 6.26)

Postmortem interval is the time between examination of body and death. It is often touted as the Holy Grail of forensic pathology. The legal importance of this interval is: (i) To calculate the time of injuries (ii) It may exclude some persons in homicidal deaths. The parameters used for estimation of postmortem interval are:

Emptying time of the stomach: Before being released into the duodenum, food stays in the stomach for a considerable period. The physical state of the food is also progressively altered by the gastric juices and movements. Therefore, its appearance and volume is taken to be a measure of the time since it was last swallowed. The last ordinary mixed meal in a normal adult stomach empties in 3-4 hours. If undigested food is present then the deceased must have died within 3-4 hours of ingestion of the last meal that can be known from the circumstantial evidence and

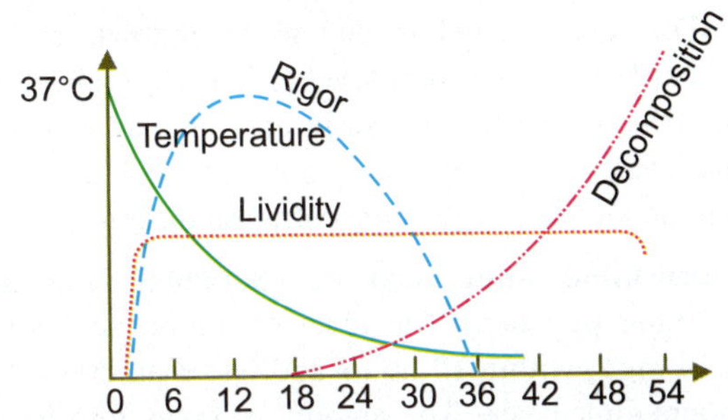

Figure 6.26: Curves for estimating time since death from various parameters

the time of death can be estimated from this. The physiological process of digestion of an average meal lasts for about 2-3 hours. According to **Modi**, it takes 4-6 hours for a meat and vegetable meal and 6-7 hours for a fatty meal. **Adelson** stated that stomach begins to empty within 10 minutes of swallowing; 'light' meal takes two hours, 'medium' meal takes 3-4 hours and a 'heavy' meal takes 4-6 hours to empty from the stomach. **Adelson** again stressed that the head of an average meal reaches the ileocaecal valves between 6-8 hours of ingestion. Milk leaves stomach rapidly whereas meat and pulses are retained for a longer time. The head of the meal reaches the hepatic flexure in about 6 hours, splenic flexure in 9-12 hours and pelvic colon 12-18 hours. Unless death was sudden and unexpected, the state of digestion or volume of stomach contents cannot be relied upon. However, when the stomach is full of undigested food it can be said confidentially that the death has occurred within 2-4 hours of the last meal.

Factors which, influence the emptying time, are: (i) Motility of the stomach (ii) Consistency of the gastric contents (iii) Osmotic pressure of the gastric contents (iv) Quantity of material in the duodenum (v) Physical nature of the meal.

The meals containing carbohydrate empty from stomach faster than protein whereas protein leaves quicker than fats. A fatty meal inhibits gastric motility. Fluids and semi-fluids leave the stomach almost immediately after being swallowed. Emotion, fear, anxiety etc. delays emptying.

Postmortem Chemistry

Blood: (i) *pH:* There is fall in pH of the blood after death due to glycolysis, glycogenolysis and accumulation of carbon dioxide and lactic acid and after 24 hours the blood become alkaline due to production of ammonia. (ii) *Nonprotein nitrogenous substances:* They are increased to the level of 50 mg% in first 12 hours after death. Amino acid nitrogen is less than 14 mg/dl upto 10 hours but rises to 30 mg/dl by 48 hours. (iii) *Enzymes*: Enzymes such as transaminases, lactic dehydrogenase, phosphatase and amylase undergoes a rapid rise for few hours after death. The level steadies for the next 2-3 days and then falls due to proteolysis. The peak level of phosphatase and amylase is within 36-48 hours whereas that of transaminase is within 48-60 hours. (iv) *Sugar:* Blood sugar level increases within 12 hours of death and rises upto

300 mg. This raised level is due to breakdown of liver and glycogen. (v) *Sodium:* Sodium level falls by 0.9 mEq/l per hour. (vi) *Urea:* Blood urea levels rise in an irregular manner due to proteolysis within 48 hours but it is never more than 100 mg% unless there is increased urea concentration during life.

Cerebrospinal fluid: CSF is examined after obtaining through lumbar puncture. The level of amino acid nitrogen is less than 14 mg% within 10 hours and less than 80 mg% during first 24 hours after death. The amount of potassium increases at a constant rate in relation to the temperature of the body during first 20 hours. The levels of creatinine are decreased to < 5 mg% within 10 hours and further < 10 mg% within 30 hours after death. **Schourup** worked out hourly change in axillary temperature, lactic acid, nonprotein nitrogen and amino acid to calculate time since death from their levels at the time of death. He introduced a formula taking an average of the results of four methods. This is a reliable method only upto 15 hours after death and is only applicable to adults. Besides this the sample of CSF should be free of blood. This formula is expected to give approximate time since death within $\pm$ 1-3 hours. The formula is given as:

$$T = \frac{36 - \text{ax T°c} - \text{antilog}\ \dfrac{\text{L.A.}}{180} - \dfrac{\text{N.P.N.} - 15}{16.7} - \dfrac{\text{A.A.} - 1}{7.35}}{4}$$

Where, T = Time since death in hours, axT°c means axillary temperature at the time of examination, L.A. = Lactic acid, N.P.N. = Nonprotein nitrogen, A.A. = Amino acids.

Schleyer in 1963 suggested that a concentration in the cisternal fluid of amino acid nitrogen not exceeding 40 mg% would indicate that death has taken place not more than ten hours previously. A nonprotein nitrogen concentration less than 80 mg% would show that more than 24 hours have elapsed since death and that creatine values under 5 mg% and 10 mg% would render probable a postmortem interval of not more than 10 hours and 30 hours respectively.

Vitreous humour: Potassium: The concentration of potassium ranges from 5- 8 mmol/L at the time of death and there is an increase in its concentration at the rate of 0.17 to 0.238 mmol/L per hour. However, it is to be noted that this relationship in estimating time since death is not linear and multiple factors like temperature, level of decomposition and urea retention in body may affect this range.

The following formulas are shown to be useful for calculating time since death using potassium concentration:

Madea's formula: PMI = 5.26 × K+ concentration - 30.9.

Sturner's formula: PMI = 7.14 × K+ concentration - 39.1.

The rise in potassium concentration occurs mainly due to diffusion from retina into the center of the globe. Also, there may be a 10% variation in the potassium concentration between the two eyes.

Hypoxanthine: Its concentration begins rising immediately after death and shows a linear pattern upto 120 hours.

Others: There is a decrease of sodium concentration at a rate of 0.9 mmol/L/hour and Chloride by 1 mmol/L/hour. Vitreous glucose starts decreasing soon after death and reaches zero value within few hours. Levels of Ascorbic and Pyruvic acid in the vitreous humour falls after death.

Pericardial fluid: Constituents are not helpful in estimating time since death.

Synovial fluid: There is a linear increase in the concentration of potassium in the synovial fluid after death which doubles within two days after death.

Examination of hair: A knowledge of the rate of growth of facial hair allows an estimate to be made of the age of the beard reckoned from the time of the last shave. Since hair ceases to grow at death, the length of the beard of dead body might then suggest the time that lapsed between death and the last shave. As there is contraction of skin towards the hair root it gives a false impression of growth of hair. Beard hair grows at the rate of 0.4 mm/day.

Changes in bone marrow cells: During life the sample of bone marrow cells is obtained by sternal puncture that shows 40% neutrophils. After death, the changes seen are: (i) *First hour of death:* Nuclei begin to swell (ii) *Within 3-4 hours of death:* Nuclei attain the size of myelocytes (iii) *Within 4-6 hours of death:* Outline of cells are distinct with vacuolation in cytoplasm (iv) *After 10 hours of death:* A syncytial mass is formed from fusion of cells and nuclear debris can be detected.

Changes in the bones: The radiocarbon dating of the bones for assessing the age of ancient remains is of interest to archeologists and not to the forensic pathologists. Radioactive carbon is formed in the atmosphere by the action of cosmic rays and a steady state is reached between the rate of its formation and decay. After death the carbon 14 contents of the remains gradually sinks and the radioactivity naturally weakens but it takes about 5,600 years to reach half its initial activity. Therefore, if the carbon 14 activity is measured and compared with what is known to exist in the body during life, a reasonable estimate can be made for the age of the remains.

Molecular approach: Several studies have tried to determine changes in molecular markers to provide more useful information for PMI. Measurable or quantifiable technique for degradation of nucleic acid molecule such as DNA, RNA, micro-RNA and protein are used to corelate the study. However, the current results have not been consistent and in-depth studies including influence of the various parameters would be necessary to verify the effective applicability to the PMI estimate both early and late postmortem period.

A. **Quantitative analysis of postmortem DNA degradation:** DNA is one of the most stable components of cells. It is believed that its degradation continues at a constant rate, regardless of the temperature and the mechanisms of death. The good stability of DNA occurs in the brain cortex, lymph nodes and psoas muscle after the 3 weeks of time (Bär *et al.,* 1988). Various Chinese forensic scholars developed multi-parametric mathematical model for PMI estimation. Methods used in assessing DNA degradation are Restriction Fragment Length Polymorphism (RFLP), flow cytometry analysis, Image Analysis Technique (IAT), Single Cell Gel Electrophoresis (SCGE), RT-qPCR analysis and by other techniques.

B. **Quantitative analysis of postmortem RNA degradation:** RNA is less stable than DNA in postmortem tissue, yet selected mRNA molecules can be detected by reverse-transcriptase PCR up to 3 days after death. A quantitative analysis of normalized transcript levels on the murine's visceral and muscle tissues identified four quadriceps muscle genes (Actb, Gapdh, Ppia and Srp72) that are significantly correlate with PMI. A mathematical model is also developed for prediction of PMI (Sampaio-Silv *et al.* 2013). MicroRNA (miRNA) can be detected in decomposed tissue as it is not easily degraded by ribonuclease, and is resistant to changes in environmental factors, can be used also for determination of PMI.

C. **Quantitative analysis of postmortem protein degradation:** Proteins tend to have unique patterns of degradation. Some proteins remain active, and others exhibit increased expression for some time after death. Proteins involved in histone modifications can be used for estimation of PMI. Study revealed muscle protein like titin, nebulin, desmin, cardiac troponin T, and SERCA1 degraded in a regular and predictable fashion which can be used estimation of PMI (Pittner, 2016). Various techniques like sodium dodecyl sulphate polyacrylamide gel electrophoresis (SDS-PAGE), Western blotting, and casein zymography can be used to analyse the time course of degradation of selected proteins.

LONG QUESTIONS

1. Discuss the immediate and early changes after death.
2. Discuss the late changes after death.
3. What are the different muscle changes after death? Discuss rigor mortis in detail.
4. How do you calculate time since death from various postmortem changes?

SHORT QUESTIONS

1. Changes in the eye after death.
2. Livor mortis.
3. Rigor mortis.
4. Algor mortis.
5. Cadaveric spasm.
6. Postmortem caloricity.
7. Adipocere.
8. Mummification.
9. Putrefaction.
10. Time since death estimation from body fluids.

MULTIPLE CHOICE QUESTIONS

1. **Cessation of circulation may be assessed by all *except:***
   (a) Magnus's test (b) Winslow's test
   (c) I card's test (d) Diaphanous test

2. **Type of curve expected during cooling of dead body is:**
   (a) Sigmoid (b) Linear
   (c) Hyperbolic (d) Parabolic

3. **The ideal place to record temperature in a dead body is from:**
   (a) Axilla (b) Groin
   (c) Rectum (d) Mouth

4. **Postmortem caloricity is seen in all *except:***
   (a) Burns (b) Tetanus
   (c) Strychnine poisoning (d) Septicaemia

5. **Postmortem staining is caused due to:**
   (a) Capillo-venous distension
   (b) Rupture of capillaries and extravasations of blood
   (c) Infiltration of blood under skin due to haemolysis
   (d) Staining of the blood vessels due to haemolysis

6. **Fixation of postmortem staining occurs in about:**
   (a) 2-4 hours (b) 4-5 hours
   (c) 6-8 hours (d) More than 8 hours

7. **Differentiating features between bruise and postmortem staining are all *except:***
   (a) Histology shows signs of inflammation in postmortem lividity
   (b) Colour of the bruise is variable depending on the duration
   (c) Postmortem staining is due to engorgement of vessels due to pooling of blood
   (d) Postmortem staining is normally present in the dependent parts

8. Rigor mortis first appears in:

(a) Heart (b) Eyelids
(c) Neck (d) Upper limb

9. Rigor mortis is developed due to:

(a) Depletion of ATP levels in the muscles
(b) Coagulation of muscle proteins
(c) Solidification of body fats
(d) All of the above

10. The onset of rigor mortis is delayed in case of:

(a) Electrocution
(b) Lightning
(c) Carbon monoxide poisoning
(d) Organophosphorus poisoning

11. As per Casper's Dictum, the rate of putrefaction of body in air compared to earth is:

(a) Same (b) Two times
(c) Four times (d) Eight times

12. In males, the last organ to putrefy is:

(a) Heart (b) Liver
(c) Prostate (d) Spleen

13. The first external sign of putrefaction in a dead body is:

(a) Distension of lower abdomen
(b) Greenish discoloration of the abdomen over right iliac fossa
(c) Peeling of skin
(d) Marbling of the skin

14. The enzyme responsible for postmortem hemolysis is liberated by:

(a) B. Cereus (b) B. Coli
(c) Streptococci (d) Cl. Welchii

15. All are true for adipocere formation *except:*

(a) Occurs in damp and moist climates
(b) Produces disagreeable rancid odour
(c) Facial features are lost
(d) Soft and waxy looking

16. In females, the last organ to putrefy is:

(a) Liver
(b) Adrenal gland
(c) Gravid uterus
(d) Nulliparous uterus

17. Delayed putrefaction of body occurs with poisoning by:

(a) Mercury
(b) Lead
(c) Arsenic
(d) Strychnine

18. The head of the meal reaches hepatic flexure in about:

(a) 4 hours
(b) 6 hours
(c) 9-12 hours
(d) 15-18 hours

19. All are true for mummification *except:*

(a) It is a modified form of putrefaction
(b) Occurred in dry, airy and warm climate
(c) The external appearance is preserved which helps in identification
(d) The average time it takes for development is 2 weeks

20. The time since death can be calculated by all *except:*

(a) Livor mortis (b) Rigor mortis
(c) Adipocere (d) Compos mentis

ANSWER KEY

1. (b)	2. (a)	3. (c)	4. (a)	5. (a)	6. (c)	7. (a)	8. (a)	9. (a)	10. (c)
11. (d)	12. (c)	13. (b)	14. (d)	15. (c)	16. (d)	17. (c)	18. (b)	19. (d)	20. (d)

7 CHAPTER

Autopsy Procedures and Exhumation

AUTOPSY

Autopsy means examination of a body after death. In India, there is provision for a complete postmortem examination. Every cavity of the body should be examined. Even if the cause of death is evident, other areas and organs of the body to be examined to find out any contributory cause of death. Complete autopsy is necessary to corroborate the evidence of the eyewitnesses and the investigations done by investigating officer since a poor autopsy can lead to miscarriage of justice.

A qualified Registered Medical Practitioner should carry out the autopsy. He should himself dissect the body and examine the organs to find out the queries asked by the Investigating Officer, most frequently the cause of death. The postmortem attendants and sweepers should be there to assist in the procedure. The term autopsy is synonymous with **necropsy**, **thanatopsy** and **postmortem**. The autopsy is of two types:

Medicolegal autopsy: It is mostly conducted at Government Hospitals or Government medical colleges/institutions. Private medical colleges/institutions can undertake postmortem examination, however, it can be conducted only with the permission of the State Government. It is conducted by a Forensic Medicine expert or medical practitioner with training in Forensic Medicine at graduation level. The request comes either from the police or SDM who is the Investigation Officer of the case. The consent of the relatives is not required. The doctor conducts a full and complete postmortem to find out the cause of death and other relevant questions asked by the Investigating Officer.

Pathological autopsy: It is conducted by the Department of Pathology and request comes from the relatives, who are the consenting party. In these cases the doctor conducts a partial autopsy of the organ or cavities where the pathologist expects to find out the cause of death.

The forensic autopsy differs from the pathological autopsy in its objectives as well as relevance. The forensic pathologist conducts the autopsy to determine the cause of death, manner of death (natural, accidental, suicidal or homicidal), the identity of the deceased if unknown and the time of death and/or injury. The forensic autopsy may also involve collection of evidence from the body that can subsequently be used to prove or disprove an individual's guilt and confirm or deny his account of how the death occurred.

The forensic autopsy involves not only the actual examination of the body at the autopsy table, but considers other aspects that the general pathologist does not consider part of the autopsy such as the crime scene, clothing and toxicological analysis. The forensic pathologist should know the circumstances leading up to and surrounding the death prior to the autopsy. The history of the case should be obtained from the investigating police officer or the subdivisional magistrate. At times the relatives or the eye witnesses can also give history.

The scene of crime should when an opportunity arises be examined and documented either with diagrams or photographs or with both. The statements of the relatives and the witnesses at the scene should be recorded by the police and should be given to the forensic pathologist. The body should be handled a very little at the scene. In cases of violent deaths, paper bags should be secured around the hands so that no trace evidence will be lost. Plastic bags should not to be used to cover the hands to avoid condensation in cold room and possible loss of trace evidence when it is moved to warm environment. The body should be wrapped in a clean, white sheet or plastic bag.

The examination of clothing for blood stains and trace evidence and correlating the tears or cuts on the clothing with bodily injuries is an important part of the autopsy. When fingerprints are to be taken for identification purposes, it should be done only after the examination of the hands.

In all gunshot deaths and severely burnt bodies, X-rays should be undertaken. This is especially important in gunshot wounds in which the bullet appears to have exited. This is because the bullet may not have exited but rather only a piece of bullet or bone may have exited. This is common with the semi-jacketed ammunition in which the jacket may remain inside the body and lead core may exit.

Aims and objectives: The aims and objectives of the postmortem examination are to: (i) Determine the identification in cases of unknown body (ii) Find out the cause of death (iii) Find out the manner of death whether suicidal, accidental or homicidal (iv) Find out the time since death (v) In newborn babies, determination of viability and cause of death (vi) Preserve the trace evidences and viscera when needed (vii) Reconstruct the accident scene from the examination of injuries by noting nature and duration etc.

Permission for autopsy: A written request must be obtained from Police Officer, not below the rank of ASI who should be the investigating officer. In cases of murder the Inspector is the investigating officer. In circumstances where the SHO/Inspector is busy and not available, he should get permission from the Deputy Commissioner to depute one junior officer for the same. The inspector should take the charge of the case once he is free. There are certain types of cases where the Magistrate holds an inquest and the request for autopsy should come from the Magistrate.

Preparation for autopsy: (i) The Investigating Officer should fill the performa 'Request for postmortem' and alongwith other inquest papers should submit the body in the mortuary. (ii) Autopsy should be done without delay. (iii) I.O. and relatives whose names are written on inquest papers should identify the body. In cases of unknown bodies, the I.O. is directed to take the photographs and fingerprints of the body and the doctor should note at least five identification marks on the autopsy report. (iv) Autopsy is conducted in the mortuary of a government hospital. At times the autopsy is carried out in the open space, or a covered area in emergency such as at the accident site in cases of mass disasters; air crash or train accident etc. (v) Mortuary should have good lightening, equipments, facility of cold storage and proper drainage system alongwith the manpower. (vi) Forensic Pathologist should take the history from I.O. and should carefully go through the inquest papers. (vii) Autopsy is done during the daytime, because of difficulty in appreciating certain colour changes in injuries and in jaundice etc. in artificial light. As per the Government of India order (2021), postmortem examination **can also be conducted after sunset (Night autopsy)**, at hospitals which have the infrastructure. However, cases such as homicide, suicide, rape, decomposed bodies and suspected foul play should not be subjected for postmortem examination during night time unless there is a law and order situation. Videography shall be done for all postmortem examination conducted during night time to rule out any suspicion and preserved for future reference for legal purpose. (viii) No unauthorized persons should be present in the autopsy room. The I.O. may be allowed if required. (ix) Autopsy is also carried out in a decomposed, mutilated, fragmented and skeletonized bodies as certain important information may still be found during examination.

Procedure of Autopsy

External examination: The external description of the body should include the age, sex, race, physique, height, weight and nourishment etc. Congenital malformations, if present should be noted. A simple listing of the articles found on the body should be noted initially such as a short-sleeve white shirt, or a long-sleeve white shirt, unbuttoned down the front, or a blood stained white T-shirt. In a case of traumatic death with significant alterations of the garments due to trauma, the clothing should be described in further detail. One should then describe the degree and distribution of rigor mortis and postmortem staining. The colour of the eye, the hair and the appearance of the eyes should be noted. Any unusual appearance of the ears, nose, or face for example congenital malformations, scarring or severe acne should be recorded. Note the presence of teeth and or presence of any dental plates. The presence of vomitus in the nostrils and mouth should be noted. Any significant scars, tattoos, moles should be noted for the purpose of identification. If there is any evidence of disease, it should be recorded. All the old injuries should be noted. Evidence of recent medical and/or surgical intervention should also be recorded.

Evidence of injuries: All recent external as well as internal injuries, whether minor or major should be described along with the age of the lesions in this section, if possible. Gun shot wounds and to a degree stab wounds should be described under the separate sections of external and internal injuries.

In gunshot wounds, if possible each individual wound should be described in its entirety before going on to a second wound. The gunshot wound should be described on the body in inches or centimeters in relation to the top of the head or the sole of the foot and to the right or left of midline. It should then be described in regard to a local landmark, such as the nipple or the umbilicus. The features of the wound that make it an entrance and that determine at what range it was fired should be described, for example abrasion collar, soot or tattooing. Pertinent negatives should also be noted. Then, the course of the bullet through the body should be described. All organs perforated or penetrated by the missile should be noted. It is useful to give an overall description of the missile path through the body in relation to the planes of the body. If the bullet exits, the exit wound should be described in relation to the entrance.

If the bullet is found, one should state where it was found, whether it is intact, deformed, or fragmented, whether it is jacketed, and the approximate caliber. A letter or number should be inscribed on the bullet. The bullet then should be placed in an envelop with the name of the victim, the date, postmortem number the location from which the bullet was recovered, the letter or number assigned to it and the name of the police station.

To describe stab wounds, one should indicate whether the weapon was single or double edged, which edge of the wound is produced by the cutting edge of the knife, the exact dimensions, and an estimation of the depth of the wound track produced. In dozens of knife wounds, it may not be possible to handle each wound separately but it should be described in groups.

Examination of clothing is to be done to locate the defects, whether they correspond to the injuries, the presence of trace evidence such as powder, soot, grease or car paint etc.

Demonstration of pneumothorax: Various methods to demonstrate pneumothorax are: (i) Skin and subcutaneous tissue are first reflected from the chest wall, by sweeping cuts through the subcutaneous tissue over the chest wall angling the blade down towards the ribs, being careful not to open the pleural cavity. The intercostal soft tissues should not be punctured and neither the pleural space be penetrated as this releases air from underlying pneumothorax. When reflection is completed to mid-axillary line, water is poured into the angle between subcutaneous tissue and the chest wall, and the intercostal tissue below the water line are pierced with the blade to detect an underlying pneumothorax, which may occur following trauma, in patients with chronic obstructive airway disease or asthma. If pneumothorax is present, air bubbles will be seen rising through the water. (ii) Before giving any incisions over the body, a wide bore needle attached to a 50 ml syringe minus the plunger is introduced into the subcutaneous tissue over an intercostal space and the syringe is then filled with water. The needle is pushed slightly deeper to enter the pleural space and the water is observed for the presence of any air bubbles. The process can be repeated on the other side also. (iii) Chest X-ray of the body to demonstrate pneumothorax should also be taken.

Demonstration of air embolism: Whenever there is possibility of venous air embolism, the following steps should be performed: (i) A plane X-ray of chest should be performed before eviscerating to demonstrate air embolism. (ii) Retina should be thoroughly examined with an ophthalmoscope for intravascular bubbles by moistening the cornea with isotonic saline to prevent interference from corneal opacity. (iii) During dissection of the neck, the large neck veins should be carefully exposed but not opened before the heart is dissected *in situ* to avoid the confusion of air introduction during evisceration. (iv) Abdomen is opened in the usual way to closely inspect the inferior vena cava for air bubbles in the lumen through its transparent wall. (v) Sternum is removed by dividing the ribs, being careful not to puncture the pericardial sac, and cutting through the sternum distal to the sternoclavicular joint. The internal mammary vessels should be clamped. The anterior pericardial sac is opened and external epicardial veins are inspected for evidence of intraluminal bubbles. The water is then introduced to fill the pericardial space. The right atrium and ventricle are incised covered in water and inspected for any air bubbles that escape. Alternatively, a water-filled syringe without the plunger is connected to a needle that is inserted into the right ventricle and the chamber of syringe is observed for air bubbles. When the presence of an air embolus is established the vena cava should be clamped and the thoracic and abdominal cavities flooded with water in an attempt to localize the source of embolism. Sometimes the intracardiac gas produced by postmortem bacterial activity may produce the appearance of a counterfeit air embolus. (vi) ***Pyrogallol test:*** 4 ml of a 2% freshly prepared pyrogallol solution is collected into two 10 ml syringes. Four drops of 0.5 M sodium hydroxide solution are added to the first syringe and the mixture should turn yellow in the presence of air. Gas is then aspirated from the right side of the heart; the needle is removed and replaced with a stopper. The syringe is then shaken and the mixture should turn brown, if air is present. In the absence of air, the solution will remain clear, indicating gas production by bacteria. The second syringe is used as a positive control by including a volume of air with the introduction of sodium hydroxide. This should also turn brown. (vii) Arterial air emboli are even more unusual and usually the result of traumatic injury such as thoracic trauma involving pulmonary veins or following air introduction during cardiopulmonary bypass. A much smaller volume of air is associated with such emboli and are much more difficult to demonstrate. Systemic emboli may be demonstrated by inspecting the intracranial vessels of the meninges and circle of Willis and then examining under water after clamping the internal carotid and basilar arteries.

Internal examination: In India due to provision of complete autopsy, the whole body is to be examined. The following types of incision are usually given depending upon the nature of the case, to open the body (Figure 7.1): (i) *'I' shaped incision:* It extends from the chin straight down to the symphysis passing either on the left or right side of the umbilicus. The umbilicus is

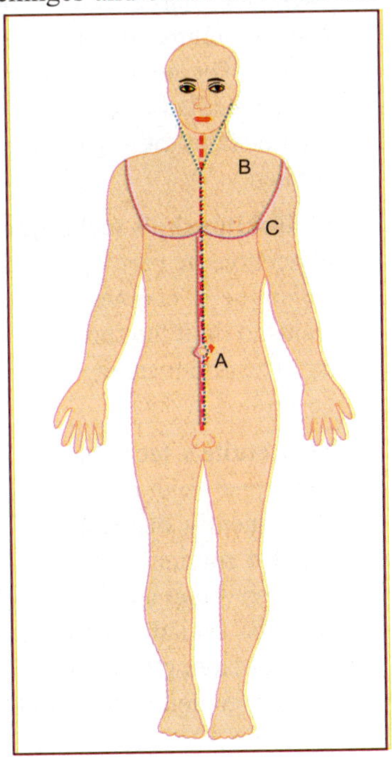

Figure 7.1: Various incisions over the body: A = I shaped, B = modified Y shaped and C = Y shaped

spared because of its dense fibrous tissue, which is difficult to stitch. (ii) *'Y' shaped incision:* The incision starts at a point close to the acromial process on both sides. It extends down below the mammary line up to the xiphoid process from where it extends down up to symphysis pubis on either side of umbilicus. (iii) *Modified 'Y' shaped:* An incision is made from suprasternal notch in midline up to symphysis pubis by the side of umbilicus. It extends from suprasternal notch to the middle of clavicle on both sides extending up to side of neck behind the ear till mastoid process. I-shaped incision is the one that is routinely employed. However, when a greater access to thoracic organs is needed then Y-shaped incision is preferred. When neck structures are to be examined, modified Y-shaped incision should be given.

The choice of opening the skull or other body cavity varies with the choice of pathologist conducting the autopsy. The major organ systems as well as organ cavities are systemically described in this section. The various organ systems and body cavities to be described are the head, neck, thoracic, abdominal and pelvic cavity as well as the biliary tract, pancreas, adrenals, urinary tract, reproductive tract and musculoskeletal system whenever the need arises.

Autopsy Dissection Techniques

The autopsy techniques used in various centres and hospitals differ very little. Therefore, the pathologist can depend on the method he masters best. Autopsy techniques may vary in the order in which the organs are removed, in the planes and lines of sectioning and most importantly in the method of removal of organs in the body.

1. **R. Virchow's technique:** In this method organs are removed one by one. First the cranial cavity is exposed and from the back, the spinal cord, followed by the thoracic, cervical and abdominal organs. This method has been used most widely. The advantage of this technique is that each organ can be studied in detail. However, the anatomico-pathologic relationships of organs are not preserved thus, cannot be studied.
2. **C. Rokitansky's technique:** This technique involves *in situ* dissection in part combined with *en block* removal. This technique is commonly preferred whenever the pathologist wants to limit the spread of infection such as HIV, hepatitis B etc. The disadvantage of this method is that the organs cannot be studied in detail.
3. **M. Letulle's technique:** In this method, thoracic, cervical, abdominal and pelvic organs are removed *en masse* but subsequently dissected as organ blocks. This technique is best for routine inspection and preservation of connections between organ and organ systems. In addition, the body can be made available to the undertaker in less than 30 minutes without having to rush the dissection. The organ blocks can then be studied in detail but the organ mass is often awkward to handle.
4. **A. Ghon's technique:** In this method the thoracic, cervical, abdominal organs and the urogenital system are removed as organ blocks. However, nowadays the modification of this technique is used where the organs are removed *en block*.

The method of evisceration should be the one with which the pathologist is most comfortable that is removing thoracic and abdominal organ blocks prior to dissection or removing each organ in sequence. Many crucial observations can be made only during evisceration.

All the organs should be weighed and a brief description of the organs with pertinent negatives should be recorded. With the pancreas, adrenals, and spleen, if there are no positive findings, use of the term 'unremarkable' as the sole description is acceptable. The term 'normal' should not be used as organs are rarely 'normal' whatever that is. The microscopic slides should be made when indicated. Samples of tissues from all major organs should be saved, but microscopic slides are often not needed in forensic cases, especially in trauma cases. The samples and viscera preserved for toxicological analyses should be noted. Finally, the opinion should be given describing briefly the cause of death in language as simple as possible.

Detailed Examination of the Neck

In asphyxial deaths, especially in hanging and strangulation, it is advisable to open the skull first and brain is taken out to drain out the blood from the neck so that the neck structures can be examined in a relatively bloodless field thus avoiding artifactual haemorrhages. The chest organs can be removed prior to neck dissection avoiding injuring the neck veins.

The modified Y-shaped incision permits a thorough examination of the anterior neck organs and removal of the tongue. The primary midline (I-shaped) incision can be extended superiorly in one of the following ways: (i) A straight incision in front of the trachea. (ii) A bilateral extension of the primary midline incision along the anterior border of the clavicles to the skin in front of the acromion process; and (iii) A bilateral incision extending the primary again along the anterior border of the clavicles but moving superiorly towards the tragus along the lateral side of the neck, ending just behind the ears. If air embolism is a possibility, the neck dissection should be altered, being careful not to injure the large neck veins. The skin and superficial tissues of the neck should be reflected to expose the underlying structures by grasping and retracting the cut border of the skin using the fingers or non-toothed forceps and making gentle horizontal slices along the dermo-subcutaneous tissue plane.

After retracting skin and muscles of the anterior chest, a pleural window should be created to detect pneumothorax by scraping the intercostals off the external aspect of the parietal pleura. This should be done on both sides of the anterior aspect of the chest, usually near the third ribs. In cases of third and fourth degree burns, it is usually necessary to make a midline incision to the chin because the tissue is contracted and indurated.

Dissection of anterior neck structures: Layerwise examination of the anterior neck structures is desirable in all cases, and is accompanied by sequential *in situ* photography in cases of suspected strangulation. The platysma muscle is inspected for evidence of bruising. The sternocleidomastoid muscles are left intact and the external jugular veins are then examined. The underlying neck muscles are then reflected in layers. First the sternal head of the sternocleidomastoid muscles is divided from the manubrium and then the more lateral clavicular head is detached. These are reflected laterally and the suprahyoid and infrahyoid muscle groups are then examined being careful not to damage any adjacent vessels and produce a false impression of significant haemorrhage. The carotid sheath containing carotid arteries, internal jugular veins and the vagus nerve is exposed after the omohyoid is reflected. The contained structures are gently mobilized and inspected for evidence of haemorrhage. All the anterior neck tissues can now be separated dividing all the structures at the thoracic inlet or further dissection can follow removal of these structures with the thoracic contents.

Dissection of posterior neck structures: Posterior neck dissection is necessary to rule out craniocervical derangement in cases of suspected suffocation in traffic accidents and is recommended in all infant deaths occurring outside the hospital. Layerwise examination of posterior neck structures is required for traffic fatalities in which there is sufficient trauma elsewhere to account for the death, or in which there is unexplained laceration of brainstem, or haemorrhage in the paravertebral fascia. The prevertebral fascia can be examined for evidence of traumatic injury, such as presence of crepitus. The fascia is then reflected from the underlying bone. The body is turned over and the superficial tissues including ligamentum nuchae is reflected from the occipital region inferiorly to the base of the neck in order to expose the underlying soft tissue.

Examination of Chest After Removing the Sternum

The costal cartilages are cut using rib cutters by sliding the lower blade of the shears beneath the cartilage close to its bony attachment to the rib and shearing through the firm tissue as cleanly as possible. In young persons, cartilages can be cut using a knife. Cartilage should be cut just medial to the rib rather than through the bone in order to avoid exposing sharp edges. Sternum can alternatively be removed by cutting through the same regions but from second rib inferiorly to the costal margin. Sternum can now be released by grasping lower end and lifting it as horizontal cuts are made upwards towards the deep surface of sternum to detached adjacent mediastinal soft tissues.

Cuts are then made using a large blade through sternoclavicular joints thus reflecting the clavicles. To localise this joints gentle manipulation of the lateral part of clavicle is done and knife is inserted into the joint with rotatory cuts to disarticulate the clavicle from the sternum. Underlying vessels are inspected before first rib is cut and then cuts are made through second rib or cartilage. The sternum can now be lifted off.

Dissection of trachea and main bronchi: Trachea and main bronchi are opened along their posterior membranous walls. In cases of aspiration and drowning, anterior incisions *in situ* may be indicated. To demonstrate clinical condition such as tracheoesophageal fistula anterior midline incision should be given.

Examination of the Heart

The sternum is removed and then the pericardial blood clots, if present should be weighed. Normal hearts and most hearts with acquired disease can be excised separately. After removal of the blood clots, the heart is weighed. The heart may be of normal size or enlarged (cardiomegaly) due to hypertrophy or dilatation or both and can involve one or more chambers. The heart is normally conical shaped but it may be globoid or irregular, as with ventricular aneurysm and one or more chambers may be abnormal in shape. The endocardium is examined for evidence of fibrosis and any evidence of premortem thrombus. The colour of the subepicardial myocardium may be gray with an old infarct, pale with chronic anaemia, and mottled or haemorrhagic, with an acute infarct or rupture. Left ventricular consistency can be firm due to hypertrophy, fibrosis, amyloidosis, calcification or rigor mortis; or soft due to acute myocardial infarction, myocarditis, dilated cardiomyopathy or decomposition.

Examination of myocardium: The myocardium is examined for fibrosis or recent infarct. The myocardial infarct is easily identifiable when it is of more than 12 hours. Between 12 and 24 hours, the infarct is dusky and shows haemorrhagic discolouration. At 1-4 days, the infarct is more obvious and shows a mottled yellow and red pattern. The infarct is more homogenous and is at first yellow then white in colour after the passage of five days. The size of the infarct, its location, the extent whether it is subendocardial or transmural and its correlation with any arterial disease is to be noted.

Evidence of ventricular hypertrophy: (i) Thickness of both ventricular walls at a point about one cm below atrioventricular valve is measured. However, any dilatation will mask the hypertrophy. The upper limits for thickness of ventricular wall is 1.5 cm for left ventricle, 0.5 cm for right ventricle and 0.2 cm for the atrial muscle. (ii) Left ventricle and septal wall are separated from the right ventricle and then weighed and the ratio is obtained.

Examination of valves: The circumference of the valve is measured with a ruler or the length of the string. The circumference of mitral valve is 8-10.5 (10 cm) and admits two fingers; tricuspid valve is 10-12.5 (12 cm); aortic valve is 6-8 cm (7.5 cm) and pulmonary valve is 7-9 cm (8.5 cm). The decrease in circumference denotes stenosis whereas increased circumference could be due to regurgitation and when the valves are incompetent. The abnormality in the measurement should always be accompanied by scarring, fusion or calcification of the valves otherwise little importance should be given to abnormal measurement.

Evaluation of coronary arteries: Coronary arteries should be inspected for calcification and tortuosity. In subjects younger than 30 years, in which the cause of death is noncardiac, the coronary arteries may be opened longitudinally. Otherwise, the vessels should be cut in cross-section at 3-5 mm intervals. Calcified vessels that cannot be readily cut with a scalpel should be stripped off the heart and decalcified for at least 24 hours before cutting. To grade coronary obstruction, a four-point system is applied, by 25% increments of narrowing in cross-sectional area. A grade-4 lesion indicates stenosis of at least 75% of the coronary artery and is considered as severe, whereas a grade-4 lesion of 90% represents **critical stenosis**. As a rule, grade-4 lesions should be documented microscopically. Depending on the number of major epicardial vessels with grade-4 lesions, a heart may have severe 1-vessel, 2-vessel, or 3-vessel disease, and its coexistence with grade-4 disease in the other three coronary arteries represents severe 4-vessel disease.

Dissection of the heart: Only two methods are practically used for routine diagnostic pathology, these are the inflow-outflow method and the short axis technique.

1. **Inflow-outflow method or following the direction of blood flow:** The technique is suitable primarily for normal hearts and the atrium is opened first on each of the side and then the ventricle is opened along its inflow and outflow tracts. The valves are cut between their commissures.

   Using scissors, the initial cut is made from the inferior vena cava to the right atrial appendage, sparing the superior vena cava with the region of the sinus node. The right ventricular inflow tract is opened with a knife or scissors from the right atrium, through the posterior tricuspid leaflet, running parallel to and about 1 cm from the posterior ventricular septum. The outflow tract is opened in a similar fashion, about 1 cm from the anterior ventricular septum extending to through the pulmonary cusp and into the main pulmonary artery. The left atrium is opened with scissors between the right and left upper pulmonary veins and then between the upper and lower veins on each side. The incision can be extended into the left atrial appendage to assess for mural thrombus. The left ventricular inflow tract is opened with a long knife along the inferolateral aspect through the left atrial wall near its appendage, through the mid-portion of posterior mitral leaflet, between the two mitral papillary muscles and then through the apex. The outflow cut travels parallel to the anterior ventricular septum and about one cm from it. This curved cut is best accomplished with a scalpel, taking care not to cut into either the anterior mitral leaflet or the ventricular septum. Scissors can be used to extend the cut across the left aortic cusp and into the ascending aorta, to one side or other of the left coronary ostium.

2. **Short axis or ventricular slicing method:** This method is of choice to evaluate ischemic heart disease as well as any other cardiac condition as the slices expose the largest surface area of myocardium. They correspond to the short-axis plane produced clinically by the two-dimensional echocardiography. The flat diaphragmatic surface of the heart is placed on a paper towel to prevent slippage and then cuts 1.0-1.5 cm thick are made with a sharp knife, parallel to the atrioventricular groove. One firm slice should be used, or two slices in the same direction, avoiding sawing motions as that leaves hesitation marks. Each slice is viewed from the apex towards the base. The basal third of the ventricle is left attached to the atria. The basal portion is then opened according to the inflow-outflow method.

3. **Other tomographic methods of dissection of heart:** For teaching purposes, the short-axis, long-axis and four chamber planes are ideally suited for demonstrating cardiac pathology: (i) *Long axis method:* The plane for long-axis method is best demarcated with three straight pins before making the cut. The first pin is placed in the cardiac apex the second in the right aortic sinus adjacent to the coronary ostium and the third near the mitral valve annulus, between the right and left pulmonary veins. The heart can then be cut along this plane, from the apex towards the base, passing through both the mitral and aortic valves. (ii) *Four-chamber method:* In this method, the heart is divided into two portions, both of which show all four chambers. Using a long knife and beginning at the cardiac apex, a cut is extended through the acute margin of the right ventricle, the obtuse margin of the left ventricle and the ventricular septum. The upper half is then opened along the ventricular outflow tracts according to the inflow-outflow method. (iii) *Base of heart method:* This method displays all four valves intact at the cardiac base and is ideal for demonstrating the relationships between the valves themselves and between the valves and adjacent coronary arteries and the atrioventricular conduction system. (iv) *Window method:* This method is used for the preparation of dry museum specimens using paraffin or other material or plastination. Heart should be perfusion fixed. Windows of various sizes can be removed from the chambers or great vessels with scalpel. The tissue blocks can then be used for histologic study. (v) *Unrolling method:* The technique is used for demonstrating opacified coronary arteries in a single plane. Following postmortem coronary angiography, the ventricular septum and free walls are unrolled by any of the three techniques; Schlesinger technique, Lumb and Hardey technique and the Rodriguez and Reiner technique. But the latter is the simplest technique of the three. The unrolling method results in considerable mutilation of the heart and is best reserved for research purposes. (vi) *Partitioning method*: Each ventricle is weighed separately for detailed assessment of ventricular hypertrophy. The epicardial fat and coronary vessels are stripped from the specimen then atria and great arteries are removed. Finally ventricular free walls are separated from the ventricular septum, the weight of each segment is now compared with the normal values. Biventricular hypertrophy may produce an abnormal ratio.

Normal ratio of LV + S: RV is 2.3-3.3:1. In left ventricular hypertrophy, this ratio is more than 3.6:1 or left ventricle with septum is more than 225 gm whereas in right ventricular hypertrophy, the ratio is less than 2:1 or right ventricle is more than 80 gm. (vii) *Examination of the conduction system:* This conduction system is examined if pathology within the conduction system is suspected. It is largely a histological process and three tissue blocks containing SA node, AV node and AV bundles are made.

Examination of the Lungs

The lung is weighed prior to the dissection. The normal lung weighs 250-400 grams each but there is a considerable variation depending on the built and sex of the individual. The weight of the lung increases with severe cardiac failure or with diffuse lung pathology. The internal examination of lung can be done by: (i) ***Dissection of the airways:*** Airways are dissected using a pair of Scissors from the medial to the lateral including all the lobes and segments opening along the branches as they are documented. The airway caliber, mucosal surface and parenchymal appearance is examined for fibrosis, consolidation, tumours, scars or cavities. Old tuberculous cavities and fungal balls can be assessed. Chronic obstructive airway disease can be assessed by how peripherally airways can be opened. The examination of airways is of considerable importance in drowning, choking and burn deaths. (ii) Pulmonary vessels can be dissected to look for the emboli and atheroma. (iii) By horizontal slicing of the lung through each lobe with brain knife to inspect the parenchyma for haemorrhages, abscesses and consolidations.

Examination of Small and Large Intestine

External examination inspecting for the surface from jejunum to rectum is done during evisceration. For internal examination the intestine is opened along the anti-mesenteric border with bowel scissors (these have hooked end to one of the arms of the blades to stop bowel from sliding off during opening and preventing accidental puncture of bowel wall). The dissection is performed in a sink in order to keep dissecting area clean and for easy disposal of intestinal contents. This part of GIT can be opened from sigmoid or rectum proximally to duodenum or jejunum distally and emptying its contents. The instestinal walls can now be examined for any congestion, haemorrhages etc.

Examination of Liver

The liver varies in weight from 1300-1500 gms. The liver may be enlarged with inflammations and neoplasms and shrunken with cirrhosis. A series of parallel vertical slices 1-2 cm apart from one side to the other are made to examine the liver parenchyma for haemorrhages, lacerations or abscesses.

Examination of Brain in Adults

Incision of scalp: First the head should be elevated using the head rest. The hair is then parted with a comb along an imaginary coronal plane connecting one mastoid over the other over the convexity. The incision is then given on one side just behind the ear lobe, as low as possible and is extended to a comparable level on the other side cutting whole thickness of the scalp using the scalpel blade (Figure 7.2). The anterior and posterior halves of the scalp are then reflected forwards and backwards respectively by short undercutting of the scalp and using a dry towel draped over the scalp edges to facilitate further reflection. The anterior flap is reflected to about 12 cm above the supraorbital ridge.

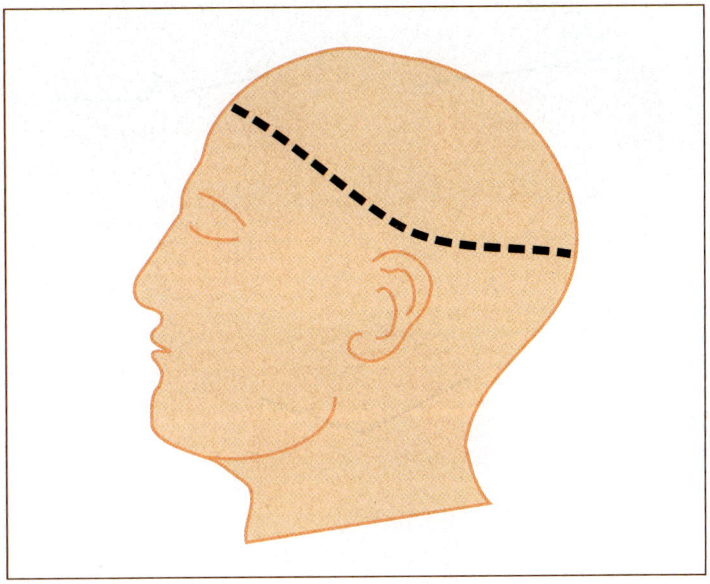

Figure 7.2: Lines for removal of scalp

Removal of skull cap: The cranium is best opened using an oscillating saw within a protective device such as plastic bag for collection of dust. The temporalis muscle should be cut with a sharp knife clearing it from the path of blade of the saw. The frontal point of sawing should start approximately two finger breadths above the supraorbital ridge and then the head is turned to the opposite side and sawing extended to the temporal point that is at the top of ear in its natural position. Finally the occipital area that is approximately two finger breadths above the external occipital protuberance is sawed. The oscillating blade should be moved from side to side during cutting to avoid deep penetration in a given area. Ideally sawing should be stopped just short of cutting through the inner table of skull that can be further detached with mallet and chisel. A hand inserted between the skull and the dura helps the blunt separation of these while the other hand is pulling the skullcap. If the dura adheres too firmly to the skull, it can be incised along the lines of the sawing and the anterior attachment of the falx to the skull can be cut between the frontal lobes. The posterior portion of the falx can be cut from the inside after the skull cap is fully reflected. Leaving the dura and underlying leptomeninges intact allows viewing the brain with overlying cerebrospinal fluid still in subarachnoid space. To obtain this view, after removal of the skull cap, the dura must be cut with a pair of scissors along the line of sawing and then reflected. The dura is then peeled off the skull cap. The superior sagittal sinus may be opened with a pair of scissors at this time. The dorsal dural flaps on both the sides can be removed easily from the brain by severing the bridging veins but in the presence of epidural or subdural haemorrhage or neoplasia, the dural flaps are left attached to the dorsal vein and can then be sectioned together (Figures 7.3 and 7.4).

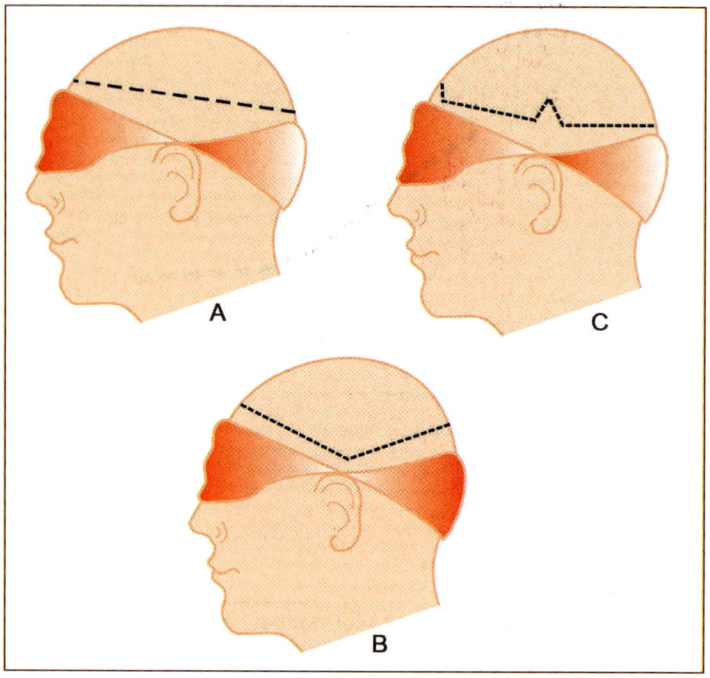

Figure 7.3: Methods of removal of skull cap

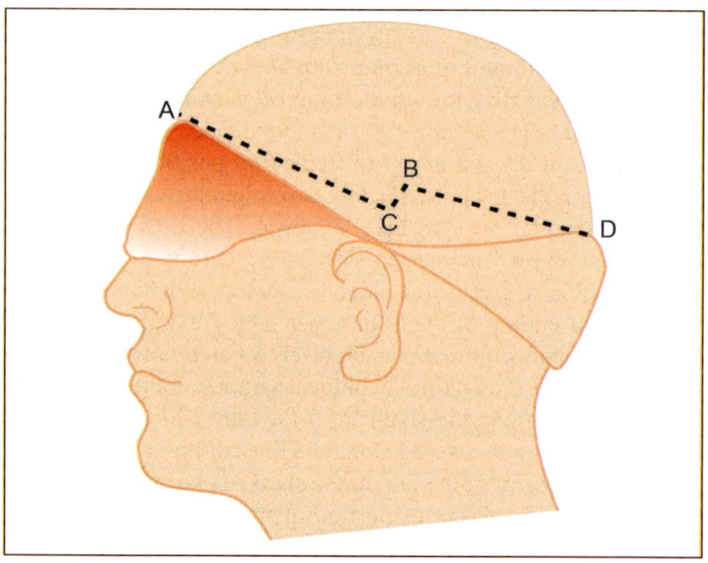

Figure 7.4: Lines along which saw cuts are made for skull cap removal

Removal of brain in adults: The brain is removed by raising the frontal lobes gently and tearing the olfactory bulbs and tracts away from the cribriform plates. The optic nerves are then cut as they enter the optic foramina. Under its own weight, the brain is allowed to fall away from the floor of the anterior fossa, supported by the palm of the other hand. The pituitary stalk and internal carotid arteries are then cut as they enter the cranial cavity. Third, fourth, fifth and sixth cranial nerves and subdural communicating veins are also severed close to the base of skull. The attachment of tentorium along the petrous ridge is cut on either side with curved scissors while the brain is prevented from dropping backwards and causing stretch tears in cerebral peduncles. Now the VII, VIII, IX, X, XI and XII cranial nerves are cut and the vertebral arteries are severed with scissors as they emerge in cranial cavities. The cervical part of spinal cord is cut using curved scissors as caudally as possible and avoiding too oblique plane. The brain is reflected back further by using the support of hand to deliver the brainstem and cerebellum from the posterior fossa without causing excessive stretching at the rostral brainstem level. The brain is pulled away from the base of skull after cutting the lateral attachment of the tentorium to the petrous bone along with the pineal body.

Fixation of the brain: The best routine fixative that allows the widest choice of stains for the nervous tissue is formalin, usually as a 10% solution. In fetuses and infants, the addition of acetic acid to the fixative solution appears to be helpful. It increases the specific gravity of the fixative and allows the brain to float in the solution; it also makes the tissue firmer without altering its histological characteristics. Fixation can be done by immersion and perfusion methods. For detailed anatomic studies, it is best to fix the brain specimen in a large amount of freshly prepared 10% formalin solution. The plastic buckets for holding 8 litres, can be used to suspend the brain to prevent distortion during fixation by passing a thread underneath the basilar artery in front of the pons. A thread can be passed under the internal carotid artery or middle cerebral arteries on both the sides, provided that no pathological lesions are suspected in these regions. Alternatively, the dorsal dura can be used as an anchoring point. However, suspension from blood vessels deforms the parenchyma less than dural suspension. The ends of the threads are tied to the attachments of the bucket handle, care being taken not to allow the specimen to touch the bottom or sides of the bucket. Formalin solution should be replaced within the first 24 hours but this is not mandatory if a large amount of fixative is used. If the fixative becomes bloody, it is to be replaced with fresh solution that prevents undue discolouration of the specimen. About 10-14 days are required for satisfactory fixation. If the brain is dissected earlier, the central portion may remain pink.

The brain can be perfused with fixative through the arterial stumps before further fixation by immersion. This shortens the fixation time and ensures adequate fixation of deeper portions of the brain. When it is necessary to dissect the brain at the time of autopsy, this preliminary fixation makes tissue harder, facilitates dissection and decreases tissue wrinkling. For the perfusion, injection of 150 ml of isotonic solution followed by 10% formalin manually with a syringe connected to a simple tubing system causes least problems.

Dissection of fresh brains: In adults the examination of brain lesions in terms of anatomic correlations with clinical symptoms can be achieved when the brain is sectioned after adequate fixation. At times the brain must be dissected in fresh state when microbiological and chemical investigations are important or when immediate diagnosis is necessary. Three to four coronal cuts through cerebral hemispheres are given leaving anatomic structures basal ganglia and upper brainstem undisturbed (Figure 7.5A). This reveals the presence of large lesions directly or indirectly by distortion of the ventricular system. The sections can then be made into primary slices of brain tissue to expose hidden but suspected lesions. The brainstem can be severed and cut into infratentorial structure and one horizontal cut through these structures is sufficient for preliminary examination. With fresh dissection of the brain, small lesions are easily missed and subtle lesions such as an early infarct can be overlooked. Every brain should be reexamined with new dissection after adequate fixation. Preliminary perfusion or cooling of the brain in a contoured support in refrigerator in about 30 minutes will increase the consistency of the brain and make regular dissection of the brain easier. The brain suspected of harbouring diffuse, roughly symmetric lesions as in cases of metabolic diseases or widespread infections may be bisected along the sagittal plane. One half may be submitted for chemical analysis or for microbiological examination while the other half is to be kept and later on sections are taken for histological examination (Figure 7.5).

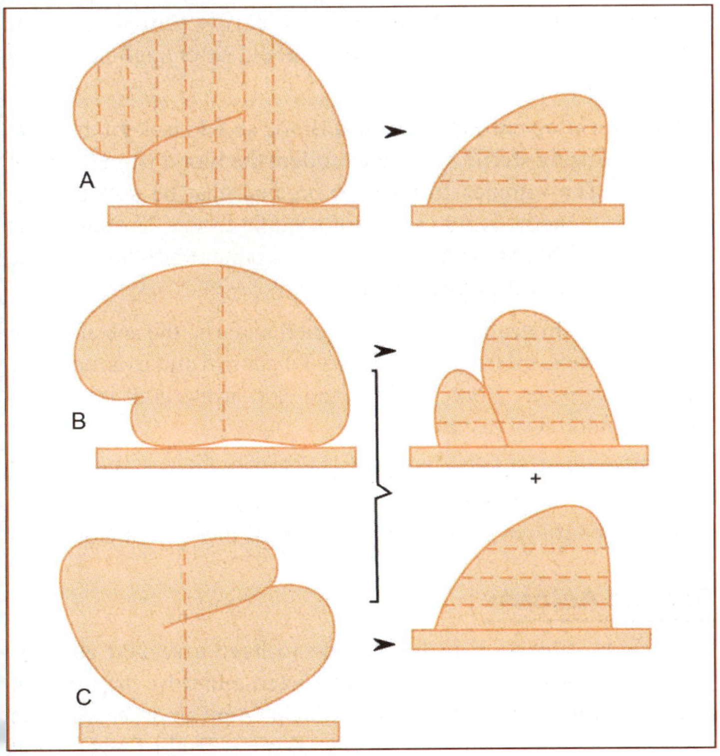

Figure 7.5: Coronal dissection methods for the cerebrum

Dissection of fixed brains: The whole brain has to be preserved in neutral-buffered 10% formalin for a period of 2-3 weeks. The external surface of the brain is carefully examined and the arteries at the base may be exposed through the tears made into arachnoid membrane. The pathologic conditions like thrombosis, embolism or aneurysm are observed. After adequate external examination the next step is to separate the cerebellum and brainstem from the cerebral hemisphere.

The brain is placed right side up that gives more stability to the specimen. The dissection may be carried out with the frontal lobes by slicing method. The preferred thickness is about 1 cm and each new cut surface is examined before another cut is made. The slices are displayed on the autopsy table on the right side of the doctor. This corresponds to viewing one's own brain from behind. There should be no overlapping of the slices displayed.

The cerebellum can be dissected on the horizontal plane on planes perpendicular to the folial orientation, the latter method gives the best histological orientation of the structures. The brain-stem is sectioned perpendicular to its axis (Figure 7.6).

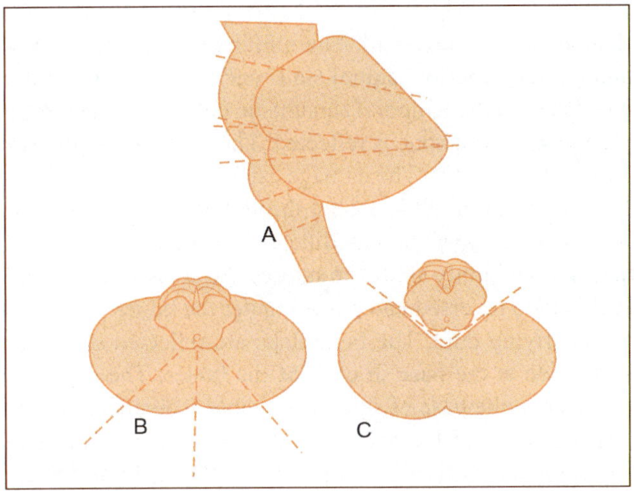

Figure 7.6: Dissection lines for brainstem and cerebellum

Pediatric Autopsy

There are various pediatric autopsy techniques being used by the pathologists. The external examination particularly of the newborn is important. The pathologist should concentrate on the search for malformations such as cleft palate, choanal atresia, stenosis and atresia of the anus and vagina. Face, ears and hands should be properly examined to look for characteristic changes in Down's syndrome and renal agenesis. The placenta and umbilical cord must be studied in all these autopsies. The esophageal hiatus should be examined *in situ*. In this age group, the skull is often difficult to separate from the dura as in adults. **Beneke's technique** is used to open the skull when the sutures are not closed and the skull bones are soft. After the scalp is reflected as in adults, the cranium and dura on both the sides are cut with blunt scissors starting at the lateral edge of the anterior fontanelle extending the incisions as shown in (Figure 7.7A to C) along the midline and

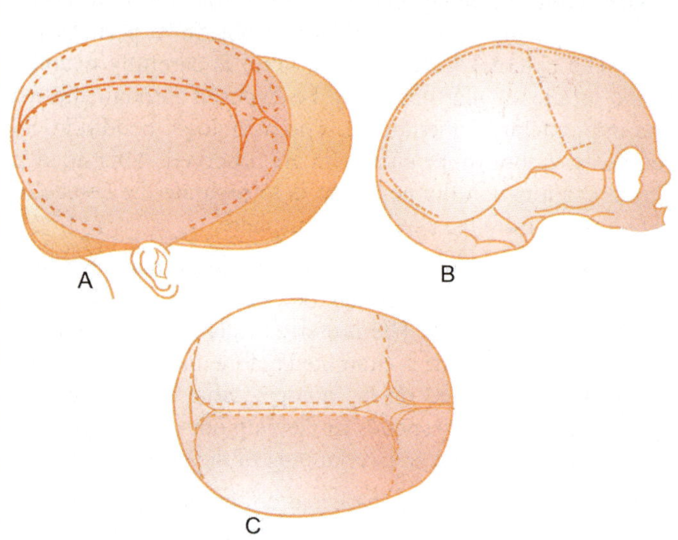

Figure 7.7A to C: Method for opening skull in fetus and neonates (Along the dotted lines)

the lateral sides of the skull. The midline strip about 1 cm wide containing the superior sagittal sinus and the falx is left and also an intact area in the temporal squama on either side, which serves as a hinge when the bone is reflected. This method usually results in damage to the brain. The damage can be minimized by infusion of 10% formalin in 70% alcohol through the neck arteries in an early stage of autopsy. In a modification of Beneke's method, the skull is incised lightly along the sutures and at the fontanelles. The scalpel is then reversed and passed under the bones to separate it from underlying dura. The bone flaps are reflected after a small nick is made at the base in each of the bones. The dura is then cut as close to the base of skull as possible. This method protects the friable brain of the infant during its removal. The damage to the brain can further be minimized if the scalp and skull are opened and the falx sectioned with the body in a sitting position and infant's head being supported by the assistant. The tentorium and vein of Galen are transacted in this position by separating the parieto-occipital lobes. The tentorium is separated and the body is suspended upside down by the assistant, the brain being cut away from the base of the skull on both the sides in this position thus minimizing the movements of the brain and hence the damage. The brain is not touched during these procedures and when all the attachment are severed, it is allowed to fall free preferably into the body of water, not on hard surface.

In infants the whole chest cavity can be opened under water in order to demonstrate a pneumothorax. In infants and foetuses **Letulle's technique** of *en masse* removal is the preferred technique in most cases so that certain rare malformations can be properly preserved for example pulmonary venous connections. Histological sections should be taken from lungs, liver, kidney, brain, thymus, placenta, umbilical cord and the free margin of falciform ligament.

Routine Sampling of Toxicological Material

The highest concentration of toxicological substances is found in dialysis and lavage fluids. The gastrointestinal tract is not the only route of entry of poisons in the body. Furthermore, if any significant period of 4-6 hours elapses from the time of ingestion until death or treatment, the poison will have passed out of the stomach. In certain cases, the poison also could have been introduced to mask a homicide. Thus, in all the cases a variety of tissues and fluids should be sampled for toxicological analysis. The knowledge of postmortem distribution of a toxic agent in different body fluids and tissues enables the forensic pathologist to distinguish inhalation poisoning from ingestion poisoning. Generally, the viscera are preserved in rectified spirit except in poisoning by carbolic acid, alcohol, phosphorus, paraldehyde and acetic acid where it is preserved in saturated solution of common salt. Rectified spirit being costly and not easily available, all the viscera are routinely preserved in saturated solution of common salt.

Blood, bile and urine should be kept refrigerated. Sodium fluoride may be added as a preservative when alcoholic intoxication is suspected (250 mg/30 ml of fluid). For longer storage periods toxicological material is best kept in deep freeze.

Laboratory Investigations

Samples for histopathological examination: The internal organs like liver, lung, brain etc. are taken for histological examination. It is not being done routinely but if after gross examination some pathology is suspected then 1-2 mm thick tissue can be removed along with normal area. It is preserved in 10% formalin or 95% alcohol. The amount of preservative should be enough not to dry the tissues inside the container.

Bacteriological examination: Blood should be kept in sterile containers using sterile syringe to collect the blood from the right ventricle. The samples from other organs must be collected by using sterile methods for culture of specific tissue. The surface is seared with a hot spatula and the area is punctured with a sterile instrument and the pulp is scraped.

Smears: In deaths due to suspected malaria, the smears from cerebral cortex, spleen and liver may be stained and examined for malarial parasites. Bone marrow and ribs or sternum is used in cases of blood dyscrasias.

Virological examination: A piece of the tissue is collected under sterile conditions and the sample is preserved in 80% glycerol in buffered saline or freezed for further examination.

Second Autopsy

There is no provision in Indian law to have a second autopsy. However, nowadays it is being conducted either by the order of a District Magistrate/senior police officer or by an order from the Court of law, though the instances are rare. Delhi Government constituted a committee in 2005 under the chairmanship of Dr P.C.

Dikshit, Dir Prof and Head, Forensic Medicine at Maulana Azad Medical College, and Heads Forensic Medicine Lady Hardinge Medical College and UCMS as its members. The following guidelines were formulated which were accepted in principle by Delhi Government:

1. The request for the second autopsy should come from the concerned SHO duly forwarded by DCP of the area to the Home Ministry.
2. The Home Ministry after scrutinizing will forward the application to the Ministry of Health who forms the board of doctors to conduct the postmortem.
3. The board will be comprising atleast three doctor's of different government hospitals having a minimum of 5 years' experience after postgraduate.
4. The I/O of the case should be atleast of the rank of Inspector.
5. Minimum honorarium to be paid to the doctors which should be decided by the Government.

The same guidelines are also applicable in cases where postmortem was done by a board of doctors.

Aim: (i) To find out the cause of death, when it cannot be opined by the doctor who had conducted the first autopsy. (ii) When the relatives are not satisfied with the cause of death, they request the higher authorities for a second autopsy done.

Procedure: Second autopsy is usually done by a board of doctors, mostly three in number, from different institutions. In these circumstances, the body is usually buried which is to be taken out from the grave. If the body has been kept in the mortuary after the first postmortem, it should be removed to the place of the second postmortem. The board should obtain a request letter/order from the competent authority along with the inquest papers. If possible the doctor who had conducted the first postmortem should be present in the theatre, so that necessary clarification or corroborations can be obtained. The interpretation of the findings of an exhumed body, that has undergone the first autopsy is very difficult because of putrefactive changes and artefacts caused during burial/exhumation, as well as the alterations made during the first autopsy. The findings should be written in detail irrespective of the fact that it correlates or contradicts with the findings during first autopsy.

During the second autopsy some new facts may come up, that may help in further investigations. If no new facts are discovered, the second autopsy will correlate the findings of the first autopsy and further doubt and allegations will come to an end.

Negative Autopsy

One of the important objectives of autopsy is to find out the cause of death as well as any contributory cause of death. Nevertheless, when the gross and microscopic findings fail to reveal any apparent cause of death, along with the examination of chemical analysis report and other relevant laboratory investigations, it is termed as negative autopsy. The rate of negative autopsy is about 5-8% of all the autopsies. Even the best equipped centres of the world have more than 5% negative autopsy rate. The possible reasons are as follows:

Inadequate history: In medicolegal autopsies, the doctors should take adequate history about the incidence. Particular references should be made about the signs and symptoms prior to death as deaths from vagal inhibition, epilepsy, laryngeal spasm, electrocution in water as well as hypersensitivity reactions may not reveal any external findings.

Lack of proper external examination: Electrical burn marks should be looked especially for the exit wounds as they are most often missed by the pathologist due to lack of experience. In addition, the needle prick marks in anaphylactic deaths are often missed. The concealed wounds may often be missed.

Improper internal examination: Faulty laboratory examination along with faulty toxicological analysis is also responsible for negative autopsies. The experience and capability of the doctors can be responsible for this.

Insufficient histological examinations: Various microscopic lesions account for death, and are liable to be missed due to insufficient histological examination.

Inadequate pathologist's training: Sudden, unexpected deaths with atherosclerotic narrowing of the coronary arteries without thrombosis or infarction may be a cause of death which is often missed by a hospital pathologist.

Obscure Autopsy

The autopsy is termed as obscure, when there is no definite or obscure cause of death. This type of autopsy creates a lot of confusion to the forensic experts. The causes of obscure autopsy are:

1. **Concealed trauma:** Concussion is a state of transient unconsciousness as a result of blunt force injury to head followed by amnesia and spontaneous recovery. Autopsy may not show any change, but in some cases petechial hemorrhages are found. Even microscopic examination does not reveal any axonal injury up to 12 hours. Injury to the cervical spine causing fracture dislocation and injury to the spinal cord can cause instantaneous death without any obvious external injuries.
2. **Cardiac lesions:** (i) In blunt force injury to heart it may stop functioning without any visible signs. (ii) Cardiac arrest can occur during or immediately following heavy exercise in which there is increase in heart rate and systolic pressure with progressive ischemia leading to cardiac arrest. (iii) Cardiac arrhythmias which, may be precipitated by emotional excitement can cause physiological asystole and may lead to death.

3. **Reflex vagal inhibition:** This can be due to pressure on neck following blows on the larynx, chest, abdomen and genital organs. When death is due to reflex vagal inhibition, there is hardly any findings at autopsy. It may occur during drowning, when the body is subjected to very cold temperature. Any manipulation of external auditory meatus may also lead to death due to vagal inhibition.

Virtual Autopsy or Virtopsy or Digital Autopsy

The concept was first proposed by scientists at the Institute of Forensic Medicine of the University of Bern, Switzerland. **Virtual Autopsy** is a word combining 'virtual' and 'autopsy' and the term **Virtopsy** was created from these two words. Virtual is derived from the Latin word 'virtus', which means 'useful, efficient and good'. Autopsy is a combination of the old Greek term 'autos' (=self) and 'opsomei' (=I will see). Thus, autopsy means 'to see with one's own eyes'. Because the goal is to eliminate the subjectivity of "autos", two terms virtual and autopsy are merged and word "autos" deleted – the term Virtopsy is created. Virtopsy is a multi-disciplinary technology that combines forensic medicine and pathology, roentgenology, computer graphics, biomechanics, and physics. The term **digital autopsy** simply means conducting autopsy in computerized environment by digital tools.

Methods: Virtopsy employs imaging methods that are also used in clinical medicine such as **computed tomography (CT), magnetic resonance imaging (MRI), Micro CT, MSCT etc.**, for the purpose of autopsy and to find the cause of the death. Computed tomography (CT) is the imaging modality of choice for two- and three-dimensional documentation and analysis of autopsy findings including fracture systems, pathologic gas collections (e.g., Air embolism, subcutaneous emphysema after trauma, hyperbaric trauma, decomposition effects), and gross tissue injury. However, it is less specific and sensitive in assessing intravenous contrast. Postmortem MRI is highly sensitive, specific, and mainly used for assessing soft tissue injuries, neurological/non-neurological trauma, contusions and hematomas. **Magnetic resonance spectroscopy (MRS)** is another technique in Virtopsy which helps in determining the metabolic concentrations in the tissues, thus helping in estimating the time of death. **MR microscopy** is a microimaging technique which is used to study the soft tissue injuries like retinal haemorrhage, electric injury to the skin, etc. **Microtomography** is used to study the weapon involved and its injury patterns. Virtopsy also provides **2D and 3D post-processing techniques**, for the synthesis of information obtained from body surface and inside the body, and thus provides the conditions for geometric records. Recording methods based on real geometric data play a powerful role in the reconstruction of injuries such as traffic injuries and falls from height. **Robotic virtual autopsy** is a multifunctional system that can perform automatic postmortem and three-dimensional surface scanning which qualitatively increase the improvement in the outcome of forensic investigations. The robotic virtual autopsy also helps in detecting the change in colour of tissue. **Postmortem angiography** is a Virtopsy technique that is helpful in visualization of the cardiovascular system that includes infusion of contrast medium with the aid of peristaltic pump and contrast medium.

Uses: (i) **Identification** by estimating age, gender, length, weight and individual features etc. (ii) **Cause and manner of death** (iii) **Timing of death** (iv) **Documentation** of foreign materials like bullet and metal fragments etc. (v) **Wound vitality** (vi) **Forensic reconstruction** (vii) **Education and research.**

Advantages: It is a non-invasive technique which is acceptable by relatives and religious communities. It is a less time consuming and aids better diagnosis. It provides contamination free sampling (poisons, infections, tissue, etc.) as there is no mutilation of dead bodies. The autopsy data can be stored digitally which can be reviewed later at any stage.

Disadvantages: The physiological senses of an autopsy surgeon like smell, texture, and colour are restricted as there is no direct contact with the dead body of the victim. There is difficulty in collection of organs for pathological examination and chemical analysis. Virtual autopsy is expensive and include high equipment and technology costs. There is problem with feasibility in using these high technology imaging devices in less developed countries.

At present, many forensic institutions around the world routinely scan corpses with postmortem CT (PMCT) or MRI before autopsy. However, the technique is not accepted by court in most of the countries. Still, it is regarded as an adjuvant but not a replacement to standard complete invasive postmortem examination. More research is required preferably showing the benefits of the virtual approach, and overcoming what obstacles the virtual autopsy may present.

As on today in India, complete autopsy is carried out in medicolegal cases. A thorough external and internal examination of all organs is carried out with opening of all the three cavities, i.e., head, chest and abdomen. There is no practice or provision of incomplete or partial or limited autopsy. There is no judicial validity yet for use of virtual autopsy. The Department of Forensic Medicine and Toxicology, AIIMS, New Delhi established the first virtual autopsy facility (Centre for Advanced Research and Excellence in Virtual Autopsy) in India.

Psychological Autopsy

Psychological autopsy is an analysis that is conducted following a person's death to reconstruct his or her mental state prior to dying (APA Dictionary of Psychology). This is based on the information gathered via structured interviews of family members, relatives or friends, personal documents (suicidal notes, diaries and letters etc.), police report and medical records. Psychological autopsy can clarify the manner of death (suicide/homicide/others), when the manner is in question. Frequently, the primary objective is often to determine definitively that the person did die as the result of a suicide. In other cases, the psychological autopsy can be a useful tool in gathering data for the purposes of suicide prevention or to better understand suicidal behaviour.

Exhumation

It is the lawful digging out of an already buried body from the grave. It is done both in civil and criminal cases. In addition when there is allegations that the proper autopsy has not been conducted or the body has been disposed off without any autopsy and any foul play is suspected, exhumation can be carried.

Civil cases: (i) Accidental death claim (ii) Insurance (iii) Liability for medical negligence (iv) Workmen's compensation claim (v) Inheritance (vi) Disputed identity cases.

Criminal cases: (i) Deaths due to criminal abortion (ii) Homicide or suspected homicide when death has been labeled as otherwise (iii) Suspicious poisoning (ii) Criminal negligence.

Rules of exhumation: The written order is obtained from an Executive Magistrate. There is no time limit for exhumation in India. The magistrate along with police officer and medical officer should report at the spot. The spot of burial is to be identified correctly. This can be done with the help of relatives and other persons related with the disposal. Even the person who had made the coffin can be called to identify the coffin. Besides, the location of the grave from some fixed objects like road, tree etc. to be noted. If the map is available, it will be of help. The entries in the register should also be seen. The relatives are allowed to stay throughout the investigations **(S. 176(4) CrPC)**.

Though, there is no time limit for exhumation in India. The period is restricted to 10 years in France whereas in Germany it is 30 years.

Procedure: After correct identification of the spot, the area should be enclosed from the public. The exhumation is carried out in the early hours as there is less of public and also the work of digging can be completed during day time.

The identified grave should then be dug carefully up to the depth of 10-15 meters and condition of soil, water content and vegetable grown should be noted down. The grave is further dug up to coffin or corpse and photographs are taken. A sketch may be drawn about the position of coffin and body. At this point it should be identified by the relatives. The plastic sheet or a plank may be lowered down to the level of the corpse. Then the corpse is shifted to plank and taken out carefully to avoid artefacts. No disinfectant should be sprinkled on the body.

In case of skeletonisation of the body, the grave is further dug and the skeleton is lifted to sheet/plank. The soil to be searched for smaller objects like bullets, teeth, hyoid bone, metallic objects. If the body cannot be transported or the mortuary is very far off then autopsy can be carried out at the spot itself. Any fluid and debris in the coffin on the body should also be collected.

Injuries if present should be carefully noted. The injuries on soft parts may get distorted or disfigured due to decomposition thus care should be taken to interpret them correctly. The possibility of artefacts during the process of digging should be excluded.

In suspected poisoning, viscera should be kept for analysis. If organs are converted into mass, then loose masses should be preserved. If nothing is found then hair, soil, teeth and bones should be preserved. About ½ kg of earth should also be collected from the top, sides, bottom of the body and kept in dry clean bottles for toxicological analysis.

A portion of coffin and burial cloths must be removed in order to exclude any possibility of contamination from external sources.

Bundle of Bones

At times some skeletal remains may be recovered from an open land, ditches, rubbish dumps etc., or a skeleton may be exhumed from a temporary grave, a burial ground, or even while new constructions. The bones should be listed and the photographs are preferably taken. The bones should be arranged in an anatomical position of articulation. If some earth, sand, dust etc. is sticking to the bones, it is to be cleaned by brushing.

General examination of bones: The bones are thoroughly examined as to whether the bones are dry, clean, brittle and whitish in colour with cartilages attached or whether they are moist and humid, yellowish or yellowish brown, with soft tissues still attached and cartilages adhering. The stage of putrefaction of soft tissues should also be noted (Figure 7.8).

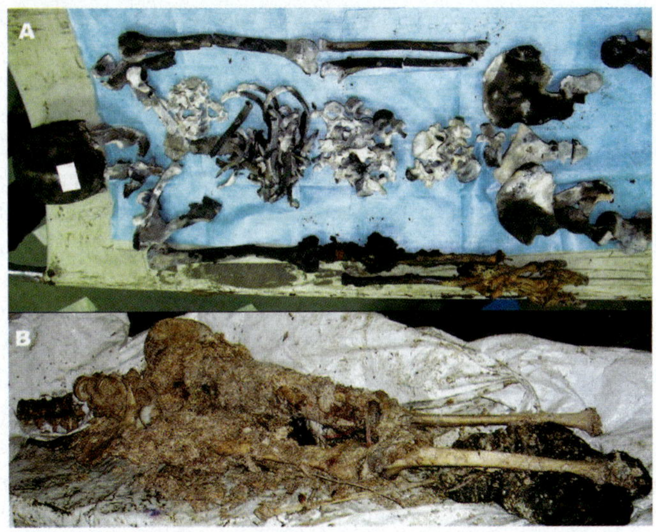

Figure 7.8: Skeletonized remains of the body

Cleaning the bones: The soft tissues can be separated by boiling in water containing sodium bicarbonate for about 6-12 hours and then brushing gently.

Examination proper: Whenever the skeletal remains or a single bone is brought for examination to the forensic expert, the following questions need to be answered:

Whether they are actually bones: Sometimes pieces of stones may be mistaken by the police officer for bones. For this, proper examination, that is looking for the protuberances, surfaces, borders and characteristics findings of bones etc. is necessary.

Whether the bones are human or animal? Human skull is commonly mistaken for that of the Chimpanzee, Gorilla or Monkey. The bones can be differentiated from that of an animal from the anatomical configurations. In an animal skull, glabella is more prominent, nasion is deeper, jaw is protruded and the cranium is small in size. In human pelvis, iliac crest and upper border of symphysis pubis lie in the same plane whereas in animals they lie in different planes due to different postures while walking. Precipitin test being species specific would be helpful when the remnants of blood are still attached to the surface of bones.

Whether they belong to one or more than one individual: The bones are arranged in anatomical position and if all the bones fit properly and anatomically and no disparity or duplication exists between the bones of contralateral side and all bones belong to same age and sex it suggests that the bones are of same individual.

Race of the person to whom the bones belong? Race of the individual can be known from **cephalic index** that is 70-75 when the skull is dolicocephalic in pure Aryans, 76-79 in mesaticephalic skull of Europeans and 80-84 in brachycephalic skull of Mongoloids. The other indices used to determine race are: (i) Brachial Index (ii) Crural Index (iii) Humero-femoral Index.

The sexing of bones give definite results only after puberty. The sex of the person can be determined from the subjective and objective parameters. The subjective parameters include the examination of different bones such as the pelvis, skull, long bones, mandible, sacrum, sternum, clavicle etc. When the bones are strong having rough surface, marked muscular markings and well marked prominences and tubercles they belong to males. The average weight of Indian male skeleton is about 4.5 kg and in an average Indian female it is about 2.5 kg. Children attain half the adult weight by about 12 years in case of boys and under 11 years in case of girls. The pelvis is the best bone used for the purposes of sexing. The objective indices for determining sex include: (i) Sciatic notch index (ii) Ischium pubic index (iii) Pelvic index (iv) Kell index.

Age of the person to whom it belongs: The age of the person can be determined from the ossification and union of the bones state of dentition, closing of sutures, state of calcification of laryngeal cartilages, sternum and hyoid bone, condition of the symphyseal surfaces of the pubic bone, changes in the sacrum and mandible, extent of wear and tear in both the jaws with ageing and changes like bony lipping, osteoporotic and osteoarthritic changes. Epiphyseal union is about two years earlier in females compared to males. The age changes after 25 years and in old age can be ascertained from the changes in the mandible, vertebra, pubic symphysis and internal bone structure and Gustafson's method.

Stature of the individual: The stature is determined fairly accurately using the long bones such as femur, tibia, humerus or radius. The tibia being the best bone is used for the purpose. Hepburn's osteometric board is used for the purpose of measuring the lengths of long bones accurately. The length is then divided by the multiplication factors as devised by Pan and Nat. The stature can also be devised by using regression formulae devised by researchers such as Dupertuis and Hadden, Karl Pearson, Trotter and Gleser.

Identifying features: The personal identity can be established from the teeth, any congenital peculiarities, any bony disease or deformities such as caries, osteoarthritis, malunited fracture, spinal deformities, supernumerary ribs and cervical ribs etc. When the skull is available, the superimposition technique can be used for superimposition of the skull over the photograph of the individual.

Nature of injury: The bones should be examined as to whether they have any sharp cuts, or any fractures implying use of blunt weapon or from a vehicle or sometimes they are gnawed by animals when the soft tissues are attached. The charred and blackened bones are suggestive of burns. But in case of intense heat of fires, the bones turn to ashes and are so brittle as to turn to powder when touched. Superficial bones when burnt will show evidence of heat fractures, charring, and cracking, splintering and calcining whereas bones lying embedded amidst thick soft tissues will show molten or guttered condition. A bone when burnt in open fire will become white but when burnt in close fire is black or ash-grey.

Time since death: The nature and circumstances of burial of the body modifies the rate of decaying of the bone. If the bones are wet and humid, and have an offensive odour, they are recent. Bodies when exposed to open air gets skeletonized within seven to fourteen days. But when the bones loose their soft tissues, the decaying odour will be lost. Because of ground water seepage, the buried bones may show increase or decrease of mineral contents, e.g., calcium phosphate, calcium carbonate etc. depending upon mineral rich content of soil. X-ray defraction studies may give an idea about the mineral content of the bone.

Following putrefaction, the bones loose their organic constituents and thus become light and brittle, dark or dark brown in colour. Such changes depend upon manner of burial (with or without coffin), the nature of soil of the grave, age of the individual etc. Usually the time taken for these to occur varies between 3 to 10 years. In case of burial in mass graves or in shallow graves without any coffin, putrefaction will occur very rapidly. Long buried bones may have chalky texture.

Bone marrow and periosteum may persist in the bones for several months often after burial. Superficially buried bones may expand or crack within few years by repeated freezing or thawing. When burial is old, the cancellous bone at the metaphysis and epiphysis may get eroded by effects of weather.

In case of fracture, the time may be judged with some accuracy by examining the callus by cutting it longitudinally. As globulin disappears rapidly, precipitin tests on 10 years old samples become negative.

Dating of human bones: Examination of the bones rarely, if ever, permits a precise estimate of the time interval since deposition in the ground. At the same time it is possible and important to decide whether they are 'ancient' or 'modern' bones that the interval is greater or lesser than 50 years. In recent years, a considerable amount of research has been carried out in an attempt to increase the accuracy of dating skeletal remains. Some of these depend on sophisticated laboratory techniques, such as radiocarbon analysis, which are difficult and expensive to perform. Radiocarbon is essentially a tool for archeologists and its forensic use is limited because of the insignificant fall in the C-14 content of bones during the first century after death. This is the stumbling block for many physical and chemical methods for bone dating, as although old samples (in excess of 100-200 years) can fairly readily be differentiated from recent bones. Discrimination between the dates of skeletal remains recent enough to be of interest to law enforcement agencies and coroners, is too poor to be of much practical use.

The environmental conditions are more potent than age in causing progressive degeneration of the bone. Even different parts of the same skeleton (and even opposite ends of the same long bone) may be quite different in their chemical and physical properties, if local changes in inhumation such as drainage, are marked. Bones in wet peaty soil may be decalcified and crumble within two decades, yet bones in dry gravel or sand may remain almost pristine for millennia.

Naked eye appearances are very deceptive, but bones with remnants of periosteum, tags of ligament or soft tissue other than adipocere are likely to be less than 5 years old, unless kept in a dry protected place. A 'soapy' texture of the surface, from residual fat, also indicates a date of less than a few decades.

The various laboratory test used for the purpose of dating human remains include the following but results of each test should be interpreted in the light of the others and with due regard to the macroscopic appearances and the fullest information of the place of concealment and any circumstantial evidence. (i) *Nitrogen content:* New bones contain 4.0-4.5 gm% of nitrogen, derived mostly from the collagenous stroma. After a variable interval following death, usually longer than 60-100 years, this declines. A value of 2.5 gm% usually indicates an age of at least 350 years. (ii) *Amino acid content:* Amino acid content is estimated by autoanalyser after acid hydrolysis of the residual protein. Up to 20 acids may be found in bones less than a century old. They then decline in number and concentration. Earlier work using thin layer chromatography suggested that proline and hydroxyproline (constituent of collagen) vanishes by about 50 years, but the more sensitive modern methods of analysis do not confirm this. (iii) *Blood pigments:* Blood remnants may be found up to a century using the most sensitive, though nonspecific tests. As benzidine have carcinogenic activity, other tests such as phenolphthalein and leucomalachite green can detect blood only up to 5-10 years, using either bone dust or the periosteal surface as the test area. (iv) *Fluorescence:* Fluorescence can be seen across the whole freshly sawn surface of a long bone under ultraviolet light for more than a century, but beyond this time, declining fluorescence is seen advancing from both the outer surface and the marrow cavity. The 'sandwich' of fluorescence progressively narrows during the first 50 years and may vanish within 300-500 years. (v) *Immunological activity:* Eluted extracts of bone when tested against animal antihuman serum gives a visible antibody-antigen reaction, either in crossovers electrophoresis or by passing diffusion in gel. Early work suggested that this persisted for 5-10 years, but recent repetition of the tests indicated that it ceases within months of death.

Cause of death: Presence of depressed comminuted fracture, cut injury or bullet wounds in the skull, fracture dislocation of the vertebral column, fracture of ribs, hyoid or any other limb bones etc. will be informative, pointing towards the cause and nature of death. Metallic poisons like arsenic, lead, antimony, mercury etc. can be detected in the bones long after death. Arsenic can be recovered even from examination of charred bony fragments. From the type and depth of cut in the bone the nature of the offending weapon can be made out.

Examination of Mutilated Bodies and Fragmentary Remains

Sometimes the mutilated bodies and fragmentary remains of the body such as one limb, part of trunk or only the head, a mass of soft tissue etc. is brought for examination by the investigating police officer. In such cases, not only the body parts are mutilated but there are chances of disfiguring the face and dismembering the limbs to destroy the identity in order to hide the crime. The body may also get mutilated by the dogs, rats, jackals, vermins specially when left exposed in open places and also by the fishes when the body is recovered from the water, to such an extent that the body remains unrecognizable even by the near-relatives. The assailants are also likely to destroy finger tips for fingerprints, tattoo marks, scars, moles and also remove jewellery, clothing and other personal belongings to further make it difficult to identify the person. The body may be burnt or incinerated. Also because of advanced decomposition, the soft tissue and viscera putrefy leaving behind the bare skeleton. The body parts may be deliberately dismembered after death and thrown off in rivers, canals, sewage holes. The body may be put in a vat of corrosive acids or alkalis to get it chemically destroyed as was in *Acid bath murder* case. The body parts may get mutilated into fragmentary remains beyond recognition in bomb explosions. The questions listed below should be answered in detail while examining the fragmentary and mutilated body parts.

Whether the remains of human or animal origin: When the head, trunk or limbs are available, it is easy to specify them to be human or animal. However, when only soft tissue with no visceral organs is to be examined, the mass of soft tissue without any preservative should be sent to the forensic science laboratory for the precipitin or antiglobulin inhibition test that is a species specific test.

Whether the parts belong to one or different individuals? When the mutilated parts fit to each other snugly and anatomically with no disparity or duplication, bearing more or less the same skin colour etc, it can be said that all the parts are of the same individual. Bones from different skeletons can be differentiated, when they show different colour emissions on exposing them to short wave ultraviolet lamp.

Do the fragments belong to male or female? If the head or trunk is available, it may be easy to determine sex from the scalp hairs, beard, moustache, pubic hairs, external genitalia, breasts etc. It is known that prostrate and non-gravid uterus resist putrefaction for a long period. In case of skeletal remains, the characteristic sex features in skull, pelvis, sacrum, femur etc. will be helpful. General configuration, remnants of cosmetics, jewelleries, clothing etc. will speak of characteristic feminine features.

Age of the person: The age can be ascertained from general development, teeth, ossification of bones, union of sutures, calcification of laryngeal cartilages, union of pieces of sternum and sacrum, changes in the symphyseal surface of pubic bone, osteoarthritic changes in the joints, graying of scalp, moustache and beard hair.

Stature: The stature can be determined from the long bones, if any.

Race: Race can be determined from the scalp hair, skin complexion, cephalic index and other anthropological features in the skull, vertebral column or other body parts.

Establishing identity: The identity can be established from the fingerprint, tattoo marks, scars, moles, deformities, congenital abnormalities if any, dental study, recent or old fractures, personal belongings of the deceased if available.

Any marks of habit or occupation: Occupational marks can help in determining the profession of the deceased.

Manner of separation of parts: This can be determined by close examination of the margins of the dismembered parts to see, whether these had been cleanly cut, sawn, disarticulated by several strikes at different levels done haphazardly or gnawed through by animals. At times the face and other body parts may be defaced and disfigured to remove the identifying features purposefully. Meticulous examination can only help to differentiate the cut in bones by sharp weapons, or sawing of long bones by sharp weapons, or surgical amputation, from gnawing of dead bones by wild animals, showing no evidence of antemortem reaction.

Time since death: The probable time since death can be ascertained from the conditions of the soft parts in relation to the stage of putrefaction.

Cause of death: It is easily determined in case when antemortem fatal injuries affecting large blood vessels, vital organs or body parts are there. Other causes are extensive antemortem burns, head injury with fracture of skull, fracture dislocation of cervical vertebra, fracture of hyoid bone or several other bones. Sometimes bullet or its fragments and part of the weapon used are recovered from the body that points towards the nature of death.

As the soft tissues decompose quickly, the injuries involving these tissues may be easily missed as in the case of neck tissues when death has been caused by compression of neck.

EMBALMING

The treatment of the dead body with antiseptics and preservatives to prevent putrefaction is called embalming. Embalming causes coagulation of tissue proteins that get fixed and hardened. It should be done as early as possible after death and for satisfactory results, preferably within 6 hours.

The main constituents of embalming fluid are formalin, sodium borate, sodium citrate, sodium chloride, glycerin etc. dissolved in water. The fluid has to be forced into the arteries for diffusion to occur into the cells and tissues through the capillaries. It can be done by hand/foot pump, stirrup pump, bulb syringe, gravity injector and motorized injectors. The injection can be continuous or interrupted with a continuous or interrupted drainage. Embalming is arterial when the fluid is injected in the arteries and then cavity embalming is done in which the fluid is injected in the body cavities. The vessel to be chosen for the arterial embalming should be preferably nearer to the heart for better results. A common method is the **'six point' injection system** in which the carotids, axillary and the femoral arteries of both the sides are used for pumping the fluid for the different body regions.

LONG QUESTIONS

1. Discuss the general procedures to be followed for a medicolegal autopsy.
2. What are the aims and objectives of conducting the various types of autopsy?

SHORT QUESTIONS

1. Negative autopsy.
2. Obscure autopsy.
3. Preservation of viscera.
4. Exhumation.
5. Embalming.
6. Examination of bundle of bones.
7. Various techniques of removal of organs.

MULTIPLE CHOICE QUESTIONS

1. During postmortem examination, when the sutures are not closed and the skull bones are soft, the techniques used to open the skull is:

(a) Beneke's technique (b) Letulle' technique
(c) Ghon's technique (d) Rokitansky's technique

2. **Virchow's method of autopsy is:**
   (a) Removal of organs one by one
   (b) Dissection after en bloc removal of all viscera
   (c) Dissecting of the organs *in situ*
   (d) Dissection of organs after en masse removal

3. **At autopsy, *in situ* dissection and removal of organs is done in:**
   (a) C. Rokitansky technique (b) Gohn technique
   (c) M. Letulle technique (d) R. Virchow technique

4. **At autopsy, pyrogallol test is helpful in diagnosis of:**
   (a) Fat embolism (b) Thromboembolism
   (c) Air embolism (d) Amniotic fluid embolism

5. **The time limit for exhumation in India is:**
   (a) 6 months
   (b) 1 year
   (c) 2 years
   (d) No time limits

6. **All are true about virtual autopsy *except:***
   (a) It is non-invasive technique
   (b) There is judicial validity for use of virtual autopsy in India
   (c) It can be used as an adjuvant but not a replacement to invasive medicolegal postmortem examination in India
   (d) The autopsy data can be stored digitally which can be reviewed later at any stage

ANSWER KEY

1. (a)	2. (a)	3. (a)	4. (a)	5. (d)	6. (b)

8 CHAPTER

Crime Scene Investigation

The objectives of crime scene investigation are: (i) To reconstruct the accident (ii) To ascertain the sequence of events (iii) To determine the mode of operation (iv) To disclose the motive (v) To uncover the property that was stolen (vi) To find out what all the criminals may have done (vii) To recover physical evidence from the scene of crime.

Evidence

Webster defined 'evidence' as something legally submitted to a competent authority as a means of ascertaining the truth of any alleged matter of fact under investigation before it. According to **section 3 I.E.A.,** evidence means and includes: (i) All statements, which the court permits or requires to be made before it by witnesses, in relation to matters of fact under enquiry. (ii) All documents produced for inspection by the courts.

Types of evidence: Evidence is of two types: (i) Testimonial and (ii) Physical evidence that may vary from fiber to a building.

Value: (i) Physical evidence is quite valuable as it can prove that a crime has been committed and helps in establishing key elements of a crime, e.g., in cases of alleged rape the victim's torn clothing and contusion over inner side of thigh are sufficient to prove a case of rape. (ii) Evidence can place the suspect in contact with the victim or with the crime scene, e.g., in a case of alleged bestiality, if an animal hair is found on the suspect's clothes it proves the contact with the animal. (iii) Physical evidence can establish the identity of persons associated with the crime, e.g., the fingerprints at the crime scene or over any articles present in the crime scene can establish the identity of the criminals. (iv) Evidence can exonerate the innocent, can corroborate the victim's testimony such as in a case of alleged rape, if the victim narrates the story alleging that the person lured her to an unknown place and mixed some sedatives in the cold drink which she drank, became unconscious and was raped. On examination and subsequent chemical analysis of the blood and urine, it has found that she was not given any sedatives. On repeated interrogation, the victim confessed of giving a false history as she was trying to falsely implicate the person. (v) A suspect confronted with physical evidence may make admissions or confessions. As in a case of murder blood stained clothes were found in the accused's possession. On grouping of the blood, it matched with that of the victim after which the accused admitted of committing the crime. (vi) It is more reliable than the eye witnesses. After several months of the crime when the eye witnesses are asked in the court of law to narrate the events, they give different versions to the same event but the physical evidences remain the same. (vii) Court's decisions have made physical evidence more important and is expected in criminal cases by courts. Moreover, the court decision depends more upon the physical evidences than that of the eye witnesses. In the recent years, more and more eye witnesses are turning hostile resulting in injustice during the trial due to lack of any physical evidence.

Collection and preservation of physical evidences: In any case of trial, the court will require the proof that the evidence that is collected at the crime scene is the same as that being produced in the court. Usually the evidences are kept in a container, tagged and identifying information is written over it such as: (i) Victim's or suspect's name, date and time of collection, case number and type of crime, brief description of the item, name of the person collecting the evidences and the name who has the custody of the item. (ii) Storage of the physical evidences has legal implications. These must be kept in a secured area prior to the transportation to the court of law and no unauthorised person should have access to it. (iii) As a general rule, sufficient samples should be collected; as much as samples that are available are to be collected. Control samples are also needed for the comparative study. (iv) Physical evidence should be handled as little as possible because too much handling may arbitrate the fingerprints and even dislodge the minute evidences like hair, fibers etc. At times forceps, gloves and other instruments may be required to handle the evidences. Contamination is a great concern and to be avoided at any cost.

First officer at the scene: Crime scenes are dynamic, rapidly changing and the first officer must be concerned with myriad of details. The actions or steps taken by him lead to a successful investigation or solution of crimes. The first officer's most important duty is to prevent the destruction or diminished utility of potential evidence that may lead to the apprehension of criminal and solution of the crime. Nothing should be changed, destroyed, added or removed to or from the scene of crime as this may mislead investigators, though the general rule of protecting crime scene cannot be applied to every case (Figure 8.1A and B). It may not be possible to preserve the crime scene in certain crimes because of their locations, e.g., when vehicular accident occurred on the road with heavy traffic on. Detailed and meticulous note taking should be adhered to. All movements should be calm and deliberate. Errors committed at the scene of crime can never be rectified. Every effort should be undertaken to preserve the crime scene as **Locard's exchange principle** states that whenever an object comes in contact with another, there is an exchange of material between them. This implies that traces from the scene can be carried on the body or tools of the criminal and traces from any of these may be left at the scene. In addition, the path followed by the criminal, objects touched by him and materials left by him serve as silent evidences against him such as fingerprints, shoe prints, blood, seminal stains, hair, fiber from clothes, broken pieces of glass, paints, scratch materials etc.

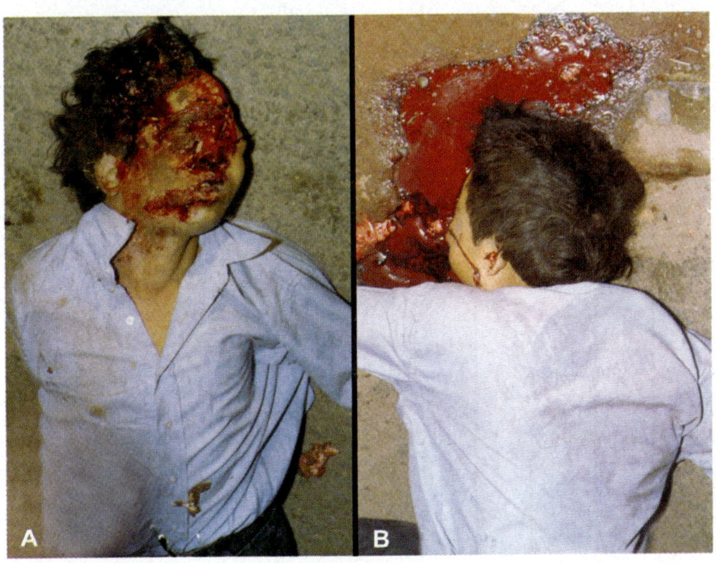

Figure 8.1A and B: Body found at the scene with bleeding from the smashed head with heavy stone

Role of the first officer before the investigating team arrives: (i) Names of the witnesses and other person who has entered the scene and who were at the scene before the arrival of the officer should be recorded. (ii) Basic facts and findings necessary to find out the cause of death should be established. (iii) Suspect and the witnesses should be kept separately. (iv) Witnesses are instructed not to discuss anything with anybody. (v) Crime scene must be protected.

The purpose of crime scene investigation is to reconstruct the events. Investigation of crime scene can be divided into two parts: (i) Photography (ii) Investigation proper.

Recording the time: The time of examining the scene of crime should be recorded. Precise noting of the time is very important. The time at which the crime was committed, the first officer was called, his arrival at the scene etc. are quite important. Track of time spent at the scene indicates the systemic way the things were done.

Entering the scene proper: Efforts should be made to observe the details and make notes on such points as doors, windows, lights, shades or shutters. Any odour as that of cigarette, smoke, gas, gun powder or perfume etc should be noted. Signs of activity like meal preparation, dishes in sink etc. date and time indicators like mail, newspaper, stopped clock, spoiled food and position of the articles should also be noted. Nothing should be removed unless essential. Position of the body should be noted, along with sketches, photographs and videography, if possible. No one should use toilets and eat or drink anything at the scene.

At times, it happens that the victim or relatives attempt to clear up the scene. Such persons would like to conceal something or want that the things should be in proper order. It is often possible to recover physical evidence on damaged items that have been thrown in the trash.

Protecting the integrity of scene: The scene should be protected from the public, other officers, press, family members and any other unauthorized access to be banned. For indoor crime scene, the door should be locked or the gate of the premises should be closed. While for the outdoor scene, one stringing rope or a commercially available tape should be used to "cordon off" the area. Vehicles and police barricades can act as physical barriers to intrusion by unauthorized people. Officers have to play a very active role in protecting the crime scene and extent of measures vary from case to case. It is important to protect crime scene proper and paths of entry and exit by criminals. If it is a very large area then local trusted citizens can be of help to protect the area. The protective measures at the scene should be taken at the earliest thus preventing the destruction of valuable evidence.

Injured persons at the scene have to be attended immediately. First aid should be given even if valuable evidence is lost or destroyed. If first aid is not essential then detailed position, photographs and sketches should be made. Hands must be examined for hairs or fibers. Dying declaration should be obtained from the injured while on the way to the hospital. In the hospital clothing to be taken charge of.

Role of Forensic Pathologist

At this point, the forensic pathologist should be called to the crime scene by the investigating agencies but it partly depends upon the local custom. At most of the places, it is better for the investigating officer to arrive first and later the doctor should be called to the crime scene. Once the doctor is at the scene, he should first stabilize the injured and make arrangements to send them to the nearest hospital. Then diagnose that the victim is dead. He along with the investigating team will collect the evidences, examine the body before transferring it to the mortuary. Examination of the scene is very important for the doctor to correlate the findings of the scene with that discerned during postmortem examination.

Diagnosis of dead persons: Diagnosis of dead at the scene is important. The body should be touched and tested for circulation, respiration, light reflex, pupillary reaction and corneal reflex. Sketch or photograph of the stains etc. should be taken and then the body is transferred to mortuary with identification tags. Each body should be sent in a separate bag.

When a suspect is found at the scene: When a suspect is found at the scene then the duty of the officer is to protect the scene. When this is not possible leave the scene in charge of a civilian till other officers arrive. The suspect should be searched and removed from the location as he may try to destroy or change the evidence.

Crime Scene Search

After collecting information about the crime scene, a quick survey should be done and actual crime scene search should be done. Various methods employed for searching crime scene are:

1. **Spiral search method:** In this method the search is started from a central point in the scene and then the single investigator walks in an outward spiral covering the whole area (Figure 8.2A).
2. **Grid method:** In this method the whole crime scene is divided into a grid and each of the grids are carefully searched for evidence. Multiple investigators can search the scene (Figure 8.2B).

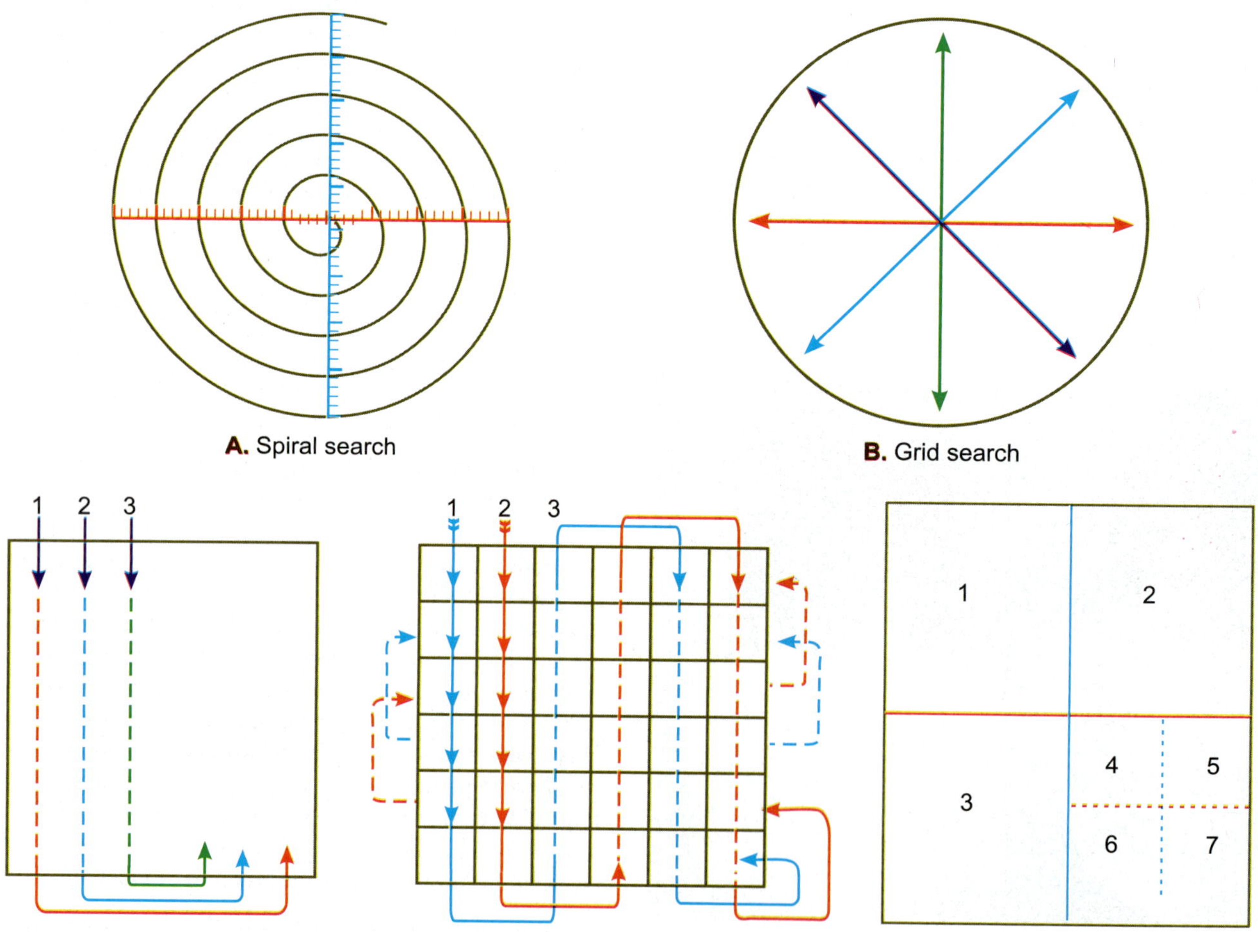

A. Spiral search

B. Grid search

C. Strip or line search

D. Quadrant or zone search

Figure 8.2: Various methods for searching the scene of crime

3. **Strip or line search:** In this method a single investigator starts searching the scene from one end and covers the whole scene in straight lines returning from side to side (Figure 8.2C).
4. **Quadrant or zone search:** In this method the whole area is divided into quadrants and each of the quadrants are searched by one or more investigators. The quadrants can be further subdivided into more quadrants as per convenience (Figure 8.2D).

Specific Crime Scenes

Traffic accidents: Evaluation of the scene should be done with a request for ambulance, fire service, forensic experts and traffic control assistance. Tow truck service should be availed to remove the damaged vehicles. First aid must be provided to all the injured.

Protecting the scene: The scene has to be protected by a patrol unit with flashing light warning and traffic flow should be arranged properly.

Witness: There are three ways to find out witnesses who can narrate the facts related with the accident. The investigator can ask "Did anyone see what happened?" or he can say "I like that witnesses should remain here". The investigator should watch the crowd while administration of first aid. Usually the teenagers and ladies are best witnesses.

Evidences: A sketch should be prepared or a photograph may be taken of the scene. Vehicle debris and broken glass etc. should be collected.

Vehicle removal: Tow truck driver is an important member. All the vehicles should be removed one by one.

Storage report: Drivers and passengers should be taken to hospital. Inventory of the vehicle should be maintained. Only engine key should go to avoid possible allegation of theft. Money and suitcase etc. should be sent with the victim. The roadways should be opened.

Statements: The passengers, drivers and public should be interviewed. Questions relevant to the accident must be asked. Statements of witnesses should be recorded. Identity of the witness should be recorded for future reference. To interview a child witness simple words and plain dress should be used rather than police dress.

Arrests: Drunken drivers should be arrested and alcoholic testing should be done.

Reporting: A report should be prepared and forwarded to higher authorities.

Collection of physical evidence: (i) *Skid marks:* They should be identified by the type of mark with its origin and termination. Measure the mark with a steel tape and not by pacing. Attempt to identify the skid marks with tyre of the vehicle. Measure the gaps, skips and deviations as they assist in locating the point of impact. If no skid marks are found write none. (ii) *Graze marks:* The length of grazing is to be measured and direction can be determined. Try to locate the point, grease, oil, water and residue around graze mark. These help in identifying the vehicle. (iii) *Debris:* Identify the type of debris and their location whether over the head lamp glass, radiator water and brake fluid etc. (iv) *Vehicle parts:* The bumpers, fenders, door handles, radio antennas etc. should be examined.

Other physical evidences: Examination of other physical evidence such as a suitcase falling from the top of the vehicle or fall and breaking of the baggage while a pedestrian is crossing the road when hit by the car. All these help in establishing the identity of the victim and reconstructing the scene of crime.

Burns: The burns can occur at any place. The room may be closed or open. The fire may have occurred outside or at any other place. Smell of inflammable substance should be taken into account. The cooking material used, condition of hair and sometimes broken bangles or weapons recovered from the scene all help in reconstructing the event. Body should be examined for pugilistic attitude and heat ruptures.

Hanging and strangulation: In these cases, the points to be noted are height of suspension, the platform height, mark on resting points or suspension or suspension points. The method of removal of the body whether by cutting the ligature or untying the knot should be noted. The pattern of knots and noose should be noted and whether the person can hang himself with it or not (Figures 8.3 and 8.4). Diagrams, sketches, photographs and videography etc. should be undertaken. Noose should be examined immediately

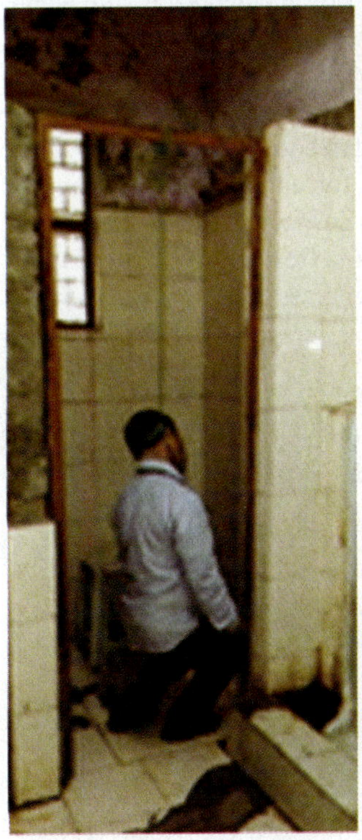

Figure 8.3: Body found at the scene in a case of hanging showing ligature around the neck

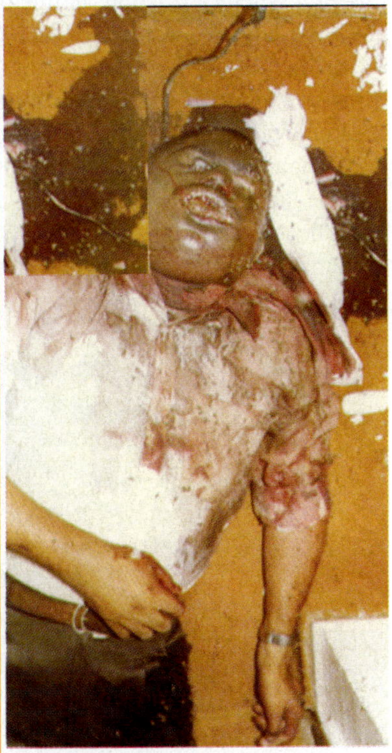

Figure 8.4: Body found at the site of crime with ligature *in situ* (ligature strangulation)

and if it is cut, the pieces should be recovered and analysed. The ground under and around the hanged person must be examined immediately. Knots in hanging case should never be undone or cut except while life saving measures are mandatory. A case of suicide at times gives a picture of homicide or a murder. On the other hand, there are cases of murder when the body has been hanged to simulate a case of suicidal hanging. In all such cases, it is important that the neck should be carefully examined along with other bodily injuries. The examination of circumstances where the crime has occurred is important. This includes noting negligible findings such as whether the room was bolted from inside or not and evidences of struggle at the scene.

Firearm: In firearm cases, clothing, injuries and surroundings must be protected. In addition, findings such as tattooing, blackening, singeing, should be protected from rain while moving the body from the scene. Hands should be protected by wrapping in polythene whereas paper bags should be used for collection of evidence.

Deaths by poisoning: In poisoning deaths, it is very rare for the investigating officer to find the presence of physical evidence at the crime scene indicating that the death was due to ingestion of some poisonous substance (Figure 8.5A). The physical evidences located at the crime scene should be noted and corroborated on examination that may sometimes indicate poisoning. In case of death from poisoning the investigation of the scene and examination of witnesses will decide the manner of death whether suicidal, homicidal or accidental. At the scene any vital clue in the form of tablets, powder, residues in bottles of medicines, wrappings, boxes, tubes, ampoules, vials and other containers if found should be preserved (Figure 8.5B). All medicine bottles, tubes, syringes and needles including the empty ones should be preserved and sent for analyses to the forensic science lab. When food poisoning is suspected, the dishes should be collected and packed (Figure 8.6). Besides, food dishes and remains of food are packed in a clean glass jar that is well sealed.

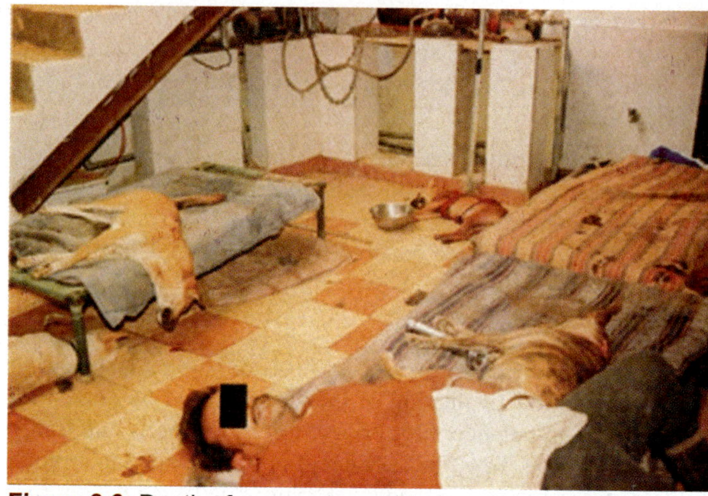

Figure 8.6: Death of a man along with dogs found at the scene in case of aluminum phosphide poisoning–Accidental death

In cases of drug abuse when syringes are found at the scene they should be recovered preventing them from contamination. The needle of the syringe is conveniently stuck in a cork to prevent it from breaking. The scene should also be searched for ampoules and vials.

Homicidal Death: A forensic medicine expert should visit the death scene of a homicide or suspected homicide. He should observe the position of the body, weapon, pattern of blood stain, external injuries on the body and the arrangement of objects in the surrounding areas (Figure 8.7). The crime may have occurred at the scene where body is found or the body may have been dumped there. Sometimes, the assailant after killing the victim, disposed of the body by burying, burning, by throwing into water, or concealing them in distant places (Figure 8.8A, B). The victim may be found dead with mouth taped, gagged (Figure 8.9A, B) and limbs tied (Figure 8.10A). Many times, the victim's face is mutilated to conceal the identity (Figure 8.10B). In case of

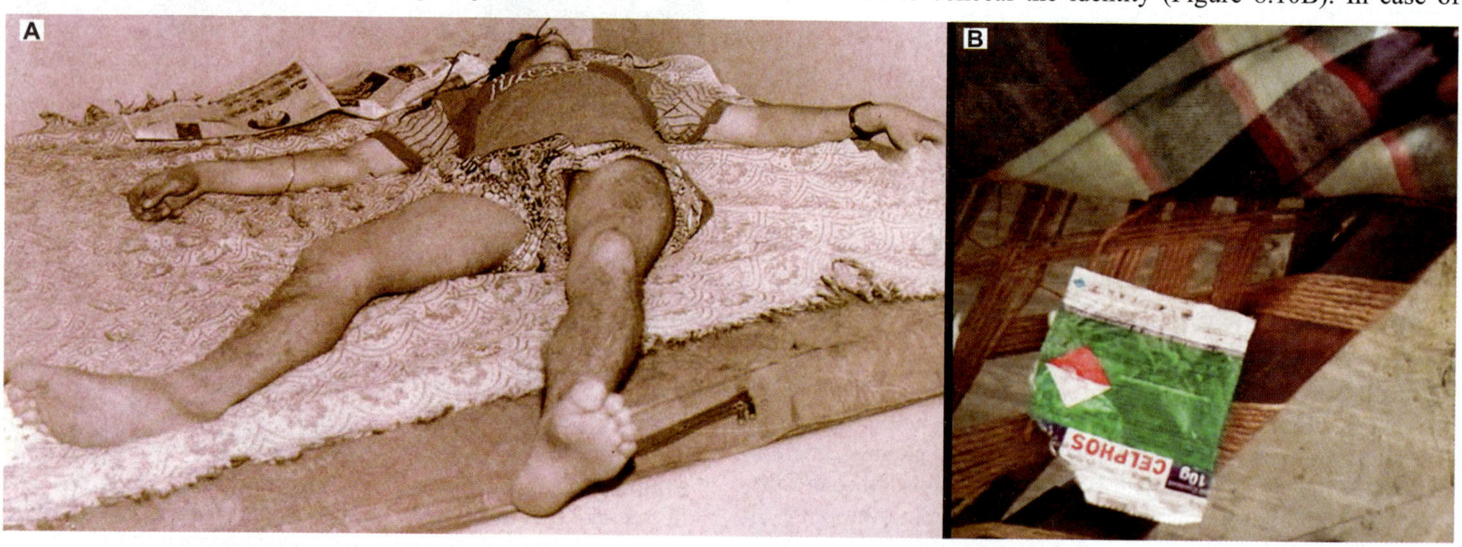

Figure 8.5A, B: Body found lying on the bed early in the morning with no external injuries (A), wrapper of Celphos at crime scene (B)

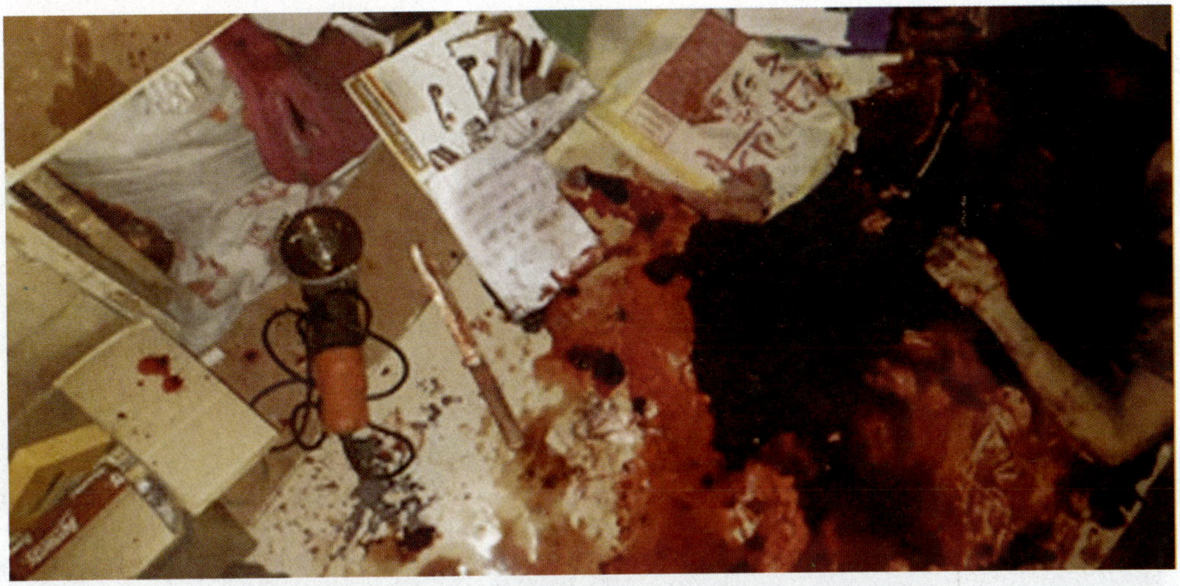

Figure 8.7: Scene in homicidal death with weapon lying on floor

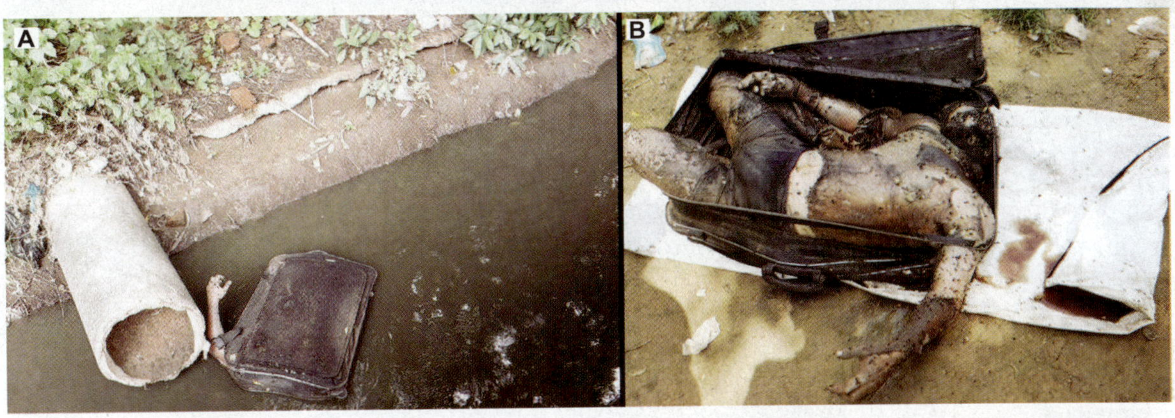

Figure 8.8A, B: Body packed in a suitcase and disposed of in a drain in a murder case

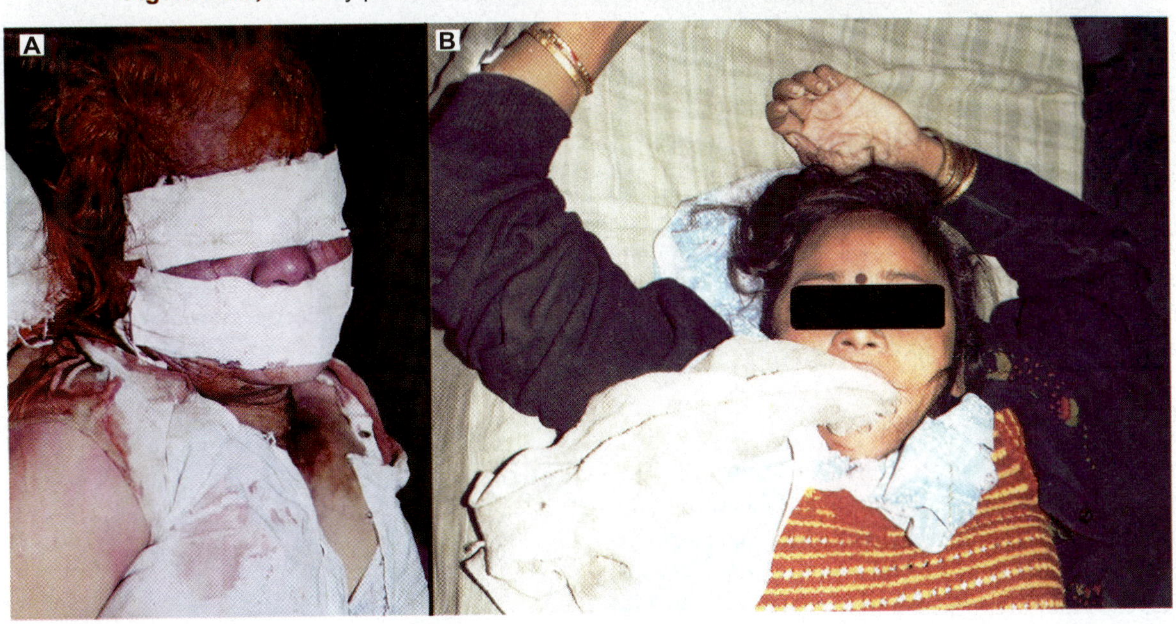

Figure 8.9A,B: Body found at the scene with strapping of eyes and mouth in homicidal death(A), gagged with cloth (B)

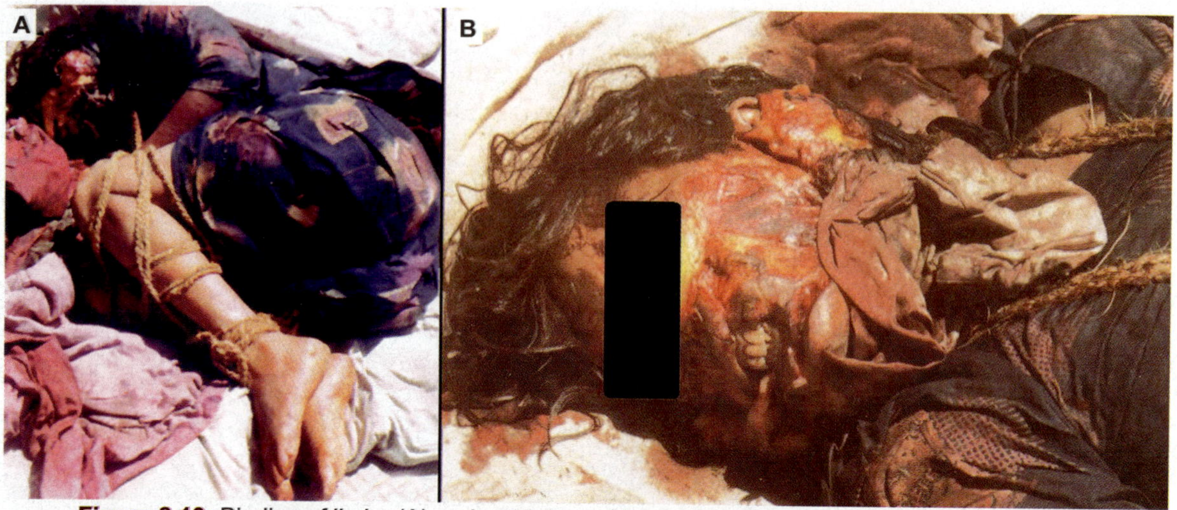

Figure 8.10: Binding of limbs (A) and mutilation of face to distort identity in homicidal death (B)

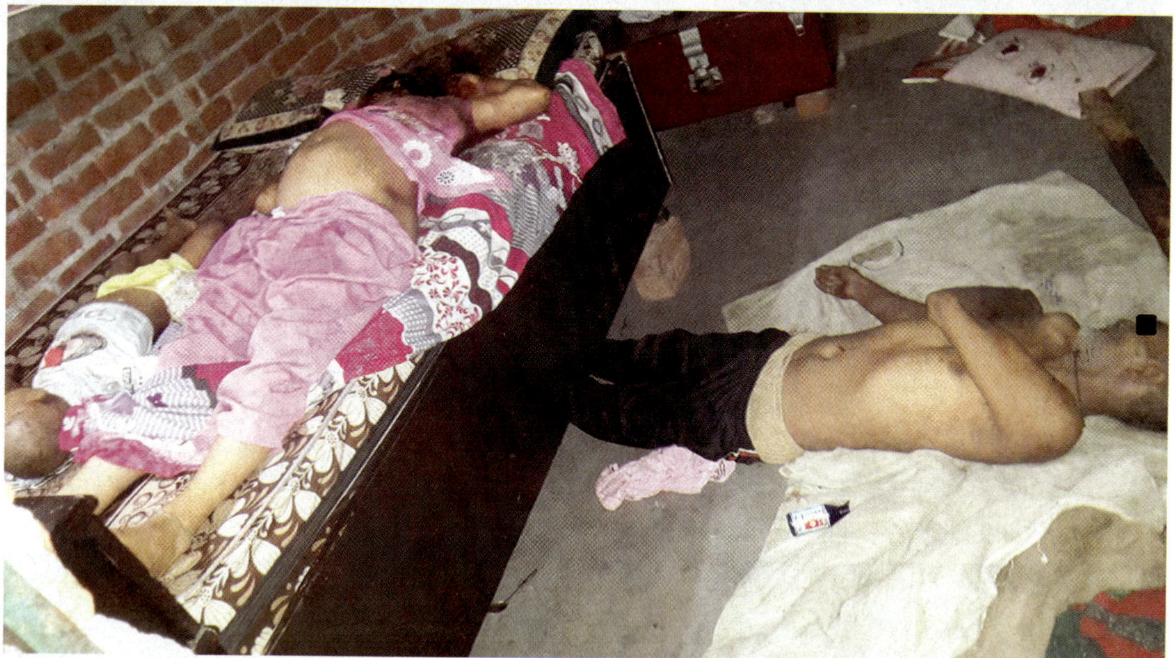

Figure 8.11: Crime scene of a Homicide-suicide (Dyadic death)–A man killed his wife and daughter by sustaining head injury with a wooden bar and later committed suicide by poisoning

homicide-suicide (**Dyadic death**), crime scene visit is important to know the circumstances of event (Figure 8.11). A thorough and complete crime scene investigation will help in proper diagnosis of the cause and manner of death.

Teamwork

Final element in crime scene investigation is teamwork. The whole system of crime scene investigation should be purposefully designed, so that nobody can operate independently. No person is more important than the other as each person has a vital role to play. Moreover, each and every person must feel empowered to do what needs to be done for the sake of justice.

LONG QUESTIONS

1. What are the objectives and usefulness of crime scene investigations?
2. Discuss the role of first officer at the crime scene.
3. What are the different findings in a crime scene?

SHORT QUESTIONS

1. Methods of crime scene search.
2. Role of Forensic pathologist in crime scene.
3. Collection and preservation of evidences in crime scene.
4. Locard's principle of exchange.

9 CHAPTER

Artefacts

Dorland's Illustrated Medical Dictionary defines an artefact as any artificial product; any structure or feature that is not natural, but has been altered by processing. In Forensic Pathology, the artefact is any change caused or a feature introduced into a body after death that is likely to lead to misinterpretation of medicolegally significant antemortem findings.

It is the duty of the pathologist to interpret the artefacts correctly. The misinterpretation may lead to: (i) Wrong cause of death (ii) Wrong manner of death (iii) Undue suspicion of criminal offense (iv) Halt in the investigation of a homicide and non-detection of murder (v) Miscarriage of justice in civil suits (vi) Unnecessary spending of time and effort as a result of misleading findings. The artefacts are divided into two groups: (i) Artefacts introduced between death and autopsy (ii) Artefacts introduced during autopsy.

Artefacts Introduced Between Death and Autopsy

Agonal artefacts: Regurgitation and aspiration of the gastric contents is a very common artefact seen in forensic practice. This may occur in natural deaths as a terminal event, from handling of the body or during resuscitation. This may result in physicians in wrongly giving aspiration of gastric contents as cause of death.

Resuscitation artefacts: The body may reveal injection marks, bruises and fractures etc. when the body is subjected to resuscitative attempts. The injection marks are usually seen in the cardiac region or on the extremities. The intracardiac injection may be associated with bruising of the heart and collection of some blood in the pericardium. The injection prick marks produced in the agonal period need to be differentiated from the marks of drug abuse.

The defibrillator applied over the body produces ring like bruises over the chest (Figure 9.1A, B). The ribs may sometimes be fractured from external cardiac massage but they do not show effusion of blood at the fracture site or in the intercostal muscles.

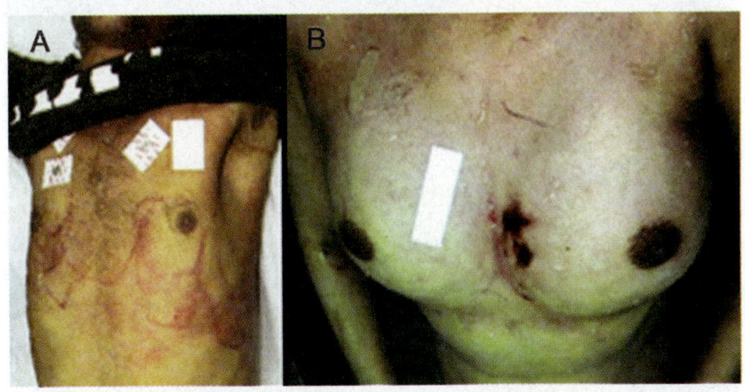

Figure 9.1A, B: Defibrillator injury mark (A) and bruise due to cardiac massage (B) over chest

Sometimes recent hemorrhages may be present in postmortem fractures. In such cases careful history of resuscitative measures is to be obtained. Evaluation of such fractures is of immense importance in deaths from violence particularly beatings and battered babies. Fat or bone marrow embolization is frequently associated with or without fractures of ribs or sternum with external cardiac massage. The positive pressure breathing apparatus used for resuscitation tend to leave the evidence of acute emphysema, occasionally with subpleural blebs, air in the mediastinum and even tension pneumothorax.

Embalming artefacts: The dimensions of the homicidal stab or gunshot wounds may be modified by the embalmer while trying to introduce the trochar through them. The multiple trochar holes may in a case of gunshot injuries may cause difficulties for the pathologist. Also, the track of the weapon or the bullet may be disturbed, creating false tracks. The surgical alteration or suturing of gunshot wounds may complicate the situation. The embalming fluids may cause confusion for the forensic scientists when analyzing the viscera for drugs or chemicals. Embalming fluids generally contain formaldehyde, methyl alcohol and sometimes other interfering compounds.

Internment and exhumation artefacts: In bodies interned for some time and later exhumed, fungus growth is common at body orifices, eyes and site of open injuries. The underlying skin is discoloured simulating bruising. While performing autopsy on exhumed bodies, the agonal, resuscitative, embalming artefacts and those resulting from handling of the body after death should be borne in mind. Skin on the dead body can be removed by friction, producing postmortem abrasion that has a yellow appearance (Figure 9.2A).

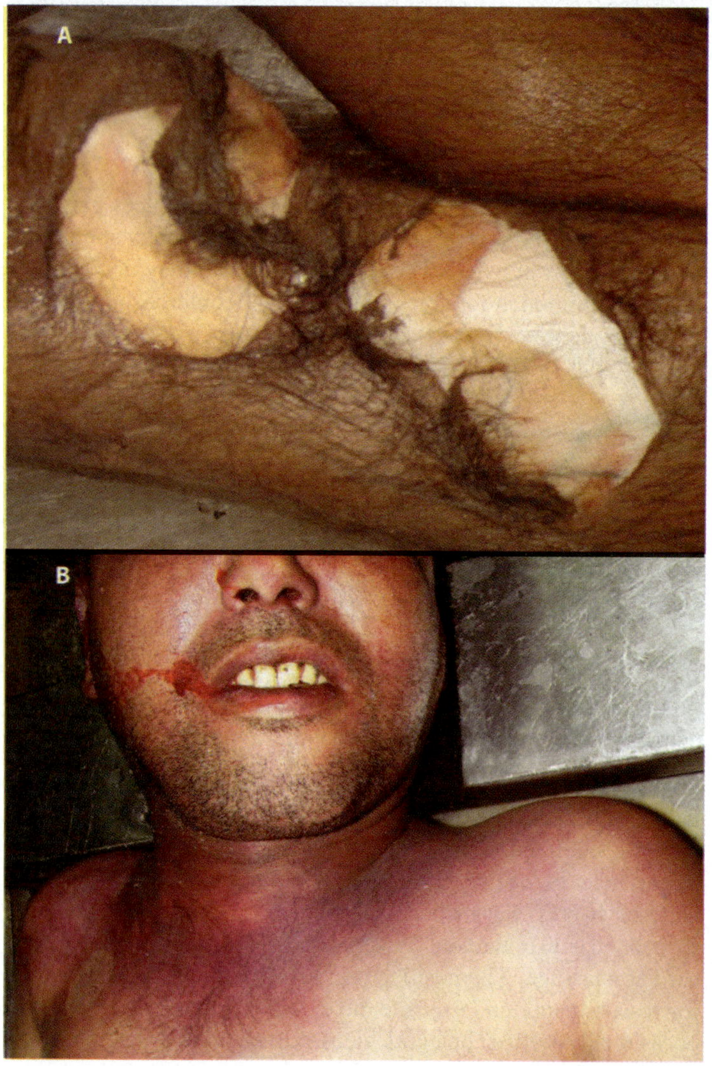

Figure 9.2A, B: Postmortem abrasion (A), Pink hypostasis on upper chest and neck due to refrigeration (B)

Artefacts related to rigor mortis and hypostasis: While handling the body the rigor may break resulting in false estimate of time of death. The onset or progress of rigor may be significantly affected by postmortem circumstances such as extreme heat or cold or antemortem conditions, e.g., extreme hyperthermia due to widespread infections. Rigor of the heart causes the stiffening of the muscles and may simulate its concentric hypertrophy.

The colour of the postmortem staining is usually purplish. Cherry red colouration may sometimes be seen in carbon monoxide poisoning. Pink hypostasis is a common finding in bodies exposed to cold temperature in an open environment or in bodies refrigerated for some time (Figure 9.2B). Localized areas of hypostasis may resemble bruises.

Decomposition artefacts: The decomposition of the body produces certain changes that may be mistakenly interpreted as pathological lesions. Advanced decomposition causes swelling of the lips, nose and eyelids, protrusion of the eyes, distension of the chest and abdomen and swelling of the extremities. These changes may lead to the false impression of the antemortem obesity. In decomposed bodies the presence of body fluids in the mouth and nose is a frequent finding. In the presence of pulmonary oedema, large quantities of such fluid may escape from the mouth and nose. This may lead to an erroneous conclusion that the person died of massive haemorrhage. Decomposition blebs are occasionally misinterpreted as vesications from burns. In a decomposed body, a deep groove may be seen around the neck if the deceased has been wearing a buttoned shirt or blouse at the time of death. These grooves often simulate ligature marks seen in strangulation cases. Even in non-decomposed bodies, bands or grooves of contact flattening in the skin of the neck of obese individual or of well nourished infants may be seen. The decomposed blood acquires a dark colour and produces appearance of congestion in the brain, lungs, right side of the heart and other parts of the body so that it becomes difficult to form the conclusion of death from asphyxia. The marks on the neck should be carefully interpreted. In some cases, marked bluish discolouration of the loops of intestine is seen. This finding may be labeled by some pathologist as that of infarcted bowel. Correct interpretation of the finding of the air in the large veins and in the right side of the heart is of great importance in medicolegal autopsies. During life air may enter the systemic venous circulation during criminal abortions, craniotomy, urethroscopy, fallopian tube insufflation, pneumoperitoneum, aortography and intravenous infusions. In cases of air embolism following abortion, air bubbles are usually found in the cavity of the uterus and its wall, the uterine and adnexal veins, the inferior vena cava and right heart, the pulmonary arteries, the left heart and the systemic arteries. The presence of gas in the right side of the heart resulting from decomposition may resemble the findings in air embolism and it may be difficult to distinguish one from the other. The analysis of the gas that is collected from the heart and brought into contact with an alkaline pyrogallol solution turns brown in the presence of free oxygen, gives support to the diagnosis of antemortem air embolism. Gas produced by decomposition will not produce this colour change.

Gunshot wounds artefacts: During the hospital stay the victim of gunshot wound may sustain additional pseudogunshot wounds. The drainage holes in the chest or abdomen, such as embalmer's trochar holes may be confused with the gunshot wounds. Surgical alteration or suturing of the wounds may lead to difficulty in evaluating the wound known as **Kennedy phenomenon.** In decomposed bodies these wounds may be greatly modified. Deliberate mutilation of the firearm injury by cutting or stabbing or sometimes, a bullet is placed deliberately inside stab injury resulted in artefact production which is called **Rayalaseema phenomenon.** The purpose is to mislead the investigation which was reported from the Rayalaseema region of Andhra Pradesh.

Toxicological artefacts: Decomposition of the biological material often causes apparent alterations in the constituents of the tissue. It is generally known that the alcohol is produced postmortem because of putrefaction (enzymatic decomposition, especially of proteins, with the production of foul smelling compounds) of the tissues and the fact that many of the bacteria can produce alcohol. However, it must be emphasized that the levels of alcohol generated by putrefaction are usually less than 100 mg%. If the levels are more than 100 mg% it should arouse the suspicion of alcohol ingestion prior to death. Decomposition is also known to cause an increase in the concentration of carboxyhaemoglobin in the blood; the increase has been reported 19-25% by various authors. Cyanide is produced by decomposition in toxicologically significant amounts; levels up to 10 mg% have been found in three months old blood.

Many substituted phenols (extremely poisonous compounds generally from coal tar) have been found in the decomposing tissues. The one that cause disturbing interference in the analysis of weak acid fractions are related to p-hydroxyphenyl derivatives.

Combustion of the body tissues and other materials associated with the burned body produces several gases. Oslen and his colleagues investigated gases generated in experimental fires and demonstrated the presence of ammonia, carbon monoxide, hydrogen cyanide, hydrogen sulphide, nitrogen, oxides of nitrogen and sulphur dioxide. Combustible material like silk and wool produces high concentrations of several of these gases because their nitrogen content is high. Some of these gases may be detected in the body tissues and the results of toxicological analysis may raise false alarms. Cyanide levels in the blood of the burn victims were reported between 17-220 mg per 100 ml.

Miscellaneous Artefacts

Fauna bites: The animal bites produce confusing changes but bears characteristic teeth marks. The rodent bites are commonly seen in bodies that are stored in a cold room (Figure 9.3A). Drowned bodies may bear the marks of injuries produced by water creatures such as fishes, crabs and may simulate stab wounds. Ant bites on the dead body cause irregular serpiginous, scalloped areas of superficial skin loss, and small punctate and scratch-type lesions which can be misinterpreted as antemortem abrasions (Figure 9.3B). These injuries are orange-pink to yellow in color and diffusely scattered over the skin surface.

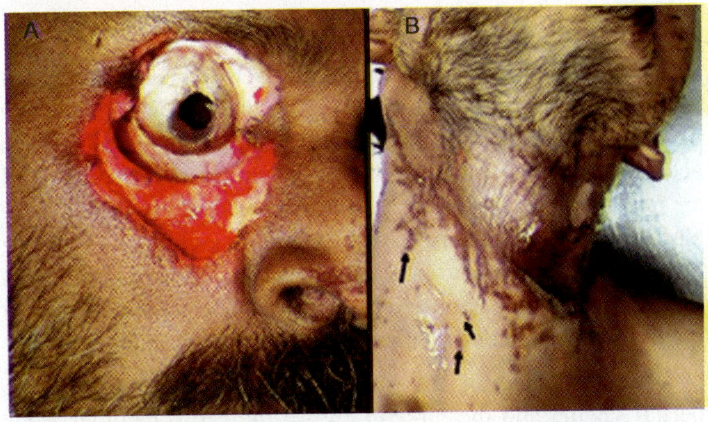

Figure 9.3A, B: Rodent bite (A) and ant bites (B)

Postmortem haemorrhage: The finding of the extravasation of blood in the tissues or even pools of blood in the body cavities does not necessarily mean that the haemorrhage was from antemortem trauma. Under normal circumstances blood in the body remains in a fluid state for a time. During this time the postmortem injury may open a blood vessel and lead to postmortem haemorrhage. The significance of blood in the pleural cavities after death has been explained to be due to substantial bleeding from wounds inflicted on the chest wall and the lung tissue.

Flattening of the convolutions of brain: Flattening of the cerebral hemisphere is invariably seen in cases of oedema of the brain caused by pathological lesions. This flattening is generalized. However, regional flattening of the cerebral convolutions is a common postmortem artefact. The parts of the brain in contact with the cranium, particularly the dependent parts show flattening and the occipital lobes show such flattening more frequently. The longer the body remains in such position and longer the time after death, the more marked is the flattening. To prevent additional artefactual flattening from contact with the container, the brains in order to be fixed should be suspended in 10% formalin by a hook passed around the basilar arteries for a period of 3 weeks before dissection.

Grooving of unci: It is widely accepted concept that the grooving of the uncus is an important accompaniment of genuine oedema of the brain from cerebral lesions. But this finding is extremely common in normal brains at autopsy, and this artefact should not lead the pathologist to a misinterpretation.

Discolouration of the liver: Blackish brown discolouration of the liver at the site of contact with the large bowel is fairly common. This is a postmortem change, the result of substances passing from the bowel to the liver and depositing sulfides in the adjacent liver tissue. Similarly bile also produces staining of the liver surface.

Artefacts Introduced During Autopsy

In the head one of the most common artefacts is the introduction of air bubbles into the vessels at the top of the brain. In the majority of cases while the dura is being pulled in the sagittal line, air gains access to the blood vessels. Likewise, postmortem introduction of air into the veins of the neck during the reflection of the skin is also very common. In cases of suspected air embolism following attempts at criminal abortion, artefactual presence of air bubbles in the vessels of the brain and neck may initiate confusion and the diagnosis of air embolism may be erroneously entertained.

While sawing of the vault of skull during the autopsy, partial sawing and the forceful pull of the cap sometimes leads to the fractures of the skull. In the already fractured skull, the antemortem fractures may be extended or additional fractures created. Postmortem tears of the midbrain may be caused during the removal of the brain from the cranium. Handling of the organs and incisions of the vessels during routine postmortem examinations often result in the extravasation of the blood into the tissues, particularly into the neck. Recognition of autopsy artefacts in cervical tissues is of special importance because they simulate antemortem bruises seen in cases of throttling and strangulation. These artefacts on neck were first described in 1951 South African forensic pathologists, Prinsloo and Gordon, hence named as **Prinsloo Gordon artefact**. Therefore, dissection of the neck should be meticulous avoiding the artefacts from seepage of blood from the neck vessels. During autopsy, when the head is allowed to fall freely over occiput, during hyperextension of the neck for removal of neck structures and also before autopsy due to careless handling of the body usually by undertakers, there can be intervertebral disc rupture at C6-C7 vertebra level causing subluxation of the spine which is called **Undertaker's fracture**.

Toxicological Artefacts

Some of the toxicological artefacts may be introduced during the autopsy caused by:

1. **Faulty technique in collecting samples:** Blood samples are sometimes drawn from the heart with a long needle and this may result in contamination of sample with gastric contents and tests particularly for alcohol may be misleading. In traumatic deaths such as those due to automobile accidents, the stomach may rupture and lead to the added likelihood of contamination. Also, alcohol is known to diffuse in significant amounts from the stomach to the pleural and pericardial cavities. During an attempt to draw blood from the heart, pericardial and pleural fluid may be withdrawn giving unreliable results.
2. **Faulty techniques in storage:** Artefacts may be introduced by cutting the organs with instruments contaminated by stomach contents or by putting the samples of tissue in contaminated containers. It is a common practice to store portions of several organs in one container. Such a practice is apt to cause alterations in true levels of the poisons because the diffusion or drainage of the blood or fluid from one organ to another may lead to an altered concentration of the poison.
3. **Use of preservatives:** The use of the preservatives can also add to the artefacts. It should be emphasized that preservatives such as EDTA, formalin, heparin and methanamine give a positive test for methanol and these should not be used as anticoagulants for blood if an analysis for methanol is required.

LONG QUESTIONS

1. What do you mean by artefacts? Discuss the different artefacts that can be commonly encountered during autopsy.
2. Discuss the artefacts produced between death and autopsy.

MULTIPLE CHOICE QUESTIONS

1. Prinsloo Gordon artefact represents:

(a) Haemorrhage on the anterior aspect of the cervical spine at autopsy

(b) Haemorrhage at posterior wall of stomach at autopsy

(c) Haemorrhage on the posterior aspect of the lumbar spine at autopsy

(d) Haemorrhage on the anterior aspect of the lumbar spine at autopsy

2. Surgical alteration or suturing of the gunshot wounds may lead to difficulty in evaluating the wound known is known as:

(a) Prinsloo-Gordon phenomenon

(b) Kennedy phenomenon

(c) Magnus phenomenon

(d) Rayalaseema phenomenon

3. Undertaker's fracture is:

(a) Fracture dislocation of C3-C4 vertebra

(b) Fracture dislocation of C4-C5 vertebra

(c) Fracture dislocation of C5-C6 vertebra

(d) Fracture dislocation of C6-C7 vertebra

ANSWER KEY

1. (a)	2. (b)	3. (d)

10 CHAPTER

Anaesthetic and Surgical Deaths

Anaesthetics are used for the management of pain in various surgical and operative procedures. Anaesthetics may in themselves result in various adverse effects and sometimes death of the patient. Various surgical procedures carry the risk of life for some of the patients. Anaesthesia may be the sole cause of death in itself and may be a contributory factor in some of the deaths. Every new technique can potentially form a new hazard that is why the lists of mishap that can occur through medical practice are unlimited.

Deaths Associated with Surgical Operation

Those directly caused by the disease or injury for which the operation or anaesthetic was necessitated: In the advanced stage of some disease, the intervening surgical procedures may be undertaken to save the life of the patient. This procedure causes death of the patient but the disease from which the patient was suffering is given as cause of death. In cases when the patient dies on the operation table itself and is brought out dead from the theatre, the relatives may demand investigations into cause of death. In those cases where the patient is of trauma, and surgical operation is done, it is not possible to separate the relative contribution of the two to the cause of death.

Those caused by a disease or abnormality other than that for which the procedure was being carried out: When the death was caused by a disease other than that for which procedure was carried out and that was known to exist before carrying out the surgical procedure, it is for the Pathologist to evaluate whether an operation is necessary. However, if clinicians did not suspect the disease and neither the facility of specialized diagnosis was available, the death is excusable. When common conditions such as hypertension, ischemic heart diseases etc. are present, they should be properly diagnosed and treated. In the aged and debilitated patients, who may be a poor risk for operation, account must be taken of the condition of their myocardium and lungs.

Surgical or diagnostic procedure mishap: Failure of surgical technique might be: (i) Inadvertent in some unusually difficult operative circumstances or some anatomical abnormality (ii) Accidental due to failure of equipment (iii) Result of error or incompetence on the part of the surgeon for which the surgeon can be sued.

Deaths Associated with Anaesthesia

Most fatalities are not related to the actual procedure but due to other factors. The fact that the death occurred during or soon after an anaesthetic by no means indicates that the anaesthetic played a significant part in the death. Anaesthetic deaths can be classified as:

Those occurring under anaesthesia, but not related to anaesthetic agent: These types of deaths can be due to: (i) Death due to injury and disease that made the operation and anaesthetic necessary. (ii) Deaths due to a disease other than that for which the operation was performed but about which the medical attendants knew before death. In this category, there is some contraindication to anaesthesia that surgeon and anaesthetist is aware of but there is presence of some other urgent injury or disease for which the operation is vital. In these cases, the risk of anaesthetic must be balanced against the risk of leaving the patient untreated. (iii) Deaths due to a disease that is unknown at the time of operation.

In an elective operation, a full clinical examination together with ancillary investigation should be made to detect any significant disease that might affect the patient during the operation. (iv) Deaths may be due to surgical shock and exhaustion in cases where there is no preexisting disease. A poor risk patient because of the condition for which operation is being carried out is more likely to be affected. (v) A surgical accident may occur under anaesthesia rarely by the inexperienced doctors under emergency situations.

Deaths as a result of administration of an anaesthetic: (i) **Overdosage of an anaesthetic agent:** The deaths that arise out of the overdosage of an anaesthetic agent are rare and usually result from ill-advised polypharmacy. To achieve Anaesthesia, the current trend is to achieve a light plane of unconsciousness with a barbiturate or a hypnotic, accompanied by the inhalation of nitrous oxide and oxygen along with small quantities of a liquid agent such as halothane. To achieve muscle relaxation, long acting muscle relaxants such as gallamine, tubocurarine or pancuronium that compete with acetylcholine at the motor end plate or short acting muscle relaxants such as succinylcholine, decamethonium iodide, which depolarize the motor end plate rendering it unexcitable to acetylcholine, are used. Both the categories result in muscle paralysis. Overdosage with long acting muscle relaxants can be treated with neostigmine while overdosage with short acting agents such as succinyl choline can be overcome by the use of prolonged artificial respiration. Anaesthetic gases cause physical and psychological dependence and are commonly used by the medical personnel. (ii) **Anaesthetic misadventure:** An anaesthetic misadventure or a critical incident is a human error or equipment failure that could have led, or did lead to an undesirable outcome, ranging from increased length of hospital stay to death when it is not discovered in time.

The anaesthetic morbidity and mortality occur from the complications of anaesthetic procedure, failure of equipment and due to some human error, such as emergencies, failure to perform a normal check, lack of skilled assistance, restricted access to patient, and inadequate supervision of the patient due to distraction, fatigue, inattention, boredom or anxiety.

Deaths that are the direct result of the administration of an anaesthetic can be due to: (i) **Acute cardiovascular failure:** This is the most common cause of sudden unexpected death due to the administration of general anaesthetic. Cardiac arrest is the usual way in which the mishap presents and it is often impossible to discover either clinically or at postmortem examination. Most cases occur under relatively light anaesthesia rather than deep unconsciousness and thus tend to occur either at the beginning or at the end of surgery. This can occur even in the hands of most experienced and careful anaesthetist. Cardiac arrest appears to be mainly neurogenic in origin and can result from any form of irritation of the respiratory tract such as intubation or laryngoscopy. (ii) **Deaths due to respiratory failure:** Hypoxia occurring during anaesthesia may be due to defects in the supply of oxygen from the anaesthetic machines, either from mechanical failure or from the inexpert manipulation by the anaesthetist. Respiratory failure can also occur due to an overdose of an anaesthetic depressing the respiratory center. Excess of premedication and the use of muscle relaxants also predisposes to respiratory failure, unless the appropriate anaesthetic procedures such as assisted respiration are carried out. Mechanical blockage in the air passage may lead to hypoxic respiratory failures due to laryngeal spasm. Regurgitation of stomach contents and other mechanical defects in the apparatus may cause hypoxia and respiratory failure. Laryngeal spasm, swabs, dentures or teeth in the airways and haemorrhage from the nasopharynx may cause or contribute to hypoxia and unless appropriate posture is maintained after an anaesthetic, the tongue may obstruct the airway in the anaesthetized patient. (iii) **Recovery phase:** During the recovery phase, hypoxia may follow anaesthetic hyperventilation. After a period of hyperventilation, the tissue carbon dioxide store being depleted, the body attempts to replenish them. The need for carbondioxide elimination is diminished, and hyperventilation results which may prove fatal. The cause of impairment to ventilation may lie at the level of CNS, peripheral nerves, the myoneural junction or even at the level of upper or lower airways. (iv) **Postoperative problems:** Adequate postoperative care must be undertaken as medical practitioners will be responsible for any danger that befall a patient due to his negligence: (a) *Respiratory insufficiency:* That occurs within 72 hours of the surgery is usually due to the preoperative pulmonary diseases. If it occurs after 4-5 days, it is due to atelectasis or pneumonia, peritonitis, pulmonary embolism or increase in energy required for breathing because of exertion (b) *Aspiration:* Aspiration of foreign material such as secretions, gastric contents, blood and food can contaminate the tracheobronchial tree. Aspiration of pus leads to multiple abscesses and that of gastric content may lead to irritation. As a result acute pulmonary oedema and chemical peritonitis may occur (c) *Atelectasis:* It frequently occurs due to the misplacement of tracheal tube into one of the bronchi or due to respiratory insufficiency (d) *Pulmonary oedema:* Pulmonary oedema may be the result of circulatory overload due to administration of excess blood, fluids or plasma expanders (e) *Pneumothorax:* Spontaneous pneumothorax may occur during operative procedures with inhalation of anaesthesia or due to rupture of an emphysematous bleb. Tension pneumothorax is dangerous as it displaces mediastinum and has a deleterious effect on the heart and blood vessels (f) *Air embolism:* Massive air embolism causes circulatory collapse by producing a frothy mixture of blood and air-bubbles within the heart chamber and causes immediate cessation of peripheral circulation. (v) **Systemic toxicity of local anaesthetics:** These are adverse effects of the absorbed drug that affect the whole body. The blood shows high blood levels of these agents. There may be allergic reactions ranging from anaphylactic shock to dermatitis. They also depress medullary centers leading to apnoea and vascular collapse. Local anaesthetics may depress the myocardium directly resulting in hypotension. (vi) **Spinal anaesthesia:** Spinal anaesthesia causes two major types of neurologic complications namely myelopathy and arachnoiditis. (vii) **Deaths due to physical fault in the anaesthetic procedure:** The failure of equipment leading to anaesthetic mishaps usually occurs in a small number of cases. Explosions are particularly common with cyclopropane or ether. Flammable liquids can cause fires. The fatalities can occur from electric shock due to defects in monitoring equipments, defibrillators or diathermies in the operation theatre.

Preventive Strategies

(i) *Training and supervision:* The inexperience, inadequate training, inadequate knowledge about a new equipment or technique and even inadequate supervision by the seniors has been cited as a cause of error. To rectify these errors, regular in-house training of the anaesthetists should be carried on. (ii) *Specific protocol development, more complete preoperative assessment and equipment and apparatus inspection:* Preoperative assessment of patients and preoperative inspection of equipment and apparatus will prevent a number of critical incidents. (iii) *Additional monitoring instrumentation and equipment and human factors improvements:* Improved standardization or arrangement of drugs in the anaesthesia workspace, and improvement in design of gas flow control knobs and breathing circuit scavenging connections are now mandated by the national standards for new apparatus.

Medicolegal Aspects

The main precipitating factors of negligence suits are failure of empathy and communication towards the patient and his relatives. To minimize the possibility of malpractice actions, the anaesthetists and surgeons should ensure the following: (i) A proper physician-patient relationship should be established. (ii) In surgical procedures, the patient should be properly identified, the type of surgery to be performed, the side on which the surgery is to be performed is important. (iii) Before carrying out surgery, an informed consent should be obtained from the patient in his own language, properly stating the detail of the procedure and the risks and disabilities associated with it. For anaesthesia, separate consent should be obtained. (iv) Preanaesthetic check-up of the patient should be properly documented. (v) It is imperative to ascertain whether the anaesthetist has acquired the necessary skill to operate it by formal training. (vi) Any preexisting natural disease such as the heart or lung disease should be properly evaluated before undertaking surgical procedures.

Autopsy Procedure, Collection, Preservation and Dispatch of Related Material Evidence in Anaesthetic and Operative Deaths

Whenever deaths occur during or shortly after the performance of a surgical operation and general anaesthetic, the pathologist must answer the following questions: (i) Was the death due to the effects of the surgical procedure or anaesthetic or is it due to the natural disease for which operation was being carried out? (ii) Would the patient have died at the time he had died, if he has not undergone through the anaesthesia or operation? (iii) Was the surgery and anaesthesia vital to save the life of the patient? (iv) Was there any defect in anaesthetic or surgical technique? (v) Was the patient suffering from any predisposing condition relating to the condition for which he was operated that made him more susceptible to death from anaesthetic or operative procedure? (vi) Was the death due to some unsuspected natural disease directly unrelated to the disease for which surgery was being performed?

During autopsy, procedures to be followed include: (i) Detailed hospital record of the patient, including full clinical and pre-anaesthetic check-up details are essential especially in anaesthetic deaths. (ii) Surgical intervention and its sequelae like sepsis, haemorrhage, oedema etc. should be noted that frequently make examination of the operative site difficult. It is sometimes difficult to distinguish defects due to postmortem changes from abnormalities existing during life. It is common for the inexperienced pathologist to misdiagnose resuscitative artefacts. The finding of gastric contents in the airway at the autopsy should be cautiously interpreted. The agonal regurgitation of gastric contents in the air passages should not be misinterpreted. (iii) There are rare instances of surgical mishap, which may not be negligence if the operating conditions were difficult. These include ligation of arteries and veins, ureters, bile ducts, perforation of large blood vessels. (iv) A full clinical history along with the consultation with the surgeon, anaesthetist and other medical staff is necessary to arrive at the best possible opinion. Sometimes the cause of death is obscure even after the autopsy. (v) Presence of preexisting natural disease such as the heart disease, respiratory insufficiency due to the lung disease and their contribution to the cause of death must be evaluated. (vi) In deaths occurring due to surgical shock and exhaustion, the pathologist must exclude or confirm surgical incompetence and also evaluate as far as possible the preexistent state of the patient. (vii) If pneumothorax, air embolism or surgical emphysema is present, it should be clearly evaluated. (viii) Surgical and anaesthetic devices such as airways, endotracheal tubes, needles, catheters etc. should not be removed prior to autopsy. (ix) A radiograph that will show a ring of oedema of oesophageal mucosa at the level of the tube along with distention of stomach and intestines, in oesophageal intubation, can check position of the endotracheal tube. (x) All the organs should be dissected and surgical sutures should be inspected. (xi) Chloroform and halothane are hepatotoxic and chloroform may cause ventricular fibrillation sometimes. Halogenated hydrocarbons cause cardiac irritability. (xii) Blood samples obtained prior to the death of the patient should be sent for analytical tests. (xiii) *Toxicological examination:* For toxicological examination following samples should be collected: (a) One lung sealed in nylon bag (b) 2 gm of fat from mesentery (c) 100 gm of cerebrum (d) 100 gm of liver (e) 100 gm of kidney (f) 10 gm of skeletal muscle (g) Urine. In case of inhaled anaesthetic specimens should be kept in containers of appropriate size to avoid empty space, are sealed and refrigerated or frozen. Alveolar air should be collected with needle and syringe by puncturing the lung under water before the chest is opened.

LONG QUESTIONS

1. What are the causes of death on the operation table? What precautions you should take to avoid such deaths?
2. Discuss in detail the autopsy procedures in anaesthetic and operative deaths. How do you collect and preserve viscera in such cases?

11 CHAPTER

Sudden and Unexpected Deaths

The definition of sudden death varies according to authority and convention. WHO defines sudden death as 'death that is unknown or sudden' and occurring within 24 hours from onset of symptoms. However, some pathologists and clinicians will only accept sudden death as the one occurring within one hour from the onset of illness. According to Gradwohl, the unexpected nature of death is more important than its suddenness. Many unexpected deaths will be sudden such as those occurring immediately upon collapse or within minutes and there may be a delay of hours or even days without a diagnosis being clinically evident. The primary objective of medicolegal autopsy in cases of sudden and unexpected deaths, including apparently accidental death is to establish cause of death.

In sudden deaths, the immediate cause is usually in the cardiovascular system.

Causes of sudden death (Figure 11.1)	
Cardiovascular system	45-50%
Respiratory system	10-15%
Central nervous system	10-18%
Alimentary system	6-8%
Genitourinary system	3-5%
Miscellaneous	5-10%

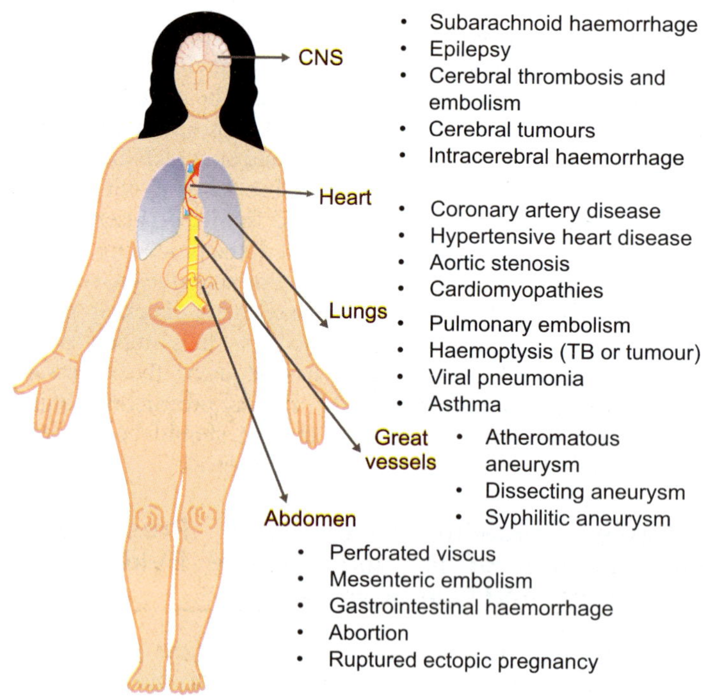

Figure 11.1: Various causes of sudden death

Cardiovascular System

In the cardiovascular system, the causes of sudden death are: (i) Coronary atherosclerosis (ii) Hypertensive heart disease (iii) Aortic valve disease (iv) Coronary circulation anomalies (v) Coronary artery diseases–polyarteritis (vi) Cardiomyopathic enlargement (vii) Congenital heart disease. Ischemic heart disease is by far the most common cause of sudden death in Western nations.

Normal anatomy of heart and coronaries: The normal weight of an adult heart varies between 275-300 gm and that of female between 225-250 gm. The atrial walls are 1-2 mm thick

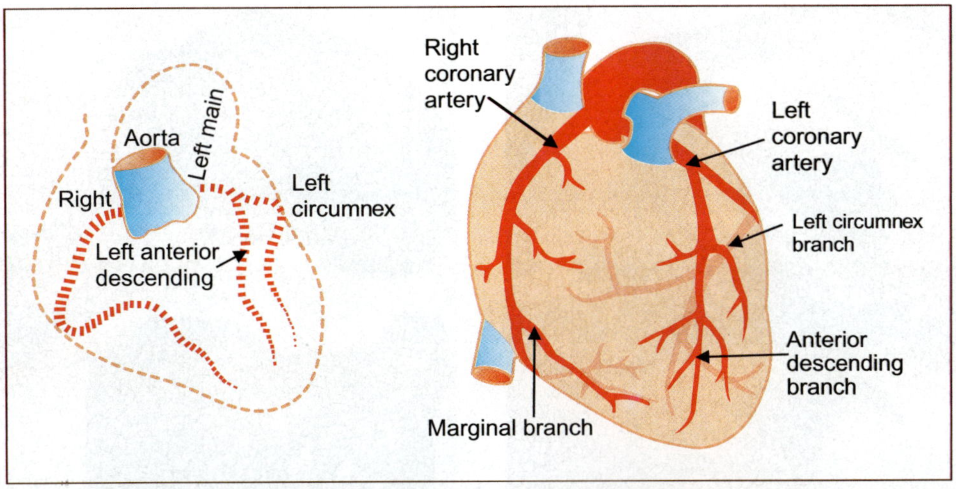

Figure 11.2: Blood supply of heart

whereas right and left ventricular walls are 3-5 mm and 10-15 mm thick respectively.

Blood supply of heart: (i) ***The left coronary artery*** arises from the left aortic sinus and the main trunk after a short course of 1 cm or less is divided into (Figure 11.2): (a) *Left interventricular (Anterior descending) branch:* This courses down the interventricular septum to reach the apex of the heart and supplies anterior aspects of right and left ventricles and the anterior 2/3rds of I.V. septum at the apex of the heart. (b) *Left circumflex branch:* It follows left A-V sulcus to reach to back of heart. It supplies small portion of the lateral aspect of left ventricle extending slightly anteriorly and posteriorly. (ii) ***The right coronary artery*** arises from right aortic sinus, passes behind the pulmonary trunk and follows the right A-V sulcus: (a) *Right marginal branch:* This branch is given off at the right border of heart and supplies the remaining anterior surface of right ventricle and posterior third of interventricular septum. (b) *Posterior descending (interventricular) branch:* The main part of right coronary artery continues at the back of the heart as posterior descending branch.

Congenital anomalies of coronary artery: Minor anomalies that usually involves the proximal coronary artery but the distal blood flow is normal (i) "High take off" when the location of the coronary ostia is 1 cm above the level of cusp margin (ii) Multiple coronary ostia (iii) Separate ostium in the right coronary sinus (iv) Third coronary artery arises from the non-coronary sinus.

Frequency of site of fatal coronary stenosis with or without thrombosis: Coronary stenosis with or without thrombosis commonly involves first 2 cm of the origin of the vessel (Figures 11.3, 11.4 and 11.5). The incidence of involvement of the branches is: (i) Left anterior descending artery also called Anterior interventricular artery 45-64%) (ii) Right main coronary (24-46%) (iii) Left circumflex (3-10%) (iv) Left main coronary (0-10%) (v) Right marginal and posterior interventricular branches are particularly immune.

Coronary atherosclerosis: Coronary atheroma may be focal, with irregular plaques. Every part of the major vessels must be examined at autopsy, with transverse cuts at no more than 3 mm intervals since few and localized atheromas may be present.

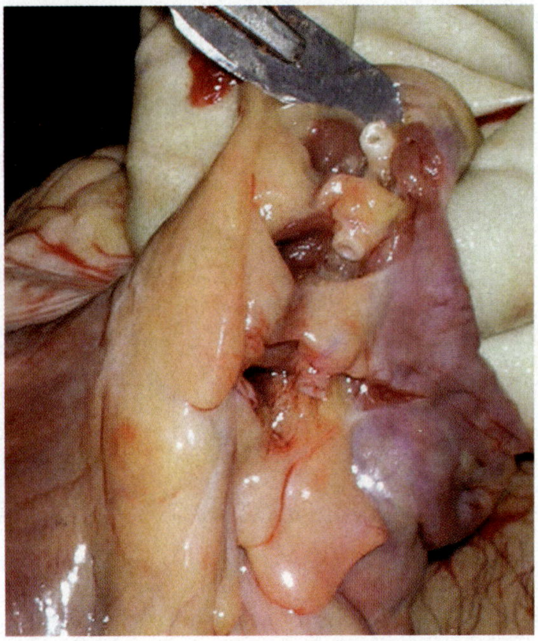

Figure 11.3: Coronary artery showing 75% blockage

Types of coronary occlusion: (i) *Simple atheroma:* Plaques are often eccentric with a central pin hole leaving a crescentic or concentric residual lumen. (ii) *Ulcerative atheroma:* This results due to breaking down of endothelium over atheromatous plaques. This is conductive to thrombus formation. (iii) *Subintimal haemorrhage:* Sudden haemorrhage resulting from rupture of tiny vessels in the wall of a coronary artery. The hematoma thus formed forces the plaque inwards to further narrow or occlude the vessel lumina. (iv) *Coronary thrombosis:* This occurs on an already stenosed plaque of atheroma with damaged endothelium. (v) *Periarteritis nodosa:* This is pan inflammatory disease of arteries of unknown etiology that affects males around fourth decade involving mainly muscular arteries of heart and kidneys.

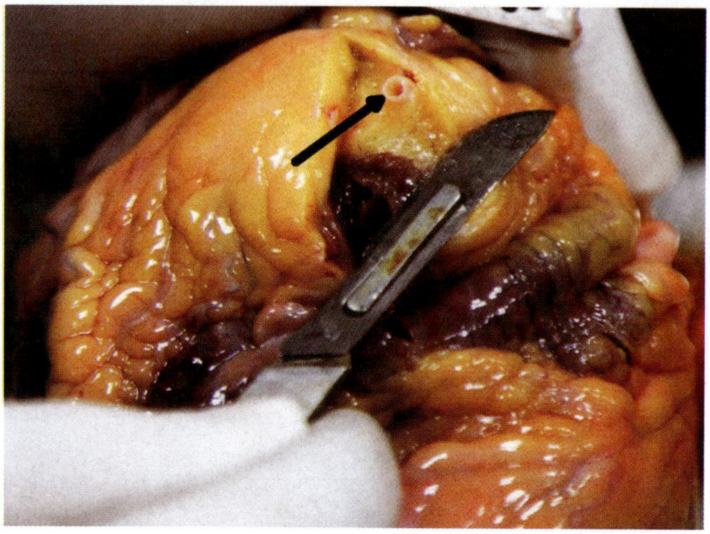

Figure 11.4: Dissection of coronary artery showing 100% patent

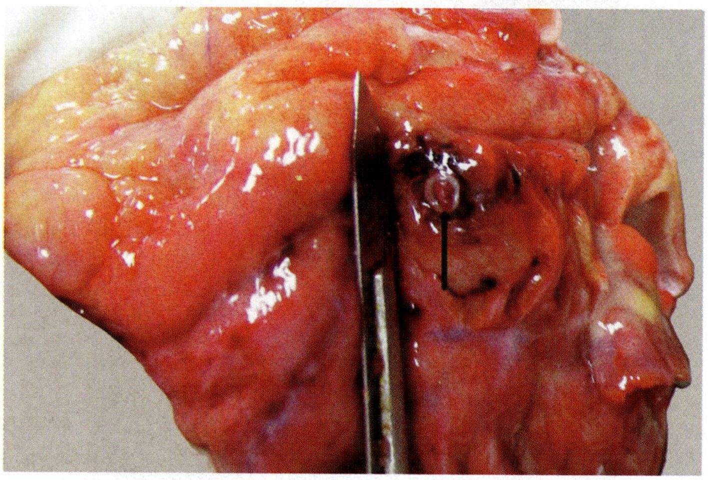

Figure 11.5: 100% Blockage of coronary artery by thrombous

Sequelae of coronary occlusion: (i) *Sudden death:* May occur at the time of occlusion or subsequently as a result of ventricular fibrillation due to damage to nodal tissue or conducting system or any other complication. (ii) *Myocardial infarction:* Myocardial infarction occurs in the myocardium distal to a complete occlusion of coronary artery in the absence of an adequate collateral circulation. (iii) *Rupture of the myocardium:* The rupture of myocardium occurs in people over the age of 60 years. It usually occurs on the 2nd or 3rd day after infarction because at this time muscle wall is soft and necrotic. The cardiac rupture results in haemopericardium leading to **cardiac tamponade** and death (Figure 11.6). The rupture almost always involves left ventricular wall. (iv) *Myocardial fibrosis:* Localized patches result from healed myocardial infarcts and are seen in areas of predilection of infarcts like distal interventricular septum, apex and the posterior wall. Diffuse fibrosis may arise from many causes like healed rheumatic carditis and are also seen in cases of long standing coronary stenosis, which are sufficient to produce

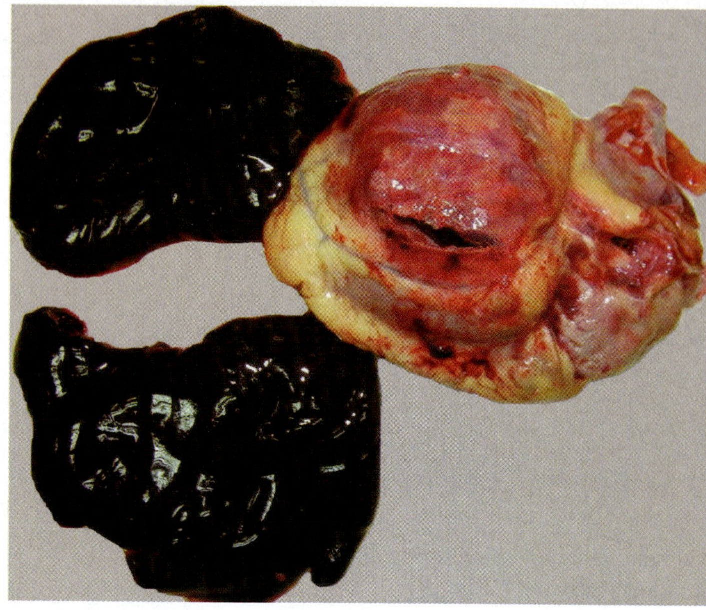

Figure 11.6: Cardiac tamponade with rupture of left ventricular wall

focal infarcts. The fibrotic patches are also seen in hypertensive heart disease or hypertrophy due to aortic incompetence (v) *Aneurysms:* Aneurysm of the left ventricle may occur if a large full thickness plaque of fibrosis becomes stretched. Rupture of aneurysm is rare (vi) *Mural thrombosis:* Thrombosis very often develops over an infarct, which reaches the endocardial surface of ventricle due to adhesion of platelets and fibrin deposition. Thrombus always poses danger of emboli (viii) *Pericariditis:* Occurs in transmural infarcts involving epicardium. Ischemic heart disease is the most common cause of pericarditis.

Myocardial Infarction

An infarct is a localized area of ischemic necrosis in an organ or tissue resulting from sudden reduction of the arterial supply or occasionally venous drainage. Myocardial infarction occurs with factors predisposing to atherosclerosis like hypertension, cigarette smoking, diabetes mellitus and familial hypercholesterolemia.

Pathogenesis of myocardial infarction: Myocardial infarction will occur in myocardium distal to complete occlusion of a coronary artery in the absence of an adequate collateral circulation. These are of the following types: (i) ***Subendocardial infarction*** involves layers of muscle adjacent to lumen of infarction. (ii) ***Intramural infarction:*** It is less common and is usually seen as satellite areas to a more extensive infarct. (iii) ***Transmural or full thickness infarction:*** It is of large extent and gives rise to both mural thrombi and pericarditis, and involves most commonly lower part of I.V. septum, apex and posterior wall of left ventricle. All transmural or full thickness infarcts involve: (a) Left ventricle with I/V septum (67-80%) (b) Right and left ventricular wall (15-30%) (c) Isolated right ventricle (1-3%) (d) Isolated left atrial (rarest of all). (iv) ***Papillary muscle infarction:***

Involvement of papillary muscle of left ventricle are common especially posterior muscles which are susceptible to ischemia.

Postmortem demonstration of M.I.: The autopsy demonstration of an early myocardial infarct has profound medicolegal implication. The age of an infarct is difficult to establish as the onset of clinical symptoms however dramatic, are often much later than the onset of the pathological lesion precipitated by a coronary occlusion.

Gross appearances: It is generally impossible to detect MI by naked eye examination within the first 8 hours after coronary occlusion and in many cases, little or no change may be apparent up to 18 hours.

On autopsy, the infarcted area of the heart on cut section looks granular and dull instead of normal moist luster when cut by sharp knife. The infarcted area shows following features: (i) ***Oedema:*** There is swelling of infarcted area and coarsely fibrillar appearance of ventricle on cutting. The muscles seem separated with a grayish opaque sheen. (ii) ***Colour:*** The colour of infarct is more pale than normal with a grayish opaque sheen. This changes to brownish purple darkening to reddish bluish yellow after 24-48 hours of occlusion. (iii) ***Tigroid appearance:*** The tigroid appearance that is alternate bands of red and pale areas is seen after 24 hours. (iv) ***Fully developed infarct:*** A fully developed infarct is yellowish with reddish marginal zones of hyperemia and is gelatinous than fibrous.

Histological methods: This conventional method is very much helpful for the detection of early myocardial infarction. However, the main disadvantage is the time required for the preparation.

Haemotoxylin and eosin staining: The paraffin embedded sections are stained with haemotoxylin and eosin and the following features are noted under microscope: (i) ***Eosinophilia:*** It is one of the most important features in the early stages not less than 6 hours of infarction. The cells are reddened and most of the cells are eosinophilic in nature along with the swelling as well as increased granularity at the same time. Eosinophilia is easily seen by the application of green filter. (ii) ***Swelling of the muscle fibres:*** The intercellular spaces are reduced due to oedema of the cells. It may occur in the large masses and at times it may be patchy in nature. It is usually associated with some degree of increased eosinophilia. (iii) ***Granularity of cytoplasm:*** This may be found easily in both transverse and longitudinal sections of muscle fibres known as cloudy swelling. At times it is a reversible phenomena. (iv) ***Corrugation:*** Dead muscle fibres may be corrugated and they may be sharply angulated in the areas where there is severe bending of the fibres. (v) ***Granularity of the cell membrane:*** Granularity occurs at an early stage before the cells begin to disintegrate as a result of necrosis. Granularity is also seen as artefact in frozen sections but when found in paraffin sections it has got some significance unless there is advanced putrefaction. (vi) ***Increase in interstitial cells:*** Increase in numbers of cells occur quite early but may also appear late. Sometimes it does not appear at all. The increase is due to wandering macrophages and the cells which cannot be distinguished from fibroblast. Polymorphs never appear in an infarction before 24 hours.

The above findings of early infarction goes on increasing as the time passes. There is increase in the necrosis of the cells with disintegration, heavy polymorph infiltration, filling of the interspaces with basophilic nuclear debris and marked vascular congestion and dilatation.

Periodic Acid-Schiff stain technique: The main purpose of this technique is to detect glycogen. It **stains the necrotic myocardium purplish pink.** The substance responsible is diastase-resistant and by histochemical analysis has been shown to be either a muco or glyco protein. It does not appear until 12 hours of onset of infarction. Thus, it has very little value for the diagnosis.

Phosphotungstic Acid-Haematoxylin technique: The above technique does not allow to detect the myocardial infarction earlier then the stains by haemotoxylin and eosin but it can demonstrate the cell death in a more clear way. The characteristic lesion is a breakup of the muscles striations, starting with a "sandy" appearance that progresses to a bizarre clumping and aggregation of the muscle. This technique is superior to haematoxylin or eosin as the infarcted areas appear in a better way.

Macroenzyme techniques: During infarction, the metabolic changes in the cells occur before any morphological changes are demonstrable. One of these changes is loss of enzymes from the cells as a result the damaged fibres are enzymatically less active. The main enzyme **dehydrogenases** may be visualized by tracing their action in a suitable substrate by means of a colour indicator.

The methods like tellurite reduction by Malic Acid Dehydrogenase and Nitro-BT method are found to be unsatisfactory because of the technical unreliability and the expense of reagent but the TTC method is of considerable practical use.

Triphenyl Tetrazolium Chloride (TTC): Transverse slices of ventricles about 5 mm thick are cut with a knife during postmortem and incubated for one hour in the staining solution of 1% Triphenyl tetrazolium chloride in a phosphate buffer at pH 8. The maintenance of this pH is very important. If the solution is on the acid side of the neutrality, no deposition of the dye will form. Moreover, if the pH rises above 8.5 the reaction will be too rapid and formazan will be deposited over the whole surface of the heart slice. Normal heart muscle with active dehydrogenases acts on the TTC to produce a **bright red formazan** compound. After the reaction has been developed with 30 minutes, the slice may be fixed in formalin which retains its colors for several weeks when kept in the dark. The real contrast appears after proper fixation. The slice so obtained may be used as the direct evidence of infarction. The technique may be very simple but needs careful supervision with occasional agitation of the solution while incubating. Postmortem interval upto two days appears to have no deleterious effect on the reaction but the slices should not be exposed to the atmosphere before incubation.

Appearance of MI with Time

In a myocardial infarct that is less than 4 hours old, no change is seen. After this period following findings are discerned:

MI < 6-12 hours old: (i) Unapparent on gross examination (ii) Oedema (iii) Slight pallor (iv) Eosinophilia within 4-6 hours; intense sarcoplasmic eosinophilia, nuclear pyknosis with contraction bands (v) Slight mottling with areas of dark discolouration (vi) Within 3-6 hours, histochemical techniques highlight necrotic area (vii) Increased cellularity (macrophages and lymphocytes) within 12 hours.

MI > 18-24 hours old: (i) Mottled and midly oedematous with bulging out surface (ii) Eosinophilia with red line on gross examination (iii) Sarcoplasmic eosinophilia with early interstitial oedema and neutrophilic infiltrate (iv) Interfibrillar oedema deepens and cellular oedema subsides as time passes (v) Better demarcated pallor lesion (vi) Tigroid appearance.

MI 36 hours to 2-4 days: (i) Soft yellow-tan core with mottled border (ii) Maximum neutorphilic infiltrate, nuclear loss and sarcoplasmic coagulation (iii) Nuclei are hollow with marked polymorphic activity in 4 days.

MI by 1st week: (i) Yellow-tan core and irregular hyperemic red-brown border (ii) Basophilic interstitial debris, early macrophage infiltration, dilated capillaries at border (iii) Disintegrated muscle fibres with fibroblast formation.

MI by 2nd week: (i) Yellow gray core and red gray border depressed cut surface (ii) Numerous macrophages with active phagocytosis, pigmented macrophages filled with lypofuscin (iii) Granulation tissue along border, ongoing phagocytosis at core.

MI by 3rd week: (i) Core becoming smaller, border becoming larger, grayer, firmer and less gelatinous, less depressed cut surface (ii) Ongoing scar formation dense at outer border dilated peripheral blood vessels, central core of necrotic tissue (iii) Removal of dead cells is complete (iv) Collagen formation starts.

MI by 4-6 weeks: (i) Marked collagen formation.

MI of > one month: (i) Firm gray-white or red-gray scar, with scar retraction, variable wall thinning (ii) Mature scar (dense collagen, focal elastin and hypercellularity) focal lymphocyte (Table 11.1).

Myocardial infarction with normal coronary arteries (MINCA) is common with a prevalence of 1% to 12% of all myocardial infarctions. Etiological factors for MINCA may include prolonged coronary spasm, coronary thrombosis with spontaneous lysis, cocaine abuse, viral myocarditis, aortic dissection, hypercoagulable states, autoimmune vasculitis, and carbon monoxide poisoning. The pathogenic mechanisms of MINCA are still unknown, but endothelial dysfunction has been suggested as a possible cause.

Coronary artery spasm (CAS) can happen both in normal as well as diseased arteries and plays an important role in pathogenesis ischemic heart disease resulting in sudden death. Autopsy in sudden death consequent to normal CAS does not reveal any infarct in myocardium or blockage in the coronary artery. Smoking is an important risk factor for development of CAS. It is mostly a disease of middle- and older-aged men and post-menopausal women. It is significantly associated with polymorphism of genes that have an antioxidant effect.

Lesions Involving Myocardium

(i) *Hypertrophy of myocardium:* Hypertrophy of myocardium (Figure 11.7) may be associated with coronary ischemia. It can occur with hypertension, valvular disease, shunts and long standing pulmonary disease. Depending on the underlying cause either one or both the sides of the heart may be hypertrophied. It

Table 11.1: Gross and light microscopical findings in a myocardial infarct

Age	Gross microscopy	Light microscopy
< 4 hours	No change	No change
4-12 hours	Slight mottling with areas of dark discolouration	Intense sarcoplasmic eosinophilia, nuclear pyknosis with contraction bands
12-24 hours	Mottled and mildly oedematous and bulging out surface	Sarcoplasmic eosinophila with early interstitial oedema and neutrophilic infiltrate
2-4 days	Soft yellow-tan core with mottled border	Maximum neutrophilic infiltrate, nuclear loss and sarcoplasmic coagulation
5-7 days	Yellow-tan core and irregular hyperemic red-brown border	Basophilic interstitial debris, early macrophage infiltration, dilated capillaries at border
8-10 days	Yellow gray core and red brown border, depressed cut surface	Numerous macrophages with active phagocytosis, pigmented macrophages filled with lypofuscin
11-14 days	Yellow gray core and red gray border, depressed cut surface	Granulation tissue along border, ongoing phagocytosis at core
2-4 weeks	Core becoming smaller, border becoming larger, grayer, firmer and less gelatinous, less depressed cut surface	Ongoing scar formation dense at outer border dilated peripheral blood vessels, central core of necrotic tissue
> 1 month	Firm gray-white or red-gray scar, with scar retraction, variable wall thinning	Mature scar (dense collagen, focal elastin and hypercellularity) focal lymphocyte

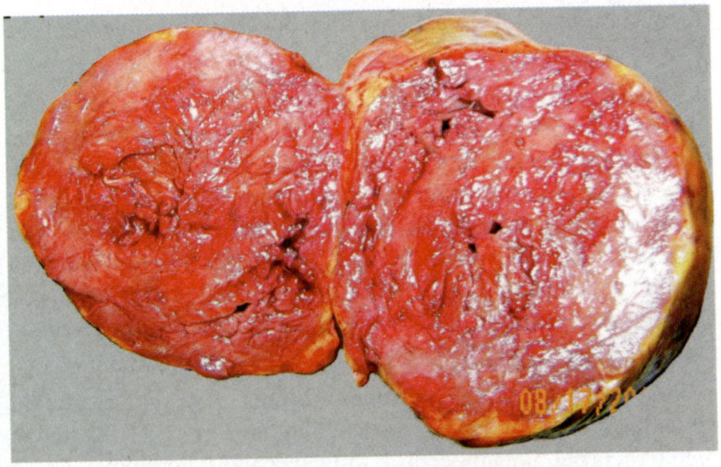

Figure 11.7: Hypertrophy of myocardium

may be familial or sporadic. Interventricular septum is enlarged and bulges into both the ventricles producing a ridge beneath the aortic valve. Sudden death is common in the familial variety. (ii) *Neoplasm:* Primary neoplasm such as rhabdomyoma are occasionally encountered. Secondary neoplasms are very rare. (iii) *Myocarditis:* Myocarditis is inflammation of the heart muscle evidenced by exudative and proliferative cellular reaction. Acute purulent myocarditis can occur as a complication of septicemia and myocardial abscesses may be produced. This is seen sometimes in deaths following severe burns with supervening infection with *Pseudomonas aeruginosa.* A pyogenic myocardial abscess as a cause of sudden unexpected death is quite unusual. (iv) *Alcoholic cardiomyopathy:* Alcoholic cardiomyopathy may result from direct toxic effect on the myocardium, general nutritional deficiencies including vitamin deficiencies and Beri Beri heart disease. The toxic alcoholic cardiomyopathy is the most common. In alcoholic toxic cardiomyopathy, the heart is overweight with hypertrophy of both ventricles. Coronary arteries are free from atheroma. On microscopic examination left ventricular wall shows scattered fibrosis. (v) *Miscellaneous conditions:* Cardiac arrest may occur with no organic disease of the heart apparent at the autopsy. A careful examination of deceased and family history can provide an evidence of preexisting disease or abnormality. A variety of minor and scarcely detectable insults to the myocardium can cause faults in the normal transmission of the heart and can cause sudden death. Sudden death can also sometimes occur in patients without any gross or microscopic abnormality of the heart who have a history of paroxysmal or sustained arrhythmia. Also, in an apparently healthy young individual overexertion can cause sudden death but preexisting cardiac conditions should be excluded for the diagnosis. (vi) Primary neurogenic shock or reflex vagal inhibition can cause cardiac arrest in the absence of any demonstrable cardiac lesion.

Lesions Involving Pericardium

Obliterated pericarditis following acute inflammatory changes can occur. Fibrinous pericarditis with blood stained fluid may result from infarction, rheumatic heart disease or uremia. These secondary effects may cause death.

Lesions Involving Endocardium

Fibroelastosis is commonly found as congenital abnormality causing death in infancy. The secondary form is associated with other congenital heart diseases. In the primary form the endocardium is thick and the changes are more diffuse. Death occurs from heart failure in first week of life in about 1/4th of the infants. Subendocardial haemorrhages are seen in cases of obstetric shock, arsenic poisoning, head injury and from infected blood transfusion. There may be severe drop in blood pressure accompanied by severe blood lesions.

Valvular lesions: Congenital valvular lesions are most commonly associated with fusion of aortic or pulmonary cusps. This may be a site of valvulitis or calcification. Valvular disease may be accompanied by long-standing medical history. Mitral valve disease can be present undetected in life. It may be associated with ball valve thrombus in left auricle and some emboli may be found in kidney or spleen.

Respiratory System

Sudden death due to respiratory tract disease in a healthy individual is rare. The main cause is hemoptysis in such cases. Death mainly results from haemorrhage or from inhalation of blood into the lungs. Haemorrhages may result from neoplasm or inflammatory lesions of the nasopharynx, carcinoma of bronchus or esophagus infiltrating adjacent tissues. Inflammatory lesions such as tuberculous cavitation, lung abscess or bronchiectasis are less common causes. An aortic aneurysm may rupture into bronchus or esophagus. Spontaneous pneumothorax rarely causes death. It most commonly results from rupture of an emphysematous bulla. Respiratory tract infections may also result in sudden and unexpected death. However, usually there is a period of some hours or a day or two preceding death. Death may result in respiratory tract infection from hypoxia due to mechanical obstruction of air passage by pus in bronchopneumonia or acute purulent bronchitis superimposed upon chronic bronchitis. Acute respiratory obstruction of the larynx may be due to local neoplasm but may occur due to angioneurotic oedema or inflammation arising locally.

Central Nervous System

Subarachnoid haemorrhage: Sudden and unexpected death due to diseases of central nervous system result from subarachnoid or intracerebral haemorrhage. Subarachnoid haemorrhage may be due to rupture of **Berry aneurysm** usually located on the **Circle of Willis** and sometimes on other cerebral arteries. These aneurysms are most commonly developmental resulting from congenital weakness of the vessel wall. Rupture of the vessel may be the result of atheromatous degeneration. Mycotic cerebral arterial aneurysm is due to damaged vessel wall by infected emboli as may arise in bacterial endocarditis. Subarachnoid haemorrhage may produce sudden collapse and rapid death. A transient rise in blood pressure for some relatively minor injury might contribute by causing damage in the already damaged tissue and by initiating the first split in the arterial wall resulting sometimes later in rupture. At autopsy, there is a massive collection of blood at the base of brain that is why it is difficult to locate the aneurysm. Multiple aneurysms may be present but are uncommon.

Intracerebral haemorrhage: Intracerebral haemorrhage may be located in either internal capsule or in brain substance, in cerebellum or pons. It is commonly seen in capsular region and rarely immediately fatal. Death may occur after a few hours or the patient may partially recover and may later on collapse due to rupture into lateral ventricle. Sometimes intracerebral haemorrhage in capsular region resulting from cerebral artery aneurysm bursts and tears through the cerebral tissue and floods the subarachnoid tissue in the base of brain.

Pontine haemorrhages: Primary pontine haemorrhages are usually single and involve hypothalamus. Secondary pontine haemorrhages may be associated with head injury and are of considerable medicolegal importance.

Cerebral thrombosis and embolism: Cerebral thrombosis and embolism may cause loss of consciousness and paresis. In cerebral embolism it is sudden and source of embolus is usually the left auricle in cases of auricular fibrillation, mitral stenosis, a valve or a mural thrombus. The embolus can originate from varying sites and the position of lesions are those supplied by cerebral arteries, basilar arteries and rarely carotid arteries.

Spinal cord haemorrhages: Spinal cord haemorrhages are uncommon and may be missed if spinal cord is not routinely examined.

Cerebral tumours: Cerebral tumours are incidental findings in small number of medicolegal autopsies. Mengiomata are the most common cerebral tumours. Rarely sudden death can occur from haemorrhage into neoplasm. The common tumour to cause haemorrhage is glioblastoma. Vascular tumours like haemangiomata may rarely bleed. Tumours themselves except meningiomata are not traumatic in origin.

Epilepsy: Sudden death in epilepsy is common. The causes of death are direct and indirect effects of seizures, epilepsy, and antiseizure therapies. Seizure related deaths include those in status epilepticus and deaths in the setting of a single seizure. Sudden death can also occur in an epileptic seizure frequently in status epilepticus from heart failure due to myocardial ischemia. Examination of brain may fail to reveal any lesion in idiopathic epilepsy. However, some evidence may be obtained from bite marks on the tongue and from the clothing for evidence of incontinence of urine and faeces. Organic diseases may precipitate epilepsy and evidence of cerebral tumors and cysticercosis should be looked for. Causes of death secondary to a seizure include trauma or drowning, severe aspiration or obstruction due to a food bolus.

Sudden unexpected death of epilepsy (SUDEP) is defined as "sudden unexpected witnessed or unwitnessed, non-traumatic and non-drowning death in a patient with epilepsy, with or without evidence for a seizure and excluding documented status epilepticus where necropsy examination does not reveal a toxicological or an anatomical cause for death (Nashef, 1997). It is a severe outcome of epilepsy and common cause of death in patients with epilepsy with incidence ranges from 0.09 to 9.3 per 1000 person-years.

Other causes in brain: Sudden death is rarely of infective origin when occasionally cerebral abscess may rupture. Rapid death has been associated with meningitis (Figure 11.8) that is meningococcal, pneumococcal, influenza and tuberculous. Acute poliomyelitis and encephalitis may be fulminant, specially when brainstem is involved. Sudden death within hours of onset of symptoms may occur in malaria. Postmortem diagnosis depends on demonstration of malarial pigment in brain, spleen, liver and kidney. The pigment must be distinguished from formalin pigment in tissues fixed for days or longer. Sudden death can also result from trypanosomiasis in which postmortem diagnosis is difficult as organisms are difficult to find in tissues. Nevertheless, the inflammation of brain and meninges with perivascular inflammatory reaction and large histiocytic cells (morula cells) are prominent.

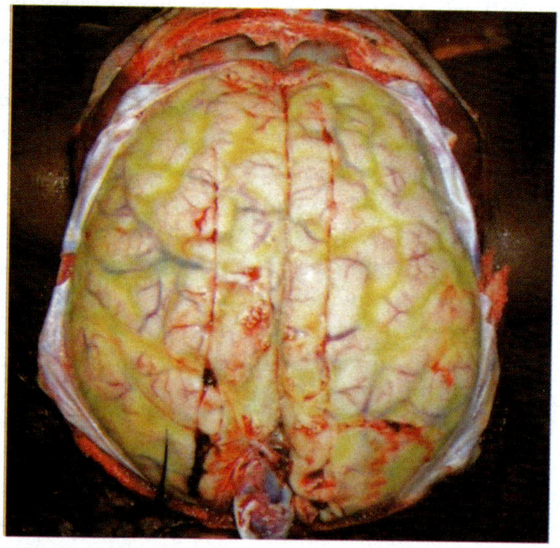

Figure 11.8: Cerebral meningitis

Alimentary System

The causes involving the gastrointestinal system that can result in sudden death are: (i) Haemorrhage into gastrointestinal tract resulting from peptic ulcer, oesophageal varices (ii) Perforation of ulcers such as peptic or typhoid (iii) Strangulated hernia (iv) Rupture of liver abscess (Figure 11.9) (v) Rupture of enlarged spleen as in malaria (vi) Intestinal obstruction (vii) Twisting of the intestinal loops (Figure 11.10).

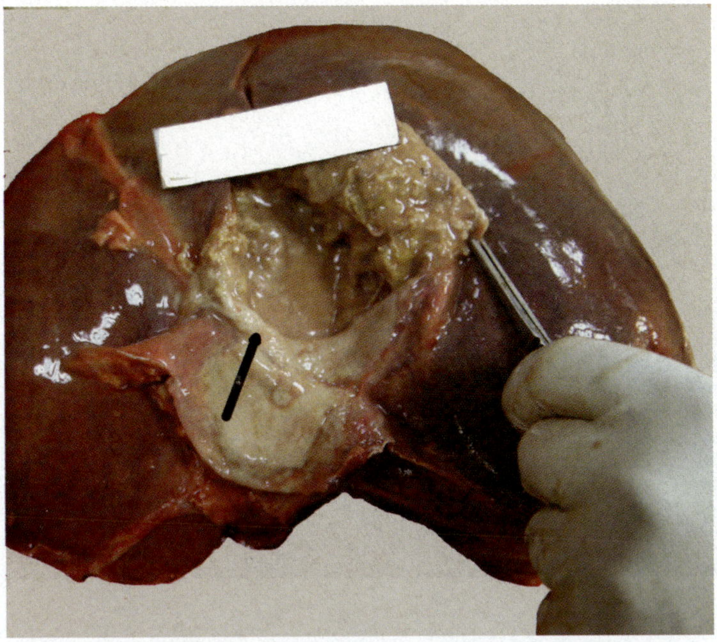

Figure 11.9: Ruptured liver abscess

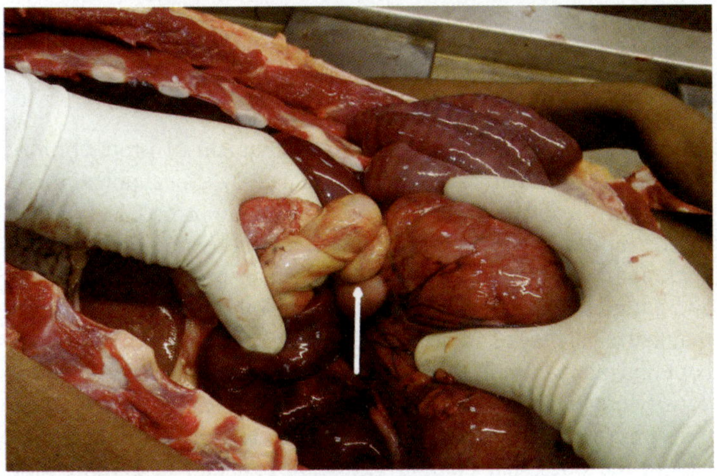

Figure 11.10: Twisted intestinal loop in volvulus

Genitourinary System

The conditions involving genitourinary system that can be the cause of sudden death are: (i) Chronic nephritis (ii) Nephrolithiasis (iii) Carcinoma of kidney and urinary bladder (iv) Uterine haemorrhages (v) Carcinoma of female genital tract eroding femoral vessels (vi) Twisting of ovary, ovarian cyst or fibroid tumours.

Miscellaneous

Many other conditions can be the cause of sudden and unexpected death such as: (i) Diabetes mellitus (ii) Cerebral malaria (iii) Vagal inhibition (iv) Drug anaphylaxis (v) Shock due to emotional excitement (vi) Mismatched blood transfusions. In these conditions, at autopsy it is difficult to ascertain the cause as the findings are non-specific such as congestion of organs and signs of hypersensitivity reactions.

LONG QUESTIONS

1. Define sudden death. Discuss in detail the causes of sudden death due to cardiovascular disease.
2. Describe the anatomy of heart and the diseases of heart that cause sudden death.
3. Describe in detail the disorders of central nervous system that cause sudden death.
4. Describe anatomy Circle of Willis and its role in sudden death.

MULTIPLE CHOICE QUESTIONS

1. **Myocardial rupture after myocardial infarction usually occurs:**
   (a) Immediately (b) On first day
   (c) 2nd or 3rd day (d) 4th and 5th day
2. **The microscopic features by histochemical techniques of myocardial infarction within 3-6 hours of attack is:**
   (a) No change (b) Loss of striation
   (c) Necrosis (d) Eosinophilia
3. **The colour of the normal heart muscle stained by Triphenyl Tetrazolium Chloride (TTC) in case of myocardial infarction death is:**
   (a) Bright red (b) Blue
   (c) Dark brown (d) Reddish blue
4. **The most common coronary artery involved in fatal stenosis is:**
   (a) Left anterior descending artery
   (b) Right main coronary artery
   (c) Left main coronary artery
   (d) Left circumflex artery
5. **The most common cause of sudden cardiac death is:**
   (a) Coronary artery disease
   (b) Cardiomyopathy
   (c) Congenital heart diseases
   (d) Trauma

ANSWER KEY ☞

1. (c)	2. (c)	3. (a)	4. (a)	5. (a)

12 CHAPTER

Mechanical Injuries

A wound is a break in natural continuity of any of the tissues of the living body. The question of examination of wounds arises in the Court of law. Mechanical injuries are the injuries that are caused to the body by physical violence.

Classification of Injuries

1. **Mechanical Injuries:** (i) *Those produced by blunt weapon*: (a) Contusion (b) Abrasion (c) Laceration (ii) *Those produced by sharp weapon*: (a) Incised wound (b) Stab wound (iii) Firearm wounds (iv) Fractures.
2. **Thermal Injuries:** (A) *Produced due to cold*: (i) Local hypothermia (a) Frost bite (b) Trench foot (c) Immersion foot (ii) General hypothermia (B) *Produced by heat* (i) *By local application of heat*: (a) Burns (b) Scalds (ii) *By general application of heat:* (a) Heat Hyperpyrexia (heat stroke) (b) Heat Exhaustion (c) Heat cramps.
3. **Chemical Injuries:** *Produced by:* (i) Corrosives (acids and alkalis) (ii) Irritants (weak acids and alkalis).
4. **Injuries:** *Due to:* (i) Electricity (ii) Lightning (iii) X-rays (iv) Radioactive substances.
5. **Legally:** (i) Simple injury (ii) Grievous hurt.
6. **Depending on Manner of Death:** *These are:* (i) Suicidal (ii) Homicidal (iii) Accidental.
7. **Wounds:** *These can be:* (i) Defence wounds (ii) Fabricated wounds.
8. **Wounds in Relation to Death:** *These may be:* (i) Antemortem (ii) Postmortem.

Mechanism of Wound Production

Moritz has described in detail the mechanism of production of wound. According to him, wound is caused by a mechanical force, which may be either: (i) *Moving weapon* (counterforce is provided by the inertia of the body) or (ii) *Moving body* (rigidity of some stationary object). Due to impact between the propelling force and counterforce, energy is transferred to the tissues of the body that causes a change in their state of rest or motion. Human body contains many complex tissues such as solidity, fluidity, elasticity, density etc. that vary in their physical properties. Therefore, there is no uniform change or effect on the body. All the body tissues except the ones that contain gases are resistant to compression forces. Mechanical force does not cause compression of the tissues but causes their displacement and deformation with the result that traction strains are produced in the affected tissues. Such strains may usually be due to forces causing simple elongation of the tissues. In addition, they may be due to other mechanisms such as bending, torsion or shearing that are more complex.

Shear Strain: Shear strain is a strain, which is produced in a body by the forceful alteration of its shape but not volume. It causes stretch in direction parallel to the plane of contact. When tenacity of an organ exceeds, it ruptures and the bones fractures.

Factors Influencing Nature and Extent of Wounds

1. **Nature of the Objects/Instruments:**
   i. ***Blow from pin pointed/sharp edged weapon:*** The force is concentrated over limited area resulting in incision or

deep penetration. The hardness and friction of divided tissues resist passage of the instrument.

ii. ***Blow from blunt objects:*** The force is dissipated over relatively large area so the damage caused to a unit of mass is less than when force is applied over a small area. A rapid transfer of energy over this small area is more likely to produce a wound than an equal amount over large area. The rapid transfer of energy is fatal than the slow transfer.

2. **Amount of energy discharged:** Kinetic energy is measured in a moving object by: $KE = ½ mv^2$, where m = mass and v = velocity.

   An object with definite velocity and definite weight have a definite amount of energy. When the mass doubles, kinetic energy is also doubled. However, when velocity is doubled kinetic energy increases four times. This indicates that the velocity has far more influence on the energy compared to the mass of the object.

3. **Conditions under which energy is discharged:** Moving objects have energy due to their movement that is directly proportional to their mass and to the square of their velocity as explained above. When moving objects are stopped suddenly on an encounter with some stationary object, the energy is dissipated at the sites of resistance, which causes various types of injuries like abrasion, contusion, laceration or incised wounds. On the other hand, if the human body is moving and encounters a stationary object, similar injuries are produced.

4. **Nature of the tissue affected:** The tissue that encounters the resistance suffers damage depending on its type as well as nature. Bones being tough undergo fractures on infliction of injury while muscles develop hemorrhages due to rupture of blood vessels in them. Soft tissues also tend to have hemorrhages or may rupture on infliction of severe force especially in cases of large organs like liver. Even, mesenteries get torn by blunt injury to the abdomen.

BLUNT FORCE INJURIES

Contusion/Bruise (Figures 12.1 to 12.4)

Contusions are collection of blood into the tissues due to rupture of blood vessels, caused by blunt trauma. It can be caused in the skin or inner organs like liver, lung, brain, kidney etc. (Figure 12.4). It is a painful swelling and is caused by crushing or tearing of subcutaneous tissue. There is no destruction of external surface in a contusion. Due to rupture of blood vessels, blood extravasates into subcutaneous tissues and the margins are blurred. The size of a bruise varies from small pinhead sized to large collection of blood in the subcutaneous tissues. The more the force is used to inflict the injury, the more is the collection of blood and the bigger is the size of the resulting bruise.

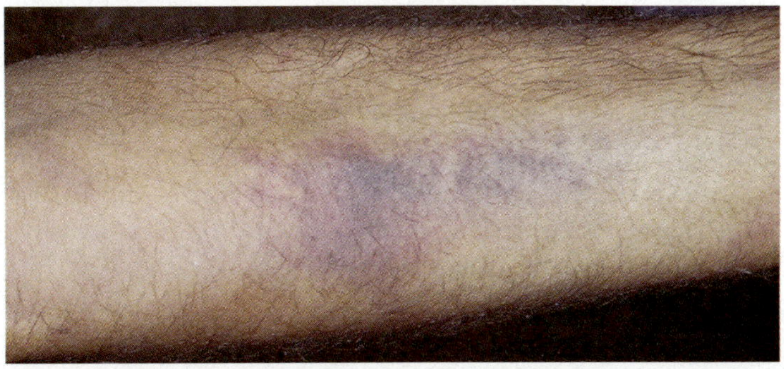

Figure 12.1: Bluish bruise over the front of forearm

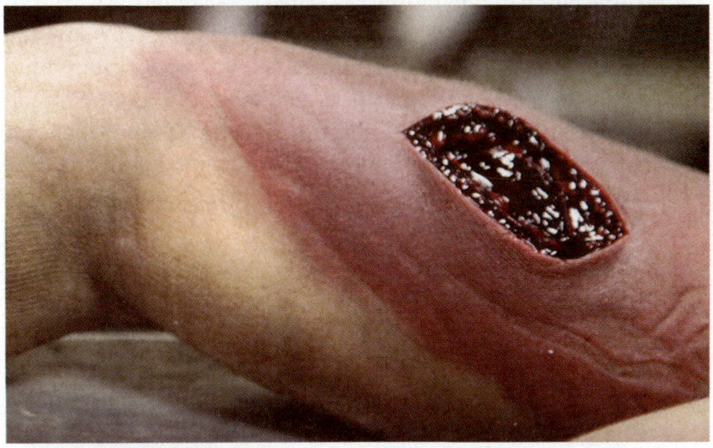

Figure 12.2: Bruise over the arm seen after incising

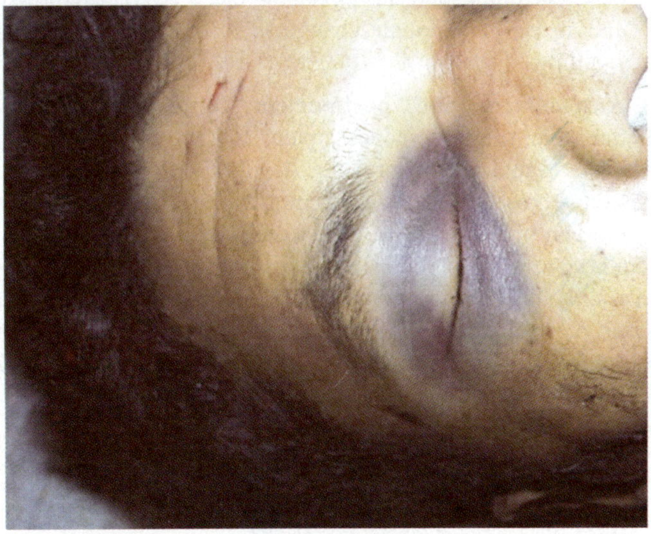

Figure 12.3: Black eye (bluish black bruising)

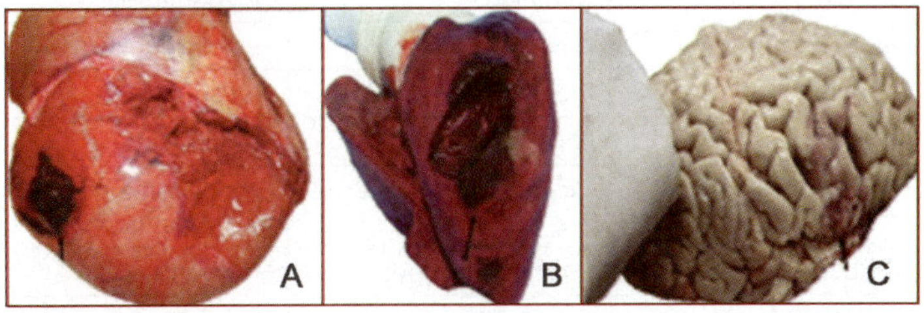

Figure 12.4: Bruises over the (A) Liver (B) Lung and (C) Brain

Factors Modifying Size and Shape of Bruise

1. **Condition and type of tissues:** The softer the tissues, more easily they are likely to bruise.
2. **Age:** The persons who are old aged tend to bruise easily because of the loss of flesh and the age related cardiovascular changes in them. The children having a softer skin and delicate tissues also get easily bruised.
3. **Sex:** Women bruise more easily because of the delicate tissues and more of subcutaneous fat.
4. **Colour of skin:** Bruising is easily visible in fair skinned people compared to the dark skinned ones though the bruised area can be felt with palpation. In an embalmed body, the bruise becomes more prominent as the embalming fluid makes the skin lighter in colour and more of blood is forced into the damaged tissues and the embalming fluid makes a dark pigment complex. Photographs are quite helpful as they can highlight even those contusions, which are not clearly visible to the naked eye.
5. **Natural disease:** The appearance of a bruise varies with the various natural diseases such as: (i) Arteriosclerosis (Bruising may occur very easily even from slight coughing or exercising). (ii) Whooping cough (In children whooping cough causes violent bouts of cough, which may cause bruising without any direct external injury). (iii) Conditions such as purpura, leukaemia, hemophilia, Vitamin C and K deficiency, phosphorous poisoning etc. lead to easy bruising and in purpura colour change is discernible without any swelling.

Antemortem and postmortem contusions: Signs of inflammation such as redness, pain, loss of function are the hallmark of antemortem bruising and in addition, extravasation of blood is present in case of antemortem injury. Colour changes can be seen only in case of antemortem injury. On microscopic examination, white blood cells are present in antemortem bruises and after about 12 hours rupture of red blood cells and the release of iron pigments occurs. A bruise has to be distinguished from postmortem lividity, congestion of organs and artificial bruise (Tables 12.1 to 12.3).

Table 12.1: Differences between bruise and P.M. lividity

Findings	Bruise	P.M. lividity
Cause	Blunt force	Engorged vessels
Cuticle	Damaged	Not damaged
Site	Any part	Dependent part
Appearance	Elevated	Not so
Edges	Ill-defined	Well defined
Cut Section	Clot cannot be washed	Blood inside vessel, easily washed
Colour	Change of colours	No change
Pressure	Gets lighter	No effect

Table 12.2: Differences between artificial and true bruise

Findings	Artificial bruise	True bruise
Cause	Juice of plant	Blunt force
Situation	Accessible parts	Any part
Colour	Dark brown	Change of colours
Margins	Well defined	Ill defined
Shape	Irregular	Shape of the weapon
Swelling, redness and ecchymosis	Not present	Slight swelling
Contents	Serum	Blood
Itching	Present	Absent
Chemical test	Present	Negative

Table 12.3: Differences between bruise and congestion

Findings	Bruise	Congestion
Cause	Blunt force	Pathological condition
Colour	Changes	No change
Margins	Diffuse, Ill-defined	Well-defined
On dissection	Extravasation of blood	Engorged vessels, blood inside

Medicolegal Significance of Bruise

1. A bruise is usually a simple injury. However, when any vital organs are involved it may amount to grievous hurt. Multiple bruises can cause death.
2. When the force is applied over the body by a weapon having definite patterns like belt, chain etc., it leaves a pattern simulating the size and shape of the object. This is called **patterned bruise** and is important from medicolegal point of view as from its examination, the type of weapon that has caused the injury can be known. This may connect the victim and the weapon besides indicating the nature of weapon. When the skin is struck by a pliable weapon like stick or cane etc., the bruise appears as two parallel lines with an undamaged area in between. It looks like a railway track or tram track, hence called **railway track bruise or railway line or tram line bruise** (Figure 12.5). The striking force at site of impact pushes the skin downwards and the traction force causes rupture of vessels at margins. However, little or no vessels are damaged by the centre of the weapon as the skin is not supported by underneath bone. When the transient impact is released, blood oozes out from the marginal vessels which gives rise to two parallel lines of bruise.
3. **Nature of weapon:** The characteristics of bruise produced by different types of weapons/objects are: (i) Hammer, closed fist produces round bruise. (ii) Rod, stick and whip produces bruise in the form of two parallel linear haemorrhages. (iii) In a broad and flat weapon like plank, the edges of plank may cause parallel lines separated by apparently normal

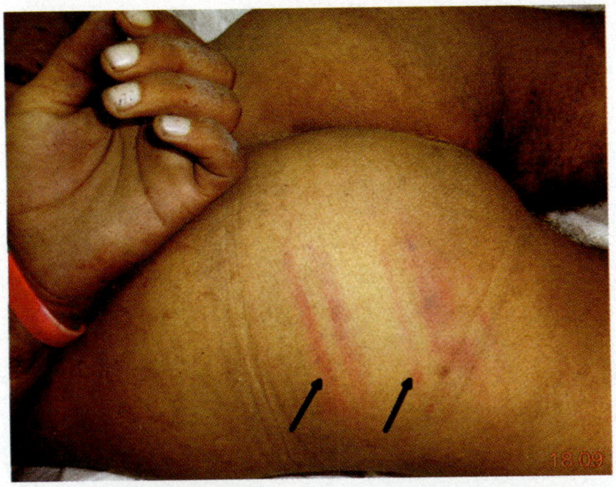

Figure 12.5: Railway track bruise

tissue. (iv) Ligature mark also forms a definite patterned bruise showing the pattern of woven, spiral ligature. (v) Elliptical patterned bruise indicates teeth bite. (vi) Tip of the shoe will also produce a definite patterned bruise. (vii) Tyre tread marks in a road traffic accident produces the pattern of the tyre.

4. **Age of a bruise:** The age can be estimated by the characteristic colour changes that the bruise undergoes with the passage of time. These colour changes are due to breakdown of RBC's and release of different pigments. The colour changes in a bruise are:

Colour of bruise	Pigment	Time
Red	Haemoglobin	Immediate (24 hours)
Blue	Deoxygenated Haemoglobin	1-3 days
Bluish black to brown	Haemosiderin	4 days
Greenish	Haemotoidin	5-6 days
Yellow	Bilirubin	7-12 days
Completely disappears	—	2 weeks

However, it is very difficult to estimate the exact age of bruise from the colour changes. Subconjunctival haemorrhages do not undergo the usual colour changes and becomes yellow from red. In old age and diseased, it takes a longer time for the various colour changes to appear. The colour changes are sustained during CO poisoning and remain bright red.

5. From the examination of bruises, the degree of violence can be estimated and the character and manner of production of injuries can be ascertained as different types of violence produces different types of bruises. In deaths due to manual strangulation thumb and finger impression in the form of bruises are seen over the neck. In sexual assault, the bruises may be present over breasts, inner sides of thigh and genitalia. From the pattern of bruises over arms, it can be known if the arms were grasped by the assailant and also the relative position of the assailant; whether front or behind can be known. If bruising is present over shoulder blades, it indicates pressure on the body against ground or some other hard surface.

6. **Delayed bruising:** The bruising at times does not appear immediately after the impact. This is due to the fact that the blood comes to the superficial layers after a delay of few hours or even days. This is known as delayed bruising and is commonly seen in abdomen, thigh etc. A **deep bruise** takes several hours to appear on the surface and very deep extravasations never appear on the surface. In casualty any injured person with no visible bruise should be advised to come after 24 hours for examination to look for any delayed bruising. Infrared photography helps in identification of such bruise.

7. **Shifting of the bruise:** Bruising may not necessarily appear at the site of impact. The blood gravitates through the loose areolar tissue to appear at a different place at the lower area. This is known as **ectopic or migratory bruise**. A few examples of bruising at sites distant from the point of injury are as given below: (a) Anterior cranial fossa fracture causes bruising of the eyes and the eyelids become black **(Racoon sign).** (b) Fracture of the middle cranial fossa of base of skull leads to accumulation of blood behind the ears at mastoid process **(Battle's sign).** (c) In case of an injury on calf muscle blood shifts in between the muscle planes to the ankles.

Abrasion

In an abrasion, there is damage of the superficial epithelial covering of skin or mucous membrane due to impact of hard surface or weapon (Figure 12.6).

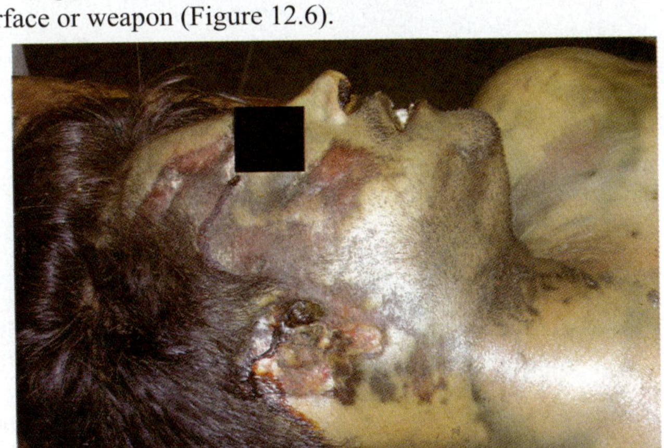

Figure 12.6: Multiple abrasions over the face

Mode of production: An impact causing friction between weapon and body surface is the most common mode of production of an abrasion. Direction of force may be horizontal or tangential causing scratches or graze abrasions or it may be perpendicular when it causes an imprint or pressure abrasion.

Features: These are superficial injuries with denudation of the epithelium. Later on a scab of dried blood is formed at the site. Gradually the granulation tissue forms beneath the scab and wound healing occurs (Figure 12.7).

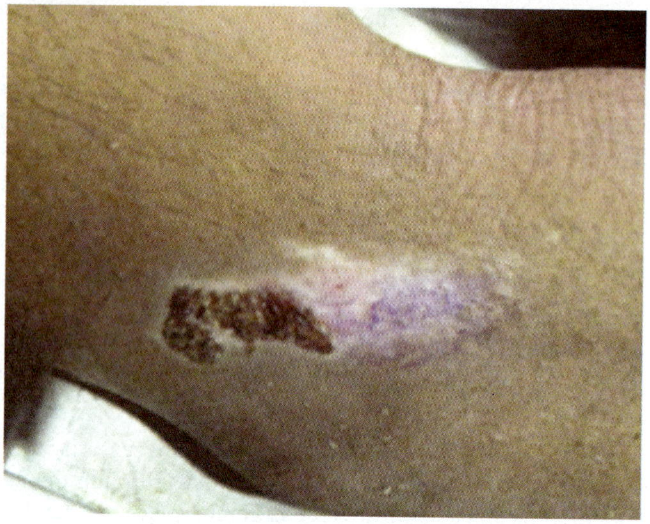

Figure 12.7: Partially healed abrasion

Types

1. **Linear or scratches:** These are caused by horizontal friction produced by pointed end of weapon (Figure 12.8). It is wider at the start and shows heaping of epithelium at the end. The features of linear abrasion depend on: (i) Type of weapon (ii) Direction of force; and (iii) Relative position of victim and assailant. Examples are scratch abrasions produced by nail marks.

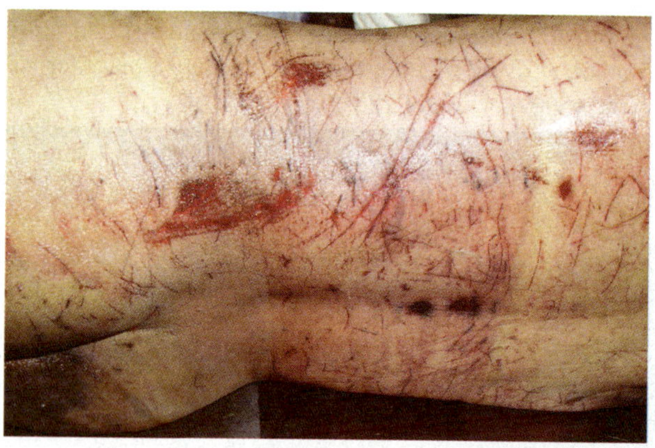

Figure 12.8: Linear abrasions or scratches

2. **Graze or sliding:** These are produced by rubbing of the skin against a rough surface of an object or ground etc. Grazed abrasions are seen most commonly in vehicular accidents (Figure 12.9). It is wider and deeper at the beginning and there is thinning at the end. Heaping of epithelium is present and indicates the direction of the force. Its size and shape have no relation to the weapon. These are also known as **Brush burns or friction burns.**
3. **Pressure:** In this type of abrasion, the force is more or less perpendicular and its size and shape depends on the part of the weapon in contact. Examples include the ligature mark in hanging (Figure 12.10) or strangulation. Teeth bite marks are also a type of pressure abrasion.

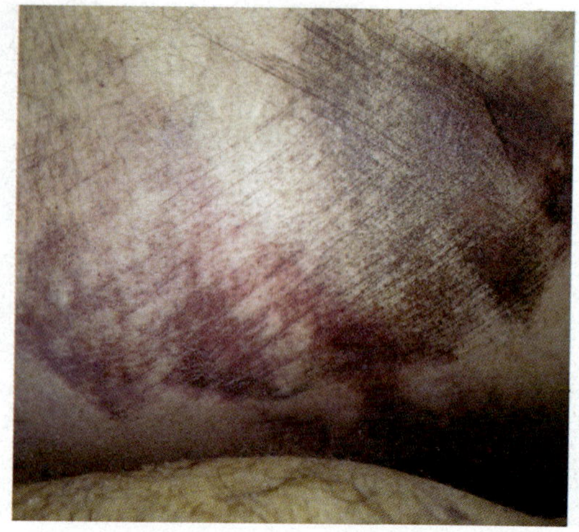

Figure 12.9: Grazed abrasion

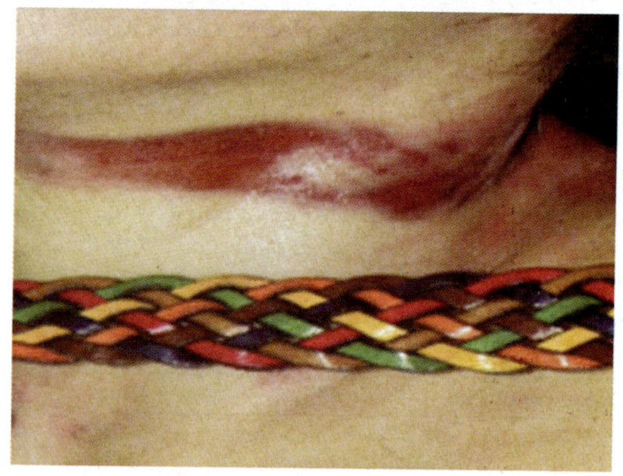

Figure 12.10: Pressure abrasion by a ligature in hanging with characteristics imprint pattern

4. **Imprint or patterned:** They reproduce the pattern of weapon causing it (Figures 12.10 and 12.11) as in vehicular accidents patterned abrasion is produced by the impact by radiator grill or headlamp. In run over accidents, the tyre marks may also produce patterned abrasions. Rough ligature material in case of hanging produces imprint abrasion.

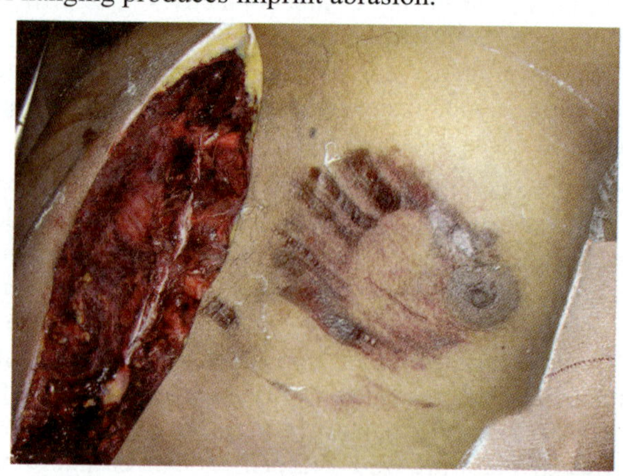

Figure 12.11: Imprint abrasion due to impact by horseshoe with effusion of blood inside the chest cavity

Medicolegal Aspects

1. They are usually simple injuries as they heal without any scar formation. Usually abrasions are not dangerous to vital organs. However, when there is involvement of underlying organs, these injuries can be dangerous to life.
2. They can be self-inflicted for levelling false charges against enemies.
3. The type of weapon can be identified from the examination of the abrasion.
4. Time of assault can be estimated by estimating the age of an abrasion. Various changes in abrasions with time are:

Time	Changes in abrasions
Fresh	Reddish and swollen, no scab
8-12 hours	Reddish scab
2-3 days	Brown scab
4-5 days	Dark brown scab
6 days	Black scab, starts falling
7-10 days	Scab completely falls off
2 weeks	Completely healed without scar formation

5. **Nature of offence:** In sexual offences, abrasion are found around breast, inner side of thighs whereas in asphyxial deaths such as throttling there are scratch abrasions resulting from nails over the neck.
6. **Postmortem abrasions:** These are yellowish parchment like and may be caused during transport to mortuary or by ant bites. Ant bites may be confused with antemortem abrasions but they are pale in appearance with multiple whitish deposits over them.
7. **Type of weapon:** It can be identified and matched with the injuries found on the person.

Lacerated Wound

When the tissues get crushed or stretched beyond the limits of their elasticity, they tear off and lead to the formation of lacerated wound (Figure 12.12A and B). The lacerated wound is caused by a blunt trauma. Thus, it may be caused in falls, in accidents, and in blows to chest, abdomen, head etc. by blunt object. The lacerations can be divided into split, stretch, avulsion and cut lacerations.

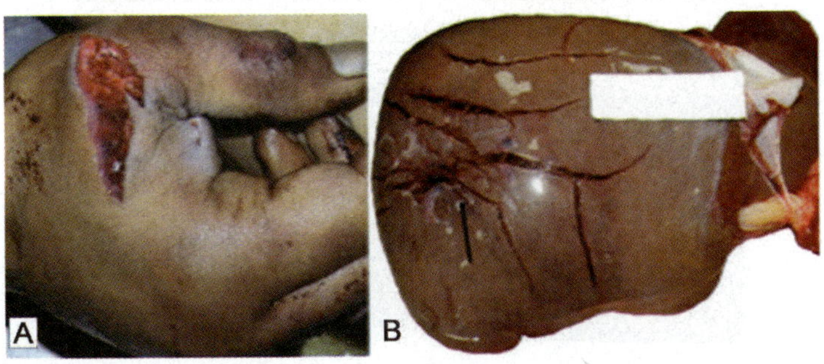

Figure 12.12: A and B: (A) Lacerated wound over the hand (B) Laceration of liver

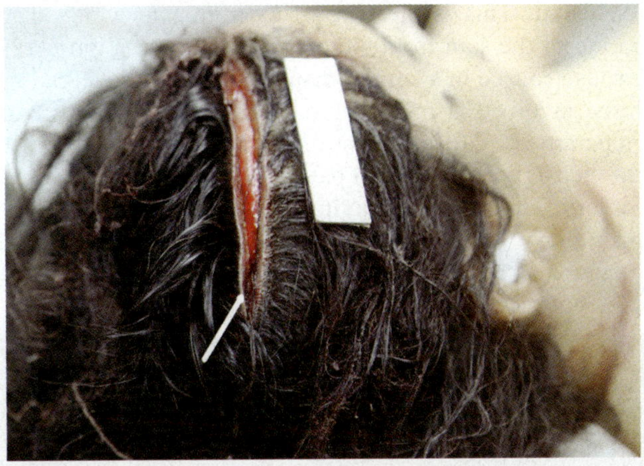

Figure 12.13: Incised looking lacerated wound on scalp

Split laceration: This is the type of laceration, which occurs due to crushing of the skin between two hard objects and leading to splitting of the skin. It is usually found on the areas of the body, which have subcutaneous bones like scalp (Figure 12.13), shin of tibia, jaw, pelvic bones and ulnar border of forearm. If these areas are hit with a hard blunt object then it may crush the skin and thin subcutaneous tissue and cause a split laceration. In these areas, the lacerated wounds may also appear clean cut and may simulate an incised wound. Such wounds are known as **incised looking lacerated wounds**. On close examination with hand lens, the edges of the wound are irregular though on naked eye they may look like clean cut wounds. This type of wounds may be wrongly interpreted by the inexperienced pathologist. These types of wounds are commonly seen on areas where skin is closely adherent to bone and subcutaneous tissues is scanty like on the scalp, jaw, pelvic bones (iliac crest) and eyebrows. The differences between incised and lacerated wound are given under Table 12.4.

Table 12.4: Differences between incised wound and lacerated wound

Features	Incised wound	Lacerated wound
Site	Any where in the body	Over bony prominences
Edges	Clean cut	Lacerated
Bruising of margins	No bruising	Present
Injury to blood vessels, nerves	Clean cut	Crushed
Hair bulbs	Clean cut	Crushed
Bleeding	More	Less

Stretch laceration: This type of laceration is caused by excessive stretching of the skin beyond which it causes tear of the skin. It is usually seen in run over accidents or in cases where a body part may be caught in the some moving machinery. These types of lacerations, if very extensive can cause a flap of loose skin and tissue. The flap can depict the direction of the force applied on the skin and can be useful in establishing the manner of the injury.

Avulsion: This is the type of laceration in which there is separation of the skin from the underlying tissue (Figure 12.14). This is also caused in a similar manner as a stretch laceration but the force involved is much more severe and the area involved is comparatively larger. The shearing and grinding forces by a weight such as a wheel of a car passing over the limb may produce such injury. This is called **flaying** of the tissue, which is a type of crush injury. Usually there is crushing of underlying muscles and fracture of bones. Internally the organs may be avulsed or completely torn off from their attachments.

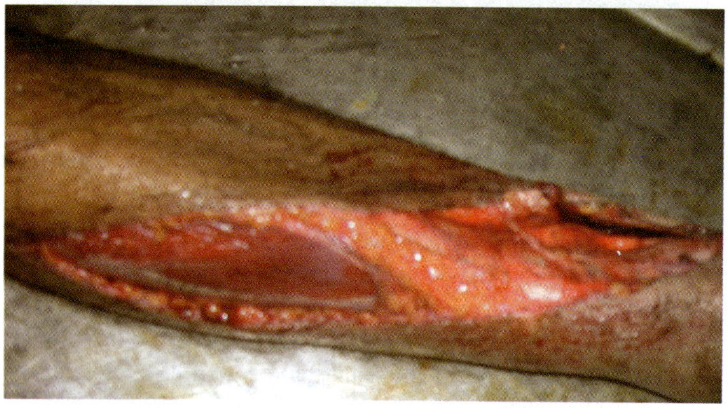

Figure 12.14: Avulsed laceration over leg

Tears: The skin and subcutaneous tissue can be teared when localized impact occur against some hard and irregular objects such as door handle of the car, protruding hinge etc.

Cut laceration: This is caused by a heavy, sharp edged weapon (e.g., axe, hatchet, chopper etc.) that causes a deep wide cut over the body tissues. The weapon cuts the skin margins, however, due to its heaviness, it crushes and stretches broad area of skin resulting in contused and irregular margins. There can be abraded margins due to rubbing of striking objects. It is a wound that can be assumed as hybrid between true laceration and true incised wound.

Characters of Lacerated Wound

The margins of a lacerated wound are irregular with bruising present all around. The deeper tissues are unevenly divided and the hair bulbs are crushed rather than being cut. The ends of the lacerations at angles from the main laceration may tear that are known as **shallow tails**. Bleeding is less in a lacerated wound compared to an incised wound as the arteries are torn and crushed irregularly thus retracting and leading to readily clotting of blood. This may not happen in scalp wounds where the temporal arteries bleed profusely. At times foreign matter may be present in the wound. From examination of lacerated wound, direction of the force can be established but the shape and size of the wound may not correspond to the instrument. Different types of weapons produce different appearances of lacerated wounds such as: (i) Blunt weapon with an edge (hammer head) produces crescentic laceration (ii) Long, thin objects (pipes, rods) produces linear lacerations (iii) Flat weapons produces irregular Y-shaped laceration.

Age of lacerated wound: It is difficult to determine the age except from the signs of healing such as formation of granulation tissue, fibroblast infiltration or inflammatory infiltrate.

Antemortem lacerations: It shows bruising, eversion, gaping of margins and signs of vital reaction.

Complications: (i) Haemorrhage, shock and death (ii) Infections (iii) Continuing pain and dysfunction of the part (iv) Pulmonary or systemic fat embolism.

Medicolegal aspects: (i) From the type of laceration, the cause of injury and rarely the shape of weapon can be known. (ii) Wound may sometimes contain foreign bodies that are helpful in locating the place of crime. (iii) Age of injury can be known from examination of lacerated wound.

Incised Wounds

The incised wounds are produced by sharp cutting weapons like knives, dagger or a razor and blade etc. Some authors restrict the term incised wounds to wounds that are longer than they are deep but some include stab wounds under this category. An incised wound that is longer than its depth is referred to 'cut' or 'slash. The knife, razor blade, sword, cleaver, panga, bottle or broken glass pieces may inflict such cuts that are typically seen in fights when the assailant strikes out with a sweeping action rather than the thrusting.

Characters: (i) Force is delivered over a narrow area of the skin by a sharp edged weapon, which causes cutting of the skin. (ii) Edges are clear, well-defined and there is no bruising (Figure 12.15A and B). The edges are usually everted but may be inverted if incision is made across a thin layer of muscle fibres that are adherent to skin for example scrotum. A serrated knife produces a saw toothed cuts on the body when the blade passes obliquely

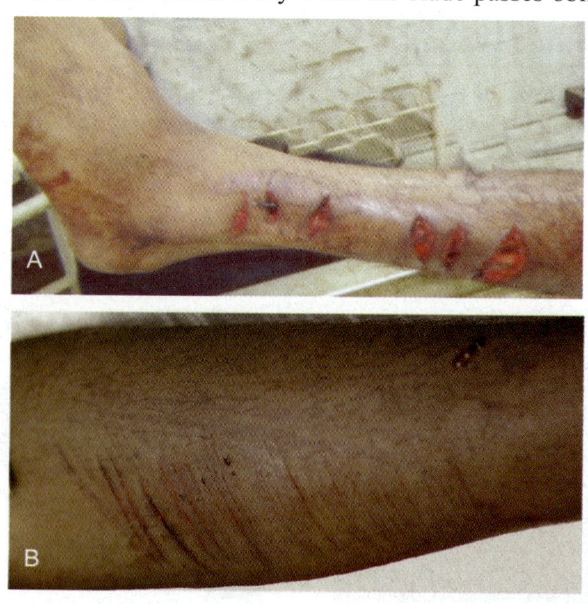

Figure 12.15A and B: Multiple incised wounds over (A) leg-homicidal (B) forearm-suicidal

or at shallow angle. In such cases depth of the wound shows no bridging tissues. (iii) Due to the elasticity of the skin, the width of the wound is greater than the edge of the weapon and the length is greater than the width and the depth. (iv) Length of an incised. wound has got no relation to the cutting edge of the weapon (v) These wounds are spindle shaped as the skin retracts due to its elasticity more so in the middle of the wound. (vi) Gaping is more if underlying fibers are cut transversely or obliquely. (vii) Haemorrhage in an incised wound is more compared to a laceration or crush injury. (viii) Wound is deeper at the start as more pressure is applied at that point than at the termination where it narrows down leaving only a superficial scratch which is known as **tailing of the wound.** The tailing of the wound can be evaluated for estimating the direction of the injury. (ix) When the weapon enters obliquely, then an oblique wound is created in which one flap is visible while the other one is undermined. This type of cut is known as a **bevelling cut.** It is usually homicidal and can be produced only by a sharp weapon and indicates the relative position of the assailant and victim. (x) ***Hesitational or tentative cuts:*** These are the cuts made by person with suicidal tendency. While attempting suicide these persons try to cut them to bleed to death. However, they hesitatingly make many superficial cuts before attempting a more deep cut. The hesitational cuts are typically multiple, superficial, parallel, uniform in depth and present on the accessible parts of the body (Figures 12.16 and 12.17).

Incised wounds are less dangerous than stab wounds as the relative shallowness of the wounds is less likely to affect a vital organ. The arms and the face are the common targets. Since the brain and chest organs are well protected by the ribs and skull, it is only the abdomen that is the target for a swung blade. A broken drinking glass is also used as a weapon, it may be broken prior to the attack to produce exquisitely sharp edges. The glass can inflict

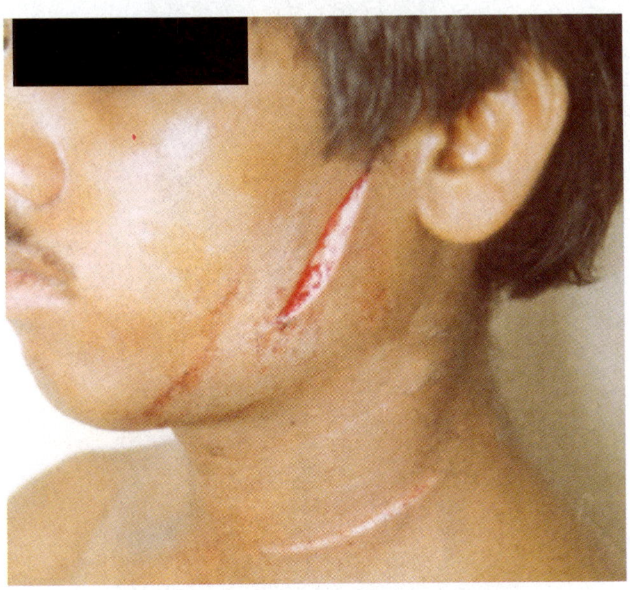

Figure 12.16: Self-inflicted incised wounds with hesitational cuts

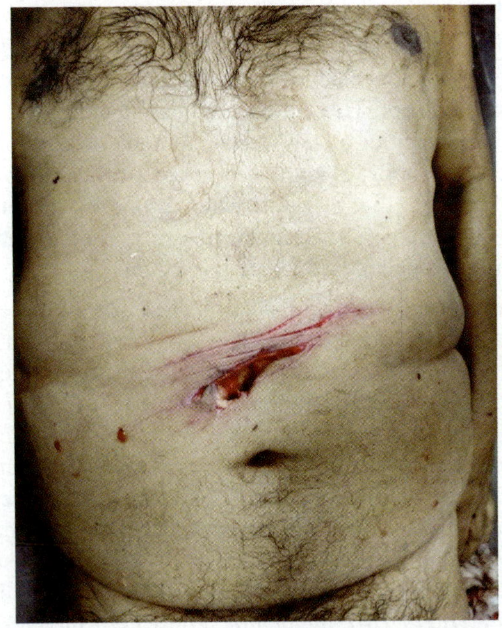

Figure 12.17: Self-stab abdomen with tentative cuts

deep wounds almost akin to a stab wound. Where a glass or bottle is used as a blunt object, it may shatter on impact with the victim's head and the resulting injuries may be both blunt and incised.

Age of incised wound: Age of incised wound can be discerned from the following features as given in Table 12.5:

Table 12.5: Age of incised wound

Age	Gross findings	Histopathological findings
Fresh	Hematoma formation	Capillary dilatation, margination and emigration of neutrophils, swelling of vascular endothelium and reactive changes in tissue histiocytes
12 hours	Edges red, swollen, adherent with blood and lymph	Reactive changes in fibroblast, monocytes in exudate
15 hours	—	Monocytes undergo mitotic division
24 hours	Continuous layer of endothelial cells cover surface with a crust or scab of dried clot	Endothelium begins to grow at edges, vascular buds begin to form
72 hours	—	Vascularised granulation tissue formation
4-5 days	—	Formation of new fibrils
7 days	Scar formation	Scar formation

The age of the incised wound delays greatly when the wound is infected.

Medicolegal aspects: (i) Incised wounds indicate the nature of weapon that it is sharp edged. (ii) Age of the wound can be calculated from various healing stages. (iii) Direction of force can be known from the tailing of the wound. (iv) Position and characteristics of the wound indicates the mode of production. (v) ***Wounds by glass:*** These are lacerated wounds but commonly resemble an incised or a stab wound. When a sharp point of the glass enters the body, it produces a wound resembling a stab wound. However, the margins when properly examined will show tiny side cuts due to irregular margins. There is presence of particles of glass penetrated inside the wound.

Manner of injuries: (i) *Suicidal*: These are multiple, parallel and are present in any specific area. They are uniform in depth and direction. The sites of election are throat, wrist and front of chest. There are initial hesitational or tentative or trial wounds. (ii) *Homicidal:* These are multiple occurring at specific area of the body. The direction is from below upwards that is quite characteristic of homicidal wound. These may be present at the back and at positions that are inaccessible to the person himself. The incised wounds produced over nose, ears and genitals are suggestive of jealously or revenge in order to cause disfiguration in cases of adultery. (iii) *Accidental:* These are usually minor and are produced while working at home or at work place. These are usually produced by sharp cutting weapon, sharp pointed weapon or sharp pieces of broken glass. These are situated anywhere over the body but commonly on hands. These wounds may be produced by mentally disordered persons.

Chop wounds or slash wounds (Figure 12.18): These types of wounds are produced by a blow with a sharp cutting edge of a heavy weapon like an axe, basola etc. In this type of injury, the dimensions of the wound correspond to cross-section of penetrating blade. The margins are sharp and may show slight abrasion and bruising with slight destruction of underlying tissue. The undermining occurs in direction from which the chop wound is made.

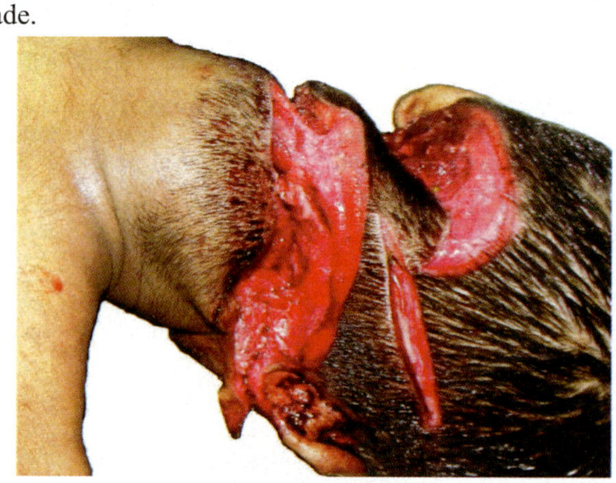

Figure 12.18: Chop wounds on neck

Non-fatal self-inflicted injuries: These types of injuries exist in persons who have some abnormality of mind leading the victim to mutilate his body and in whom the injuries are inflicted for motives of gain. Some mentally disordered persons may inflict many small wounds upon themselves, which may be in addition to the actual cause of death. The arms may be covered with scores of parallel superficial incisions from a knife, razor or broken glass. They may cross each other in groups and are more frequent on the non-dominant side, usually the left. Another well recognized injury is self mutilation of the genitals, almost invariably by men who are paranoid schizophrenics. The penis, testis and scrotum may be removed and death occurs from intractable haemorrhage in such cases.

Self-inflicted injuries, usually non-fatal unless some complication has arisen, may be motivated by some form of gain. The most common is fabrication of injuries to simulate an assault, either to divert attention from the person's own theft or to arouse sympathy. Fabricated accidental injuries are usually a form of malingering, as in armed forces, or in fraudulent attempts to obtain compensation. In other cases the injured may claim that a specific person assaulted him.

Features of self-inflicted incised wounds (Figures 12.19 and 12.20): (i) Cuts are usually superficial but occasionally may penetrate the full thickness of the skin, but not in sensitive areas such as face. The injury is rarely dangerous to life unless infected. (ii) Incised wounds are regular with an equal depth at origin and termination unlike serious wounds that tend to be deeper at the start and tail off to the surface. (iii) Cuts are multiple and parallel

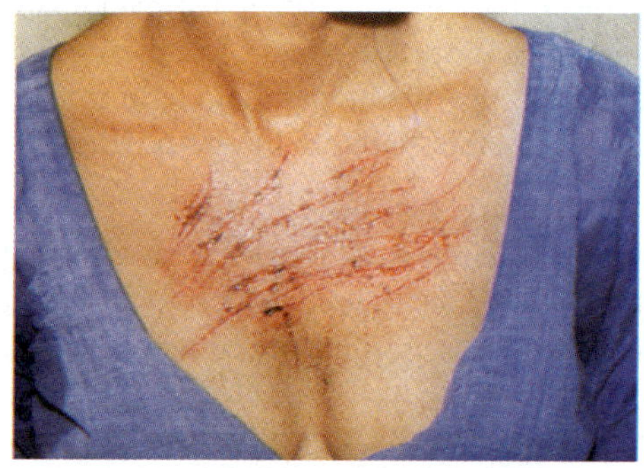

Figure 12.19: Multiple self-inflicted injuries

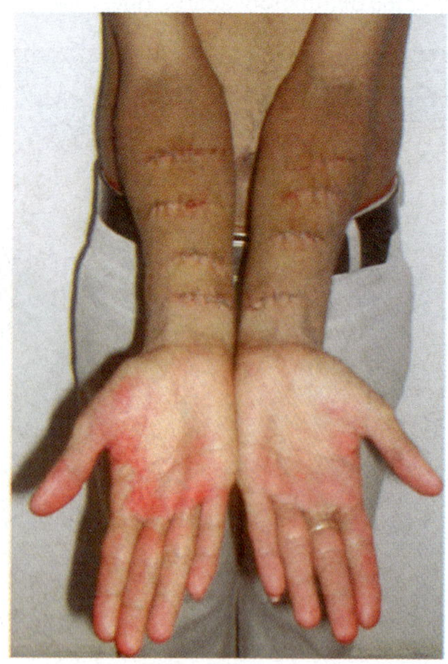

Figure 12.20: Self-inflicted incised wound over forearm

and avoid the sensitive areas like the eyes, lips, nose and ears, usually being drawn on the cheeks and the jaws, temples and forehead, sides of neck, chest, shoulders, front and back of arms and forearms, back of hands and thighs. This is inconsistent with an attack by another person, as the victim is unlikely to stand still to allow these multiple delicate and uniform injuries to be carefully executed. (iv) In the right handed person, most of these injuries are on the left side, especially side of face and left hand. (v) When the incisions are on the covered area, the relevant garments may show either no cuts or if there are cuts they do not match the injuries in position or direction. Various sites of election used for inflicting injuries by the suicides are given in Figure 12.21.

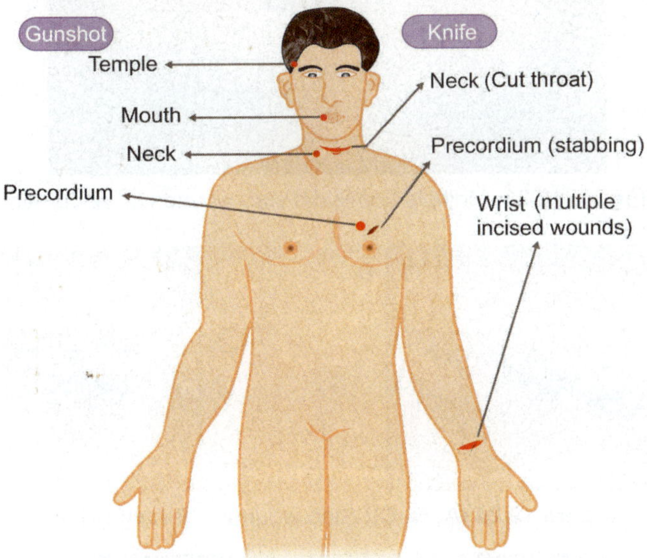

Figure 12.21: Various sites involved in suicides

Cut Throat Wounds

Suicidal cut throat wounds: Cut throat wounds are commonly suicidal in manner and have a number of tentative cuts (Figure 12.22A). If successful, there will be one or more deep incisions superimposed, which may destroy some of the previous shallow cuts. The classical description of the cut throat is of incisions starting high on the left side of the neck below the angle of jaw, which pass obliquely across the front of the neck to end at a lower level on the right. This assumes that the victim is right handed, the obliquity being reversed in a left-handed person. The cuts are said to be deeper at their origin, becoming shallower as they cross the throat, tailing off into surface cuts at the extremity but commonly the cuts show no variation at the either end. Most suicides raise their chin to provide a better access to the throat, so that the skin is stretched out when cut. This tends to cause straight-edged incisions, rather than the jagged cut that is seen when a knife is drawn over the loose skin. Throwing back the head moves the carotid bundle under the protection of the sternomastoid muscles and if cuts are confined to the centre of the front of the neck, only the larynx or trachea may be damaged, rather than large blood vessels.

Homicidal cut throat wounds (Figure 12.22B): Cut throat wounds are also homicidal in manner when there are no tentative cuts. The wound is more deep and may be found any where on the neck.

Atypical cut-throat injuries: Cases have been reported where there is absence of hesitation cuts in suicidal deaths and presence of multiple superficial wounds near the incision wounds in homicidal wounds.

Accidental cut throat wounds (Figure 12.22C): Accidental cut throat wounds are rare. It can happen in vehicular or industrial accidents. There can be other injuries over the body due to accidents. No tentative cuts present.

Cause of death in cut throat wounds: Death from a cut throat depends on the nature and extent of local damage to the neck. (i) **Severe haemorrhages** from the jugular veins, or less often the carotid arteries, may lead to death from exsanguination. (ii) If the larynx or trachea is opened, then even relatively minor haemorrhage from local vessels may cause **blockage of airways** by blood and clot, though many slashed air-passage victims survive. (iii) A rare cause of death is **air embolism** caused by

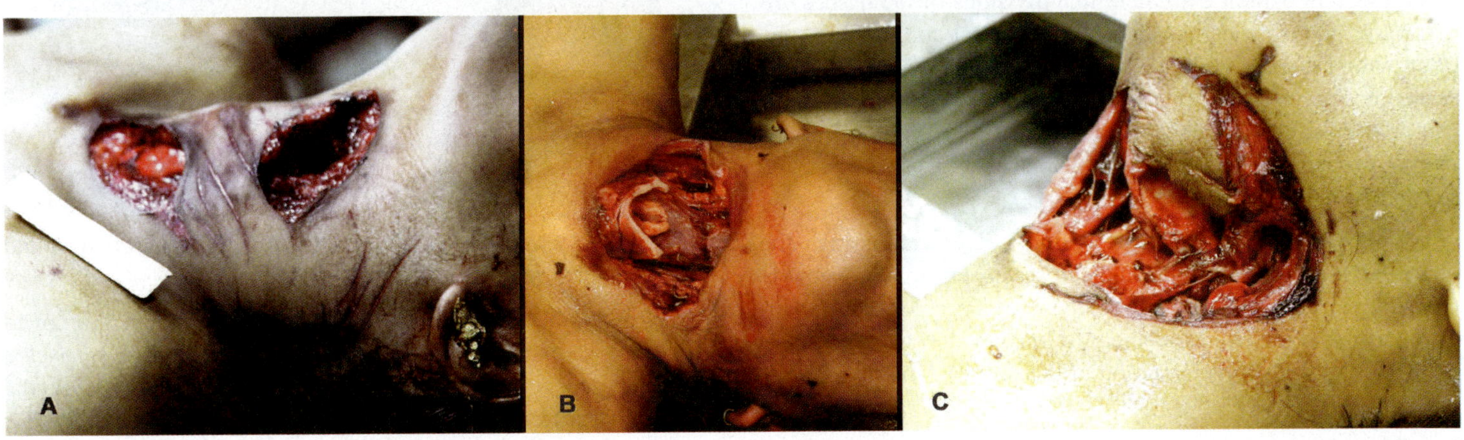

Figure 12.22 A to C: (A) Suicidal cut throat wound with hesitation marks (B) Homicidal cut throat wound (C) Accidental cut throat wound in RTA

aspiration into cut jugular veins while standing or sitting with the neck at a higher level than the thorax. Many suicides either use multiple methods of suicide or may sometimes abandon the pain of cut throat for some other mode such as poison, burns or fall from height.

Stab or Punctured Wounds

A stab or punctured wound is a wound that is deeper than it's length and width (Figures 12.23 and 12.24). Sharp pointed objects such as a knife, dagger, nails, needle, spear, arrow, screwdriver etc. cause it. A stab wound can be produced by (i) Driving the object into the body; or (ii) Falling against the object. A punctured wound is called **penetrating wound** when it enters the body cavity and once it passes through and through it is called a **perforating wound** (Figure 12.25). In a perforated wound, the entry is larger with inverted edges while the exit is smaller with everted edges. Though a stab wound may penetrate only the skin and subcutaneous tissue, more commonly fatal wounds are encountered in the practice of forensic medicine.

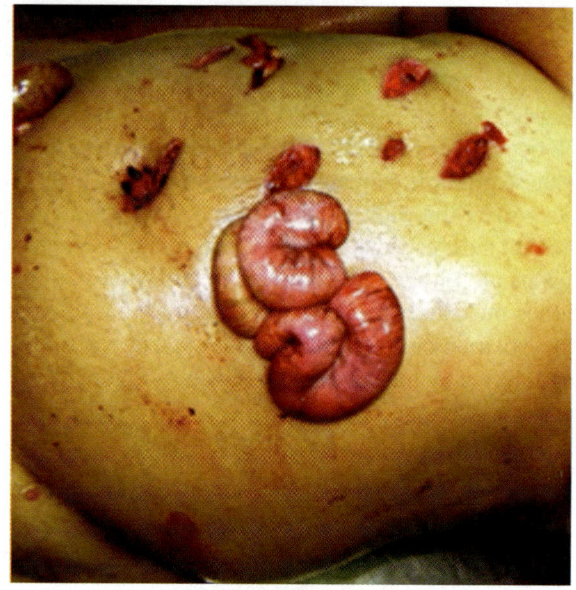

Figure 12.23: Multiple homicidal stab wounds on abdomen

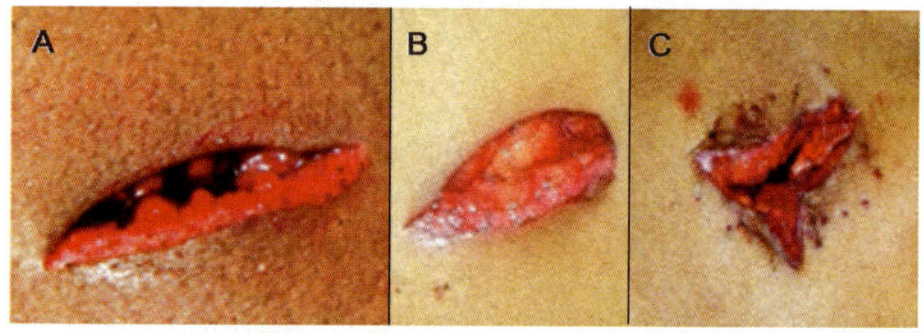

Figure 12.24 (A, B, C): Stab wounds showing gaping

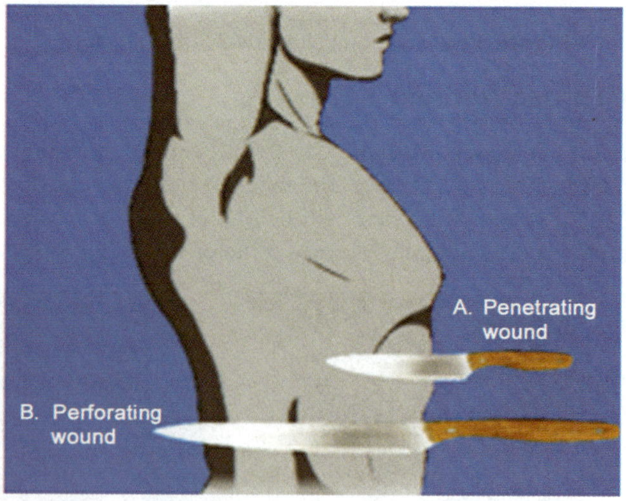

Figure 12.25: Schematic diagram showing (A) Penetrating wound (B) Perforating wound

Nature of stabbing weapon: Most commonly, the knives are employed in producing a stab wound and their physical features are quite important in shaping the wound. The examination of the knife should include following: (i) Length, breadth and thickness of the blade of knife (ii) Whether the knife is single edged or double edged (iii) Whether the blade especially its extreme tip is sharp (iv) In a single edged knife, the nature of the back edge (v) Face of the hilt guard adjacent to the blade (vi) Is there any grooving, forking or serration of the blade (vii) Note whether any foreign material is sticking to the blade such as blood stains.

Besides the knife, certain knife like weapons are used for stabbing including scissors, chisels, razor blades, swords and even sharpened screwdrivers. In addition, larger cutting instruments such as axes, choppers, *parangs*, machetes, shears, hayknives have been used as stabbing weapons. Spiked instruments such as ice-picks, hayforks, case-openers cause a typical looking wound. Some of these weapons are exquisitely sharp and the wounds made by them exhibit extremely fine divisions of the tissues. To razor and razor blades may be added surgical and craft knives, often with a disposable blade. Equally sharp is broken glass and sometimes porcelain. Both sheet glass and smashed glass utensils can provide edges that equal or exceed surgical scalpels in their cutting ability. Smashed china cups and mugs can also provide sharp cutting edges.

Characteristics of stab wound: By examining the characteristics of stab wound, the forensic expert can provide opinion on: (i) Dimensions of weapon (ii) Type of weapon (iii) Taper of the blade (iv) Movement of knife within the wound (v) Depth of the thrust (vi) Direction of thrust (vii) Amount of force used.

Dimensions of the weapon in relation to characteristic of stab wound: The dimensions of the knife may be a vital part of investigation of a homicide when the weapon has been removed from the scene by the assailant. The examination of the suspected weapons recovered from the site, may indicate whether the dimensions are consistent with the injuries found on the body. For this purpose, the injuries found on the person of the victim should be thoroughly examined under the following headings:

Length: Length of a stab wound is slightly less than width of the weapon due to elasticity of skin. It is measured to the nearest of a centimeters. In most instances, the wound will have gaped across the centre, to form a long ellipse. The extent of gaping will depend upon the anatomical situation, for example over joints or in the axilla or groin, and whether the axis of the stab is in line with or across the tension of **Langer's lines** (Figure 12.26) or underlying muscle bundles. The length of the wound should be again measured after opposing the edges that more accurately approximates the length when the blade was *in situ*. The length will be more if lateral movement of the weapon or the body occurs. When the knife is withdrawn the elasticity of the skin causes it to retract, making the wound smaller than when the blade was inside the body.

Breadth: The breadth is the second dimension on the surface of the body. The breadth varies depending upon the site of the injury. The breadth of a stab wound over the abdomen will be different from that over the chest or thigh.

Depth: It is the length of the track and is the greatest dimension of the injury. In a patient, the injury should not be probed as there is danger of dislodging a clot causing more hemorrhage during life or it may cause a false track to be formed. Depth is equal to or less than the length of the blade producing it. Depth is greater on yielding surface such as anterior abdominal wall, rib cage and chest in young individuals. The depth of the wound and the force required depends on: (i) *Nature of the weapon*: A sharp, slender weapon will pass more easily through the body while a blunt pointed weapon will require more force to penetrate the body. (ii) *Part of the body*: Soft body parts like abdomen can be pierced easily while parts with underlying bone like skull cannot be pierced and sustain only superficial cuts. (iii) *Age and bodily built of the injured:* Healthy adults with muscular bodies are less likely to sustain deeper injuries while children and females who have softer skin can sustain deep penetrating injuries with small amount of force.

Margins: The margins of a stab wound are clean cut when produced with a sharper weapon. The margins are irregular in case a blunt pointed weapon such as a screw driver is used. A hilt mark of the knife may be seen at the angles of the wound indicating that the full length of the weapon has entered.

Shape: If both the angles of the wound are acute, it has been caused by a double-edged weapon. While if one angle is more

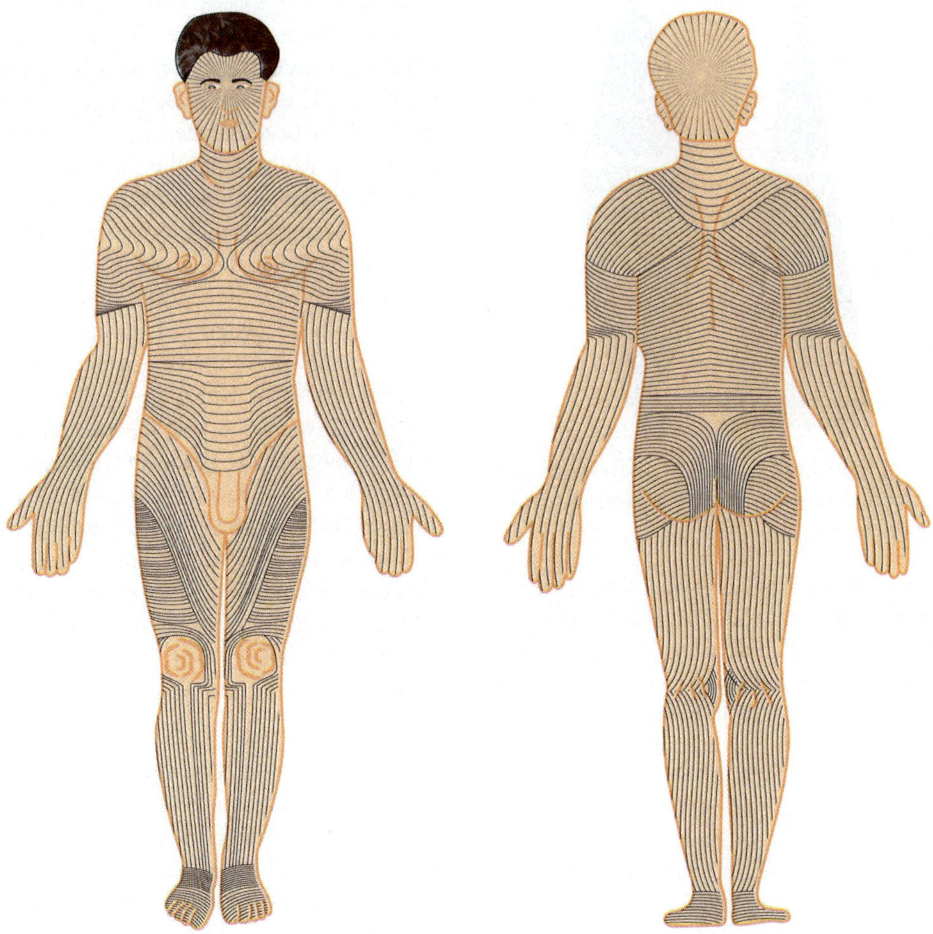

Figure 12.26: Cleavage lines of Langer

acute than the other, the weapon is a single-edged. A stab wound that cuts the **cleavage lines of Langer** transversely or obliquely will gape. A stab wound that runs parallel to the cleavage lines will be slit like. Shape of the wound usually corresponds to the weapon used but it varies at different parts of the body. Single edged weapon may form a triangular, wedge or tear drop shaped wound in which one angle is acute and the other angle is obtuse (Figure 12.27 A and B). However, when the weapon enters parallel to the cleavage lines, even though single edged it can produce wound with two acute angles. Because of initial penetration by the knifepoint, it first produces a dermal defect with sharp angles at each end. Double-edged weapon can cause elliptical, slit like wounds in which both angles are acute (Figure 12.27C). Round object or a spear may cause a circular wound. A round blunt pointed object may cause a circular wound with ragged margins whereas square weapon causes cruciform injuries. Ice-pick or screw driver causes injuries like small bullet holes and two "A" or "V" shaped stab wounds can also be seen. In a homicidal stab wound, the knife may be pulled upwards and downwards during insertion or withdrawal and the length of the wound is more than the width of the blade.

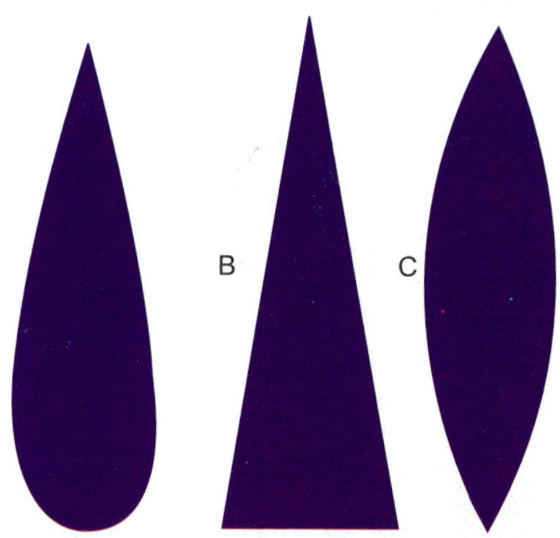

Figure 12.27A to C: Single edged weapon produces (A) tear drop or (B) wedge shaped wounds whereas doubled edged weapons produces (C) spindle shaped wounds

Direction: In solid organs the track is better seen. The principal direction is noted first and then the others such as backwards and to the right. One external wound and two or more internal wounds may be caused, if the weapon is taken back and again pushed. In a perforating wound entrance, track and exit indicates the direction of the wound. To know the track of the wound it should not be probed with a metal probe, instead a pliable tubing should be used or a radiopaque dye should be injected and then X-ray is taken to reveal the complete track. As far as the direction of the wound is concerned the pathologist should take care of the differences in the position of internal organs as measured at autopsy in a supine body compared to their position in the living that is often in an upright position. In the chest and abdomen the relationship of various organs varies with the stage of respiration.

Tapering of the blade: The wound size depends on the taper of the blade. If the taper of blade is inserted to 4 cm, the length of the wound is that of the width of the blade whereas in case of blade showing tapering at 8 cm level, the wound will be correspondingly longer. When the blade edges become parallel the wound size will remain constant for further penetration of the knife. If the tapering blade perforates, the exit wound is smaller compared to entry wound.

Movement of the knife within the wound: When the knife is stabbed directly into the body and withdrawn along the same track then the size of the wound will indicate the minimum width of the blade at the maximum depth of penetration. A knife that is thrust into the body may itself move or the body may move against it before it is withdrawn. This relative movement may extend the wound in a linear fashion or there may be twisting of the blade in the wound. In the latter case, the resulting skin incision may be V-shaped or is totally irregular. A single stab can also produce multiple skin wounds such as stab over the arm that enters the superficial tissues and then reenters the chest wall.

Depth of the thrust: To assess the length of the weapon the depth of the stab wound is important. Certain points should be observed. This varies with the following factors: (i) When the knife is driven inside the body upto the hilt, depth of the wound when measured at autopsy may be greater than the true length of the blade. This is quite common in the injuries on abdomen and rarely chest because the impact of stab may indent the chest or abdominal wall so that the tip of the knife penetrates tissues that apparently should have been out of the reach. This particularly happens when hiltguard of the weapon impinges on the skin. (ii) *Direction of thrust:* Determination of the direction depends on the appearance of the skin wound and the track in deep tissues. Where a knife penetrates the skin with the plane of the blade at appreciably less than a right angle to the surface, the wound is often undercut being shelved so that subcutaneous tissue is visible below one edge of the wound. Where the knife is plunged in obliquely but the plane of the blade remains perpendicular to the surface, no such shelving can be seen at the site of the wound though it may just be visible at the end of the wound. The track of the stab wound can provide further information on to the direction. Attempt have been made to delineate the track of the stab wound before dissection either by filling the defects with the radiopaque fluid before taking X-rays or by filling by the plastic or even metallic substance that will harden to form a cast. These methods have a very little advantage over routine dissection method.

Estimation of the degree of force used in stabbing: The assessment of force used in the stabbing is subjective and cannot be quantified in any satisfactory way that is meaningful to the court of law (i) Tissue most resistant to the knife penetration is the skin followed by muscle apart from the bone or calcified cartilage. (ii) For skin penetration, the sharpness of extreme of knife is the most important factor. The cutting edge of the knife once the knife is penetrated has no significance. (iii) In achieving penetration the speed of approach of knife is important as when a knife held against a skin and steadily pushed requires more force than the same knife launched against the skin like a dart. (iv) It is difficult for the knife to penetrate a lax skin compared to a stretched skin. The chest wall is easy to penetrate by sharp knife as there is stretching of intercostal spaces. (v) Thickness of the palms and soles is tough to penetrate than the rest of the body. (vi) When the knife penetrates skin rapidly as when the body falls or runs on to the blade, the knife does not need to be held rigidly in order to prevent it being pushed backwards. (vii) Uncalcified cartilages such as costal cartilages are easily penetrated by sharp knife. Calcified rib and bone provide a resistant barrier but a forceful stab from strong, sharp knife can easily penetrate sternum, skull or rib.

Medicolegal aspects: (i) Shape of the wound may indicate the type of weapon. (ii) Depth will indicate force of penetration as in homicidal injuries more force is used compared to suicide. (iii) By the direction and dimensions of the wound, the relative position of the victim and assailant can be known. (iv) Age of injury can be evaluated. (v) Position and number of injuries can indicate whether it is homicidal, suicidal or accidental (Table 12.6). (vi) If broken fragment of the weapon is available it can identify the weapon.

Table 12.6: Differences between suicidal and homicidal stab wound

Findings	Suicidal stab wounds	Homicidal stab wounds
Position of wound	Accessible parts	No fixed site, vital parts
Grouping of wounds (Deep and superficial)	Arranged	Irregular
No. of main wounds	Usually One	Multiple
Direction	In right handed persons, left to right	Any direction
Severity	Mostly superficial, 1-2 fatal	Mostly severe an extensive
Defence wounds	Absent	Present
Secondary injuries	Absent	May be connected with fight
Weapon	Present	Absent
Clothes	Not damaged	Damaged
Motive	Domestic worries, disappointment in love	Revenge, robbery, sexual assault

Defence Wounds

Usually limbs are most commonly used to protect oneself from assault as a result of which defence wounds may be produced over the body of the victim. These indicate that victim was conscious, partially mobile and not taken completely unawares. Classically defence wounds are produced over back of forearms that are used to protect vital areas such as eyes, face and head. In addition, while protecting genitals, the injuries may be sustained on thighs. In blunt weapon attack or from fists, bruise may be produced commonly on outer parts of forearms, back of hands, wrist and knuckles. The size and shape may correspond with attacking weapon/object. This may be accompanied by fractures. Palmar side of forearm may also receive blows when arm is held in front of face. Defence bruises and abrasions from kicks or blows may occur on the thigh. In sharp weapon while seizing the weapon injuries may be received on flexures of phalanges on one or all fingers. Defence wound between web of base of thumb and index finger is quite common while trying to grab blade (Figure 12.28). They are also present in firearm injuries.

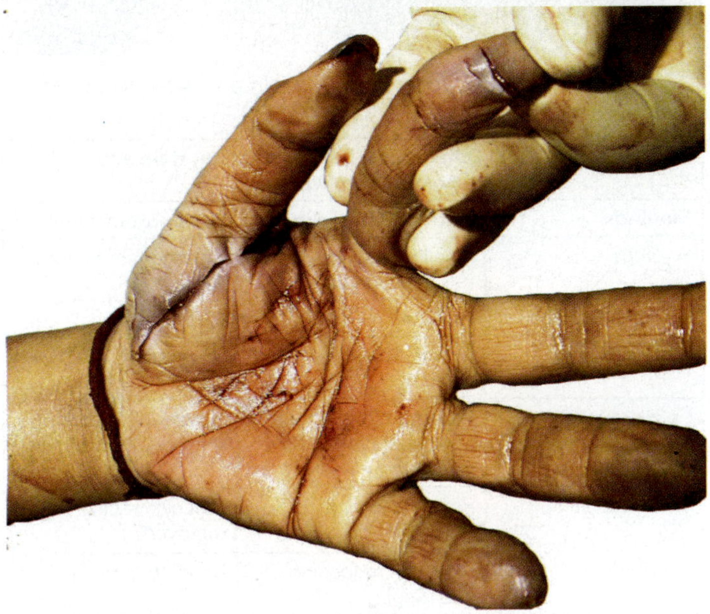

Figure 12.28: Multiple defence wounds over palm and fingers

Railway Injuries

Railway injuries are quite common in countries with many 'level crossings' where a public road crosses a railway track with either no barrier at all or with only a flimsy lifting pole. Few rail passengers are killed or injured in moving trains compared with accidents on railway property. Track workers may be run down and some may die from electrocution from overhead cables. The person to commit suicide lays himself in front of an approaching train. Decapitation is the most common injury (Figure 12.29) with features of local tissue destruction, usually with grease, rust or other dirt soiling of the damaged area. In railway accidents the viscera should be analysed for alcohol and other drugs as suicides often employ multiple methods for committing suicide. Sometimes the individual is killed and the body is thrown over the railway track to mimic an accident but in such circumstances, the presence of coexistent injuries such as strangulation mark over the neck will be evident.

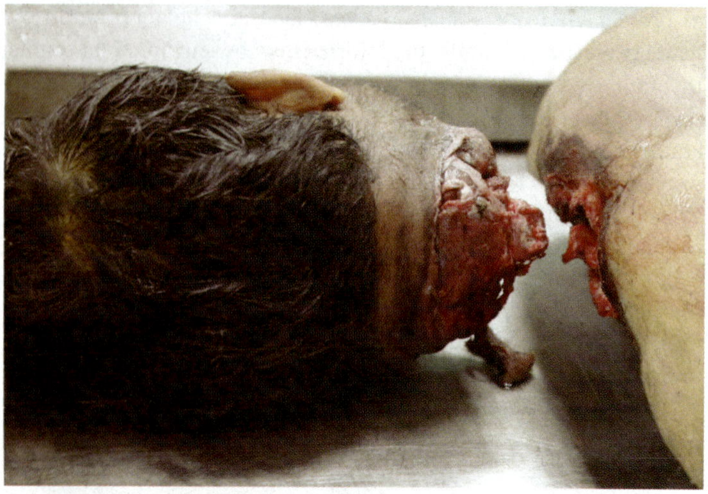

Figure 12.29: Decapitation of head in a railway accident

Tables 12.7: Differences between antemortem and postmortem wounds

Findings	Antemortem wounds	Postmortem wounds
• Edge	Swollen, everted, retracted, gaping	Antemortem features Absent
• Haemorrhage	Profuse	Slight, venous
• Spurting	Arterial flow, over clothing	No spurting
• Extravasation of blood	Staining of the edges of wound, cannot be removed by washing	Not deeply stained, removed by washing
• Coagulation	Firm and difficult to wash	Soft clot easily removed
• Vital reaction	Swelling, reddening and repair	No such process
• ↑ Enzyme reaction (Esterase, acid phosphates)	Can be seen	No such reaction

Injury Report

The patient in a medicolegal case should be examined by the doctor for preparation of medicolegal case report after receiving a written requisition from the investigating police officer. The preliminary details of the patient should be noted such as: (i) Name (ii) Age and sex (iii) Address (iv) History (v) Brought by (vi) *Identification marks:* Two permanent identification marks preferably on exposed parts of the body that would help in identification of the victim in court of law should be noted. (vii) *Consent:* An informed consent of the patient should be recorded describing the procedure along with its risks and consequences. The doctor can be charged of assault if examination is attempted without prior consent. The consent should then be signed or the thumb impression applied by the patient in presence of a witness preferably third party. The signature of the witness should also be recorded.

The injury report should describe the following in detail: (i) General physical examination noting the vitals of the patient as well as his systemic examination. (ii) Examination proper that includes: (a) nature of each injury (b) size, shape and direction of the injury (c) part of the body on which injury is present (site) (d) whether injury is simple or grievous (e) type of weapon used (f) whether weapon is dangerous or not. (iii) *Opinion*: The opinion should include the nature of injury, whether it is simple or grievous, the time passed since the infliction of the injuries, the type of weapon producing it. At times it is difficult specially in head injury cases to opine whether it is simple or grievous. In such cases the doctor can opine after necessary investigations and keeping the patient under observation. In addition, if any investigations are mandatory such as radiological examination in firearm cases, preservation of blood for grouping, examination of clothing should be mentioned in the report itself. Finally the report bears the signature of the doctor along with the date.

LONG QUESTIONS

1. Discuss in detail the injuries caused by a blunt weapon. Enumerate the differences between lacerated and incised wound.
2. How can you classify injuries? What are the features of stab wound?
3. How will you proceed to make an injury report?

SHORT QUESTIONS

1. Abrasion.
2. Contusion.
3. Laceration.
4. Stab wounds.
5. Age of incised wound.
6. Self inflicted injuries.
7. Cut throat wounds.
8. Chop or slash wounds.
9. Defence wounds.
10. Railway injuries.

MULTIPLE CHOICE QUESTIONS

1. The colour of the postmortem abrasion is:

(a) Red (b) Yellow
(c) Black (d) Reddish-brown

2. The exact age of the abrasion can be ascertained by:

(a) Histological method (b) Histochemical method
(c) Naked eye examination (d) None of the above

3. Colour of the subconjunctival haemorrhage changes from red to:

(a) Blue (b) Green

(c) Yellow (d) Black

4. In cases of stab wounds:

(a) Depth is more than length and breadth

(b) Length is more than depth

(c) Breadth is more than length

(d) All dimensions are equal

5. The colour of the bruise becomes green on:

(a) 2nd day (b) 3rd day

(c) 4th day (d) 6th day

6. The depth of an incised wound is:

(a) Equal throughout

(b) Deeper at the beginning

(c) Deeper at in end

(d) Uneven throughout

7. Which of the following is not an example of pressure abrasion?

(a) Ligature mark in hanging

(b) Ligature mark in strangulation

(c) Finger nail marks

(d) Teeth bite

8. A reddish scab is formed in an abrasion in about:

(a) 2-3 hours (b) 6-8 hours

(c) 8-12 hours (d) 12-24 hours

9. In an incised wound:

(a) Breadth is more than length

(b) Length is more than depth and breadth

(c) All are equal

(d) Depth is more than breadth

10. Latent bruises can be detected by:

(a) Colour photography (b) UV light

(c) Oblique light (d) Infrared light

11. The direction of a stab wound indicates:

(a) Type of weapon

(b) Force of penetration

(c) Relative position of assailant and victim

(d) Stretching of the tissues

12. Blunt force injury will produce incised looking wounds over:

(a) Forehead (b) Mandible

(c) Shin of tibia (d) All of the above

13. Stretch lacerations are caused due to:

(a) Run over vehicular accident

(b) Grinding force by a weight

(c) Injury by axe

(d) Injury by pieces of glass

14. Defence wounds are found in cases of:

(a) Accidental injuries (b) Homicidal injuries

(c) Suicidal injuries (d) Self-inflicted injuries

15. Tentative cuts are seen in:

(a) Homicide (b) Fall from height

(c) Suicides (d) Accidents

16. Lacerated looking incised wound may be seen in:

(a) Head (b) Scrotum

(c) Ankle (d) Knee

17. A person has been brought in casualty with stab wounds by a double-edged knife. The shape of wound is likely to be:

(a) Wedge shaped (b) Oval

(c) Triangular (d) Elliptical

18. Tyre marks seen on the body in run over vehicular accidents is classical example of:

(a) Ectopic bruise (b) Shifting bruise

(c) Latent bruise (d) Patterned bruise

19. Fishtailing of the entry wound of a stab wound is caused by:

(a) Single edged knife (b) Double edged kitchen knife

(c) Pointed ice pick (d) Iron rod

20. Which injury denotes the weapon best?

(a) Stabbing (b) Contusion

(c) Laceration (d) Abrasion

ANSWER KEY

1. (b)	2. (d)	3. (c)	4. (a)	5. (d)	6. (b)	7. (c)	8. (c)	9. (b)	10. (d)
11. (c)	12. (d)	13. (a)	14. (b)	15. (c)	16. (b)	17. (d)	18. (d)	19. (a)	20. (a)

13 CHAPTER

Road Traffic Accidents

Road traffic accidents account for majority of deaths worldwide. These occur on the road between the vehicles or a vehicle with pedestrians. It accounts for about 44% of the total accidental deaths in India. The pattern of injury and fatality varies depending on whether the victim is a vehicle occupant, a motorcyclist, a pedalcyclist or a pedestrian. The most common form of accident is between a vehicle and a pedestrian.

Mechanism of injury

The mechanism of road traffic accident is thoroughly studied by **De'Haven**. (i) Injuries to tissues result from a change of rate of movement that is acceleration or deceleration. A constant speed has no effect, however rapid it may be. The change of speed is the main culprit, rather than its absolute speed. He has found that the severity of injury to a vehicle occupant is directly proportional to the degree of acceleration or deceleration force. (ii) Change of rate is measured by 'gravities' or 'G' forces. The amount that the human body can tolerate depends on the direction in which the force acts. Deceleration of the order of 300 G can be tolerated without any injury and even forces of 2000 G can be survived for a short period provided it acts at right angles to the long axis of the body. The G formula is used to calculate the main force (impact of deceleration force) involved in an accident:

$$G = \frac{V2 \times 0.0039}{D}$$

Where G = Force exerted by gravity.

V = Velocity of the vehicle in km/hour.

D = Stopping distance in metres.

0.0039 is a mathematical conversion factor. (If V is in mph and D is in feet, then C becomes 0.034). (iii) Tissue damage produced will depend upon the force applied per unit area both during acceleration and deceleration (iv) In frontal impact the vehicle does not arrest instantly but deforms from the front thus there is always a deceleration distance and time, however small. (v) $PS = \frac{1}{2} MV^2$, where

P = Deceleration force: This is the force acting on the person when brakes are applied and the speed of the vehicle starts decreasing.

S = Linear deceleration distance: This is the distance between the point when the brakes were first applied and the vehicle comes to a complete stop.

M = Mass of car.

V = Velocity of the car at the time of applying the brakes.

Primary Factors in Accidents

These factors are the most important ones in the causation of the accident. The factors can be both human as well as environmental.

Human factors: These are age, sex, educational status, medical conditions, fatigue, psychological factors and lack of body protection.

Environmental Factors

(i) *Relating to road:* Defective narrow roads, defective layout of cross roads and speed breakers, poor lighting, lack of familiarity. (ii) *Relating to vehicle:* Excessive speed, old and poorly maintained roads, large number of two or three wheelers, overcrowded buses, low driving standards. (iii) *Other factors:* Bad weather, inadequate enforcement of existing laws, mixed traffic (slow and fast moving, pedestrians, animals etc.). Both the human and environmental factor lead to increased vulnerability as well as risk situation leading to accidents.

Road Traffic Injuries

Large varieties of injuries are sustained by persons involved in traffic accident and by detailed examination of these injuries it is possible to reconstruct the accident. These may help in confirming or refuting the evidence of eyewitness. Further it may be possible to identify the hit and run accidents. The injuries can be:

Primary impact injuries (Figures 13.1 and 13.4): Primary impact injuries are the injuries caused to the first body part struck by the vehicle. In these injuries, the part of body involved, i.e., right or left side, front or back, depending upon the position of person in relation to vehicles when struck, i.e., whether crossing the road or walking with or against traffic. The injuries will be further modified depending on whether both feet are on the ground or one is raised and the firmness or otherwise of either or both feet. The relative heights of various parts of the vehicle, i.e., bumper, radiator, door handles etc. and the pattern of these parts of the vehicle if found on the body of the individual in the form of injuries help in identification of vehicle. For reconstruction of accident, it is better to discuss injuries only in relation to one type of motor vehicle as the models keep on varying all over the world and from year to year.

Secondary impact injuries: Secondary impact injuries are the ones caused by further impact by the vehicle (Figures 13.2 and 13.4).

Secondary injuries: These are injuries received by the victim on striking the ground (Figures 13.3 and 13.4).

If the person is struck from behind with the feet fixed, primary impact will be on the back of legs and fracture occurs if the feet are fixed. At the same time the buttocks and back will come in contact with the car and the person is pushed forward. It may cause fracture dislocation of lumbar or thoracic spine. If the person is struck from behind and feet slide forwards, the whole body may fall forwards and have a secondary impact of the head against the windshield, causing shattering of the wind shield and head injuries. Alternatively, the body may be thrown into air or to one side with resultant secondary injuries from striking the ground, i.e., on head and other parts of the body. If the person is facing the vehicle, he may receive intra-abdominal injuries and injuries to the chest wall. The victim may get injured from the bumper over the front of legs resulting in characteristic fracture of tibia, rarely fibula can be fractured or both of them can be fractured simultaneously **(bumper fracture).** The fracture fragments are wedge shaped and

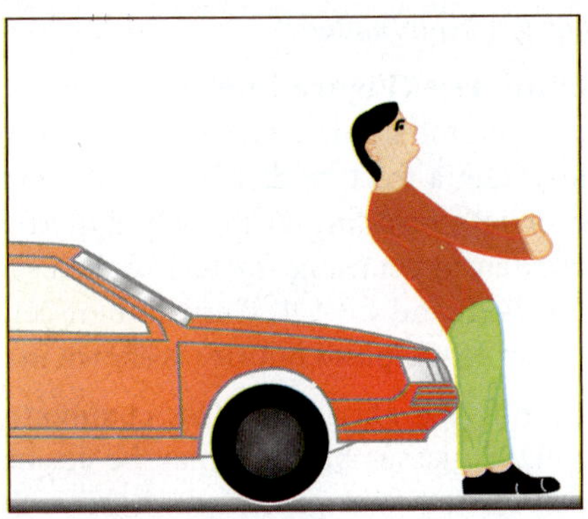

Figure 13.1: Pedestrian hit by a vehicle onto back of legs (Site of primary impact injuries)

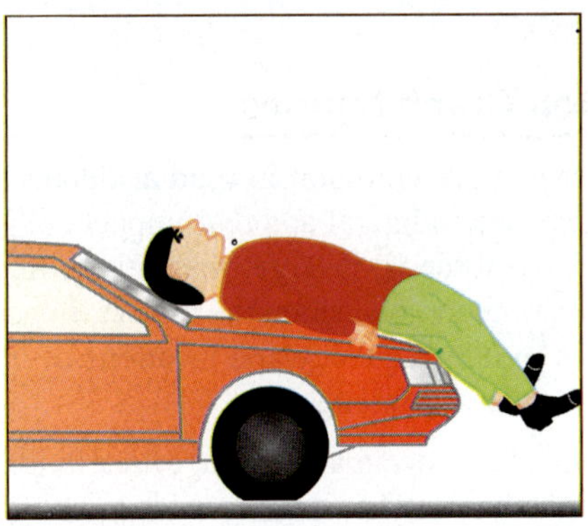

Figure 13.2: Pedestrian getting further hit by the vehicle (Site of secondary impact injuries)

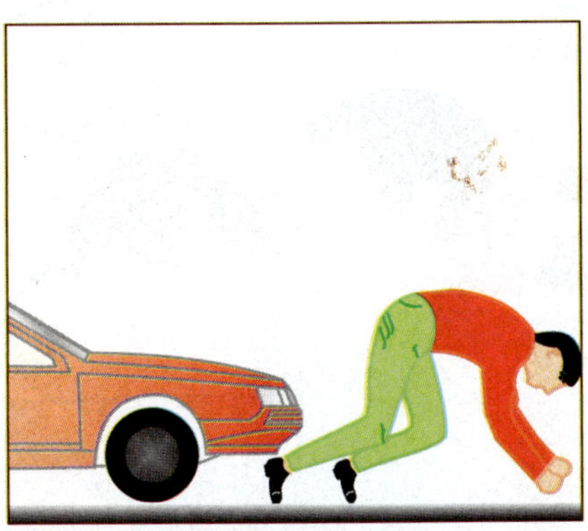

Figure 13.3: Pedestrian falling on the ground after getting hit by the vehicle (Site of secondary injuries)

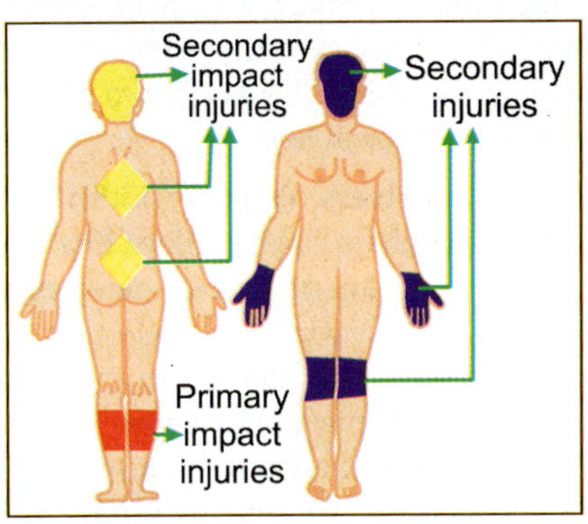

Figure 13.4: Sites of primary impact, secondary impact and secondary injuries

are displaced forwards. Frequently bumper injuries are present at different levels on the two legs or absent on one leg which suggest that the person was walking or running when struck. An impact against a mudguard or headlamp may result in a fracture of pelvis or fracture dislocation of sacroiliac joint.

If the person is struck on hip on its side, the initial impact will be against leg and produce bruises. However, the other injuries will depend if the foot was fixed or sliding forwards. Additional injuries like bruising of elbow and fracture of ribs may occur from striking the different parts of the vehicle. Victim will then receive secondary injuries on striking the ground. In a glancing blow from the side of a car in cases where driver attempts to avoid a direct impact, injuries to projecting parts of body such as elbow, shoulder or hips may take place. Penetrating or tearing wounds caused by protruding objects of the vehicle such as door handle etc. may occur. When the vehicle travels at a greater speed, the pedestrian may be thrown at height and fall on the vehicle roof and sometimes on the road behind the vehicle. In them the head is injured by direct impact with vehicle and by striking the road. Both impacts produce fracture involving almost all parts of the skull, especially those with underlying extensive injuries of the brain.

In road traffic accidents, the injuries are caused to the occupants while they are inside the vehicle **(non ejection crash injury)** or when thrown out of the vehicle **(ejection crash injury)** or both.

Non-Ejection Crash Injuries

Frontal impact is more common in road accidents, the occupant may also be exposed to lateral and rear impact collisions. During lateral impact, the force is of larger magnitude, for there is very little of the car structure to cushion the impact. In general, there is little difference in the frequency and locations of injury between rear seat and front seat passengers.

Injuries to vehicle occupants is important in identifying their positions in the vehicle at the time of accident including the driver and the persons in the front seat.

Injuries to front seat passengers: The front seat passengers are injured by the primary impact. The head, abdomen, knee and chest are injured. The head, knee and the chest are injured as they hit the steering wheel and the dashboard of the car while the abdomen is injured by the seat belt.

Injuries to car drivers (Figure 13.5): Driver has the advantage of a momentary appreciation that an accident is inevitable and he avoids full impact of steering wheel on the chest or of the head against windshield. He may sustain sprains or fractures of the wrist or if he attempts to apply brakes, fracture of femur or the pelvis takes place. Movement of the seat forwards and the steering wheel backwards may cause crush injuries, i.e., fracture of ribs and sternum, splitting of aorta, crushing of heart, liver, spleen, kidneys etc. Imprints of brake or accelerator pedal designs on the sole of driver's shoe may be found.

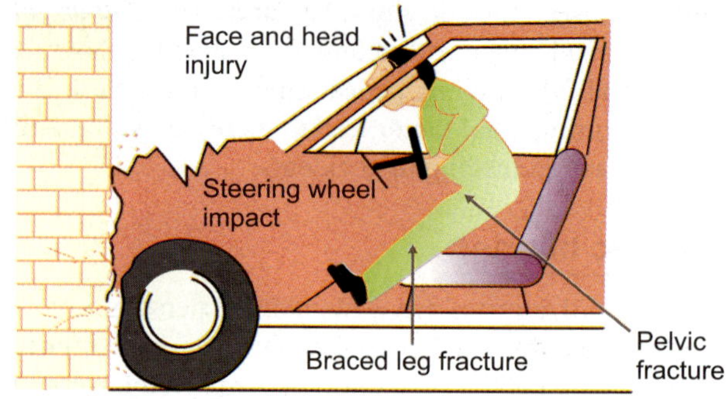

Figure 13.5: Various points of injury to unrestrained driver in deceleration impact

Driver may impact the chest on the steering wheel or the upper abdomen on the wheel rim leading to fracture of the sternum, laceration to heart and splitting of the aorta. Lung roots may be pressed against the wheel rim and may also crush the spine, liver, spleen or the kidney. The throat may be crushed by top of steering wheel. The head or face may impact on a shattering windscreen. In such cases, asphyxia may result by inhalation of blood. Whole of skull may be thrust down to cranial spine. Drivers or passengers may sustain 3 or 4 sliding forward motions off in seat and may also split one or both patellae or crush the knee joint and fracture femur or pelvis. If car overturns the person may be pinned to ground or crushed leading to traumatic asphyxia. He may be burnt or get asphyxiated.

Whiplash injuries (Figure 13.6): The driver and front seat passengers may split the head or face on a shattering windscreen and may even sustain a fracture dislocation of cervical vertebrae due to impact or jerk resulting in initially hyperflexion of neck and then hyperextension causing fracture of the cervical vertebra at the level of C2-C3 and C3-C4. Curvature of cervical spine at various speeds during whiplash injuries is shown in (Figure 13.7).

Injuries from flying glasses are less common due to use of safety by laminated glasses but face may be cut or damaged by impact. The risk of front seat passengers is more than drivers or back seat passengers.

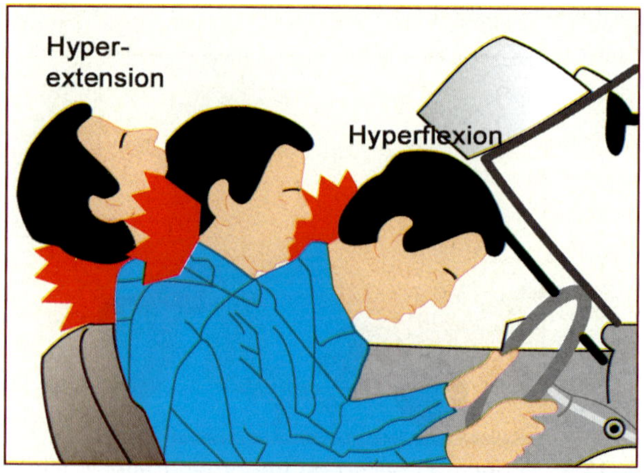

Figure 13.6: Mechanism of whiplash injury

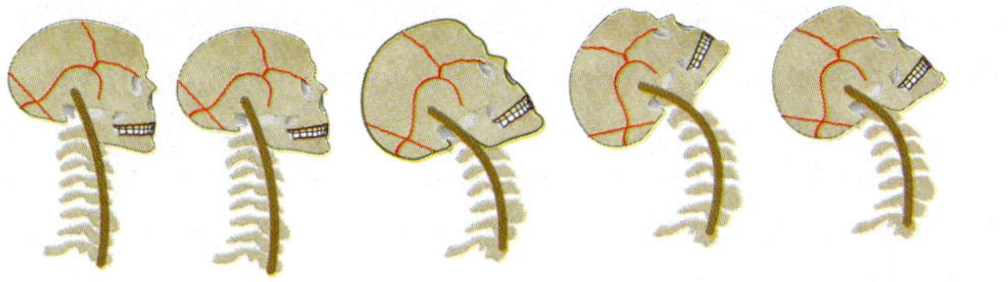

Figure 13.7: Curvature of cervical spine during whiplash injury

Injuries to back seat passengers: They receive the injuries due to striking the side, or top of the vehicle or back of the front seat.

Ejection Crash Injury

Ejection is second only to the steering wheel as a major cause of injury. Ejection is largely dependent on whether the door springs open at the time of crash. The door may open sometimes and person may fall out. This occurs most commonly in roll-over accidents. In ejection fatalities, one frequently encounters severe multiple injuries, any one of which may be responsible for death. Head alone or in combination with chest and abdomen is injured in 2 out of 3 cases. Chest and abdomen alone or in combination is seen in more than half the cases. Fracture of ribs is seen in 2/3rd of cases. Various ejection crash injuries are: (i) Fracture of ribs (66.6%) (ii) Laceration of liver (33%) (iii) Injury to soft tissues and other abdominal viscera (50%) such as heart, lungs, spleen or kidneys. Traumatic asphyxia can occur when vehicle overturns and the occupants may be pinned and crushed. Rarely occupants may be burnt or asphyxiated while in the interior of the car.

Injuries to Pedestrians

Pedestrian when hit by a car at speeds of over 23 km/hr can be scooped on the car and suffer from head injuries when hit against the windscreen and later fall off sideways (Figure 13.8). In addition, when a pedestrian is struck by the car, he may project forwards or is lifted onto the car (Figure 13.9). Both primary and secondary impact injuries occur as the person is thrown to ground or may be crushed and run over. Bumper of the car causes injuries below the knee, the radiator hits the pelvis and the abdomen is hit by the fender. It has been found that the pedestrians sustain fracture of legs in about 25% cases while in 40% cases there is injury to chest and abdomen. The fracture of ribs and injury to heart and lungs are the most common form of injuries.

Injuries to Bicyclist

If caused by an automobile, injuries may be similar to those sustained by a pedestrian except that the impact will be lower on the body or only against to some part of bicycle itself. The secondary injuries may be more severe due to greater distance to fall. When a person travels by a bicycle and is hit by a vehicle

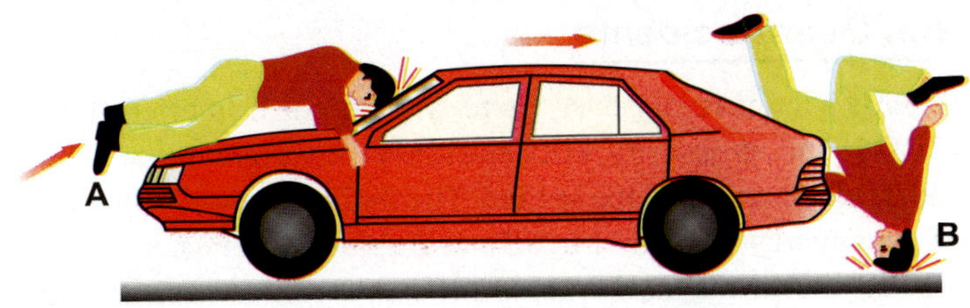

Figure 13.8: Pedestrian when hit by a car at speeds of over 23 km/hr can be (A) scooped on the car and suffer from head injuries when hit against the windscreen and later (B) fall off sideways

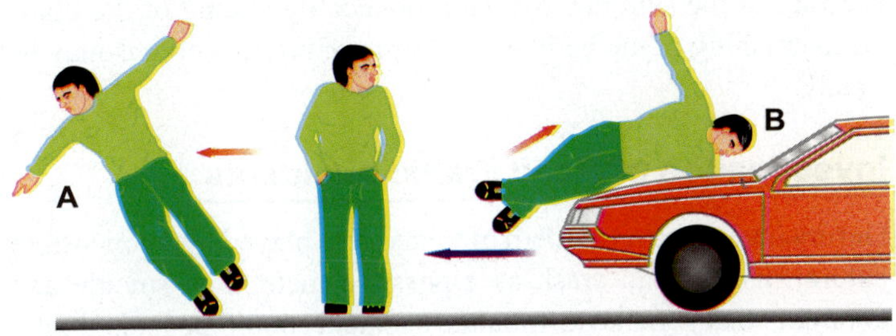

Figure 13.9: When a pedestrian is struck by the car, he may (A) project forwards or (B) lifted onto the car

fracture of bones, severe soft tissue injuries and bicycle spoke injury is produced particularly in children. Injuries due to running over may be present.

Injuries to Motorcyclists or Scooter Riders

Usually occurs by running in front of a vehicle from one side to other. The motorcycle is hit and the person is thrown violently on the ground. At times they are thrown beneath a vehicle and crushed like any pedestrian. These result in most of the cases from being struck with a motor vehicle. The primary and secondary impact injuries are seen similar to the pedestrian being hit by a vehicle. Secondary injuries will occur from striking the ground and on occasions being dragged with the vehicle. The same type of injuries are found in pillion passengers. Classical injury in motorcyclist and pillion passengers is fracture of skull usually from secondary impact on the ground. Temporal and parietal bone fracture, fracture of base of skull and contrecoup injury to the brain are seen. Temporoparietal fractures are common which usually extends across the base of skull through pituitary fossa. The transverse basal skull fracture across the floor of the skull especially a 'hinge' fracture is called **'the motorcyclist's fracture'**. Crash helmet reduces friction of head against the ground and although the head injuries may be less, there will be other effects such as broken neck or fractured ribs or limbs with internal visceral injuries. One type of injury peculiar to motorcyclists and scooter rider in collision with the rear of the truck when the vehicle will pass underneath the back but the head of rider impacts against the tailboard.

Run Over Accidents

When a victim is run over, there will be crush injuries (Figure 13.10A) and its severity will depend on the weight of the vehicle and its clearance from the ground. The findings would be presence of tyre marks (Figure 13.10B) and grinding abrasions. There will be skin avulsion, burning of the skin due to heat produced by sliding of the body, deep crushing of the trunk or limbs with rupture of internal organs, flattening deformities of the head, chest or pelvis. When a child is run over by a vehicle, fracture may not be produced due to elasticity of partly cartilaginous skeleton. Burning of the skin due to heat produced by sliding of the body. Deep crushing of the body with rupture of internal organs may be found.

Investigation of Road Traffic Accidents

During investigation, pattern of injury, role played by a concurrent natural disease and crash as a possible method of suicide and homicide that is made to simulate accident should be looked into. The role played by intoxicating drugs should also be analysed. The incidence of accidents resulting from the natural death of a sober driver has been estimated to be less than 6 per 100,000 motor vehicle collision. This possibility must be kept in mind where bodily injury is minimal or absent and damage to the vehicle is limited.

Hit and run: These cases require very thorough investigation of the scene as well as clothing worn by the victim (Figure 13.10C). Detection of patterned injuries, paint or metal fragments, grease, dirt or glass particles may provide the only evidence capable of leading to the identification of the responsible vehicle. More accurate information relating to mechanisms of injury will be obtained resulting from impact of human body upon the vehicle interior (or in case of pedestrians, the vehicle exterior).

Factors to be Investigated: (i) Pattern of injury and of death in various groups of road users. (ii) Time interval between accidents and death. (iii) Cause of injury in relation to specific parts of the vehicle. (iv) Direction in which force acts on the human body to produce injury. (v) Levels of human tolerance to dynamic loads applied to different parts of the body. (vi) Effectiveness of various safety design features in terms of reduction in frequency and severity of injury.

Procedure of accident injury investigation: It is the same for all classes of road users whether they be vehicle occupants or pedestrians or motorcyclists. Research team is interdisciplinary and consists of medical scientists, engineers, professional photographers etc. and it requires cooperation of hospitals, police, garages, motoring public etc. The standard procedure for investigation consists of: (i) Medical interview and medical examination of injured persons (ii) Follow-up study of vehicles (iii) Interview of police officers concerned with the accidents and other witnesses (iv) Writing up the accident in detail (v) Analyses of results when number of accidents reaches an adequate level.

Procedure of medical examination of casualties: (i) Undertaken usually in hospital (ii) Patient's informed consent is obtained (iii) Clinical and radiological findings are obtained (iv) All injuries are classified according to their severity as minor, moderate (v) Exact site of injuries and nature recorded on diagrams (vi) Colour photographic record made (vii) In case of fatalities, postmortem examination with details of all injuries, time elapsed between injury and death and an assessment of the cause/s of death are recorded. Follow-up study of vehicle: (i) Enquiry into accident and examination of the vehicles as it is necessary to reconstruct with reasonable accuracy the events of accident in relation to both the vehicle and movement of occupant. (ii) Whether using on the spot techniques or retrospective techniques, a three-phase investigation of the accident circumstances is undertaken. (iii) Reporting police officer and other witnesses are interviewed. (iv) Accident site is examined. (v) Vehicles are subjected to careful scrutiny.

Using retrospective techniques: Certain basic data can be obtained from reporting officers regarding the accident which will

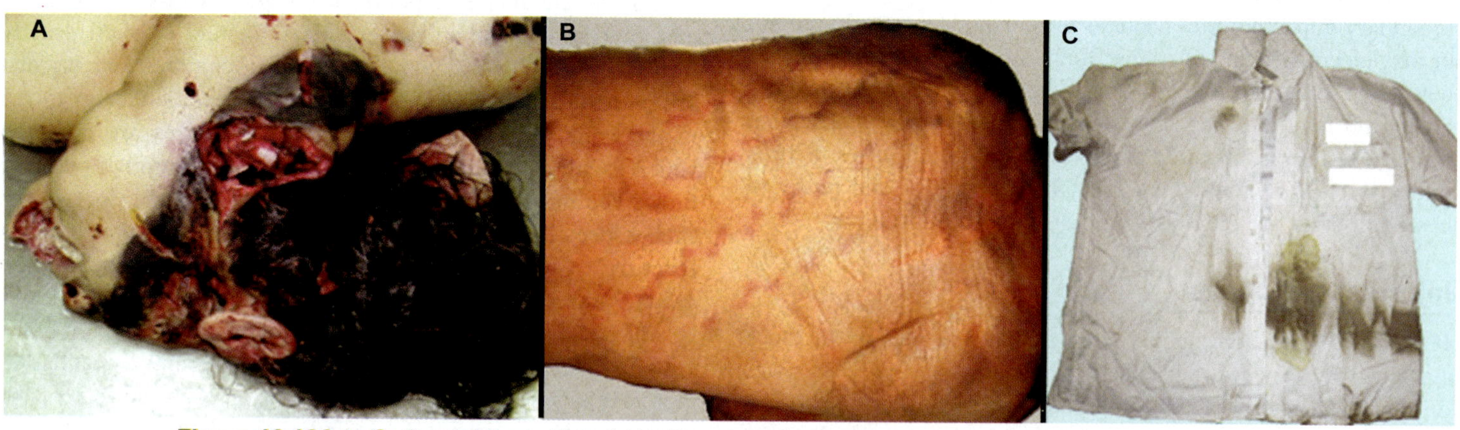

Figure 13.10A to C: Crush injury of head (A), Tyre mark back of trunk (B) and Grease mark over shirt (C)

include: (i) Directions in which various vehicles were traveling (ii) Final positions of vehicle after the accident (iii) Rough estimate of pre-accident speeds (iv) Evidence of ejection or trapping of occupants.

Examination of scene: It is useful for reconstruction of accident for interpretation of wounds and the mode of dying. Dragging marks, which are superficial and extensive, suggest that the victim had been dragged and is not ejected. Measurements of the leg fracture and other body injuries from the heel of the feet may help in identification of suspect vehicle in hit and run cases.

The bumper fracture may be compared with the suspected car by measuring the height of bumper from the road. Diagrammatic representation of injuries is quite useful. All injuries cannot be interpreted but patterned injuries should primarily be considered. Specimens should be collected for alcohol, barbiturates and antihistaminic drugs. Any foreign material like glass, paint or oil found on clothing, skin or the wound should be collected. The vehicle itself may give evidence of contact in the form of blood, flesh, hair, fragments of clothing, damage and signs of attempt to clean or repair.

Reconstruction of the crash: Overinterpretation of the postmortem findings is undesirable, since it must be remembered that it is usually impossible to attribute a specific causative mechanism to each and every injury on the victim's body. Patterned injuries by virtue of their location are vital to the accident reconstruction like the circular abrasion on the driver's chest or face from the impact on the steering column or steering wheel or the impact of the head light on the thigh of a pedestrian struck by an automobile. It is advisable to collect blood and urine samples for alcohol in vehicular accidents. A driver who is not a property controlled diabetic or epileptic or suffers from cardiac disease is potentially dangerous on the road. He is liable to unexpected impairment of consciousness. Also a driver who smokes more than 20 cigarettes in a day is considered to be living at a physiologic altitude of 8000 feet and impaired oxidation has striking effects on visual acuity at low levels of illumination.

Promotion of Safety Measures

For prevention of accidents, proper safety measures should be devised. If accident is a disease, education is a vaccine. Safety education must begin with students itself. Belief that accidents are inevitable must be curbed in the minds of drivers. Drivers should be trained for safe driving and proper maintenance of vehicle. Young people must be educated regarding risk factors, traffic rules, safety precautions and first aid.

Primary Preventive Measures

Primary preventive measures are devised to improve the driving condition and also to reduce the driving fatigue to avoid accidents. Primary care includes planning, organization, emergency care services for the trauma patient and management of trauma. Emergency care should begin at the accident site and anytime during transportation and should conclude in hospital emergency department.

Elimination of causative factors: Accidentology deals with accident research and involves gathering precise information about extent, type and other causes of accidents, seeking ways to make environment-evaluating efficiency of content. These include: (i) Investigating new and better methods of altering human behaviour (ii) Improvement of roads with better road designs for better safety (iii) Proper road lights to minimize accidents (iv) Imposition of speed limits (v) Marking of danger points (vi) Reduction of electric voltage (vii) Provision of fireguards (viii) Traffic lights and traffic signs should be visible from a distance and not be hidden behind a tree (ix) Self-diagnosing on board computers (x) Driver while driving should avoid talking on a cell phone. High volume music may divert attention. He should avoid talking to the other occupants.

Accidents are a matter of chance, safety is not. Thus, proper safety measures must be devised to minimize the chances of road traffic accidents. These can be broadly of three types: (i) ***Leather clothing and boots:*** Leather clothing reduces risk of extensive superficial soft tissue injury. Leather belts protect lower legs and feet from injuries. (ii) ***Child locks:*** Children should remain seated when they are in vehicle. They should be prohibited to take front seats of cars. Child locks should be present in the cars. There should be provision of central locking of all 5 doors. (iii) ***Electronic power steering:*** It uses less than half the power consumed by an ordinary power assisted steering. This steering does not suffer from loss of power assistance due to leakage. Electronic sensors in these provide varying levels of power assistance at different speeds for better maneuverability and greater control. These are electronically controlled and incorporates self-diagnosis in case of any problems.

Other measures include: (i) For total comfort of the driver and occupants, full flat reclining front seats as well as reclining rear seats should be there. (ii) Upright design, low side steps, high seats and wide opening doors for easy entry and exit. (iii) Better air-conditioning to reduce the fatigue of driving in temperate climates to minimize irritability arising out of heat and carbon monoxide emanating out. (iv) Bernoulli's flaps on the undersurface of cars makes it to be driven sticking to the undersurface. (v) Shock absorbers with wide diameter shockers struts allow to drive smoothly over the worst roads. (vi) Wide tread tyres ensures surest road grip and the safest drives. (vii) Power brakes and anti-lock brakes. (viii) Strengthened body shell. (ix) Antiglare windscreens, glasses and mirrors. (x) Large vertical headlamps, good quality headlights, improved design of tail lights and high quality wide windscreen. (xi) Improved engine design for smooth and effortless pickup. Besides these measures, new safety features are being introduced that include:

Lane departure warning system: This system warns drivers when they are about to leave a lane unintentionally.

Adaptive cruise control: This system prevents the driver from getting too close to the vehicle in front of them by applying brakes automatically if the distance is too little.

Pre-crash warning: This system detects a possible collision and warns the driver. If the driver fails to react, the advanced versions of the system can activate the brakes and even turn the steering wheel.

Secondary Preventive Measures

These are measures to reduce fatalities if accident has occurred. These are:

1. **Airbags and window bags:** These minimize the injuries to head and face in case of an accident.
2. **Collapsible and energy absorbing steering column:** These steering wheels collapse on impact thus minimizing steering wheel impact injuries to the chest and abdomen.
3. **Helmets:** Helmets in case of two wheelers minimizes the impact to head in case of an accident. Safety helmets reduce the risk of head injury by about 30% and reduces fatalities by about 40%. Helmet reduces friction of the head against the ground. It makes deceleration force less by allowing the protected head to skin across the ground rather than come to an abrupt halt. They prevent damage to scalp and skull fracture to a great extent. Full-face helmets are very popular among two-wheeler riders. Egg shelled helmet may lead to fracture of spine or strangulation by the strap. Occasionally when helmet is pinned or crushed, the chin strap may be drawn upwards and cause strangulation.
4. **Seat belts:** These reduce the number of fatalities and non-fatal injuries by about 50%. In India, they have been made compulsory for all four-wheelers. These are of following types (Figure 13.11): (i) *Safety belts 1 or 2 point:* Almost all of these are lap-strap and shoulder diagonal type. Diagonal only type has a disadvantage of slipping out from the hold and causes whiplash injuries. Simple lap-strap can be dangerous to aorta and they are now fitted in aircrafts only. (ii) *3 point safety belt:* They provide for a better hold and avoid the impact of driver or other occupant to the front in case of sudden deceleration. (iii) Other are diagonal plus lap strap types that are commonly used in cars. (iv) There are shoulder harness and crotch strap that are more complex types and are fitted only in light aircrafts, gliders and racing cars. The seat belts: (a) Hold the occupants back against the seat thus preventing the forward projection against steering wheel, windscreen and corner "A" frame. Thus, head is prevented from smashing through the glass. (b) Restraints the occupants within the vehicle preventing ejection during bursting opening of the door thus preventing serious injury and death. (c) Extend the deceleration time and distance by substantial stretching of the fabric of belt which lengthens a few centimeters during a violent arrest.

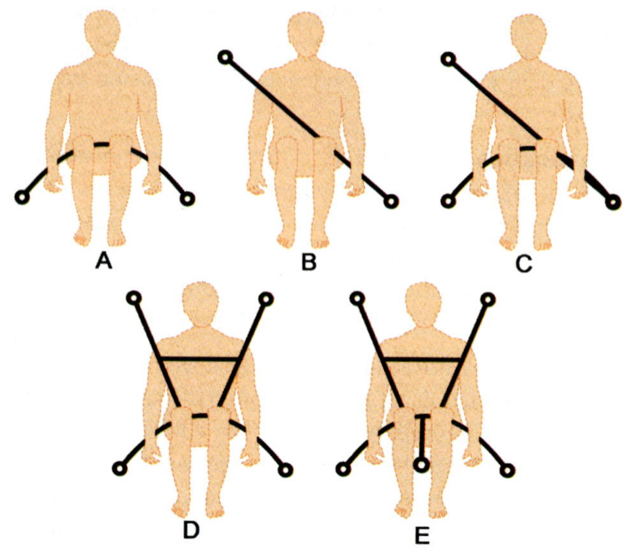

Figure 13.11: Different types of seat belts (A) Simple lap strap (B) Sash strap (C) Three-point (D) Shoulder harness (E) Five-point harness

Seat belt syndrome: With abrupt deceleration, the seat belt compresses the contents of the abdominal cavity and ruptures the musculature of abdominal cavity and often of left hemidiaphragm. The shear forces applied against adjacent structures lead to the bowel injury. Such forces cause bowel transection, particularly near points of fixation, such as iliocaecal valve and the **ligaments of trietz.** Perforation of ileum, caecum and sigmoid colon is common due to compression of intra-abdominal viscera. Presence of abdominal wall contusion associated with paralytic ileus should raise a suspicion of significant intra-abdominal injury. Also fracture of lumbar spine results. The injuries caused by the seat belt depend upon the type of belt present: (i) *Lap belt:* It causes injury to the lumbar spine, spleen, pancreas, uterus, urethra and iliac artery. (ii) *Shoulder restraints:* If shoulder restraints are used then various injuries occur such as fracture of the ribs, cervical spine, lumbar spine and sternum. Deep organ lesions involving the larynx, liver, spleen and kidney can be found. (iii) *Three point belts:* They cause a pattern of injuries which includes fracture of ribs, sternum and clavicle. Abdominal injury leading to jejunal or duodenal perforation is seen. Contusions and abrasion on the chest, shoulder, neck and back may also be seen underlying the position of the seat belt.

Other preventive measures: (i) High penetration resistant windscreen glass. (ii) Sturdy design of vehicle to absorb front and rear impact through crumple zones. (iii) Side impact beams and bars in front and rear door to take up the impact. (iv) Anti-roll bars are net like pillar or strongholds in case of rolls during accidents and prevent the collapse of whole structure. (v) Laminated windshields are designed to prevent the shredding of glass in case of impact and if it displaces then it gets stick to the place only. (vi) Fire proof paints and upholstery prevents fire from spreading.

(vii) Trail hazing head lamp technology. (viii) High beam assist. (ix) Personalized voice safety alerts. (x) Powered drivers' seat with memory. (xi) Anti-lock braking system (ABS) with electronic break distribution (EBD). (xii) Tyre pressure monitor. (xiii) Front and rear parking sensor. (xiv) 360° cameras with bling spot monitoring. (xv) Electronic stability control. (xvi) Driver fatigue warning. (xvii) Advanced driver assistance system. (xviii) Rear cross traffic alert and avoidance technology. (xiv) Automatic emergency braking. (xv) Forward collision warning. (xvi) Lane keep assist and departure prevention.

Tertiary Measures

These include enabling speedy salvage and rescue in case of accidents using cellular phones, audio system, global positioning system and computers.

Medicolegal Aspects of Road Traffic Accident

Most of the accidental deaths are caused by automobiles but it may be occasionally used to commit crime like planned killing, accident faked to conceal crime, victim killed by other means and thrown on the road or victim killed by other means and dead body burnt in a car. Suicide with automobile is difficult to prove but following events may be useful: (i) History of previous suicidal attempts and recent threat to commit suicide (ii) History of depression recently or in the past (iii) History of domestic quarrels or financial crisis (iv) Evidence of speeding (v) Impact with a tree or bridge usually on the front of vehicle in its center (vi) Single occupancy of the car (vii) Absence of evidence of applying brakes (viii) Recovery of suicidal note (ix) Imprint of the gas pedal pattern on the driver's shoe sole and the absence of skid marks leading to the site of collision are believed by some to be suggestive of suicide, because they indicate that the driver was accelerating his vehicle at the time of impact.

Natural death at the wheel versus death from injuries: Natural disease like coronary artery disease may lead to an accident and sudden unexpected death of a driver. Driver suffering from uncontrolled diabetes or epilepsy is a potential danger on the road. In case of pedestrians, cardiovascular diseases, cerebrovascular diseases, poor vision or impaired hearing may all lead to accidents. In these cases, only a complete autopsy can provide a right answer as to whether the persons died of accidental injuries or naturally. Sometimes death occurs after a considerable time lapse. After examination of injuries it is important to give opinion in such cases whether the death was entirely natural or directly or indirectly related to injuries specially if injuries were minor.

Alcohol and other drugs: Alcohol impairs driving ability and increases the risk of an accident as well as severity of its consequences. Alcohol is the direct cause of 30-50% of road traffic accidents. Though the legal limit is 30 mg % in India but impairment can result at blood level of 50 mg % and accident risk increases at 50-80 mg % level. Drugs like barbiturate, amphetamines and cannabis impair driving ability.

Driving under the influence of drugs or alcohol or both remains a major socioeconomic problem in modern society. Drug use should be considered when driver's behavior is suggestive of alcohol consumption but tests of his blood or breath for alcohol are negative. This particular category of driver should be tested by standard methods of drug screening for barbiturates, amphetamines or other drugs that might explain the disorderly behaviour. The alcohol intoxication contributes to a traffic fatality both by impairing judgment, coordination and vision before the accident and by interfering with the evaluation and interfere with the treatment of injuries sustained at the time of crash. The most important investigation in road accidents is the determination of the degree of intoxication present. The concentration of blood alcohol should always be determined in the driver of a vehicle, in the pedestrian injured or killed in the accident and in the passenger of the vehicle involved with accident.

LONG QUESTIONS

1. Discuss the various types of injuries sustained by a pedestrian in vehicular accidents.
2. Discuss the modern safety measures in the vehicles.
3. How you will proceed to investigate the vehicular accidents along with the reconstruction of the scene?

SHORT QUESTIONS

1. Different types of seat belts.
2. Seat belt syndrome.

MULTIPLE CHOICE QUESTIONS

1. Bumper fracture mostly involves:

(a) Tibia and fibula
(b) Pelvis bone
(c) Fracture dislocation of C5-C6 vertebra
(d) Fracture dislocation of C6-C7 vertebra

2. Motorcyclist's fracture is a:

(a) Depressed fracture of frontal bone of skull
(b) Hinge fracture of base of skull
(c) Comminuted fracture of skull
(d) Fracture dislocation of C6-C7 vertebra

ANSWER KEY ☞

1. (a)	2. (b)

14 CHAPTER

Firearm Injuries

Firearm: It is any instrument or device that propels a projectile by the expansile force of the gases generated by combustion of an explosive substance. These are arms of any description designed or adapted to discharge a projectile or projectiles of any kind by the action of any explosive or other forms of energy.

Forensic ballistics: It is the science concerned with the investigation of firearms, ammunition and problems arising from their use. It is divided into:

Interior ballistics: It is the study of forces of propulsion within the firearm.

Exterior ballistics: It is the study of flight of projectile after its exit from the firearm.

Terminal or wound ballistics: It is the study of the interaction of the projectile with the target.

Classification of Firearm Weapons

1. **According to the condition of barrel:**
   (a) *Smooth bore (Shotguns):* (i) Single barreled (ii) Double barreled (iii) Slug shot gun (iv) Pump action.
   (b) *Rifled weapons:* (i) Long barrel (Semi rifle, shoulder rifle) (ii) Short barrel rifles and Hand guns (<22" Carbine, >22" Pistol and revolver) (iii) Machine guns.
   (c) *Country made firearms* (*katta* or improvised firearms): They are mostly 12 bore smooth guns.
   (d) *Air rifle and pistols.*
2. **According to the muzzle velocity:**
   (a) Low velocity (Up to 1200 ft/s).
   (b) Medium velocity (Between 1200-2500 ft/s).
   (c) High velocity (more than 3000 ft/s).

Parts of Firearm Weapons

In general, a firearm consists of:

1. **Barrel:** It is a long hollow steel cylinder in which the propellant charge is placed. It is long in rifles and shot guns and short in revolvers and pistols. The lumen is known as **bore.** The rear end where the cartridge is inserted is known as the **breech end** and the front end where the bullet comes out is the **muzzle end.** The guns in which the missiles are loaded at the breech end is known as **breech loaders**. Most of the modern weapons are of this type but in those firearms where missiles are loaded at the muzzle end as known as **muzzle loaders**. These weapons are of primitive variety and are rarely found nowadays. The breech end may have a chamber to accommodate the cartridge and may carry an extractor to help in removing the cartridge case after firing.
2. **Action:** This consists of a bolt, a striker or hammer and a trigger. The breech block is a metal which seals the breech end of the barrel when the firearm is closed. It can be reopened to insert a new cartridge. It is generally pierced in its centre to accommodate the **firing pin.** The trigger is a lever that is situated below the block and is operated by a finger pressure.

3. **Grip or butt:** This is the part of the gun which is normally gripped in the hand in the long barreled weapons. The butt is elongated and is shaped to fit against the shoulder. However, in hand guns this part is gripped in hand. A **magazine** is a spring loaded container carrying a number of cartridges. It is attached to the forestock of rifle, carried as a tubular magazine in a repeating shot gun and lodged in a grip of a pistol.

Mechanism of Operation

The operating mechanism is almost same in most of the firearms. Usually a firearm is first loaded then cocked and lastly fired, when the trigger is pulled. This releases a firing pin which strikes the percussion cap and detonates the chemicals in the primer. The detonation of the primer ignites the main propellant charge after passing through the vent and results in rapid formation of expanding hot gases at a very high pressure. The pressure of these gases rises up to the maximum and forces the missile out of the barrel with high velocity. At the same time the base of the cartridge case is forced backward against the breech block.

The velocity of the missile as it comes out of the muzzle end known as **muzzle velocity** depends upon many factors like amount of powder, bullet weight, the accuracy with which the projectile is sealed and amount of combustion of the powder. The velocity gradually decreases as it strikes the target which is known as **striking velocity.** The release of the projectile is accompanied by some amount of flame, hot gases, soot particles, unburnt grains of powder, grease and wadding. The fire cartridge case that is emptied after firing is left which has to be removed manually or automatically ejected.

Range of the Firearm

It is the distance where the energy or area of presentation of the missile drops to such a value as to be ineffective for penetration into the human body. In shotguns, it is about 40 yards whereas in rifled firearms it is up to 2000 mts. However, variations do exist in the range.

Improvised or country-made firearm *(Desi Katta):* These are firearms made out of steel tubes and mostly smooth 12 bored unlicensed weapons used by criminals in India. The muzzle velocity in a country-made firearm weapon is about 500 feet/ seconds.

Smooth Bore Weapons (Shotguns)

In smooth bored weapons, the bore or the inner surface of the barrel is uniformly smooth. The projectile in shotgun may be either a single pellet or pellets. Shotgun has a barrel length of 55-72 cm. They are effective up to 30-40 yards.

Types of shotguns (Figure 14.8): Shotguns are divided into the following types depending on the length of the barrel, the loading and the number of barrels: (a) (i) Long barreled (Musket) (ii) Short barreled (Carbines), (b) (i) Muzzle loading (ii) Breech loading, (c) (i) Single barreled (ii) Double barreled (iii) Multi-barreled (iv) Pump action (v) Slug shot gun. In majority of cases, shotguns are double barreled with two barrels placed side by side.

Paradox gun: It is firearm having initial part of barrel as smooth while last part (muzzle end) as riffled.

Gauge or Bore

It is measured by internal dimension of the barrel and is given in decimals of inch or millimeters. The bore of a smooth bore weapon is measured in this way up to 1.27 cm. For larger bore, the size can be determined by the total number of lead balls made out of one pound (454 grams) of lead that fits the barrel. In England and USA barrel diameter is measured in inches and in Europe in millimeters.

Twelve bore gun: It is the gun whose diameter is same as that of a ball of lead of such a size that 12 lead balls are made from one pound of lead that fits into the barrel; = 0.729 inch = 18.52 mm.

Choking

The terminal few centimeters of the bore near the muzzle end is slightly constricted in some of the shotguns. The degree of constriction is in thousands of an inch and the degree of choking may be as shown below. Choking varies from full choke (minimum dispersion) to true cylinder (maximum dispersion).

Degree of choke	% pellets that would remain inside a 30-in circle at 40 yds	Constriction in	
		Inch	mm
Full choke	70%	0.04	1.00
Three quarter choke	65%	0.03	0.75
Half choke	60%	0.02	0.50
Quarter choke	55%	0.01	0.25
Improved cylinder	50%	0.0003-0.0005	0.075-0.125
True cylinder	40%	0	0

Choking of the smooth bored weapons lessens the spread of shot, enhances the explosive force and increases the velocity of the shot and thus increases the range.

Rifled Firearms

Rifled firearms have 2-20 spiral grooves at the inner side of the barrel usually 6 in number. Rifle is a gun with long barrel and the bore varies from 5.6 to 7.7 mm (0.22 to 0.303 inch) decimal of an inch. The range of firing is about 1000 metres.

Caliber is the distance between two opposite lands as shown in the Figure 14.1.

Advantages of rifling: (i) It gives spin in its long axis (ii) To impart rotatory motion to the bullet (iii) It increases the power of penetration (iv) Prevents from wobbling when travels in the air (v) Stabilizes the bullet (vi) Ensures greater accuracy and longer range.

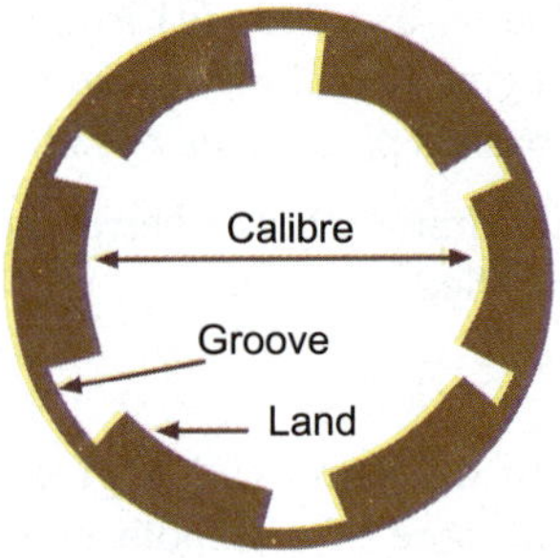

Figure 14.1: Cross-section of rifled firearm showing lands and grooves

Classification of Rifled Firearms

Shoulder rifles: These can be of following types depending on the manner in which the action operates a cartridge in the chamber for firing (i) Slide action (ii) Bolt action (iii) Lever action (iv) Semiautomatic.

Hand guns: These are fired from the hands: (i) *Pistols:* Cartridge is directly loaded into the chamber by a magazine. In the pistols, single shot is discharged repeatedly (Figure 14.3). (ii) *Revolvers:* This can be used with one hand. The cylindrical magazine rotates immediately in rear of the barrel. It has rotating cylinders or drum that has 5-9 chambers from which the cartridges are fired. Each cartridge is in a separate chamber (Figure 14.2 and Figure 14.4).

Automatic guns: These will continue firing repeatedly as long as the trigger is held back. Machine guns are truly automatic guns. These continue to fire through the action of gases of previous explosion and of ejector and recoil spring.

Semiautomatic guns: These are self loading guns in which discharge is utilized for ejecting the fired cartridge case, reloading and for cocking the action so that the weapon is automatically rendered ready to fire again. The trigger is pressed anew for every shot that is fired. A magazine of 6-14 cartridges are used depending upon the model and the caliber.

Military rifles: Muzzle velocity is 800 meters/second, killing range is 3000 meters and the bullet rotates at about 3000 revolutions/second. A service rifle needs about 5 pounds of pressure to release the pin whereas revolver needs 3 to 5 pounds of pressure to release the pin. The shape, weight, muzzle velocity and the medium through which the bullet passes determines its range and the effect on the target. There cannot be accidental discharge as safety catch locks the trigger. Different countries have different types of service rifles with magazines and bolt actions of varied forms.

Air pistols and Air rifles: In these weapons compressed air is used to fire lead slugs. In some of the weapons liquid CO_2 is used as propellant. Here the mass of the pellet and velocity is low and usually minor injuries are caused. Serious injuries can be caused at short range. The missile is single and fired with a rifled barrel. They are usually regarded as safe weapons. However, the modern air rifles can fire a bullet up to .22 with accuracy up to ranges of at least 50 yards.

Pen guns: These are used in teargases but can be modified to fire ordinary cartridge.

Zip guns: It is crude home-made rifled firearm that is used to fire single shot.

Stud guns: These guns are used to fire metals studs into wood, concrete or steel.

Common features of a riffled firearm shown in Figure 14.5.

Primers

The purpose of the primer is to ignite the powder or propellant charge. Primers are ignited by impact of gun's firing pin. These are small metal cups containing the priming mixture. Primer cups contain priming mixture and an anvil are so placed that blow of the firing pin on the primer cup crushes the priming compound (lead peroxide, lead Styphnate and barium nitrate) against the anvil center and ignites it which then flashes through the **flash hole** (vent) and ignites the powder charge.

Shotgun cartridge consists of the following as shown in the Figure 14.6: (i) Retaining cardboard disc (ii) Shots (iii) Cardboard disc (iv) Felt wads (v) Cardboard disc (vi) Propellant charge (Black, smokeless and semi-smokeless powders) (vii) Primer battery cup consists of mixture of lead peroxide and barium nitrate and the anvil (viii) Rim of metal cylinder (ix) Percussion cap.

Cartridge of rifle consists of metal cylinder with a flat base. The base has a projecting rim which are known as **rimmed cartridges** used in revolvers. Rimless cartridges are used in pistols. Detonator cap acts as an igniter that fits in a circular hole in the center in cases of center fire cartridges. Detonating composition could be in the rim in rimfire cartridges like in revolvers (Figure 14.7). Distant end of the cylinder lightly fits into the bullet which has a core of lead or lead alloy with outer hardened envelop of steel or brass with a thin cuprous-nickel coating or aluminum. The propellant charge is between detonator cap and bullet.

Bullets

Traditional bullets are made of soft metal like lead and antimony is added to provide hardness. Those usually known as round nose soft bullets are used in rifles and revolvers. The bullet is short and round in pistols and revolvers and elongated with pointed ends in rifles. Various types of bullets are (Figure 14.9):

Jacketed bullets: These are of two types: (i) *Full metal jacket bullet:* A tough, heavy jacket covers all but the base where soft exterior is exposed. The tough jacket is made of steel, copper, nickel and zinc. (ii) *Semi-jacketed bullet:* It is provided with a relatively thin but tough jacket which covers the base and cylindrical portion of the bullet leaving the nose partly or fully exposed.

Mushroom bullets: These bullets are more serious types of semi-jacketed bullets, which are meant to expand like mushroom on impact due to the soft nose, which is not jacketed.

Dum Dum bullets: These types of bullets are open at the base but the point is covered with the jacket. When it strikes

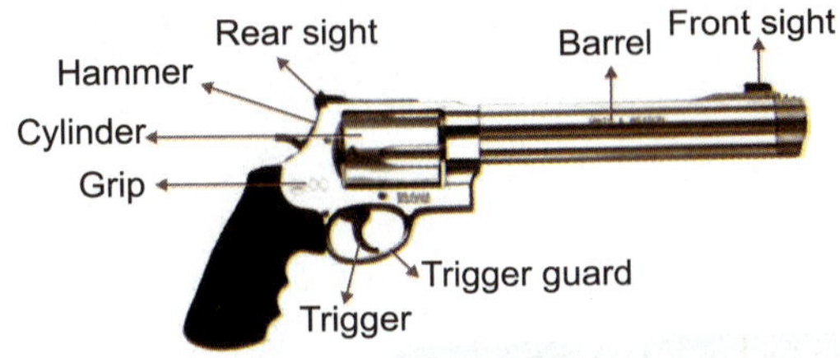

Figure 14.2: Different parts of revolver

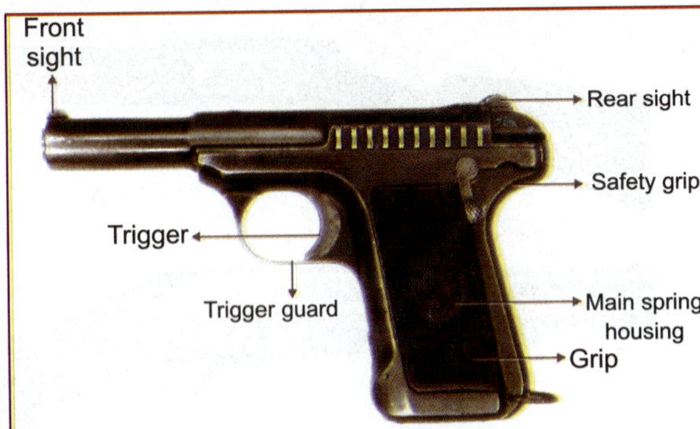

Figure 14.3: Different parts of pistol

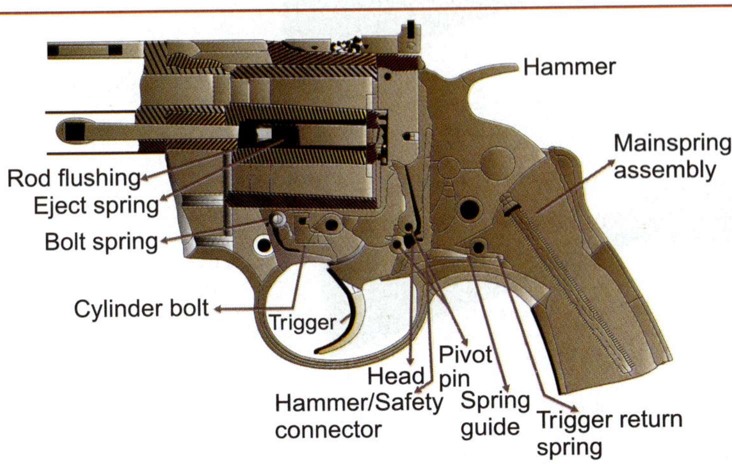

Figure 14.4: Inside view of a revolver

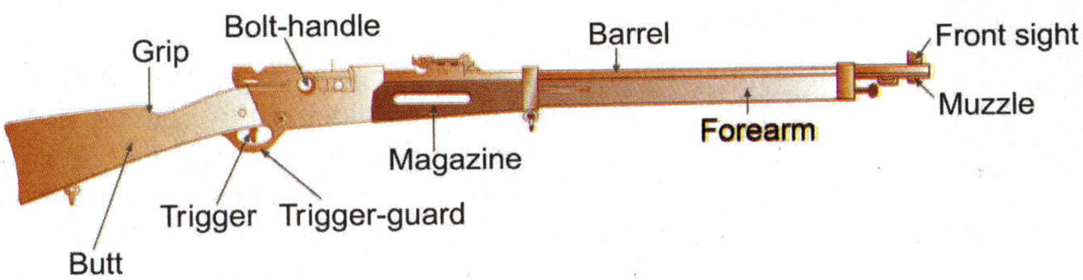

Figure 14.5: Different parts of rifle

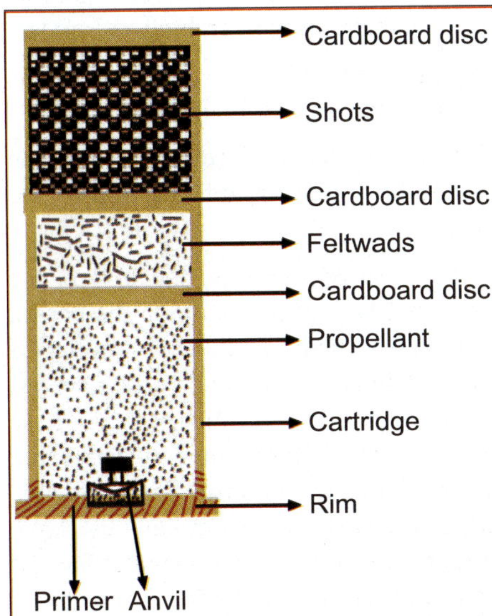

Figure 14.6: Different parts of shotgun cartridge

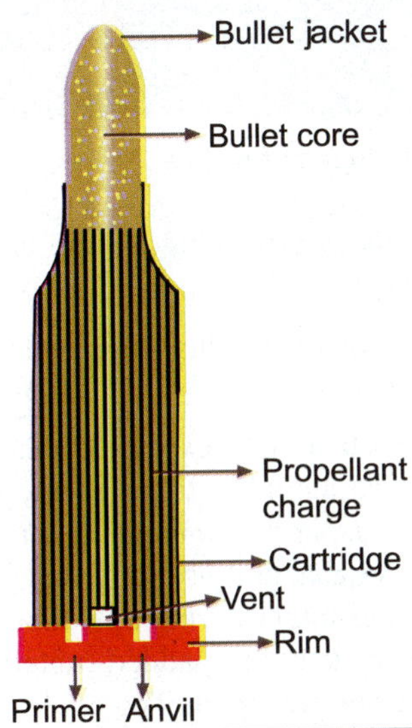

Figure 14.7: Different parts of cartridge of a rifled firearm weapon

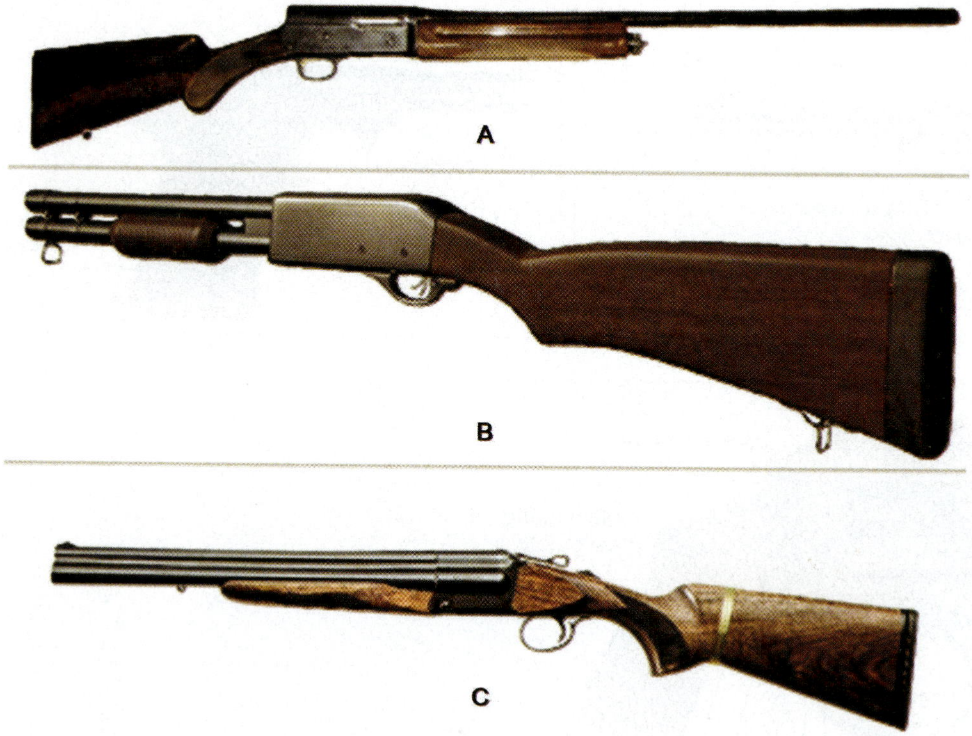

Figure 14.8A, B, C: Shotgun single barreled (A), Double barreled (B) and Triple barreled (C)

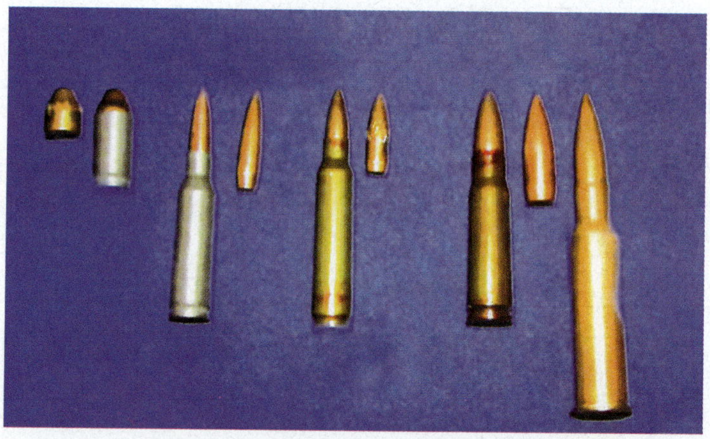

Figure 14.9: Different types of bullets

an object the lead at the point expands producing a large entry wound. They are not in use nowadays.

Frangible bullets: They are made of iron that fragments on impact and completely disintegrates.

Explosive bullets: These are filled with explosive charge and may explode while handling; care should be taken at autopsy if these bullets are expected. Ultrasound technique must be avoided. The doctor should wear goggles and use long handled instruments to manipulate the missiles either during operation or autopsy. The removed bullet should be kept in a padded container to protect it from excess impact during transport. The explosive bullets produce a greater destruction of the tissues because of the fragmentation of the bullets so the wound produced is larger than the usual one.

Plastic bullets: These are plastic cylinder of PVC (Polyvinyl chloride), 38 mm in diameter, 10 mm long and weighs about 135 gram. It is fired from a smooth bore weapon and the effective range is about 50 to 60 meters. They are used for riot control but may cause serious injuries if hit from near distance. They cause fracture of the skull, damage to eyes and even fracture of the limb bones and ribs depending upon the distance from which it is fired. It can also cause contusion and laceration of liver, lung and spleen.

Crime bullet: Any type of bullet found in the body of the victim is kept as evidence and is known as crime bullet.

Test bullet: This is the bullet that is fired from the same weapon that has been used for committing the crime for comparison with the crime bullet.

Primary markings: In all rifled firearms, the bullets are slightly larger than the barrel and as it passes through the barrel, its sides are marked by the rifling pattern (calibre, number of lands and grooves, direction of twist of the lands and grooves, and widths of the lands and grooves) of the barrel. These markings on the bullet which are called **class characteristics** that may indicate the make and model of the firearm. If an evidence bullet and test bullets fired from a suspect firearm have the same class characteristics, the firearm examiner can conclude that the evidence bullet could have been fired from the suspect firearm.

Secondary markings: While passing through the barrel of the rifled firearms, the surface of the bullet is also grooved by the random imperfections and irregularities on the inner surface of the barrel itself producing **individual characteristics**. These irregularities are due to adherence of the particles of the bullet to the bore when the shots are fired and results during manufacturing process. These markings are caused by **metallic fouling**.

Comparison microscope is used for comparing the crime bullet and the test bullet for the primary and secondary marking. If an evidence bullet has the same class characteristics and matching individual characteristics as test bullets fired from a suspect firearm, it can be concluded that the bullet was fired from the suspect firearm.

Powders (Propellant Charge)

The word 'powder' means dry particles reduced to fine dust. The gun powders used in various ammunitions are not fine dust particles but granular. These are of the following types:

Black powder: Black powder comprises (i) Potassium nitrate (60-75%) (ii) Sulphur (10-20%) (iii) Charcoal (2-8%). Powder grains are black, coarse and fine. It burns with production of much heat, flame and smoke. One gram of powder forms 3000-4500 cc of gas that is CO_2, CO, N_2, H_2S, hydrogen and methane all at a very high temperature. The granulation size of the black powder controls the degree of its strength and speed of burning. Large grains of black powder are much harder to ignite than fine grains. It is designated as FG, FFG, FFFG depending on the size of grains and more the number of 'F' more finer are the powder grains. Fine grains travel up to 60-90 cms or more.

Smokeless powder: It comprises either:

i. **Single base** contains nitrocellulose or gun cotton.
ii. **Double base** contains both nitrocellulose and nitro-glycerine.
iii. **Triple base** contains nitrocellulose, nitroglycerine and nitroguanidine and 1 gm of powder yields 12,000-13,000 c.c. of gas.

Nitrocellulose is a powerful explosive that is formed by the action of nitric and sulphuric acid on cotton or any other cellulose. It is a granular powder coated with graphite giving it a dark gray colour. Nitroglycerine is colourless, oily liquid and is one of the strongest known explosives.

Semismokeless powder: It is comprised 80% black powder and 20% smokeless powder.

Examination of the Scene of Crime in Firearm Deaths

The following points should be noted while examination of the scene of crime in firearm deaths: (i) Handle the body as little as possible. (ii) Hands should never be tried to be opened with force. (iii) Fingerprints should never be taken at the scene as this may result in wiping out of the fibers, hairs and powders from the fingers and introduction of some new materials. (iv) Police officers often handle the firearm weapons with their hands which may get contaminated with primer residue; barium or lead. (v) Before transportation of the body to the mortuary, paper bags should be placed over the hands to prevent loss of trace evidence. Plastic bags should not be used as condensation of moisture will occur in the refrigerator which will wash away the residue and may make fingerprints more difficult to obtain. Whole body should be wrapped so that there is no loss of trace evidence and contamination is avoided by the transporting vehicle. (vi) Sketch of the site and the body should be drawn and photographs should be taken. (vii) Before the autopsy examination, clothes should not be removed. (viii) Radiological examination is done for locating the bullet or pellets. (ix) Wounds should not be probed as this may lead to the formation of false track. (x) Radiopaque dye is poured into the wound and X-ray is taken to know about the track of the bullet. (xi) To recover primer residue from the hands, swabs moistened in acid or by using adhesive material should be used. (xii) Any other trace evidence recovered from the body or the site should be properly preserved. (xiii) After all this, fingerprints should be taken. (xiv) Clothing is now examined. (xv) Photographs should be taken showing the relationship of the body with the other landmarks. A close up view is then taken and most people prefer to take a third view also in between the other two. (xvi) In doubtful cases wounds should be excised and retained for analysis either by EDX or FAAS. (xvii) Bullet should be handled carefully with a cotton wool pack during autopsy in order to avoid making extra markings or fingerprints.

Handling of the Body After the Examination of the Scene

Examination of clothing: (i) Body should be disrobed with care. (ii) Clothing should not be torn or cut. (iii) Try to find out the bullets, if any in the clothing. Then the number and location of bullet holes in clothes is described in relation to the distance from the collar, seams, pockets etc. Several holes may result from a single bullet due to presence of creases in the garment there by simulating more than one shot. (iv) Findings of evidence of close range firing should be looked for. (v) Extent of soot and gunpowder distribution should be noted as this helps to compare with test shot pattern to evaluate the distance. (vi) Size of shot in the garment and whether the fibers of fabric are inwards or outwards should be noted. (vii) All the injuries, condition and extent of bleeding from them should be noted. (viii) Photography of pertinent findings is often helpful but does not replace a good description. (ix) Clothing should be dried, sealed and handed over to the police for laboratory analysis.

Autopsy Examination

In addition to general information that is applicable to every autopsy protocol, in a victim of gunfire the following observations should be included: (i) Description of clothing should be given detailing the tear over the clothing corresponding to the body injuries. (ii) Pertinent findings regarding bullet wounds should be noted. Their appearance should be described in detail for easy correlation with the bullet recovered and fixing up of responsibility. (iii) The autopsy surgeon should recover the bullet from the body preferably with gloved hand and no sharp/pointed instruments not to be used for handling of bullet. Scratching to the bullet should be avoided as subsequent examination of it helps in firearm identification. (iv) Samples should be kept for toxicological analysis when coexistent poisoning is suspected. (v) Blood on gauze piece should be preserved for blood grouping and cross-matching. (vi) Hand washings should be kept in saline soaked cotton swabs for evaluating gunpowder residues. (vii) Opinion regarding cause and time of death should be given.

Autopsy file should also include adequate police report with a concise description of the scene where the body was found with the help of the photographs and sketches.

Pertinent findings regarding bullet wounds: (i) Note the number of entrance and exit wounds and grazes (ii) All the wounds should be numbered (iii) Location of wound from a fixed landmark should be described (iv) Sketch and photographs should be taken.

External evidence of injuries: (i) Wounds are to be described regarding their shape; satellite, oval, round, slit like or jagged (ii) Size and site of abrasion collar to be noted (iii) Wounds are never incised until the measurements are taken.

Internal evidence of injuries: (i) Describe wound track in anatomical order (ii) Injuries are best documented following the track of hemorrhage (iii) X-rays must be taken to locate the bullet.

Firearm Wounds

Firearm wounds simulate that produced by a burning pointed stick. Glancing wounds produced by the firearm may simulate incised or lacerated wound. Before describing injuries produced by firearm weapons, abrasion collar, contusion collar, blackening and tattooing needs description.

Abrasion collar: When the bullet strikes the skin, it first indents then stretches the surface and after that it perforates the skin. During the stretching period, the skin comes in contact with the high speed spinning bullet as a result of which the skin surface is abraded, known as *abrasion collar* (Figure 14.10). It is found surrounding the entry wound. The abrasion collar uniformly surrounds the entry wound when the bullet strikes the skin at right angle but it can also be elliptical depending on the angle at which the bullet strikes the skin. If the bullet strikes obliquely from the right side then the abrasion collar will be on the right side of the wound not on the left side. In these cases, usually some amount of contusion is also present along with the abrasion known as **contusion collar**. The abrasion collar is usually 2 to 3 mm wide. The abrasions become reddish brown when it dries.

A black coloured ring known as **grease or dirt collar** is seen as a narrow ring surrounding the entrance wound and is sharply outlined. This is due to the removal of substances from the bullet when it passes through the skin. This phenomenon is also known as **bullet wipe**. The dirt collar is less common if the bullet is a jacketed one. The abrasion collar surrounds the dirt collar.

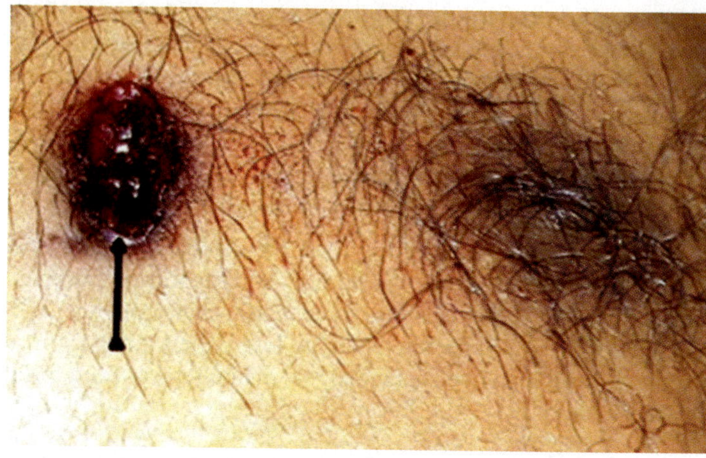

Figure 14.10: Rifled firearm entry wound over the chest showing abrasion collar

Medicolegal aspects: (i) Presence of abrasion collar indicates that it is entry wound (ii) Abrasion collar indicates the direction of firing.

Tattooing (Figure 14.11): Tattooing is an antemortem phenomenon that consists of unburnt and partially burnt powder particles embedded in and under the skin through the force of their impact. It cannot be wiped off and is seen only when the weapon is near enough for the powder grains to strike with force. When the range increases to the point that the powder particles do not embed themselves but still leave a visible mark, it is called **stippling.** At autopsy, it is necessary to examine the shape and size of the skin markings as a reflection of the shape and size of the powder grains of which they are made. Postmortem tattooing appears grey or yellow in colour and it can be wiped off easily.

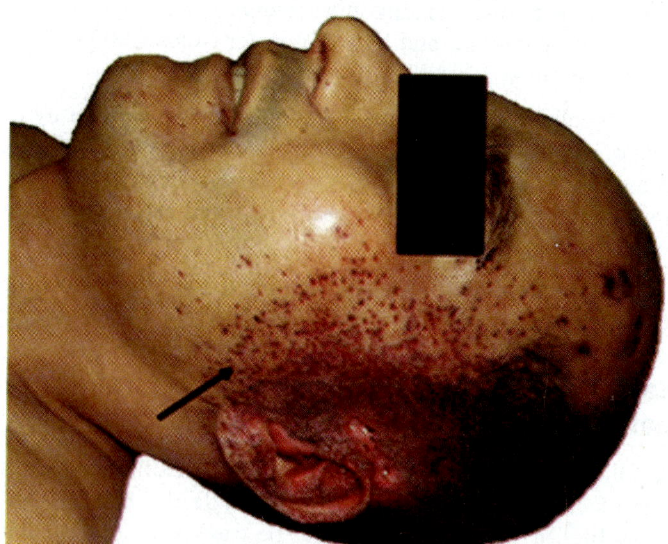

Figure 14.11: Rifled firearm entry wound showing tattooing

Deposition of powder soot (Blackening) (Figure 14.12): The deposition of powder soot producing blackening depends upon: (i) *Range:* As range increases, size of powder zone will increase and the density will decrease. (ii) *Propellant:* Some powders burn more readily than the others. (iii) *Angle of muzzle:* If the angle of muzzle is perpendicular then there is a circular wound while if the angle is oblique then an oval wound is produced. (iv) *Length of barrel:* The range of soot deposition varies with the length of barrel. The approximate soot range in a 6" barrel is 30 cm whereas it is 25 cm and 20 cm in a 4" and 2" barrel respectively. (v) Caliber of the weapon. (vi) Type of weapon. (vii) Target material whether it is bloody or non-bloody.

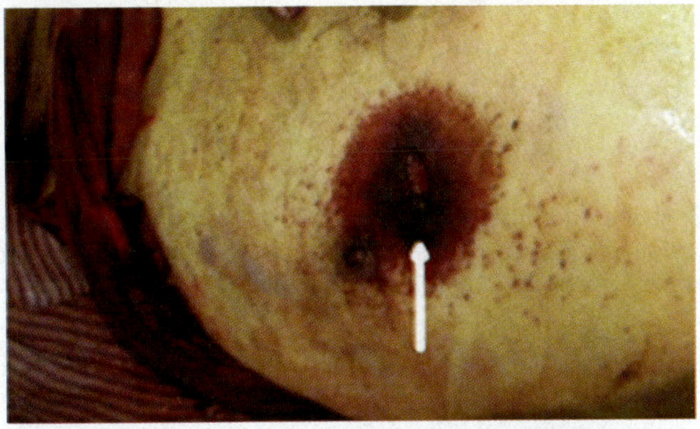

Figure 14.12: Blackening in a riffled firearm entry wound

Appearance of Wounds by Shotguns (Figures 14.13 to 14.18)

In shotgun wounds, the mass enters like a single bullet. The wound is irregular, contused and scorched. Wad and gas rupture

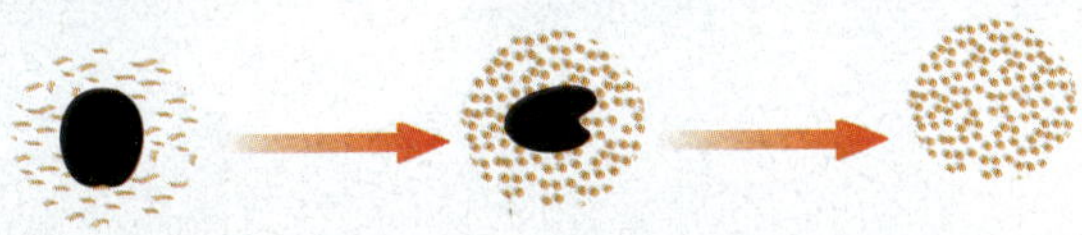

Figure 14.13: Shotgun firearm entry wound at various ranges

and lacerate the tissue. Unburnt powder is present in the wound. The wound is circular in shape, if the pellets strike the body at right angle. If it is a covered body part, there will be no effect of burning, tattooing or blackening. In the skull, irregular hole that may be accompanied by fissured fractures running from its margins is present. The appearance of injuries depends on the distance of the shot: (i) ***Within 6":*** Carbon monoxide may be present in the blood and the damaged tissue. Skull is less disrupted than at the contact range. The pellets have a cutting action and a clean hole is produced. (ii)***1-3 feet:*** Irregular single wound is produced due to loosening of the pellets. (iii) ***1 mts:*** The pellets start spreading and there is a central mass of pellets with a few satellite pellet injuries. (iv) ***2 mts:*** The pellets spread in a diameter of 5 cm with the central mass gradually decreasing and satellite pellets increasing in spread. (v) ***4 mts:*** Almost all the pellets are present separated

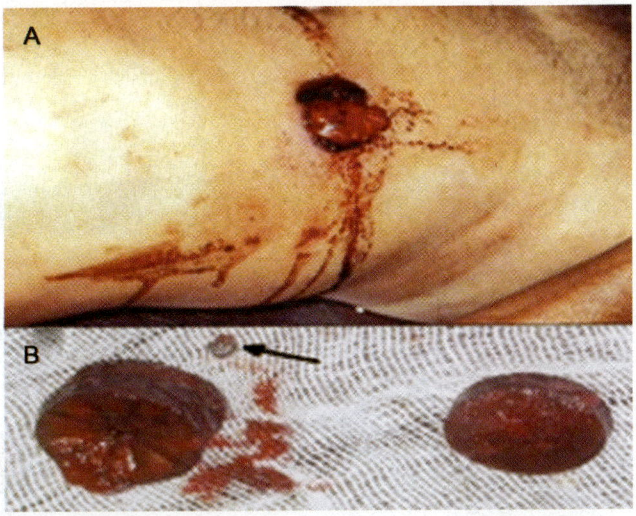

Figure 14.14A, B: Near contact shotgun firearm entry wound over abdomen (A) and Wads and pellet (arrow) recovered from the abdomen (B)

from each other and the central mass is no longer seen. (vi) ***20 mts:*** Beyond about 20 meters the pellets lose their energy and only penetrate the skin and beyond 30-40 meters they cannot even penetrate the skin.

Contact wounds: (i) ***Size and shape of the wound:*** Size of the wound is equal to the bore of the weapon and may be even smaller. The edges are crenated. (ii) ***Soiling and burning:*** In tight contact, skin forms a seal around the muzzle, preventing much escape of gas and soot so that soiling and burning is minimal or absent. The recoil that takes the muzzle away and if not pressed firmly, gas and soot escapes sideways. (iii) ***Muzzle impression:*** Muzzle impression may be there and is due to deep contusion from the effects of the blast. (iv) ***Carbon monoxide:*** It differentiates entry wound from the exit. CO gas deposition is more at the entry than exit, and also causes cherry red discoloration of the wound track. (v) ***Contact wounds over the bone:*** Over the bones, as gases cannot dissipate, muzzle imprint is there. In addition, there is cruciate wound due to splitting of the skin caused by the gases separating the skin over the bone.

Close range: The appearance of shotgun wound within 12 inches: (i) ***Shape of the wound:*** The wound is circular in shape, when the weapon is held at right angles and elliptical when it is held in a slanting position. Depending on the size of the pellets, there can be nibbling or crenation of edges. The margins are inverted and surrounded by an abrasion collar. (ii) ***Singeing of hairs*** that is clubbing appearance of hair around wound. This is due to melting of keratin and then solidification on cooling. (iii) ***Burning of skin*** unless protected by head hair. Hyperemia and even blistering may be present. (iv) ***Cherry red discolouration*** of tissues within and around the wound due to deposition of carbon monoxide. (v) ***Smoke soiling or soot deposition*** due to deposition of carbon particles. (vi) ***Tattooing*** is due to partly burnt and unburnt propellant flakes and grains. It produces small reddish brown or orange red punctate lesions on the skin. Unburnt flakes

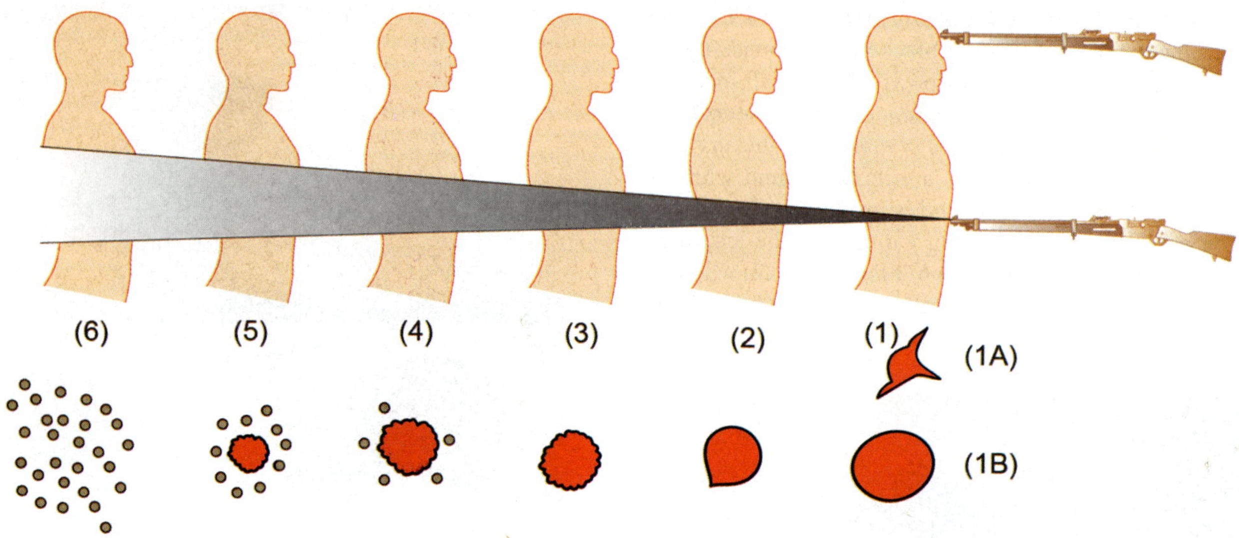

Figure 14.15: Appearance of shot gun wounds with increasing range: (1A) Split wound from contact over bone (1B) Round contact wound (2) Wound at closed range upto 30 cm (3) Rat hole wound from 30 cm-1 meter (4) Satellite pellet holes above 1 meter (5) Diminishing central hole with increasing shot spreading (6) No central hole above 10 meters with uniform spread of shot

are due to nitrocellulose, which are small glistening particles. (vii) Any felt or cardboard wads will be seen inside the wound.

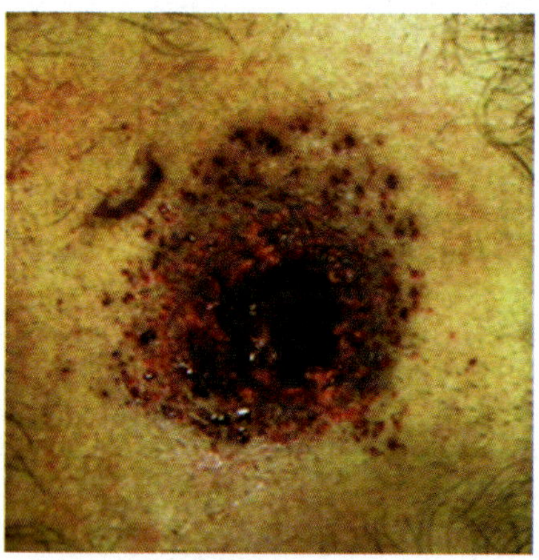

Figure 14.16: Rat hole appearance of shotgun entry wound with tattooing

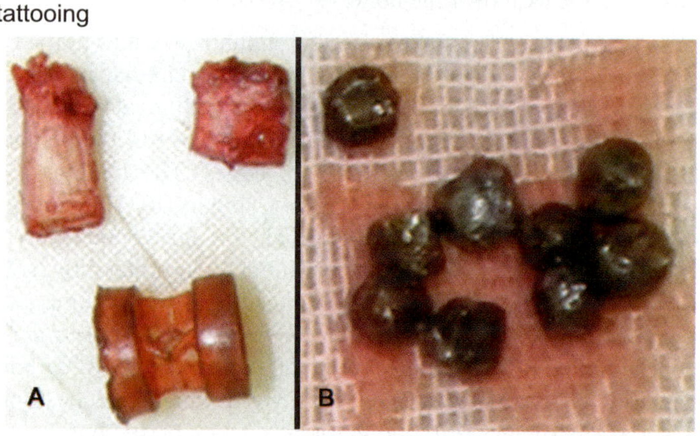

Figure 14.17A and B: Wads (A) and Pellets (B) of short gun recovered from the body at autopsy

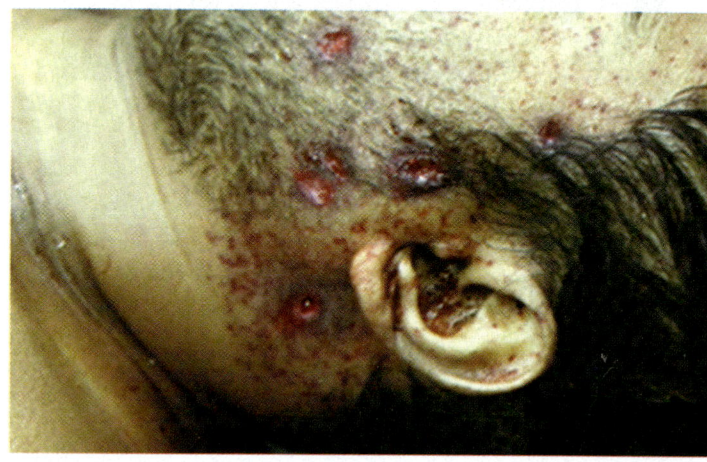

Figure 14.18: Multiple pellet wounds with tattooing due to shotgun

Short to mid-range (6"-6 feet): The findings are similar to that of close-range discharge except that soot soiling is less and will disappear at over 8-16 inches and with increasing distance the edge of wound will be abraded and crenated (**Rat hole**) specially with large shot. In addition, with increasing distance the pellet holes will progressively increase around the main wound. Soot soiling is present at 20-40 cm. Tattooing may persist somewhat further and it heals completely if the patient survives. Hair singeing is seen up to 12" and soot soiling up to 20". Single hole persists till 1 meter or 3 feet.

Mid to distant range (>2 meters): No burning and no smoke staining is there but powder tattooing is rarely present up to 5 meters. The wads may penetrate the skin and can produce a second lacerated wound and can also bruise the skin. As the distance increases, the spread of pellets increases and the rat hole diminishes in size. The range of firing can be calculated by the **rule** that is:

Diameter of spread in inches is roughly equal to the range in yards; for example if the spread of the pellets is in an area of 5" then the range of fire is 5 yards or 1/3rd of the spread in cms = range in meters, e.g., if the spread is in area of 18 cm, the range of fire is from a distance of 6 meters.

Distant range (More than 6-10 meters): At a distance more than 6-10 meters, there is no central hole, no burning, no tattooing and no smoking. The effective range is up to 30-50 meters.

Exit wound: Usually no exit wounds are produced in injuries by shotguns except in cases of: (i) Contact wounds (ii) Tangential wounds which are just piercing soft part of body and have to pass through very small section of body tissues (iii) Thin part of the body such as neck, extremities where there is little intervening tissue. In exit wounds, there is no tattooing, burning, singeing and blackening and the margins are everted.

Billiard ball ricochet effect: At close range, when the shots are bunched while striking the main target such as skin or clothes, they strike one another. Then they spread out in a wide pattern while passing through the body. As a result, the shots are spread widely and they suggest a greater range then actual. This type of spread may also be seen when the shots strikes some intermediary object such as wall, door, window before targeting the victim. Radiological examination is important as it will provide a true picture of the range of fire. When the range of fire is great enough then only the shots spread out before striking the main target.

Balling or welding of shot: Balling of shotgun pellets results in conversion of shot into a compact mass that moves *en masse* up to several meters. This is usually caused by faulty manufacture or from the use of old ammunition. It can also be due to hand loading of cartridges when too much powder is used or the wads inserted are incorrect or sealing pressure on the wads is too high. Most commonly, it is due to pouring of paraffin wax into the cartridges after removing the outer cardboard or by replacing some of the pellets by a larger ball bearing which is held in place with wax. The wound produced by balling of shots is a circular or oval entrance wound, 5-10 mm diameter and widespread, small circular punctures.

Appearance of Wounds by Revolvers and Automatic Pistols

Wounds of entrance: Depending on the distance of muzzle of firearm from the body, the entrance wounds are divided into: (i) Contact wounds (ii) Close range wounds (iii) Near shot wounds (iv) Distant shot wounds. In revolvers and automatic pistols, flame extends upto 8 cm; smoke upto 30 cm, unburnt and partially burnt powder grains and metallic particles can travel upto a distance of 60-90 cm.

The appearance of entrance wound depends on: (i) Amount of smoke, flame and unburnt and partially burnt powder grains (ii) Distances travelled by them (iii) Type of gun powder (iv) Amount of powder load (v) Weight of projectile (vi) Type of firearm (vii) Tightness and fitting of projectile in gun barrel.

Contact wounds: The wound depends on whether the muzzle is firmly pressed, making a tight seal or has loose contact with the body like backward jerk or revolving and whether there is presence of any clothing between muzzle and skin. Small circular wounds at soft parts and cruciate, satellite and linear wounds are produced on the bony parts of the body. A muzzle impression may be seen in cases where the muzzle is tightly applied to the body. The skin may swell up if there is a bony area beneath the skin like on the skull. No burning, blackening or tattooing is seen around the entrance. On loose contact, burning and soiling in the immediate vicinity of the muzzle may occur.

Back splatter: Contact wounds may cause blood and tissue fragments to enter the muzzle for several centimeters called 'back splatter'. This is due to momentary suction effect after the pressure of the gas blast subsides due to rapid cooling of the barrel. This seems to aspirate material such as piece of skin, hair and adipose tissue into the muzzle. Sometimes, blood and tissue may soil the hands and arms of the person firing the gun. This is of considerable forensic importance.

Point blank (very close range): Circular wounds are produced and abrasion collar as well as grease or dirt collar is present. There is extensive burning, singeing, blackening and tattooing due to the large amount of flame, smoke and unburnt carbon particles.

Close range (flame range)–within 5-8 cm: When there is short distance between muzzle and body surface, the wound will vary according to the type of ammunition used. Wound will invariably be circular as tearing due to gas intrusion is unlikely to occur. The edges may be inverted and at times level up or everted due to the rebounding gases. Abrasion collar is present. Within few centimeters, burning with singeing of hair is present. Clubbing of hair is there and hyperemia around the wound and some bruising can occur. It is more evident as postmortem interval increases. Soot or smoke soiling and powder tattooing is present.

Near shot range (12-18"): It is the range of powder but outside the range of flame that is up to 90 cm. It is due to absence of flame so there is no burning but singeing is present due to hot gases. Tattooing is also present in these cases.

Distant shot: A shot which is fired from a distance more than the range of powder and smoke is considered as distant shot. In these cases, the entrance wound is often smaller than the bullet and is surrounded by an inner grease collar and outer abrasion collar. The margins will be inverted and there will be no burning, blackening or tattooing (Figures 14.19 and 14.20).

Exit wound (Figure 14.21A, B): Exit wound may be stellate, circular, cruciate, elliptical, crescent or star shaped (more common on scalp). At times these may be slit like bullets get deformed as when struck by a bone. This is more common on head and shoulders. In contact wounds and at very close range, exit wound is smaller than wound of entrance. However, as range increases the size of exit wound also increases. Exit wounds do not show any burning, blackening, tattooing, abrasion or contusion collar.

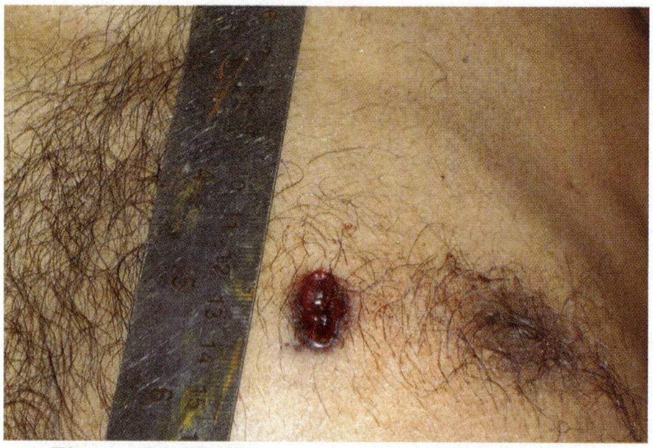

Figure 14.19: Firearm entry wound over chest

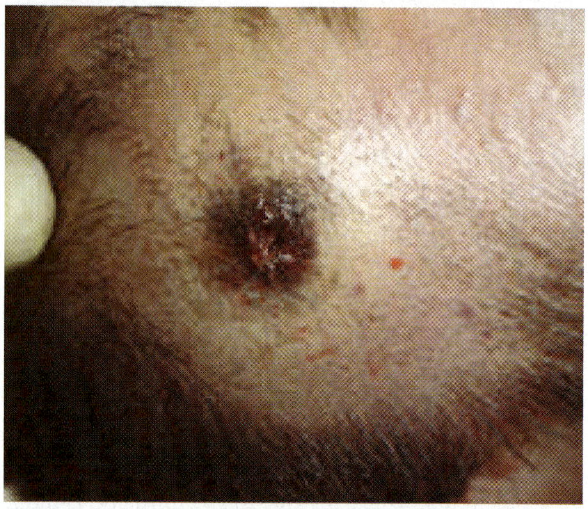

Figure 14.20: Entry wound over right temporal region

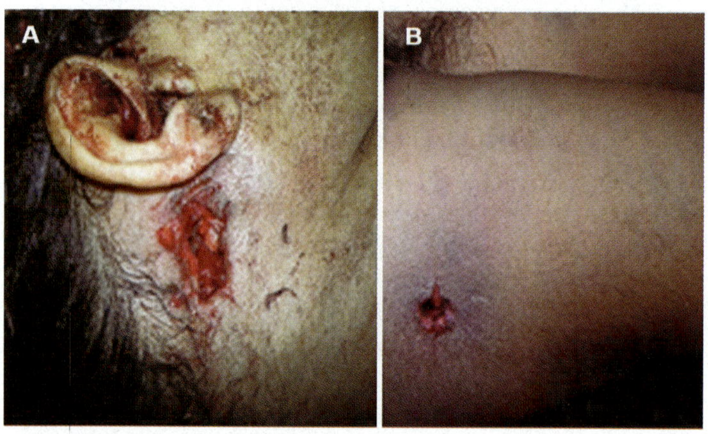

Figure 14.21A, B: Firearm exit wound over the right temple (A) and right arm (B)

The edges are everted, torn or puckered with pieces of contused, haemorrhagic subcutaneous fat or muscle protruding out of the defect. Sometimes even the bullet may protrude out of an exit wound.

Variations in shape and size of exit wounds: (i) When bullet tumbles in the body and fails to exit nose-end first (ii) When the bullet is deformed (iii) When the bullet exits as many pieces after breaking up in the tissues (iv) When the fragments of bone are blown out of body alongwith bullet (v) When the unsupported skin at exit tends to tear and break into pieces.

Shored (supported) exit wound: When the exit wound is over supported skin, it is circular or nearly circular defects that is surrounded by a margin of abrasion similar to an entry wound. The shored exit wounds are produced (i) When bullet is fired at long range (ii) Bullet fired through clothing (iii) In a firearm with small calibre when it is discharged in contact with skin at a point where bone is not immediately below the skin surface (iv) When firm object such as belt, waist band of trousers, collar, brassiere or tie is pressed against the body at site of exit wound (v) When body is leaning against a hard surface such as wall, back of chair, table, floor, bed, mattress etc. when the person is lying down.

Medicolegal aspects of exit wound: From the exit wound we can know (i) Direction of firing (ii) Position of victim while firing (iii) Number of bullets that are remaining in the body.

Wounds from Rifled Firearm

The wounds are similar to that produced by pistol or revolver. However, these produce more damage. In a rifled firearm, flame extends upto 15-20 cm, unburnt powder grains and small metallic particles upto 75 cm and smoke upto a distance of 30 cm from the muzzle. These may produce unexpected results and vary quite considerably. Usually entrance and exit wounds are of the same size and shape when the bullet is not touched by a resistant structure such as bone. Hence, in firearm contact wound of skull, sometimes there is large entrance wound (Figure 14.25). Sometimes, there may be extensive explosive effects and severe lacerated exit wounds even though not touched by a resistant structure.

Entrance wound is usually smaller than the diameter of bullet with depressed edges and is surrounded by a reddish zone that becomes brown on drying. Along the track of bullet there is bruising of deeper tissues. When the bullet strikes at an angle, skin may split or turned up. When it strikes a bone in its tract, extensive shattering and comminution of bone takes place. When bullet strikes an angle, exit wound is a lacerated wound and can vary from the size of 2.5 cm to the size of palm of hand. The fragments of bones that are driven out may produce several small holes around the exit wounds. Appearance of rifled firearm entry wounds at various ranges are shown in Figure 14.22.

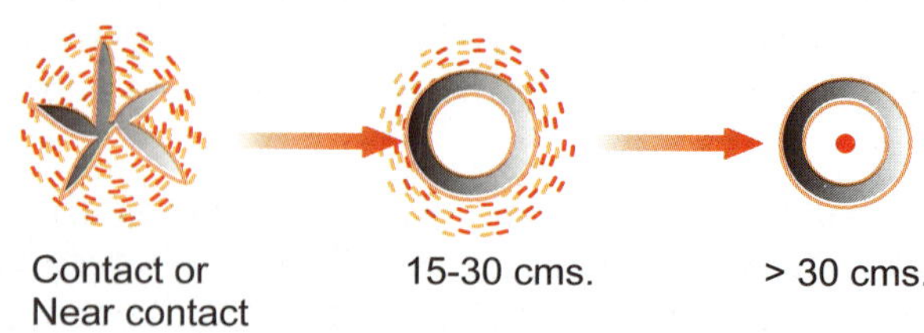

Figure 14.22: Rifled firearm entry wound at various ranges

The differences between entry and exit wound in rifled firearms are shown in Table 14.1.

Table 14.1: Differences between the entry and exit wounds

Features	Entry wound	Exit wound
Edges	Inverted	Everted
Bruising (Abrasion/ grease collar)	Present	Not present
Burning	Present	Absent
Tattooing	Present carried into the wounds	Absent
Tissue	Cherry red	Not such
Lead ring (Metal ring)	Around the wound seen on X-ray/micro chemical examination	Absent
Size	Smaller except contact wound	Larger
Wound on skull	Chipped in words	Bevelled and everted
Blackening	Present	Absent
Fibers or clothes	Turned in	Not so
Wound track	Bright pink due to carboxyhemoglobin in near discharge	Not so
Spectrography	More metal is found	Not so

Effects of Firearms on Skull

In the skull, the wound of entrance shows a punched-in hole (clean cut) on the outer table (Figure 14.23A). As the inner table remains unsupported, the chipping of the bone occurs resulting in beveling appearance (Figure 14.23B). In firearm exit wound, the inner table of the skull shows clean cut margin (Figure 14.24A) and the outer table shows beveling appearance (Figure 14.24B).

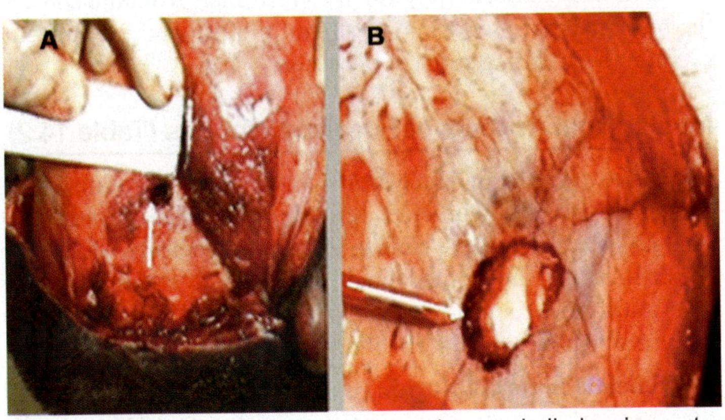

Figure 14.23A,B: Firearm entry wound over skull showing outer table clean cut margin (A) and beveling of inner table (B)

Fissured fractures often radiate from the hole. The piece of bone from the entry wound is driven inside the cranial cavity that causes brain injury and is often lost in the track. The dura mater shows irregular tears. On the other hand, at the point of exit the inner table shows clean cut hole and the beveling appearance is found on the outer table. The exit wound is larger due to the

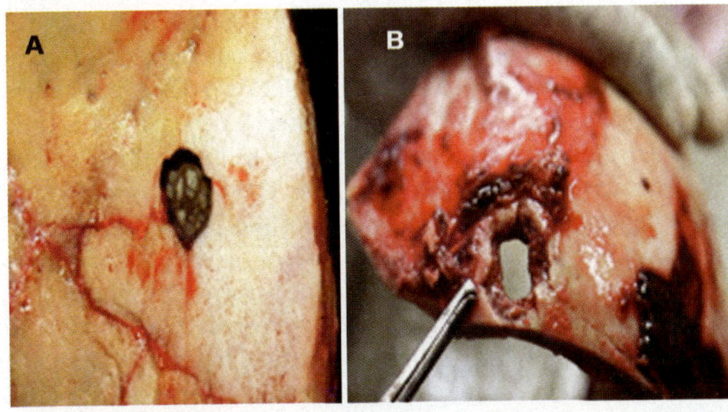

Figure 14.24A, B: Firearm exit wound on skull showing inner table clean cut margin (A) and beveled outer table (B)

deformity and tumbling of the bullet upon entering the skull. At times fractures are present from the exit wound. The size of the beveling is useful in the assessment of the angle of fire. In contact wounds shattering of skull wound occurs (Figure 14.25).

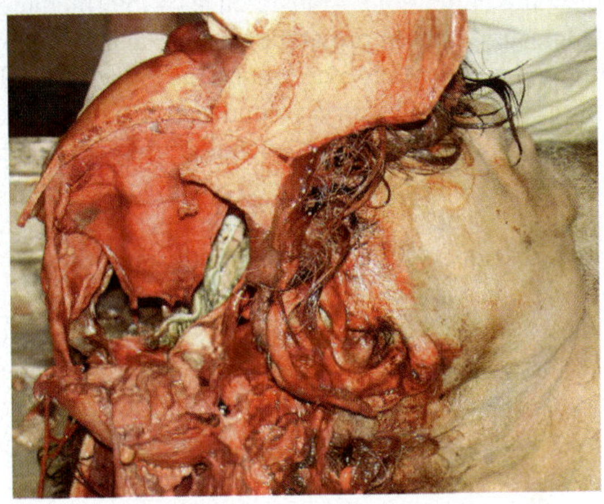

Figure 14.25: Firearm contact entry wound

Puppe's rule: It determines the sequence of shots when several bullets have struck the cranium. Even this rule is applicable to the multiple blunt forces striking the skull causing the fracture. The rule was developed by **Madea** in relation to bullet injuries. It depends on the observation of the fracture lines either when they intersect each other or when they intersect a cratered lesion. Thus, one can determine which crack was formed first. This rule states that when two fracture lines intersect each other, the second fracture line never crosses the first one.

Peculiar Effects Produced in Firearm Wounds

Atypical entrance wound: (i) For a few microseconds after bullet leaves the muzzle (up to 50 meters in pistol and 150 meters in rifle), there may be **tail wobble** or **tail wag.** This is partly responsible for causing great damage. (ii) Gyroscopic effect of the bullet diminishes as it reaches the end of its flight until it begins to wobble then to tumble and produces large atypical entrance wound. (iii) ***Yawning bullet:*** The bullet instead of travelling nose-on travels in an irregular fashion is called yawning bullet. (iv) ***Tumbling***

bullet: During its motion when the bullet rotates end-on-end it is called tumbling bullet. (v) Stippling or tattooing on the skin may be altered by the use of silencers. Muzzle breaks, flash hiders also alter this effect. (vi) ***Ricochet bullet:*** A ricochet is a missile that is deviated from its course by striking an intermediate object. Such missiles are commonly deformed. The degree of deformity varies depending on the: (a) Texture of the bullet (b) Angle of impact (c) Intermediary object. The path of ricochet bullet is quite unpredictable except over the surface of water where the angle of incidence is equal to the angle of reflection. A bullet wound can be caused intentionally by calculating its angle. In no other case, the injury by ricochet is inflicted intentionally. The entrance wound can be round or elliptical or keyhole or irregular shape and large. In injuries caused by ricochet bullet, abrasion collar, burning and blackening is absent. **Yuw-Er Yong** reviewed the pattern of injuries in ricochet gunshot incidents and revealed that, in a close-range, pseudo-stippling or pseudo-gunpowder tattooing, pseudo-soot blackening and tumbling abrasions can be seen on the skin surrounding the bullet hole. Transference of intermediate surface materials and fragmented projectiles may cause satellite injuries resembling gunpowder tattooing around the bullet hole. However, pseudo-stippling around entry wound can also be observed in non-ricochet incidents like due to bullet fragmentation, bullet perforation of an intermediary object such as glass, postmortem insect bites etc. There is also less significant bullet wipe on the margin of Ricocheted bullet holes as some bullets' surface contaminants are lost while ricocheting. Internal ricochet may occur when a bullet strikes hard tissue. In such cases, a postmortem computed tomographic (CT) imaging is helpful in localizing a bullet and its fragments in the body and characterizing the wound track. In 20% of the skull injuries ricochet occurs. *Medicolegal importance:* Missiles have to be examined for possible foreign material inclusions such as intermediary substance and entrance wounds produced by ricochet. It is not necessarily different from that produced by ordinary bullet although it may assume a bizarre shape due to deformity of the missile. (vii) ***Bullet graze or slap:*** When the bullet hits the target at so acute an angle that it does not perforate the skin. In such cases, grazing or slap wound is produced that appears in the form of reddish brown, elliptical or triangular, elongated furrow or abrasion. In a bullet graze or slap, adjacent skin may be ecchymosed and the underlying dermis may sometimes be involved. (viii) ***Bullet strikes sternum:*** Travels between rib cage and skin, and it may come out at the back causing minor injuries.

Single entrance and multiple exit wounds: This may occur in case of piggyback bullets. Also, in case of injury by automatic firearms many bullets may enter through the same entrance and come out from different exits. Also, at times a bullet may enter the body and then fragment on impact with bony parts and the fragments may exit from different points.

Bullet strikes the skull but does not enter it: This scenario occurs when the bullet hits from a far distance. The bullet looses its energy and on hitting the skull either causes a bruise or just pierces the skin and fails to penetrate the skull. The bullet may graze or rub the top and sides of skull. Entry and exit wounds are seen over the scalp in such cases that are about 2-3 cm apart and the skull between the wounds show a gutter like impression (**gutter wound**). This wound may be oval or elongated. However, when bullet strikes skull at an angle, due to impact on the bone, it may rarely deviate its path and produces continuous wound under the skin and does not penetrate the skull.

Multiple wounds of entrance and exit from a single shot: It may be seen at times and the clothing is very essential to assess the direction of the shots in such cases.

Entrance wound but no bullet or exit wound: It could be due to following reasons: (i) Bullet entered in the stomach and got vomited out (ii) It has been coughed out of the trachea (iii) Bullet entered the gastrointestinal tract and from there, passed out in the faeces (iv) Bullet comes out through the same wound.

Unexplained bullets in the body (Tandem bullet or Piggy Back bullet): It is the bullet that comes out one after the other and this may result from the use of faulty ammunition, faulty barrel or due to loaded firearm that was unused for several years.

Kennedy phenomenon: It is an artefact that is due to surgical alteration or suturing of gunshot wounds, the evaluation of such wounds becomes difficult on autopsy.

Bullet embolism: When fired the bullets may enter inside a big vessel and are lodged at a distance causing embolism.

Concealed firearm wounds: They are usually seen inside the mouth, nostrils, over inner canthus of eye, axilla, external auditory meatus, rectum and vagina. They may not be detected if the body is covered with blood or blood clots thus obscuring the injuries.

Souvenir bullets: They are the bullets that are retained inside the body without producing any harmful effect and they are not even removed during surgical operation.

Medicolegal Aspects of Firearms Wounds (Table 14.2)

Whenever there is an allegation of accidental shooting in an attempt to mask a homicide, test firing at different ranges to produce a target pattern similar in size and density of shot to victim's injury should be done. This enables the investigator to evaluate the circumstances and thereby test the alibi of the individual who claims the shooting was accidental.

Suicidal firearm injuries: (i) Rarely females opt this method for committing suicide. The suicide note or threatened note may be found at the site and forgery of suicide note is a remote possibility. There is evidence of preparation for committing suicide at the scene. The weapon is invariably found at the scene usually near or on the deceased's body. However, the person can fling the gun away from its body when he collapses or his body may slide a few feet from the weapon. While conducting autopsy, the pathologist should measure the arm of the person to find out whether he can

Table 14.2: Differences between suicidal, accidental and homicidal firearm wounds			
Features	**Suicide**	**Accident**	**Homicide**
Site	Head, side of temple, centre of forehead, under the chin, over the heart and rarely epigastrium	Any area	Any area
Shot distance	Contact or very close range	Close or very close range	Any range, usually distant
Direction	Upward or backward (consistent with self firing)	Any direction	Usually upward
Number of wounds	Usually one	Usually one	Any number
Powder residue over hands	Present	Present	Absent
Weapon	Found at the scene	Found at the scene	Not found at the scene
Scene of crime	Usually in his own house with no evidence of disturbance or struggle	May be indoors or outdoors in the marriages/parties	Any place and there is evidence of disturbed scene and struggle
Victim	Usually males	Usually males	Any sex
Cadaveric spasm	Present rarely with weapon found firmly grasped	Not so	Not so

reach the trigger or has used an implement. (ii) Weapon when found in hand (cadaveric spasm) is the hallmark of suicide but the absence of weapon does not exclude suicide. (iii) Ownership of the gun should be ascertained; although a person may be murdered by his own gun but in suicide it's very unusual to use other person's gun. (iv) Fingerprints on the gun, if exclusively of the deceased suggest suicide. However, if mixed, there may be possibility of an attempt to prevent suicide. (v) Posture of the body and its relationship to the surroundings should be noted in the forms of sketch and photographs. (vi) If the clothes are removed and have no tears or holes, it suggests suicide. (vii) If the site of entrance wound is on accessible sites such as temple, forehead and mouth, it suggests a planned suicide. (viii) Contact wounds have a very strong presumption of planned suicide. If the wound deviates by an inch from the center of forehead, it should be cautiously interpreted. (ix) Hands should be examined for powder grains and swabs should be preserved for nitrates. Presence of burns and soiling of hands with blood is absent in homicides. (x) A single shot indicates suicide although multiple shots are also known but they are usually homicidal. (xi) In decomposed and burnt bodies, X-ray of the body is done that will reveal whether the pattern of shot injuries were produced by the person himself to commit suicide.

Homicidal firearm injuries: (i) *Site of the body:* If firearm injury is on an inaccessible part of the body like back, it is homicidal. However, deviation from normal suicidal injury raises suspicion of homicide but it does not follow that an entrance wound at the back of head is always homicidal. There is a case of a Portuguese student who shot himself at the back of head with shotgun. Usually, the wound at center point between ear and back of head is suicidal. (ii) If the range of firing is outside that of self-infliction, it is presumptive evidence of homicide unless special steps had been taken by victim to effect suicide at a distance. This can be corroborated with the circumstantial evidence of arrangements he had made to make it simulate homicide. The contact wounds are presumptive of suicide but this may not be always the case. In homicidal injuries, patient may be incapacitated by disease, drink or drugs or shot while he was sleeping. Toxicological and drug analysis of blood and viscera would be quite informative in such cases.

There are certain medicolegal questions pertaining to deaths due to firearm injuries such as:

Is the injury caused by the discharge of firearm? This can be deduced from the: (i) Appearance of the clothing (ii) Entrance and exit wounds (iii) Bullet tracks; and (iv) Presence of bullets and pellets in the clothes or on the body.

What kind of weapon fired the shot? The kind of weapon is determined by: (i) Size, shape and composition of the bullet (ii) Examination of the cartridge, shot and bullet left in the body or found at the scene of crime (iii) Stains on the clothes of black or smokeless powder (iv) From the examination of primary and secondary markings on the bullets.

From what distance and direction was the shot fired? (Table 14.3): Range of firing is determined by the presence or absence of flame effect, smoke and tattooing etc. When the range is greater, it can be approximated from the appearance of wounds and penetration of bullets. At close range, while the shots are bounced they strike one another upon impact on the primary target such as skin or clothing of the victim and spread out in a wide pattern as they continue on into the body. This produces a wide dispersion of the shot and may lead to the conclusion of a greater range of fire than that actually occurred. The same holds true if the shot strikes any other intermediary object such as a door or window before reaching the victim. The range of firing can also be determined from concentrated pattern of antimony around the bullet hole. Test fires are useful in such circumstances. The direction of fired shot depends upon: (i) Posture of the body at the time of impact (ii) Position of entrance and exit wounds (iii) Possibility of deflection of bullet (iv) Position of abrasion collar.

Table 14.3: Distribution of flame, smoke and tattooing produced at various distances in shot guns and rifled firearm weapons

Effects produced	*Shot gun*	*Pistols*	*Revolvers/Rifles*
Flame	Up to 30"	2-3"	6-8"
Smoke	1-meter	24"	12"
Tattooing	1-2 meter	24"	24-30"
Cards	2-3 meter	—	—
Wads	4-6 meter	—	—

If multiple wounds of entrance and exit are present, could they have been produced by a single bullet? It is possible for a single bullet to cause multiple wounds of entry and exit. For instance, if the bullet strikes the body from the side, it may enter the arm, come out and then enter the chest or abdomen and again comes out thus producing multiple wounds.

If multiple wounds are present, are they from same or different weapon? Examination of wounds, bullets etc. is necessary for conclusive opinion.

When was the firearm discharged? If black powder has been used then hydrogen sulphide may persist in the barrel for a few hours, if breech is closed. Gun powder washings are alkaline and contain nitrite sulphate and thiosulphates etc. Smokeless powder produces grey deposits that neutralize in distilled water. It contains nitrites and nitrates but no sulphates. The peculiar smell of mixture of gases stays for several hours.

A. **Color tests**

(i) ***Dermal nitrate test (Paraffin test):*** This test was in vogue earlier to determine if a subject had discharged the firearm. The residues deposited on the palm and web of the suspect's hand were removed for testing either by ordinary paraffin cast or simply by swabbing with cotton soaked with normal saline. This was tested for nitrates using diphenylamine reagent. This test is now obsolete as it is given by common oxidizing substances and non-incriminating materials like fertilizers, cigarettes, urine etc.

(ii) ***Harrison and Gilroy test:*** This is a qualitative chemical test designed in 1959 by Harrison and Robert Gilroy to detect gunshot metallic residues like barium (Ba), antimony (Sb), and lead (Pb) in the firearm discharge. However, test was not adopted widely because of its marginal sensitivity.

B. **The modern instrumental methods used for this purpose are:**

(i) ***Neutron activation analyses:*** This is a chemical method to identify traces of elements present in the hair, nails, soil, glass pieces, paints, gunshot residues and drugs. This method is based on the detection and the measurement of characteristic radioisotopes formed by irradiation in a nuclear reactor. The neutrons bombard the atoms of the elements that are present in specimen. Some of the nuclei of the atoms capture neutrons and become radioactive. This radioactivity is measured with a detector connected to an analyser. This method is helpful only when samples for comparison are available. In discharge of a firearm, the residues from the suspect's hand are removed by swabbing the back of hand with cotton swab moistened with 5% nitric acid.

(ii) ***Atomic absorption spectroscopy:*** The analytical system utilizes high temperature to vaporize the metallic elements of the primer residue and to detect and quantitate them for: (i) Identifying holes in clothes, tissues, wood as bullet holes for the presence of lead, antimony, barium and copper. (ii) Determining the common origin and bullet fragments of shotgun pellets found at different places from the concentration of lead, antimony, arsenic copper silver and from the alloys. (iii) Determining from the presence of lead. Antimony and barium on hands whether or not the person has fired a gun.

(iii) ***Scanning electron microscope (energy dispersive X-ray analysis):*** This can detect even the most minute traces of gunshot residues that are found on the suspect's body. These gunshot residues comprise chemical substances that burn and produce gases providing for the velocity for the bullet. During the process the metal such as antimony, barium, copper, lead are also sprayed out and gets deposited on the clothes, hands and face of the suspect.

How long did the victim survive? It depends upon the cause of death such as: (i) Shock and hemorrhage (ii) Injuries to vital organs (iii) Septicemia and other complications.

How much activity could the person perform following the injury? It depends upon the site of injury and organs involved such as: (i) If the bullet destroys motor area or spinal cord there will be immediate incapacitation. (ii) If laceration of heart and aorta occurs the person is immediately incapacitated. (iii) If medulla is involved, death is instantaneous. (iv) Bullet wound of the brain involving non-vital regions may allow the patient to carry out some work. (v) Amount of blood loss is not excessive death may not occur immediately.

Suicide, homicide or accident: To decide homicidal, suicidal, accidental manner of death the circumstantial evidence, autopsy findings and the circumstances of shooting should be corroborated.

Number of shots: In automatic weapons, pressure is released till one becomes unconscious or the first shot may not be lethal. It is very important to distinguish multiple exit wounds from those of the entrance. Single missiles can disintegrate to produce multiple exit wounds. '*Secondary missiles*' like portions of broken bone, buttons and clothing may produce exit wounds. The curious results are seen if the bullet is split by bone into two fragments; one fragment recovered from the brain and the other ricochets back through another wound at a higher level.

LONG QUESTIONS

1. Discuss the injuries caused by a firearm. How will you estimate the distance and the type of weapon from which the shot was fired?
2. What is ballistics? Discuss the injuries caused by a rifled firearm from a close range.

SHORT QUESTIONS

1. Shotgun wounds.
2. Gunshot wounds.
3. Puppe's rule.
4. Abrasion collar.
5. Grease collar.
6. Tattooing
7. Choking of a shotgun.
8. Caliber of a firearm.
9. Primer mixture.
10. Ricochet bullet.
11. Differentiate between entry and exit wound.
12. Neutron activation analysis.
13. Atomic absorption spectroscopy.
14. Dermal nitrate test.

MULTIPLE CHOICE QUESTIONS

1. Smokeless (single base) powder consists of:
(a) Nitrocellulose (b) Nitroglycerin
(c) Nitrites (d) Nitro B.T.

2. Billiard ball ricochet effect is seen in cases of fire by:
(a) Service rifle (b) Semi-automatic rifle
(c) Shotguns (d) A.K. 47

3. A wound produced by a ricochet bullet is:
(a) Small and round (b) Large and elongated
(c) Triangular with tattooing (d) Square with blackening

4. The black gun powder consists of the following *except:*
(a) Sulphur (b) Charcoal
(c) Potassium nitrate (d) Nitroglycerin

5. Abrasion collar is present at the entry wound caused by:
(a) Revolver (b) Rifle
(c) Pistol (d) All of the above

6. Dermal Nitrate test is done to detect:
(a) Blood stains
(b) Gun powder
(c) Nitric salt poisoning
(d) Nerve gases poisoning

7. In a firearm entry wound, blackish discolouration is due to:
(a) Unburned powder (b) Flame
(c) Smoke (d) Hot gases

8. Bevelling of the inner table of skull is found in:
(a) Firearm entry wound (b) Firearm exit wound
(c) Drowning (d) Head injury by blunt force

9. X-ray examination in firearm cases helps to:
(a) Locate the bullet which has not exited
(b) Locate metallic fragment along with path
(c) True pathway of a bullet for evidence
(d) Know the distance of firearm discharge to the target

10. Harrison and Gilroy test is used in cases of:
(a) Hanging (b) Firearm
(c) Thermal burns (d) Electrical burns

11. A gun having initial part of barrel as smooth while last part as rifled, referred as:
(a) Musket (b) Air gun
(c) Paradox gun (d) Stud gun

12. Stellate wound is produced with firearm in:
(a) Contact shot (b) Close shot
(c) Near shot (d) Distant shot

13. Presence of the following is found with shot gun fire only:
(a) Primer (b) Wads
(c) Gun powder (d) Bullet

14. During autopsy the bullet should be removed preferably with:
(a) Toothed forceps (b) Gloved hand
(c) Using magnet (d) Using glass rod

15. Range of firearm injury can be determined by all *except:*
(a) Examination of clothes
(b) Presence of singeing of hair
(c) Presence of bullet in the skin
(d) Dispersion of pellets in the skin

16. Following test is not useful to detect metallic deposits from body in firearm injury:
(a) Neutron activation analysis
(b) Harrison Gilory test
(c) Atomic absorption spectroscopy
(d) Paraffin test

ANSWER KEY

1. (a)	2. (c)	3. (b)	4. (d)	5. (d)	6. (b)	7. (c)	8. (a)	9. (a)	10. (b)
11. (c)	12. (a)	13. (b)	14. (b)	15. (c)	16. (d)				

Chapter 15

Regional Injuries

HEAD INJURIES

Anatomy of scalp: The scalp extends from the top of forehead in front to the superior nuchal line behind. Laterally it projects down to the zygomatic arch and external acoustic meatus. It consists of five layers: (i) Skin (ii) Subcutaneous tissue (iii) Occipitofrontalis and its aponeurosis (iv) Subaponeurotic areolar tissue; and (v) Pericranium (Figure 15.1).

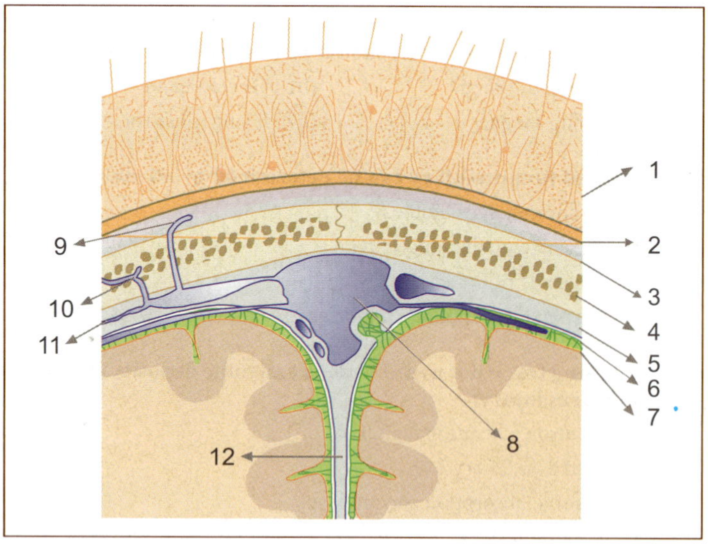

Figure 15.1: Coronal section through scalp, skull and brain: (1) Subcutaneous fibro-adipose tissue (2) Epicranial aponeurosis (3) Pericranium (4) Parietal bone (5) Dura mater (6) Arachnoid mater (7) Pia mater (8) Superior sagittal sinus (9) Emissary vein (10) Diploic vein (11) Neuropial vein (12) Falx cerebri

Injuries to Scalp

The usual range of abrasion, contusions and laceration may be inflicted though a modifying factor that is presence of brain, which may deflect a tangential blow or partly cushion a direct impact. In hair-covered areas, care must always be taken at autopsy to palpate the scalp in any case in which there is possibility of injury that may otherwise be missed. When a lesion is found or suspected, the hair must be carefully shaved away to expose the scalp for further examination and photography.

Bruising of scalp: Bruising may be difficult to detect until the hair has been removed. Marked swelling is a common feature of extensive bruising, as the liberated blood cannot extend downward because of the rigidity of underlying skull. In addition to frank bleeding beneath the scalp, marked oedema may occur after injury and the layers of the scalp may be greatly swollen and thickened by jellylike infiltration of tissue fluid. Bleeding under the scalp (Figures 15.2 and 15.3) may be mobile. A bruise under anterior scalp may slide downwards to appear in orbit. Similarly, a temporal bruise may later appear behind the ear. As with bruises elsewhere, those under the scalp may be obvious immediately after infliction or their appearance may be delayed either during life or as a postmortem appearance.

Laceration of scalp: Laceration of scalp bleeds profusely and dangerously and even fatal blood loss can occur from an extensive scalp injury. The injury that is most gross is avulsion of a large area of scalp (Figure 15.4). This may happen when hair is entangled in machinery while working in industries. Scalp injuries may bleed profusely even after death, especially if head is in dependent position. Severe blows from shaped object such

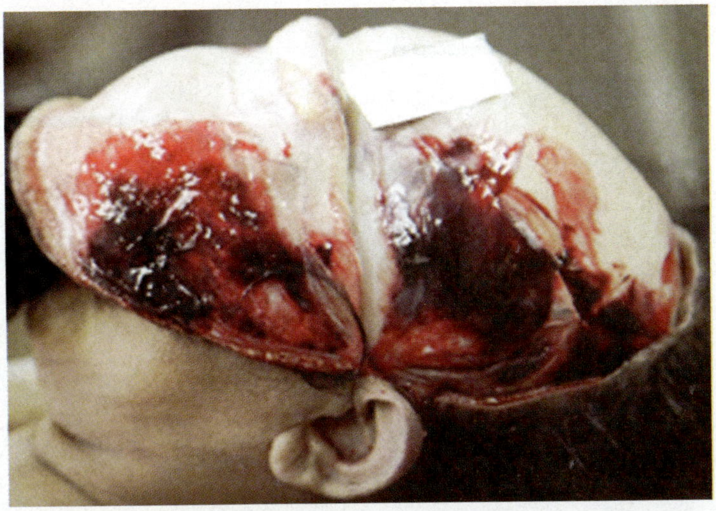

Figure 15.2: Effusion of blood underneath the scalp

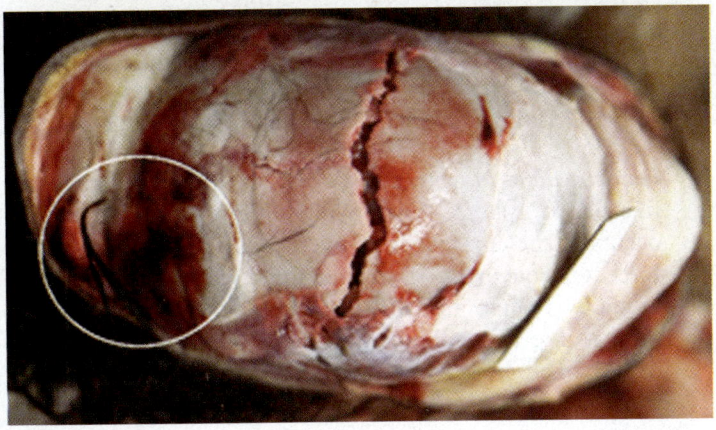

Figure 15.3: Effusion of blood underneath the scalp with diastatic fracture of skull

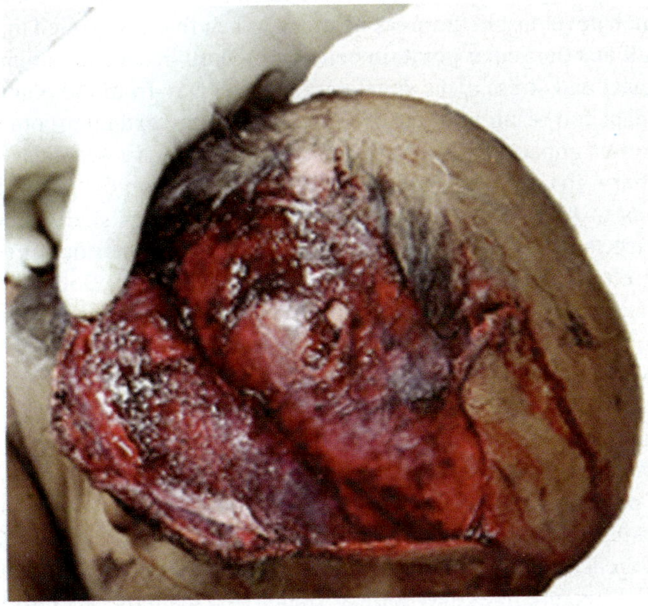

Figure 15.4: Avulsed lacerated wound of scalp

as hammers or heavy tools may reproduce the profile of weapon totally or in part. A circular faced hammer may punch a circle but more often only an arc of circle is seen. In such cases, position of edges that digs in most deeply may give an indication of the angle of blow. A major problem in scalp injuries is differentiation between incised wound and laceration. Close examination using a lens if necessary will show that this blunt laceration has (i) Bruised margins, even though this zone may be narrow (ii) Head hair crossing the wound are not cut (iii) Fascial strands, hair bulb and perhaps small nerve and vessels are in the depth of wound.

Scalp injuries from fall: From the fall, the injuries usually involve the occipital protuberance, forehead or the parieto-temporal area and are not possible on the vertex even from a considerable height. Falls from standing position can occur if the person is drunk, in an assault and during some illness (fit/faint).

Complications of scalp injuries: (i) Deep bruise may take a longer time to appear and heal (ii) An infected lacerated wound may cause infection of superior sagittal sinus through the emissary veins.

Black eyes: Black eye (Figure 15.5) is also called periorbital hematoma and may be the result of: (i) *Direct violence:* It may be associated with abrasion or laceration of upper cheek, eyebrow, nose or other part of the face. (ii) *Gravitational seepage:* An injury to front of scalp and also on or above the eyebrow leads to gravitational seepage of blood beneath the scalp into the eyelids. (iii) *Percolation of blood:* This results from fracture of anterior cranial fossa of skull, is often a contrecoup injury caused by fall on to back of head leading to secondary fracture of paper-thin bone of orbital roof.

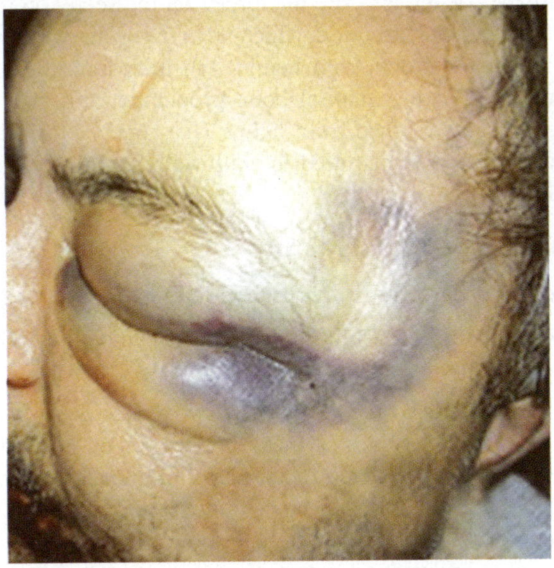

Figure 15.5: Black eye in a case of head injury

Anatomy of Skull

Adult skull consists of two parallel, thin tables of compact bones; outer being twice thicker than inner, separated by soft cancellous (spongy) bone containing bone marrow. The term 'diploe' is used to describe this cancellous bone within the flat bones of skull (See Figure 15.1). The diploe starts forming at 4 years of age. Before this age, it is a thin compact and elastic bone. This zone is interrupted at suture lines and vanishes where the bone is particularly thin especially in floor of skull. Greater wing of sphenoid, petrous temporal, sagittal ridge, occipital protuberance and glabella are the strong parts of cranium. The thin areas are parietotemporal, lateral frontal and lateral occipital zones. The temporal bone is the thinnest with a thickness of 4 mm and occipital is thickest, in midline it may be more than or equal to 15 mm. The frontal and parietal bones are about 6-10 mm in thickness.

Fractures of Skull

Fatal brain damage can occur even with an intact skull. Thin skull is less likely to be fractured as it is flexible and can return to normal after distortion like that of infants. It is rare for the skull fracture itself to be dangerous but the concomitant effect of transmitted force upon cranial contents makes it dangerous. The presence of skull fracture is an indication of the severity of force applied to the head. Postmortem and antemortem differentiation is difficult in the absence of soft tissue. The fracture of skull can occur either by direct or indirect violence.

Direct violence: The forces act directly on the bone to produce a fracture such as: (i) Compression of foetus during forceps delivery or clinical use of a cranioclast (ii) Moving object like stone or bullet strikes the head (iii) Head crushed under wheels of a moving vehicle in road traffic accident (iv) *Punch drunk syndrome.*

Indirect violence: Here the forces act indirectly on the skull through some other structure, which receives primary impact such as: (i) Fall on buttock from height transmits force through the vertebral column to occipital bone producing ring fracture (ii) Blast explosions of face from below (iii) Heavy blows on chin when the force is transmitted to skull with resulting fracture of base of skull.

Mechanics of Skull Fracture

Rowbotham has described direct and indirect injuries to skull.

Direct injury to skull: Direct injuries can be due to local or general deformation such as:

1. *Fractures due to local deformation (Struck hoop analogy):* When skull receives a focal impact, there is momentary distortion of the shape of cranium. Infants skulls are more pliable and flexible and more liable to deformation. Due to this more distortion occurs than the more rigid adult skulls. The area under the point of impact bends inwards, contents of skull being virtually incompressible, a compensatory distortion or bulging of other areas occurs called the **struck hoop analogy** (Figure 15.6). Skull is more susceptible to traction forces than the compression, so convexities fracture during distortion of 'struck hoop' (Figure 15.7).

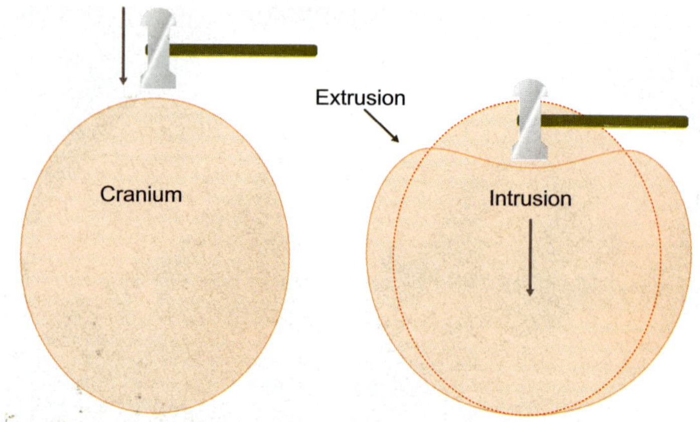

Figure 15.6: Illustration of 'struck hoop' analogy of impact on the skull

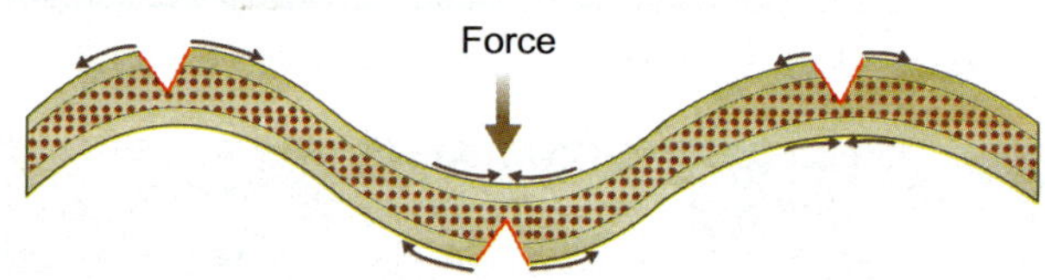

Figure 15.7: Fracture during the distortion of the 'struck hoop'

2. *Fractures due to general deformation:* Skull is compressed like elastic sphere. When skull is deformed, compression occurs on the concavity of curved bone and tension (tearing) force on convexity. If tearing force exceeds the limit of elasticity, fracture results. The inner table will fracture where skull is indented and outer table will fracture at the margins of deformed area. If forces are great enough, comminuted fracture occurs.

Indirect injury to skull: Here, the forces act away from the body that is chin, feet and buttocks resulting in skull fracture. (i) **Gurdijian** gave the hypothesis for the purpose of linear fracture, which develops, in the areas of stress. When force is applied to the skull at a particular point, in bending of skull occurs at a point of impact and stress areas develop at places away from the point of impact and result in linear fracture, which may extend to join the point of impact. These stress areas may be primary, secondary or tertiary. (ii) A heavy impact on the side of the top of head often leads to fracture of the vault running into base of skull usually across the floor of middle cranial fossa along the anterior margins of petrous temporal to enter the pituitary fossa. (iii) Sometimes, fractures are initiated at a distance away from the point of impact due to compensatory deformation but running usually back towards the impact site. In major injuries, this fracture may often cross the floor of skull to form a hinge fracture. (iv) A blow or fall onto the occiput may produce a fracture passing typically vertically or obliquely downward just to the side of midline of posterior fossa commonly reaching foramen magnum and causing ring fracture. (v) When severe local impact causes focal and general deformation, combination of depressed fracture and radial fracture lines may form a 'spider web' pattern. (vi) ***Puppe's rule:*** When two or more separate fractures occur from successive impacts and meet each other the later fracture (Y) will terminate at, that is not cross, the earlier fracture line (X) which naturally interrupts the cranial distortion which proceeds fracturing (Figure 15.8).

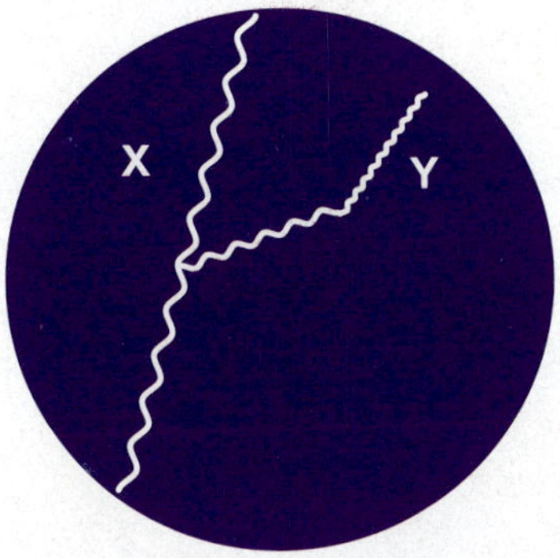

Figure 15.8: Puppe's rule

Types of Skull Fracture

1. **Linear (Fissured fracture) (Figure 15.9):** Linear fracture is commonly missed radiographically and is found at autopsy. The fracture is straight or curved lines often of considerable length. They either radiate out from a depressed zone or arise under or at a certain distance from impact area from bulging deformation. It usually involves either table of skull, sometimes both inner and outer. The fractures are common in weak unsupported areas like temporal, frontal, parietal and occipital. The fracture line may extend towards foramen magnum to the base of skull, across the supraorbital ridges or into the floor of skull which is called **'motorcyclist's fracture** (Figure 15.10). In children and young adults, a linear fracture may pass into a suture line and causes a 'diastasis' or opening fracture of the weaker seam between the bones. The fracture is direct or 'stepped'.

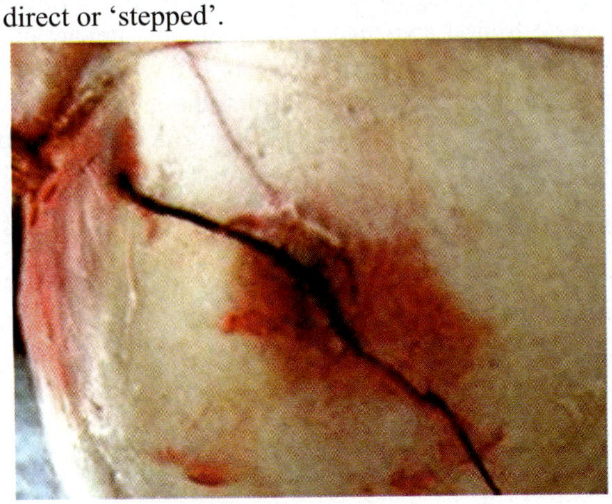

Figure 15.9: Linear fracture of vault of skull

2. **Diastasis (Sutural fracture Figure 15.3):** It is a linear fracture, which in children and adults passes into a suture line and cause diastasis or opening of weaker seam between sutures. The most commonly involved suture is sagittal and even the metopic suture may reopen. This type of fracture is common in child abuse syndrome.

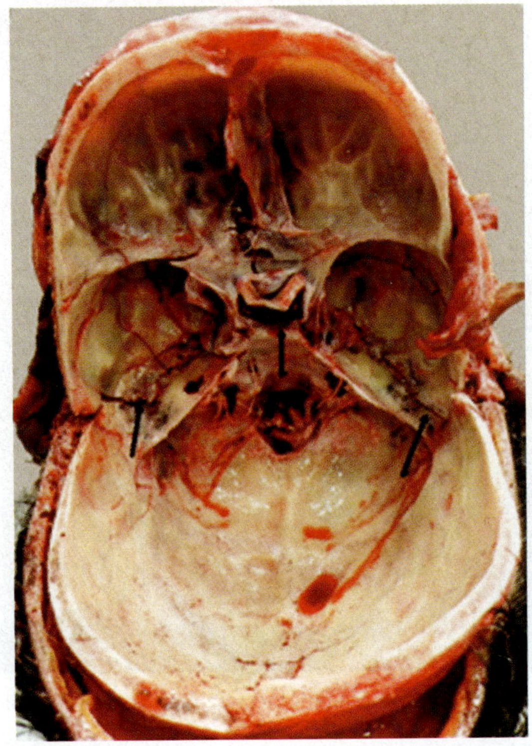

Figure 15.10: Fracture of base of skull into anterior and posterior halves (Hinge fracture)

3. **Ring fracture (Figure 15.12):** Occurs in posterior cranial fossa and foramen magnum. It is most often caused by fall from height on to the feet or buttocks. If kinetic energy of fall is not absorbed by fracture of legs, pelvis or spine, impact is transmitted up the cervical spine. This may be rammed into the skull, carrying a circle of occipital bone with it.
4. **Pond or Ping-pong ball or Indented fracture:** The pond fracture is shallow depressed fracture forming a concave 'pond'. The fracture is more common in pliable bones of infants. Depression occurs in absence of fracture akin to distortion produced by squeezing a table tennis ball.
5. **Comminuted (Mosaic/Spider web fracture) (Figure 15.11):** A comminuted depressed fracture may also have fissures radiating from it forming a spider web or mosaic pattern. This results when severe local impact causes focal and general deformation of the skull.
6. **Depressed fracture (Signature fracture) (Figures 15.13 and 15.14):** When the focal impact is severe, it causes outer table to be driven inwards and unless absorbed in the diploe, inner table will be intruded into cranial cavity with all the dangers of direct damage to the contents. Sharp-edged weapons such as heavy knives and axes may cause this type of fracture. The deepest part of the depression will indicate where the weapon first struck, there may be 'terracing' of the margin.
7. **Gutter fracture:** When a part of thickness of skull bone is removed to form a gutter, e.g., in oblique bullet wound. Sometimes, it is associated with irregular depressed fracture

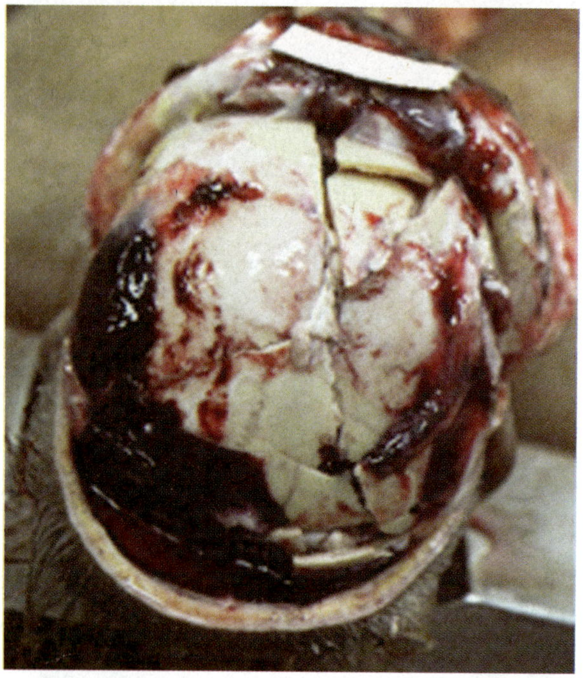

Figure 15.11: Comminuted fracture of vault of skull

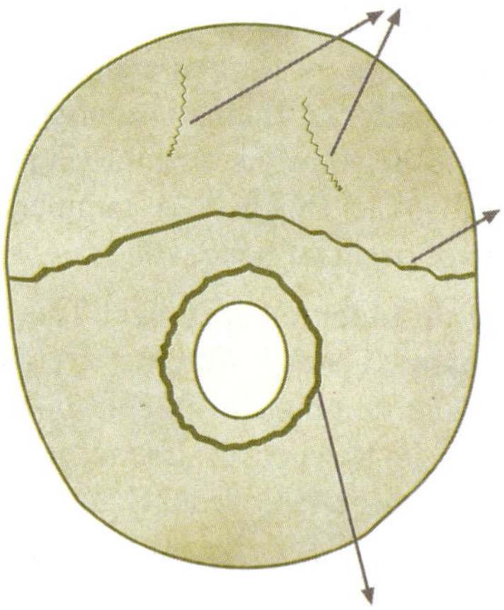

Figure 15.12: Different fractures of base of skull

of the inner table, compressing the underlying dura mater and brain.

Force Required for Causing Skull Fracture

(i) Tensile strength of adult skull is 100-150 psi and compressive strength varies from 5000 to 31000 psi. A force of about five foot-pounds can cause a simple fissured fracture of the skull. Falling to the ground from an erect posture develops at least 60 ft./lb and can easily produce skull fractures. A small stone or golf ball weighing about 100 gms may cause a linear fracture or when thrown with moderate force against the temporal bone. (ii) The adult head

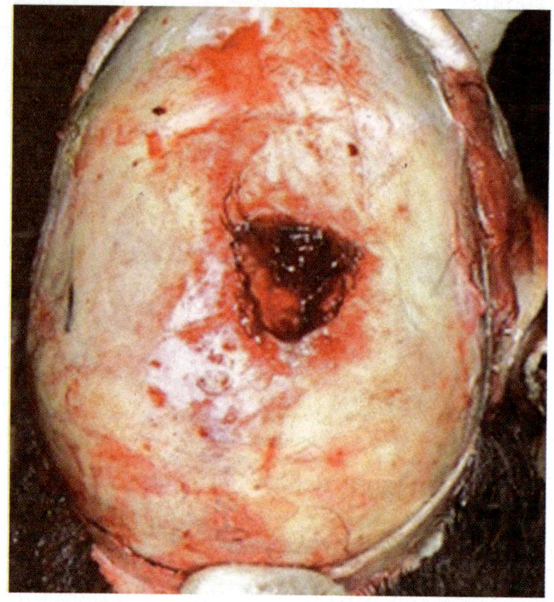

Figure 15.13: Vault of skull showing depressed fracture

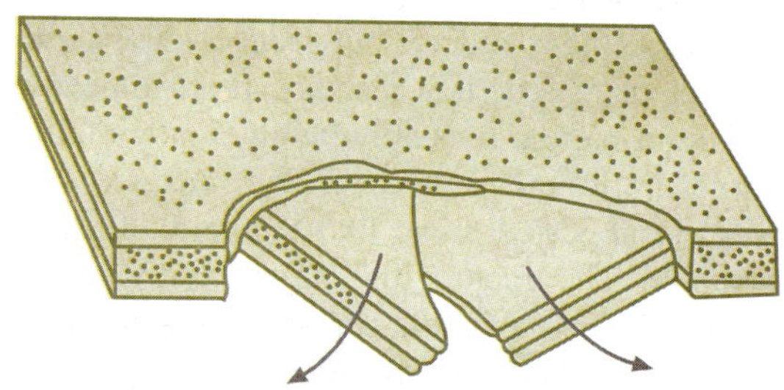

Figure 15.14: Depressed comminuted fracture of skull

weighs 3-6 kgs averaging 4.5 kgs, when falling through about one meter so frontal area strikes hard surface, impact energy of about 35 ft/lb develops that can cause one to two linear or mosaic fracture. Great variations occur in this, the area of skull struck, the thickness of the skull, scalp and hair, direction of impact all affect the outcome.

Complications of Fracture of Skull

1. **Injury to brain:** The fracture of the skull causes the injury to the brain that is dangerous to life.
2. **Haemorrhage:** If fracture passes through embedded meningeal artery haemorrhage results that is fatal.
3. **Traumatic epilepsy:** Late effect of depressed fracture of skull is traumatic epilepsy that usually manifests as tonic or clonic fits, which may be difficult to differentiate from idiopathic epilepsy. Usually when fit starts one or two years after major head injury in otherwise fit individual then the diagnosis is easy. There is usually a depressed fracture impinging on underlying cortex often in parietotemporal area. It is more common in open head injuries with infection.
4. **Infections:** Infections following skull fractures can be by

(i) Direct spread through compound fracture (ii) By spread from nasal cavity when fracture of cribriform plate is allowed communication to anterior fossa; and (iii) By spread from fracture that involves a paranasal sinus such as frontal or ethmoid or from the mastoid air cells or middle ear cavity.

Traumatic Intracranial Haemorrhages

The intracranial haemorrhages are of the following types:

Extradural Haemorrhage

Bleeding between inner surface of skull and dura mater is least common of three types of brain membrane haemorrhage. It is also known as epidural haemorrhage. According to Rowbotham, only 3% of head injuries have epidural haemorrhage. The dura is closely applied to the interior of the skull except in the posterior fossa, that is why extradural bleeding does not occur over the skull floor. Most extradural haemorrhage is associated with fractures of the skull. About 10% of extradural haemorrhage is associated with subdural haemorrhage. The usual site is unilateral in a parietotemporal area caused by the rupture of middle meningeal artery that runs between the dura and the skull (Figures 15.15 to 15.17).

Hume Adams suggests that a minimum volume of 35 ml is needed before clinical signs are apparent though other writers suggest 100 ml is usually the minimum associated with fatalities. Leakage of high-pressure arterial blood strips back the underlying dura with progressive accumulation of a hematoma. When bleeding is venous, the hematoma rarely reach a large size as pressure is insufficient to tear back much of dura. The clinical signs of an epidural haemorrhage are clinically those of a **lucid or latent interval**, as there may be recovery from the initial phase of concussion before. Typically, the patient recovers consciousness from the initial trauma only to slip back into a progressively deepening coma. Sufficient blood accumulates to cause raised intracranial pressure and consequent relapse into unconsciousness. In Rowbotham's series, the range of latent interval was from two hours to seven days, but most were apparent after 4 hours. Extradural hematomas are surgical emergencies that if not drained will produce uncinate herniation, tonsillar herniation, medullary compression, respiratory arrest and death rapidly.

Heat haematoma: This artefact mimics an extradural haemorrhage, when head has been exposed to severe external heat sufficient to burn the scalp and perhaps skull. Blood may be extruded from diploe and venous sinuses into the extradural space to produce a 'heat haematoma'. It contains about 100-120 ml of blood. This haematoma is brown and friable and adjacent brain shows hardening and discolouration from heat. The haematoma shows honeycomb appearance and is pink in colour due to high levels of carboxyhaemoglobin. Level of carboxyhaemoglobin in the haematoma in cases of fire can give us the idea about whether the bleed is true extradural haematoma due to blunt force/surface impact or is heat haematoma. If level of carboxyhaemoglobin

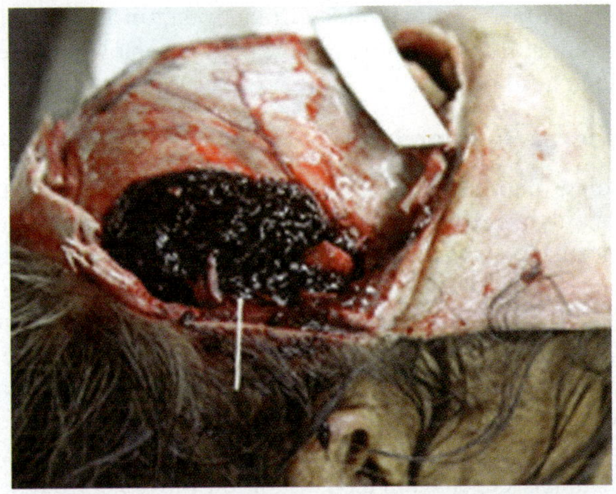

Figure 15.15: Extradural haemorrhage right temporoparietal area of cerebrum

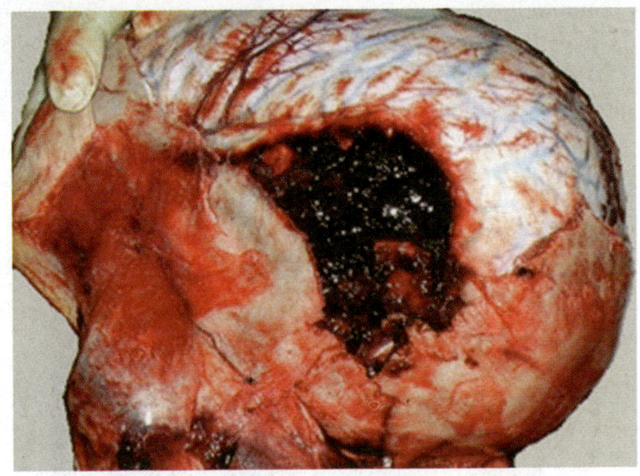

Figure 15.16: Extradural haemorrhage over left parietal area of cerebrum

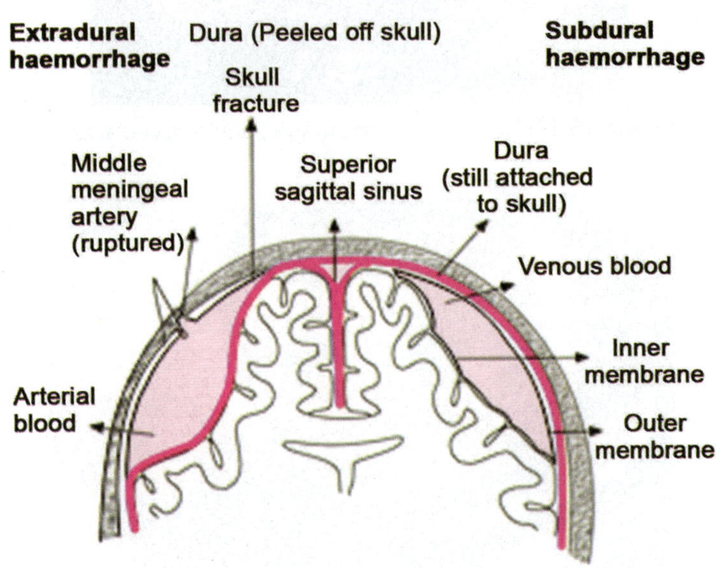

Figure 15.17: Formation of subdural and extradural haemorrhage

is same in both haematoma and blood, then it is probably heat haematoma. If there is little or no carboxyhaemoglobin the bleed is due to head injury.

Subdural Haemorrhage

Bleeding into relatively wide space between the dura and arachnoid membrane is much more common than extradural haemorrhage. It results from the rupture of the bridging veins that connects the venous system of the brain to the large intradural venous sinuses (Figure 15.17). Because the brain, in its bath of CSF, can move within the skull but the venous sinuses are fixed, the displacement of brain that occurs in trauma can tear some of these delicate veins at the point where they penetrate the dura. It is less often associated with fracture of skull. As subdural haematomas depend for their origin on movement of the brain rather than the direct application of force, they are the reflection of inertial rather than impact forces. Consequently, they occur most commonly where the freedom of movement is the greatest, that is over the convexities of the hemispheres (Figures 15.18 and 15.19). They are relatively uncommon where little relative movement is possible, such as the posterior fossa.

Subdural haemorrhage can occur at any age but is common at extremes of lives. Subdural haemorrhage with long bone fracture is typical of child abuse as seen by Caffey. In old people, these haemorrhages exist in chronic form. The condition is always due to trauma. In alcoholics and people with bleeding diathesis, minimal trauma can start the bleed. The lesion is traditionally classified into acute, the subacute and the chronic.

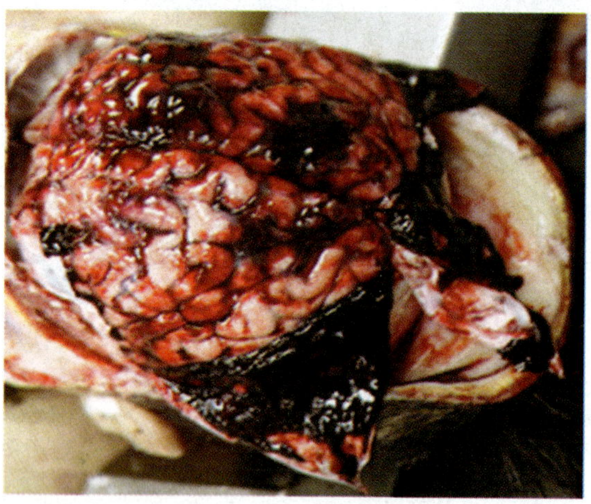

Figure 15.18: Subdural haemorrhage parieto-occipital area

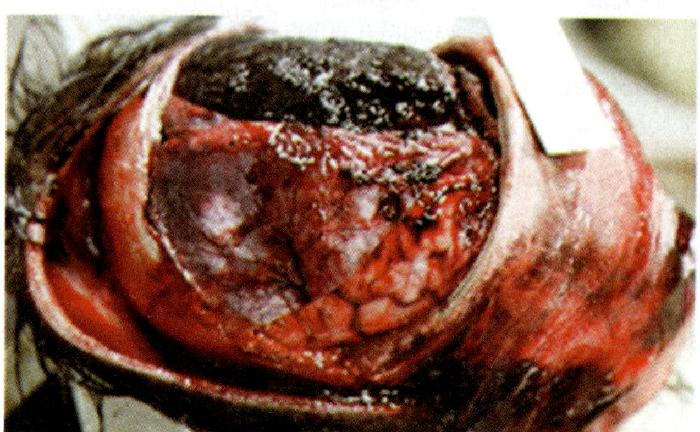

Figure 15.19: Subdural haemorrhage over left cerebral hemisphere

Acute subdural haemorrhage: The classical feature is presence of lucid (latent) interval. Since the bleeding in acute subdural haemorrhage is of venous origin and at lower pressure, onset of symptoms is delayed. The lesion is manifested by gradual decline in level of consciousness and focal signs rarely.

Chronic subdural haemorrhage: Older people and chronic alcoholics are commonly the victims of chronic subdural haemorrhage. In these patients, there is usually some atrophy of brain and consequent upon this, an increased range of movement of the brain within the skull. Thus there is a higher risk of rupturing the bridging veins and bilateral subdural haematomas may develop slowly following an insignificant or unnoticed trauma. As they develop relatively slowly, the brain is able to accommodate to their mass effect. Thus these haematomas produce much greater cerebral distortion and herniation than acute subdural hematomas before symptoms and signs develop.

Gross appearance of subdural haemorrhage varies with age. Recent lesions up to several weeks old are tan or brown with gelatinous membrane covering the surface. The contents are thick but liquid and may have area of redder more recent bleeding. An older haematoma up to months or even a year old is firmer with a tough membrane around both surfaces, resembling a rubber hot water filled with jelly or oil. The contents are liquid and may be brown or even straw coloured. Sometimes, variegation in colour is seen due to bleeds of different ages. Many subdural bleeds in old people are small and do not give rise to any neurological defects. Hence, the mere finding of such small lesion at autopsy should not be used to provide cause of death.

The chronic hematoma may become large and press down on cerebral hemisphere sufficiently to dent or distort the surface. This may progress and give rise to sign of hippocampal and cerebellar tonsillar herniation and dangers to vital center in the brainstem. The chronic hematoma arises from the center lesion, which after an interval becomes sheathed in a capsule of connective tissue. The mechanism of enlargement is controversial and the theories put forward are: (i) One theory is repeated bleeding from new blood vessels that enter the mass as part of healing process; and (ii) Other theory involves osmosis, in which because the center of haemorrhage commonly liquefies forming haemorrhagic fluid that osmotically attracts into it CSF from outside the capsule.

Dating of Subdural Haemorrhage

- **Gross appearance:** (i) Within few hours reaction to subdural bleeding begins when cellular infiltration begins from dural surface. (ii) A subdural haematoma gradually changes colour from dark red to brownish colour, first being apparent not before five days and sometimes not obvious for 10-12 days. (iii) Discrete surface membrane becomes obvious by 2nd week. (iv) Liquefaction of contents occurs after more than 3 weeks. (v) After one month, a firm capsule forming a cystic cavity containing a dark brown watery fluid is formed.

- **Histological appearance:** A delicate **neo-membrane** histologically composed of thin-walled capillaries and fibroblastic granulation tissue, grows from periphery to cover outer surface of the clot during next few days and weeks. If no further enlargement occurs, this capsule becomes more and more fibrous. According to **Crompton** the presence of a membrane firm, enough to be picked off with forceps makes subdural haemorrhage at least 12 days old. There are claims made for accurate dating of subdural haematomas by histological criteria as given by **Monro and Meritt.** They are briefly summarized under Table 15.1.

Table 15.1: Histological dating of subdural haematoma

Time	Histological appearance
With 36 hours	Fibroblasts appear at margin of clot
By 4 days	Neo-membrane adjacent to dura is few cell thick
5-8 days	Membrane well established; fibroblast migrate from it into the clot. After 5 days, hemosiderin laden phagocytes are present which may be stained with Perl's reaction
By 8 days	Membrane 12 to 14 cell thick, visible to the naked eye after few days
By 11 days	Strands of fibroblast subdivide the clot
By 15 days	Membrane also present on the under surface of clot and outer neo-membrane is half to one third the thickness of dura. Inner membrane is still only half thick
1-3 months	Membrane has lost many fibroblastic nuclei and becomes hyaline
6-12 months	Membrane is thick and fibrous resembling the dura

Subarachnoid Haemorrhage (Figures 15.20 and 15.21)

The third type of brain haemorrhage bleeding is even more common than subdural haemorrhage. It is usually associated with extradural or subdural haemorrhage, sometimes it can occur as

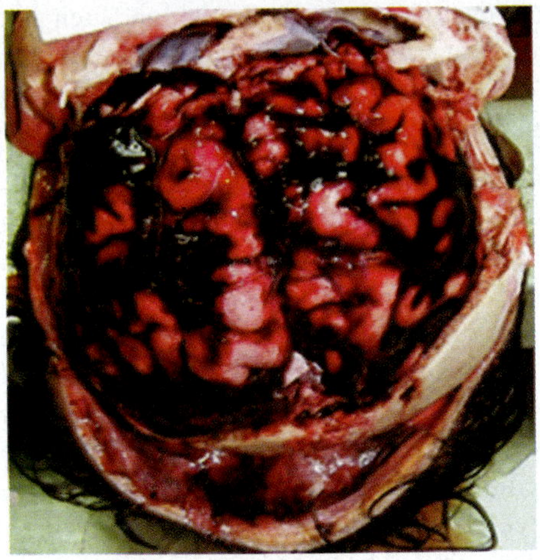

Figure 15.20: Subarachnoid haemorrhage over bilateral cerebral hemispheres in road traffic accident

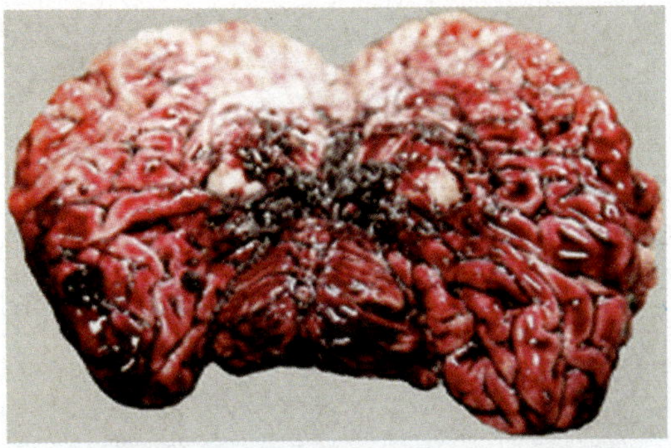

Figure 15.21: Subarachnoid haemorrhage over base of brain due to ruptured aneurysm

pure lesion. It sometimes occurs as a result of natural disease especially as rupture of vascular malformation of several types.

Appearance and mechanism of formation: The appearance of subarachnoid haemorrhage caused by trauma varies greatly according to the nature and extent of injury. When it is secondary to laceration of the brain or extensive cortical contusions then its localization and severity depends upon primary injury. When it arises from a blunt impact, then its position is not a good localizing sign. Blood in the subarachnoid space mixes with CSF, which dilutes it and makes it less ready to clot and allows more mobility. Hemolysis turns CSF into xanthochromatic yellow and within weeks the blood disappears. There may be some residual brown or yellow staining of pia or arachnoid.

Intracerebral Haemorrhage (Figures 15.22 and 15.23)

Traumatic intracerebral haemorrhage is primarily occurring at the time of impact or soon afterwards; others are secondary and caused by changes in intracranial pressure. In the cerebral hemisphere, deep haemorrhage can be caused by coup or contrecoup mechanisms and may be situated anywhere in the hemisphere. They may rupture into ventricular system or through overlying cortex with resulting intracerebral haemorrhage. Whether a scalp injury (such as fall) was responsible for cerebral haemorrhage or whether sudden stroke caused by a natural cerebral haemorrhage resulted in fall is to be answered during autopsy examination.

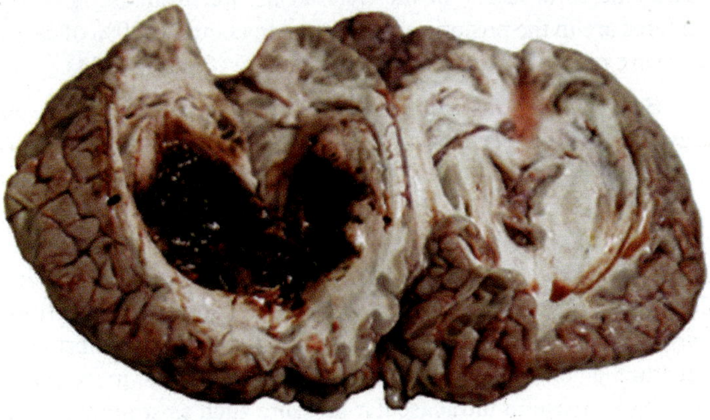

Figure 15.22: Intracerebral hemorrhage

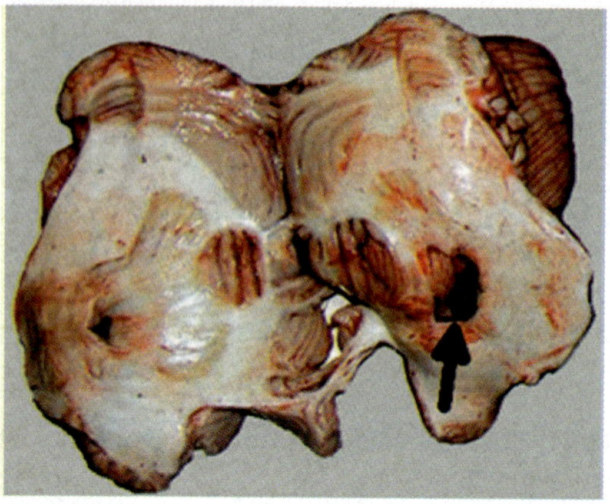

Figure 15.23: Fourth ventricle bleed in a case of road traffic accident

Non-Traumatic Intracranial Haemorrhage

Spontaneous subarachnoid haemorrhage: The hypertensive haemorrhages result from the rupture of microaneurysms called Charcot-Bouchard aneurysms that form at the bifurcations of small intraparenchymal arteries. Bursting destroys the aneurysm responsible for the haemorrhage and the adjacent brain tissue. These aneurysms are seen in increasing number in the arteries of the brain with age and length of history of hypertension. The major sites of hypertensive haemorrhages are the putamen (55%), lobar white matter (15%), thalamus (10%), pons (10%) and cerebellar cortex (10%).

Bleeding into subarachnoid space is usually the result of rupture of an aneurysm or rarely an arteriovenous malformation. Aneurysms can be (i) Developmental (Berry, congenital) (ii) Arteriosclerotic (fusiform) (iii) Inflammatory (mycotic); and (iv) Traumatic.

Berry aneurysms are the most common variety accounting for 95% of the aneurysms that rupture. They occur at the bifurcations of major cerebral arteries. The most common sites that account for about 85% of all ruptured berry aneurysms are at (i) Junction of carotid and posterior communicating arteries (ii) Anterior communicating artery (iii) Major bifurcation of the middle cerebral artery in the Sylvian fissure. Remaining of the ruptures are in the posterior circulation. In about 20-30% of cases, there are multiple berry aneurysmal rupture (Figure 15.24).

Berry aneurysms are also called congenital aneurysms but they are not present at birth. They develop because there is a discontinuity in the smooth muscle of the media of the carina of arterial bifurcations. The arterial wall bulges out through the muscular defect to form a thin-walled saccular fundus, composed of only fibrous tissue in which there may be additional local degeneration and calcification. Laminated blood clot and fibrin may be deposited on this attenuated wall. This insubstantial structure is like an inflated balloon, and ruptures in activities causing increase in intravascular pressure such as straining while defecation, lifting heavy weights and sexual intercourse.

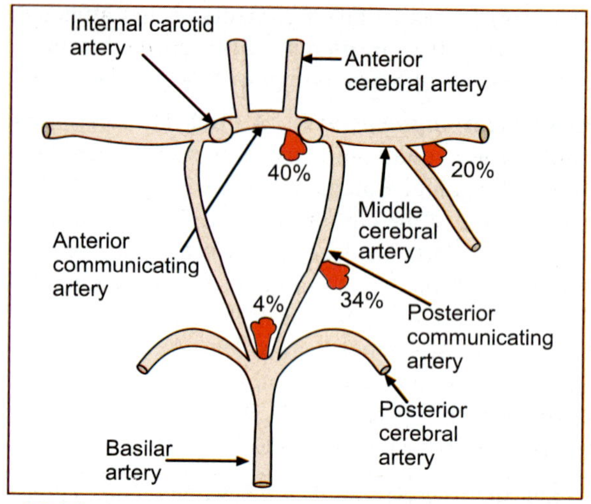

Figure 15.24: Common sites of berry aneurysms in the circle of Willis

Mixed subarachnoid and CNS haemorrhages: These mixed haemorrhages result from (i) Arteriovenous malformations (ii) Cavernous angiomas (iii) Capillary telangiectasis.

Medicolegal Aspects of Brain Haemorrhage

Ruptured berry aneurysm and trauma: Several variation of this exists. Most commonly, an assault is rapidly followed by signs of subarachnoid bleeding and subsequently death. When the blow to the head is hard then it is easy to prove that trauma led to the rupture of berry aneurysm, but when the blow is not so heavy then the evidence is not so convincing. The complicating factor is that most assault occur in conditions when both the aggressor and victims are physically and emotionally active, so that adrenal response is likely to be present. Muscle tone, heart rate and blood pressure increase and it is likely that raised internal blood pressure in a weak aneurysm is a far more potent reason for rupture than a blow on the head. A second possibility is that already leaking aneurysm may have a rapidly developing neurological even behavioral abnormality that led him to conflict with another person or into dangerous physical position, such as fall or traffic accident. However, at autopsy, it may not be able to distinguish the sequence of events and the aneurysmal rupture may be blamed on the trauma instead of the reverse.

Subarachnoid haemorrhage and alcohol: A high blood alcohol is said to facilitate bursting of an aneurysm because it dilates cerebral blood vessels and increases blood flow. The fibrous wall of an aneurysm is incapable of dilating; neither can major basal arteries do so to appreciable degree, as they possess little muscle. However, there is no evidence that alcohol is associated with completely natural subarachnoid haemorrhage from a ruptured aneurysm, though intense physical activity such as sports or coitus certainly does predispose to rupture. Moreover, alcohol increases the chance to fight producing trauma and leading to subarachnoid haemorrhage. Due to unsteady gait, there are always chances of fall.

Head injuries in boxers: Persons who indulge in boxing are at the risk of both acute and chronic damage to their brain. The acute injuries are less common but occur during or soon after fight itself. The most common lesion is a subdural haemorrhage. Extradural bleeding almost never occurs.

Most attention has been paid to the chronic changes in boxer's brain, which is very common and give rise to what is generally known as **punch-drunk syndrome**. Due to repeated blows by boxers, the victim presents with findings that may be mistaken for drunkenness. It is also known as **Dementia pugilistica.** The length of time a boxer is involved in fighting is more important than number of serious traumatic events he has suffered. There are both anatomical and microscopic lesions. Grossly affected brain may show some cortical atrophy and slight hydrocephalus. Throughout the brain substance, there may be scars and patches of gliosis. These persons also suffer from development of an Alzheimers like condition, with neuro-fibrillatory tangles throughout cerebral cortex and brainstem though no senile plaques are present.

VERTEBROBASILAR ARTERY INJURY

It has been recognized that blows to the side of the neck can give rise to fatal subarachnoid bleeding because of tearing or dissection of intrathecal course of vertebral artery allowing blood to track along the upper part of the vessel and enter the cranial cavity where the artery penetrates the dural membrane of the foramen magnum. Basilar artery and internal carotid artery can also give rise to the syndrome. The injury is manifested as skin bruising and bleeding into the deep neck muscles.

Mechanism of vertebral artery trauma: The vertebral artery is injured due to (i) Overstretching of atlanto-occipital membrane and (ii) impact on muscles overlying the transverse process of upper cervical vertebrae.

The damage to the vertebral artery occurs at the following places: (i) In the canal within the first cervical vertebrae (ii) Just below the axis, in the space between transverse process of axis and atlas (iii) As it emerges from the exit of the canal in the atlas (iv) Within the subarachnoid space in the foramen magnum.

The most vulnerable points for trauma are: (i) At the penetration of dura (ii) At exit from Atlas and transverse process; and (iii) In osseous canal in atlas.

The demonstration of intracranial bleeding from the vertebrobasilar system is difficult since while removing the skull and brain at autopsy, the damage to vessels occurs causing artifactual bleeding.

Autopsy findings: (i) When an external bruise is seen on the side of the neck in a case of fatal assault such as from a fist, shoe or blunt weapon, the possibility of vetebral artery injury should be borne in mind. (ii) When there are circumstantial evidences suggesting subarachnoid haemorrhage, vetebral artery damage should be suspected. (iii) Usually an external injury is absent but on dissection of neck, there is bruising of subcutaneous or deep tissues of neck. (iv) Radiographs of the anteroposterior and lateral view of the upper cervical region should be taken. These would reveal fracture of transverse process of the atlas vertebra, if rarely present. (v) Before search for vetebral artery damage is made, brain should be examined for berry aneurysms or other vascular haemorrhages in cases of substantial subarachnoid haemorrhages. (vi) Postmortem angiograms can be taken, if facilities exist. (vii) When the facilities for radiography and angiogram do not exist, upper cervical region is dissected to search for vertebral artery damage. (viii) Upper cervical spine is exposed by a posterior approach by making spine free of muscles. The spine should then be sawn till fourth cervical vertebra. The block of bone is cut out of the floor of the posterior cranial fossa. This block is decalcified by prolonged immersion in 10% formic acid. After a week, lateral parts of transverse process can be shaved. The block is again decalcified for further one week. The artery can now be exposed by shaving transverse processes.

Cerebral Injuries

The brain may be injured: (i) By direct intrusion of foreign object such as a penetrating weapon, either bullet or fragments of skull in a compound fracture. (ii) By deformation of the brain in closed head injury. Rotatory movement is the main culprit in causing brain damage. No actual blow or fall need be suffered by the head to cause severe and even fatal brain damage. It is the change in velocity, either acceleration or deceleration with a rotational rather than solely axial element that leads to damage.

Cerebral Lacerations and Cerebral Contusions

They are most often found in those areas of the brain where cortex is most likely to be exposed to irregularities in the internal profile of skull. The undersurface of the temporal lobes and the orbital surface of the frontal lobes suffer most often.

Cerebral contusions (Figure 15.25): They occur where blunt trauma crushes or bruises brain tissue without rupturing the pia. The most common sites of contusions are either (i) Directly

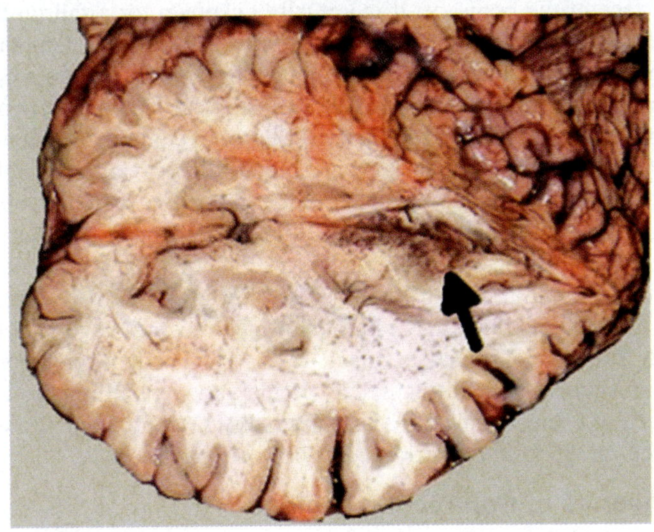

Figure 15.25: Haemorrhagic contusion seen on dissection of brain

related to the trauma, in which case they may be coup or contrecoup lesions; or (ii) Indirectly related, occurring at points where the brain as it moves, can strike the irregularities on the inner surface of the skull such as the lesser wing of the sphenoid, and the orbital ridges that produces contusions at the frontal and temporal poles and on the orbitofrontal gyri. Contusions usually affect only the crowns of the gyri, leaving the depths of the gyri intact, but there is often substantial attenuation of the underlying white matter that extends under adjacent intact cortex. In ischemia, cortical lesion is usually more extensive than the damage to white matter. Histologically, acute contusions show foci of haemorrhagic gray matter that is subsequently removed by macrophages leaving an irregular yellow-brown crater with a floor of reactive glial tissue and often some leptomeningeal fibrosis.

Cerebral lacerations: These are tears in the brain tissue produced by more severe blunt trauma that is often accompanied by other damage such as fractures and local haemorrhage and necrosis. Resolution of lacerations is similar to that of contusions, except that it results in an irregular, yellow-brown gliotic scar that involves not only the cortex and meninges but also deeper structures.

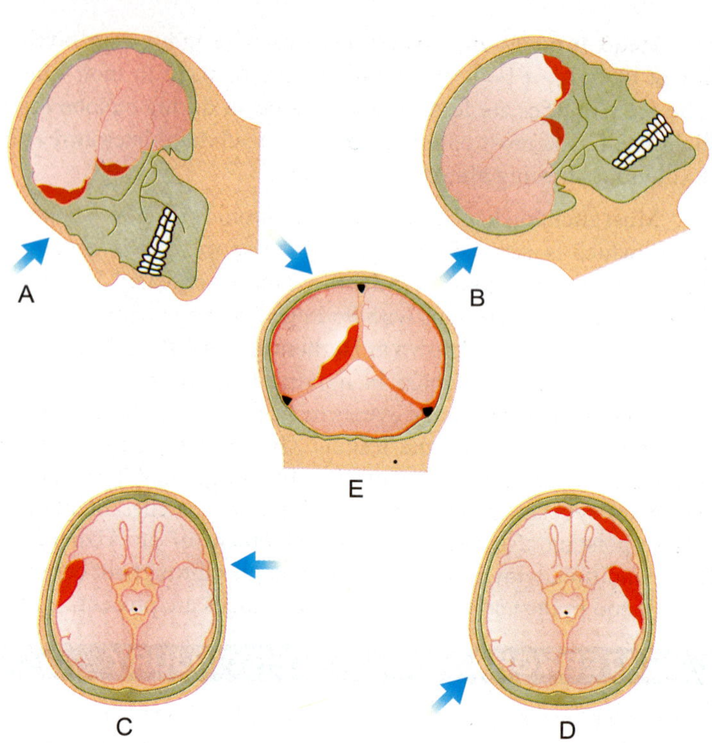

Figure 15.26: Mechanism of coup and contrecoup injuries of the brain (A) Coup frontotemporal contusions from falls on the frontal region (B) Contrecoup contusions in the same location from fall on the back of the head (C) Contrecoup contusion of lateral aspect of the temporal lobe from impact of head on opposite side (D) Contrecoup injury of the frontotemporal region from fall on the opposite parieto-occipital region (E) Diffuse contrecoup 'contusion' of medial temporo-occipital region from impact of fall on parietal region

Coup and Contrecoup Damage

Coup (blow impact) means injury that is located beneath the area of impact and results directly from impacting force. **Contrecoup** means that the lesion is present in an area opposite to the side of impact.

The following practical points should be considered (Figure 15.26): (i) Sometimes only contrecoup lesion is there with no coup damage at all. (ii) There need not be any fracture of skull, even in presence of coup and contrecoup lesion. (iii) Most common sites for contrecoup injury is in the frontal lobes. It is often at the tips of frontal poles and may be symmetrical, if a fall on occiput has occurred. (iv) In temporal and parietal impacts, the contrecoup lesions are likely to be diametrically opposite on the contralateral surface of the brain. (v) It is virtually unknown for a fall on the frontal region to produce occipital contrecoup. (vi) In a temporal impact, the contrecoup damage may not be on contralateral hemisphere but on opposite side of ipsilateral hemisphere from impact against the falx cerebri. (vii) Degree of contrecoup damage may be severe, sufficient to cause blood-filled cavitations in the deep cortex and underlying white matter especially in frontal lobes and tips of temporal lobes. (viii) With severe frontal contrecoup from a fall on occiput, the transmitted force may be sufficient to fracture the thin bone of the floor of anterior fossa. Such cracks in the roof of orbits may allow meningeal haemorrhage to seep into orbits and appear as **black eyes.** (ix) Though contrecoup contusion is classically caused by deceleration of a falling head, it can also occur when a fixed head is struck. (x) Contrecoup lesions occur in the form of cortical contusions or lacerations.

Theories of Contrecoup Lesions

Various theories for such type of injuries are:

Struck Hoop theory: Due to the elasticity of skull, the flattening of the skull result at the point of impact resulting in compression of skull so that skull assumes an ovoid shape shortly and thus damage is caused to the opposite side of the impact on brain.

Russell's theory: Sudden displacement of brain towards impact site due to brain reacting as jelly mass and potential space is developed on opposite side, injuring the vessels and resulting in subdural and cortical injuries.

Gaggio's pressure gradient theory: At the moment of impact, there is positive pressure on the side of impact and negative pressure on opposite side; this bursts the vessels on the other side.

Holbourn shear strain theory (Rotational force theory): Contrecoup lesions are chiefly due to local distortion of blow that causes shear strains due to pulling apart of constituent particle of brain.

When the moving head is suddenly decelerated by hitting a firm surface, contrecoup injury results, e.g., striking head on ground directing fall. The sudden arrest of head results in brain that is still in motion striking the stationary skull.

Rawling's theory of bony irregularities: Irregular bony prominences particularly orbital and cribriform plate, lesser wings of sphenoid contuse or lacerate base of frontal lobes and tips of temporal lobe sometimes with fracture of orbital plate. A blow at the front of head may damage inner and lower parts of back of brain by contact with the edges of tentorium leading to brainstem injury and pontine haemorrhage.

Fall on the side of head producing contusion on the opposite side of the brain is due to formation of cavity or vacuum in cranial cavity on the opposite side of impact as brain lags behind the moving skull. The vacuum exerts a suction effect that damages the brain.

Moritz radiating wave theory: Energy of impact in a hollow organ propagates by radiating waves along the meridional lines that damages as they leave the site of impact and converges as they approach the opposite side.

Concussion

It is a transient paralytic state due to head injury, which is of instantaneous onset, does not show any evidence of structural cerebral injury and is always followed by amnesia from actual moment of accident. There may be evidence of depressed medullary function. Rate of change of velocity of head is important in producing concussion. It is extremely common and true concussion lasts for seconds or minutes. At autopsy, there is no macroscopic damage; though sometimes there is slight cerebral oedema and scattered nonspecific petechial haemorrhages. Shear stresses are instrumental in causing neuronal damage. Concussion is followed by **post-concussion state** characterized by headache, unsteadiness and anxiety. Retrograde amnesia is almost inevitably associated with concussion and it may also be transient. Though commonly only of minutes duration, it can extend to several days before head injury. However, there is often a later recovery of much the lost period, the memory of events immediately before the incident rarely return. The most acceptable hypothesis is **diffuse neuronal injury.** Histologically, extensive diffuse lesions are demonstrated as disruption of axon from shear and tensile strain, leading to bulbous and clubbed appearance.

Cerebral Oedema

Cerebral oedema leads to death because it compresses vital centers of brain. It may result from a local phenomenon around any laceration, contusion and infarct. Generalized cerebral oedema is common after head injury in children. Oedema is most common cause of raised intracranial pressure seen more often than localized space occupying such as hematoma and tumour. In cerebral oedema, the amount of fluid in the brain mainly in the white matter increases and total weight of brain increases by 100 gms.

Autopsy features of cerebral oedema (Figure 15.27): The weight of the brain is increased to more than 1450 gms. The dura is stretched and tense and the brain is bulging. The gyri are pale and flattened and there is thinning of grey matter. The sulci are filled and as a result, the cerebral surface is smooth. The cut surface is pale. In children, ventricles may be reduced to slits. Severe oedema causes large volumes of cerebral hemispheres to press

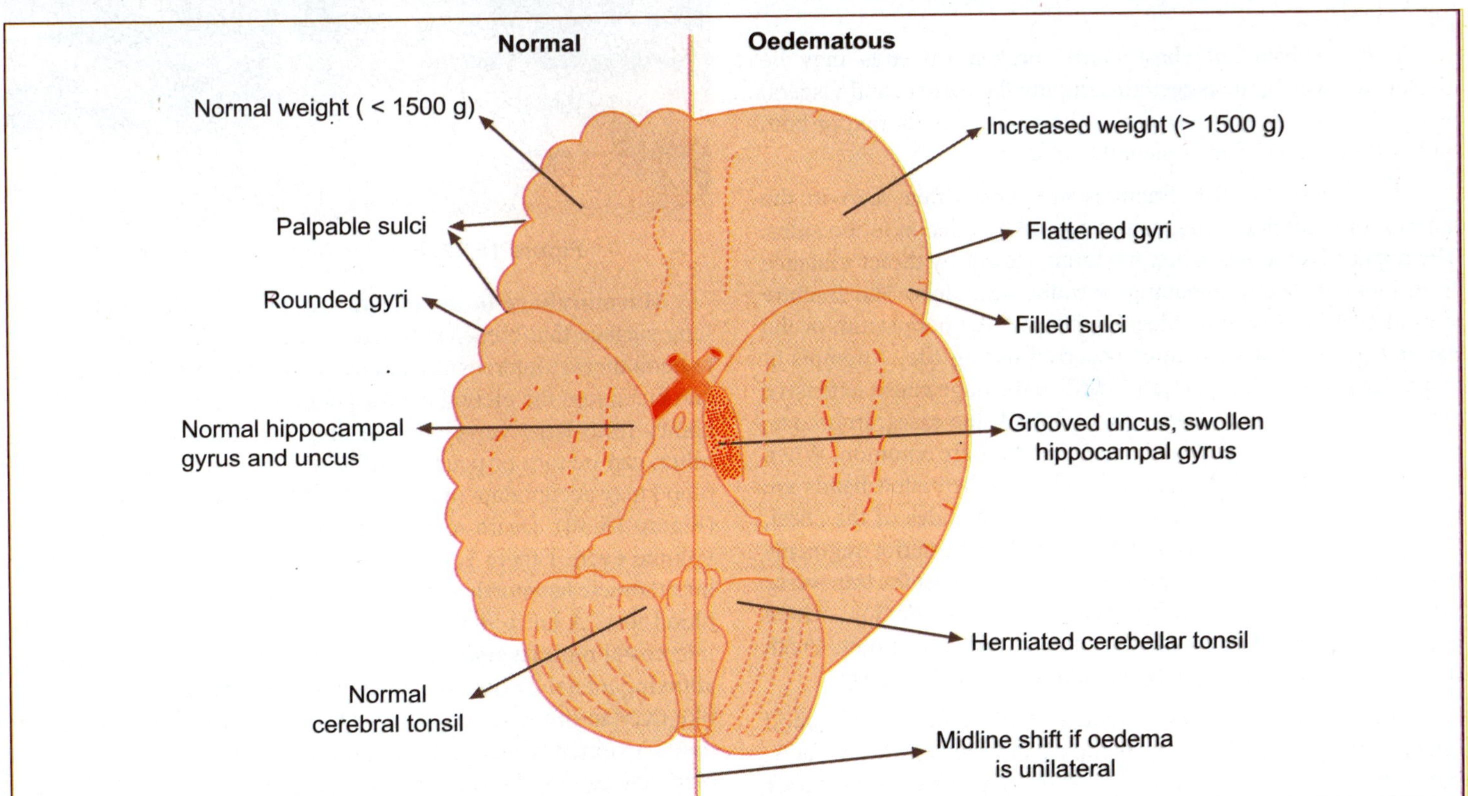

Figure 15.27: Features of cerebral oedema

down upon tentorium that herniates through midbrain opening. In addition, there are findings of uncal herniation.

CHEST INJURIES

The thoracic and abdominal viscera are most vulnerable to the penetrating injuries by the knife to the lower lateral wall of the thorax that may enter the pleural as well as the peritoneal cavity. The stab wounds of the heart may also involve the diaphragmatic and upper abdominal injuries. The stomach may often be penetrated.

Injuries to the chest wall: The integrity of the chest wall can be compromised either by severe mechanical failure of the rib cage or by the penetration of the pleural cavities. Rib fractures commonly occur but may embarrass respiration when they are multiple and thus prevent expansion of the thorax; their broken ends penetrate pleura and lungs or when the pleural and muscular pain limits respiratory effort.

Flail chest: The flail chest occurs when there are multiple bilateral fractures of most of the ribs and also of sternum. The rigidity of rib cage is lost and attempts at expanding the thoracic volume during inspiration are impaired. The loose section is sucked inwards during inspiration, is called paradoxical respiration. In this condition dyspnoea, cyanosis and progressive hypoxia results that is incompatible with life. The flail chest is caused by: (i) Frontal impact in motor vehicular accidents where the victim is thrown against the steering wheel or fascia (ii) In stamping accidents where the shod foot is applied violently to the supine body.

In any substantial chest injury, broken rib ends may be displaced inwards, the jagged tips ripping the parietal and visceral pleura. This may cause a pneumothorax or haemothorax, or both with formation of bronchopleural fistula.

Rib fractures: Rib fractures are most often seen in the anterior or posterior axillary lines caused by falls on to the sides. The upper ribs are less often fractured, except by direct violence from kicking, heavy punching or traffic accidents. The fracture sites almost always show bleeding beneath the periosteum or the parietal pleura if the fractures occurred during life. Attempts at resuscitation especially external cardiac massage cause extensive rib fractures (Figure 15.28) in about 40% of the cases. In infants, especially victims of child abuse, rib fractures are common. When an infant is squeezed from side to side, as when adult hands are clamped in each axilla or lower on the lateral sides of the chest, the hyperflexion can easily break ribs in their posterior segments usually near their necks. The ribs are levered against the transverse processes of the vertebrae by excessive anterior flexion, which explains the tendency to fracture in paravertebral gutter. Fresh fractures will be obvious both on radiography and autopsy.

The sternum may be fractured with effusion of blood underneath (Figure 15.29) by stamping or other frontal impacts, but far more force is necessary than with ribs. If posterior displacement of a fragment occurs, the underlying heart or great vessels may be severely damaged.

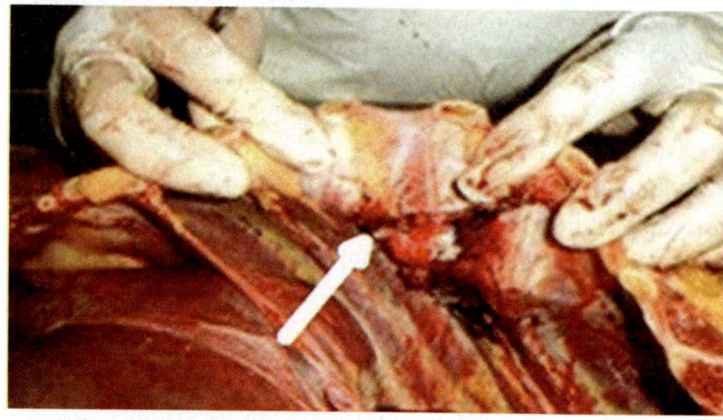

Figure 15.28: Fracture of ribs

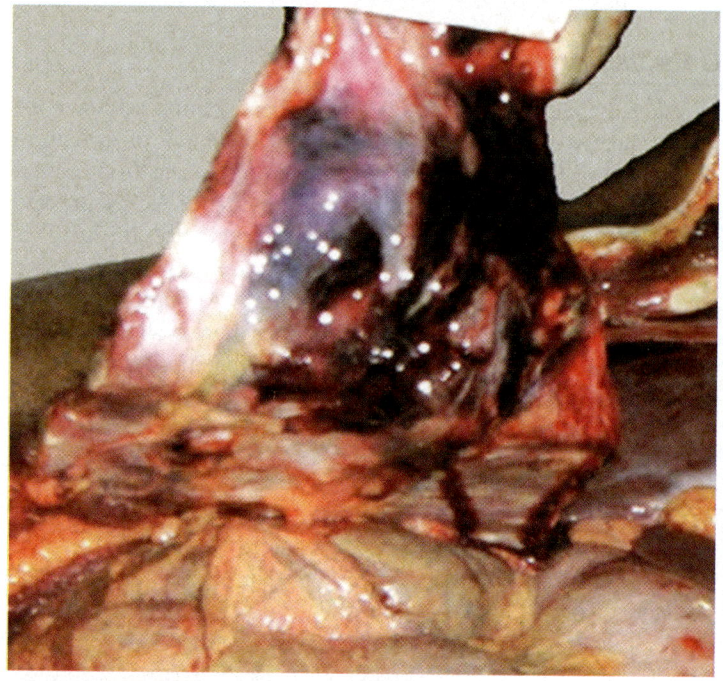

Figure 15.29: Effusion under the sternum

Haemorrhage in the chest: Any injury to the chest wall or lung surface that breaches blood vessels and the pleura can lead to hemothorax. Intercostals and less commonly mammary arteries can bleed into the pleural cavities but most massive haemorrhage comes from large vessels in the lung or mediastinum. The lung hilum can be torn or penetrated by stab wounds. Several liters of blood may accumulate in the chest, either as liquid or clot, or both (Figure 15.30). Death may occur from loss of circulating blood volume even if there is relatively little external bleeding. Many intrathoracic haemorrhages may be fatal with virtually no external blood loss. A knife that passes obliquely into the chest through intercostal muscles may puncture a great vessel or heart chamber allowing a fatal cardiac tamponade or hemothorax, yet the valve-like overlap of the tissues after withdrawal of the blade may seal up the external wound almost completely and prevent significant bleeding, especially as the blood inside the chest is not under any appreciable pressure. In a gunshot wound also, if the wound is uppermost after death, the bleeding can be virtually absent.

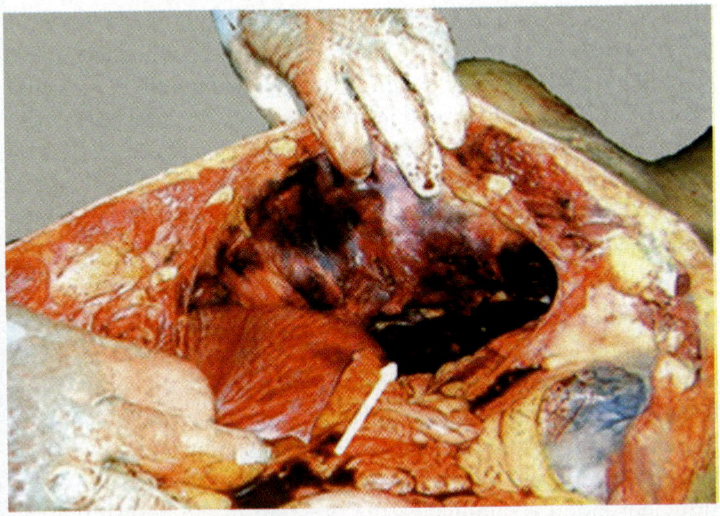

Figure 15.30: Blood in peritoneal cavity due to in injuries to chest wall

Infections in the chest: Infection following a chest wound is uncommon in forensic practice as most deaths occur from haemorrhage within a relatively short time before infection sets in. Cellulitis, pleural inflammation and empyema may supervene due to use of some dirty weapon or clothing or some foreign material being carried into the wound.

Pneumothorax: Pneumothorax is of following types:

1. *Simple pneumothorax:* Where a leakage through the pleura allows air to enter the pleural cavity but where the communication rapidly closes. The lung partly closes and the air is soon absorbed. If the communication remains open, then a bronchopleural fistula ensues with air in the pleural cavity, but is not under pressure. It will bubble out at autopsy when 'water test' is attempted. **Radiology** is the best to demonstrate this type of pneumothorax.
2. *Tension pneumothorax:* When the leak in the pleura or rarely the chest wall has valve-like action, air is sucked into the pleural cavity at each inspiration, but cannot escape on expiration. This pumping action leads to a tension pneumothorax, which causes complete collapse of lung onto its hilum and a mediastinal shift to opposite side. This type can be demonstrated at autopsy by penetrating an intercostal space under water and also by radiological examination.
3. When an injury of the chest wall communicates with the pleural cavity, a sucking wound may form with direct passage of air from the exterior. This type is seen in military surgery and is complicated by haemorrhage and infection.

A common traumatic cause of pneumothorax is a stab wound of the chest that allows direct communication with the exterior, though usually the layered skin and intercostal muscles close the track when the weapon is withdrawn. Natural diseases such as ruptured emphysematous bulla, a tuberculous lesion at lung periphery or a tear at the site of fibrous pleural adhesion can also cause pneumothorax.

Injuries to the lungs: The lung injuries can be of following types:

Bruising of the lungs: Bruising of the lungs (Figure 15.31) can occur in open as well as closed injuries to the chest. The lungs can be contused at the site or opposite the site in any substantial impact to the chest. Deceleration injuries are seen in falls and traffic accidents commonly along the posterolateral surfaces where a vertical line of subpleural bruising occurs. The outline of the ribs may be imprinted in lines of contusion on the pleural surface of lungs. Severe bruising may cause subpleural blood blisters. In all severe chest injuries the central parts of the lungs may show bleeding with actual haematoma formation.

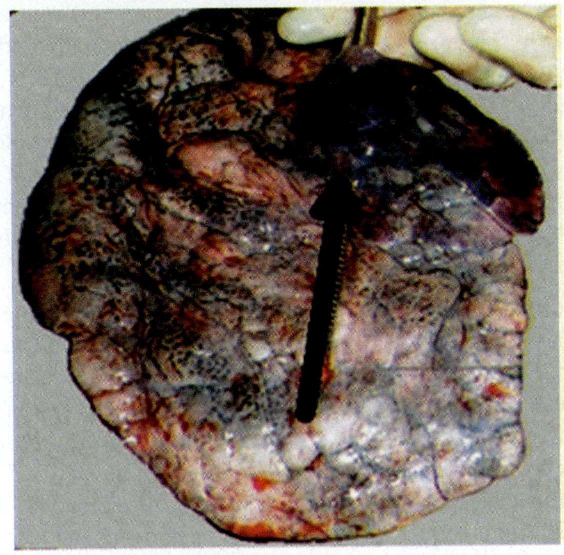

Figure 15.31: Contusion of lung

Laceration of the lungs: Lacerations of the lungs can result in blunt injuries with detachment of lobes or parts of a lobe. The hilum may tear and the pulmonary ligament below the hilum is a frequent site of haemorrhage. Vessels in the hilum especially pulmonary veins or those more peripherally, may be ripped, causing severe intrapleural or mediastinal haemorrhages.

Penetrating injuries of the lungs: Penetrating injuries of the lungs are commonly produced by the knives. The wounds may penetrate lung parenchyma, large vessels or through and through causing severe damage to heart and great vessels.

Blast injuries to lungs: Lungs are the most vulnerable organ to blast injuries.

Injuries to the Heart

The heart is vulnerable to both blunt and penetrating injuries.

Penetrating injuries to the heart: A stab wound of chest that penetrates the heart is a common homicidal wound. Sometimes the sternum is penetrated by a forceful blow that reaches the underlying heart but most stab wounds enter via the intercostal spaces, or through a rib or costal cartilage. Rarely, an upward stab from the abdomen reaches under the costal margin to penetrate the diaphragm. The right ventricle is often injured by a stab wound as it presents the largest frontal area, but the anterior interventricular septum and the left ventricle are also vulnerable. A shallow stab wound may enter the myocardium and does not reach the lumen of the ventricle. In such a case there may be little disability unless a coronary vessel is severed, which may either cause death from myocardial insufficiency, if a major artery is transacted or from cardiac tamponade.

In the thin right ventricle the knife passes more often leading to copious bleeding in the pericardial sac even though the intraventricular pressure is relatively low because thin wall is unable to close the defect by muscle overlap and contraction. Whereas in the left ventricle, the contraction of the layered thick wall may partly or wholly seal the wound and there is slight bleeding. Cardiac tamponade can result if the drainage from the pericardial wound is less than the leakage from the ventricle. The wounds in the right ventricle are more dangerous than that in the left ventricle due to absence of muscular self-sealing effect. The stab wounds of the heart are mainly through and through with knife entering one wall and emerging from the other.

Blunt injuries to the heart: The blunt injuries to the heart result in road traffic accidents, fall from height and in stamping assaults. Multiple rib and sternal fractures result with or without flail chest. In a child due to pliable thorax, heart can be damaged in an intact rib cage. Fatal blunt damage to the heart may occur, without a mark on the skin or thorax or damage to rib cage. The cardiac injuries are usually seen on the front of the organ, especially right ventricle. Rarely posterior bruising and laceration can occur if the heart is compressed against the thoracic spine as in stamping assaults and steering wheel impacts (Figure 15.32). In gross injuries such as aircraft crashes the whole heart may be avulsed from its root.

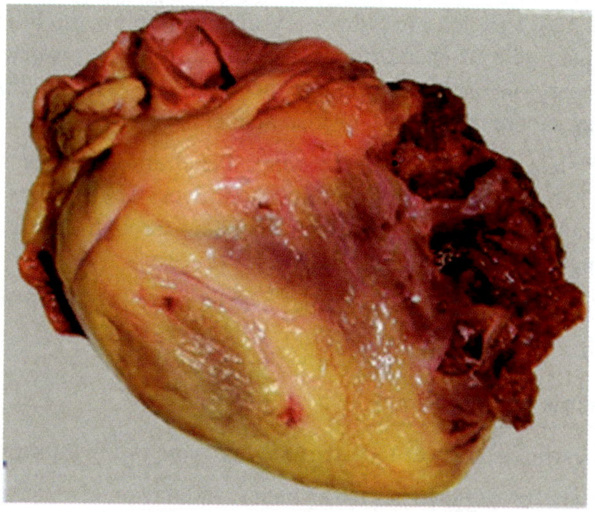

Figure 15.32: A lacerated heart

Haemopericardium: Haemopericardium or bleeding into the pericardial sac may occur from the surface or the cavities of the heart, or from the intrapericardial segments of the roots of the great vessels, particularly the aorta and the pulmonary artery. Haemopericardium may result from: (i) Ruptured myocardial infarct (ii) Ruptured dissecting aneurysm of the aorta (iii) Chest injury such as stab injury. When the damage has been caused by the stab injury that has perforated the pericardial sac, bleeding can escape into the pleural cavities, mediastinum or even the abdomen when diaphragm has been perforated. Death usually occurs from haemorrhage.

Cardiac tamponade: Cardiac tamponade is the condition when blood accumulates in the pericardial sac faster than it can escape, either because the bleeding rate exceeds the drainage or because the exit hole in the pericardium becomes blocked by blood clot. In cases where the bleeding is from a contusion or laceration of heart, there is no escape route from the sac. When sufficient blood accumulates, the pressure in the pericardial sac increases and begins to prevent the passive filling of the atria during the diastole. The cardiac output falls, as does the systemic blood pressure and the venous pressure rises. If unrelieved the death will occur with collection of about **400-500 ml** of blood.

Injuries to Great Vessels

Injuries to aorta: Aorta is the most vulnerable vessel that suffers in injury in deceleration trauma from both road and air accidents and falls from height. When the thorax is suddenly decelerated, the heart being relatively mobile in the chest, attempts to continue in the original direction. This causes severe traction on the root of the heart with complete or partial rupture of the aorta in the descending part of its arch. In falls from height, the lesion is the result of abdominal and thoracic viscera being forced caudally by the abrupt deceleration while landing on the feet or buttocks. Rupture commonly occurs almost constantly at a point 1.5 cm distal to the attachment of the ligamentum arteriosum. The lower thoracic aorta is closely bound to the anterior longitudinal ligament on the front of the dorsal spine, until it reaches the termination of the arch, where it curves forwards. This appears to be the weak point and transaction occurs at this level, sometimes so cleanly that it looks like a surgical incision. The tear is annular and at right angles to the axis of the aorta. Sometimes, there may be multiple parallel intimal tears near the main transaction, called the **'ladder-rung tears'**. In deceleration trauma, these incomplete tears, that affect the intima and media only, may be found without major transactions.

Injuries to pulmonary artery: The pulmonary artery may be damaged by depressed rib cage and sternal fractures in stamping assaults and steering wheel impact in vehicular accidents. The pulmonary artery and vein branches may also be damaged in the root of the lung, where hilar tears are not uncommon. The great vessels are often involved in penetrating injuries, notably stab wounds. Stab of the upper part of the chest may pass directly into the arch of the aorta, especially on the right side of the sternum. Stabs that are too high or are directed too laterally puncture the chambers of the heart and may penetrate the ascending aorta or pulmonary artery. If the wound is below the reflection of the pericardium, a haemopericardium and cardiac tamponade may result.

ABDOMINAL INJURIES

Abdominal injuries can be of two types:

Closed/blunt injuries: These types of injuries usually result from increased abdominal pressure and cause dysfunction of chest and abdominal organs. They can occur in: (i) Road traffic vehicular accidents due to the impact of steering wheels. It was quite common when the use of safety belts or air bags was not popular or due to a carriage wheel passing over the abdomen. (ii) Crush accidents that result from crushing between the two vehicles, crushing between a vehicle and a wall, railway accidents and industrial accidents. (iii) Blow by blunt weapons or by kicking, stamping, heavy punching occurs in homicides, assaults and child abuse. The liver, spleen, intestine and mesentery are most vulnerable internal organs to be affected. (iv) Fall from heights.

Open or penetrating injuries: They may result from cutting or stabbing weapons, firearms, horns and claws of animals or fall over sharp projecting object. These are dangerous injuries and sometimes death may occur without any injury to abdominal viscera. Sharp pointed weapon injuries to peritoneum, intestines or soft viscera may be produced by penetration with slight force. The injuries may be fabricated for charge of assault such as superficial incised wounds. Homicidal injuries are the most common whereas suicidal stab wounds are rare that may result from **Japanese Hara-kiri method** when the victim falls forwards on ceremonial sword and tries to disembowel himself. Intestines and mesentery are the major targets and are often involved in multiple wounds. The cause of death in such cases is due to sudden cardiac collapse due to fall in intra-abdominal pressure. Liver and spleen bleed extensively with resulting haemoperitoneum. Stomach is more commonly involved in chest stabs passing downwards through the diaphragm.

Features of Abdominal Injuries

Bruising of abdominal wall (Figure 15.33): Bruising in muscle tissues without any external violence can occur in tetanus and strychnine poisoning whereas discrete bruising on abdominal skin may result from kicks that produces scuffed bruised abrasion if tangential unless protected by clothing and in cases of child abuse where fingertip/knuckle bruises from holding, forcibly gripping or lifting the child, on the side of the abdomen or along the maxillary lines of chest. Usually abdominal wall escapes gross injury by transmitting force of violence to more resistant organs inside the abdominal cavity, which gets injured due to protective clothing and owing to the large surface area of abdomen. Laceration of abdominal wall with protrusion of coils of intestine can result in run over accidents under the wheels. Blow on upper/central

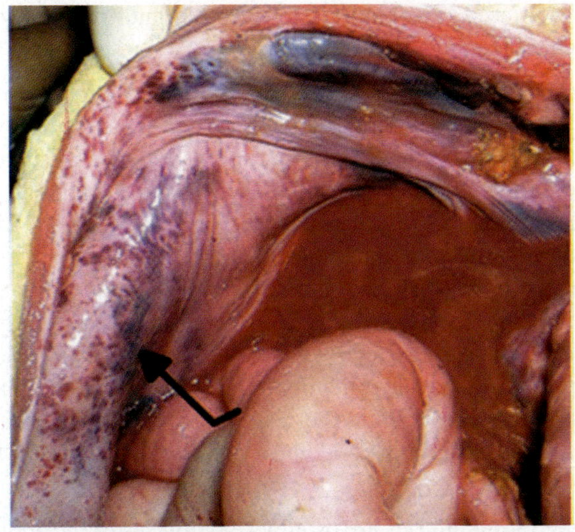

Figure 15.33: Abdominal wall bruising

(epigastric region) of abdomen has an inhibitory action on the heart through reflex action on solar plexus. Bleeding may be subcutaneous from initial area of impact to more diffuse involving large area of abdomen. Injury to epigastric artery causes severe haemorrhage. Extensive bleeding into peritoneal cavity may result from rupture of the solid viscera or from bleeding from the mesenteric vessels.

Bruising or rupture of stomach: The stomach is less vulnerable than the intestines and are lacerated by heavy blows in upper abdomen when full of fluid or food or the penetrating injuries.

Intestines and mesentery (Figure 15.34): External bruising of the gut and vascular mesentery when being crushed against the prominent lumbar vertebra in the midline. Mesenteric lacerations

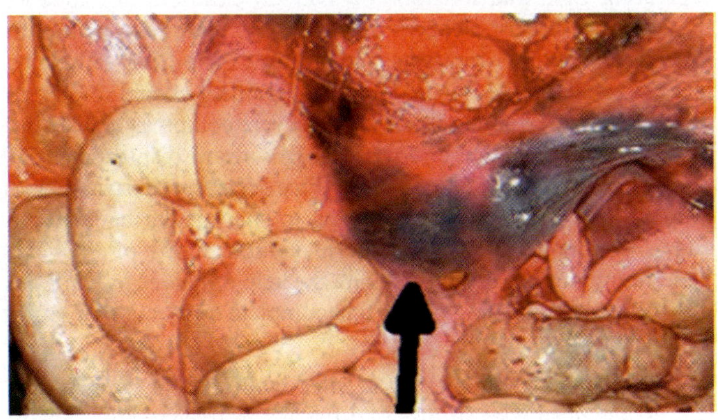

Figure 15.34: Bruising of mesenteries

occur in traffic accidents and assault. Bruising or tearing of central part of mesentery occurs while compression against the lumbar spine occurs towards the intestinal margins. Duodenum or jejunum is more vulnerable to transaction compressed against the spine especially in children from heavy blows to central or upper abdomen cutting through the third part of duodenum. Colon is rarely injured. The injuries to intestine and mesentery cause intractable bleeding.

Injuries of liver (Figure 15.35A): The rupture of liver results from the penetrating as well as non-penetrating injuries. The non-penetrating type of injuries may occur in abdominal trauma, fall from height, crush from wagon, and road traffic accidents from the impact of driver on rim/center of steering wheel or by unrestrained passenger being thrown against the face. The pedestrian can receive such injuries as primary impact from the vehicle or secondary damage by being thrown to the ground. External cardiac massage, sudden contraction of abdominal muscles such as during epileptic fits, lacerations by the fractured ends of ribs may perforate the diaphragm. In infants abdominal injuries may be found in child abuse syndrome and during breech delivery.

Penetrating injuries are usually stab injuries of the abdominal walls over the front, back or sides of lower part of chest. The liver is frequently injured due to its large size and weight, friable consistency and fixed and exposed position. The liver may be injured by forcible impact over the lower parts of right side of the chest, upper parts of right side of abdomen from the front, back and the sides. The right lobe of liver is injured five times more frequently than the left due to its size and position. The convex surface and anterior margin gets involved. Anterior surface and inferior border is more commonly involved. Ruptures can vary from superficial linear tears on convex upper surface to oblique to anteroposterior and rarely transverse. The tears are 1-2 inches deep and may pass through the entire substance of organs. There is complete transaction of organs when greater force is applied. There may be subcapsular tears or subcapsular haematoma. Liver is involved in 40% of multiple injuries. Lacerations may range from shallow splits confined to capsule to deep laceration separating right and left lobe of liver. In children, one lobe of liver may lie in peritoneal cavity, as it is more prone to being run over in road traffic accidents. According to ***Kindling et al.***, the lacerations along the line of falciform ligament occurs in drivers and passengers of automobiles due to severe compression causing bursting of organs; due to upward or downward displacement of liver. The satellite lacerations or fractures occur in pedestrians. The bruising of liver is usually localized to subcapsular haematoma and is common in newborn due to complications of delivery. Penetrating injuries are caused with the help of knives by multiple thrusts; limited bleeding occurs and complete transaction of organ may occur.

The puncture of liver by needles while taking liver biopsy causes haemorrhages in diseased liver. The liver is more easily lacerated if enlarged and fatty as in alcoholics. The rupture of the liver cause haemorrhage and shock and immediate death occurs especially if portal vein or vena cava is injured. The liver abscess may rupture causing septic infection and if patient survives for long time, infarction results. The lacerations of liver can be of the following types: (i) Transcapsular over convex surface under the site of impact, the portal vein or inferior vena cava may be involved and profuse haemorrhage results. (ii) Subcapsular over the convex surface under the site of impact. (iii) Distortion can cause laceration over the superior or inferior surface. (iv) Contracoup involving the posterior surface. (v) Whole organ ruptures in vehicular accidents and gunshot injuries. Large subcapsular haematoma ruptures after several days following muscular exertion or violence. Fatal pulmonary embolus may result from liver tissue emboli.

Rupture of Spleen (Figure 15.35B): Spleen is most vulnerable to injuries by blunt force and considerable crushing and grinding force is required like passing of carriage or motor car over the body; railway accident crushing, fall from height, foreign body piercing accidentally the pulp and by stabbing or cutting. Normal spleen may rupture by the broken ends of fractured ribs, severe kicks or blows by blunt weapon over lower part of right side of chest and in mechanical or industrial accidents. Enlarged spleen may weigh up to 2 kgs, is 32.5 × 17.5 × 6.0 cm, and is liable to rupture from fall or slight violence. Spontaneous rupture of spleen can occur during bouts of coughing, sneezing, vomiting or straining particularly if the spleen is abnormally mobile. When the spleen is diseased from malaria, infectious mononucleosis, kala azar and glandular fever it enlarges and is more friable and the incidence of rupture increases. It may also rupture spontaneously in pregnancy. The spleen can rupture due to compressive force

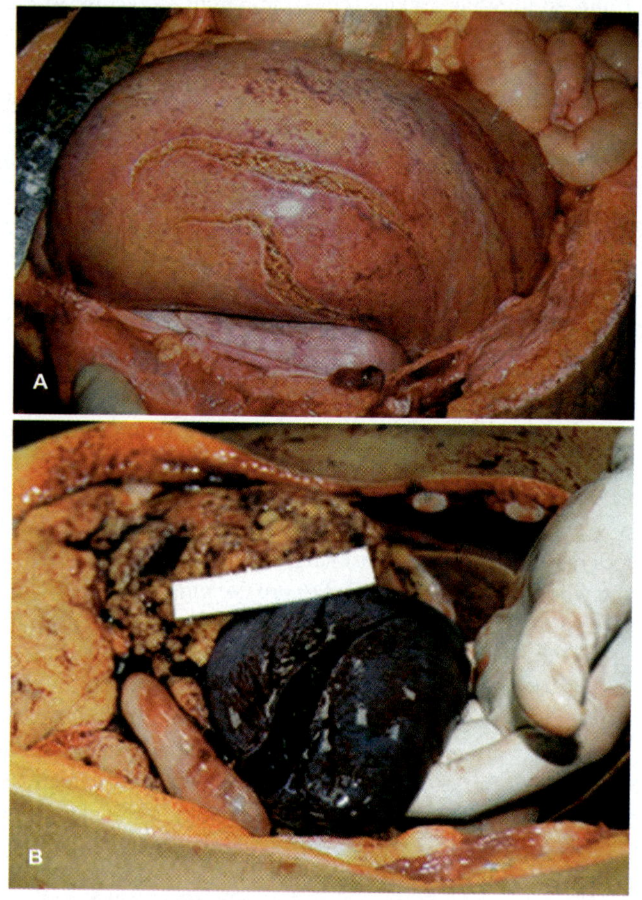

Figure 15.35A and B: Laceration of liver (A) and laceration of spleen

resulting from laceration of the surface or whole of it and traction force tearing spleen from pedicle and penetrating injuries. Concave or inner surface is the most common site of rupture and death occurs from haemorrhage. The injuries may vary from the large lacerations of capsule most often on lateral surface running up to the hilum to multiple lacerations traversing the surface almost bisecting the organ. However, complete detachment from the hilum is uncommon. Subcapsular haematoma if capsule is intact and substance ruptured causes delayed death as capsule prevents excessive bleeding and is disrupted with sudden muscular exertion.

PELVIC INJURIES

In severe trauma, the pelvis undergoes various fractures as well as dislocations such as: (i) When there is application of great pressure to the front of abdomen or pubic area such as in run over by the wheel, the pelvis is splayed open, symphysis pubis separates and one or both sacroiliac joints also dislocate. (ii) When an impact occurs from the side, superior and inferior pubic ramus are fractured with dislocation of sacroiliac joint on the side of impact. (iii) In circumstances of fall from height on to the feet, due to transmission of force up the legs, both the sacroiliac joints may dislocate and even one or both femoral head may also be driven into acetabulum. When the hip joints remain intact, the pelvic girdle may fracture and sacroiliac joints may dislocate. (iv) Due to a kick or heavy fall on to the base of spine, fracture of sacrum or coccyx may result. (v) Empty bladder is rarely injured in trauma but a full bladder gets injured from blows, kicks and other blunt trauma. Other pelvic organs are quite protected from blunt injuries. (vi) Male urethra may be injured as a result of direct trauma such as falling astride a solid object like a gate or being kicked in the crutch, due to being compressed against the undersurface of the pubis. (vii) External genitalia may suffer injuries especially scrotum is quite vulnerable to severe bruising resulting from kicks. Scrotum and vulva may suffer injuries from falling astride on objects and in vehicular accidents. Various types of pelvic fractures encountered in medical practice are described in Figures 15.36 to 15.39.

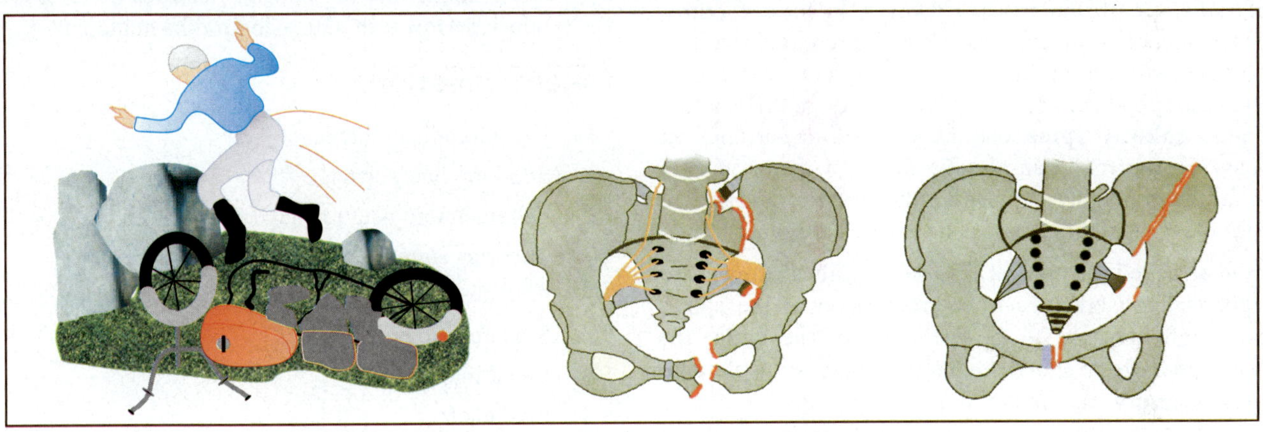

Figure 15.36: Vertical shear fracture (Malgaigne fracture)

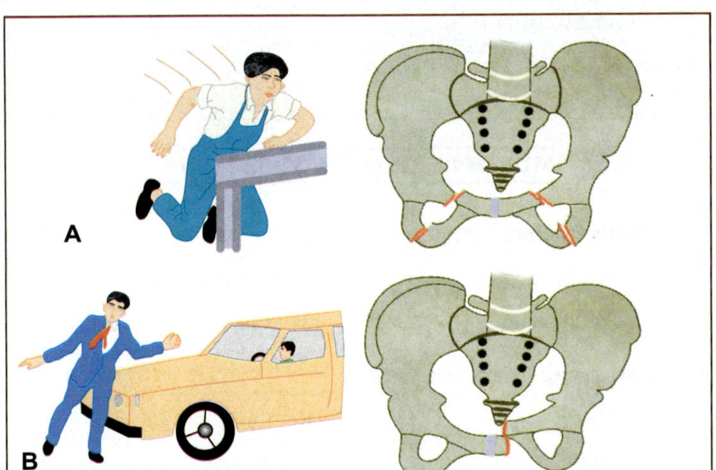

Figure 15.37: Fracture of pubic rami (A) straddle injury (B) lateral compression injury (overlapping pelvis)

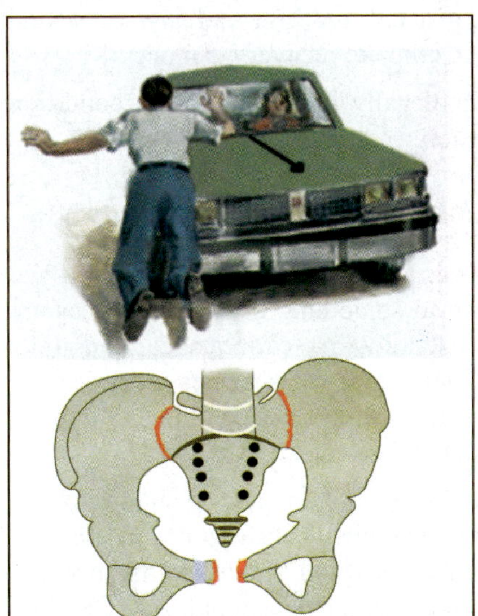

Figure 15.38: Anteroposterior compression fracture of pelvis (Open book fracture)

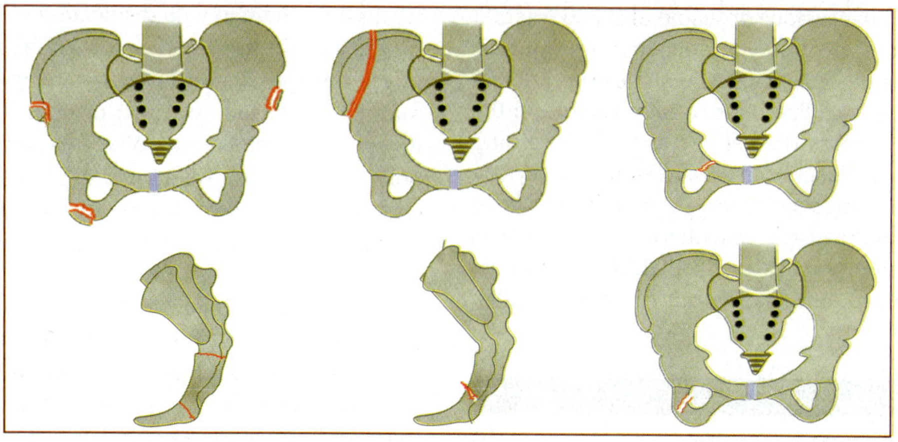

Figure 15.39: Fracture of pelvis without disruption of pelvic ring

RAILWAY SPINE OR ERICHSEN'S DISEASE

Sir John Eric Erichsen (1866), observed persistent symptoms (somatic, cognitive, emotional, motor, or sensory) in trauma victims of railway collision cases. However, in these victims, no objective evidence of injuries was seen. He reported that this was due to **concussion of spine** that showed organic pathology, inflammation the spinal cord but no spinal fracture or dislocation. This is called **railway spine** due its frequent occurrence in rail accidents. However, it can also be found in motor vehicle collisions, fall from height, aeroplane accident cases and severe blow to back etc. It is often known as **Erichsen's disease.**

Erichsen arranged the clinical features of railway spine into three categories: (a) Cerebral—from progression of the spinal meningitis or inflammation to the meninges of the brain; (b) Spinal—back pain from spinal meningitis; and (c) Referable to the limbs—sensory and motor impairments "giving rise to peculiarity and unsteadiness of gait". The signs and symptoms are: headache, memory impairment, poor concentration, sleep disturbances, anxiety, back stiffness and pain, hearing problems, extremity numbness, pain in hand and arm and loss of sexual desire, incontinent bladder. Complete recovery can occur.

Railway spine is medicolegally important as the condition leads to claim of compensation.

Crush Injury and Crush Syndrome

Crush injury is the injury caused as a result of direct physical crushing of the muscles due to something heavy. The cases are commonly reported after natural (e.g., earthquake, land-slide, tornadoes, tsunami) or man-made catastrophes (e.g., wars, terrorist attacks), conventional causes, such as building collapses, road traffic accident, accident at work etc.

Crush syndrome is defined as traumatic rhabdomyolysis with systemic and local complications. Crushing of muscle cells releases myoglobin, potassium, sodium, calcium, magnesium, phosphate, acids, enzymes like creatine phosphokinase (CKMM) and lactate dehydrogenase (LDH), etc into the circulation, leads to metabolic derangement and acute kidney injury.

LONG QUESTION

1. Discuss injuries caused by impact of a blunt weapon to the head. Enumerate the peculiar features of various types of injuries. How will date subdural haematoma?

SHORT QUESTIONS

1. Extradural haemorrhage.
2. Subdural haemorrhage.
3. Subarachnoid haemorrhage.
4. Theories coup and contrecoup injuries.
5. Fractures of skull.
6. Signature fracture.
7. Lucid interval.
8. Flail chest.
9. Abdominal injuries.
10. Injuries to liver.
11. Fractures of pelvis.
12. Railway spine.
13. Crush syndrome.

MULTIPLE CHOICE QUESTIONS

1. Pond's fracture is seen in:

(a) Infant (b) Adolescents
(c) Young man (d) Elderly

2. Contrecoup injury is seen in:

(a) Heart (b) Lung
(c) Brain (d) Kidney

3. Gutter fracture is due to:

(a) Sharp weapon (b) Blunt weapon
(c) Firearm injury (d) Heavy object

4. **Which is called the signature fracture in a medicolegal injury case?**
   (a) Linear fracture (b) Ring fracture
   (c) Depressed fracture (d) Suture fracture

5. **Holbourn's hypothesis explains the mechanism of damage to:**
   (a) Liver (b) Heart
   (c) Brain (d) Lung

6. **A 45-year-old male with history of road traffic accident was brought dead to the casualty. At autopsy, the pathologist noted two linear fractures over the left parietal bone with fracture line meeting with each other. To know the sequence of fractures (First one and second one) which rule is applied?**
   (a) Young's rule (b) Ashley's rule
   (c) Mc Naughten's rule (d) Puppe's rule

7. **Lucid interval is observed in:**
   (a) Subdural haemorrhage
   (b) Subarachnoid haemorrhage
   (c) Intracerebral haemorrhage
   (d) Extradural haemorrhage

8. **Concussion can be differentiated from alcoholic intoxication:**
   (a) Retrograde amnesia
   (b) Abusive talkative behaviour
   (c) Confused memory
   (d) Sober behaviour

9. **Shearing damage is seen in:**
   (a) Heart (b) Liver
   (c) Spinal Cord (d) Brain

ANSWER KEY

1. (a)	2. (c)	3. (c)	4. (c)	5. (c)	6. (d)	7. (d)	8. (a)	9. (d)

Explosion Injuries

Explosions are commonly reported in both military and civilian setup. Usually explosions occur as an act of terrorism, fireworks, household explosions, industrial accident, motor vehicular accidents. Explosions by terrorist have increased dramatically over the last decade. Today, explosion injury is a leading cause of civilian deaths worldwide.

Mechanism of Explosion

An **explosion** is the instantaneous transformation of a solid or liquid into a gas, releasing tremendous kinetic and heat energy. Pressures of 1000 tons/inch^2 (150,000 atm.) and the temperature of 3,000°C can be generated in an explosion. The overpressure from the blast generally follows a well-defined pressure/time curve, called a **"Friedlander wave",** (Figure 16.1**).** There is an initial near instantaneous spike in the ambient air pressure which quickly decays and is followed by a negative pressure wave that sucks debris into the area. Explosions produce several effects by blast waves, blast winds, and thermal injury etc. High-order explosives produce a strong supersonic pressure wave, known as the **blast wave or shock wave**. A **blast wind** is the flow of superheated air that follows the blast wave.

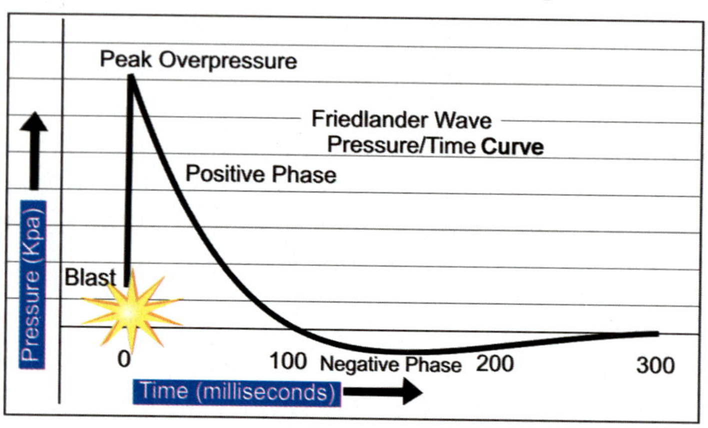

Figure 16.1: Friedlander wave

Classification of Explosives

Explosives can be classified based on the materials use such as (i) **High-order explosives (HE)**, e.g., Dynamite, trinitrotoluene (TNT), Nitroglycerin, C-4, Semtex, Ammonium Nitrate Fuel Oil (ANFO). Blast wave is produced by HE. (ii) **Low-order explosives (LE)**, e.g., Gun powder, pipe bombs and petroleum-based bombs. No blast wave produced by LE.

The Explosive and incendiary (fire) bombs are further classified based on their source (i) **Manufactured (military)** explosives are quality tested weapons, exclusively HE-based and produced in mass scale (ii) **Improvised explosive devices (IEDs)** are illegally obtained manufactured weapons, used outside its intended purpose, produced in small quantities and may be composed of HE, LE or both.

Classification of Blast Injuries

The blast injuries can be classified according to the forces causing the injury. There are four main types of blast injuries namely **Primary** (effects of blast wave)**, Secondary** (effects of projectiles/shrapnel)**, Tertiary (**effects from fall from blast winds) **and Quaternary** (effects of burns, asphyxia, and exposure to

Table 16.1: Characteristics of blast injury			
Category	**Mechanism**	**Body part affected**	**Types of injuries**
Primary blast injury	Caused by impact of the over-pressurization wave with body surfaces, Characteristics of HE blasts	Air filled organs are most susceptible, e.g., lungs, GI tract and middle ear	• **Blast lung** • **Blast ear** – Tympanic membrane rupture and middle ear damage • **Blast brain** – Injury to brain parenchyma even without direct injury to the head • **Blast eye** – Perforation of the globe of the eye • **Blast belly** – Abdominal haemorrhage and perforation
Secondary blast injury	Caused by flying debris and bomb fragments	Any body part	• Penetrating ballistic (fragmentation) or blunt injuries • Eye penetration (can be occult)
Tertiary blast injury	Results from individuals being thrown by the blast wind	Any body part	• Fracture and traumatic amputation • Closed and open brain injury
Quaternary blast injury	All explosion-related injuries, illnesses, or diseases not due to primary, secondary, or tertiary mechanisms – Includes exacerbation or complications of existing conditions	Any body part	• Burns (flash, partial and full thickness) • Asthma, COPD, or other breathing problems from dust, smoke, or toxic fumes • Angina • Hyperglycemia • Hypertension

toxic inhalants) **blast injury** whose characteristics are mentioned in Table 16.1 and Figure 16.2.

Primary Blast Injury

Primary blast injury is caused by blast wave which spreads concentrically from the blast center in a round wave of very high pressure, the velocity of this shock wave soon decreases to about the speed of sound in air (1120 fps). It is many times faster near the explosion and as the distance from the explosion is increased the pressure component lasts longer. Blast wave can knock a person down, move objects and causes demolition of buildings. On the heels of the blast wave there are winds that can displace objects at considerable distances. Post blast wave can knock buildings down. Ground shock is a complex train of shock waves that is similar to earthquake.

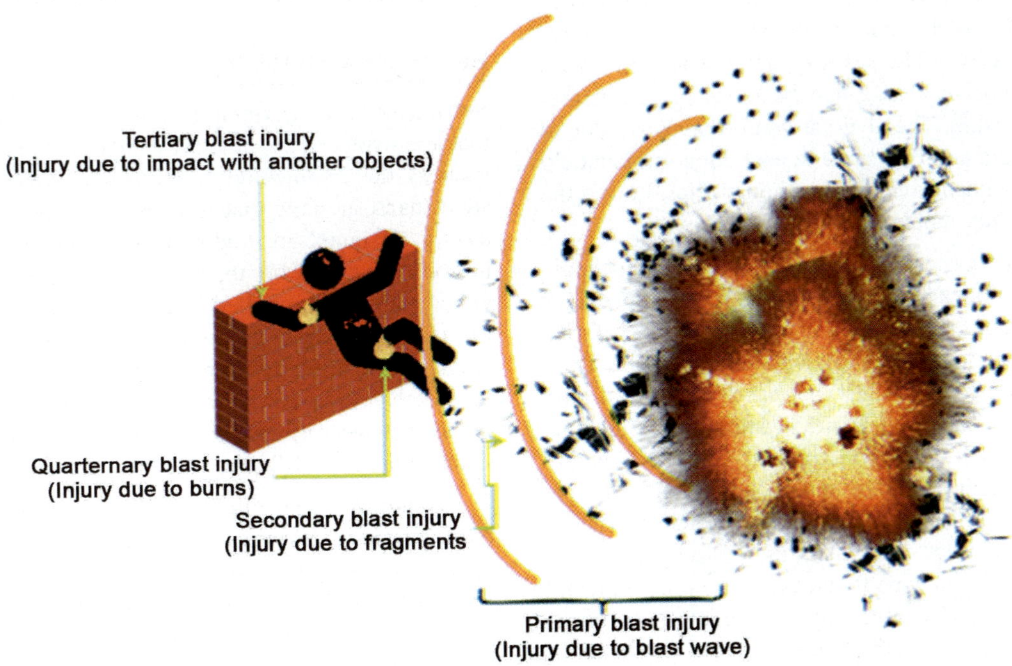

Figure 16.2: Classification of blast injury

Biophysics of air blast injury: Shock wave strikes the body surface and the part of it is deflected, a part reflected and the rest of it is absorbed. The shock wave passes through the homogenous organs like heart and thigh and solid organs but does not damage them. The organs that contain air are very vulnerable, e.g., in its passage through non-homogeneous lungs, there is considerable damping of wave achieved by the movements of lung tissue. Acceleration of parts of different density and compression and expansion of alveoli as pressure wave passes through them are thought to be among the causes of lung damage. Also, the shredding and bursting effect that occurs when a pressure wave breaks out of liquid medium of lung tissue into gaseous medium of the alveolus. Structural damage due to shock wave is confined to air or gas containing organs such as ears, lungs and segments of large bowel. Effects of air blast diminishes rapidly as the distance from the explosion increases.

Tissue damage due to air blast: The blast wave being a sound wave damages the ear and the damage depends on: (i) Intensity of the blast (ii) Its proximity to the source (iii) Orientation of axis of external auditory canal to wave front (iv) Duration of exposure (v) Awareness of explosion (vi) Protection by any object.

Effects of air blast on ear: (i) Hyperemia of intact tympanic membrane (ii) Punctate bruising of intact tympanic membrane (iii) Rupture of tympanic membrane at an overpressure of 5 psi, results in bleeding into middle ear (iv) Damage to the cochlea that is more frequent than tympanic membrane rupture (v) Sudden severe deafness with period of recovery during which acuity for all frequencies is depressed (vi) Slight haemorrhage into scala tympani near round window (vii) Haemorrhage into basal coil of cochlea and in fundus of internal meatus (viii) Prominent symptoms are tinnitus, sensorineural and conductive deafness.

Effects of air blast on lung: Lung lesions **(blast lung)** of the air blast are due to direct impact on the body wall of pressure component of shock wave. The severity of lung lesions varies from the size of explosive charge and becomes greater nearer the victim to the explosion. The alveolar hemorrhages are due to tearing of alveolar septa and they arise in each lung immediately after explosion, if patient survives for few hours. Blast lung is the most common fatal injury among initial survivors.

Autopsy examination reveals subpleural haemorrhagic patches of purple red colour and of varying size. These hemorrhages are scattered at random, cross the lung surface in line of ribs and are grouped near anterior and costophrenic margins. Lung sections reveal discrete hemorrhages that are more central than peripheral and the rest of the lung tissue is patchily oedematous. On microscopic examination, alveoli contain haemorrhages and oedema fluid, the alveolar septa are not discernible and there is emphysematous dilatation of alveolar ducts. The haemorrhages are seen in the bronchioles and interstitial tissue. The pink staining fluid and red cells may be found between epithelium and lamina propria is infiltrated by neutrophils. Direct blows by bomb fragments debris on chest bruise the lungs.

Effects of air blast on gastrointestinal tract: The injuries to GIT are inconstant. The haemorrhages beneath the peritoneum of gut, mesentery and omentum vary in size. They are usually seen as small punctate spots, over extensive areas of intestine. They extend circumstantially as annular bands occurring mainly over the caecum, colon, small intestine and stomach. The stomach and small intestine are less frequently affected. There is no correlation between the abdominal haemorrhages and peak pressure or impulse of blast wave.

Effects on other organs: Other organs such as liver, kidney and spleen are uncommonly injured showing haemorrhages or rarely a laceration. No specific changes are seen in the brain. **Zuckerman** described haemorrhages around nerve roots of thoracic spine and posterior column of spinal cord and oedema around central canal.

Clinical effects of air blast: The person receiving the blast is shocked, is pale, cyanotic and restless. The blood pressure falls, pulse is rapid and thready. There is chest pain, widespread crepts and haemoptysis.

Blast (Shell) shock: The blast shock is psychogenic war neurosis and the symptoms of anxiety are produced. There is confusion, muscular and mental weakness, stammering and jerking, hysterical blindness, numbness and paralysis.

Causes of death: (i) *Suffocation:* Death from suffocation occurs from extensive pulmonary haemorrhages in an hour of explosion and there is copious bloody froth in air passages. (ii) *Systemic air embolism:* It is the result of air gaining the pulmonary veins after blast damage to the lungs. In animals, air has been found in lethal quantities in coronary arteries, left chamber of heart and basal arteries of brain. Air embolism might account for those deaths that occur soon after explosion and no obvious pathologic changes can account for death. (iii) Blast shock (iv) Injuries.

Secondary Blast Injury

Secondary blast injuries are caused by debris and bomb fragments that are displaced by the blast wind of the explosion. The material such as the fragmented containers of explosive, metal case of shell, hand grenade that is meant to expel **missiles** and missile casing designed to fragment into lethal shrapnel can cause injuries. In a nail bomb, large nails are bound round the stick. Other materials propelled by explosion are remains of explosive material and debris of surroundings namely earth, brick, plaster, wood and dust. Larger fragment penetrates deeply. The fragments accelerate more slowly than associated gases, lag behind blast in early stages and tend to be more damaging at a distance with kinetic energy of $1/2\ mv^2$.

Common basic injury due to fragments of explosion is a **triad of small lesions (Marshall's triad); bruises, abrasions and punctate lacerations** with tattooing on skin (Figures 16.3 to 16.6). Abrasions and bruises are small 1-10 mm in diameter and puncture lacerations are up to 3 cm in diameter surrounded by an irregular zone of bruising and abrasion. Large lacerations due to larger fragments can perforate neck damaging carotid arteries

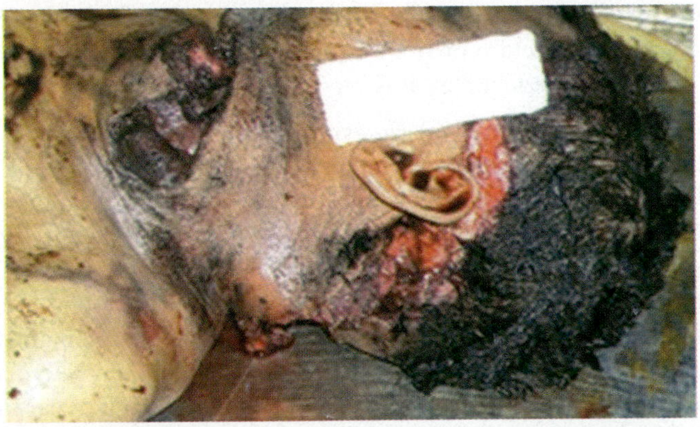

Figure 16.3: Triad of injuries with singeing of hair in a case of blast of an AC compressor

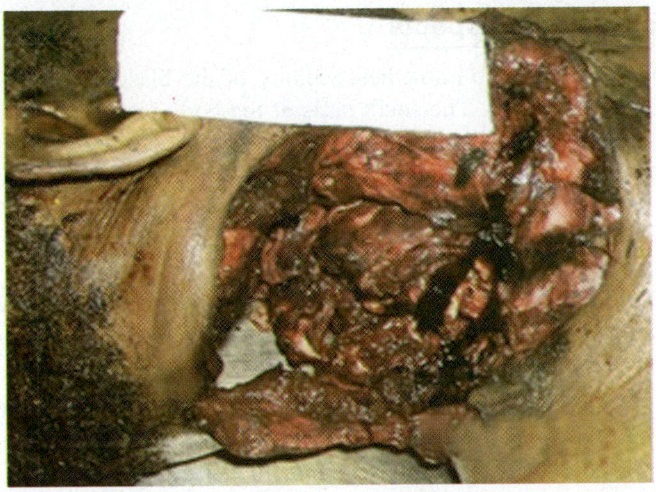

Figure 16.4: Blast injury over the neck due to blast of a compressor of AC

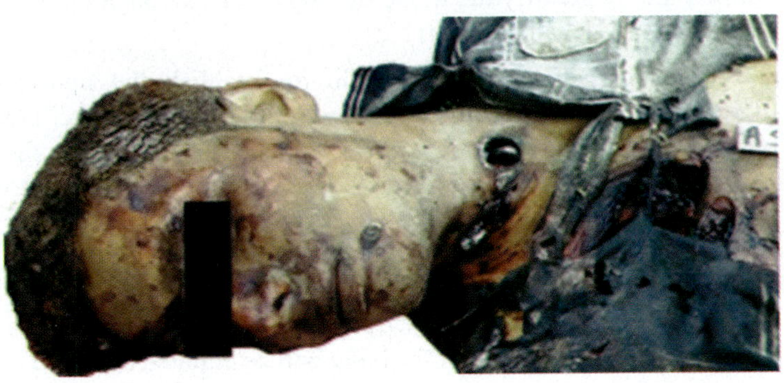

Figure 16.5: Blast injury over the neck and chest due to blast of a compressor of AC

or airways. Perforation of chest and abdomen results in internal organ injury. The dust propelled from the explosion is large in amount and when driven into skin produces uniform tattooing and skin darkening. Fragments of minute size can penetrate soft tissues of the body quite deeply. The distribution and pattern of bruises, abrasion and punctate lacerations helps to determine relationship of victim to explosion. Secondary blast injuries are more common

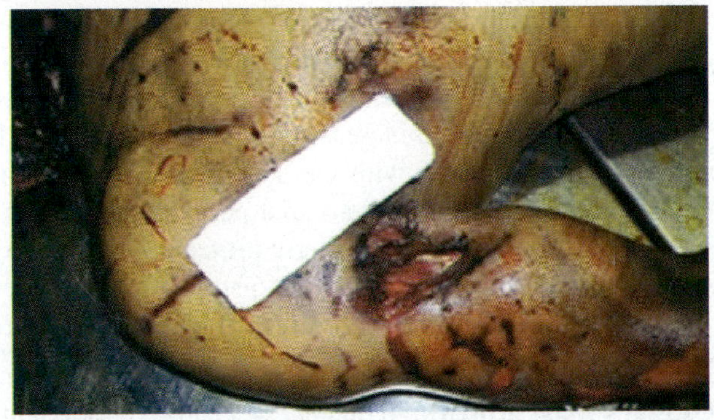

Figure 16.6: A triad of laceration, contusion and abrasion in AC compressor blast

than primary blast injuries. Secondary blast injuries are the most common cause of mortality in victims of an explosion.

The severity, distribution and pattern of injuries can be compared. Those carrying a bomb have their arms and midriff blown; the one carrying the bomb in his lap or car receive injuries on the pelvis. The explosion at ground level produces more of leg injuries whereas explosion at the side have more of side injuries than other types of explosion. The fragments and debris of explosion may cause an eye injury.

Tertiary Blast Injury

Tertiary blast injuries are caused when the person in displaced through the air and impacts on another object by the blast wind, or when a structure collapses and causes injury to the person. There can be blunt force trauma or penetrating injury, if victim is propelled and the striking structure that enters the body.

Injuries from falling masonry: The demolished building by an explosion may lead to injuries caused by collapsing masonry. The body and clothes are soiled by dust from brick, cement or plaster. The cause of death in these cases is traumatic asphyxia and the findings are purple discolouration of upper parts of body, patchy haemorrhages of skin and conjunctiva, oedema of conjunctiva and congestive haemorrhages of nose and ear.

Quaternary Blast Injury

Quaternary blast injuries are comprised all injuries that are not included in primary, secondary, or tertiary blast injury categories. Quaternary blast injuries can be caused by fire, fumes, radiation, biological agents, smoke, dust, toxins and environmental exposure. Psychological impact of the event resulting in exacerbation of anxiety, depression and can lead to post-traumatic stress disorder (PTSD).

Poisoning by fumes: Toxic fumes are harmful in an enclosed space and mining accidents with greater damp

Effects of Flame and Radiant Heat

The temperature rises to 3000°C and momentary flame contact causes burns. Radiated heat burns people outside this range.

The burning effect of radiated heat depends on the total thermal energy received and the rate at which the energy is supplied. The rate of heat transfer depends on the duration of explosion. Thermal explosion received increases directly with the weight of the explosive and inversely with the square of distance from it. The flash burns produced affect an area perhaps the face or one side of limb and spares the area that are protected by the clothing and solid objects. Areas are dry and reddish brown or parchment like. The individual has to be within feet of an ordinary bomb to sustain heat burns.

Quinary blast injuries: Kluger *et al.* (2007) reported the 5th blast injury pattern in the person immediately after the explosion. This is due to systemic inflammatory response in the persons which is unrelated to their injury complexity and severity of trauma. The hyperinflammatory state manifested as hyperpyrexia, sweating, low central venous pressure, and positive fluid balance. The early hyperinflammatory state can be partly explained by the unconventional materials used in the manufacture of the explosive.

Immersion Blast

Immersion blast refers to blast effects of an explosion in water experienced in wartime by those who abandon the sinking ship. Injury can be expected within 150 feet of a 300 lb charge of TNT exploding at a depth of 50 ft. The physical changes are similar to those accompanying an explosion in air. Explosion converts the charge into gas of a very high temperature and pressure, which expands pushing the surrounding water radically. Pressure of underwater explosion might be 1000 psi. The pressure waves pass through the solid tissues unimpeded. Injuries are found predominantly in GIT and less constantly in the lungs. Most of the lung injury is due to pressure transmitted from abdomen through the diaphragm. There is pain abdomen, abdominal rigidity and tenderness, occasional testicular pain, nausea, vomiting with blood and bloody diarrhoea. No external injury marks are seen over the trunk.

Solid Blast

Solid blast refers to a wave of energy that spreads through a rigid structure when an explosion is detonated near it and people in contact with its structure can be injured. Steel construction of tanks and warships conducts shock wave well and causes solid blast injury. An explosion beneath tank or ship causes initial movement of small displacement by very swift acceleration. Person standing in deck of ship could blow, bones can break and skin and subcutaneous tissue may burst causing compound fracture. The solid blast injuries are predominantly skeletal with fracture of calcaneum, lower end of tibia and fibula. The situation depends on subject's position; those standing receive injuries to lower limbs and those seated in chair suffer from fracture of vertebral column. The skin of ankles and feet are bruised and lacerations of ankle and weight bearing surface of heel occurs. The knee joint may be dislocated and rarely fractured. The fractures of femur and pelvis occur rarely. Fracture of spine is more common and 9th thoracic or 4th lumbar vertebra are involved.

Autopsy findings: (i) *Haemorrhage:* There is haemorrhage beneath the peritoneum, mesentery and intestinal mucosa. The submucosal haemorrhages account for blood found in the lumen of the gut, haemetemesis and melena. The haemorrhages are multiple and in majority are upto 3 cm in diameter and the intestinal walls are oedematous. (ii) *Perforations:* The perforations found in the small and large intestine are circular, half to one inch in diameter with prolapsed mucous membrane. They can occur anywhere but the anterior mesenteric border of ileum and outer side of caecum are the sites of predilection. The gas filled bowel segments are vulnerable to pressure of more than 250 psi.

Medicolegal Aspects

The persons in the immediate vicinity of the blasts are literally blown into pieces. The small parts of the body may be scattered over a wide area. If someone is carrying the bomb or in cases of landmine explosions the victims are blown up. The body parts of the individuals who died as a result of explosion should be collected by the trained persons otherwise mistakes are liable to be committed. The internal organs are less frequently found at the scene of explosion. In cases of small explosions, the limited body parts are blown up and, in all cases, the mangled remains are heavily soiled.

When there is a blast in the civilian, the number of victims should be counted. Within 200 yards the areas must be searched for the parts that are usually scattered due to explosions. The parts thus recovered must be washed in water and carefully examined. The non-human tissue must be identified and discarded. If it is not possible to identify the tissue by naked eye examination then precipitation test can be done.

The segregated parts will help to establish the number of victims. Pieces of scalp, skin, jaw, joints and hands etc. are put in separate heap. Thus, skin must be kept according to the colour and likewise the hair should be segregated according to the colour length and texture. The joints are to be marked whether they belong to left or the right side of the body. The sex can be determined from the genitalia, hair and breast tissue. At times the help of the microscopic study will be required. From the above data the minimum number of the body will be counted but there is always is chance for more number of bodies.

The identification of the bodies can be done by visual inspection after washing the parts recovered. The evidence of the lay people must be expected with caution because the deformity of the skull or facial injuries may be a misleading factor. The clothing is to be identified by the relatives. The most important thing is taking the fingerprints and matching with the records available specially in cases of the terrorist and criminals. In other cases, the fingerprints will be matched with some article of use at home. The dentician and the denture found at the scene may also be recovered and matching to be done. Other points like the tattoo marks, scars and old fractures are also helpful to identify the victims.

LONG QUESTION

1. Describe the autopsy findings in cases of explosion deaths.

SHORT QUESTIONS

1. Blast lung.
2. Effects of air blast on ear.
3. Immersion blast.

MULTIPLE CHOICE QUESTIONS

1. Which of the following is most likely to be affected by shock wave in cases of explosion injuries?

(a) Liver (b) Lungs
(c) Heart (d) Kidneys

2. Which of the following is not a diagnostic injury in bomb explosion (Fly Missiles)?

(a) Bruises (b) Abrasions
(c) Puncture lacerations (d) Fracture of bones

3. Common organ affected in primary blast injury, *except:*

(a) Stomach (b) Lungs
(c) Eardrum (d) Liver

4. Secondary injuries in a case of bomb blast is caused by:

(a) Blast wave (b) Flying debris
(c) Impact of forceful blast wind (d) Heat or radiation

5. In case of a bomb explosion, most of the casualties are caused by:

(a) Primary blast injuries (b) Secondary blast injuries
(c) Tertiary blast injuries (d) Quaternary blast injury

6. In case of a bomb blast, psychiatry injury and post-traumatic stress disorder are classified under:

(a) Primary injuries (b) Secondary injuries
(c) Tertiary injuries (d) Quaternary injuries

7. Triad of injuries indicates bomb explosion is:

(a) Bruises, abrasion and punctuate lacerations with tattooing of the body
(b) Contusion, grazed abrasion and fracture of bones
(c) Fracture of bones, patterned bruises and punctuate lacerations with tattooing of the body
(d) Compound fractures, patterned bruises and multiple sharp injuries

ANSWER KEY ☞

1. (b)	2. (d)	3. (d)	4. (b)	5. (b)	6. (d)	7. (a)

17 CHAPTER

Fall From Height

Fall is dropping down from a height of relatively high position by the force of gravity. International classification of diseases (ICD 10) gives a range of heights like slipping or stumbling through to the falls from the cliff. During fall the potential energy due to height is converted to kinetic energy under the influence of gravity. At impact some of the energy is imparted to the body resulting in injuries. Falls may occur at the ground level or from some height.

Falls at Ground Level

Causes of fall: (i) Mechanical due to slipping on polished surface or rugs or due to some faulty footwear (ii) Cardiovascular accidents (iii) Postural hypotension (iv) Intake of alcohol or hypotensive drugs.

Injuries resulting from fall on ground level: (i) *Fractures:* Femur (In old people, commonly), Colles' fracture, Pott's fracture, humeral fracture, pelvic fractures. (ii) Internal organ injuries, retroperitoneal haemorrhage resulting from pelvic fracture, rupture of liver and spleen and bruising of intestines. (iii) Injury to head leading to subdural haemorrhage.

In such cases speculation arises as to whether femoral fracture has antedated the fall as this fracture can occur spontaneously due to bone rarefaction and poor blood supply.

Fall From Height

The fall from height may vary from high rising building to ladder, chairs, tables or staircases. The falls are common in the middle aged from the windows or accidentally in children or suicidal commonly in adults.

Epidemiology of the Fall

Age and sex distribution: Falls are more common in extremes of ages. The range extends from children falling from the cots through to elderly slipping on ice or at home. The falls in middle aged persons are usually due to accidents related to work or suicidal. Females are more vulnerable to suicidal falls whereas males are more prone to falls in their late adulthood.

Geographic distribution: Places near high rise buildings and high bridges are the preferred sites for suicidal attempts. For these sites considerable distances may be travelled to their chosen sites.

Coexisting psychiatric conditions: Suicidal jumping makes a considerable proportion of those who die from fall in whom psychiatric conditions are common. More than 50% people have some pre-existing psychiatric illness or heavy drug over dosage. In the elderly, coexisting medical problems also contribute to increased incidence of fall.

Velocity of fall: For a fall on to the earth from a height, the acceleration is due to gravity 'g' and velocity 'v' after a fall from height 'h' is given $V = \frac{1}{2}$ gh.

It is true for a fall in vacuum but in actual position air drag, clothing, body surface area, human body flexibility and non-homogeneous mass distribution come into play. The error may vary from 5-7% for jumps up to height of 23 metres.

Factors Influencing the Pattern of Injury

1. **Height:** A direct relationship exists between height fallen and survival. It is also correlated with the extent of injury as

measured by injury severity score. The height of fall of about 11 metres, results in pelvic damage and when the height is more than 15 metres, multiple rib fractures result. When a person falls or jumps from height, trajectory is downwards and outwards. However, the distance the body strikes the ground is variable.

2. **Orientation:** Orientation of body at point of impact is important in determining injury pattern and mortality. In majority of falls, vertical landing with feet first is common and the next common being with head first. In all falls, lower limbs are almost exclusively injured. In side impacts and in feet first impact, mainly upper limbs are injured due to secondary impact.
3. **Surface impact:** The surface on to which a body falls determines the pattern of deceleration and energy exchange. On a relatively yielding surface, such as a safety net, the energy is given up slowly, but on a relatively unyielding surface such as concrete, time of deceleration is shorter and hence the forces on the body are much great.
4. **Deceleration:** Quicker the body is brought to rest, greater will be forces acting on it. Deceleration depends upon the weight of the body, surface of impact and energy dissipation, i.e., bouncing back. Duration of deceleration is extremely short, in milliseconds. A fall onto concrete results in a very rapid onset of deceleration or a high jolt factor. At impact body comes to a halt and in doing this, it must give up the kinetic energy. The magnitude of kinetic energy and the way in which it is dissipated determines the changes to body tissue. If certain tolerance limits are exceeded, injury results. The body turns and twists in an unpredictable manner during the fall.

A person falling 15 metres, attains a speed of 17 m/s. When falling from high building, the displaced air tends to act as the cushion, which drives the body from the wall. A simple fall can result in a body impact some distance from the foot of the building that is not an evidence of push or deliberate jump.

Injury Pattern From Fall

The injuries due to fall from height can be direct or indirect.

Direct injuries: These are immediately anatomically related to the point of impact. As a result of the injury resulting from direct impact on head, head is suddenly decelerated and brain tends to continue falling because of its momentum. Brain is suddenly pressured against the skull at the site of impact and a corresponding negative pressure is present on the opposite surface of brain. In more severe falls, the head is accelerated prior to impact and deformation of skull occurs. It results in massive fracture often with laceration of scalp with extrusion of brain and fracture of vault and base. Other injuries on various parts of head can be:

1. *The top of the head:* Injuries are severe and the character and extent will depend upon the surface or object against which impact takes place and they depend on the distance fallen. Other injuries such as fracture of spine, limbs or chest will usually be present. The point of impact against a hard flat surface, e.g., concrete will be indicated by a bruised laceration overlying fissure fractures of skull following direction of lines of force.

   Impact against blunt protruding object such as sharp corner of furniture will produce a localized depressed fracture of skull with comminuted or radiating fissure (Figure 17.1).

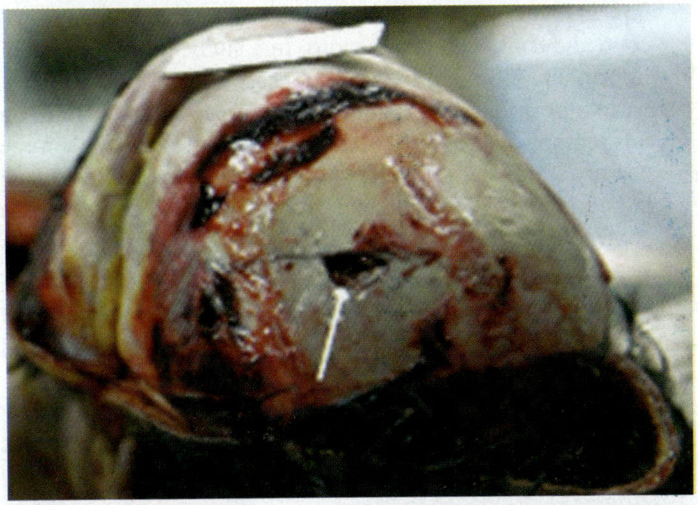

Figure 17.1: Depressed fracture with radiating fissure of skull

2. *The side, back and front of head:* These may occur from simple falls from erect position and depends upon the part of the head striking the ground that is related to direction of fall. The usual injury is bruise situated just above and behind either ear with or without abrasion or laceration of scalp.

   On a flat surface, fissure fracture occurs parallel with the line of impact and usually run through the middle fossa in to pituitary fossa, sometimes to opposite side. Anterior and posterior fossa may also be involved.

   Ring fracture of base of skull separates rim of foramen magnum from the rest of the base. It occurs in fall from height landing on feet or buttocks thus driving vertebral column into the skull.

   The leg bones (tibia) are sometimes driven through the side of the feet. The major blood vessels near their junction with the heart are severed. The inner lining of carotid arteries shows small horizontal tears. Heart may be driven through the pericardial sac and the diaphragm may burst and expose ventricle or may be torn from its pedicle.
3. *Fall on the back of head:* The inertia of brain produces a positive acceleration pressure over the fronto-orbital region and negative acceleration pressure over the occipital and cerebellar regions of brain. This pressure lasts until the deformation of skull at the site of impact reaches its maximum. Since with the onset of this deformation the brain

becomes displaced towards opposite side as two positive forces act on the fronto-orbital cortex.

At the site of impact, the positive force of deformation is diminished by the existing negative acceleration pressure that is why contrecoup contusions are formed in falls on head. The degree of acceleration does not depend on the height of fall. It may be greater and produce more damage in a fall from sitting position than from standing position. In fall from high buildings, brain and skull accelerate at the same rate; no acceleration pressure develops within the skull prior to the impact that is why skull may be totally fractured with minimal coup and contrecoup contusions. In a study, the variations of impact due to fall on the back of head were: (i) Fall on right parieto-occipital area resulted in contrecoup contusions on left temporal lobe. (ii) Fall on cerebellar region with force of impact traveled forward causing contrecoup contusions in pons and in gyri. (iii) Fall on lower surface of occipital region showed intermediary coup contusions in tegmentum of pons.

Indirect injuries: From the forces transmitted through the body or from its deceleration. As a result of fall on feet, axial skeleton may break up at number of points (Figure 17.2A, B) and ring fracture results (Figure 17.3).

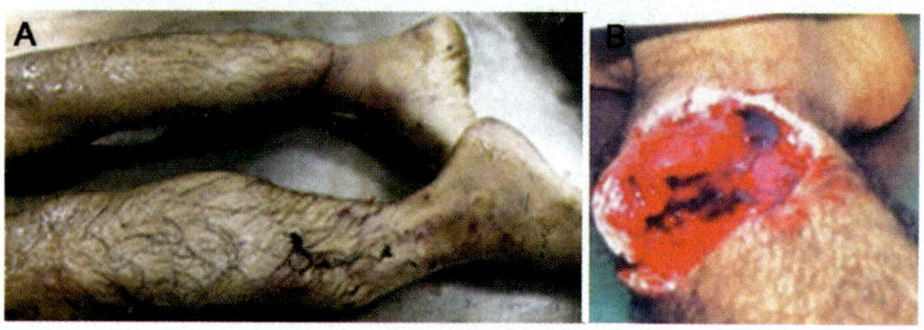

Figure 17.2A, B: Fracture of bones at lower leg (A) and Laceration with fracture of calcaneum at ankle joint (B) due to fall on feet

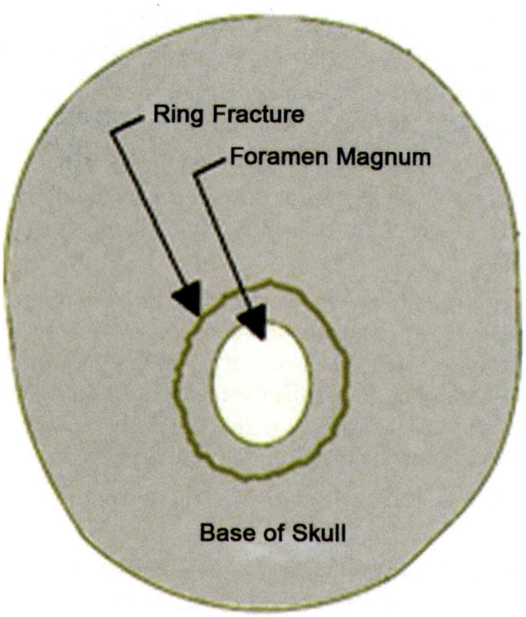

Figure 17.3: Ring fracture at the rim of foramen magnum due to feet first fall

Fractures of Skull

Goonetilleke classified the pattern of skull fracture fatalities into five groups: (i) Fracture of vault, including depressed fracture (Figure 17.4A, B) (ii) Fracture at the level of brim of a hat (iii) Fracture of the base only (iv) Extensive fracture of the vault and base (v) Ring fracture at the rim of foramen magnum.

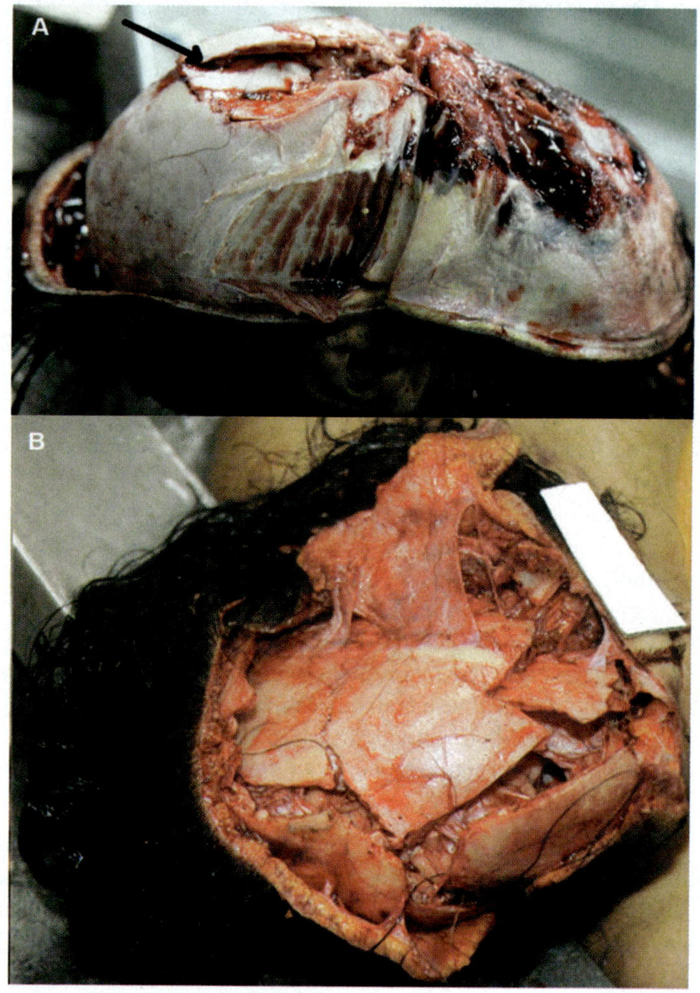

Figure 17.4A, B: Depressed fracture of vault (A) Extensive fracture of vault and base (B)

The first four patterns of skull fracture are attributed to direct head impact, either primary or secondary. The ring fracture is associated with **feet first fall** and is attributed to indirect fracture, the deceleration force being transmitted up the spine to atlanto-occipital joint.

The scalp can absorb 20 J of energy and 18-55 J forces can cause skull fracture. The extensive damage could be caused due to small increase in energy beyond that needed to produce linear fracture.

Injury to brain: A range of intracranial injury varying from the extradural, subarachnoid and subdural bleed to brain laceration or contusion results. It is clear from many reports that brain injury may be present without skull injury and vice versa. Brain and skull injury offer the poorest correlation with height fallen but the severity of brain injury correlates well with probability of mortality.

Other Injuries Resulting From Fall

Rib fractures: The ribs are prone to fracture through direct force and break at the point of impact. Anterior impact produces indirect stress concentration at posterolateral angle of the rib, and laterally because of posterior curvature and caudal angle of ribs.

Cardiac and pulmonary contusion and laceration: Cardiac contusion and laceration are frequently involved in extreme falls. Any chamber may be affected, the atria is more commonly injured in indirect injury without rib fracture. Pneumothorax and haemothorax are commonly associated with thoracic trauma. Pneumothorax in presence of rib fracture is explained by rupture of visceral pleura.

Diaphragmatic injury: Diaphragmatic injuries are infrequent in falls related to deceleration. The mechanism involved is the relative upward movement of the abdominal contents, forced up against the diaphragm as a result of impact to abdomen or deceleration (feet first or head first) as abdominal contents oscillate up and down on impact.

Abdominal viscera: Damage to solid viscera such as the liver and spleen are common from fall from height in excess of 12-15 metres. Liver is more commonly involved than spleen with multiple laceration. These injuries are usually coincident with severe overlying trauma to bony thorax but in most cases indirect shear mechanism are involved.

Medicolegal Aspects

The death that occurs due to fall from height must be carefully evaluated. Majority of the cases are either suicidal or accidental in nature but there may be allegations that the person was thrown or pushed from high rise buildings. Therefore, injuries over the body must be evaluated thoroughly while the intervening object should also be kept in mind.

1. **Suicidal:** When the person commits suicide by jumping from the building, the body is usually found at a distance from the baseline of the building. In these cases, usually the person lands on foot and he is expected to get injury involving both the feet alongwith the fractures, fracture of the pelvic bones that may be pushed upwards. Even at times, there may be fractures of base of skull (Ring fracture) due to transmission of force.
2. **Accidental:** In cases of accidental falls the body is found very close to baseline unless there is rolling of the body on landing and usually there is injuries to the head, chest and abdomen.
3. **Homicidal:** If the person has been pushed or thrown from the building the body may be found a little bit away than that of the accidental fall though the injuries may be more or less similar to accidental fall. However, there may be defence wounds on the body during quarrel or fight while the person is pushed down. The position of the body after the fall also depends on the weight of the body as well as the surface of landing.

Autopsy Findings

(i) Before deciding the nature of crime one has to visit the scene of crime and examine the location and height of the building, presence of any intervening objects, presence of boundary wall at the edge of the roof and the site and nature of injuries over the body. (ii) While interpreting injuries over the body following factors should be considered: (a) Body orientation on forces of impact (b) Distribution of forces of impact (c) Age of the patient.

LONG QUESTION

1. Describe and discuss injuries related to fall from height.

18 CHAPTER

Dysbarism and Barotrauma

DYSBARISM

Dysbarism consists of those disturbances in the body exclusive of hypoxia and air sickness that result from existence of a pressure differential between the total ambient barometric pressure and the total pressure of dissolved and free gases within the body tissues, fluids and cavities.

Classification of dysbarism: Dysbarism has been classified by **Adler** as: (i) *Those due to hyperbarism:* Result from an excess gas pressure over that within the body fluids, tissues and cavities. This is noted during the descent. (ii) *Hypobaric effects:* Result from excess of gas pressure within the body fluids, tissues and cavities over ambient gas pressure, that is noted during ascent.

Injuries From Hyperbarism (Barotrauma)

Physical effects related to increase in atmospheric pressure are referred to as barotraumas. It occurs most frequently underwater. The pressure of underwater environment is always greater than that of atmosphere. When pressure of air or gas in body cavity differs from surrounding tissues, problems of dysbarism arises. The failure to maintain equality of pressure between body and surroundings may be due to the: (i) Weakness of the individual himself (ii) Inadequacy of the protection available to him or his equipment (iii) Mishandling of the equipment by other people.

When an individual inhales a lungful of air and plunges into aquatic environment, as he descends into water, chest pressure increases with increasing depth and the volume of air in lungs is decreased as air pressure increases. At about 100 ft, the total respiratory volume may be reduced to residual volume and with increasing descent air in the lungs is at constant volume and pressure but pressure of pulmonary circulation and tissue wall continues to increase. Thus a pressure difference is created resulting in pulmonary oedema by fluid transfer from the alveolar capillaries into alveolar spaces leading to vessel rupture and haemorrhage, the air pressure increases than that of tissues that results in pulmonary tissue rupture and air escapes into interstitial tissue or pleural cavity or be drawn into circulation. High altitude decompression sickness has symptoms similar to those of Caisson disease but the two differs in circumstances of development and progression of the process.

Syndromes of Barotraumas

Pulmonary barotraumas: This can manifest as pneumothorax, interstitial emphysema and air embolism causing chest and abdominal pain, nose bleeding, haemoptysis, coughing and cyanosis. Immediate recompression is mandatory to shrink the embolic bubble mass. The clinical effects of air embolism depend upon the actual site namely, convulsions, visual changes, spastic/flaccid paralysis, tingling in the limbs and vertigo.

Barotalgia: The second location where injury from barotraumas can occur is in middle ear where air pressure differs from that in the external ear and nasopharynx. If air pressure in middle ear cannot be kept in equilibrium with that of nasopharynx for example because of inflammation of eustachian tube, eardrum may bulge inwards resulting in stretching, pain, haemorrhage, and ultimately perforations. This occurs in sudden descents from high places such as mountains or in landing of an aircraft, and in diving. In diving this is more of a problem but acute pain prevents diver to go deep enough as it produces the perforation in his ear. If an individual is wearing a tight fitting cap, air may be trapped in external canal.

Barosinusitis and barodontalgia: Divers experience vertigo or dizziness under water and those with sinusitis or polyps of nasopharynx may experience a painful condition owing to pressure variations between surrounding tissue and sinuses. Small pockets of gas resulting from fermentation in the roots of teeth may shrink during compression and the space becomes occupied by blood or fluid with increased pressure and pain when the diver returns to the surface.

Intestinal complications: As a result of increased volume of gaseous content of intestinal tract, continued fermentation may produce additional gas which will cause abdominal distension, discomfort and embarrassing flatulence upon return to the surface.

Nitrogen narcosis and oxygen poisoning: Despite the chemically unreactive nature of some noble gases at certain pressures they display all typical properties of anaesthetic agents. Nitrogen makes up about 79% of the air we breathe, produces euphoria followed by narcosis. With alcohol, the effect of nitrogen is greatly enhanced. Usually upon release of pressure, excess nitrogen leaves tissues and recovery is complete. Helium is used in place of nitrogen in breathing mixtures which allows for deeper diving potentials.

Hyperemia (Oxygen poisoning): The effects may result from prolonged exposure to low oxygen concentration or brief exposure to very high tensions (1500 mm Hg). *Acute oxygen poisoning* is much more common danger in diving. Convulsions are reported if divers have breathed pure oxygen at a pressure of 4 atm. At depths greater than 25 ft pure oxygen is not currently used. Mechanism of oxygen poisoning includes an excessively high partial pressure of oxygen. In *chronic oxygen poisoning*, irritant effect on lung tissue from smaller excess pressure for a considerable time may be there.

SCUBA Diving Fatalities

SCUBA is a Self Contained Underwater Breathing Apparatus. The diver is supplied by one or more tanks strapped to his back, which enable him to remain submerged for indefinite periods of time.

Snorkeling: The hazards are similar to that of swimming. It refers to diving apparatus that has mouthpiece at one end and the other end of the tube remains above the surface of water unless the diver submerges, when the spherical float attached to it keeps the water from entering it. The diver holds his breath for the length of time he remains underwater. These fatalities are contributed by four basic groups of factors: (i) *Panic in minor emergencies such as:* (a) Loss of a mouthpiece or face mask (b) Entrapment in kelp or gill net (c) Poor judgment in estimating distance from safety. (ii) *Improper use or maintenance of equipment:* (a) Insufficient servicing (b) Use of defective components (c) Occasionally regulators are defective (d) Water may be inhaled instead of air. (iii) *Acute alcoholism:* Due to alcoholism, judgments are impaired and inhibitions are lost. (iv) *Organic diseases:* Cardiovascular diseases especially severe coronary sclerosis. Hypoxia is associated with increased susceptibility to the effects of alcohol, impairment of coordination of muscular activity and decreased perception of depth and colour.

Hazards of SCUBA diving: These include drowning, barotraumas, bends (Caisson's disease), acute pulmonary oedema, emphysema, pneumothorax and air embolism. In SCUBA diving, frequently there is entrapment of air within the lungs on rising from depths producing fatal or nonfatal extra-alveolar air syndrome. Air escapes from alveoli and may result in interstitial emphysema, pneumothorax and air embolism. It is caused by disproportionate expansion of air containing alveoli compared to the adjacent fluid filled vascular changes during too rapid an ascent.

Water accident investigation team (WAIT): The medicolegal investigation technique for water accidents is developed by Noguchi. It consists of forensic pathologist and his medical or paramedical support team, diving expert (may be a medical officer who has sufficient experience in hyperbaric medicine). The work of this team is coordinated by means of a liaison officer. Every SCUBA fatality should be thoroughly documented and investigated as to what happened, circumstances surrounding the death and what recommendations should be made to prevent such incidents. The training should be improved and licensing and maintenance of diving gear is important to prevent such fatalities. A coordinated effort should be made with active sports diving equipment manufacturers.

Medicolegal autopsy in fatal water accidents including SCUBA deaths: (i) Do not remove any mask or gear from the divers, as equipment should be examined for flaws such as absence of a weight belt. (ii) Photograph the tank and send it to proper testing facility. (iii) Leave wetsuit undisturbed until the autopsy begins. (iv) Document the time of notification, arrival time and diving time. (v) Conversations with witnesses such as skipper, other divers and diving instructions are important. (vi) Photograph the body in position in which it was found underwater (face down, face up) as soon as possible. (vii) Note the condition of the body especially rigor mortis. (viii) There should be minimum disturbance of the position of the remains, diving gear, wetsuit and safety equipments. (ix) Transfer the body to the examining room without delay to prevent artefacts being increased by putrefaction.

External examination: The external examination should be conducted from top of head to tips of toe without missing any surface of skin as: (i) Evidence of squeezing or pressure of skin. (ii) Eyelid, conjunctiva, sclera, neck and thoracic wall should be examined for subcutaneous emphysema. (iii) *Radiological examination:* X-ray of chest in standing position will indicate a fluid level in chest cavity or presence of pneumothorax or pneumomediastinum. Radiographs of knees will show nitrogen bubbles in the joint, indicating a long diving period. (iv) In case of air embolism, air samples should be removed with a syringe lubricated by oil for gas chromatography and electron mass spectrometer analysis of gas components. >95% nitrogen indicates nitrogen narcosis (In case of massive air embolism from rupture of lungs, O_2 to N_2 ratio would be 20 : 80%) (a) While giving skin incisions, never overlook small air bubbles coming out from subcutaneous tissue (b) Blood is generally fluid, not coagulated (c) Heart need not be opened underwater (d) It is more important to measure total amount of air in heart chambers to find out air embolism. (v) Stomach contents must be examined for presence of food, drugs or alcohol.

Injuries Relating to Low Atmospheric Pressure (Hypobarism)

The barometric or atmospheric pressure at sea level is above 760 mm Hg. This pressure is referred to as standard or 1 atm if temperature is 0°C. The effects of hypobarism are related to its causation by:

Evolved gas types: Gases are evolved and form bubbles when with a rapid decrease in ambient pressure, tissues saturated with a dissolved gas may become supersaturated. Nitrogen is implicated in most of the cases but oxygen and carbon dioxide may also form and cause dysbarism. In the body nitrogen is transported in simple solution according to Henry's law. It enters into and is removed from the body by establishment of equilibrium between nitrogen pressure in the alveolar air and venous blood and another between tissues and arterial blood. During an ascent, ambient nitrogen pressure is decreased and nitrogen transport is directed towards its removal from the lungs. Nitrogen in tissue, then being higher in pressure than that of arterial blood, is transported to blood then to alveolar air and is expired.

As only a small amount of nitrogen can be transported by a given amount of blood, the rapid reduction in ambient pressure results in super saturation of the tissues with the resultant bubble formation. Nitrogen bubbles can form in any tissue including blood and are characterized by bends and chokes. **Bends** are joint pains caused by evolved gas bubbles within the joints. **Chokes** are characterized by cough, chest pain and dyspnoea due to pulmonary evolved gas as well as mediastinal emphysema from evolved gas bubbles.

CNS symptoms are caused by evolved gas pressure on or in the brain as well as embolic phenomenon. CNS disturbances are produced due to evolved gas bubbles under the skin. *Microcirculatory phenomenon* are produced due to bubble pressure on nerves and blood vessels.

Trapped gas types: Gases may be trapped in hollow viscera, teeth or body cavities with resultant pain and possibility of ruptures. Gases may be trapped in sinuses, middle ear, teeth, joints, beneath skin and intestinal tract.

Factors effecting clinical manifestations of hypobarism: (i) Age. (ii) *Obesity:* Fatty tissue contains less blood than muscular tissues and nitrogen is five times as soluble in fat as in muscle. (iii) Exercise, because of concomitant increase of tissue metabolic carbon dioxide. (iv) Rate of ascent. (v) Attained altitude during ascent. (vi) Increased tissue pressure of nitrogen prior to ascent. (vii) *Recent SCUBA diving:* United States has adopted the 'Rule of 12' to cover the circumstances in which hypobarism occurs at lower altitudes, if individual has been SCUBA diving for 12 hours, 'No flight above 12,000 ft for 12 hours following a SCUBA dive of 12 ft or more'. Physiological reason for this rule is that enough time must be allowed at sea level, breathing air to complete respiratory wash out of the excess nitrogen stored in the tissues during the dive. (viii) *Lower ambient temperature:* Occurs with great frequency because of decreased nitrogen transport associated with peripheral vasoconstriction due to cold. (ix) Total dissolved gas tension. (x) *Previous injury:* Bubbles tend to form at the sites of recent injuries. (xi) *Repeated exposure:* Individuals having one such attack of dysbarism is prone to another episode.

Clinical features: (i) *Bends:* Onset follows the ascent with a variable lag period. It includes joint symptoms, pain in muscles and long bones. The areas involved are first the knee then shoulder, elbow, wrist, hand and finger in decreasing order. The features are not serious and may be relieved in descent. (ii) *Chokes:* Are characterized by substantial distress, non-productive cough, respiratory distress, sense of apprehension and suffocation. The chokes are more serious than the bends. They result from bubble formation and accumulation in the pulmonary capillaries or from the effects of extravascular mediastinal bubbles exerting pressures on mediastinal contents and adjacent pulmonary tissue. It may be solitary manifestation of hypobarism and may accompany the bends. Chokes are found later than bends in the flight and become progressively disabling. Cough and substantial distress are markedly aggravated when an attempt is made to take deep breath resulting in decreased pulmonary ventilation, then hypoxia, syncope and collapse. Onset of chokes demands: (a) Prompt attention (b) Return to normal pressure by way of descent to lower altitude (c) Termination of flight of aircraft (d) Removal from low pressure chambers. (iii) *CNS involvement:* Vision is disturbed and there is disturbance in orientation. This is related to bubble size and location of lodging in the arterioles and capillaries of the brain, indicate mandatory hospitalization. (iv) *Skin manifestation:* Are due to pressure on dermal nerve endings and subdermal emphysema revealed by crepitation on palpation. (v) *Rapid and explosive decompression:* They result from mechanical failure of aircraft pressurization system. (vi) *Explosive decompression:* Loss of pressure is less than a second in explosive decompression and more than a second in rapid decompression. The eardrums are ruptured in the absence of basal skull fractures. Microscopic examination of lungs will reveal presence of bone marrow emboli resulting from non-fatal injuries sustained before ground impact.

LONG QUESTION

1. Discuss injuries caused by exposure of humans to high pressure environment.

SHORT QUESTIONS

1. Barotalgia.
2. Barodontalgia.
3. SCUBA.
4. Dysbarism.

19 CHAPTER

Thermal Injuries

HYPERTHERMIC INJURIES

Hyperthermia can cause systemic as well as localized injuries to the body. A delicate balance between heat loss and heat dissipation maintains thermal homeostasis. To maintain it both environmental and internal heat of the body are involved. Internal heat is generated by the oxidation of heat produced during rest that is the basal metabolism of the body. Environmental heat that comes from the sun and its effect is influenced by: (i) Moisture content of the air (ii) By its wavelength (iii) Spectral distribution (iv) Absorption by ozone and dust (v) Reflection and absorption by skin (vi) Clothing worn by the individual. Both the internal and environmental heat is measured in calories. A **calorie** represents the quantity of heat needed to raise a kilogram of water from 0°C to 1°C.

Exogenous or No Febrile Hyperthermia

The human body reacts to an environmental elevation of temperature by reducing thermogenesis and by increasing heat dispersion. Thermogenesis is decreased by reduction of metabolic rate to the minimal required for the vital functions and thermodispersion is achieved by: (i) Peripheral vasodilatation (ii) Profuse sweating (iii) Evaporation converting sweat to water vapour. All these factors are affected by the high humidity and lack of air movement. The diseased states due to the effect of excessive heat are divided into four categories in progressive order of severity:

Heat Cramps (Boilers Room, Miners Cane Cutters)

The painful spasm of the voluntary muscles especially of the extremities and abdominal wall is produced during or after physical activity in a hot environment. The predisposing factors such as ill-health and intake of alcohol results in depletion of salt that are the main causes of heat cramps. The cramps are severe, paroxysmal and affect the muscles of legs, arms and abdominal wall. Flushing of face and dilatation of pupil occurs. Administration of physiologic saline brings about dramatic relief. Prophylactically, salt tablets can be used to combat heat cramps.

Heat Syncope

Heat syncope is a circulatory phenomenon induced by posture and/or exercises.

Heat Exhaustion

Heat exhaustion results from dehydration and salt depletion producing the following symptoms: (i) Intense thirst (ii) Nausea, vomiting and headache (iii) Mental fogginess (iv) Dizziness (v) Irritability (vi) Incapability to work (vii) Fainting (viii) Peripheral vascular collapse (ix) Sweating (x) Temperature may or may not rise (xi) Skin is not dry (xii) Oliguria (xiii) Death results from heart failure.

Thermogenic Anhydrous

Thermogenic anhydrous is also known as **Desert syndrome or Anhydrite heat exhaustion**. It occurred in some soldiers who were separated during the summer in American desert. The features are most likely that of heat exhaustion. After profuse generalised sweating for several days, perspiration ceases suddenly in all parts of the body below the neck region and persists in face and neck. Eruption of prickly heat rash is seen known as *miliaria profunda*. The condition is not uncommon in Bengali children, tanker personnel reforming from Persian Gulf.

There is no suitable explanation for this. There is hyperkeratotic plugging of sweat glands leading to functional failure of sweat apparatus or a combination of both.

Heat Stroke

In heat stroke, there is complete absence of sweating and the body temperature is raised to 106°F or 41°C. In the environmental heat stress, absence of any other cause of pyrexia constitutes heat hyperpyrexia. Several workers have pointed out that heat stroke can occur at lower temperatures also. A temperature of 32ºC with 100%, humidity may lead to heat stroke. The features of heat stroke include hot and dry skin, increased depth of respiration, pulse is raised to 160-180/min and there is severe asthenia. Cerebral deficit produces convulsions, delirium, stupor and coma. When there is hypotension, increased urea concentration and raised potassium levels then prognosis is bad. Urine shows proteins and casts. Serum iron and bilirubin levels are raised due to liver damage. SGOT is raised due to liver and muscle damage. The first 24 hours are critical and death usually occurs within a week.

Autopsy findings of hyperthermic deaths: Autopsy findings in hyperthermic deaths are similar to those in cardiac failure. These are: (i) Visceral haemorrhages and congestion in heart, liver, lungs and kidneys are present due to thrombocytopenia, decreased plasma fibrinogen concentration and decreased prothrombin levels causing hepatic damage. (ii) Haemorrhage also occurs due to increased capillary fragility due to anoxia and circulatory collapse. (iii) Patients who survive for more than 24 hours show lobar pneumonia, acute tubular necrosis, centrilobular necrosis, adrenal necrosis and haemorrhages. (iv) Heart shows subendocardial haemorrhages, changes in the muscle fibers and the chambers are dilated. (v) Brain is congested and oedematous; convolutions are flattened and scattered petechiae are found in the walls of the third ventricle and floor of the fourth ventricle. (vi) Cerebellar changes are more rapid and in the form of oedema of Purkinje layer and swelling, degeneration and reduction of Purkinje cells. (vii) Those who survive longer show rarefaction of granular layer along with oedema of hypothalamic nuclei. (viii) In the brain, the heat dissipation center (preoptic and supraoptic area) and the heat conservation and production center (occipito lateral portion of hypothalamus) are usually affected.

Medicolegal aspects of hyperthermia: (i) All hyperthermic deaths are accidental. (ii) Autopsy examination is done to rule out any other cause of death or contributory cause of death.

HYPOTHERMIC INJURIES

The term systemic hypothermia is used to indicate cooling of the human body below 35ºC (95ºF). It can be classified as mild hypothermia (temp. 35-32°C), moderate hypothermia (temp. 32-28°C) and severe hypothermia (temp. <28°C). This occurs when the loss of heat exceeds the production.

Causes of hypothermia: (i) Hypothermia caused by exposure to severe cold possibly with exhaustion is called **environmental hypothermia** that depends on environmental factors. (ii) Hypothermia under the influence of drugs and alcohol affecting the generation or conservation of body heat. (iii) Hypothermia caused by climatic conditions with some disease affecting the body resistance. (iv) Hypothermia ending fatally in connection with therapeutic procedure that has some medicolegal importance.

Types of hypothermia: (i) Dry cold hypothermia (ii) Immersion hypothermia.

Accidental hypothermia: It is produced during: (i) Hiking or skiing expeditions (ii) In ship wrecked (iii) People falling in ice water; or (iv) When there is insufficient heating facility in the room.

Immersion hypothermia: In immersion hypothermia, the loss of heat is three times more than that due to exposure to dry cold air. Water conducts heat 25 times faster than dry air. Insulating air between skin and water is 1/10th than that of skin and air. Women endure cold water better than males due to body fat. Human body is able to retain body heat in water up to 22ºC and below 16ºC, survival time decreases sharply. Immersion hypothermia is more fatal as there is rapid loss of heat.

Diagnosis of Hypothermia

Clinical signs and symptoms: Body temperature preferably oesophageal (rectal temperature is also satisfactory) should be taken. Clinically three phases are produced: (i) Body temperature is 37ºC-32ºC with shivering and vasoconstriction. (ii) Body temperature is 32ºC-24ºC and body response to production of heat grossly disappears. (iii) Body temperature is below 24ºC, body cannot withstand the heat loss and general paralysis is produced.

Clinical features in children: In children features produced are cold skin, redness of face, subcutaneous oedema, scleroma, muscular stiffness, feeble cry, inability to suck, cutaneous and mucosal lesions are uncommonly present. Convulsions are also seen in some cases.

Clinical features in adults: In adults the features produced are red patches over the skin, pallor of skin, subcutaneous oedema of the face, stiffness of neck muscles, mental disorders, pulse is decreased and irregular with hypotension and slow respiration.

Laboratory findings: (i) E.C.G. is mandatory and following findings are discerned: (a) Occurrence of 'J' wave (b) Widening of QRS complex (c) Prolongation of PQ interval (d) Inversion of 'T' wave (ii) Hyperglycemia (iii) Raised blood urea and lactic acid levels (iv) Haemoconcentration (v) Serum amylase levels are increased.

Causes of Death

The mechanism of death in hypothermia is: (i) Cessation of circulation preceded by ventricular fibrillation; the dangerous level of temperature for ventricular fibrillation is 26ºC-30ºC though people have survived at a much lower temperature. (ii)

There is decreased supply of oxygen to the central nervous system with resulting hypoxia of the brain cells.

Autopsy Findings

(i) Postmortem staining is red or pink due to antemortem binding of oxygen to haemoglobin and its postmortem diffusion through the skin. (ii) Rarely, the skin is white that is why hypothermic deaths are called the **'white deaths'.** (iii) Spots of bluish discolouration are seen on the hands, elbows and knees. They are minor frostbite lesions. (iv) In the gastric mucosa, small, multiple dark-brown spot may be observed which is called **Wischnewski spots.** (v) In the heart, there is dilatation of right atrium and ventricle and congestion of vena cava. (vi) Trachea contains frothy and sanguineous fluid. (vii) Lungs are congested, oedematous and shows haemorrhages. (viii) Bronchopneumonia is a frequent complication. (ix) Liver and spleen are congested (x) Gastric mucosal erosions occur in 72% of cases. (xi) Kidney shows acute tubular necrosis. (xii) Fat deposition occurs in the cardiac and skeletal muscles and there is focal myocardial necrosis. (xiii) There can be haemorrhagic synovial membrane and bloody discolouration of synovial fluid **(inner knee sign).** (xiv) Viscera should be submitted for blood alcohol and toxicological analysis. (xv) Histological examination of skin shows oedema and hyperemia of the dermis with occasional inflammatory cell infiltration.

Paradoxical undressing: In some hypothermic deaths, the body is found in fully or partially naked condition despite low environmental temperature (usually below 29°C). This contrasting behaviour of removing clothes by the victim is due to diminished mental capacity resulted from changes in peripheral vasoconstriction in severe hypothermia. This situation may arouse suspicion of violence like homicide or sexual assault. Descloux *et al.* (2017) reported a case of suspected paradoxical undressing associated with subarachnoid haemorrhage resulted from ruptured cerebral aneurysm (non-hypothermia case).

Hide and die syndrome or Terminal burrowing: In some hypothermic deaths, the body is found in small and enclosed space such as underneath the bed or other objects (hidden position). This behaviour of the victim is imitating a primitive, burrowing-like behaviour of protection, as seen in hibernating animals. The hypothesis for this behaviour is either due to mental confusion or a terminal primitive reaction pattern, i.e., an autonomous behaviour triggered by the brainstem in the final state of hypothermia. This situation also may arouse suspicion of violence like homicide or sexual assault.

Treatment

(i) Rewarming by warm water (40-42°C); but never rewarm the patient by exercise or intense dry heat or fire as it leads to gangrene (ii) Blisters should not be pricked (iii) Antibiotics should be given to combat infection (iv) Alcohol and tobacco is to be avoided as they hamper the peripheral blood flow.

Local Cold Injuries

1. **Chilblains (Acute perineo):** Chilblains can be categorized as a first-degree frostbite. The skin is red or bluish as there is capillary congestion and mild inflammation. As a rule, complete recovery occurs without residual deficit.
2. **Chronic perineo:** Chronic perineo presents with reddish flat nodules in the skin, seen commonly in the women involving the lower limbs. There is ulceration, haemorrhages and scarring. These lesions become activated in the cold weather. The microscopic findings include skin atrophy, dermal fibrosis, panniculitis, angiitis, and sclerosis of arterial walls.
3. **Cold panniculitis:** This can be produced with local application of ice. There is inflammation and necrosis of the underlying adipose tissue. The children are most commonly affected because the fat of the children contains more saturated fatty acids than that of adults. The finding could be of interest in a battered baby syndrome as deliberate exposure of an infant to cold develops panniculitis.
4. **Immersion foot and trench foot:** Immersion foot and trench foot usually occurs at a temperature above 0°C most commonly when the temperature is between 5-8°C. Wetness is an important contributory factor. There is necrosis of fingers and toes. Obliterating angiitis causes severe gangrene and loss of tissue.
5. **Frostbite:** Frostbite occurs due to exposure to dry cold as well as following immersion at temperature below 0°C (usually -2.5°C). It is commonly seen in mountaineering and polar expeditions. It is of superficial type when only the skin is affected and deep type when subcutaneous fat, muscles, nerves and bones are affected. Degrees of frostbite and their manifestations are given below in Table 19.1.

Table 19.1: Degree of frostbite and their manifestations

Degrees of frostbite	Features
First degree	Redness and oedema of skin
Second degree	Only epidermis is affected, there is blister formation
Third degree	Skin and subcutaneous tissue is necrosed
Fourth degree	Total loss of tissue in the exposed area including muscles and bone

THERMAL BURNS

Burns: These are injuries that are produced by the application of dry heat such as flame, radiant heat, and some heated solid substance like metal or glass to the surface of the body resulting in tissue destruction. Injuries caused by friction, lightening, electricity, UV rays, infrared light, X-rays and corrosive chemical substances are also classified as burns for medicolegal purposes.

Microscopically, the epithelial cells are elongated and flattened that are deeply stained with haematoxylin and eosin.

There are small haemorrhages in the deeper layers and vacuoles are also seen.

Scalds (Figure 19.1): These are moist heat injuries produced by the application of a liquid to the body at or near its boiling point or in its gaseous form (steam). Water at 60°C for 10 seconds at vulnerable parts produces scalds. In scalds, immediately redness appears whereas blister formation may occur within a few minutes. When the skin of blisters is removed it will leave a pink, raw surface and later on the exposed dermis gets brownish, dry and hardened. Scalds do not produce singeing, blackening and charring of skin. However, it produces soddening and bleaching which may later change to dirty white colouration. The degrees of scalds are: (i) *First degree:* There is erythema due to vascular paralysis. (ii) *Second degree:* Due to increased capillary permeability blister formation occurs. (iii) *Third degree:* There is necrosis of dermis.

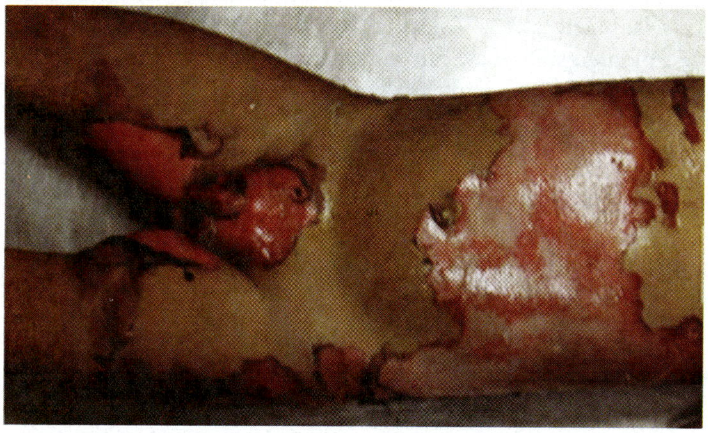

Figure 19.1: Scald burn over lower chest, abdomen and inguinal region of a child

In scalds, usually the injuries limited to the area of contact where it is more severe. However, due to splashing the areas of scalding appear large. Due to streaks of liquid that run downwards there may be formation of lines of blisters. Liquids that are sticky such as oils, syrup and tar produce severe scalding than hot water. Usually there is an edge corresponding to the limits of contact of fluid that is sharply demarcated. Scalds leave much thinner scars and cause less contractures and disfiguration. Moreover, blisters are surrounded by hyperaemic zone with redness and swelling of papillae in the floor. The blister fluid contains white and red blood cells. Antemortem blister formation is to be differentiated from postmortem blisters that does not show reddening and zone of hyperaemia. When any inflammable liquid such as kerosene and petrol is used there will be signs of trickling on some parts of the body.

Causes of death: In scalds death usually results from (i) Shock (ii) Hypovolaemia due to loss of fluid volume (iii) Fluid and electrolyte disturbance (iv) Secondary infection (v) Asphyxia due to obstruction of airways by oedematous respiratory tract mucous membrane resulting from inhalation of steam.

Medicolegal aspects: (i) Scalds are usually accidental that result when the hot water bottle, boilers bursts or splashing of hot fluid while cooking and when sauce pans or kettles fall over children. Occasionally children may suck spouts of kettles containing hot liquid that causes oedema of mucous membrane of mouth and respiratory tract and glottic oedema (ii) Scalds are rarely suicidal (iii) Homicidal scalding is also quite rare (iv) Sometimes boiled water or any other liquid may be thrown over the person to cause injuries.

Varieties of Burns

The burns are produced at a minimum temperature of 44°C for 5-6 hours and at 65°C for two seconds. External appearances vary with the nature of the substance used to produce the burns such as: (i) *Highly heated solid body or molten metal:* It produces blisters and reddening of the corresponding size. When kept in contact with the part, the destruction and charring occurs. Cuticle is found blackened and dry with shriveled appearance. Hair is singed and distorted. (ii) *Burns by flame:* These burns may or may not produce vesication but the singeing and blackening is always present. The hairs are curled, twisted, blackish, breaks off or are totally distorted. (iii) *Kerosene oil and petrol:* Produces severe and sooty blackening of the parts, and have a characteristic odour. (iii) *Explosion in coal mine and gun powder:* Causes extensive burns and tattooing due to deposition of particles and splinters or fragments are present in the tissues. (iv) *X-rays and radiation*: The injuries vary from redness to dermatitis with shedding of hair and epidermis with pigmentation of the surrounding skin. Nails show degenerative changes and wart like growth. Severe exposure may produce vesicles and pustules. The scars radiate in shape with surrounding pigmentation. (v) *U-V rays:* Erythematic and eczematous dermatitis and vesication are seen. (vi) *Corrosive substances:* The corrosive substances produce ulcerated patches, line of redness is absent and there is no singeing of hair. (vii) *Electrical:* The characteristic electrical entry and exit mark is present. (viii) *Lightning stroke:* The lightning injuries are linear in shape present in moist creases or skin folds. Arborescent markings like branches of tree on the chest are present due to staining of the tissues by haemoglobin from lyses of red cells. Lightning is always accidental and there is history of rain with thunders. True burns occur beneath the metallic objects that the person is wearing or carrying.

The differences between the burns due to dry heat, moist heat and chemicals are as given in Table 19.2.

Preternatural combustibility: During life gases from anus can cause partial burning but during putrefaction, inflammable gases are ignited if a flame is nearby. These gases are hydrogen, hydrogen sulphide and methane. It is very rare and complete combustion does not occur.

Classification of Burns

The burns are classified depending upon how deeply and severely they penetrate the skin and underneath tissues:

Table 19.2: Differences between the burns caused by dry heat, moist heat and chemicals

Features	Burns	Scalds	Chemical burns
Cause	Flame, heated solid objects	Steam or liquid	Corrosive chemicals
Site	At and above site of contact	At and below site of contact	At and below site of contact
Splashing	Absent	Present	Present
Skin	Dry, shriveled and charred	Sodden and bleached	May be destroyed
Vesicles	At the circumference of the burnt area	Over burnt area	Very rare
Red line	Present	Present	Absent
Color	Black	Bleached	Distinctive
Charring	Present	Absent	Present or absent
Singeing	Present	Absent	Absent
Ulceration	Absent	Absent	Present
Scar	Thick and contracted	Thick and less contracted	Thick and contracted
Clothes	Burnt	Wet not burnt	May be burnt, stains on clothes

1. **Dupuytren's classification:** Guillaume Dupuytren, a French military surgeon classified burns into six degrees: (i) First degree (Erythema) (ii) Second degree (Vesication with blister formation) (iii) Third degree (Destruction of superficial skin) (iv) Fourth degree (Destruction of whole skin) (v) Fifth degree (Destruction of fascia and muscles) (vi) Sixth degree (Charring involving vessels, nerves, bones).
2. **Wilson's Classification:** (i) Epidermal (Dupuytren's first and second degree) (ii) Dermo-epidermal (Dupuytren's third and fourth degree) (iii) Deep (Dupuytren's fifth and sixth degree).
3. **Hebra classification:** Same as Wilson's. However, the symbol degree is used (Three degrees) (i) First degree (Epidermal) (ii) Second degree (Dermo-epidermal) (iii) Third degree (Deep).

Other classification used such **Evan's classification** that categorized burn into: (i) Superficial (involves epidermis only), (ii) Partial (involves both epidermis and dermis) and (iii) Full thickness (extend beyond dermis). **Muir and Sutherland** also classified burn injuries into three degrees upon the degree of dermal involvement (i) Superficial partial thickness (ii) Deep partial thickness and (iii) Full thickness burn. Wilson's classification is used by the forensic medicine experts in routine practice.

Dupuytren's classification: ***First degree:*** Erythema and redness is present that disappears in few minutes. First degree burns are painful. Signs of superficial inflammation are present. Mild irritants can also produce the features of first degree burn. It may last for several days when cuticle peels off but leaves no scar. They disappear after death due to gravitation of blood to the dependent parts. It involves superficial layer of epidermis.

Second degree: This type of burns consists of acute inflammation and blister formation. These blisters are to be distinguished from blisters produced by strong vesicants like cantharides. Blisters can also be due to decomposing fluid and urine and faeces when subjected to warmth in old bed ridden patients. In deeply comatose patient, bullous formation may be there. Blackening and singeing of the hair is present in second degree burns. On healing, no scar formation occurs but only some light staining of the skin remains.

Third degree: There is destruction of cuticle and part of true skin that appears horny and dark. There is exposure of nerve endings and much pain is produced. Scar formation occurs but no contraction is seen as scar contains all the elements of a true skin

Fourth degree: In fourth degree burns, whole skin is destroyed. Slough is yellowish brown and parchment like that separates on the 5th or 6th day. The burns are not very painful.

Fifth degree (Figure 19.2): The penetration of the deep fascia and muscles occur and great scarring and deformity results.

Sixth degree: The bones and nearby organs are involved in sixth degree burns. These burns can still be compatible to life, if the initial shock is overcome.

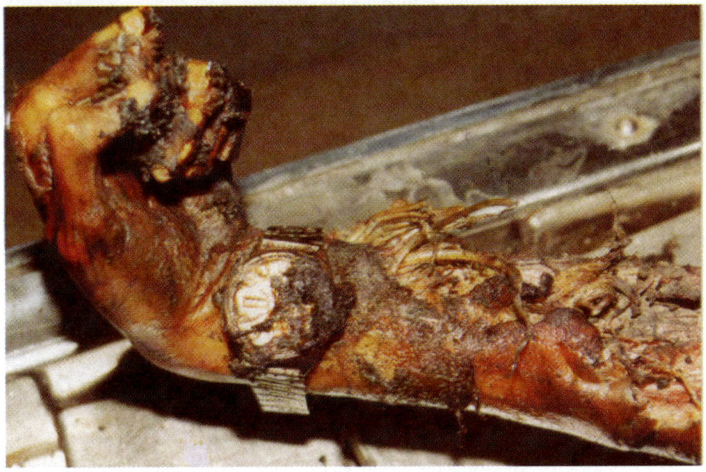

Figure 19.2: Deep burns over forearm and hand

Factors Influencing the Effects Produced by the Burns

1. **Degree of heat:** House fires at temperatures more than 650°C do not completely burn the adults. For cremation, incineration is done at 900-1000°C and only ashes about 1-1.5 kg and bone fragments remain after incineration.
2. **Duration of exposure:** Duration of exposure influences the burns produced.
3. **Body surface area involved in the burns:** The estimation of the burn surface area in adults is calculated by the **Wallace Rule of Nine.** In children the burn surface area can be calculated by the **Lund and Browder chart.** If the burn surface area is more than 15% in an adult and 10% in a child, the loss of circulating blood volume must be replaced else hypovolemic shock may develop. Patients with superficial burns involving 50% of the body surface area can survive.

   Wallace Rule of Nine: To calculate burn surface area in adults 9% is given to each body part and 1% to perineum as given below: (i) 9% for head and neck (ii) 9% for each upper limb (iii) 9% for front of chest (iv) 9% for back of chest (v) 9% for front of abdomen (vi) 9% for back of abdomen (vii) 9% for front of right lower limb (viii) 9% for front of left lower limb (ix) 9% for back of right lower limb (x) 9% for back of left lower limb (xi) 1% for perineum.

   In children, the burn surface area is calculated using **Lund and Browder chart** (Table 19.3 and Figure 19.3). Age of the children as an additional factor is considered while calculating the body surface area.

   Rule of Palms: The surface area of palm including fingers constitutes approximately 1% of total body surface area (TBSA) and palm excluding fingers constitutes approximately 0.5% of TBSA according to conventional method. It can be used for rough estimation of burn surface area calculation for small and patchy burns in children and adults; however, it varies according BMI, gender, ethnicity etc.
4. **Age:** The fatality caused by the burns depends upon the age of the victim. Children and old people are more susceptible to the burns. In children about 50-60% burn is fatal, in a person of about 40 years of age, about 40% is fatal whereas in old age only 10% can be fatal.
5. **Sex of the person:** Women are more susceptible than men.
6. **Site of the body involved:** The burns are more dangerous when involving the face, chest or genitals.

Table 19.3: Estimation of body surface area of burns

	Age group (in years)			
Burnt area	**1-4**	**5-9**	**10-14**	**Adults**
Head and neck	19%	15%	13%	9%
Upper limbs	19%	19%	19%	18%
Lower limbs	15% × 2	17% × 2	18% × 2	18% × 2
Front of chest	8%	8%	8%	9%
Back of chest	8%	8%	8%	9%
Front of abdomen	8%	8%	8%	9%
Back of abdomen	8%	8%	8%	9%

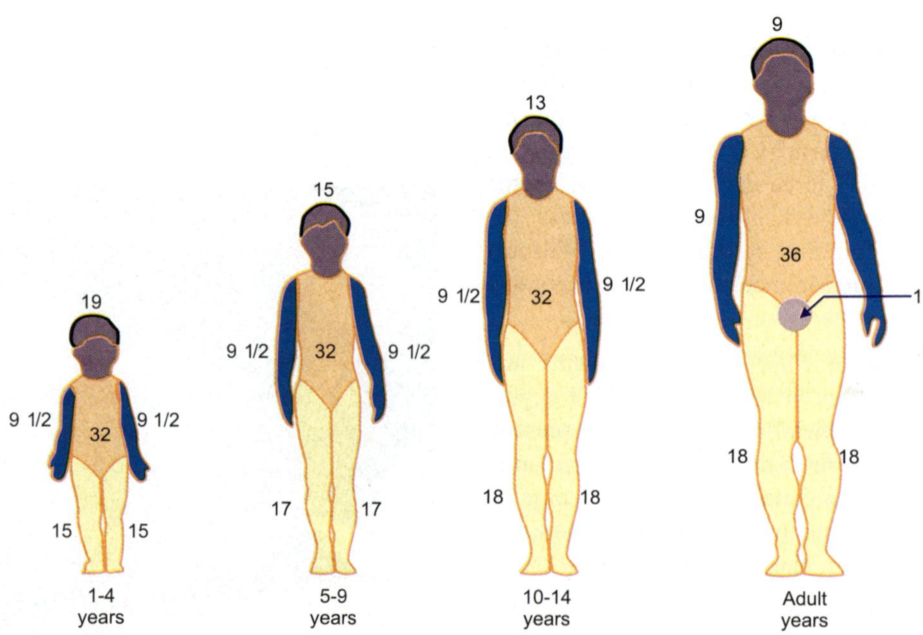

Figure 19.3: Estimation of body surface area in burns in children (Lund and Browder chart) and adults (Rule of nine)

Causes of Death in Burns

(i) ***Primary shock***: Due to the severe pain caused by burns. (ii) ***Secondary shock***: From hypovolemia due to fluid loss from the surface of burns within first 48 hours. (iii) ***Toxemia***: Within 3-4 days due to absorption of toxic metabolites from the burnt tissue. (iv) ***Septicemia:*** Sepsis of infected burns results in death within 5-6 days (Figure 19.4). (v) ***Biochemical disturbances***: This also occurs due to loss of fluid and tissue destruction, e.g., hypokalemia. (vi) ***Acute renal failure:*** This develops on 3-4th day due to necrosis of lower nephron. (vii) ***Glottis and pulmonary edema:*** This occur in massive house fires or fires in buildings when the person dies at the spot itself. Edema of glottis and lungs results from inhalation of CO and CO_2. (viii) ***Suffocation:*** Inhalation of smoke containing carbon monoxide, cyanide gas, lack of oxygen, and free radicals and non-specific toxic substances. (ix) ***Accidents:*** These may occur while attempting to escape from a burning house or by injuries resulting from falling masonry, timber or other objects over the body.

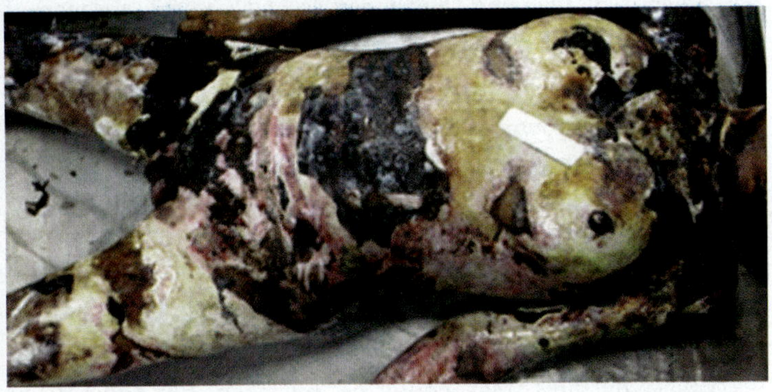

Figure 19.4: Infected burns over the body with deposition of yellowish green pus

Determination of Cause of Death

To determine the cause of death one has to establish whether the victim was alive at the time of fire.

1. **Differences between antemortem and postmortem burns:** The differences are shown in Table 19.4. However certain points need to be discussed. These are: (i) Presence of CO in the blood is suggestive that the person was alive at the time of burns. However, its absence does not exclude it. It is absent in flash fires such as explosions, chemical plant fires or warfare etc. (ii) As a rule, flames that hit the face are liable to cause death rapidly due to oedema of airways and suffocation. (iii) Toxic effects of inhalation of combustion products of some synthetic material like plastic furniture, upholstery cause rapid death. (iv) Phosgene, chlorine, cyanides and nitrogen oxides aggravate the anoxic effects of carboxyhaemoglobin. (v) Carbon monoxide is generated by the combustion of household material. Carbon monoxide level varies in a dead body depending upon age and health of the victim. (vi) Fatal level is usually 50-70% carbon monoxide saturation but in the presence of lung and cardiac diseases death occurs at a much lower level. (vii) Infants and children build up the carbon monoxide level quickly due to increased respiratory rate. As a result, the children die before the parents when sleeping in same room. (viii) In a foetus, diffusion of CO across the placental barrier has conflicting opinion. (ix) Black soot particles get deposited over the mouth and nostrils. Soot frequently extends to the lungs and at times may be found in the esophagus. The soot can be spread as a thin film on a white paper and examined with the naked eye and then under the microscope. The trachea and other airways show congestion. (x) There is blister formation over the joints and any other parts of the body in second degree burns. These blisters are to be differentiated from those formed in CO and barbiturate poisoning and deep coma.
2. **Fat embolism:** Presence of fat droplets in blood vessels of the lungs must be interpreted with care as it occurs due to fat embolism. This is to be differentiated from the similar finding in blunt force injury and physicochemical alterations of fat in the blood.
3. **Heat fractures (Figure 19.5):** Fractures of extremities due to shrinkage of muscles occurs. Skull fractures are seen on either side of skull above the temples and are sometimes bilateral and no displacement of the outer table occurs. It consists of several lines radiating from a common center. It

Table 19.4: Differences between antemortem and postmortem burns

Features	Antemortem burns	Postmortem burns
Line of redness	Present; absent if death is immediate	Absent
Redness	Base is inflammed and swollen; contains protein and chloride; inflammatory reaction is present	Base is dry and yellow; contains air and no protein or chloride but at times traces may be seen; inflammatory reaction is absent
Vital reaction	Positive	Negative
Enzymes	SH group increased, mucopolysaccharides are present. Following enzymes show an increase in the peripheral zone Nonspecific esterases—1 hour Lucein amino-peptidases—2 hours Acid phosphates—3 hours Alkaline phosphates—6 hours	Mucopolysaccharides are absent. There is no increase in any of the enzyme groups

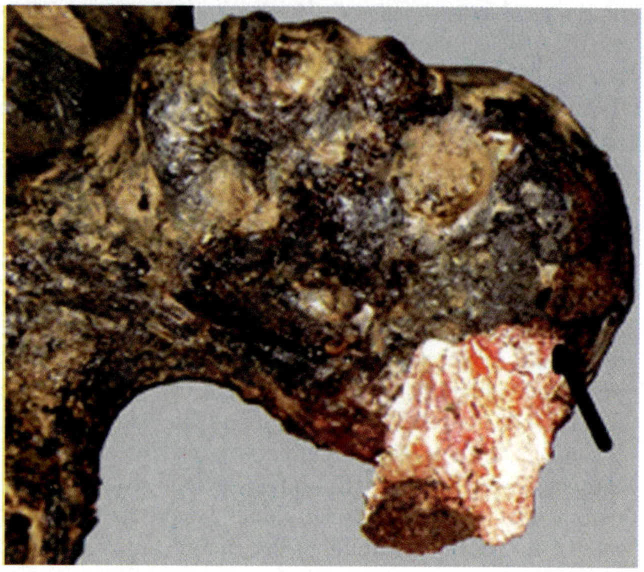

Figure 19.5: Extensive burns with heat fracture of skull with brain tissue coming out through it

is commonly produced by bursting effects with brain tissue coming out due to steam pressure within the skull. The cracks are limited to the outer table. The skull fractures due to burns should be differentiated from the fractures due to blunt force. Heat fractures do not involve the sutures of the skull even in young individuals with open sutures. The bone becomes brittle due to direct effect of heat. Blood and marrow are expressed from the skull bones by heat that accumulates between dura and the bone that clots and thereby formation of heat haematoma occurs.

4. **Heat haematoma (Figure 19.6):** Heat haematoma is soft, friable clot that is pink in colour and shows **honeycomb appearance**. It is 2-15 mm thick and contains 100-120 ml of blood. There is charring of the skull. The distribution of heat haematoma is related to the charring of skull. The diploic veins and longitudinal sinus is involved. The brain

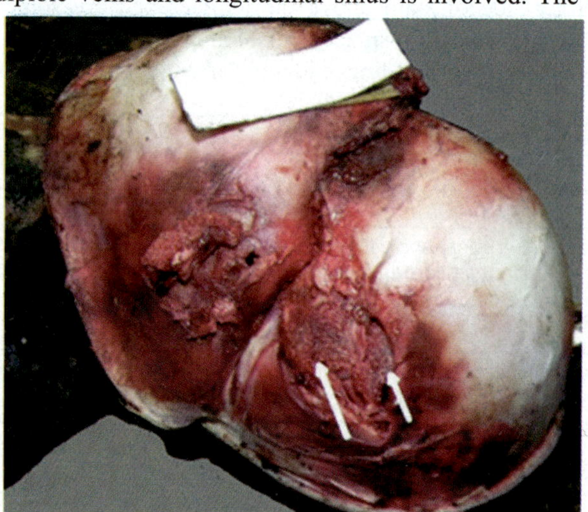

Figure 19.6: Heat haematoma-honeycomb appearance

is shrunken, firm and yellow to brown due to cooking and the dura is leathery. Heat haematoma should be differentiated from extradural haematoma. Extradural haematoma is found over the temporoparietal region of brain due to rupture of middle meningeal artery. It is always traumatic in origin and does not have a cherry red colour or honeycomb appearance.

5. **Subdural haematoma:** Subdural haematoma in burn victims develop due to the injuries and not by the effects of the flame. This clot should be submitted for chemical analysis as positive alcohol level in subdural clot indicates that the victim is habitual to alcohol because the peripheral blood alcohol may have metabolized but subdural clot still contains it.
6. Due to the effects of heat, blood is pressed out of the lung tissue into the airways, mouth and nostrils suggesting injury.
7. **Heat ruptures:** Splitting of the skin due to heat should be differentiated from antemortem cuts and slashes by the absence of bleeding, intact nerves and vessels, absence of bruising and irregular margins.
8. **Curling ulcer:** The stress ulcers secondary to systemic burns are known as Curling ulcers. Curling ulcer due to inflammation and ulceration of Payer's patches develops on the 7-10th day of the burns most probably due to thrombosis of the vessels. The common site of stress ulcer are gastric body and fundus, however can also be observed in the antrum and duodenum.
9. Anus is occasionally dilated due to shrinkage of peripheral tissue by heat that could be mistaken for sodomy or homosexuality. In putrefaction also due to formation of gases the abdominal pressure is increased and dilatation of anus occurs that may be mistaken for sodomy.

Autopsy Findings (Figures 19.7 and 19.8)

The aim of the postmortem examination is to establish identification of the victim and cause of death, whether the person was alive at the time of incidence that is whether the burns are antemortem or postmortem, time since death, age of the burns and whether the burns are accidental, suicidal or homicidal are also to be established. The postmortem examination in deaths due to burns when the period of marriage is less than seven years is to be conducted by a board of two doctors. In addition, vide order of Government of N.C.T. the autopsy is to be conducted by two doctors when the age of the married woman is less than thirty years.

Establishment of Identity: (i) Identification of the victim is carried out according to the general outline but certain principles are peculiar to the victims of fire. (ii) Length and weight of the charred body are unreliable as dimensions are altered due to desiccation of the tissues resulting in skull fractures and pulverization of the intervertebral discs. Body length may be shortened by several

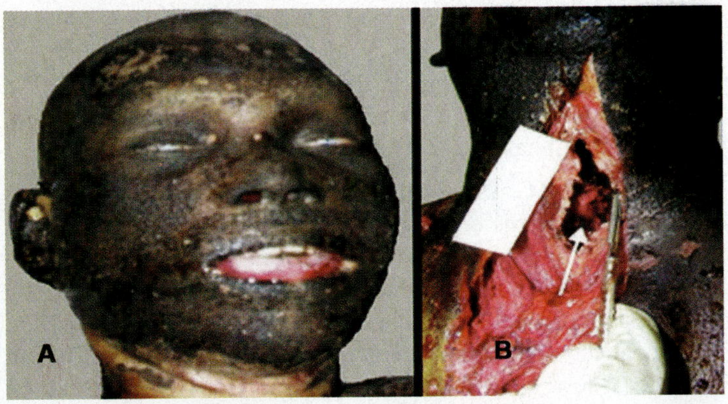

Figure 19.7A and B: Burn injuries over the face showing blackening and protrusion of tongue (A) Shoot particles inside the trachea (B)

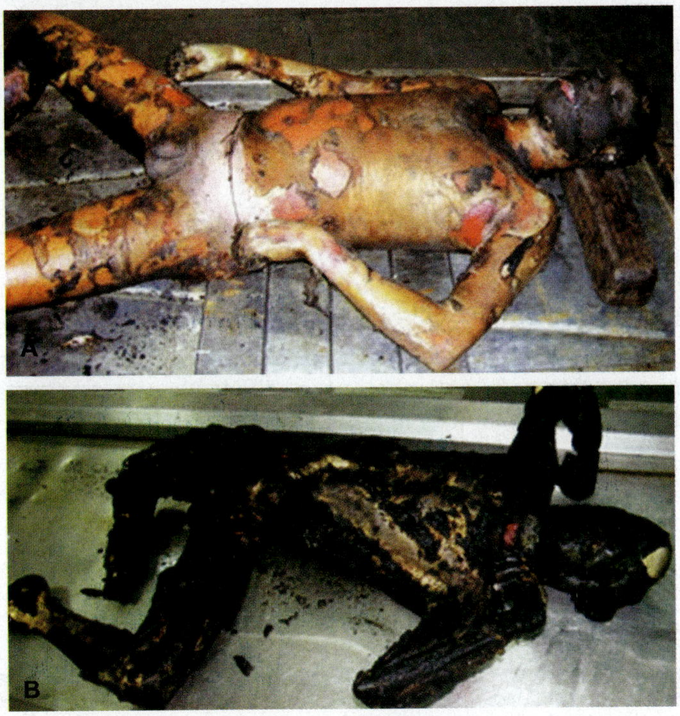

Figure 19.8A and B: Body showing pugilistic attitude and extensive burns covering 100% of the body surface area, note the erythema suggestive of antemortem burns

inches and weight is reduced to about 60%. (iii) Body features are changed and skin is tightened and contracted. An ear is reduced to 2/3rd of its original size. Eyes show cataract formation due to coagulation of proteins in lens even at 150 °F. (iv) Identification marks on the body like scars, tattoos, moles etc. may be destroyed. Removal of superficial layers of skin by wiping or rubbing makes tattoo better. (v) Degloving occurs due to deposition of fluid between the layers of skin that is used to obtain fingerprints. This is to be differentiated from deaths due to decomposition or immersion. (vi) Surgical scars such as missing appendix and mastectomy can be diagnosed at autopsy. (vii) Bones, pelvis and teeth can help in identifying the age, sex and race of the deceased. (viii) *Sex of the victim:* It is identified from the presence of genitalia and breast tissue. Internally, sex can be identified from the organs such as prostate and uterus. (ix) *Age of the victim:* Estimation of age from breast tissue is misleading as heat causes fluid loss that leads to shrinkage, erection and firmness regardless of the age of the person. (x) *Race of the victim:* The skin is brown or mottled in Negroes and in them dark gray deposit of melanin in the arachnoid membrane in the medulla oblongata, base of frontal lobe, olfactory bulbs etc. is seen on microscopical examination. (xi) *Complete X-ray of the body:* It is done to detect old fractures, bony abnormalities, foreign bodies etc. (xii) *Dental examination:* X-ray of the teeth to identify metal pins in root canal treatment and fillings. Teeth examination is difficult when the teeth are fragmented or there is deposition of smoke and soot. When heat contractures have tightly locked the jaws; in such cases the teeth can be examined after disarticulating the mandible and excising the upper jaws. (xiii) Pathologist should look for the patches of intact skin under tight clothing, belts, brassiere or buttoned collar. On the ankle and wrist as the victim may be tied with strings or ropes before burning. Ligature marks may be present on the neck. At times, skin and hair in the armpits are spared and gums are also preserved.

External findings: The buttocks and armpits are usually spared from burns. The body will show burn areas accompanied with blackening that is characteristic of burns from kerosene or petrol. Erythema of burn area is characteristic of antemortem burns. There is finding of peeling of skin.

Pugilistic attitude: Pugilistic attitude results due to the coagulation of muscle proteins due to excessive heat and flexors muscles are more affected (Figure 19.8A and B). Pugilistic attitude is also known as **Boxer's attitude/fencing attitude/ defence attitude.** It is not an antemortem phenomenon and can be produced after death also.

Hair changes due to burns: There are light hair changes at different temperatures such as gray hair at 250°C attains brassy blonde and brown hair at 400 °F for 10-15 minutes attains a slight reddish hue.

Heat ruptures: These are produced by splitting of soft parts at the joints. They may be confused with the incised or lacerated wounds. Can be differentiated from them by the absence of bleeding; presence of intact vessels and nerves; irregular margins and absence of bruising and other vital reactions.

Internal findings: The internal findings such as heat haematoma can be recognized by the presence of soft, friable clot. It is pink in colour due to the presence of carboxyhaemoglobin and honeycomb appearance.

Age of the burns: The question arises as to when the burns were caused and whether several burns were caused simultaneously. Formation of cicatrix and deformity takes time depending on the amount and extent of infection. The following features help in finding out the time of burn (Table 19.5).

Table 19.5: Changes in burns with time

Features	Time
Redness	Immediate
Vesication	1-2 hours
Exudates begins to dry	12-24 hours
Dry brown crust formation	48-72 hours
Pus formation	48-72 hours (not before 36 hours)
Superficial slough separates	4th-6th day
Deep slough separates	15 days
Granulation tissue begins to cover Formation of cicatrix and deformity	More than 15 days Several weeks or months

Medicolegal Aspects

Suicidal burns: Suicidal burns are very rare among men but common in women. The victim may commit suicide by burning due to disappointment in love, being tired of domestic worries or chronic diseases. At times, suicidal note is recovered and the room is locked from inside. Dowry deaths are caused using this method commonly that occurs in young brides who are unable to bring dowry or due to harassment by the in-laws leading to abetment to suicide. Self-immolation is also employed sometimes to protest like Mandal Commission, *Sati* system.

Homicidal burns: Homicidal buns occur in the following circumstances. Bride burning by the in-laws is common. The master and sometimes stepmother or stepfather applies hot *chimta* over the private parts, hands or thighs etc. of the servants and children. As a punishment for infidelity, cigarettes are applied to produce burns that can be circular, or triangular in shape. The victim may be burned after he is murdered by strangulation or by any other manner to conceal the crime. Homicidal burns are also produced to torture a criminal to extort information or as a punishment for infidelity. In addition, burns, scalds or electrical injuries may be produced in child abuse cases. Acids or old bulbs may be thrown on the face out of jealousy or disgruntled behaviour. At 1000-1100°C, complete burns are produced but house fires can occur at 700°C causing charring of the body.

Accidental burns: Accidental burns result while the person is drugged, diseased or drunk. When the house is on fire, while sleeping in winter, cooking, during epileptic fits, or children may fall into fire while playing. Scalds are usually accidental due to application of hot water bottles or when water from the boiling kettle falls on the victim. Lamps or stoves may explode and cause burns.

Self-inflicted burns: Self-inflicted burns are caused for the charge of false accusation.

Dowry deaths: Dowry death is also known as bride burning. For burning a bride, fire accelerant such as kerosene and petrol can be used by the husband and in-laws. **Dowry Prohibition Act 1961** was amended in 1983, 1984 and 1986. According to **section 3** of Dowry Prohibition Act as amended in 1986, taking dowry is an offence and **section 4** implies demanding dowry is an offence. A new prescribing punishment for dowry deaths **S. 304B I.P.C.**, **S. 498A I.P.C.** and **S. 34 I.P.C.** (more than one person acting with common intent) has been enacted.

S. 304B I.P.C. Dowry death: Where death of the woman is caused by any burns or bodily injuries or occurs otherwise than under normal circumstances within 7 years of her marriage and it is shown that soon before her death she was subjected to cruelty or harassment by her husband or any relative of her husband for, or in connection with any demand for dowry, such death shall be called "dowry death", and such husband or relative shall be deemed to have caused her death.

S. 498A I.P.C.: Husband or relative of husband of woman subjecting her to cruelty: Whoever, being the husband or the relative of the husband of a woman subjects such woman to cruelty shall be punished with imprisonment for a term which may extend to 3 years and shall also be liable to fine.

S. 113B I.E.A: If cruelty or harassment before the death of woman is related to 'dowry demand', dowry death shall be presumed.

S. 176 Cr.P.C.: Magistrate inquiry shall be conducted in dowry death cases. Postmortem will be conducted by the two doctors where the period of marriage is within 7 years. Duty of the public is to inform the police who will take the necessary action.

S. 201 Cr.P.C.: Causing disappearance of evidence of offence or giving false information to screen offender. In cases of Capital offence, punishment with imprisonment for 7 years or fine.

S. 202 Cr.P.C.: Intentional omission to give information of offence by person bound to inform. Punishment with imprisonment for 6 months, fine, or both.

S. 203 Cr.P.C.: Giving false information regarding an offence committed. Punishment with imprisonment for 2 years or with fine or with both.

ELECTRICAL INJURIES

Factors Influencing Electrical Injuries

The factors that affect production of electrical injuries and shock are:

Voltage or tension: Voltage is less important than the amperage or intensity. (i) *Low voltage (< 50 volts)*: It is used for therapeutic purposes and rarely causes accidents. Low tensions of A.C. can cause fatalities. Tension as low as 25 volts passes through heart and can cause deaths. (ii) *Medium voltage (< 500 volts)*: This voltage predisposes to prolonged contact because the victim grips and holds on to the conductor. It really depends upon amperage rather than voltage. The typical 'Joule burn' cases are related to "Hold on" cases. The agents commonly responsible are hand tools, overhead lines, switchgears and lamps etc. Most fatalities occur at 220-250 volts that is the usual household supply.

(iii) *High voltage*: It is the voltage in thousands and the death does not occur necessarily. Life can be saved depending upon the time of exposure to this voltage.

Amperage (Intensity): It is the most important factor in electrocution. It is the cause of "hold on" to conductors that is the cause of serious local damage and fatal shock. It is given by: A=V/R; Where V = Voltage, R = Resistance of the conductor. Contact with the current at 1mA causes tingling sensation. As amperage rises, it is a more painful experience. Normal healthy man can tolerate up to 21.6 mA but 'hold on' occurs at 8-9 mA. Women are less tolerant, the maximum level is 14 mA and 'hold on' occurs at 6 mA. Danger increases when the amperage is between 100 mA to 4 A. Above 4 A, it arrests cardiac fibrillation; this is the principle of treatment with a defibrillator. High voltage with low amperage is less dangerous than moderate voltage with high amperage.

Density of the current: Density of the current depends upon the following: (i) Dry or moist skin: Dry skin of the palm have the resistance of 1-2 million Ohms. Sweating reduces the resistance from 30,000 ohm to 2500 Ohm. (ii) When moistened with water or saline the density of current further drops between 1200-1500 Ohms. (iii) Charges in skin due to current is less than 380 Ohms but once it is burnt, resistance of the skin rises and that may cause a break in the circuit.

Resistance of the body: It plays an important part in causing effects of electrocution. Effects will be modified according to the part of the body that comes in contact with the current. Resistance is greatest on the palms (of the labourers) and least on the inner sides of thighs. Average resistance of various body areas and tissues is: (i) Skin is 500-10,000 Ohms (ii) Mucosa is 1500-2000 Ohms (iii) Bone is 9,00,000 Ohms (iv) Vascular areas like cheek are better conductors and most of the current passes through the blood vessels.

Insulation: Stout rubber gloves and rubber boots in good condition gives considerable protection. Therefore, all the tools used in electricity should be adequately insulated.

Contact with electric supply: Electrocution is normally the result of direct contact with 240 volts A.C. and closer the contact, greater is the danger especially when it results in 'hold on', glancing touch or fall followed by a break in the circuit. High tension currents throw or repel violently and the death may be due to the fall. Broad and good contact reduces the skin resistance from 100,000 Ohm to 1000 Ohm. Indirect contact with high-tension current results in arcing and direct flow of current in an indirect fashion such as while urinating on a high-tension conductor. The area of contact modifies external appearances such as: (i) Conductor involving small surface area such as the end of a rod or wire produces circular hole in the tissue and simulates bullet injury. (ii) Wire wound around wrist produces linear grooves. (iii) A broad conductor closely applied may not leave any mark. (iv) In electrocution in a bath, flow of current occurs without generation of heat and no external injuries are produced.

Duration of contact: Longer the contact, greater is the damage. There is formation of electric mark, blister formation, charring of the tissues, Joule burn and destruction of tissues with exposure of muscles and bones.

Site of contact: Electrical injuries on the face and arms are serious whereas those on the palms are less serious. When the path taken by the current is from left hand to leg, 2-3 times more current is passed to the heart compared to the path taken from right hand to leg. Various paths taken by the current are shown in Figure 19.9.

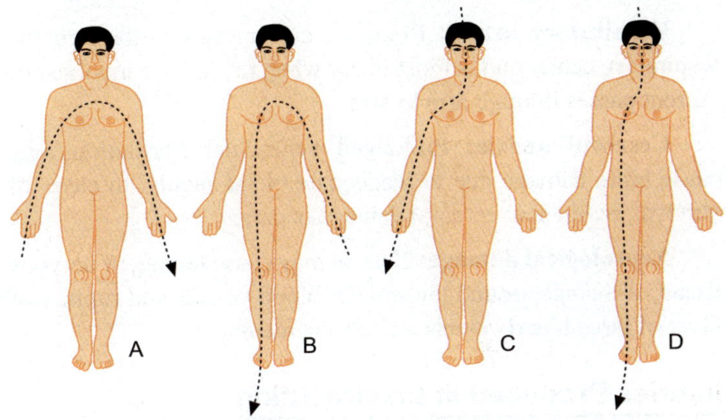

Figure 19.9: Various paths taken by the current: A-Hand to hand, B-Hand to feet, C-Head to hand, D-Head to feet

Kind of electrode: **Jellineck** found that area of contact did not determine the severity of shock but others believe that it is important.

Kind of current: A.C. is more dangerous than D.C. and the numbers of cycles in A.C. are important. The rate of: (i) 40-150 cycles/second is dangerous (ii) 50-60 cps is the critical frequency (iii) At frequencies more than 1700 cps, heart becomes 20 times more tolerant (v) D.C. only causes a single convulsion or contraction, usually thrown the person away from the electrical source.

Personal idiosyncrasies: Individual personality, physical condition and existence of mental or bodily distress influence the effect of shock.

Presence of diseases: Cardiac diseases may predispose to electrocution even at low tension current.

Anticipation of shock: In anticipation of shock, the individuals can sustain current better.

Sleep: Sleep increases the resistance to an electrical current.

Important factor: Net effect of the current depends on Voltage × Duration—Tolerance and alertness.

Mechanism of Electrocution

Ventricular fibrillation: **Prevost and Botelike** first described ventricular fibrillation in 1899. It is an important factor in low and medium voltage currents. Ventricular fibrillation is not always associated with loss of consciousness or respiration. Some individuals can also walk about before they die. Cyanosis is not seen in these cases.

Tetanic asphyxia: Low or medium voltage current passing through the chest of 20-30 mA can induce tetanic contraction of the extrinsic muscles of respiration and death from mechanical asphyxia. Cyanosis is present in these cases. Production of Joule burn at the point of contact may lower the resistance thus increasing the amperage above the critical level at which the ventricular fibrillation occurs.

Respiratory arrest: Route of current passes through the respiratory center and is most likely when the head is involved or current passes through arm to arm.

Cerebral anoxia: Prolonged ventricular fibrillation may cause brain damage due to inadequate blood supply. In cases of survival, permanent cerebral damage occurs.

Neurological damage: Current may cause tearing of nervous tissue, shrinkage around the smaller blood vessels and rupture of layer of large blood vessels and elastic membrane.

Injuries Produced in Electrocution

Low and Medium Tension Injuries

The electric burn/mark (Joule burn): The electric mark is found at the point of entry mostly associated with the thermal burns. The typical mark is usually absent. The mark may be trivial at times. Rarely, there may not be any mark, but it only indicates inadequate search by the pathologist rather than the absence of mark. The electric mark is specific for contact with electricity but not a proof of electrocution as an electrocution mark can be produced even after death. However, when the mark is present, there is strong presumption of death due to electrocution.

Features: The mark is in the form of round or oval, shallow crater bordered by a ridge of skin 1-3 mm high, partly or fully around its circumference (Figures 19.8 to 19.11). The floor is lined by pale, flattened skin. Ridge pattern is preserved but due to flattening ridges are broad and scarcely above the general level. At times, there is breach in the continuity of skin that should be differentiated from broken blister. The skin is pale and hyperemia is present beyond the mark. The shape of the conductor or part of it determines shape of the electric mark. When the conductor is rod like wire or flex, round or oval mark is produced. Contact with the long axis of wire produces linear mark or groove whereas contact with the end of the wire produces a deep hole into muscles or bone that needs to be differentiated from the bullet injury.

When contact is more prolonged, skin shows biscuit or brown tint that on further contact produces charring due to burning. Flash burn is the term that distinguishes it from the changes caused by exogenous heat following contact with high voltage. Electric mark are usually found on the exposed parts of the body and more commonly the palmar aspect of hand especially the tips of index finger and thumb in the hands of electricians. It can be

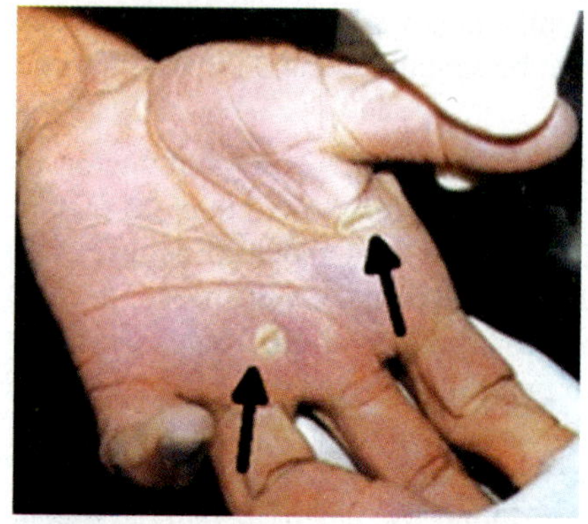

Figure 19.8: Electrical entry wound over the palm, note the pale, depressed base and raised margins

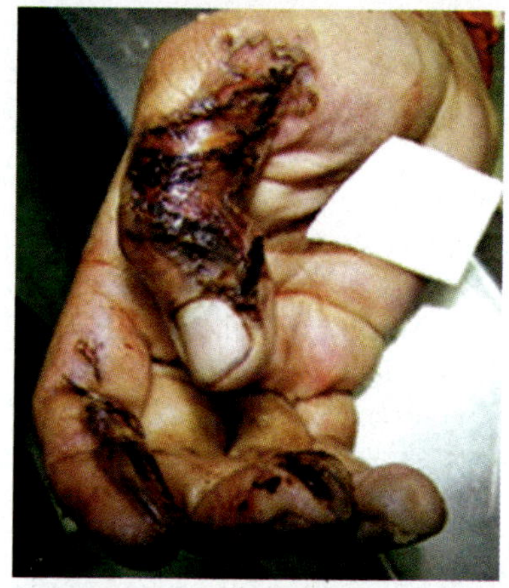

Figure 19.9: Electrical entry wound over fingers

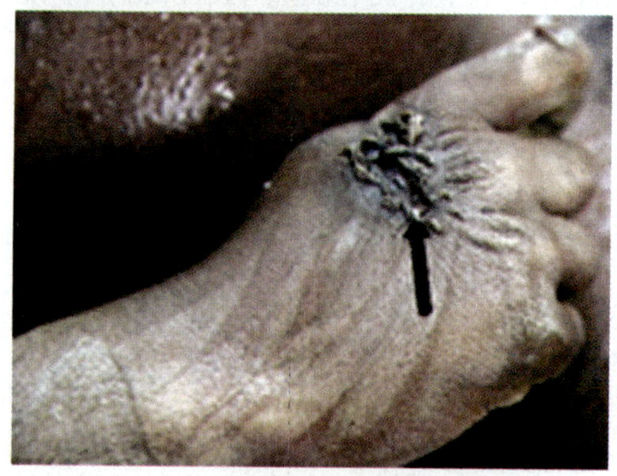

Figure 19.10: Electrical entry wound over dorsum of hand

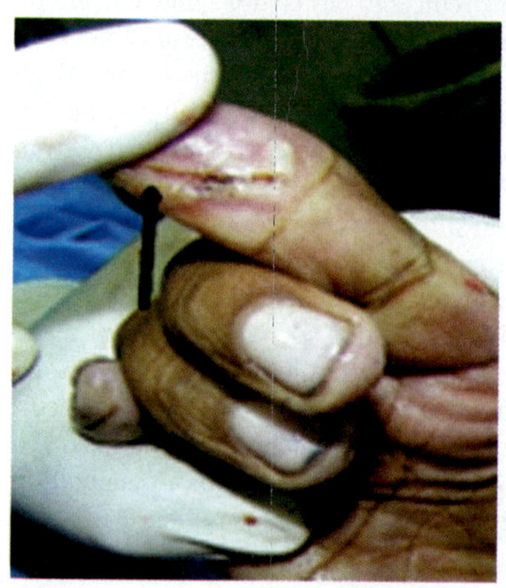

Figure 19.11: Electrical entry wound showing no extravasation underneath on dissection

present anywhere on the body and can be produced beneath the intact clothing that may be undamaged by thermal heat such as shoulder or thigh. The Joule burn is produced by the conversion of electricity into heat within the tissues, the so-called **endogenous burns**. Heat generated in the skin (corium) and subcutaneous tissue causes the fluid to boil to produce blisters by prolonged process and the steam thus generated bursts through the skin.

High-tension injuries (Exogenous burns): High-tension injuries are either due to direct contact or indirectly by arcing of the flash (Figure 19.12). As much heat is generated in the arcing of the flash and there is knock down by sudden increase of local atmospheric pressure, multiple discrete lesions due to arcing are produced with the blast effect. These are called **crocodile burns** (Figure 19.13). When someone climbs on to an electric pole for suicide or theft of cable, there are chances of arcing when the person comes nearer to the conducting wire. Distance between person and cable leading to arching is related to voltage. At the voltage of 5000 voltages, the distance between the individual and the person should be 1 mm and at 1,00,000 voltages there should 35 mm distance for arching (**Mueller** cited by Simonin, 1955).

Although flash burns are extensive and severe and they may be exaggerated from ignited clothing, direct contact causes gross destruction of soft tissues, charring of bones or fusion of bone into pearl like bodies and sequestration of dead bones that are seen radiologically as '**bone pearls**' or '**wax drippings**'. In flash burns due to revitalization of tissue, healing may take a long time even upto 6 years.

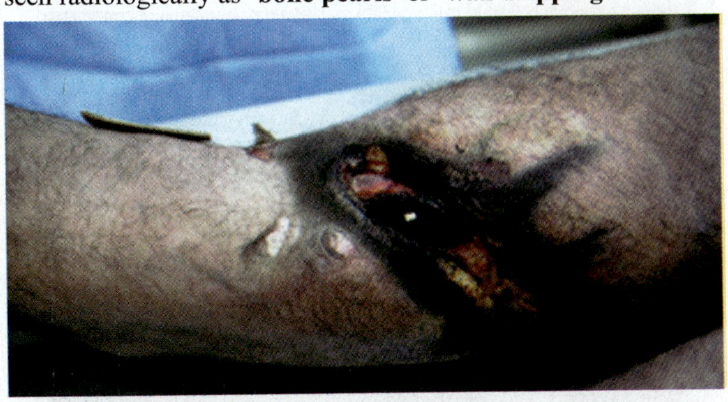

Figure 19.12: Electrical contact burn with flash burn/spark burn

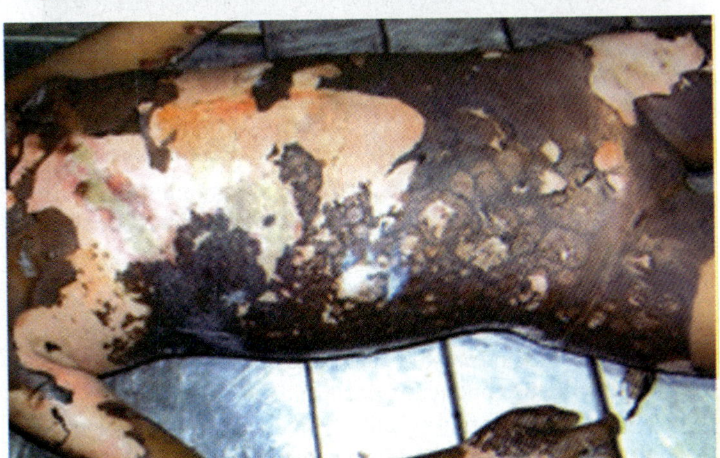

Figure 19.13: Crocodile burn in case of electrocution

Exit mark: Exit mark is variable in appearance and has some of the features of electrical entrance mark (Figures 19.14 and 19.15). Exit mark causes more disruption of tissues and is seen as splits in the skin where the skin has been raised into ridges by the passage of current. Splitting may be continuous or interrupted. There is honeycomb appearance of damaged tissue, which is seen microscopically.

Metallisation: Metallisation is a specific feature of electrocution and lightning stroke, seen more commonly and completely in the latter conditions. The following features are encountered: (i) Face of the victim may become darkened brown and black. (ii) Colour of the skin varies with the nature of the conductor; if the conductor is iron, the skin is black or brown and when the conductor is copper; the skin is yellow brown or blue. It is due to volatilization of the metal particles that are driven into the skin. (iii) Small gray green areas are present in the floor of the electric mark and the face of the brass becomes pitted and dull. It occurs in low and medium voltages.

Metallisation is detected by low magnifications on histological examination and chemical examination. Metallic

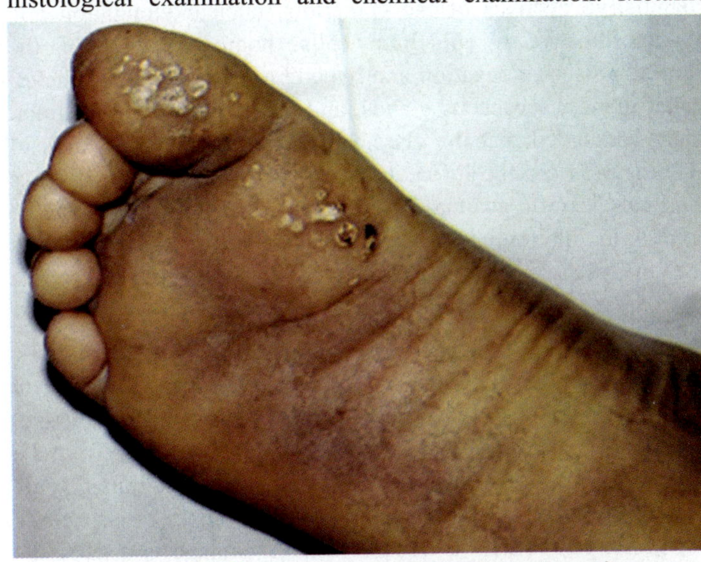

Figure 19.14: Electrical exit wound over the sole

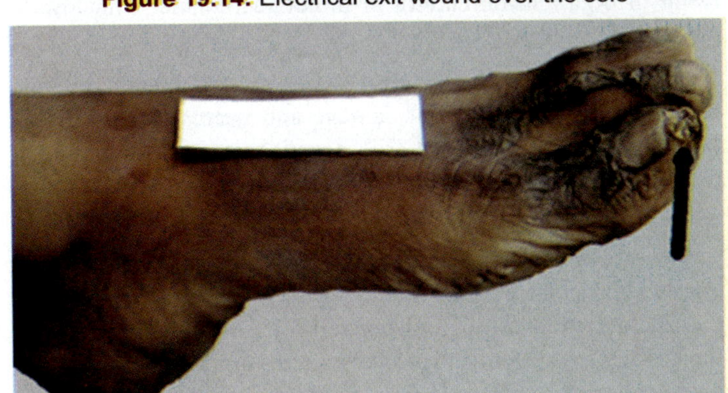

Figure 19.15: Electrical exit wound over great toe

deposit is invariably present and for this acroreaction test should be done. It is useful even in advanced putrefaction. A positive test is a proof of electrocution. Depending on the composition of the conductor, metallic deposits are mainly in the superficial layers of the skin and hair follicles as seen on histological examination.

Acroreaction test: A microchemical test for metals devised by **Skalos** in 1944 for the identification of electric marks. It is based on the solubility of metals either in the hydrochloric acid or nitric acid. Iron, aluminum, zinc and nickel are soluble in hydrochloric acid except copper whereas all of the above except iron are soluble in nitric acid. Metal of the electric mark is dissolved with the acid and this solution is kept on a filter paper with the reagent, the colour change will occur. When iron is the metal, over the filter paper add a solution of potassium ferrocyanide and the blue coloration will indicate iron.

Microscopic examination: Microscopic features of electrocution mark are not very specific. **Behera *et al.*** (2020) studied antemortem electrical (AME) and postmortem electrical (PME) burn marks with the help of histopathology. The slides were stained with haematoxylin-eosin stains and the parameters studied were intraepidermal and subepidermal separation, coagulative necrosis of the epidermis, nuclear elongation and hyperchromasia of epidermal cells, homogenization of the dermis, nuclear elongation and hyperchromasia of hair follicles, sweat glands, sebaceous glands, and blood vessel endothelium. They concluded that the classical histopathological features of electrocution cannot differentiate between AME and PME burn marks but careful evaluation of grading of these changes can be helpful in differentiating them. The histopathological changes seen in electrical burn marks are mainly due to the physical effect of the heat produced by the electric current within the skin.

Description of electrocution injuries: In these injuries, confusion may arise because the forensic pathologists constantly describe the effects of electric shock as burns. It is better to call the mark of electricity as electric mark and distinguish it from the effects of a flash that produces burns akin to flame burns. Joule burn is produced by same mechanism that causes electric mark but prolonged contact is needed. Visible damage is usually the result of high-tension current or prolonged contact with low or medium tension current.

Delayed effects of electrocution: (i) Gangrene and haemorrhage due to arterial damage and necrosis of the tissue (ii) Damage to spinal cord (iii) Aseptic necrosis and resultant depression of the bone marrow (iv) Angina pectoris or myocardial necrosis (v) Eye injuries resulting in cataract and optic atrophy.

Cause of death in Electrocution: (i) Most of the deaths occur due to ventricular fibrillation ending in cardia arrest. It is due to passage of current through myocardium or endocardium affecting the conduction system and producing arrhythmia. (ii) Respiratory arrest can occur when the current pass through the thorax causing paralysis of diaphragm and intercostal muscles. (iii) Other causes of death can be due secondary injury from non-electrical trauma, e.g., blunt force trauma due to fall and flash burns.

Autopsy Findings

(i) Electric burn mark (joule burn) are the pathognomic features when low and medium voltage current is involved. Proof of electric mark is obtained by histological and photochemical (Acroreaction) examination. (ii) High-tension currents cause gross thermal injuries that are the result of direct contact, flash over, or thermal burns. (iii) Circumstantial findings are corroborative in cases of electrocution. (iv) In electrocution in a bath, the following findings are present: (a) No external injuries are present over the body (b) On examination of the scene, live wire is recovered (c) Exclusion of other cases of death such as natural disease and poisoning etc. is to be ruled out. (v) Other non-specific findings may be present such as cyanosis of the face, petechial haemorrhages over the face, pleura and pericardium. (vi) Viscera is congested and lungs are intensely congested and oedematous. (vii) Heart is dilated due to fibrillation. (viii) Froth is present over the mouth and nostrils. (ix) *Postmortem electric mark*: Electric mark unaccompanied by hyperemia can be produced even after death. It is possible to produce changes in the skin, which resemble electric mark by applying Bunsen burner or a glowing wire (Figure 19.16). In electric mark, acroreaction is positive but this is negative in thermal burns.

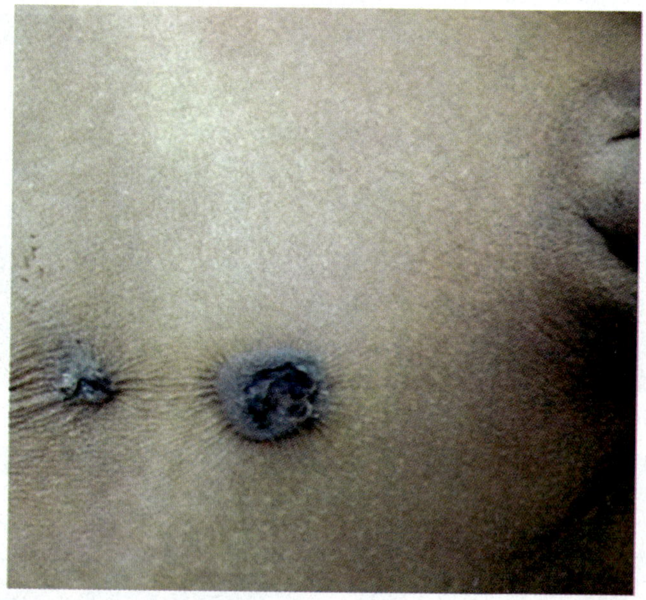

Figure 19.16: Postmortem electrocution burn mark (Electrocution burn mark produced after death) having similar characteristics of antemortem electrocution burn mark

Judicial electrocution: Death penalty is carried out in an electric chair in USA. The condemned man is strapped to a wooden chair and one cap like electrode is put on the shaven scalp, moistened with the conducting paste and the other is applied to the right lower leg. A current of 2000 volts and 7 amperes is passed through the body. After tetanic spasm and loss of consciousness, the same current is passed for a second time for one minute.

Medicolegal Aspects

Electrical burns are usually accidental resulting from defective appliances or negligence in the equipment. They may be produced from application of live wire during convulsive therapy of mentally diseased patients. Homicidal electric burns may occur during theft and suicidal electric burns are rare.

LIGHTNING STROKE

Lightning stroke is a flash of lightning due to an electrical discharge from the cloud to the earth. The electric current is direct with a potential of 1000 million volts or more. At the track of current much energy is liberated most of which is converted into light. The highest points attract the lightning stroke. Dry skin and dry clothes are bad conductors whereas wet clothes and wet skin are good conductors.

Signs and symptoms: (i) Unconsciousness (ii) In non fatal cases, giddiness, ringing in the ears and headache develops (iii) Conjunctivitis, clouding of cornea, cataract and retinal haemorrhage (iv) Loss of memory (v) Paralysis and titanic convulsions (vi) Deafness or dumbness etc. develops.

Autopsy findings: The following effects are produced: (i) Direct effect from electrical discharge passing to the earth surface produces '**flash burns**'. Mechanical effect due to force of displaced air and compression effect due to air movement in its return wave produces the changes. (ii) Clothes are usually torn or burnt at the point of entry or exit. At times, clothes are thrown at a distance. There can be exceptions when clothing is not damaged even if the person has been killed. Conversely clothing may be damaged without any damage to the person. (iii) Blast like lesions are produced comprising a triad of contusions, lacerations and rupture of organs.

Burns Due to Lightning

These are linear burns 3-30 cm or more in length and 0.3-2.5 cm in breadth involving the moist creases and folds of the skin called **filigree burns or arborescent markings** (Figure 19.17). These are superficial, thin, irregular and tortuous markings in the skin like a tree due to minute deposits of copper in the skin. They indicate the path taken by discharge and are due to breakdown of RBC within the capillaries of the skin and escape of haemoglobin. They disappear in 1-2 days if person survives.

The surface burns in case of lightning are true burns and occur beneath the metallic objects worn or carried by the person that are fused by the flash. Internal findings are not very characteristic and the cause of death is due to paralysis of heart and respiratory center.

Medicolegal Aspects

(i) Death is accidental. (ii) Appearance left on the body by lightning stroke sometimes closely resembles those produced by criminal violence. (iii) When the body is found in an open field, history is characteristic and there is fusion or magnetization of the metallic substance.

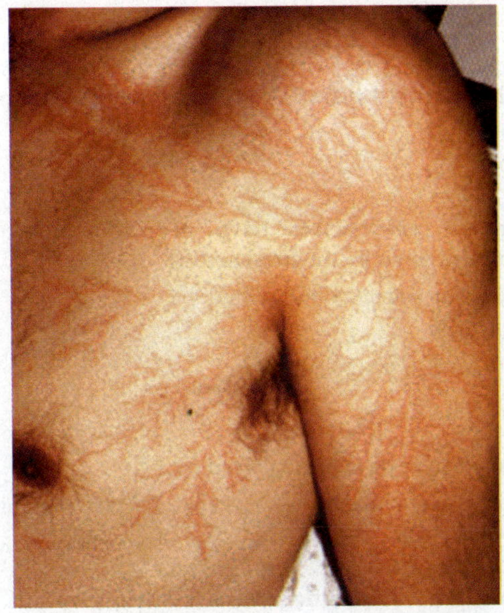

Figure 19.17: Filigree burns in lightning

Burns Due to Radiation

The radiation can be categorized as (i) Nonionizing radiation, e.g., radiowave, microwave, infrared light, ultraviolet light (ii) Ionizing radiation, e.g., X-rays, gamma rays. The incidence of fatal burns due to radiation is rare. A sunburn is the most common type of radiation burn caused by the sun's ultraviolet (UV) rays or by exposure to artificial sources of UV rays such as tanning beds. Many times, burns due to radiation occurred during radiation therapy or medical imaging. The severity of burns depends upon the dose, frequency, total surface area, and location of the radiation. The clinical features include redness of skin, itching and or burning sensation, blister formation, ulcerated lesions, skin pigmentation, degenerative changes in fingernails etc.

LONG QUESTIONS

1. Discuss injuries caused by electric current. Enumerate the differences between the burn injuries caused by flames, hot liquids and chemicals.
2. Define and classify burns. Discuss the various medicolegal issues in deaths due to burns.

SHORT QUESTIONS

1. Hypothermia.
2. Hyperthermia.
3. Filigree burns.
4. Joule burns.
5. Rule of nine.
6. Pugilistic attitude.
7. Heat fractures.
8. Arborescent markings.
9. Differences between antemortem and postmortem burns.
10. Differences between burns and scalds.

MULTIPLE CHOICE QUESTIONS

1. Frost bite occurs when the body is exposed to a temperature of:
(a) -10°C (b) -5°C
(c) -2.5°C (d) +4°C

2. Vesicles in antemortem burn are differentiated from a postmortem burn by the presence of:
(a) Chloride and albuminous fluid
(b) Chloride
(c) Plasma and WBC in fluid
(d) Air

3. Heat hyperpyrexia is precipitated by:
(a) Increased humidity (b) Decreased humidity
(c) Hypotension (d) Hypercalcaemia

4. Which of the following degree burn is very painful?
(a) 1st degree (b) 2nd degree
(c) 3rd degree (d) 4th degree

5. Rule of Nine is applied for calculation of:
(a) Degree of shock (b) Surface area affected
(c) Fluid required (d) All of the above

6. Heat rupture shows:
(a) Irregular margins
(b) Ruptured vessels in the floor
(c) Clotted blood in the wound
(d) Smooth and even margins

7. Pugilistic attitude is seen in cases of:
(a) Hanging (b) Lightning stroke
(c) Heat stroke (d) Burns

8. Arborescent marks are seen in:
(a) Firearm wounds (b) Burns
(c) Lightning

9. Heat haematoma is:
(a) Extradural (b) Subdural
(c) Subarachnoid (d) None of the above

10. Filigree burns are seen in:
(a) Electrocution (b) Lightning
(c) Bomb blast (d) Chemical burns

11. Following are the methods used to classify burns *except:*
(a) Hebra (b) Wilson
(c) Rokitansky (d) Dupuytren

12. Hypothermia is diagnosed when core body temperature falls below:
(a) 37°C (b) 35°C
(c) 32°C (d) 30°C

13. Lund and Browder chart are useful to calculate the body surface area of the children, in which additional factor incorporated is:
(a) Age of the victim
(b) Stature of the victim
(c) Body weight of the victim
(d) Body water content of the victim

14. A 2 years child presents with burns over head and neck and upper limbs. Total body surface area involved in burn is:
(a) 38% (b) 27%
(c) 32% (d) 34%

15. A 25-year-old male child sustained burn injury due to fire. Body parts involved in burns include both upper limb, head and neck and perineum. What is the percentage of the body surface area involved?
(a) 18% (b) 27%
(c) 28% (d) 25%

16. Gastric ulcers occurring due to systemic burns have been named as:
(a) Curling's ulcer (b) Cushing's ulcers
(c) Karolin's ulcer (d) Marjolin's ulcer

17. "Bone pearls or wax drippings" are seen in X-rays of bones in cases of:
(a) Electrocution (b) Hypothermia
(c) Exhumed dead bodies (d) Intrauterine fetal death

18. 'Joule burn' is produced by:
(a) Electrocution (b) Gas stove
(c) Lightning (d) Burning matches

19. A burnt body of a driver is found near a burnt car. Which of the following suggests that the person was alive at the time of burning?
(a) Black soot in the upper airway
(b) Paltauf's haemorrhage
(c) Blisters on the skin are present
(d) Dermis contains abundant fat globules

20. All are true about pugilistic attitude *except:*
(a) Occurs due to coagulation of protein
(b) Seen only in antemortem burns
(c) Seen both in antemortem and postmortem burns
(d) Also known as Boxer's attitude

ANSWER KEY

1. (c)	2. (a)	3. (a)	4. (a)	5. (d)	6. (a)	7. (d)	8. (c)	9. (a)	10. (b)
11. (c)	12. (b)	13. (a)	14. (a)	15. (c)	16. (a)	17. (a)	18. (a)	19. (a)	20. (b)

20 CHAPTER

Mass Disaster

Mass disaster is commonly defined as the death of more than 12 victims in a single event. It is the number of deaths that exceeds the capacity of the local death investigation system to handle it. In certain parts of the world, nature is frequently responsible for mass disaster with flood, hurricanes, avalanches or earthquakes killing hundred to thousand to more of the people. In these nearly enormous disasters, when whole communities are wiped out, there can be very little detailed investigations. The task would be far too great and the most that could be attempted would be identification of some of the dead bodies. Examination of the bodies of the victims by pathologists is necessary for two main reasons: (i) To identify each dead body and to establish the cause of death for legal purposes so that a death certificate can be issued. (ii) To discover evidence relating to the investigations of the disaster itself like obtaining sample for toxicological analysis where appropriate. (iii) To find out the cause of the disaster itself, e.g., bomb or detonator fragments that may be embedded in the bodies of the victims.

In many disasters, the extent of damage to bodies and their clothing by traumatic forces or by fire is such that specialized examination of the bodily remains is necessary to establish the identity. It is therefore considered highly desirable that from the outset very close liaison could be established between the police and the pathologist, to carry out postmortem examination.

Scandinavian practice provides for the appointment by a Prefect of Police of an identification commission including a policeman, a doctor usually a pathologist) and a dentist, whenever the need arises by reason of mass disaster or crime. This commission collects evidence of identity of the bodies recovered, each member working in his own field of competence and jointly it reviews all the evidence and determines whether or not in each the evidence warrants a particular identity being assigned to a particular body. In India, no such practice is followed and collection of evidence at the site as well as shifting the bodies to the morgue is the role of the police officials. The cooperation of pathologist and the police can be conveniently considered in three phases.

First Phase (At the Accident Site)

Priorities in the initial stages of the post-disaster situation will generally be self-evident. There may be survivors to be rescued. All possible means should be used to save life without unduly endangering rescuers from the various continuing dangers that may exist, e.g., fire. When no further lives can be saved, situation should be taken stock of.

Evidence should be preserved that may contribute both to their identification and to the investigation of the accident itself in the widest sense. The first task should be to: (i) Locate bodies (ii) Label them with a number (iii) Photographing them *in situ* (iv) Preparing a plan of the disaster site showing the main pieces of wreckage and position of the bodies is clearly more appropriate in the context of an aircraft accident than, say a hotel fire, for in the latter a written record of which numbered bodies were found in which rooms might be considered sufficient (v) Exact location of a body at a disaster site may prove to be very important, whatever the disaster (vi) Work of identification of the bodies should be undertaken (vii) For accident reconstruction from medical evidence, bodies are labeled, photographed and a record made of their precise position (viii) Record each body and place it in a suitable container for transfer to the mortuary. Make sure that things belonging to one body are not assigned to another. Polythene sheeting can be used for covering it. It should be semitransparent to see the numbered label attached to a body without need for further labeling to facilitate carrying. (ix) *Media room:* A temporary room may be constructed and news regarding the victims may be provided to the press as well as relatives periodically. (x) *Counselling room:* The counsellers to be there for counselling of relatives of the victims and if not possible at the site then near the mortuary counselling should be carried out.

Second Phase (In the Mortuary)

In the mortuary accommodation and in particular refrigeration are likely to be problems following any major disaster. Bodies should be dispersed to numerous small mortuaries but preferably a building of suitable size to be designated a temporary mortuary, for a coordinated investigation, where there is sufficient space and light can be used. In certain types of mass disaster, where identification is not difficult and evidence in the bodies cannot contribute in anyway to a reconstruction or explanation of the accident, only external examination may be required.

When as is the rule in aircraft accidents, a full autopsy is required from the point of view of accident investigation itself, then better facilities such as a properly equipped autopsy room becomes essential.

It is ideal to have in close proximity an autopsy room, refrigerated mortuary accommodation, an area for embalming and casketing room for interviewing relatives and viewing bodies, if necessary and a suitable room for use as a communication headquarters. The ideal is likely to be most closely approached when there has been pre-planning by the appropriate local authorities (in particular the police) before a disaster situation of medium to considerable magnitude occurs, with decisions having been taken in advance about what accommodation could be brought into use in the event of a disaster of particular size.

The procedures in the mortuary should be a matter for team work involving at least a pathologist and a police officer, usually a forensic odontologist and occasionally other specialists such as a radiologist, when appropriate to the particular circumstances and conditions of the bodies.

It is always important to count the number of bodies recovered. This is easy enough when there has been little or no mutilation and fragmentation, but when the traumatic forces of the accident have been severe, the total number of items of human remains recovered may far exceed the number of persons killed: (i) ***Primary identification*:** A term that could apply either to the first clue to identity discovered in a given instance, whether it be strong or insubstantial evidence, or to the most valuable clue, judged in retrospect, when all evidence has been adduced. The categorization of pieces of evidence as primary or secondary is probably of little practical consequence that is to seek routinely from the outset to establish identity by all or several of the different means and not to rest content unless identity has been established and confirmed by at least two different means if at all possible. (a) *Visual identification* is the standard method used by police to establish the identity of a dead body. Visual identification of facial features can be reliable when a body is intact or little damaged externally; the effect of burns in a disaster reduces its value considerably (b) *Photographs* of distinctive clothing, personal possessions or physical characteristics may be recognized if facial features are damaged. Initial and subsequent photography is essential to make a photographic record to relate, body, site and cadaver numbers. After initial photography clothing and jewellery must be removed from the body, examined and catalogued. This is primary for identification purposes. (ii) ***Examination of clothing:*** Evidence of vomit, blood or stains upon clothing may prove useful. Any marks on clothing like manufacturer's label or laundry marks also prove valuable. Examination of clothing is necessary to find out any damage to clothing due to the accident sequence or bomb explosion. (iii) ***External examination:*** To determine: (a) Sex (b) Height (c) Weight (d) Hair colour (e) Location and abundance of hair (f) Colour of eyes and skin (g) Any anatomical, surgical and traumatic scars (h) Tattoos or birth marks (i) Abnormalities such as congenital or acquired. (iv) ***Injury sustained*** during the accident related to cause of death. (v) In case of blast injuries, trace evidences may be preserved. (vi) ***Radiographic examination:*** (a) Ideally, complete set of skeletal X-rays should be taken for each victim (b) In case of suspicion of sabotage, full skeletal radiography is required (c) Radiographs are helpful in identification in case of extremely burnt body and they are also helpful in revealing the presence of articles embedded deeply in charred muscle that may be overlooked otherwise (e) A permanent record of bone injuries are obtained that reduces the time spent in assessing and recording these during autopsy. (vii) ***Full internal autopsy:*** Evidence relevant to identification will be collected such as: (a) Surgical absence of internal organs (b) Presence of postsurgical states like gastroenterostomy (c) Evidence of preexisting disease (d) Any internal injury (e) Precise cause of death. (viii) ***Histological examination:*** During autopsy, specimens of certain organs and tissue will be collected for routine histological examination in 10% formal saline and 1% sodium fluoride for fluids like blood or urine. Tissue specimens containing metal fragments for chemical analysis should be deep-frozen and for histological examination preserved in 10% formalin. Histological examination may reveal a disease relevant to consideration of impaired function if the body is that of operating crew or expectation of life, should medicolegal problems for compensation arise. (ix) ***Fingerprints:*** They should be taken after the autopsy when all possible evidence has been collected from examination of the body. Fingerprints are of limited value in identification of victims of aircraft accidents due to nationality of most of passengers being in question. (x) ***Dental examination:*** At the end of the autopsy, dentist should make an examination of the jaws and teeth; value of dental evidence in identification has become widely recognized after the work of Scandinavian forensic odontologist such as Strom, Keiser Nielson and Gustafson (a) A positive identification can be made when there are a number of points of similarity as between teeth missing and points of matching in restorations by a particular tooth and surface and when there are no incompatible inconsistencies

(b) Minimum number of points of similarity (7 or 8) are required for a confident identification, but each case must be judged on its merits by forensic odontologist (c) A tooth present in a cadaver recorded as extracted in a known person, or an intact tooth in the body recorded as having been filled in the known person's chart, is an incompatible inconsistency; it can only be disregarded in the face of overwhelming forceful evidence that the inconsistency is due to miscasting of some other artefact perhaps in the telegraphed transmission of the dental notes or chart (d) In the context of mass disaster in which traumatic forces are severe the value of the dental charts is reduced and the value of radiographs is enhanced (e) It is quite common for a body to have retained one or two fragments of jaw, perhaps with one or two teeth. These teeth may have a restoration or two, but they may be commonly filled teeth and a chart may be quite inadequate in its detail of the size of the restorations for the evidence to be strong enough to form the basis of identification. If an antemortem radiograph of the relevant part of the dentition is available, it may prove to be of greatest possible value for comparison with the postmortem radiograph of the fragments recovered (f) Above references to dental evidence as a means of identification have been primarily in connection with the comparative approach of this work, this is most appropriate in the field of aircraft accidents when the names of all the persons involved in the accident are nearly always known with a considerable degree of certainty (g) When a completely unknown body is found, or when mass disaster involves quite unknown persons, is usually the case in a department store fire or railway disaster, the reconstructive value of dental evidence is more often utilized. The teeth may reveal much about its owner, his/her country of origin, perhaps from a characteristic restorative work, his/her occupation such as notching of upper incisors may occur in hair dressers, for example and the teeth may be a good guide to age. One of the main problems in the field of international forensic odontology has been the lack of a common dental nomenclature. **Freehold and Lysol** reviewed the various systems used by dentists in various countries in 1962. These authors emphasized the possibilities of combustion after a mass disaster involving people of many nationalities, when dental information is received in telegraphed form. At the International Dental Federation meeting at Bucharest in 1970, new **two-digit system** was proposed and adopted for recommendation for international use. (xi) **Other means of identification** such as: (a) Multivariate analysis of race in cranium (Stewart 1970) and cephalic index (b) Identification of scars of parturition and other pubic symphyseal changes in skeletal remains of female (c) Neutron activation analysis of hair are also used.

Last task to be performed in the mortuary is the examination of any fragments of bodies, with, so far as possible, matching of those fragments with the bodies from which they originated.

Not only many clues to identity be found in separated fragmented remains, but occasionally important evidence about the cause of the accident can be ascertained.

Third Phase (Comparison of Records and Identification)

Identification of bodies depends upon accurate information about those who are believed to have been involved. When the persons killed are of the country in which the disaster occurs, it is probable that normal police communication system is the best for collection of required information. During recent years, the need for practical record forms in the context of a mass disaster has come to be appreciated, Australian Police, Interpol has produced a disaster victim identification form.

The forms, which have evolved from 15 years of practical experience by those pathologists who have worked in the Royal Air Force Aviation Pathology, Department of Haltom consists of four different coloured forms and a white one. Two of the coloured forms are for the males, other two for the females; white form is for missing persons. One of the coloured forms is for external feature of the body and the other is for autopsy findings. These are kept in transparent envelop upon completion and since they are coloured, on single sheets of paper, the subsequent exercise of matching records and 'proving', the identification of bodies is much more simplified. In India no such forms are available and all the information related to identification should be recorded in a postmortem report.

Review of Evidence and Accident Reconstruction

In some disaster the pathological examination of bodies of victims, can achieve beyond proving evidence leading to identification and confirmation of an obvious cause of death. Comprehensive pathological investigation can help a great deal to reconstruct the accident, sometimes to the extent of revealing the cause, though more often helping to encode possible causes. Sometimes a serious disease is revealed as a likely cause of an accident.

Routine toxicological tests on the tissues of human bodies also reveal a cause of death (like CO poisoning in disaster due to navigational error). Injuries in passengers and their correlation with damage to seat structures and other solid structures is also helpful in knowing the relative safety of different parts of aircrafts/other vehicles and how to improve them to prevent such disasters.

LONG QUESTION

1. How will you investigate a case of mass disaster? What measures will you undertake for proper identification of persons involved?

SHORT QUESTIONS

1. Preservation of trace evidences in mass disaster.
2. Methods of identification in burnt bodies.
3. Autopsy procedures in mass disaster.

21 CHAPTER

Trauma and Disease

The relationship between trauma, work stress and disease assumes importance mainly for two reasons: (i) ***Compensation:*** Under the Workman's Compensation Act, provision is made for disabilities suffered as a result of occupationally acquired diseases or industrial accidents while at work, provided the worker himself was not negligent or responsible for the injury. In cases of death without any medical attention and when the possibility of disease seems remote, a question arises whether the ill effects of work conditions or previous injury suffered while at work could be responsible for death. (ii) ***Insurance:*** A person who has insured himself for accident only. Some life insurance policies include a double indemnity policy; the sum payable is doubled if death is due to accident.

When these matters become subject of investigation, a medical officer is called upon to examine the person: (i) To assess disability or degree of physical damage: A very thorough examination is essential; if necessary the worker may be kept under observation to assess degree of disablement either temporary or permanent. Most important aspect is evaluation of whether the disabilities claimed and observed are consistent with the injury received. **Malingering** means a deliberate attempt on the part of the patient to deceive the doctor. The person may malinger and make false claims or he may have developed neurosis after the accident. (ii) To perform an autopsy to interpret the relationship of disease or trauma to death. The medical officer should analyze the data carefully and opine on the relative role of trauma and disease to death. Just because a given episode of stress, exertion or trauma was antecedent, the assumption of cause and effect relationship is not necessarily warranted.

The association of trauma and preexisting disease is most often met in fatal cases, where an injury or alleged injury has been sustained by a person with substantial natural disease. The problem then is to evaluate whether: (i) Death was due entirely to injury and would have occurred whether or not the disease was present. (ii) Whether the death was due entirely to disease and would have occurred at that time irrespective of the injury. (iii) Whether the two processes in combination has caused death.

Trauma and Infection

Bacteria being the normal inhabitants of external environment gain entry to the injured tissue and set up local infection. The bacteria may also be present on the object producing injury.

Wounds associated with extensive crushing of tissue are more likely to be infected. Penetrating wounds involving deeper tissues are more susceptible to contamination than superficial wounds. Pathogenic microorganisms are commonly present in the blood of normal individual **(benign bactericidal)**. Usually these bacteria are quickly disposed off by the host defences and do not elicit any signs or symptoms of disease. Concurrently due to the stress of trauma and lowered resistance, these transient bacteria can easily migrate into the wound, setting up localized infection. Since the time elapsing between the contamination of the wound and the reaction of the host is variable the question may arise: (i) Whether the infection occurred in coincidence with the original trauma **(primary infection).** (ii) Whether the infection occurred subsequently to original trauma as a result of accidental implant of bacteria, e.g., following application of contaminated dressings **(secondary infection)**.

The concept of aggravation applies well to the situation in which trauma in association with accident or assault affects a preexisting infection, disturbing the local defence mechanism and thus transforming a relatively innocuous process into a life threatening situation, e.g., dislocation of an infected teeth resulting from blow to the face or to the abdomen leading to the development of peritonitis from perforation of gastric or duodenal ulcer.

Trauma and Heart Disease

Injury to any part of the body may predispose to myocardial infarction with or without coronary thrombosis, if the injury is sufficiently severe to cause hypovolaemic shock and coronary arteries are previously narrowed by atherosclerosis. In such a case, the injury causes circulatory failure and myocardial infarction occurs during the period of shock. Diagnosis is to be confirmed by clinical and laboratory tests in the living and appropriate findings at autopsy in the dead.

If the disease is present months before trauma, only a direct blow to the chest will damage heart and dislodge an atheromatous plaque leading to subluminal haemorrhage proving that the trauma has caused death from myocardial dysfunction. Actual death may not occur soon after trauma because period of hypertension will precipitate MI and death. Even threatening the person can cause cardiovascular changes and sudden rise in blood pressure that can rupture the atheromatous plaque.

Two basic situations are most likely to find access to the Courts of Law: (i) ***Direct injury to heart:*** When the heart has been perforated or lacerated by a penetrating object (flying missile or sharp object) or has been bruised or crushed by a violent impact against the chest, the ensuing death or disability can reasonably be attributed to injury. Contusion of heart is a common complication of steering wheel injuries in car collisions. As a general rule, the cause and effect relationship is substantiated by the absence of a symptom free period, and if the victim dies, unmistakable evidence of cardiac damage is found at autopsy. Blunt trauma to chest can cause a broken rib to bruise the myocardium or one of the coronary arteries, causing a blood clot (thrombus) to form in the lumen of the damaged blood vessel. In this situation, the casual relationship between the injury and the ensuing heart failure may remain a matter of speculation unless the sequence of events can be proved at postmortem examination. (ii) ***Indirect heart injury:*** It is more difficult to prove as after injury to heart, ECG changes occur due to arrhythmias, overactivity, increased sympathetic tone or excessive release of catecholamine.

A severe injury to any part of the body is usually associated with loss of blood and destruction of the tissue with resulting low blood pressure, decreased blood volume and slowing of blood flow that results in shock leading to clotting of blood (thrombus formation) that may result in thrombosis of coronary artery and myocardial ischaemia and death.

Mechanical injury causes increased coagulability of circulatory blood that results in coronary artery thrombosis, cardiac instability and death. A casual relationship between the trauma and post traumatic increase in blood coagulability and resulting coronary thrombosis can be accepted if laboratory evidence can be presented that following trauma, blood coagulability was greater than normal and that the manifestations of coronary thrombosis developed a few hours or at the most a day or two after the injury.

More difficult to assess is heart failure or any other cardiac disorder occurring in an individual with antecedent history of heart disease as an indirect effect of trauma. Anxiety, pain, anger or fear associated with severe injury impose an extra load on heart leading to heart failure.

Whenever the coronary circulation is impaired the extra work imposed on the heart by conditions of anxiety may contribute to an angina attack as well to a host of acute changes in heart rhythm such as paroxysmal tachycardia, arrhythmias, flutter and fibrillation. These are regarded as evidence of vasomotor instability or autonomic imbalance.

Any attempt to recognize a casual relationship between the aggravation of the cardiac disorder and the trauma includes the following criteria: (i) Trauma must be of some significance. This is indicated by the disappointing but realistic observation that death does not always find a suitable explanation in detectable lesions at autopsy. This occurrence is particularly well documented in the case of blunt head trauma. (ii) Symptoms must develop shortly after the event that precipitated the episode of cardiac distress.

The weakness of the concept in this case rests in the fact that sometime may elapse between the establishment of the disorder and the ability of the physician to demonstrate the existence by clinical and laboratory methods.

Since heart failure occurs in the natural course of events of any cardiac condition and this may be sudden and unexpected, not infrequently the situation arises that the critical event occurs while the patient is walking or driving a vehicle.

Injury concurrent to heart failure raises the question whether the fall and the ensuing injury precipitated the cardiac condition or whether the sudden failing of the heart was responsible for the loss of consciousness, the fall and the injury. As a general rule, if the injury was sufficiently severe to be considered incompatible with life and it can be shown to occur before death, the death can be attributed to the injury. Conversely, if the injury was of minor nature, and the heart condition at autopsy provides an adequate explanation at death, the death can be attributed to the cardiac condition. Following injury bacteria may gain entry to blood stream, lodge and grow in heart valves and give rise to acute bacterial endocarditis.

Occupational Trauma

As defined by effort at work, occupational trauma can precipitate death by giving rise to circulatory overloading or by aggravating previously existing disease such as coronary atherosclerosis, or aortic aneurysm. Narrowing is sufficient to explain death and a clot or acute obstruction is not necessary. Death from partial coronary stenosis is commonly precipitated by some exertion resulting in a greater demand of blood, the pumping action of the heart and oxygen demand of the muscle of the left ventricle. Climbing stairs, working a hand pump, and lifting a weight may precipitate such deaths.

If the deceased at the time of such deaths was engaged in some such work as a part of his employment, then a claim of compensation may succeed. Cardiac conditions which predispose to acute heart failure following physical exertion or excitement and which frequently result in sudden death include syphilitic arteritis with or without aortic valvular insufficiency and hypertensive heart disease usually with coronary atherosclerosis.

Trauma and Post Traumatic Psychosis

In the absence of acute brain damage, nearly all post traumatic mental disturbances represent both an aggravation of preexisting latent psychosis, primarily dementia praecox (schizophrenia) and Mania Depressive Psychosis (MDP). In a general sense, injury comes to play the role of a precipitating factor.

It is generally accepted that the relation between injury and true post traumatic psychosis rests on the demonstration that: (i) Patient had been a mentally well adjusted person prior to injury. (ii) Injury has produced organic damage to CNS. (iii) Injury regardless of the location was of such magnitude as to reasonably threaten the very existence of the victim of the injury. (iv) Injury was of a nature to affect the structure or function of certain parts of the body to which emotional importance is attached such as genital organs, breasts, eyes, face and hands etc. (v) Victim was obsessed about the outcome from the time the injury was sustained. (vi) Psychosis developed within a reasonable time after the occurrence of the injury. (vii) Psychotic thoughts had a positive relationship to the assault or accident that was responsible for the injury.

Trauma and Nervous System

It is difficult to refute completely the direct cause and effect relationship between: (i) Head injury and meningitis (ii) Head injury and epilepsy (iii) Head injury and psychosis (iv) Head injury including occupational stress and rupture of a congenital cerebral aneurysm.

Intracerebral haemorrhage can occur due to violence alone without any evidence of disease or blood vessels. Head injury can cause death due to subarachnoid haemorrhage due to rupture of Berry aneurysm in the Circle of Willis that can rupture spontaneously also. A ruptured aneurysm can occur after a fight or assault also. Very small aneurysm may be destroyed by bleeding, which may not be recognized at autopsy. Following trauma, there may be absence of rupture of Berry aneurysm due to rupture of vertebral arteries in the transverse process of atlas vertebra by the kick or blow over the side of the neck.

To attribute trauma as a cause of death for disease or disability, following criteria should be satisfied: (i) Disease must not have been present before the injury but developed after injury was sustained, e.g., meningitis following violence to the head with or without physical damage. (ii) Disease is such as to be compatible with the nature of trauma ascribed to it, e.g., meningitis following violence to the head with or without physical damage. (iii) Length of interval (latent period) that elapsed between injury and development of disease is compatible, e.g., tetanus developing 3-10 days after injury sometimes 2-3 weeks after the injury. (iv) Disease does not develop spontaneously, e.g., tetanus.

Trauma and Pulmonary Embolism

It is almost always due to impaction of thrombus, which has been shifted from thrombosis of leg veins, pelvic thrombosis and post-puerperal embolus. It is a well-known complication of trauma. When leg is the site of injury, it occurs more commonly and takes two weeks after the injury.

Main aim of the doctor is to tell that initiation of leg vein thrombus occurred after the injury. Histological dating to correlate with injury can be done. There can be pulmonary infection leading to death after injury. Pulmonary infection occurs within the first few weeks after injury. During intervening period when the patient is immobilized and respiratory distress occurs, a connection is established.

Trauma and Alimentary System

Whenever a history is obtained of blow to the abdomen, the patient should be kept under observation until all likelihood of a ruptured abdominal viscous can be dismissed. A blow to the epigastric region can cause death by inhibition of heart through reflex action on the celiac plexus without leaving a mark externally or to the viscera. The result of the trauma to bowel may be very serious. Perforation of peptic ulcer leads to rapid death; this gives rise to compensation claims when death occurs due to some abdominal injury at work. Perforation of lower small intestine and large intestine are usually not followed by intense shock similar to the shock of peptic ulcer perforation and may not cause death if timely surgical aid is available.

The liver is easily lacerated and ruptured especially if it is fatty, congested, enlarged or diseased. However, death may not occur immediately. Sometimes bleeding occurs between the liver and its capsule that is the subcapsular hematoma. Serious symptoms become apparent only when the capsule ruptures. The damage is often fatal due to bleeding from the organ into peritoneal cavity. A kick or punch on the upper abdomen may injure the duodenum and pancreas and cause death within a few days from resultant chemical peritonitis. External injury to the abdominal wall may not always be visible in such cases.

Trauma and Malignancy

Trauma may occasionally cause cancer. The occurrence of estrogenic sarcoma and development malignancy in a scar tissue after injury has been documented. Cancer on rare occasions develop at the site of long standing unhealed wound of the skin or in the scarred skin provided the trauma that was responsible for scar formation was definitely something more than a single mechanical injury, e.g., severe burns, X-rays burns and chemically inflamed lesions like varicose ulcer and chronic sinus tracts e.g. draining of a chronic osteomyelitis sinus, which may cause skin cancer adjacent to the site of continued irritation. In accepting trauma as a cause of cancer, the following criteria based on **Ewing's postulates** must be satisfied: (i) Tumor site prior to injury was normal. (ii) Injury was sufficiently severe to disrupt continuity of tissues at the site of injury and so initiate a reparative proliferation of cells. (iii) Tumor followed injury within a reasonable length of time. (iv) Tumor is of same histological type that might reasonably develop as a result of regeneration and repair of specific tissues that received the injury. (v) Exact nature of the tumor can be established by clinical, X-ray and microscopic examination. (vi) Tumor must have originated in the part of the body that has sustained the injury. (vii) It must develop within a certain period of time between a minimum of 3-4 weeks and maximum of 3 years after receipt of injury. Some investigators have increased upper limit to 10-20 years.

No organ in the human body is there in which the development of a cancer has not been attributed to trauma. Most frequently implicated are breasts, testes and bones.

Occupational Cancer

Exposure to arsenic, asbestos, chrome, nickel and other metals, aromatic amines, azo-compounds and an endless list of other organic substances for which the ability to produce cancer is substantiated by controlled experiments. Industrial or occupational cancer rests on the concept that exposure to chronic irritants may provide in the targeted tissues a background that is favorable to the development of a tumor. Mechanical trauma can provoke such a situation but among the irritants, it represents a statistically minor factor far surpassed by the chemical, physical and biologic agents that crowd the environment.

SHORT QUESTIONS

1. Ewing's postulates.
2. Trauma and heart disease.
3. Trauma and infection.

MULTIPLE CHOICE QUESTIONS

1. Ewing's postulate is to establish relation between:

(a) Magnitude of force with fracture of bone.
(b) Site of trauma with new cancerous growth at that site
(c) Level of blood alcohol with sudden death
(d) Nature of crime with degree of punishment

2. To find out a relationship between trauma and malignancy, the postulates should be satisfied:

(a) Ewing's postulates (b) Wallace's postulates
(c) Widmark's postulates (d) Ema's postulates

3. A 20-year-male fell from stairs and sustained fracture of femur of one side. After two days, he suddenly develops breathlessness. It is suggestive of

(a) Asthmatic attack (b) Pneumonitis
(c) Pulmonary embolism (d) Congestive cardiac failure

ANSWER KEY ☞

1. (b)	2. (a)	3. (c)

22 CHAPTER

Medicolegal Aspects of Injuries

Injury (S. 44 I.P.C.): Any harm whatever illegally caused to a person in body, mind, reputation or property.

Hurt (S. 319 I.P.C.): Bodily pain, disease or infirmity caused to any person. In English Law, hurt is defined same as battery infirmity is the disease or weakness due to administration of any poison or even alcohol.

Assault (S. 351 I.P.C.): An attempt, offer or threat to apply force to the body of another in a hostile manner. It is basically an attempt to offer with force and violence, a corporal hurt to another.

Battery: Battery is an assault brought to execution. It is more than an attempt to do a corporal hurt to another. It is an actual injury to a person. Every battery includes the assault, the distinction is only of the degree.

Simple Injury

Simple injury is defined as which is neither extensive nor serious and heals without leaving a permanent scar.

Grievous Hurt (S. 320 I.P.C.)

The following eight clauses are included:

1. **Emasculation:** It means loss of masculine power and the term is only applicable to males. The loss of power can be due to direct trauma to genitalia leading to amputation of the organ. However, even if one testis with intact male organ is present, it cannot be called emasculation. If both testes are removed before puberty, impotency is the rule, but if they are removed after puberty, potency is retained. Trauma to lumbosacral region leads to loss of masculine power indirectly.
2. **Permanent privation of sight of either eye:** The gravity of such injury lies in its permanency because it deprives a person to use its organ of sight and also disfigures him. Causing the permanent loss or impairment of vision in either eye is considered as grievous hurt. Examples include corneal scarring, retinal detachment etc. Permanent loss doesn't mean that it should be incurable.
3. **Permanent privation of hearing of either ear:** Causing permanent loss or impairment of hearing of either ear is considered as grievous hurt. Rupture of the tympanic membrane or injury to auditory nerve due to a blow to the head or pouring hot liquid into the ear or due to a blast effect will be considered as grievous heart even if there is partial hearing loss.
4. **Privation of any member or any joint:** Causing loss of function or anatomical separation of any body part is considered grievous hurt. A **member** means any organ or tissue capable of performing a distinct function in the body. It includes eyes, ear, nose, hands, legs, etc. If the joint becomes permanently stiff and normal function is not possible, then it can be called grievous hurt.
5. **Destruction or permanent impairing of power of any member or joint:** During life, the use of limbs and joints are very essential to discharge normal functions. Their deprivation causes lifelong crippling and makes the person defenceless and his life becomes miserable. If any joint is destroyed so as to cause loss of its function or there is damage to any other organ or part of the organ, causing loss of its function is grievous hurt. The damage should be permanent. It causes great hardship to the person in maintaining normal life.

6. **Permanent disfiguration of head or face:** Permanent disfiguration of face or head region is considered as grievous hurt. This depends on the nature of impact of the injury on the person involved. Even a small scar on a young girl may be considered as grievous while a large scar on an old aged man may not be considered as grievous hurt. Other examples include cutting of nose, ear etc.
7. **Fracture dislocation of a bone or tooth:** Fracture of either outer or inner table of the skull is taken as a fracture. If a wound of any depth didn't cut the bone or fracture it, it is not considered as a fracture. It is not necessary, that the bone should be completely fractured through and through. Even all fractures including the hairline fractures are considered as fracture for this particular section. It is not necessary that there should be displacement. Dislocation means displacement. Mere looseness of the tooth doesn't amount to dislocation. It has to be proved that originally the tooth was not loose and there is a fracture or dislocation as a result of injury.
8. **Any hurt which endangers life, which causes its sufferer severe bodily pain or makes him unable to follow his ordinary pursuits for a period of 20 days:** Under this clause any injury which is endangering life or causing severely body pain to the person or the person is not able to carry on with his ordinary pursuits for a minimum period of 20 days, it is considered as grievous. Whether an injury is dangerous or not, it is to be assessed from the clinical condition at that moment. It is the prerogative of the examining doctor to label an injury as 'dangerous to life' depending on the condition and vitals of the patient. Thus it can be said that all dangerous injuries are grievous but not vice versa. It is very difficult to ascertain that the patient is suffering from severe bodily pain for a period of 20 days. For this, the attending physician has to evaluate the nature and site of injuries, method of treatment and presence of infection. The treating physician must try to elicit the pain rather than to ask the patient whether he/she is having pain. For this clause '**ordinary/daily pursuits**' means acts which are a daily routine in every human being's day-to-day life like eating food, taking bath, going to the toilet etc. A simple inability to attend the office or work even for period longer than 20 days is not considered enough for this clause to categorize the injury as grievous.

HOMICIDE

The word "homicide" is derived from the Latin word *homo* and *cide. Homo* means "man" and *cide* means "I cut". Thus homicide is the causing of death of a human being by a human being, i.e., death through human agency. Death from an accident such as falling or slipping is not homicide but if such fall or slip is caused by human agency it will amount to homicide. Homicide may be lawful or unlawful. **Lawful homicide** may again be classified as (1) Excusable homicide and (2) Justifiable homicide.

Unlawful homicide: It may be classified as: (i) Culpable homicide not amounting to murder (ii) Murder (iii) Homicide by a rash and negligent act that is not culpable.

Culpable Homicide (S. 299 I.P.C.)

Whoever causes death by doing an act (i) With the intention of causing death, or (ii) With the intention of causing such bodily injury that is likely to cause death, or (iii) With knowledge that he is likely by such act to cause death, conducts the act of culpable homicide. This section defines culpable homicide which is a wider offence than that of murder. The offence of culpable homicide as defined in this section involves the doing of an act (including illegal omission) (A) With the intention of causing death; or (B) With the intention of causing such bodily injury as is likely to cause death; or (C) With the knowledge that it is likely to cause death and if death results from any of them the offence of culpable homicide is committed. Thus, the guilty intention in (A) and (B) above and the knowledge that the act is likely to cause death as in (C) are the main ingredients of the offence. Further this section enacts that the doing of an act which causes death is culpable homicide if it is (A) With the intention of causing either: (i) Death or (ii) Such bodily injury as is likely to cause death, or (B) With the knowledge that death is likely to be caused by such act. Thus (A) and (B) being alternative it is seen that culpable homicide may be committed without any intentions on part of the accused if he has knowledge that death is likely to result from the act. **'Knowledge'** implies consciousness a mental act, a condition of the mind which is incapable of direct proof. The word **'likely'** means probably. The knowledge required by this clause is the knowledge that the act is likely to cause death. The word likely implies higher and lower degrees of probabilities of risk. On the question of knowledge much depends on the intellectual capacity of the individual. Even an illiterate person will realise that a blow with an axe in the region of abdomen can cause death or injury resulting in death. On the question of intention, it is stated that the man in law must be held to intend the natural and ordinary consequences of his acts irrespective of object at the time of doing such act.

Explanation 1: The first explanation reproduces the English rule that an injury which accelerates the death of a dying man is deemed to be the cause of death, if he knows that the condition of the deceased was such that his act was likely to cause death. When the injury inflicted is such as to cause death but that results from rupture of organs such as spleen or liver and the accused had no knowledge of his ailment, the offence is not culpable homicide.

Explanation 2: It deals with refusal of medical treatment for injury inflicted which could have averted death as being a defence to the charge cannot be sustained. That is because the accused is responsible for the natural consequences of his conduct and the fact that the natural consequences could have been averted by artificial means is no answer. The fact that if an operation had been conducted within half an hour after the infliction of the injury and that consequently his life could have been saved could not be valid defence to the charge of culpable homicide.

The *mensrea* or mental element in culpable homicide is intention or knowledge towards the consequences of his conduct. There are three kinds of *mensrea*: (i) An intention to cause death (ii) An intention to cause dangerous injury (iii) The knowledge that death is likely to result.

The prosecution is not bound to establish motive for a crime, but evidence of motive may be adduced and considered. The mere absence of motive can be of no assistance to the accused when the offence could be proved by the prosecution. Otherwise in the absence of intention or knowledge as envisaged by section 299 I.P.C. the offence committed may be one of grievous or simple hurt.

MURDER (S. 300 I.P.C.)

Whoever causes death by doing an act (i) With the intention of causing death or (ii) With the intention of causing such bodily injury as the offender knows to be likely to cause the death of the person to whom the harm is caused or (iii) With the intention of causing the bodily injury and such bodily injury intended to be inflicted is sufficient to cause death in ordinary course of nature or (iv) With the knowledge that the act is imminently dangerous that it must in all probability cause death.

Differences between culpable homicide and murder: There is real distinction between culpable homicide and murder. Broadly speaking, the offence is culpable homicide if the bodily injury intended to be inflicted is likely to cause death. It will be murder if such injury is sufficient in the ordinary course of the nature to cause death. When the question of intention arises, such intention has to be gathered from what he does. Where the injury deliberately inflicted is more than its being merely likely to cause death but sufficient in the ordinary course of nature to cause death, the higher degree of guilt is presumed.

Clause (1): In order to attract the provisions of clause (1) of section 300, the prosecution has to prove that the very act that was done by the accused was done with the intention to cause the death of the victim. The intention also includes the foresight of certainty. A question of intention is always a matter of fact. Once intention of causing death is proved, culpable homicide amounts to murder unless any of the exceptions are applied. Intention can be rarely proved by direct evidence, when facts are so intervened determining whether it is culpable homicide and then finding out separately whether it amounts to murder may not be convenient.

Intention can also be inferred from the acts of the accused, namely nature of the weapon used, the part of the body where injury is inflicted and the force of the blood etc.

Clause (2): This clause deals with cases where the intention is to kill the person even though the injury is not fatal in the ordinary course of nature but is fatal in the case of that particular person, by reason of the knowledge of accused as regards the physical infirmity, disease of the person's subnormal state of health and his special physical condition. It requires not the intention to cause death but only the intention of causing such bodily injury as is likely to cause death of the person to whom the harm is caused. Here both the elements of 'intention' and 'knowledge' are required to be proved that is the intention to injure and the knowledge about the consequences of injury relating to a particular victim. The 'knowledge' imparts a certainty and not merely probability.

Clause (3): The third clause of section 300 speaks of an intention to cause bodily injury which is sufficient in the ordinary course of nature to cause death. Emphasis here is on the sufficiency of injury to cause death. **Sufficiency** is the high probability of death, depending upon the nature of weapon used, or the part of the body where the injury is inflicted or both. If the injury is not such as would be sufficient to cause death, i.e., if the probability is not so high, the offence will not fall under section 300 but will fall under section 299 or even a lesser offence.

Supreme Court in the case of **Virsa Singh vs. State of Punjab**, observed that to bring the case under this part of the section the prosecution must establish objectively: (i) That a bodily injury is present (ii) That the nature of injury must be proved (iii) It must be proved that there was an intention to inflict that particular bodily injury (iv) That the injury inflicted is sufficient to cause death in the ordinary course of the nature (this is purely objective).

Once these four elements are established by the prosecution, then the offence is described under section 300. It does not matter that there was no intention to cause death. It does not even matter that there is no knowledge that an act of that kind is likely to cause death. Once the intention to cause the bodily injury is actually found to be present is proved, the rest of the inquiry is purely objective, and the only question is whether as a matter of purely objective inference, the injury is sufficient in the ordinary course of the nature to cause death. Thus where no evidence or explanation is given about why the accused thrust a spear into the abdomen of the deceased with such force that it penetrated the bowels and the coils of the intestines came out of the wound and that digested food oozed out from cuts in three places, it would be perverse to conclude that he did not intend to inflict injury that he did.

Clause (4): Clause (4) of section 300 is usually applied to cases where the act of the offender is not directed against any particular person. There may even be no intention to cause harm or injury to any particular individual, but it is the result of a general disregard for human life and safety. What this clause contemplates is the imminently dangerous act which must in all probabilities cause death. This clause deals with cases where an act which is dangerous is done, without any intention to kill a particular person but with knowledge that death is very likely and that such act is done without any excuse. Example include: (i) Number of persons set upon one and hit him on his head with *lathi*, it is murder and necessary intention must be presumed. (ii) Several persons took part in assaulting a man who dies from cumulative effect of their assault.

S. 302 I.P.C. Punishment for murder: Whoever commits murder shall be punished with death or imprisonment for life and shall also be liable for fine.

S. 307 I.P.C. Attempt to murder: Whoever does any act with such intention or knowledge and under such circumstances that if he by that act caused death, he would be guilty of murder and shall be punished with imprisonment for a period of 10 years and also fine. If only hurt is caused life imprisonment or like before attempts by life convicts shall be punished with death.

Essentials for the criminal attempt: (i) An existence of an intent on the part of the accused to commit a particular offence (ii) Some steps were taken towards it after completion of preparation (iii) Steps must be apparently though not necessarily adopted to the purpose destined (iv) It must come dangerously near to success (v) It must fall short of completion of ultimate design.

S. 321 I.P.C. Voluntarily causing hurt: Whoever does any act with the intention of thereby causing hurt to any person, or with the knowledge that he is likely thereby to cause hurt to any person and does thereby cause hurt to any person, is said "voluntarily to cause hurt".

S. 322 I.P.C. Voluntarily causing grievous hurt: Whoever voluntarily causes hurt, if the hurt which he intends to cause or knows himself to be likely to cause is grievous hurt, and if the hurt which he causes is grievous hurt, is said, "voluntarily to cause grievous hurt".

Explanation: A person is not said voluntarily to cause grievous hurt except when he both causes grievous hurt and intends or knows himself to be likely to cause grievous hurt. But he is said voluntarily to cause grievous hurt, if intending or knowing himself to be likely to cause grievous hurt of one kind, he actually causes grievous hurt of another kind.

Example: A, intending or knowing himself to be likely, permanently to disfigure Z's face, gives Z a blow which does not permanently disfigure Z's face, but which cause Z to suffer severe bodily pain for the space of twenty days, A has voluntarily caused grievous hurt.

S. 323 I.P.C. Punishment for voluntarily causing hurt: Whoever except in the case provided for by section 334, voluntarily causes hurt, shall be punished with imprisonment of either description for a term which may extend to one year, or with fine which may extend to one thousand rupees, or with both.

S. 324 I.P.C. Voluntarily causing hurt by dangerous weapons or means: Whoever, except in the case provided for by section 334, voluntarily causes hurt by means of any instrument for shooting, stabbing or cutting, or any instrument which, used as weapon of offence, is likely to cause death, or by means of fire or any heated substance, or by means of any poison or any corrosive substance, or by means of any explosive substance or by means of any substance which it is deleterious to the human body to inhale, to swallow, or to receive into the blood, or by means of any animal, shall be punished with imprisonment of either description for a term which may extend to three years, or with fine, or with both.

S. 325 I.P.C. Punishment for voluntarily causing grievous hurt: Whoever, except in the case provided for by section 335, voluntarily causes grievous hurt, shall be punished with imprisonment of either description for a term, which may extend to seven years and shall also be liable to fine.

S. 326 I.P.C. Voluntarily causing grievous hurt by dangerous weapons or means: Whoever, except in the case provided for by section 335, voluntarily causes grievous hurt by means of any instrument for shooting, stabbing or cutting or any instrument which, used as a weapon of offence, is likely to cause death, or by means of fire or any heated substance, or by means of any poison or any corrosive substance, or by means of any explosive substance, or by means of any substance which it is deleterious to the human body to inhale, to swallow, or to receive into the blood, or by means of any animal, shall be punished with, imprisonment for life, or with imprisonment of either description for a term which may extend to ten years, and shall also be liable to fine.

S. 304A I.P.C. Causing death by negligence: Whoever causes death of any person by doing any rash and negligent act not amounting to culpable homicide shall be punished with imprisonment up to 2 years or with fine.

To impose criminal liability under section 304 A I.P.C., it is necessary that the death should have been the direct result of a rash or negligent act of the accused and that the act must be the proximate (not remote) and efficient cause without intervention of another's negligence and with no intention or knowledge.

Distinction Between Rash Act and Negligent Act

Rash act: The criminality lies in running the risk of doing such an act with recklessness or indifference as to the consequence.

Criminal negligence: Criminal negligence is the gross and culpable neglect or failure to exercise the reasonable and proper care and precaution to guard against injury either to the public generally or to an individual.

COMPLICATIONS OF INJURIES

Serious bodily injuries, from whatever cause, may either lead to virtually instantaneous death from destruction of vital organs and structures or may cause delayed death from complications of the original injury. This delay may be short, as in torrential haemorrhage or acute respiratory failure or it may be progressively longer stretching for hours, days, weeks or even years. Some of the most difficult problems in forensic pathology and some of the most arduous testimony and cross examination in the Court of law concerns deaths from which post-traumatic complications are disputed as being causative factors. The various complications of injury resulting in death are discussed in this chapter.

SHOCK

Shock commonly called circulatory collapse may develop following any serious assault on the body's hemostasis such as profuse haemorrhage, severe trauma or burns, extensive myocardial infarction, massive pulmonary embolism, or uncontrolled bacterial sepsis. Shock constitutes widespread hypoperfusion of cells and tissues due to reduction in the blood volume or cardiac output, or redistribution of blood resulting in an inadequate effective circulating volume. Incident to the perfusion deficit, there is insufficient delivery of oxygen and nutrients to the cells and tissues and inadequate clearance of metabolites. The cellular hypoxia induces a shift from aerobic to anaerobic metabolism, resulting in increase in lactate production and sometimes lactic acidosis. While at the outset the hemodynamic and metabolic derangements are correctable and induce reversible injury to cells, persistence of worsening of the shock state leads to irreversible injury and death of the cells. The shock is classified into the following types (Table 22.1):

Primary or Neurogenic Shock

Primary or neurogenic shock is a reflex neurovascular disturbance immediately after an injury. It results from exciting factors such as pain, grief, anxiety, emotions, stress etc. Even a site of blood may cause this type of shock and is common after massive haemorrhages. The reactions are due to symapthetico-adrenal stimulation with its resulting systematic effects. There is sudden reduction of venous return to the heart due to pooling of blood in the splanchnic and peripheral vascular bed from neurogenic vasodilatation. The sudden rise of blood pressure can precipitate complications like intracerebral haemorrhage from rupture of arteriosclerotic cerebral vessels or Berry aneurysm and rupture of dissecting aneurysm of aorta. Minor stimuli or injury over the receptive spots having receptor nerve endings forming the afferent pathway for reflex action by inhibitory vagus nerve causing vagal inhibition result in sudden death from neurogenic shock. Rapid death can occur especially in persons with chronic cardiac lesions.

Clinical Features of Neurogenic Shock

(i) Tremors and anxiety (ii) Pallor (iii) Cold clammy extremities (iv) Sighing respiration and repeated yawning (v) Dilatation of pupils (vi) Rapid pulse and slightly raised blood pressure.

Diagnosis at Autopsy

(i) There is history of sudden death resulting from blow or injury over the receptor areas (ii) Person is usually of emotional temperament, severely ill, feeble, an old person or young child (iii) Findings of fatal injuries, poisoning and natural diseases should be ruled out.

Secondary or Haematogenic Shock

The circulatory disturbances develop gradually after infliction of injuries. It is more serious and fatal.

Pathogenesis

The reduction in effective circulatory volume can result from loss of blood or plasma at the site of injury and peripheral capillary dilatation or increased capillary permeability. Due to changes in this hemodynamic mechanism, there is diminution of effective circulatory volume, diminished venous return to the heart, decreased cardiac output and diminished supply of oxygen to the tissues. This tissue anoxia results in the disturbance of intracellular and anaerobic glucose metabolism leading to increased production of lactic and other acids that causes disruption of lysosomes and release of lytic enzymes with resulting cell death. The reduced production of ATP causes reduced protein synthesis, disturbance in transport mechanism and cell membrane permeability. The continuing tissue anoxia causes interference with enzyme systems leading to metabolic acidosis, water and electrolyte imbalance and renal insufficiency. If there is superadded gram negative endotoxaemia circulatory failure may be enhanced by increased capillary permeability or widespread peripheral vasodilatation.

Reversible or compensated shock: The compensatory body mechanism try to fight this by producing arteriolar vasoconstriction and increased peripheral resistance by increasing levels of circulating catecholamine, cortisol, aldosterone and angiotensin and secretion of ADH hormone. As a result, arteriolar constriction may try to improve the venous return to heart and circulating blood volume. With appropriate treatment the compensatory mechanism reestablish the circulation and the patient is recovered. This type of shock is reversible or compensated shock.

Decompensated or irreversible shock: In the decompensated or irreversible shock, the compensatory mechanisms fail to prevent deterioration of hemodynamic mechanisms as a result the condition of patient worsens with ensuing death. This irreversible

Table 22.1: Classification of shock

Types	Clinical condition	Principal mechanisms
Cardiogenic shock from interference of heart function	Myocardial infarction, heart rupture, arrhythmias, cardiac tamponade, massive pulmonary embolism	It is due to the failure of myocardial pump resulting from intrinsic myocardial damage, extrinsic pressure or obstruction outflow
Hypovolaemic, also known as haemorrhagic or traumatic shock	Massive haemorrhage (10-20% of total blood volume) and loss of fluid in as in vomiting, diarrhoea or burns	Blood or plasma volume is inadequate
Septic	Gram negative bacteremia-endotoxic shock or gram positive septicemia	There is peripheral vasodilatation with pooling of blood and cell membrane injury with DIC
Primary or neurogenic shock	Anaesthesia and spinal cord injury	Parasympathetic inhibition or sympathetico-adrenal stimulation of the circulation; peripheral vasodilatation with pooling of blood

shock occurs in massive myocardial infarction, bacterial sepsis and repeated haemorrhage and is due to many factors such as: (i) Due to persistent reflex vasoconstriction, cellular hypoxia and acidosis occurs. (ii) Generalized vasoconstriction may injure gut mucosa helping in the absorption of proteins and bacterial products with resulting bacterial endotoxaemia that causes motor atony and peripheral pooling of blood. (iii) Due to falling circulation, tissue anoxia is produced that disrupts lysosomes in the cells and release of hydrolases and thus further tissue damage. (iv) Due to vasoconstriction after injury, the renal anoxia, splanchnic anoxia is produced that results in the production of vasodepressor material in the liver, spleen and kidneys. This causes peripheral vessels to become refractory to adrenaline. This is followed by vascular atony with capillary dilatation and peripheral pooling. (v) Due to formation of minute capillary thrombosis of the injured capillaries from hypercoagulability.

Hypovolaemic or Oligaemic Shock

It results from diminished blood volume caused by: (i) Loss of blood or plasma resulting from traumatic injuries, burns or surgical operations. (ii) Loss of fluid as in diarrhoea, vomiting and adrenal insufficiency. (iii) Due to generalized vascular permeability and peripheral vasodilatation there is escape of fluid in tissue spaces resulting in withdrawal of blood into these vessels from the general circulation.

Clinical Features

(i) Generalized weakness (ii) Profuse respiration with cold clammy skin (iii) Dilated pupils (iv) Tachycardia and tachypnoea (v) Diminished pulse pressure.

Autopsy Findings

The findings are nonspecific with generalized capillovenous engorgement and widespread petechial haemorrhages in different areas of body. There are findings of tissue oedema and necrosis of visceral organs.

THROMBOEMBOLISM

Thrombosis: It is the formation of clotted mass of blood within the non-interrupted cardiovascular system is termed thrombosis and the mass itself a **thrombus.** Thrombi may diminish or obstruct vascular flow causing ischemic injuries. Thrombi may diminish or obstruct vascular flow causing ischemic injuries to tissue and organs, or become dislodged or fragmented to create the emboli.

Emboli: These are defined as a detached intravascular physical mass that is carried by the blood to a site distant from its point of origin. 95% of all emboli consist of mass of blood clot dislodged from an intravascular thrombus. Other less common form are globules of fat, bubbles of airs, debris of amniotic fluid, particles of normal tissue such as bone marrow and brain, some abnormal tissue such as malignant brain cells and aggregates of bacteria or even parasites. Embolic phenomenon can be an added risk associated with surgical operation procedure, trauma and non-traumatic natural disease.

External embolism: External embolism can be due to a: (i) Foreign body (bullet from firearm) or (ii) Foreign material (I.V.) that is: (a) Oxygen (by accident) (b) Air (by accident/injection) (c) Solid particles (drug addicts from I.V. injections) (d) Solid particles (suicidal and therapeutic injections).

Internal embolism: Most emboli are derived from the thrombi. Thrombosis may be due to vegetations or clusters of bacteria (septic thromboembolism). It can be: (i) Fat embolism (ii) Bone marrow embolism (iii) Amniotic fluid embolism.

Thrombus may be of arterial or venous origin. Arterial thrombi may arise from: (i) Left auricle and appendage especially in mitral stenosis and atrial fibrillation (ii) Mural thrombus mainly from left ventricle (iii) Thrombus dislodged from aorta or from aneurysms (iv) Vegetations from valves due to subacute bacterial endocarditis or ulcerative endocarditis.

Venous emboli may result from sudden immobilization for even a short period of time may result in bilateral phlebothrombosis in calf veins. Most common sites of thrombosis are in deep femoral vein, posterior tibial vein and popliteal vein. The factors predisposing to leg vein thrombosis after an injury that is traumatic lesions of lower extremity especially fractures of long bones are: (i) Local tissue damage causing injury to the veins (ii) An increase in clotting time of blood which is maximum at two weeks after the injury (iii) Immobility and bed rest (iv) General debility especially in the old leading to poor general circulation and cardiac output.

Thrombus is more common in veins than the arteries and usually develops in thigh and leg veins (Figure 22.1A). Thrombus usually develops in 10-20 days (usually a week after the trauma). It may be seen in pelvic vessels and rarely in jugular veins. The thrombus is detached in part or whole, and travels to pulmonary and other veins such as venous plexus of the dura mater, subclavian veins, axillary veins, external and internal iliac veins, prostatic veins, uterine veins and ovarian veins. All these veins develop bland thrombi after traumatic injury. Bullet wounds and stab wounds of carotid arteries may injure intima and a thrombus may develop at the site. The thrombus is to be differentiated from postmortem clot. The thrombus is pale gray in colour and tangled fibrin strands are present (Figure 22.1B). It is often attached to the underlying vessel wall. It shows the perfect casts of the vessels in which they are located. **Postmortem clots** are rubbery, gelatinous coagulum that lacks fibrin strands and attachment to

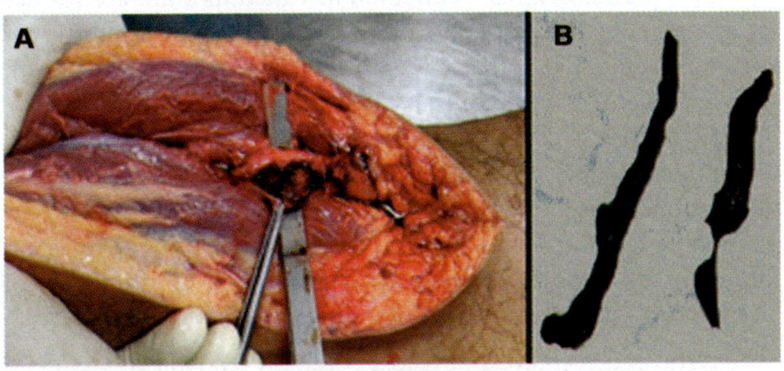

Figure 22.1A, B: Thrombus in the popliteal vein at autopsy (A) and the removed thrombus (B)

the underlying wall. It is uniformly dark red, slippery, soft, lumpy moist clot **(black currant jelly)** or pale, bright yellow **(chicken fat).**

As a result of thromboembolism, massive infarcts may result but may not be seen if death has occurred rapidly. When a large embolus obstructs the bifurcation of pulmonary artery or one of its branches (Figure 22.2), an immediate acute dilatation and failure of right side of heart occurs **(Acute Cor pulmonale).** Unusual types of pulmonary embolism are sometimes produced by trauma: (i) Fragments of bone marrow may be found as emboli in smaller branches of pulmonary artery, usually follow fracture of bone containing marrow. (ii) Fragments of liver parenchyma may enter torn hepatic veins after blunt force injury to liver and may be carried as emboli. (iii) Laceration of brain accompanied by tearing of venous sinuses may lead to pulmonary embolus. (iv) Foreign bodies may enter veins or arteries and are transported as emboli, e.g., a bullet.

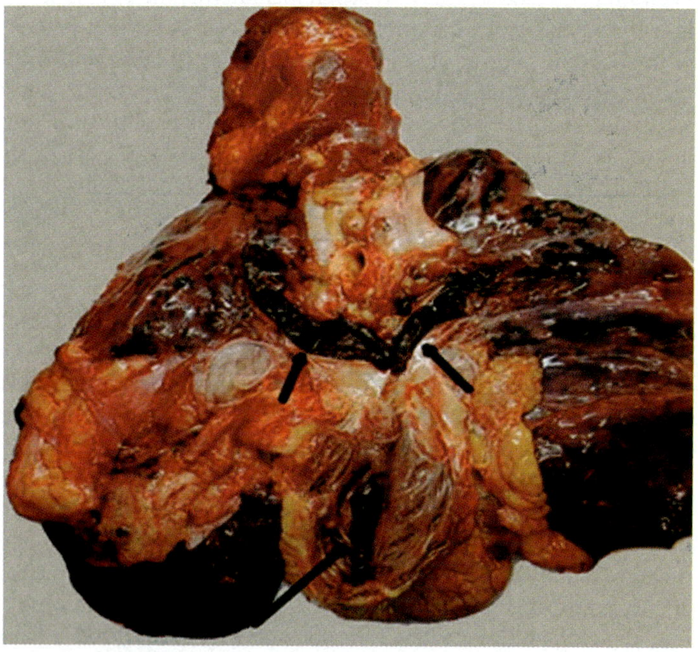

Figure 22.2: Thrombus in the right ventricle and both left and right pulmonary artery at autopsy

Pulmonary Air Embolism

Pulmonary embolism is a condition in which thrombi are formed in the walls of the pelvic and leg veins and such thrombi break away and embolise to the lungs. Although the thrombosis is the primary event, the embolus itself usually consists of a tube of thrombus with a central core of clotted blood. When it reaches the lung, its effect depends on its size, small ones are carried to the periphery of the lung and causes **pulmonary infarcts.** Large emboli reach the bifurcation of pulmonary artery completely blocking the blood circulation. Most common sites of thrombosis are in deep femoral vein, posterior tibial vein and popliteal vein.

Intravenous route is the most common recognized source of entry especially during therapeutic injection. For a serious result, two main factors are required; either positive pressure or negative pressures usually at a site near the heart. In any event there must be an adequate amount of air, at least 60 ml or more. Systemic air embolism occurs when an air in sufficient quantity enters a vein of the pulmonary system and is carried through the left side of the heart to block arterioles and capillaries in different parts of the body especially brain and heart. One to two ml of air may be enough to produce death because air travels directly from the lungs to the left side of the heart, from which it can be forced into coronary or cerebral arteries. Death from air embolism occurs within a few minutes, not delayed beyond 45 minutes. Air entering the venous system is carried to the heart and pulmonary arteries, which causes mechanical obstruction of the pulmonary arterial vasculature. This causes churning of blood and air producing froth. The churning can result in development of complexes of air bubbles, fibrin, platelet aggregates, erythrocytes and fat globules thus further occluding the vasculature, which causes death. This occurs most commonly in penetrating wounds of chest, crush injuries of the chest and surgical procedures upon thorax. Other circumstances under which such accidents occur are: (i) During transfusion when positive pressure is being used. (ii) During surgical operations especially during those on neck and chest when negative pressure will produce a 'suck-in' effect. (iii) During craniotomy in the sitting up position. (iv) Operations on nasal air sinuses. (v) Incised and penetrating wounds of the neck and chest involving jugular and subclavian veins. Fatal accidental oxygen embolus may occur during an operative procedure. (vi) Intravenous drug addicts inject foreign bodies at the time or following subsequent surgical procedures, e.g., metallic mercury embolism. (vii) A wound of sagittal sinus inside the skull. (viii) Injection of air under pressure in fallopian tube to test the patency. (ix) Injection of air or fluid mixed with air or soapy water in the pregnant uterus for procuring abortion. (x) Caesarean section, version or manual extraction of placenta may introduce air into the uterus. (xi) Crush injuries of chest. (xii) Subclavian vein catheterization. (xiii) Positive pressure ventilation in newborn infant. (xiv) Artificial pneumothorax and pneumoperitoneum. (xv) Air encephalography. (xvi) Caisson's disease.

Autopsy Diagnosis

Thromboembolism should specially be suspected when death occurs after a week of trauma. This is seen in up to 65% of such patients who die after a week of trauma. The thrombus can be demonstrated by inserting a flexible wire with blunt terminal knob inserted in femoral vein (i) If air embolism is suspected, head should be opened first and surface vessels of brain examined for gas bubbles, which must be prominent and definite and not the segmental break up of blood in the vessels with collapsed segments in between. (ii) Avoid pulling the sternum and ribs to avoid creating negative pressure in the tissues, which may result in aspiration of air into vessels. (iii) Before handling thoracic organs, the pericardium is opened, heart is lifted upwards and the apex is cut with a knife. (iv) Left ventricle is filled with frothy blood, if air is in sufficient quantity to cause death. (v) If the right ventricle contains air, the heart will float in water. (vi) Air embolism can also be demonstrated by cutting the pericardium anteriorly and grasping the edges with hemostat on each side. (vii) Pericardial sac is filled with water and heart is punctured with the scalpel and twisted a few times. Bubbles of air will escape if air is present. (viii) Amount of air can be measured by placing inverted water filled graduated glass cylinder, with the mouth of cylinder in pericardial sac. (ix) Oxygen in heart indicates air embolism because it is not present in appreciable quantity if gases were those of decomposition. Frothy blood resembling air embolism can be found especially in right ventricle due to handling of heart before it is opened at autopsy, putrefaction, as a postmortem event and artificial respiration in dying or recently dead. (x) Skull vault should be removed without puncturing the meninges. (xi) Internal carotid and basilar arteries are ligated before the brain is removed. (xii) Meningeal vessels should be examined for visible air bubbles. In acute cases, gas bubbles will be visible within the cerebral arteries but not in the cortical veins. (xiii) Brain should be submerged in water and ligature should be released. Then the vessels are cut and slightly compressed to watch for air bubbles. (xiv) An air tight, water filled glass syringe with a needle can be used to collect gas from blood vessels, heart or cavities.

Dating of pulmonary embolus: For dating an embolus, veins along with the thrombi and the muscles around it are excised as a sample for routine histopathological examination. This tissue can be processed and fibrin can be demonstrated by phototungstic acid-haematoxylin stain and Martius Scarlet Blue stain. With phototungstic acid-haemotoxylin acid stain the changes are:

- *First day:* Purplish strands of fibrin.
- *Four days:* Thicker strands and sheets of fibrin.
- *Two weeks:* Fibrin strands are dark purple.
- *By twenty-fifth day:* Fibrin begins to be absorbed.

With scarlet blue stain, initially the fibrin is seen as pink coloured that becomes scarlet in about a week.

Diagnosis of Air Embolism

Radiological examination of the whole body will detect large quantities of air. Ophthalmoscope will detect air bubbles in retinal arteries. The gas collected from heart on addition of alkaline pyrogallol solution will become brown in the presence of free oxygen and indicates antemortem air embolism.

Bone Marrow Embolism

Emboli can always be found in the lungs in cases of death from severe multiple injuries such as that seen in aircraft disasters, their presence may be of value in determining the rapidity of death. Fat will also be present in the lungs.

Amniotic Fluid Embolism

It is one of the leading causes of sudden death during labour and during abortion. Vernix and fat can be demonstrated in the lungs and cardiac vessels.

Fat Embolism

Fat embolism is caused by: (i) Fracture of a long bone namely, femur and pelvic bones. (ii) An injury to adipose tissue which forces liquid fat into damaged blood vessels. (iii) Injecting oil into circulation, e.g., in criminal abortion. (iv) Occasionally due to natural disease without trauma as in sickle cell anemia, diabetes, following blood transfusion, fatty change seen in liver as seen in chronic alcoholics, septicemia, steroid therapy, acute pancreatitis, osteomyelitis, decompression sickness (Caisson's disease), in too rapid ascent to high altitudes without functional pressurized cabin or under simulated flight conditions in decompression chambers and in burns.

Two factors favours pulmonary fat embolism: (i) Fixation of walls of veins, e.g., in clavicular and pelvic regions, the upper dorsal spine and dural membranes. (ii) Suction effect of the respiratory movements and heart's actions on such veins as the jugular, subclavian and vertebral has a tendency to create a negative pressure in the vessels during phase of inspiration.

Presence of fat droplets in the blood stream indicates that the injury was produced during life, except in case of burning, advanced putrefaction and charring after death. Large amounts of liquefied fat are derived from fat cells. When cardiac massage is done, fat enters the blood vessels even if the circulation has stopped. If during resuscitation, the sternum or ribs are fractured bone marrow embolism is seen in the lungs.

Clinically: The phenomenon presents as sudden loss of consciousness usually after a period following the traumatic accident, which need not in itself be serious such as a fractured tibia and fibula.

Autopsy Diagnosis

Droplets of fat should be demonstrable in the peripheral viscera notably vessels of kidneys and brain. There are petechial haemorrhages in organs and punctate haemorrhages in the white matter of brain.

HAEMORRHAGE

Bleeding may occur externally through a lacerated or incised wound or through trachea, bronchi, oro-nasal passages, ears, vagina, urethra or rectum. The contusions result in internal bleeding from rupture of vessels and bleeding into body cavities; pericardium, peritoneum, pleura and cranium. The amount of total blood volume, the rapidity and site of bleeding governs its fatality: (i) When the leakage is slow the body can compensate for the loss of far greater volume, by adjustment of vascular bed and by restoration of blood volume by transfer from other aqueous compartments. (ii) As far as site is concerned, the small quantity of bleeding into the brainstem is likely to be fatal whereas the same volume exuded into the pleural cavity would be of little consequence. (iii) Bleeding usually begins at the time of injury with a momentary delay at the instant of infliction. Due to transient spasm of local vessels from the stimulus of the injuring object, blood may hesitate for a second or so before welling out in sharp cuts of skin. Then the bleeding continues until normal hemostasis plugs the vessels. (iv) In some injuries involving arteries, the musculoelastic vessel may retract and its wall invaginates, so that an immediate seal prevents copious haemorrhage. (v) Sometimes gross injuries such as amputation of limb by railway wheel may be devoid of significant bleeding because the crushing effect may combine with arterial wall retraction to seal the cut vessel. (vi) Failure of hemostasis is a hematological matter but it has medicolegal significance if a surgery is performed on some one who has a haemorrhagic diathesis either from natural disease or from anticoagulant treatment.

Delayed bleeding is seen: (i) In road traffic accidents when liver, spleen or lung may be injured within their capsules or covering membranes that may initially remain intact. A subcapsular hematoma of the liver may grow even larger due to continues bleeding stripping more capsule from the parenchyma. Eventually, a blister may rupture with bleeding into peritoneal cavity. (ii) Trauma can weaken the walls of an artery or vein leading to a false aneurysm that can rupture later on. An arteriovenous fistula may also rupture. (iii) Infections at the site of trauma can involve vessels in the vicinity so that an abscess or cellulitis can lead to secondary haemorrhage when the vessel wall is eroded. (iv) It is sometimes difficult to know that how much of the haemorrhage found at autopsy may be accounted for by postmortem bleeding. Except in serous cavities such as pleura or peritoneum, or externally from the body surface, in most cases this is a small proportion of that which leaked under arterial pressure during life, due to the tissue pressures opposing passive bleeding. (v) A hemothorax from a ruptured aorta may amount to several litres and much of this is in the form of a large clot. In this case any postmortem addition will not affect its interpretation.

INFECTION

Infection used to be common after wound infection before the advent of antibiotics. Criminally inflicted wound that were not dangerous to life may become fatally infected so that an assault becomes a homicide. Purulent wound infection from Gram positive cocci, Gram negative bacilli, anaerobes such as *Clostridium perfringens* and the other more common organisms is the most frequent. Tetanus and anthrax are also dangerous. The forensic relevance is to prove the chain of causation between the original injuries and death from intercurrent infection. There may be medicolegal issues such as failure to give or delay in giving antibiotic cover which have both civil and criminal consequences. A criminal assault that ends in death because of a neglected infection does not exonerate the perpetrator from all responsibility, even though there has been a *novus actus interveniens* in the form of defective medical treatment.

ADULT RESPIRATORY DISTRESS SYNDROME

Adult respiratory distress syndrome develops following severe lung injury, such as gross impact upon the thorax or blast injury from explosion, or from aspiration of gastric contents, infections, toxins, systemic shock, irritant gases, near drowning and many other causes. As a result, the lung epithelium may suffer 'diffuse alveolar damage'.

Clinical Features

(i) Marked dyspnoea (ii) Progressive respiratory failure, leading to hypoxaemia.

Autopsy Findings

At autopsy the lungs are hard and retain their shape after removal, having a 'dry-oedema' appearance, being almost double in weight in some instances.

Histopathological Findings

Pathologically the lungs show a stiff oedema that progress to a rigid, infiltrated lung if survival is long enough. Histologically the initial changes are shedding of type I pneumocytes with intra-alveolar exudates, the formation of hyaline membrane and patchy alveolar haemorrhage. This destructive phase is then replaced after a few days with a proliferative stage, when Type II pneumocytes begin to fill the alveoli and a mononuclear response infiltrates the interstitial areas. The alveolar proliferation organizes, if survival continues, and eventually pulmonary fibrosis develops.

RESPIRATOR LUNG

This condition is similar to adult respiratory distress syndrome developing when a patient dies after an appreciable period of mechanical ventilation. It may appear within a few days, but usually supervenes after many days or weeks on a ventilator. The lungs are stiff and rigid which though heavy does not usually appear obviously oedematous. Microscopically, proteinaceous fluid and a mixture of proliferative cells may be seen in the alveoli.

RENAL FAILURE

Renal failure is a common sequel to extensive muscle damage or to burns affecting considerable areas of skin. When the muscle is crushed, severely torn or otherwise rendered ischemic, where there are excessive burns, or where poisons such as mercuric salts or carbon tetrachloride are given, destruction of the renal tubular epithelium may be seen. A similar change occurs during postmortem autolysis. In burns and muscle damage, the tubules may also be blocked with brown casts of myoglobin and these two changes of distal tubular necrosis and the casts were thought to cause profound oliguria and anuria often associated with trauma and burns. In biopsy as opposed to autopsy material, the tubular damage has been found to be minimal and the casts may be a sequel to reduced infiltration rather than to tubular damage, so the validity of acute tubular necrosis as an explanation of renal failure following trauma has been questioned.

DISSEMINATED INTRAVASCULAR COAGULATION

DIC is a consumption coagulopathy associated with the blood clotting mechanism. It follows a whole range of traumatic, infective and other acute events. There is an abnormal activation of the coagulation process within the blood vessels caused by many factors related to the blood itself, the vessel walls and to blood flow. Damaged tissue from trauma and burns can trigger thromboplastin initiated coagulation–entry of tissue cell elements, especially from erythrocytes; brain and placenta are particularly potent. Particulate matter such as microorganisms or microemboli of all types (including fat and air emboli, especially those from decompression) can precipitate coagulation via Factor XII. Vascular endothelial damage and stasis of flow can have a similar effect. Whatever the cause, the fibrinogen is consumed and fibrin precipitated in vessels, leading to both vascular obstructive effects and to haemorrhagic diathesis from depletion of the coagulation system. Platelets are also consumed, adhering to the fibrin thrombi. Fibrinolysis is activated and there is a dynamic contest between intravascular coagulation and its removal.

After death there can be postmortem fibrinolysis, which lessens the ease with which fibrin deposits can be detected. Staining techniques are also an imperfect method of visualizing the fibrin so a careful search must be made in autopsy histology for fibrin remnants. Lungs, liver, kidney and adrenals are most likely organs to yield positive results. Microvascular obstruction leading sometimes to frank infarction as well as reduced function together with bleeding forms major dangers of DIC in forensic context.

SUBENDOCARDIAL HAEMORRHAGE

Subendocardial haemorrhages were specifically studied in the 1930 by **Sheehan** in cases of abortion and acute haemorrhages associated with pregnancy. They were formerly known as 'Sheehan's haemorrhages' and are a striking feature of many autopsies especially on victims of severe trauma: (i) These are well marked haemorrhages seen under the endocardium of left ventricle, on the interventricular septum and on the opposing papillary muscles and adjacent columnae carnae of the free wall of the ventricle. (ii) These are flame shaped, confluent haemorrhages, not petechial, and tend to occur in one continuous sheet rather than patches. The bleeding is in a thin subendocardial layer, but when severe may actually raise the endocardium into a flat blister that can be palpable on the smooth septum. (iii) The mechanism of production is obscure, but they are commonly seen: (a) After sudden, profound hypotension from shock resulting from severe haemorrhage (b) When there is intracranial damage from head injuries, cerebral oedema, surgical craniotomy or large intracranial tumours and sudden intracranial decompression (c) In obstetric conditions such as deaths from antepartum or postpartum haemorrhage, ruptured ectopic gestation, abortions and ruptured uterus often reveal these lesions (d) Poisonings especially heavy metal poisoning, particularly arsenic.

The common factor seems to be sudden hypotension and if the intraventricular pressure drops precipitously, the existing blood pressure in the coronary system is then unsupported across the endocardium by an equal pressure within the ventricular lumen, so that rupture of superficial vessels occurs. There being flaws in this theory, one being the common incidence in intracranial lesions. These haemorrhages are known to be a part of Virchow's triad of 'pulmonary oedema, gastric erosions and subendocardial haemorrhages' seen in head injuries and cases of raised intracranial pressure.

SURVIVAL PERIOD AFTER WOUND

During an investigation, a forensic pathologist is often asked the probable time interval between the fatal injuries and death. The pathologist should never give a dogmatic answer unless the nature and severity of injuries are obviously incompatible with continued life or activity. The doctor should always give opinion with caution as victims sometimes survive for long than expected. A person whose brainstem is destroyed by a penetrating injury or whose aortic arch is completely transacted, will be inactive and clinically dead almost immediately. But extraordinary instances of survival have been recorded when the frontal lobes are damaged or the abdominal aorta was crushed by a railway wheel. In the more usual stab injury, head injury, cut throat or firearm wounds, the forensic pathologist must try to assess the nature of severity of the physical damage and relate that to the age, health and environment of the victim. Other than injuries to the brain or to a large blood vessel, most other injuries can rarely be declared to have caused sudden death or rapid loss of function. A senile old lady, or someone with severe cardiac or respiratory disease is less likely to survive multiple injuries for as long as the robust young person, though if the nature of injury is grossly life-threatening, these factors make little difference. In criminal cases, it may be a point of some importance to decide whether the victim could have continued fighting, have resisted, ran away or even have inflicted injuries on someone else before collapsing and dying. In the adrenaline response of 'fight or flight', the shock element of pain is greatly suppressed in an assault and only the sheer physical and hemodynamic sequelae of injury will eventually lead to a slowing down, then collapse and death: (i) A wound in the left ventricle can partly seal itself by the contraction of muscle around the defect and victim will collapse only when sufficient blood has leaked into the pericardium to form cardiac tamponade. (ii) Wounds of the right ventricle are often more rapidly fatal as, although the pressure of contained blood is less, the thinner wall is not so effective in preventing the leak. (iii) Head injuries present many paradoxical instances of prolonged survival, depending on the part of brain injured. Frontal lobes are remarkably resistant to damage as it is generalized impact rather than focal damage to this area that does the most harm. (iv) A cut artery will lose blood faster than a vein of the same general size, especially if it is only partly severed so that it cannot retract. Other factors such as possibility of air embolism in cut jugular veins might alter the situation. The heart is less vulnerable than great thoracic vessels in many stab wounds. Where a wound has transacted a major coronary artery, prolonged survival is unlikely, as is one that interrupts a major branch of the conducting system.

Most issues of such nature revolve around periods of a few minutes, the perimortem or agonal time when few morphological signs are available. The accepted wisdom of wound dating is that polymorph leukocytes begin to appear in the wounded tissue within minutes, but can happen even several hours after death as all leukocytes do not become immobile with cardiac arrest. The death being a process is conventionally taken to be the moment of cardiac arrest and thus collapse of blood pressure and cerebral circulation, the cells of the body are still alive and remain so for variable time–only minutes in the case of neurons, but leukocytes and muscle cells survive for many hours and connective tissues such as fibroblast for days. Thus it is unreasonable to expect dramatic changes within minutes in skin wounds, until progressive hypoxia alters biochemical processes and enzyme activity. Leukocytes may be motile for more than 12 hours and can aggregate around chemotactically active material such as gastric content around the air passages. This makes the vital reaction a dubiously valid phenomenon in perimortal period. If the survival is longer, then both gross and histological changes of 'vital reaction' such as thrombosis, inflammation, infection and healing may be useful, but they usually require hours or even days of survival to appear.

TIMING AND HISTOPATHOLOGY OF WOUNDS

Clinical timing of wounds: It is not possible to determine the exact age of a wound by naked eye examination because the intensity of local inflammatory reaction varies. Under normal conditions, the features of the wound with the passage of time are given in Table 22.2.

Table 22.2: Clinical timing of wounds

Time	Features
After 12 hours	Edges of the wound are red and swollen
After 24 hours	Small wound may show scab
After 36 hours	Epithelium around the edge of the wound begins to grow
4-5 days	Epithelization of small clean wounds may be complete

A small wound may show scab formation after about 24 hours and pus formation appears after about 36-48 hours, if septic and does not heal for days or weeks of sloughing of surrounding tissue. Vascular endothelium shows distinct proliferative changes. During 24 hours, vascular buds are given off from minute vessels at periphery and in 36 hours a complete network of new capillary vessels seen. In the living body the damaged tissues imbibe the extravasated blood. The wound edges gape and become swollen after a lapse of about 12 hours. Later on signs of inflammation and of healing dominate the picture. Haemorrhages even with abundant fibrin formation are no longer reliable indicators of antemortem origin of wound.

Microscopical examination of the wounds: Because of the uncertain and variable results of the naked eye examination, it is important to study injuries microscopically that reveals. The findings are: (i) Leucocytic reaction is the earliest histological sign of inflammation. (ii) Appearance of a few leukocytes in the wound periphery does not justify the diagnosis of a vital reaction because these cells are regular component of the connective tissue. (iii) Margination and limited migration of leukocytes may occur in tissues in response to injury even after somatic death. (iv) First leukocytes to pass into the tissues are polymorphonuclear neutrophils. (v) Monocytes appear before a lapse of about 12 hours but later than neutrophils. (vi) Exudation reaches its maximum intensity within 48 hours of the injury. (vii) Epithelial growth is clearly visible on 3rd day. (viii) Fibroblasts show reactive changes within a few hours. They begin to undergo division within about 15 hours after injury and granulation tissue develops within at least three days. (ix) New collagen fibrils appear within 4-5 days of injury. (x) A fibrous tissue scar may appear within a week in small wounds.

Wound Healing

Wound healing is described as an epimorphic process by **Needham** namely a form of regeneration in which there is development in situ of portion lost. It shows two main phases:

Regressive phase: It is subdivided in order of occurrence of wound closure, demolition of damaged cell and differentiation of cells to provide new tissue for the process of repair.

Progressive phase: It is divided into three phases: the formation of repair tissue, growth of repair tissue and differentiation of repair tissue.

All these stages overlap and vary in different organisms and even in different parts of the same organism. The series of events in response to the initial injury generally follow a definite order and the two main phases described above are generally subdivided in descriptions of wounds in human tissues into four periods **(Douglas, 1963).** (i) ***Phase of traumatic inflammation***: It lasts from one to three days after wounding when fibrin and dilated capillaries appear histologically. (ii) ***Destructive phase***: It varies from 4-6 days and is characterized by numerous leukocytes and macrophages. (iii) ***Proliferation phase***: It lasts from 4-14 days and is characterized by the presence of fibroblasts around capillaries and some metachromasia of tissue ground substance. (iv) ***Maturation phase***: This phase is gradually reached over many months. Collagen formation is accompanied by decrease in number of fibroblasts and there is progressive increase in tensile strength of the wound. Phase 1 and 2 are lag phase in which no proper repair occurs.

Histochemical Examination of Wounds

Enzyme histochemistry methods are applied for the study of wound healing. Enzymes are proteins that catalyze biologic reactions. Thus demonstration of enzymes could reveal earlier reaction than could visualization of the resulting morphologically demonstrable changes. Healing is an example of enzymatically-catalyzed processes in the organism on which its life depends. Histological examination is based on the production of microscopically visible reactions by applying chemical tests to tissue sections prepared for microscopic study. For histological and histochemical examination: (i) Wounds or their parts are excised with their surroundings about ½ an inch in each direction. (ii) One half of the tissue block is fixed overnight in neutral 10% formalin at 4°C for demonstration of esterase and phosphatase activity and for histological examination. (iii) Other half is fresh frozen with isopentane chilled with dry ice; the frozen specimen is subjected to histochemical methods for detecting adenosine phosphatases and amino peptidases.

The demonstration of enzymes in situ depends on their action on a specific substrate in the presence of other substances with which one of the decomposition product resulting from enzyme activity will form an insoluble deposit at the site of enzyme action. If this deposit is not already coloured, it is rendered visible by the use of suitable chemicals. That is, an increase in enzyme activity appears as an intensified colour and a decrease in enzyme activity as a declining stainability.

To summarize the results, two zones can be demonstrated around antemortem wounds (Figure 22.1). (i) ***Central (superficial) zone:*** It is in the immediate vicinity of the wound edge and is 200-500μ deep, shows decreasing enzyme activity. It should be considered as an early sign of imminent necrosis. The regressive phenomenon in this zone may be called **negative vital reactions**, since no such decrease in enzyme activity is observed in the wounds inflicted after death. (ii) ***Peripheral zone:*** It surrounds the central zone, is 100-300 μ deep and has increasing enzyme activity. It represents adaptive defence mechanisms of the local connective tissue cells as an enzymatic response to injury. The increase in enzyme activity in this zone is called **positive vital reaction,** since there are no such changes in postmortem wounds.

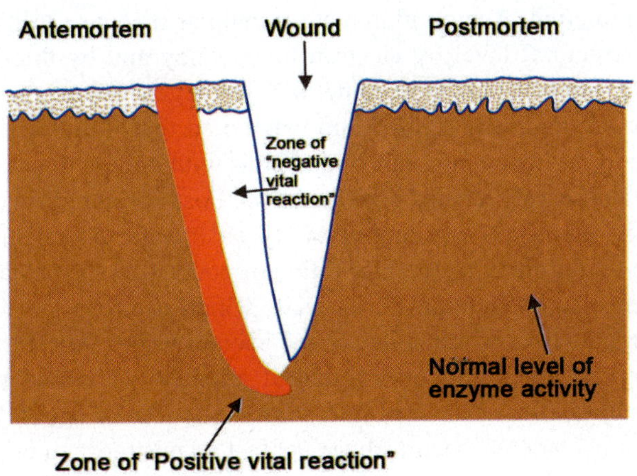

Figure 22.1: Difference between the enzyme activity in antemortem and postmortem wound

Histochemistry of an antemortem wound: Activity of adenosine triphosphatases and esterases increases as early as about one hour after injuries and the activity of aminopeptidases increases in about two hours whereas activity of acid and alkaline phosphatases increases in about four and eight hours respectively (Figure 22.2). Histochemical vital reactions are recognizable several days after death.

Mucopolysaccharides in wound healing: Acid mucopolysaccharides disappear from vital wounds and reappear during healing process. They also disappear from vital bruises, abrasions and electric marks but remain present in the antemortem hanging and strangulation marks. This suggests that the alteration in vital wounds and bruises are mainly the consequence of haemorrhage into the connective tissue.

Distribution of histochemically identified substance in two main components of skin:

RNA: By pyronin methyl green/ribonuclease method, in the epidermis, RNA is moderately intense in basal cells and becomes less so in the squamous cells showing inverse relationship to degree of keratinization. In skin wounds, a great increase in concentration of this substance is noted when there is active regeneration at the edges of a healing wound. It generally reaches the peak of activity when cells have bridged the central gap.

DNA: By Fuelgen method it is shown in lower squamous and basal cells to comprise faint purple granules of uniform size normally and confine it to the nucleus.

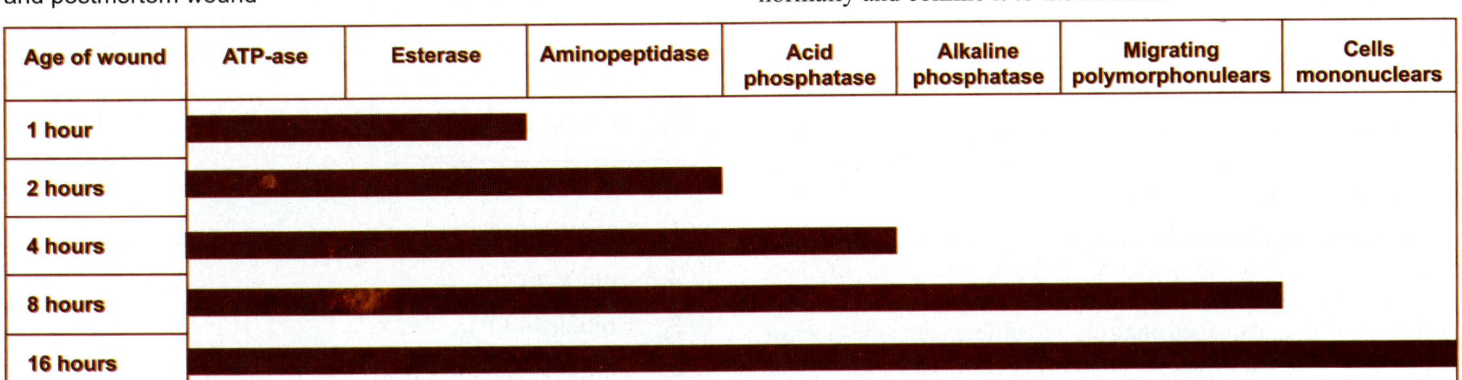

Figure 22.2: Changes in enzymes as seen histochemically in the first hours after wounding

Glycogen: By Periodic Acid Schiff/diastase method, an inverse relationship is shown to the degree of maturity of the epidermal cells being aggregated in basal cell layer and virtually absent in keratinized epithelium. Sulphydryl and disulphide group shows an inverse relationship to each other, the presence of S-S groups being noted when keratinization is almost complete.

The study of distribution of these components has not proved to be of any practical assistance in evaluation of wounds for forensic purposes. An increased reaction for RNA, glycogen and sulphydryl groups is noted in actively regenerating epithelium.

Connective Tissue Histochemistry

Fibroblasts: Fibroblasts show increased RNA content in the cytoplasm and prominent glycogen and metachromatic granules showing some alkaline phosphatase activity.

Mucopolysaccharides: Mucopolysaccharides disappear from vital bruises, abrasions and electric marks but remain in the antemortem hanging and strangulation marks that were suggested to be due to the consequence of haemorrhage into connective tissue in case of vital wounds and bruises.

Fibrin: With Mallory's phototungstic acid haematoxylin and Lendrum's acid picric Mallory method, haemorrhages in human tissue are shown as: (i) *4-12 hours*: Network of fine fibrils. (ii) *>24 hours:* Coarse fibrils. (iii) *>4 days:* Small concentrated areas appear. (iv) *>2 weeks:* Solid areas predominate. (v) *>1 month:* Granular areas appear among solid areas. (vi) *At 4 months:* Only granular appearance.

Platelets: Thrombosis has been recognized as an essential reaction to injury and was regarded by earlier writers as an unequivocal sign of antemortem infliction. Four stages are distinguished as platelet adherence, aggregation, degranulation and disruption. They are associated with formation of fibrin and platelet plug that is mixed fibrin red cell leukocyte mass and extension of thrombus. Agglutinated platelets arrest haemorrhage in normal skin by rapidly sealing the mouths of all cut vessels larger than capillaries.

Elastic tissue: Haemotoxylin and eosin stains the elastic tissue; normal elastic fibers are pink and others are blue gray with pink granules. Toluidine stains as deep blue green and normal elastic fibers as colourless. From a microscopic examination of elastic fibers in skin, it is possible to differentiate between antemortem wounds where these are wave like and postmortem wounds when they are straight.

Pigments: Phagocytosis of red corpuscles is well marked after 48 hours; formation of hemosiderin after 24 hours and formation of hematoidin within some 80 days.

Disc electrophoresis: Distribution of esterases was compared using disc electrophoresis in the cathode area. Two of these fractions showed up more intensely in antemortem skin wounds compared with undamaged controls. No difference in the esterase pattern was distinguished in undamaged skin and postmortem wounds.

Biochemistry of Wounds

Although enzyme histochemical methods have considerably shortened the indeterminable period after wounding but the study of last hour before death is very challenging. Histamine and serotonin (5-hydroxytryptamine) are vasoactive amines known to participate in an acute inflammatory process especially in the earliest phase after injury. The minimal increase of free histamine content occurs within 20-30 minutes and of serotonin in 10 minutes of injury. These additives have been conducted in experimental investigations of skin injuries as well as autopsy materials. About 2 gm of injured skin sample is removed and an equal size of control sample is taken from neighbouring intact skin of the corpse. The subcutaneous fat is removed from the samples before further processing and the free histamine and serotonin in the wound samples are compared with those of control samples.

Immunofluorescence Techniques

Fibrin in certain tissue lesions does not stain by standard techniques in the generally accepted manner. Sections from these fibrin clots were shown to react specifically with fluorescent-labeled rabbit antihuman fibrin antibodies. Also fluorescent antibody method was used to demonstrate fibrin in leukocytes in areas of fibrin accumulation. Acute inflammatory cellular response to fibrin at ultrastructural level by electron microscopy and by fluorescent microscopy using rhodamine antifibrinogen in experimental work on dogs was studied and was noted that fibrin is either a network of heavy interweaving strands with orange fluorescence or less intensely stained delicate fibers. Postmortem fibrin cannot be distinguished with any certainty on morphological grounds from vital fibrin. A large proportion of postmortem subcutaneous haemorrhages undergo fibrinolysis, which destroys the formed fibrin networks within a day of the haemorrhage. Therefore well preserved fibrin networks found at autopsy performed two to three days after death appear to point to the vital or agonal origin of a subcutaneous haemorrhage against its postmortem origin.

LONG QUESTIONS

1. How can you classify injuries and estimate the time of injuries?
2. Discuss in detail the grievous hurt.

SHORT QUESTIONS

1. Grievous hurt.
2. Simple injury.
3. Section 44 I.P.C.
4. Thromboembolism.

MULTIPLE CHOICE QUESTIONS

1. **The minimum amount of air required for fatal systemic air embolism is:**
   (a) 60 ml (b) 100 ml
   (c) 150 ml (d) 200 ml

2. **Hurt means any bodily pain, disease or infirmity caused to any person defined under section:**
   (a) 319 of I.P.C. (b) 320 of I.P.C.
   (c) 321 of I.P.C. (d) 322 of I.P.C.

3. **All are grievous injury *except:***
   (a) Fracture of skull (b) Facial disfiguration
   (c) Avulsion of nail (d) Stab injury of heart

4. **A 28-year-old male got eye injury during a quarrel. There was cornea injury and impairment vision which was corrected later on by keratoplasty. Legally this injury amounts to:**
   (a) Simple injury (b) Serious injury
   (c) Grievous injury (d) Dangerous injury

5. **Voluntarily causing grievous hurt by dangerous weapons or means is described in:**
   (a) S. 323 I.P.C. (b) S. 324 I.P.C.
   (c) S. 325 I.P.C. (d) S. 326 I.P.C.

6. **A person convicted under section 304A can have punishment of imprisonment up to:**
   (a) Two years (b) Five years
   (c) Seven years (d) Ten years

7. **All are grievous hurts *except:***
   (a) Dislocated shoulder
   (b) Incised wound on abdominal wall without peritoneal injury
   (c) Nasal bone fracture
   (d) Permanent disfiguration of face

8. **Which of the following is a grievous injury?**
   (a) Extensive lacerated wound on the forehead
   (b) 6 cm × 4 cm laceration present over scalp
   (c) 6 cm × 2 cm bruise present over extensor aspect of forearm
   (d) Abrasion present at the back of trunk

9. **A person beaten up but having no fracture or dislocation and is hospitalised for 20 days is considered grievously injured?**
   (a) Even if there is no other injury
   (b) If during the twenty days he is in severe body pain or unable to follow his ordinary pursuits
   (c) If during the first ten days he is in severe body pain but later on could follow his ordinary pursuits
   (d) Even if has sharp injury over abdomen without penetration of peritoneum

10. **Which of the following indicates that the wound in a hospitalized woman typist hit by 'lathis' admitted for 20 days was grievous?**
    (a) She is not able to recognize
    (b) Wound does not heal completely
    (c) Incised wound over scalp
    (d) She is not able to do her daily routines

ANSWER KEY ☞

1. (a)	2. (a)	3. (c)	4. (c)	5. (d)	6. (a)	7. (b)	8. (a)	9. (b)	10. (d)

23 CHAPTER

Torture and Custodial Deaths

TORTURE

The Webster dictionary defines torture as anguish of body or mind; something that causes agony or pain, to punish, coerce or afford sadistic pleasure.

The oppression of the Nazi regimen during the Second World War prompted the UNO to come out with Universal declaration of Human Rights (1948), followed by an International agreement of civil and political rights (1966) and a declaration on the protection of all persons from torture and other cruel, inhuman or degrading treatment or punishment (1975).

In 1975, World Medical Association adopted a declaration called **Declaration of Tokyo** that defined torture as, "A deliberate, systemic or wanton infliction of physical or mental suffering by one or more persons acting alone or on the orders of any authority to force another person to yield information, to make a confession or for any other reason." This declaration clearly expressed that a doctor must in no way, for any reason take part in the practice of torture or other forms of cruel, inhuman or degrading procedures as the doctor's role is to alleviate the distress of his fellow persons and no motive whether personal, collective or political shall prevail against this higher purpose. Though this definition is considered by many as the most authoritative as far as doctors are concerned, it has few drawbacks, namely: (i) It is applicable only in content of detention and imprisonment and not in other situations where torture could take place. (ii) There is no distinction as far as severity or aim of torture is concerned. (iii) Unethical experimentation with human subjects has not been covered under this declaration. (iv) It is implied that torture can be perpetrated only by others and not by self. No guidelines have been offered for self torture.

Classification of Torture

(i) That done on the person by his consent (ii) That done by others (without consent) that can be further subclassified as that committed on an innocent person or on a person who is not innocent (criminals or terrorists).

Reasons for Torture

The reason for torturing a person varies from country to country and time to time depending on the availability of weapons, circumstances and the motive for the crime. In the earlier days, the basic purpose of the torture was to get information or confession; to spread terror in the society or a country; to destroy a personality; to take revenge and to get a testimony incriminating others.

Types of Torture

Torture can be physical or psychological.

Types of injuries in torture: Though virtually any type of injury can be inflicted deliberately to extract information, punish or degrade the victims, but the repetition of a particular injury, such as **tram line bruises** from beating, is suspicious. The following types of injuries are commonly produced in the victims of torture.

Beating: It is one of the most common forms of torture and can take various forms, varying both with the weapon used and the part of the body injured. The blows may be inflicted with a fist, foot, shoe or some weapons such as whip, a *lathi*, metal or wooden bars, clubs, batons, rifle butts or belts may be used. Many of these weapons produce a characteristic single or double edged linear bruise. The bruise may be line of confluent petechial haemorrhages or a continuous mark of red skin. The **'tram line' bruise** is a double line of parallel marks with a pale unbruised zone between them, caused by the impact of a rectangular or circular-sectioned object. The bruising may be intradermal, when it reproduces the pattern of the weapon well. If a leather whip with, for example, plaited thongs is struck against the skin, the pattern may be imprinted clearly on the skin. Buckles on belts and other recognizable artefacts may occasionally be useful in identifying the weapon. Where the bruising is deeper, no such pattern is likely. The skin may be broken causing abrasions or lacerations and if full thickness is breached, healing will cause scars, which may even be recognizable as **tram lines**.

Repeated beating leaves multiple overlapping and criss-crossing marks that have a generally similar orientation that indicates that the attacker stood in a relatively fixed position to the victim. The use of multi-thonged whip will leave a series of marks with same orientation as above. Back is the most common target but whipping and beating may be applied to the buttocks, thighs, front of chest, breasts and abdomen, lower legs, soles of feet and even perineum and genitals.

Beating of the soles of feet with canes or rods **(falanga)** is extremely painful and debilitating a torture rooted in antiquity. The tough tissues and thick fascial planes of the foot do not readily reveal bruising, though it may be found on deep dissection in victims who have been killed by some other means.

If injuries were inflicted months before the examination, little or nothing may be found unless the skin was broken, when scarring will have taken place. Sometimes however, faint red lines will be seen in pale skinned people and hyperpigmentation along the lines of injury in the dark-skinned.

Burns are also commonly caused as a means of torture and they may either be the actual cause of death or visible as recent or scarred evidence of previous torture. All kinds of burns may be suffered such as from molten rubber dripped onto victims from motor tyres suspended overhead, hot irons applied to the skin, ignited kerosene soaked rags wrapped around the limbs and numerous burns from cigarettes passed on to the skin. The findings of burning **motor tyre necklace** and shadow areas indicating direction of contact where molten liquids have been dripped from above onto a bound victim may be seen on examination of the victim.

Cutting and stabbing wounds are also quite common and may be caused by a variety of weapon but knives and bayonets are commonly used. The chest and upper arms are the favourite sites for infliction of injury. The old stab wounds from knives and bayonets may be recognizable as elliptical scars many months or years after the infliction.

Blunt injuries and clubbing are quite common, either to cause death or as forms of abuse. The head is the most common target, but the legs and knees are also often struck. Blows on the back and sides of neck may result in subarachnoid haemorrhage due to damage to vertebrobasilar artery.

Suffocation and drowning are not commonly employed practices but nonfatal practices such as **wet submarining** (repeated dipping of the victim's head under water or even in foul liquid such as sewage water) is a well-known method of abuse. Such practices may cause death from drowning or if the victim survives, pneumonia may develop. **Dry submarine** is a partial suffocation by enveloping the head in an opaque plastic bag which is more a means of disorientation than physical torture but may eventually prove fatal.

Electrical torture is also quite commonly employed method of abuse. Either mains voltage of 110 or 240 volt is used, that can cause fatal cardiac arrhythmias and local burning. A magneto delivering high voltage is painful but not lethal and will not leave any significant marks over the skin owing to its low amperage. Electrical current may be applied anywhere on the body but the genitals especially the penis and scrotum and the female nipples are the favored sites. The term **'Buzzer'** is used for a torture method in which the individual is repeatedly shocked using wires or other conducting objects that are attached to parts of the body like eyes, ears, genitalia, soles of feet etc.

Injuries to ears may occur as a result of ***telefono*** (repeated slapping of the sides of head and ears by open palms of the assailant). Very rarely injuries to the inner ear and rupture of tympanic membrane may be demonstrated on autopsy.

Suspension: It is a common method of torture victims hung by the wrists or other body parts. When the individual is suspended by the wrists after the hands are tied at the back, it is called **'strappado'** or by the obsolete term **'Palestinian hanging'**. The victim can be suspended upside down from the knees, placed over a dowel or bar, with wrists bound to the ankles, is called **'Parrot's Perch'**. In such cases abrasions, bruises and chafing marks may be found at ligature sites.

Shooting is a common means of execution or nonfatal punishment but not a method of torture. **Knee-capping** where opponents and suspected traitors are shot either through knee joint or lower thigh, perpetrated in Northern Ireland.

Sexual abuse is commonly seen even multiple rapes in women that will leave some of the physical signs.

Management of torture victims: First and foremost is the diagnosis of torture by taking a proper history, complete examination including the general physical examination, examination of the injuries and proper investigation including the radiological examination and bone scintigraphy. The treatment of the victim is an important aspect by providing the physical and psychological treatment simultaneously and treating the victim and his family. The victim should not be reminded of torture and proper rehabilitation is necessary.

Medicolegal and Ethical Aspects of Torture

(i) Freedom from torture is among the human rights contained in the United Nations, Universal Declaration of Human Rights.
(ii) Doctors are obliged by the Hippocratic Oath, not to use their

professional knowledge in order to harm their patients. (iii) Geneva Declaration of the World Medical Association reconfirmed this obligation and precludes any medical involvement in the practice of torture.

In spite of this the doctors are at the risk of being involved in the practice of torture directly or indirectly: (i) As a humanist citizen (ii) As a participant in the process of torture by coercion by society, government or terrorists, or sometimes unknowingly becoming a part of it and with his own desire (iii) As victims of torture themselves, e.g., Chile, Turkey.

Participation of doctors in torture: The doctors can participate in torture in various ways, namely: (i) Evaluating the victim's capacity to withstand torture (ii) Supervising torture through provision of medical treatment, if complication occurs (iii) Providing professional knowledge and skills to the torturer (iv) Falsifying or deliberately omitting medical information when issuing health certificates, or autopsy reports (v) Administering torture by directly participating in it (vi) Remaining silent in spite of the knowledge that abuse have taken place.

The most vulnerable doctors are military doctors, police and prison doctors, those in Government jobs and forensic medicine specialists. These experiences led to the adoption of a special declaration on the doctors in torture at the World Medical Assembly in Tokyo in 1975, known as the '**Tokyo Declaration**'. These are: (i) Doctor shall not countenance, condone or participate in the practice of torture or other forms of cruel inhuman or degrading procedures, whatever the offence of which the victim of such procedures is suspected, accused or guilty and whatever the victims' belief or motives and in all situations including armed conflict and civil strife. (ii) Doctor shall not provide any premises, instruments, substances or knowledge to facilitate the practice of torture or other forms of cruel, inhuman or degrading treatment or to diminish the ability of the victim to resist such treatment. (iii) Doctor shall not be present during any procedure in which torture or other forms of cruel, in human or degrading treatment is used or threatened. (iv) A doctor must have completed clinical independence in deciding upon the case of a person for which he or she is medically responsible. (v) Doctor shall in all circumstances be bound to alleviate the distress of the fellowmen and no motive whether personal, collective or political shall prevail against this higher purpose. (vi) Where a prisoner refuses nourishment and is considered by the doctor as capable of forming an unimpaired and rational judgment. Concerning the consequences of such voluntary refusal of nourishment he or she shall not be fed artificially. The decision as to capacity of the prisoner to form such a judgment should be confirmed by at least one other independent doctor, the consequences of the refusal of nourishment shall be explained by the doctor to the prisoner. (vii) The WMA will support and should encourage the international community, the national medical associations and the fellow doctors to support the doctor and his/her family in the face of threats or repraisals resulting from a refusal to condone the use of torture or other forms of cruel inhuman or degrading acts.

Statement by the International Union of Psychological Science (1976): "No psychologist in the exercise of his/her professional functions should accept instructions or motivations that are inspired by considerations that are foreign to the profession." It requests each member of society to make certain that it has enacted a code of ethics and to take those actions required by its code against any member guilty of such abuses against human rights.

Principles of Medical Ethics (United Nations 1982) relevant to the role of health personnel particularly physicians in the protection of prisoners and detainees against torture and other cruel, inhuman or degrading treatment and punishment as given by United Nations in 1982 are the following: (i) Health personnel particularly charged with the medical cases of prisoners and detainees have a duty to provide them with protection of their physical and mental health and standard as is afforded to those who are not detained or imprisoned. (ii) It is a gross contravention of medical ethics as well as an offence under applicable international instruments for health personnel particularly physicians to engage actively or passively in acts which constitute participation in complicity in incitement to or attempts to commit torture or other cruel, in human or degrading treatment or punishment. (iii) It is contravention of medical ethics for health personnel particularly physicians to be involved in any professional relationship with prisoners or detainees, the purpose of which is not solely to evaluate, protect or improve their physical and mental health. (iv) It is a contravention of medical ethics for health personnel particularly physicians: (a) To apply their knowledge and skills in order to assist in the interrogation of prisoners and detainees in a manner that may adversely affect the physical or mental health or condition of such prisoners or detainees and which is not in accordance with the relevant international instruments (b) To certify, or to participate in the certification of fitness of prisoners or detainees for any form of treatment or punishment that may adversely affect their physical or mental health and which is not in accordance with the relevant international instruments, or to participate in any way in the infliction of any such treatment or punishment which is not in accordance with the relevant international instruments. (v) It is a contravention of medical ethics for health personnel particularly physicians to participate in any procedure for restraining a person or detainee unless such a procedure is determined in accordance with purely medical criteria as being necessary and for the protection of the physical or mental health or the safety of the prisoners or detainee himself of his fellow prisoners or detainees or of his guardians and it presents no hazard to his mental or physical health. (vi) There may be no derogation from the foregoing principle on any ground whatsoever including public emergency.

Declaration of Hawaii World Psychiatric Association (1983): The declaration states that "The psychiatrist must never use his professional possibilities to violate the dignity or human rights of any individual group". If the patient or some third party demands actions contrary to scientific knowledge or ethical principles the psychiatric must refuse to cooperate.

World Conference on Human Rights (1993): The conference states that "Freedom from torture is a right which must be protected under all circumstances, including in times of internal or international disturbance or armed conflicts".

The Human Rights Act (1993): In the United States, the Human Rights Act has the principal aim to curb violation of any of the rights, including safety from torture of the individuals of this country.

The victim of torture may either suffer from injuries or may die because of injuries and therefore such cases should be carefully and thoroughly examined, reported to the police or the magistrate and treated. A proper examination may help in establishing or disproving the charge of torture both during the examination of injury and autopsy.

S. 330 and 331 I.P.C. deals with crime and punishments of voluntarily causing hurt and grievous hurt for the purpose of extorting confession or any information which may lead to the detection of an offence or misconduct. The person shall be punished with imprisonment up to 7 years with fine for voluntarily causing hurt and imprisonment up to 10 years with fine for voluntarily causing grievous hurt.

CUSTODIAL DEATHS

Custodial deaths are those occurring while a person is either in the custody of police or is an inmate of a prison. A meticulous autopsy is needed to confirm or dispel the allegations that an act of commission or omission on the part of custodians has led to, or contributed to, the death. It is sometimes helpful to the pathologist to visit the scene of the death, especially if it was caused by hanging or some form of mechanical trauma.

Situations under which death may occur in custody: The death may occur during or soon after the arrest by the police officers during physical struggle, especially when the police officers are attempting to control or overpower the resisting offender. The offender may also threaten the police officers with a knife, gun or blunt weapon and the police have to subdue him either by sheer physical force, truncheons or riot sticks or by the use of firearms. The arrest of a drunken offender poses many problems.

Causes of Deaths During Arrest

Traumatic asphyxia when several policemen fall upon a resisting offender to overpower him.

Arm locks or neck holds applied by police officers to resisting persons are other causes of deaths during arrest. The arm lock is applied either from behind or with the head of the offender tucked under the police officer's arm against the waist. The dangers are compression of the front and sides of the neck and death can occur either from reflex cardiac arrest or cerebral ischemia during carotid compression or asphyxia from airway obstruction, though the latter is unlikely to be the sole mechanism.

Blunt injury may occur from the use of fist, arm or leg and by use of a weapon such as a truncheon, riot stick or pistol butt. Any type of blunt injury may be received. Head injuries may occur during a scuffle from falls either against the ground, or against a wall or other obstruction. A heavy punch in the face may cause nasopharyngeal bleeding that can block the air-passages, especially in a person affected by alcohol. A blow on the sides of the neck can cause reflex cardiac arrest or a subarachnoid haemorrhage from vertebrobasilar artery damage. A backward blow from the point of an elbow can be damaging, if it strikes the face, neck or abdomen. Kicking and stamping are unusual, but not uncommon in custodial deaths. A blow in the abdomen can be fatal if delivered with sufficient force. Though in an adult a fist blow is not very likely to cause serious damage, it can in a very younger person. The use of the elbow, knee or a head butt can deliver extreme force, especially from a fit, muscular police officer as well as from the offender.

Alcohol is a frequent cause of death in custody and also it is major factor in provoking aggression and violent resistance. When blood alcohol levels rise to above 350 mg/100 ml there is an increasing risk of coma and central respiratory depression. At lower blood alcohol levels there is still the risk of aspiration of vomitus and choking on gastric contents. At autopsy, this aspiration should be distinguished from the common agonal phenomenon. Where an otherwise healthy person dies with a high blood alcohol concentration in these circumstances, then gross blocking of the trachea and bronchi with vomitus can be accepted as the cause of death. Alcohol also attributes to accidents during custody, especially head injuries resulting from falls on the ground, falls down steps and stairs. Falls onto a hard surface are often on the occiput and the frequent finding of frontal and temporal contrecoup brain damage at autopsy is good evidence of a deceleration injury rather than an assault with a weapon. Some falls may occur during custody or in transit from the site of arrest to the police station and the police is often blamed for allowing or causing the injury. Drugs such as amphetamine, cocaine or hallucinogen may also lead to physical damage. Drugs are commonly available within prisons and overdose and hypersensitivity deaths are occasionally seen.

Suicides in custody are quite common. Most police forces deprive the prisoner of any objects that could be used to hang himself in the cells such as belts, braces, cord or even bootlaces. In addition, the police cell may be specifically designed to avoid any convenient suspension points, such as bars, hooks, internal door handles. Nevertheless, prisoners regularly manage to find some means of killing themselves as hanging can be successfully accomplished by traction on the neck at low levels and need not occur at high suspension points, so prisoners have killed themselves by attaching ligatures to bed-heads, chairs and other unlikely objects in the cell. At autopsy homicidal hanging should be ruled out by the absence of signs of struggle and other injuries resulting in death. The person at times may be hanged after killing to simulate suicide. The situation is fully assessed preferably by a visit to the scene with the body at the site.

Natural deaths may occur from purely natural causes, usually of cardiovascular origin and no objective proof can be provided when the emotional and physical upset of being arrested and confinement may have affected the blood pressure and heart rate sufficiently, by an adrenaline response, to have precipitated an acute cardiac crisis in the presence of severe preexisting disease. The presence of diabetes, epilepsy, asthma or other diseases that can potentially cause sudden or unexpected death should be sought for by medical history and autopsy appearances.

Investigations of torture and custodial deaths: (i) All deaths in custody should be examined with care to ensure that the guardians are cleared of any suspicion of ill-treatment. (ii) Torture and custodial deaths are confirmed by circumstantial and corroborative evidence. (iii) Victim is usually in detention in or some form of custody. (iv) Such types of death are usually involved with the non-cooperating attitude of the authorities that are hostile to impartial injury. (v) Cases are handed over to the responsible authorities such as Red Cross, Amnesty International, Physicians for Human Rights. (vi) There is usually delay in the process before a victim is being brought for examination, the injuries may have healed and body may have decomposed. Body is sometimes disposed off early. (vii) Causes of deaths in torture or custodial deaths may be sepsis, haemorrhage, internal organ injury and even sheer exhaustion.

Recommendations of the National Human Rights Commission (NHRC) in Custodial Deaths and Torture: Commission requires all District Magistrates/Superintendents of the Police to report any instance of custodial death or rape directly to the commission within 24 hours of occurrence and failure to send such reports would lead to a presumption by the commission that an effort was being made to suppress the occurrence. It was made clear that third degree methods in investigation should not be used. Commission also recommended insertion of a section 114 (B) in the I.E.A.1872 to introduce a rebuttable presumption that injuries sustained by a person in police custody may be presumed to have been caused by a police officer. The recommendation of the Indian law commission that section 197 Cr.P.C. to be amended to obviate the necessity of governmental sanction for the prosecution of police officer where a prima facie case has been established in an enquiry conducted by a session's judge, of the commission of a custodial offence was endorsed. There should be a mandatory enquiry by a session's judge in each case of custodial death, rape or grievous hurt. In addition, commission believes that the arrested person being held in the custody is entitled, if he so requests to have a friend, relative or any other person who is known to him, or likely to take an interest in his welfare, to be informed that he has been arrested and told of where he has been detained. Compensation due to the next of kin of those who have died in custody should be the liability of not just the state government but of the offending police officials themselves.

NATIONAL HUMAN RIGHTS COMMISSION GUIDELINES FOR POSTMORTEM EXAMINATION

Magisterial inquiry: A magistrate inquest under section 176 Cr. P.C. to be held in all cases of custodial deaths.

Additional inquest procedure: While conducting inquest, proper assessment of "Time since death" shall be done during first examination of the body at the scene. A trained police officer or medical officer shall record the rectal temperature and ascertain the status of the rigor mortis. These observations as well as the time of its recording shall be recorded in the inquest report which would be helpful to the doctors conducting postmortem examination later.

Model postmortem report form: A model postmortem report form has been designed by NHRC to ensure quality and standardised post mortem report across the country.

Precautions to be taken: Before transportation of the dead body, both hands of the deceased need to be wrapped in white paper bags and the body should be covered in special body bags having zip pouches. The clothings of the deceased should not be disturbed before postmortem. At postmortem, the clothings should be examined, collected, sealed by the doctor and should be sent for further examination at the concerned forensic science laboratory. The findings of cloth examination should be incorporated in the postmortem report. In case of alleged firearm deaths, the body should be subjected to radiological examination (X-rays/CT scan) before postmortem. The autopsy should be conducted in a natural light and a Forensic medicine expert should conduct the autopsy.

Videography: The purpose of the videography during postmortem examination is to (i) Record the detail findings especially pertaining to injury marks and violence which may suggest custodial torture. (ii) Supplements the findings of postmortem examination by videographic evidence so as to rule out any undue influence or suppression of material evidence. (iii) Facilitate an independent review of the postmortem examination report at later stage, if required.

During postmortem, the voice of the doctor including his narration of prima facie observations should be recorded. Details regarding the name of deceased, general particulars of deceased and particulars of requisition of autopsy also should be recorded on the video. The video cassette should be immediately sealed after autopsy and dispatched to the inquest authority who in turn send it to commission.

Photography: Multiple coloured photographs (20 to 25) covering the whole body should be taken. Few photographs should be taken before removing the clothes. Photographs should be taken after incorporating postmortem number, date of examination and scale for dimensions in the frame of the photographs itself. A good quality camera with 10X optical zoom and minimum 10 mega pixels should be used. While taking photographs, the camera should be held at right-angle to the object being photographed.

Both videography and photography should be done by a person trained in forensic videography and photography.

The photographs should include (i) Profile photo-face (front, right lateral and left lateral views), back of head. (ii) Front of body (upto torso-chest and abdomen) and back. (iii) Front and back of upper extremity. (iv) Front and back of lower extremity. (v) Focussing on each injury/lesion-zoomed in after proper numbering the injuries. (vi) Internal examination findings (2 photos of soles and palms each, after making incision to show absence/evidence of any old/deep seated injury).

In case of firearm death, the injuries should be described in relation to the distance from heel, from the midline and distance from each other which will help later in reconstruction of events.

Viscera analysis: Viscera can be kept for toxicological analysis in some cases. However, the viscera report takes some time in coming and therefore the postmortem report and other documents should be sent to commission without waiting for the viscera report. The viscera report should be sent subsequently as soon as it received.

Submission of reports: The postmortem report, videography and inquest papers must be sent to the commission within 2 months of incident.

Family Violence

It is the physical, sexual and psychological violence that occurs in the family, including battering, sexual abuse of female children in the household, dowry-related violence, marital rape, female genital mutilation and other traditional practices harmful to women, non-spousal violence, and violence related to exploitation. It is also called **domestic violence.**

Any one can be affected by family violence, regardless of their age, gender, sexual identity, cultural background, ability, religion, wealth, status or location. According to the World Health Organization (WHO) 1 in every 3 women across the globe experience physical and/or sexual violence in their life time. As per National Crime Record Bureau (NCRB), in year 2019, domestic violence figures at the top in violence against women and majority of cases were registered under 'Cruelty by Husband or His Relatives'.

As per National Human Rights Commission, domestic violence is considered as violation of human rights. The commission issues advisory for combating such violence and promoting women's rights in general.

THE PROTECTION OF WOMEN FROM DOMESTIC VIOLENCE ACT, 2005

The Act came into force from 26 October 2006. It is a civil law with criminal procedures to ensure effective protection and immediate relief to victims of violence of any kind occurring within the family. The Act recognizes a woman's right to live in a violence-free home.

Salient Features

1. The Act defines **domestic violence** for the first time in Indian law which is in consonance with the UN Model Legislation on Domestic Violence. It includes not only physical violence but also other forms of violence such as sexual, verbal, emotional or economic abuse. Harassment by way of unlawful dowry demands to the woman or her relatives would also be covered under this definition.
2. **Aggrieved person** means any woman who is, or has been, in a domestic relationship with the respondent and who alleges to have been subjected to any act of domestic violence by the respondent (section 2(a)).
3. **Respondent** means any adult male person who is, or has been, in a domestic relationship with the aggrieved person and against whom the aggrieved person has sought any relief or any male or female relative of the husband or male partner of a married woman or a woman in relationship in the nature of marriage (section 2(q)).
4. **Domestic relationship** means a relationship between two persons who live or have, at any point of time, lived together in a shared household, when they are related by consanguinity, marriage, or through a relationship in the nature of marriage, adoption or are family members living together as a joint family (section 2(f)).
5. **Protection officer** means an officer appointed by the State Government (Section 8(1)). The officer preferably should be women and qualified. The duties and responsibilities of the protection officer includes filling domestic incidence report, providing shelter home, medical facilities and legal aid to the victims. The officer shall be under the control and supervision of the Magistrate (Section 9).
6. **Service providers** means any voluntary association registered under appropriate law or other assistance registered as a service provider for the purpose of this Act (Section 10). A service provider registered under sub-section (1) shall have the power to: (a) Recording of domestic incident report in the prescribed form and forwarding to the Magistrate and the protection officer (b) Getting the aggrieved person medically examined and forwarding to the Magistrate and the protection officer (c) Ensure that the aggrieved person is provided shelter in a shelter home (d) No suit, prosecution or other legal proceeding shall lie against any service provider for action in good faith.
7. **Information to protection officer and exclusion of liability of informant (Section 4):** (a) Any person who has reason to believe that an act of domestic violence has been, or is being, or is likely to be committed, may give information about it to the concerned protection officer. (b) No liability, civil or criminal, shall be incurred by any person for giving in good faith of information for the purpose of sub-section (a). The information/complain can be given to police officer or magistrate.

8. **Duties of medical facilities (Section 3):** If an aggrieved person or, on her behalf a protection officer or a service provider requests the person in charge of a medical facility to provide any medical aid to her, such person in charge of the medical facility shall provide medical aid to the aggrieved person in the medical facility.
9. **Relief available (Sections 14, 15, 17, 18, 19, 20 21, 22):** A woman can seek a protection order, monetary compensation, residency order, custody order, free legal services, medical aid and counselling with the help of the protection officer or service provider. The magistrate may issue the protection order. Woman cannot be evicted from the shared household and if evicted can seek immediate relief. The custody of children may be granted to the victim as required, with visiting rights to the respondent, if necessary.
10. **Proceedings to be held *in camera* (Section 16):** If the Magistrate considers that the circumstances of the case so warrant, and if either party to the proceedings so desires, he may conduct the proceedings under this Act *in camera*.
11. **Penalties:** (a) *Penalty for breach of protection order by respondent* shall be punishable with imprisonment upto one year, or with fine upto Rs 20,000, or with both (Section 31). The offence is cognizable and non-bailable (b) *Penalty for not discharging duty by protection officer* shall be punishable with imprisonment upto one year, or with fine upto Rs. 20,000, or with both (Section 33).

LONG QUESTIONS

1. Discuss the autopsy findings in a case of death due to torture.
2. How to investigate a case of custodial death?

SHORT QUESTIONS

1. Torture.
2. NHRC guidelines for custodial deaths.
3. Falanga.

MULTIPLE CHOICE QUESTIONS

1. **Producing impairment in hearing by beating both ears simultaneously is called:**

   (a) Telefono (b) Baton

   (c) Submarine (d) Falanga

2. **Covering and tying of plastic bag over the head in custodial torture is called:**

   (a) Falanga (b) Dry submarine

   (c) Telefono (d) Cold torture

3. **Beating of the soles of feet with canes and rods in custodial torture is called:**

   (a) Dry submarine

   (b) Telefono

   (c) Wet submarine

   (d) Falanga

ANSWER KEY ☞

1. (a)	2. (b)	3. (d)

24 CHAPTER

Asphyxial Deaths

GORDON'S CLASSIFICATION OF DEATH

Gordon in 1944 postulated that vital functions of the body depend upon the availability and utilization of oxygen by the body tissues and tissue anoxia finally leads to cardiac failure and death. It is a classification that lays stress on the pathogenesis in different forms of death of medicolegal importance. It is brought about in following four ways:

1. **Anoxic anoxia:** Defective oxygenation of the blood in the lungs: (i) *By obstruction to air passage:* Suffocation, smothering, overlaying (ii) *By obstruction to the passage of air down to the respiratory tract:* Drowning, choking, throttling, hanging and strangulation (iii) Excessive compression of the chest and abdominal wall (iv) Primary cessation of respiratory movements causing respiratory failure as in narcotic poisoning, electrical injury (v) Inhalation of carbon dioxide and inert gases.
2. **Anaemic anoxia:** Reduced oxygen carrying capacity of the blood as in acute poisoning due to CO, chlorates, nitrites.
3. **Histotoxic anoxia:** Depression of the oxidative process in the tissues as in hydrocyanic acid poisoning.
4. **Stagnant anoxia:** Insufficient circulation of the blood in the tissue as in traumatic shock, heat stroke, acute irritant and corrosive poisoning.

The term **asphyxia** is commonly applied to a variety of conditions in which interference with respiratory exchange occurs to a greater or lesser degree. Many of these conditions vary so greatly in their physiological mechanisms and in their pathological appearances they present that the use of the term is best avoided, whenever possible. It is usual to divide the effects of asphyxia into a number of stages: (i) Stage of inspiratory dyspnoea with deep and forceful respiration, cyanosis lasting for a minute or so. (ii) Stage of expiratory dyspnoea with spasmodic efforts at expiration. During this stage, the consciousness is lost, pupils are dilated and blood pressure is raised. (iii) There is fall of blood pressure, pulse is increased and spontaneous defecation occurs. The erection of penis and ejaculation of semen may occur. (iv) Respiratory movements cease except for terminal irregular occasional respiration. Heart continues to beat for 10-15 minutes.

MECHANICAL ASPHYXIA

Mechanical asphyxia is a term applied to circumstances in which mechanical interferences to the respiration occurs that either: (i) Impedes access of air to lungs; or (ii) Reduces blood supply to head and neck; or (iii) Causes sudden cardiac arrest due to stimulation of carotid sinus with resulting vagal reflex mechanism. The examples of mechanical asphyxia listed in Figure 24.1.

It is doubtful if there are any constant postmortem changes produced by the direct effect of anoxia upon the tissues except the appearance of cyanosis. There are abnormal appearances of respiratory obstruction in the form of local effects of the constricting agent, raised intravascular pressure and terminal heart failure.

Classical Signs of Asphyxia

The classical signs of asphyxia are nonspecific and can occur in deaths from other causes.

1. **Cyanosis (In Greek meaning 'dark blue') (Figure 24.2):**

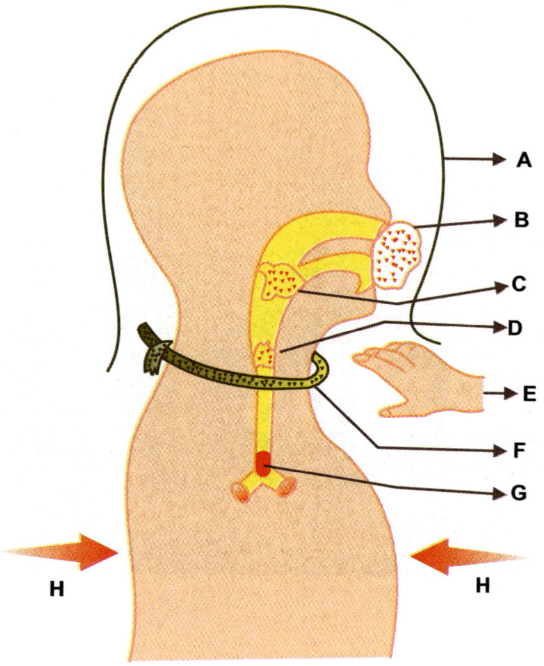

Figure 24.1: (A) Impermeable plastic head cover (B) Pad over mouth and nostrils (suffocation) (C) Gag in pharynx (gagging) (D) Foods bolus or an object in larynx (choking) (E) Manual strangulation by hands (throttling) (F) Ligature of hanging or strangulation (G) Blockage of trachea with food/vomitus (aspiration) (H) Pressure on chest (traumatic asphyxia)

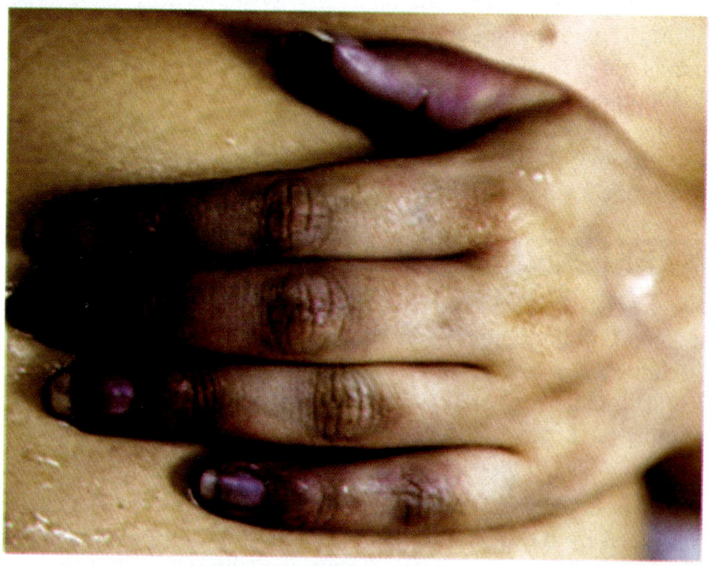

Figure 24.2: Bluish discolouration of nails in asphyxia

Significance of cyanosis in a cadaver must be evaluated very critically. Cyanosis depends upon the absolute quantity of oxyhaemoglobin and reduced haemoglobin in red cells. The normal pink colour of well-oxygenated blood may change to purple or blue when oxygen is lacking. Cutaneous cyanosis depends upon absolute amount of reduced haemoglobin, rather than amount of reduced oxyhemoglobin. There must be at least 5 gm% of reduced haemoglobin before cyanosis becomes evident, irrespective of total amount of haemoglobin. In constriction of neck, cyanosis almost invariably follows congestion of face, as venous blood contains much reduced haemoglobin. After perfusion to head and trunk, it is directed back to tissues that becomes bluer as blood accumulates. When the airway becomes blocked, then impaired oxygenation in the lungs leads to a diminution in the oxygen content of tissues, which leads to darkening of organs and tissues and accentuates the cyanosis of face.

This depends upon complete or substantial obstruction of the airway or restriction of respiratory excursions of the chest. If the body is examined within few hours of death, presence of intense cyanosis is of some significance. The loss of oxygen of cadaveric blood is very variable, but certainly after 24 hours the appearance of cyanosis may be due entirely to postmortem changes. Absence of cyanosis within few hours of death does not necessarily signify that cyanosis was not present at death. Terminal cyanosis is common in many forms of death and its presence is seldom of much use in the diagnosis of respiratory obstruction.

2. **Congestion:** Visceral congestion is due to capillovenous congestion and is the result of susceptibility of capillaries to hypoxia. This results in dilatation of capillaries with stasis of blood in the dilated capillaries and the venules. Systemic and pulmonary congestion and dilatation of right side heart are signs of asphyxial death. Their significance should be treated with greater reserve than the presence of cyanosis. There is considerable redistribution of blood in the cadaver under the influence of gravity and to some extent by rigor mortis. The effect of these factors also depends upon the fluidity of blood after death.

   Right ventricular dilatation and pulmonary congestion are common to many forms of death and by no means specific for death from interference with respiration. Conversely, when death is due to blockade of airway, one may fail to find this phenomenon. Furthermore, the size of heart chambers can alter with rigor mortis and so the amount of blood in the pulmonary circulation. Congestion immediately above a mark on the neck may be of great significance in the diagnosis of the cause of the mark.

3. **Fluidity of blood:** At one time, it was thought that fluid blood in the cadaver was an indication of asphyxia. The presence of fibrinolytic enzymes in the cadaver has been established, so fluidity depends upon fibrinolysin and the amount of fibrinolysin depends upon the rapidity of death rather than the nature.

4. **Pulmonary oedema:** Some degree of pulmonary oedema is common but not invariable in deaths associated with anoxia. It is debatable whether it is due to heart failure or increased capillary permeability. It has little or no value in the diagnosis of death due to respiratory obstruction. It is common in many modes of death. In anoxial deaths oedema of anything more than a minor degree indicates that death has not been very

rapid. Lungs should be weighed properly to know the extent of oedema.

5. **Pulmonary haemorrhages:** Large submucosal haemorrhages in pharynx especially over the dorsum of cricoid is due to direct trauma of this part against anterior surface of spine. Submucous venous plexus at this site is made of very large thin walled vessels and rupture of these vessels is due to severe venous congestion. These haemorrhages are also found in variety of deaths unconnected with trauma.

6. **Petechial haemorrhages (Figures 24.3 and 24.4):** In the year 1866, **Tardieu** a French police surgeon described when he found them beneath the pleura and pericardium. He was of the opinion that these haemorrhages were the pathognomic of mechanical asphyxia. Later on, these haemorrhages were known as **Tardieu's spots.** Injuries to the walls of the epithelium may result in the development of petechial haemorrhages. Until 1944, **Lime and Gordon** questioned their significance as they had found it in many forms of death. In 1953 **Gordon, Trevor and Trice** also found it in secondary shock and natural cases. In 1955, **Gordon and Mansfield** questioned their antemortem origin as they commonly developed after death and were found during autopsy. In 1955, **Shapiro** again opined that some of these are spontaneous postmortem artefacts and disappeared in a short period. This disappearance was confirmed and depicted in the year **1981 by Zaini** and **Knight** who considered them to diminish when intravenous pressure is reduced in major pulmonary vessels at autopsy. They found that it was difficult to distinguish between true and false petechiae by naked eye examination. Only one third of these haemorrhages are true and two thirds are false. These false haemorrhages were due to intrapleural venous channels air blisters, thickened pleural plaques and dust pigments. They are mostly unrelated to mechanical asphyxia. Tardieu spots develop from: (i) Increased venous stasis causing congestion leading to increased pressure causing rupture of the vessels (ii) Increased permeability due to hypoxia.

   Tardieu spots are usually pinhead, but vary in size and shape. They may be scanty, detectable under low magnification or may be numerous like measles rash involving the skin of the face and eyelids, beneath the conjunctiva etc. These are most prominent in the visceral pleura and epicardium. The most common site in the heart is atrioventricular fissure whereas in the lungs it is the base and interlobar fissure. Examination of petechial haemorrhages for evidence of injury and its severity should be done.

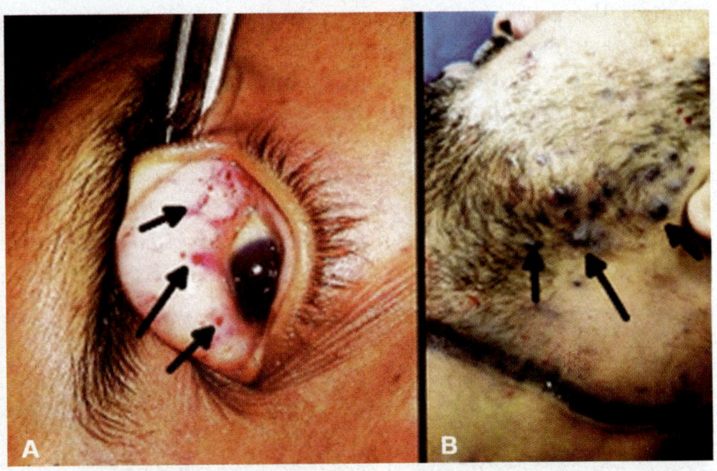

Figure 24.3A, B: Petechial haemorrhages in conjunctivae (A) and over face (B)

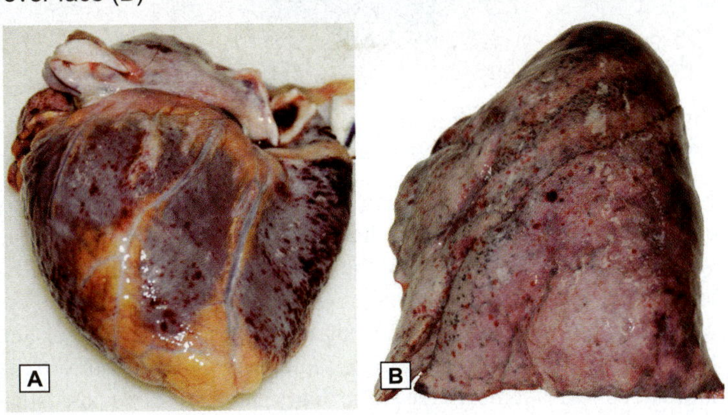

Figure 24.4A, B: Petechial haemorrhages over heart (A) and lung (B)

7. **Stasis haemorrhages:** These haemorrhages may be seen beneath the mucosa of larynx in the subglottic space and above the level of constriction of the ligature as in homicidal strangulation. These are produced by venous stasis leading to rupture of the capillaries.

   These can be seen in: (i) Coronary deaths (ii) In terminal stages of asphyxia (iii) Various diseased states (iv) Epilepsy (v) Electrocution (vi) Metallic poisoning. The haemorrhages found in diseases are small with greater distribution and more in number. Blood examination may reveal the underlying cause but laboratory findings may be misleading.

8. **Sudden cardiac arrest:** There are cases where these findings such as petechial haemorrhages, cyanosis, congestion etc. are present but death is rapid and diagnosed as sudden cardiac arrest as that in café coronary. In **Knight's** experience, 50% of his cases where death occurred from mechanical asphyxia, cause was sudden cardiac arrest, as the cyanosis, haemorrhages or congestions were absent. These cases were deaths resulting from karate blows to the neck, mugging and drowning. Sudden death might occur due to cardiac arrest and accurate history of the circumstances of the death is important. Sudden collapse and loss of consciousness is the outstanding feature. Heartbeat or breathing may continue for 15-30 seconds and there might be atrial fibrillation. An important factor is evidence of surprise, emotion, apprehension or fright. Alcoholic intoxication is commonly present. If no injury or slight injury is present over the body then the diagnosis of acute cardiac arrest is made.

Classification of Asphyxial Deaths

1. **Hanging:** (i) *Mode of hanging:* (a) Judicial (b) Sexual (Autoerotic) (c) Lynching (homicidal hanging) (ii) *Manner of hanging:* (a) Suicidal hanging (b) Homicidal hanging (c) Accidental hanging (iii) *Position of noose:* (a) Typical hanging (b) Atypical hanging (iv) *Position of feet:* (a) Complete hanging (b) Partial hanging (partial standing, sitting, reclining or kneeling position.
2. **Strangulation:** (i) Ligature strangulation (ii) Manual strangulation (throttling) (iii) Mugging (iv) Garroting (v) Bansdola (vi) Palmar strangulation (vii) Strangulation with bend of knee/elbow (viii) Foot strangulation.
3. **Suffocation:** (i) Smothering (a) Overlaying (b) Burking (ii) Gagging (iii) Choking (iv) Café coronary (v) Traumatic asphyxia.
4. **Drowning:** (i) Dry drowning (ii) Wet drowning (iii) Secondary drowning (iv) Immersion syndrome.

HANGING

Hanging is a form of asphyxial death, which is caused by the suspension of the body by a ligature that encircles the neck, the constricting force being the weight of the body. Asphyxia in hanging is secondary to compression or constriction of the neck structures by a noose or other constricting band tightened by the weight of the body.

Types of Hanging

Complete hanging: This is the type of hanging when the constricting force is the weight of the body as the body is fully suspended in air (Figure 24.5A, B).

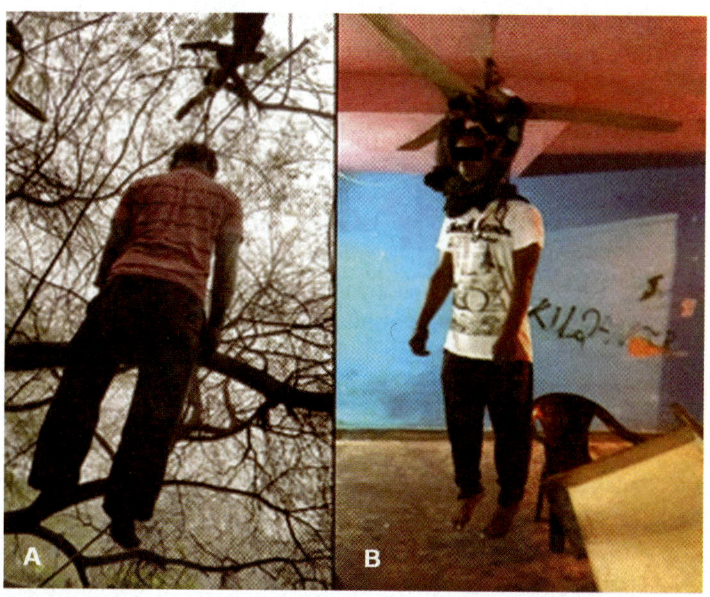

Figure 24.5A, B: Cases of complete hanging–body not touching the ground

Partial (incomplete) hanging: In this type of hanging, the constricting force is the weight of the head (about 5-6 kg) and the lower part of the body such as toes, feet, knees or buttocks touches the ground (Figure 24.6A, B, C).

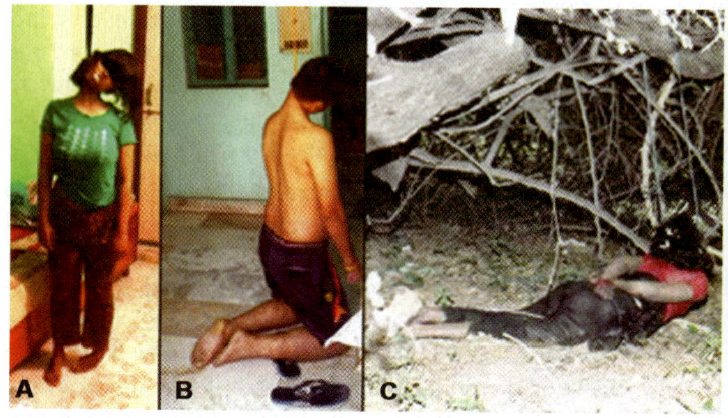

Figure 24.6A, B, C: Cases of partial hanging with body parts touching the ground in different positions–Standing (A), kneel down (B) and prone position (C)

Ligature mark: On the neck, ligature mark will be in the form of a furrow. This furrow, as a rule, does not completely encircle the neck, but slants upwards, towards the knot, fading out at the point of suspension that is the knot. If the knot is under the chin, the site of the knot may be indicated by an abrasion or indentation beneath the chin. The clarity and configuration of the ligature mark depends upon the material used. The ligature mark produces a groove or furrow, which may be pale, yellowish or yellow brown and look like parchment due to drying of the abraded skin (Figure 24.7A). It is usually inverted 'V' shaped with the apex of the 'V' at the knot (Figure 24.7B). Impression

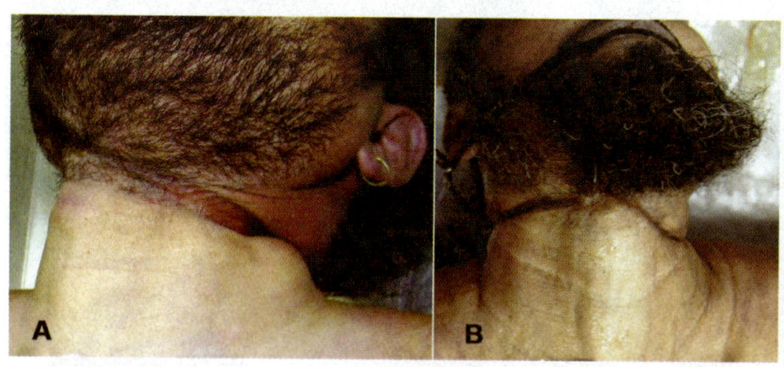

Figure 24.7A, B: Cases of hanging showing brownish, parchment like ligature mark (A, B) and inverted 'V'-shaped ligature mark (B)

of the knot may be found, depending upon its position. Along the edges of the depression, a thin line of congestion or haemorrhage will be seen above and below the groove at some point, usually at the deepest. Ecchymosis and slight abrasion in the groove are rare. Ecchymosis alone has no significance but it is important to establish whether hanging is antemortem or postmortem. Abrasions with haemorrhage are strongly suggestive of suspension taking place during life. There may not be any visible mark due to beard, long hair, clothes intervening between the ligature material and the neck. Decomposition obliterates ligature mark. It may disappear after several hours when the loop is removed.

Position of ligature mark: In 80% cases, ligature mark is present above the thyroid cartilage, in 15% at the level and in 5% it is present below the thyroid cartilage (common in partial hanging). The width of the groove is about or slightly less than the width of the ligature material. A definite pattern may be seen but when fresh, the ligature mark is less clear. After drying it becomes well marked.

On microscopical examination, in case of antemortem hanging signs of vital reaction are present in the neck structures. The absence of vital reaction however does not exclude an antemortem hanging.

The appearance of the furrow over the neck varies with the following factors:

1. **Type of ligature material:** In hanging, a simple slipknot type of noose is typically used. The noose is constructed from anything that is handy. Most common are ropes, dupatta, sari, electrical cords, wires, strings, belts and any piece of cloth or any other material that is available at that moment. Even in jails or prisons, the convict may use his own clothes to hang. The usual point of suspension is the side of the neck, followed by the back or front. At the time of suspension, the noose typically slips above the larynx, catching under the chin. A rope will give a deep, well-demarcated, distinct furrow, often with a mirror image impression of the weave of the rope on the skin. This furrow initially has a pale yellow, parchment appearance, with a congested rim. With time, the furrow dries out and becomes dark brown. A rough ligature material like coir rope or nylone rope can produce **rope burns** (Figures 24.8A, 24.21A). Friction of rope against the skin generates considerable amount of heat leading to second degree burn and blister formation (Figure 24.8B). It is a feature of antemortem hanging. If the ligature material is a soft material, the ligature mark may be poorly defined, pale and devoid of bruises and abrasions. In some cases, the lower margin of the groove (ligature mark) is pale with upper margin red due to postmortem congestion of vessels. A soft broad cloth such as a towel, *dhoti* or *scarf* may show faint or no ligature mark over the neck (Figure 24.9A, B). In majority of suicidal hangings, the ligature consists of a single loop and mark. If the noose is a belt, it will produce two parallel ligature marks, as the upper and lower edges of the belt will dig into the skin. Less commonly, ligature consists of two loops. This results in two furrows which may be parallel, overlap at points or follow two completely different paths, for example, one oblique and other horizontal (Figure 24.10 A, B). The two loops may pinch the skin between them, producing a haemorrhagic strip of skin. If a soft noose is used and the body is brought down by cutting the ligature shortly after death, no marks of ligature may be present on the skin. The groove will be narrow, deep and distinct when a thin and hard ligature is used. The mark becomes more prominent when it has been suspended for long. When the ligature is broad such as *dupatta,* strip of cloth, *sari,* the furrow will be broad and shallow.

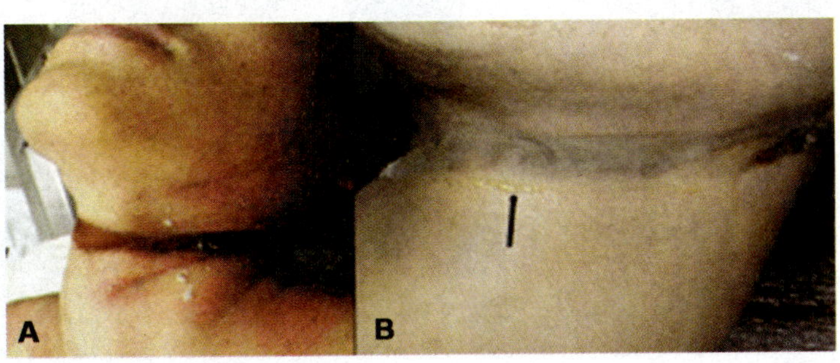

Figure 24.8A, B: Rope burns (A) and blister formation at the margin of the ligature mark (B) in hanging

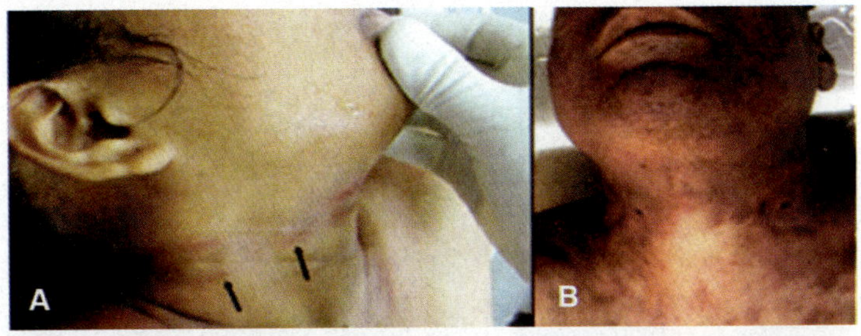

Figure 24.9A, B: Faint ligature mark (A) no visible ligature mark (B) in hanging cases

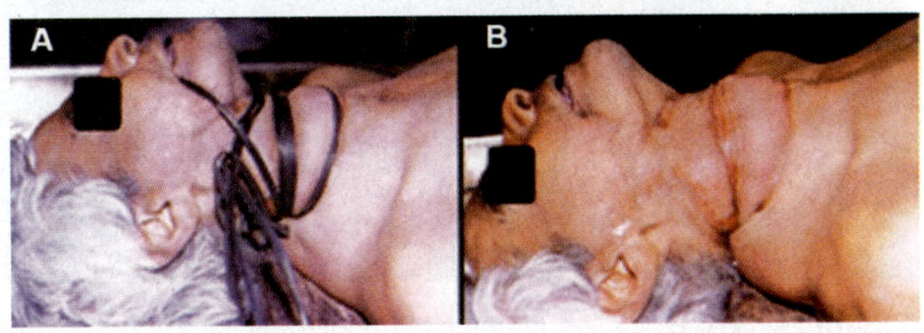

Figure 24.10A, B: Ligature mark in the form of multiple furrows in hanging

2. **Point of suspension:** Usually, the ligature mark is deepest opposite the point of suspension. In addition, rarely there may be scratch abrasions above and below the ligature when the victim tries to undo the noose during terminal stages.
3. **Type of hanging:** When the hanging is complete, the ligature mark is more prominent while in partial hanging there may be little or no mark at all.
4. **Tightness of ligature:** When the ligature is tightly present around the neck, the mark is more marked.
5. **Time of suspension:** The longer the body remains suspended the deeper is the ligature mark.
6. **Position of the knot:** The main force to the neck is applied opposite to the point of suspension. When the knot is present over the occipital region **(typical hanging)** (Figure 24.11A, B) the front of the neck shows a prominent ligature mark. When the knot at any other point it is known as **atypical**

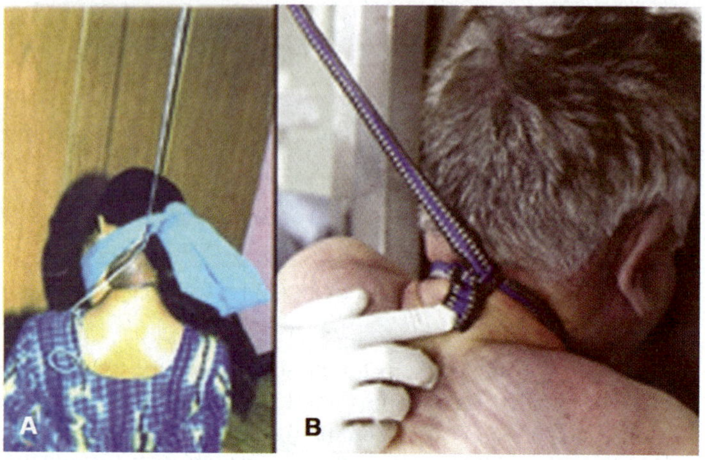

Figure 24.11A, B: Cases of typical hanging with knot at the occiput

hanging (Figure 24.12A, B). Absence of knot on the noose in hanging is rare (Figure 24.13).

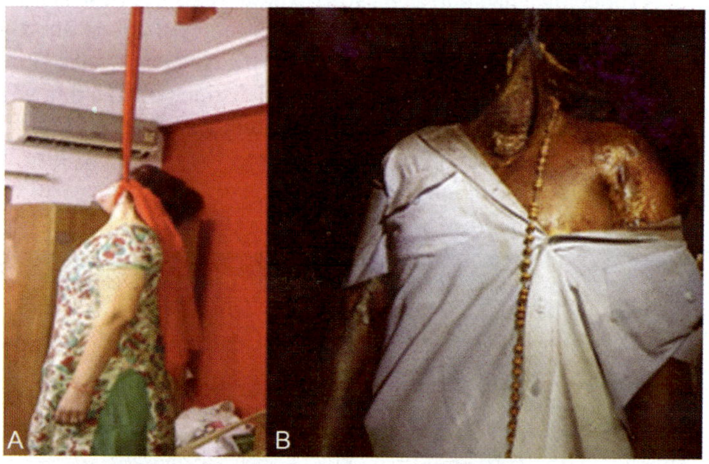

Figure 24.12A, B: Cases of atypical hanging with knot at the side of neck (A) and front of neck with partial decapitation by ligature (B)

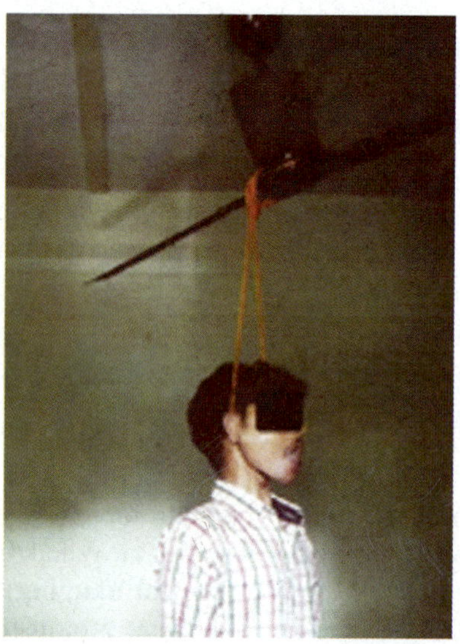

Figure 24.13: Absence of knot in ligature in hanging case

7. **Slipping of ligature:** It may cause a double impression of a single turn of ligature material. Occasionally, the ligature can be slipped over to the face and mark may be present (Figure 24.14A, B).

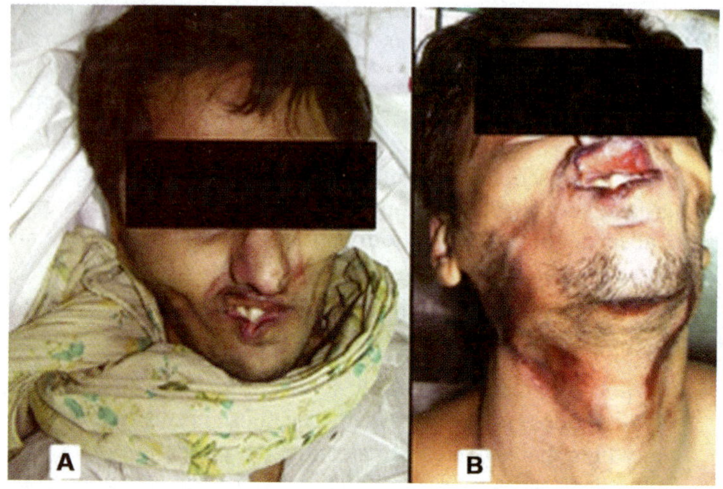

Figure 24.14A, B: Slippage of ligature over the face (A) and injuries over lower face (B) in suicidal hanging

8. **Knot:** Usually a simple slipknot is made to produce a running noose fixed by granny or reef knot. At times simple loop is used. It is placed either on sides or over occiput, but rarely under chin. Knot is higher than the ligature. Removal of the noose is done by cutting the noose away from the knot and ends are tied with string/wire.
9. **Padding below the ligature on neck:** In suicidal hanging (Figure 24.15A) and during autoerotic asphyxial activity, protection of the neck by padding may occasionally occur, possibly to reduce the pain from ligature compression or to prevent chafing. The ligature mark may be masked or not visible in such case. The victim may also insert own fingers between the ligature and the neck (Figure 24.15B). This can

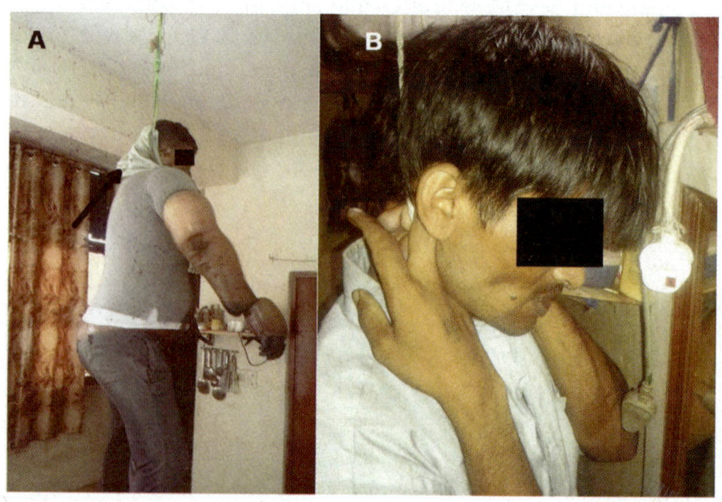

Figure 24.15A, B: Padding below the ligature (A), hands underneath the ligature (B) in suicidal hanging

produce a very unusual pattern injury with the ligature mark on either side of the neck interrupted by vertical marks due to the position of the fingers. Irregular scratches may occur from agonal movements of a victim's hands in suicidal hanging (Byard *et al.,* 2015).

In most hangings, the face is pale and tongue is protruding and is black due to drying (Figure 24.13) except in partially suspended individuals where the noose is tightened only by the weight of the head or the torso. In these instances, while venous drainage is completely occluded, the blood supply of the vertebral arteries continues in part producing congestion of the face and petechiae. Blood will pool in the dependent areas of the body, usually the forearms, hands and legs secondary to gravity. With time punctate haemorrhages and Tardieu's spots due to hydrostatic rupture of the vessels will be seen.

Prior to the removal of the noose from the neck, it should be described in detail as to the nature and composition, width, mode of application, location and type of knot. After removal of the noose, the ligature mark on the neck should be described in detail. One should describe the location of ligature mark over the neck in relation to anatomical landmark, direction of the furrow as obliquely upward or horizontal, continuous or interrupted, its colour and dimensions and whether there is distinct imprint of the pattern of the ligature over the neck.

Causes of death: Death in hanging is due to compression of the blood vessels of the neck such that insufficient amount of oxygenated blood reaches the brain. Obstruction of the airway can also occur and is due to either compression of the trachea or, when the noose is above the larynx, elevation and posterior displacement of the tongue and floor of the mouth. Blockage or compression of the air passages is not necessary to cause death in hanging. A number of individuals have hanged themselves with the noose above the larynx and a permanent tracheostomy opening below. As only a small amount of pressure is sufficient to occlude carotid arteries, quite commonly one can hang oneself in sitting, kneeling or lying down position. The weight of the head (10-12 lb) against a noose is sufficient to occlude the carotid arteries and cause death. Fracture of the neck plays virtually no role in non-judicial hangings. It is extremely rare and is usually seen only in individuals with advanced degenerative diseases of cervical spine such as osteoarthritis, accompanying complete suspension of the body, a sudden drop, and frequently obesity or very old age.

Causes of immediate death: In hanging immediate death can be caused by the following mechanisms:

1. **Asphyxia:** Ligature forces the root of tongue against the posterior wall of pharynx, and folds the epiglottis over the entrance of larynx to block the airway. A weight of 15 kg is required to compress the trachea to cause asphyxia.
2. **Venous congestion:** Jugular venous cerebral circulation can be stopped with a pressure of 2 kg on the neck.
3. **Cerebral anemia:** Carotid arteries require a pressure of 4-5 kg to stop the flow of blood in them while vertebral arteries require 30 kg of pressure.
4. **Reflex vagal inhibition:** Vagal sheath or carotid bodies when compressed can get stimulated and cause vagal inhibition of the heart causing it to stop.
5. Fracture dislocation of cervical vertebrae leading to injury to the spinal cord. As a result, there is ascending oedema that affects the vital centers in the medulla.

Causes of delayed death: In hanging delayed death occur due to the following reasons: (i) Aspiration pneumonia (ii) Infections (iii) Hypoxic encephalopathy (iv) Oedema of lungs (v) Encephalitis (vi) Cerebral abscess.

Autopsy Findings

External Findings

General findings: Typical asphyxial signs are present in about 50-60% of all hangings. These are: (i) Neck may be stretched and elongated and rarely may be severed from the body if the weight of the body is too heavy and the fall is from a greater height. (ii) Head is bent opposite to the knot. (iii) Face is usually pale but at times it may be congested and swollen. Swelling disappears when the ligature is cut down. (iv) A dried rivulet of saliva often runs from a corner of the mouth down the chest, which is an indicator of antemortem hanging. It is caused due to the stimulation of salivary glands by the ligature. The salivary stain may dribble over to the face, neck and sometimes chest (Figure 24.16). (v) Blood tinged fluid may be present in the nostrils. (vi) Petechiae on the skin and conjunctiva are present. (vii) Signs of asphyxia are more marked when the noose is high up in the throat. (viii) If only veins are obstructed there is engorgement of head and

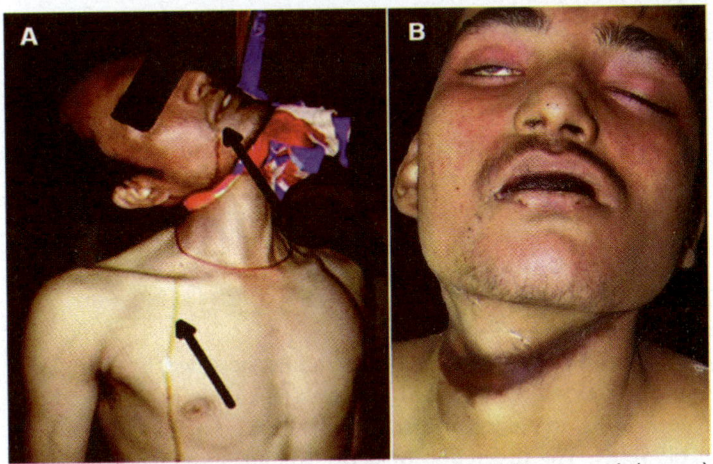

Figure 24.16A, B: A case of hanging showing salivary mark (arrow) over the angle of mouth and chest (A), Le Facies sympathique–closed eye on the side of knot and opened eye with dilation of pupil opposite side (B)

neck. (ix) Eyes are protruded and firm due to congestion or may be closed and the pupil is dilated. (x) Tongue is swollen, coming out between the lips. Tip may be black due to drying and may be clenched between the teeth (Figure 24.7A). (xi) Slight haemorrhage or bloody froth is sometimes seen caused by congestion in the lungs and pulmonary oedema. (xii) In the head sometimes haemorrhages are present due to rupture of engorged vessels. (xiii) In the middle ear haemorrhages may be seen due to rupture of the small blood vessels. (xiv) Penis may show semen drops coming out of the urethral meatus. (xv) Lower limbs show hypostasis (Figure 24.17) due to the prolonged hanging posture and are an indicator of the duration of hanging and later on seen on the back when the body is laid down. (xvi) In few cases **postmortem petechial haemorrhages** may be seen in the lower limbs. These haemorrhages are differentiated from the Tardieu's spots, being larger in size and bilaterally symmetrical. They are due to rupture of capillaries in lower limbs due to pressure of accumulated blood.

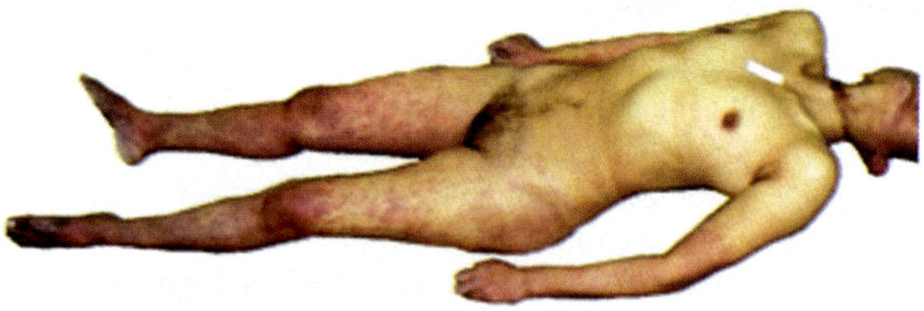

Figure 24.17: Hypostasis in lower part of both limbs in hanging

Local findings: (i) Ligature mark over the neck (ii) Usually, except for the ligature mark, no other injuries are present over the body. However, when other injuries are present they should be carefully interpreted whether they are self-induced, occurred during convulsive phase preceding death, produced when body was brought down, during attempted resuscitation, when the swinging body contacted other objects or were produced by a second party in a homicide.

Differential Diagnosis of Ligature Mark

(i) Skin folds on the neck of infants simulate a ligature mark, especially after refrigeration of the body has caused coagulation of the subcutaneous fat. (ii) Swelling of the neck due to decomposition and jewellery of the neck or clothing causing the ligature mark.

Internal Findings

The dissection of neck structures should be ruled by following two considerations: (i) Need for an extensive exposure; and (ii) Necessity of avoiding artefacts from seepage of blood from the neck veins. The dissection of neck structures should be done *in situ* in a relatively blood free field after the cranial cavity, chest and abdomen is opened and the organs removed. **Schrader (1940)** drew attention to artefacts and recommended that neck should be drained of blood by removing the brain and dissecting heart followed by the dissection of neck structures done *in situ*.

On examination of internal structures of the neck in 83 consecutive cases prospectively by **DiMaio**, no injuries (Figure 24.18) were seen in more than 50% of the cases. Absence of petechiae in most hangings is because there is complete obstruction of the arterial system, so there is no pooling of blood in the head, no increased pressure and thus no petechiae. The fractures of the hyoid bone and thyroid cartilage are considered antemortem when there is blood at the fracture site. Tissues under the mark are dry, white and glistening. Ecchymosis may be seen in the muscles.

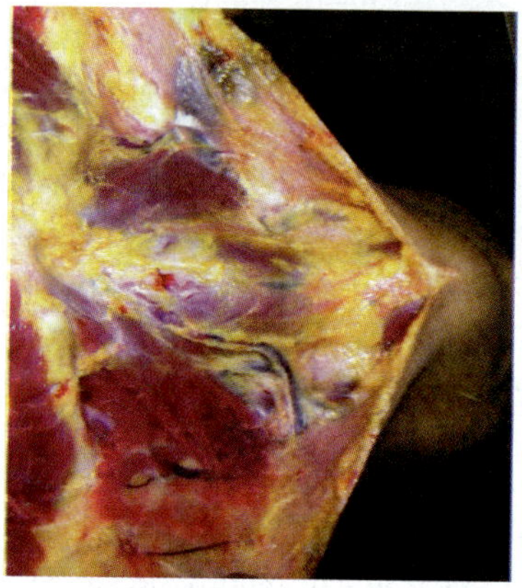

Figure 24.18: Absence of extravasation of blood in the soft tissues of neck in a case of hanging

Neck muscles, the sternomastoid and platysma are ruptured in about 10-15% cases if considerable violence is involved during hanging. Carotid artery may show transverse tear in the intima (**Amussat's sign**) (Figure 24.19). This is due direct compression of the artery by the rope and indirect stretching because of the gravitational drag produced by the weight of the body. It is a nonspecific finding in hanging and can also be found in blunt neck trauma, extreme overstretching, or whiplash-injuries. In long drop tears may be seen at different places. Vertebral artery may show rupture at place. Hyoid bone is fractured in 15-20% cases but it is rare below the age of 40 years due to elasticity of cartilage and the mobility of joints. It is more common above 40 years and is usually found at the greater horn and junction of inner 2/3 and outer

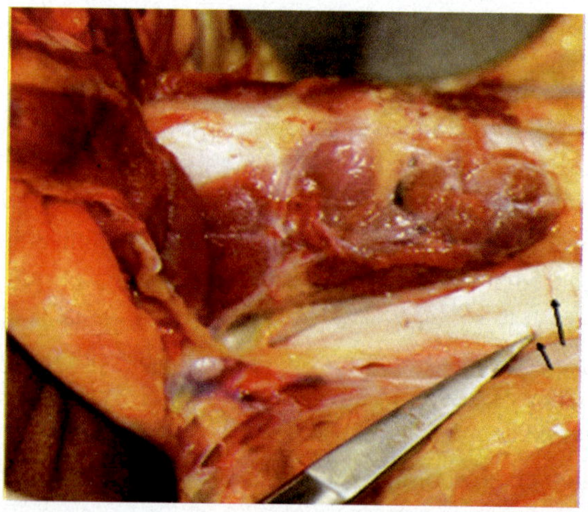

Figure 24.19: Arrow showing transverse tears (arrow) in the intima of carotid artery (Amussat's sign)

1/3. Thyroid cartilage is fractured in about 40-45% of the cases. Superior horn is fractured or the thyrohyoid ligament is torn. Visual inspection reveals petechial haemorrhages over the epiglottis, trachea and larynx. Abdominal organs are congested and in the brain subarachnoid effusions are commonly seen. **Simon's bleedings** are stripe-like haemorrhages present on anterior aspect of the intervertebral disks of the lumbar part of the spinal column in hanging. It may be due to the traction force on the spine resulted from free suspension of the body and agonal convulsions. These are considered as typical sign of vitality in cases of hanging, but more frequently present in complete suspension than in cases with incomplete suspension. However, these are also not specific for hanging, can also be present in cases of traffic accident injuries, falls from heights, drowning, hypothermia and putrefaction.

Diagnosis of Antemortem Hanging

(i) Presence of antemortem ligature mark with vital reaction. (ii) ***Le facies sympathique***: Eyes on the side where the knot presses cervical sympathetic trunk remains open with dilated pupil. It is an important sign of antemortem hanging. (iii) Saliva dribbling mark from the angle of mouth. (iv) Ecchymosis of larynx or epiglottis. (v) Extent of fracture of thyroid cartilage and hyoid bone. (vi) Rupture of intima of carotid vessels. (vii) Emission of seminal fluid is quite common in antemortem hanging.

Crime Scene Examination

Examination of the scene of crime is very important and has to be done carefully. The body should not be cut down so that proper photographic documentation can be made. The important points, which must be observed, include the posture of the body, any signs of violence in the area like disturbance of articles etc. The noose should never be cut from the body but left intact for transport with the body to the morgue. The ligature material has to be examined carefully for the texture and the knot etc. When the noose is removed from the neck, the knot should not be untied. The noose should either be slipped off the head or cut opposite to the knot with the cut ends secure with the tape or string. The height from which the body is suspended should be measured and the platform that was possibly used by the victim must be noted. Sometimes when the ligature is broken, the body may be found lying on the ground. In such cases, the part of the noose around the neck should be properly secured and the other part that is left attached to the ceiling fan, hook or rod of window or doorknob should be removed and compared with the part around the neck.

Critical Evaluation

(i) At times when the person is attempting suicide and the first attempt fails he may fall down and sustain injury. The victim then tries a second attempt with another rope at another place and may be found with bleeding and injuries. The scene may also be disturbed in such cases with blood present at places. The injuries on the body of the person may be misinterpreted as struggle marks. Careful evaluation of the crime scene is required in such cases to arrive at a conclusion. (ii) When a person hangs with a rope then it leaves its groove marks on the hook or beam, which is used to tie the rope. The groove mark has to be carefully observed for the pattern of the cord on it and must be matched with the width of the cord. If some clothing or hair comes in between, then the mark may not be visible. (iii) Dead persons can show grooves on the neck which can be confused with hanging grooves. Such marks are caused by clothing like tight collar or a tight necklace etc. These marks disappear after decomposition while a ligature mark does not decompose as easily as there is little blood in the skin underneath leading to much reduced bacterial growth. (iv) Murder by hanging is very rare and is usually possible in children, unconscious persons and those who are unable to defend themselves. (v) Persons who have committed suicide by hanging may show other injuries which in themselves could be fatal. (vi) When the body is hanging free but there is no jumping point in the vicinity such as chair, table, step etc., there is every reason to suspect murder. In such cases scene must be examined for marks of climbing over trees and development of postmortem staining over the lower limbs. If staining is present on the back of a freely hanging body it signifies that person has been killed first and then hanged. Wrinkles on the clothes may indicate that limbs were previously bent. (vii) Presence of material evidence on the clothes such as leaves, twigs of plants, soil, dust that is not present at the scene of hanging must be noted. In addition, the observations such as presence of blood, urine and saliva flowing in the wrong direction should arouse suspicion of crime. If the knots and noose present around the neck are such that it is not possible for the individual to make them should raise suspicion of crime. (viii) In a right-handed person, knot is usually on the right side and any reversal should raise suspicion of homicide. (ix) Autopsy rarely reveals whether the hanging is suicidal or homicidal. It is the duty of the police officer to correlate the course of events.

Medicolegal Aspects

Hanging can be suicidal, homicidal and at times accidental.

Suicidal hanging: Hanging is one of the most common method used for suicide. Virtually all hangings are suicidal in nature unless proved otherwise. In India, it is quite popular and the most common method of suicide, more common amongst males. The person finds it as one of the easiest and surest methods of death. Hanging is known as painless mode of death. The person hangs himself with any long ligature material available that is tied to a ceiling fan, roof, window etc. There may be a fixed loop or a knot. The individual usually hangs himself in an isolated area and when hanged in his house, the room in such cases is bolted from inside. A handwritten suicide note may be found at the scene or on the body of the deceased. Now-a-days, the victims use various electronic devices or social media to express their suicidal thoughts instead of conventional methods, before committing suicide which is called an **e-suicide note** (Behera *et al.*, 2014). All these suicide notes can help in confirming the manner of death as suicide.

In suicidal hanging, occasionally, to prevent change of mind, the individual may tie his/her hands or legs **(bound limbs)** (Figure 24.20A,B). Rarely, there can be co-occurrence of **masking** (Figure 24.20C) or **gagging.** The reason for covering of mouth or gagging could be to prevent shouting for help. All these findings suggest that the person is determined to die. Cases have been reported in suicidal hanging with face mask *in situ* during corona pandemic (Figure 24.20D). There can be suspicion of homicide or accidental

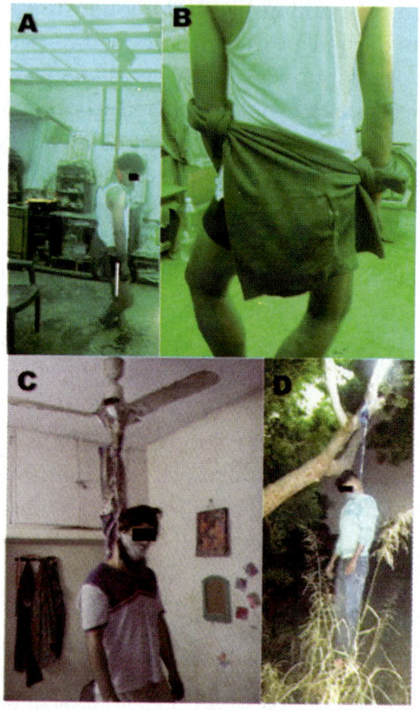

Figure 24.20A-D: Binding of both hands (A,B), Masking of face (C) and masking during corona pandemic (D) in suicidal hanging cases

autoerotic deaths in these situations. Apart from the characteristic ligature mark, **periligature injuries** on neck due to rope burns and nail marks, may present around the ligature mark *Mohanty et al.* (Figure 24.21A, B). Injuries may be present on the other parts of body **(associated injuries)** in a suicidal hanging victim reported by the author. This could be found in different situations, e.g., during convulsive movements of the body and striking with the

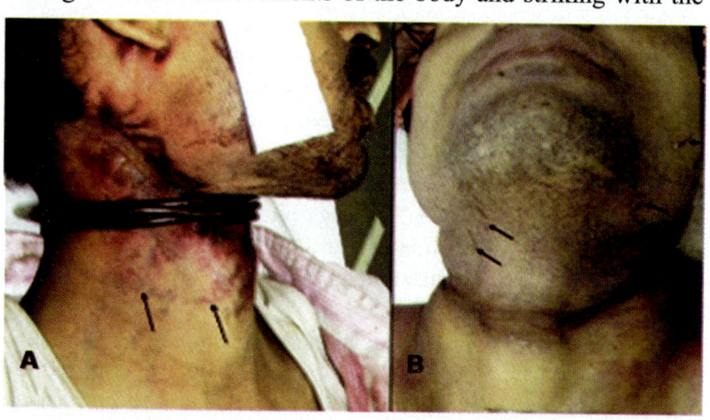

Figure 24.21A, B: Rope burns (A) nail marks produced by the victim himself (B) in suicidal hanging cases

surrounding objects at the time of hanging, during transportation to the health facility, during resuscitation, self-inflicted injuries or inflicted by another person before hanging etc. A crime scene investigation, detailed history and thorough autopsy should be done for confirmation of manner.

Dyadic deaths comprise deaths occurring simultaneously or one after another in two or more people, either with an agreement or without one. It includes both **homicide-suicides** and **suicide pacts.** Hanging is a common method used by the perpetrator to end his/her life after killing the victim in homicide –suicide deaths. Suicide pact is an agreement between two or more persons in which they decide to end their lives together at the same time by their own separate actions. Cases have been reported by the author in which one of the victims or all victims committed suicide by hanging by using the same ligature or different ligatures (Figure 24.22).

Homicidal hanging: Homicidal hanging is extremely rare. It can be a possibility in cases where the victim is a child, an unconscious person or a very frail person unable to defend himself. It would virtually be impossible for one of two healthy males, equally matched physically, to hang the other unless the victim was beaten unconscious or rendered helpless by alcohol or drugs. In the first instance, one would suspect homicide by virtue of the injuries on the victim. In the second scenario, or if the victim was rapidly subdued by two or more stronger assailants, there might not be any other marks on the body but for the noose mark or possible contusions of the arm inflicted while being forcibly restrained by the assailants. If there were also a marked disproportion in strength between the assailant and the victim such as an adult and a child, it would also be possible to hang the

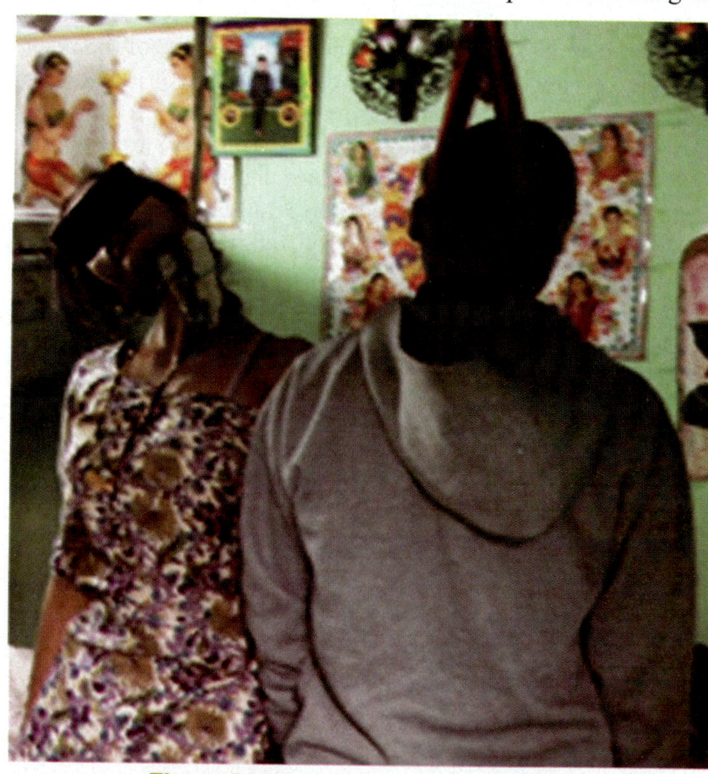

Figure 24.22: Suicidal pact by hanging

victim without any marks of violence. In addition, an individual might be first strangled with ligature and then hanged. In this case, the ligature mark over the neck would not have classic inverted V configuration of hanging. Although there are cases on record of suicidal hangings involving incomplete suspension, where the noose mark overlaid the larynx and was horizontal, not sweeping upward to the point of suspension in an inverted V configuration. To rule out any violence that might not be visible and to make sure that the individual was not drugged, in all alleged homicidal hangings, a complete toxicological screen should be performed. If there are signs of violence then it may be homicidal in nature. Circumstantial evidence is of value in these cases. When an unruly mob hangs a person in public, it is called **lynching.**

Accidental hanging: Accidental hangings usually involve children who are playing while simulating judicial hanging get entangled in a rope. Boys playing in gardens while jumping from trees get their clothing caught in the branches and are accidentally hanged. Adults engaging in the practice of **sexual asphyxia** may be accidentally hanged. The chin may be suspended from the steering wheel of a vehicle. In cases of a fall from a staircase, a person may get his neck caught in the railing and hang. An intoxicated person may accidentally hang himself from the arm of a chair. Rarely an infant accidentally hang himself from a pacifier placed around his neck on a cord or are entangled in a toy placed above his crib.

Judicial hanging: Judicial hanging is the term used when convicted criminals are hanged. It is a method of execution practiced in many countries including India. The person's face is covered with a dark mask and he is made to stand over trapdoors that open downwards. The noose is put around the neck with the knot placed on the left side of the jaw, close to chin. This position knot is officially used because there is less chance of slippage, however, submental position of knot is the most effective. A trapdoor is sprung and the prisoner falls a specific distance determined by his weight. For an effective hanging, the victim's neck should be subjected to a constrictive force of 126 pounds. The platform is at a height allowing for a fall of about 5 meters. If he falls an insufficient distance (<1 m), he strangles rather than break his neck and if he falls too far (>5 m), he is decapitated. As the person falls there is a sudden jerk to the neck causing fracture dislocation at the 2nd to 3rd cervical vertebral level or sometimes at the atlanto-occipital or atlantoaxial joint with transaction of the cord. In properly performed judicial hangings, the victim abruptly stops at the end of his fall when his head is jerked suddenly and violently backward, fracturing his spine. In case of submental knot position, the hyperextension of neck resulted in traumatic spondylolisthesis of axis vertebrae (C2), called **Hangman's fracture,** a term coined by Schneider *et al.* It is a bilateral fracture of the pedicle of C2 vertebrae associated with anterior subluxation or dislocation of the vertebral body. However, it is rarely seen. The neck is at times lengthened and may be severed in some cases and the neck vessels are torn transversely. There is immediate unconsciousness leading to death though the heart may continue to beat for 8-20 minutes. In addition, there are muscular contractions of the facial muscles, twitchings and convulsions of the limb and trunk, and violent respiratory movement of the chest. The doctor is required to authenticate a person as "fit to be executed" and to certify him or her dead at the end of the execution. The postmortem of the body is conducted as per the guidelines laid down by the Supreme Court in the landmark judgment of Shatrughan Chauhan vs Union of India.

STRANGULATION

It is a form of asphyxia, which is caused by constriction of neck by a ligature without suspending the body. It is mainly of two types (i) Ligature strangulation; and (ii) Manual strangulation. Nevertheless, other types may also be encountered as given before.

Medicolegal Aspects

(i) Whether death is due to strangulation can be ascertained from the general features of asphyxia mainly on the head and neck that are strongly presumptive of strangulation deaths; the ligature mark around the neck, internal findings in the neck and circumstantial evidence. (ii) Manner of death in strangulation can be discerned from:

Homicidal strangulation: Strangulation is a common form of murder and is seen in adult women usually combined with sexual acts. Single turn of ligature with one or more knots, at the front or sides of neck is usually found. If two or more knots are present with each turn of ligature then homicide is almost certain. Abrasions are usually seen due to movement of the ligature in the neck during struggle by the victim. Evidence of struggle may be absent in cases as in weak and frail individuals especially children or when the victim is attacked suddenly or made unconscious earlier by trauma or drugs.

Strangulation should be taken as homicidal unless proved otherwise. The observations which can prove to be of value in establishing the nature of the injury include ownership of ligature and the possession of the ligature material with the suspected person. Unusual ligatures may indicate a particular occupation of the assailant. Looseness of the ligature or missing ligature is a near definite sign of homicidal strangulation. If the mark does not correspond with the ligature material recovered, it is also indicative of homicidal strangulation. Circumstantial evidence is of value in deciding doubtful cases.

Accidental strangulation: Children may accidentally get entangled in ropes during play. An infant may be strangled with a string attached to a log tied to the crib. Intoxicated persons may get accidentally strangulated by their necktie, scarf or collar etc. In industry belts, ropes and parts of clothing may be caught in rollers or parts of moving machinery and cause strangulation. Umbilical cord inside the uterus may also accidentally strangulate the foetus. Though it is rare but has been reported in the literature. In addition, women may get their *dupatta* entangled in the moving wheel of cycle rickshaw or motorbike and it may tighten around the neck sufficient to cause strangulation.

Suicidal or self-strangulation: Self-strangulation by ligature is uncommon. Various methods for tightening the ligature are employed by the victims. Number of knots, tightness, method of knotting should be considered. The ligature material can be used like a tourniquet by the victim.

A person can have one or two knots before consciousness is lost. Some arrangement is always made to keep the ligature tight. A cord may be tied around and twisted by stick working as a lever. When consciousness is lost, the grip is released, but ligature will not become loose, as it gets arrested against the shoulder or chin. When a running noose is applied to neck, a weight is attached to the free end of the rope at the end of the bed on which the patient is lying. Signs of venous congestion are very well marked above the ligature and very prominent at the root of the tongue due to slow tightening of ligature and no draining of postmortem blood.

Injuries are less marked on the body of the person as less force is used. No signs of struggle are seen. Ligature is found *in situ*. Application of ligature with several turns whether closed with half knot or complete knot is consistent with suicide. Single turn of a broad ligature of rough cloth, closed with a half knot also indicates suicide.

Opinion is given based on the ligature material recovered, the way it was tightened, absence of marks of violence on the body. Examination of surroundings with finding of the body at a lonely place, presence of suicidal note and whether the room is locked from inside or not etc. are helpful in pointing towards the manner of death.

Pseudo strangulation: In persons having short neck, depression mark similar to ligature mark is produced after death due to the folds of skin. Even in infants and children with short neck, similar marks are produced after death. In decomposed bodies, the tight collars or other clothing produce grooving similar to ligature mark. All these are examples of **Pseudo ligature marks** (Figure 24.23A, B) and can confuse with ligature mark in strangulation. Dissection of neck will reveal absence of abrasions or underneath bruising of tissue.

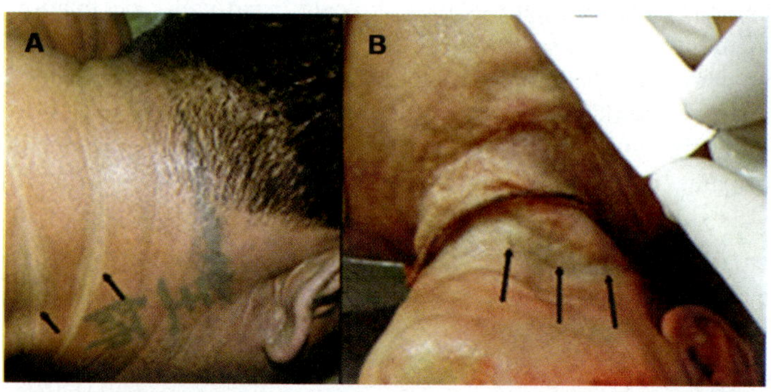

Figure 24.23A, B: Neck fold in adult (A) and infant (B)–Pseudo ligature marks at autopsy

LIGATURE STRANGULATION

In ligature strangulation, the pressure on the neck is applied by a constricting band that is tightened by a force other than the body weight. This is the type of strangulation in which a ligature material is used to compress the neck and the assailant applies the constricting force without suspending the body. Usually a U-shaped ligature is pulled around the neck from behind though multiple turns of the ligature material are often used. Virtually all cases of ligature strangulation are homicides and suicides and accidents are rare. Females are predominantly involved.

Ligature mark: The ligature used in ligature strangulation may range from electrical cords, ropes, telephone cords, sheets and neckties. The appearance of the ligature depends on the nature of ligature, amount of resistance offered by the victim and the amount of force used by the assailants. When the ligature used is soft material, the ligature mark may be faint, barely visible or even absent in children or incapacitated adults. When a very thin ligature is used, the mark appears as deep mark and encircles the neck.

Facial findings (Figure 24.24): The face and neck above the ligature mark are markedly congested with confluent petechial haemorrhages in the sclera and conjunctivae. Fine petechial haemorrhages over the face especially in periorbital area are seen. The findings of congested face, congestion, petechiae and haemorrhages in the sclera (Figures 24.25A and B) in ligature strangulation are due to the fact that unlike hanging there is no complete occlusion of the neck vessels. The blood continues to enter the head from vertebral arteries and the venous drainage is very less. This results in increase intravascular pressure, congestion and rupture of vessels.

Causes of death: Death in these cases is due to asphyxia, cerebral anoxia, vagal inhibition and fracture dislocation of cervical vertebrae. By far the most common cause is asphyxia caused due to elevation of the larynx and tongue, which closes the airway at the pharyngeal level. If extreme pressure is applied by the assailant then the trachea or the larynx itself may be blocked and cause asphyxia. Cerebral anoxia is caused by compression of the blood vessels in the neck and if the pressure is moderate then it may cause only the compression of the veins leading to venous congestion. Vagal nerves can get stimulated and cause depression of the heart to cause death. Fracture dislocation of the cervical vertebrae is a very rare finding but may happen in case of thin and frail person who is attacked by a very strong assailant.

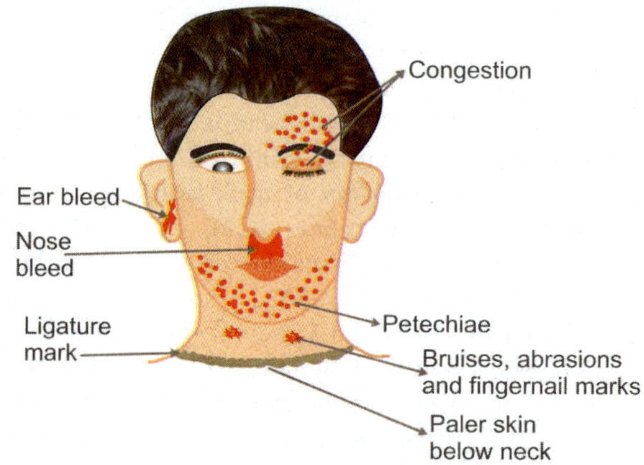

Figure 24.24: Facial findings in strangulation

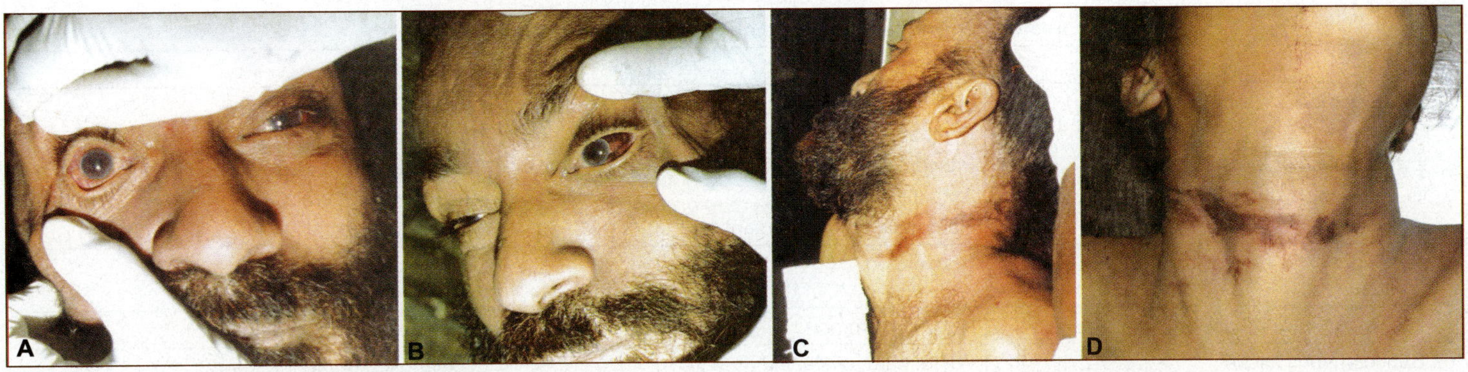

Figure 24.25A-D: Findings in ligature strangulation (A) Congestion of sclera (B) Subconjunctival haemorrhage (C and D) Ligature mark (horizontal, over thyroid cartilage) over neck

Autopsy Findings

External findings: The ligature mark is usually a well-defined depressed mark present at the middle or lower part of the neck (Figure 24.25C and D). The mark may encircle the neck fully but is most prominent at the front and the sides of the neck. It is usually transverse but may be oblique if the victim has been dragged by the assailant for some distance. The base of the mark is usually reddish when a soft ligature has been used. However ligature material such as cords, rops and wires cause abrasions of the surface that on drying becomes hard yellowish brown and parchment life. Sometimes exudation of tissue fluid may dry and from stiff film. Usually adjacent to the ligature mark petechial haemorrhages are present that are suggestive of its antemortem nature. Commonly a narrow zone of reddening and congestion is found immediately above and below the groove of ligature mark. This occurs due to squeezing out of blood under pressure. Besides this scratch abrasions are found near the ligature mark. These abrasions are usually linear, irregular or crescentic. In all cases of suspected strangulation, fingernails of the deceased should be examined for fragments of skin and blood. For this during autopsy examination, scraping and debris inside the nails and if available whole fingernails should be preserved. Depending upon the type of the ligature material its pattern in the form of ligature mark is found over the neck.

Internal findings: Haemorrhages are found in the muscles and soft tissues underneath the ligature mark. If severe force is used carotid artery tear may be present. Fracture of hyoid bone and thyroid cartilage may be seen. Hyoid fracture is seen in inward compression, which can be bilateral while outward compression such as in hanging gives rise to anteroposterior compression fracture of the greater horn at the junction with the body.

Avulsion fracture may be seen due to muscular overactivity without there being direct injury to the hyoid bone. They are called **traction (Tug) fractures.**

The differences in findings between hanging and ligature strangulation are enumerated in Table 24.1.

MANUAL STRANGULATION (THROTTLING)

It is asphyxia produced by compression of the neck manually, i.e., human hands. The mechanism of death is occlusion of the blood vessels supplying blood to the brain. Occlusion of airway probably plays a minor role in causing death. Virtually all manual strangulations are homicidal in nature.

Suicidal throttling: Suicide by throttling is impossible as when the pressure by the victim's own hands is sustained for a sufficient time to cause unconsciousness, the hands relax and the victim recovers.

Accidental throttling: The application of one or both the hands to another person's throat can cause sudden death from vagal inhibition. This may occur in unintentional circumstances brought on by touching, grasping and demonstration of affection such as during intercourse, or during physiological experiments. This is theoretically possible but highly improbable and suspicious. The mechanism of death in this case would be an arrhythmia produced by stimulation of the carotid sinuses. The carotid sinus is a focal area of enlargement of the common carotid artery at the point it bifurcates into the external and internal carotid arteries. The compression or stimulation of the carotid sinuses causes an increase in blood pressure in these sinuses with resultant bradycardia, vasodilatation and hypotension. Pressure on the common carotid artery below the sinuses reduces blood pressure within the sinuses by reducing the amount of blood flowing into it. This mimic decreased blood supply from haemorrhage and shock causing tachycardia, vasoconstriction and hypertension. This explains the fact that why in some cases of throttling if the hands are lower down over the neck there is tachycardia, vasoconstriction and rise in blood pressure.

Homicidal throttling: Death resulting from asphyxia consequent upon manual strangulation raises the suspicion of homicide. This method is employed when the victim is an infant, a child, or woman. Healthy adults can be throttled only when they are under the influence of drugs or other intoxicants, are stunned or the attack is sudden. Throttling is a common method of infanticide.

Table 24.1: Differences in findings in hanging and strangulation

Features	Hanging	Strangulation
• Ligature mark:		
i. Shape	Oblique	Transverse
ii. Complete or incomplete	Incomplete	Complete
iii. Level of thyroid	Above thyroid	Below or over thyroid
iv. Base	Hard, pale and parchment like	Soft and reddish
• Abrasions and ecchymoses at the edge of ligature	Uncommon	Quite common
• Bruising of neck muscles	Not very common	Very common
• Subcutaneous tissue	White, hard, glistening	Ecchymosed under the mark
• Hyoid bone fracture	Very common	Less common
• Carotid artery damage	May be seen	Rare
• Thyroid cartilage fracture	Rare	Common
• Fracture of larynx and trachea	Rare	May be found
• Facial congestion and petechiae	Pale	Marked with petechiae
• Protrusion of tongue	Less common	More common
• Asphyxial signs	Less marked	More marked
• Bleeding from nose, mouth and ear	Less common	More common
• Salivary stains	Present	Absent
• Neck	Stretched or elongated	Not stretched or elongated
• Lungs	No bulking	Congested and oedematous
• Subpleural hemorrhage	Less common	More common
• Semen discharge	Common	Not very common
• Bullous lesions of lungs	Not present	Present

Autopsy Findings

External findings (Figure 24.26A to C): The situation and extent of bruise on the neck will depend upon the relative positions of the assailant and victim, manner of grasping the neck and degree of pressure. Bruises are produced by tips and pads of fingers, are oval or round and of the size of digits (1.5-2 cm). The size may be altered due to bleeding underneath the skin. The grip can be produced by right hand with thumb on right side of neck and fingers on left side and vice versa of the assailant. Finger marks may be present obliquely, separately or clustered together. Both hands are commonly used with the thumb of one hand and finger of other hand present over both the sides. Strangulation is easier for assailants with big hands on victims with small necks. Signs of struggle or bruises may be found anywhere, not definite to say whether the attack was from behind or from the front. Bruises

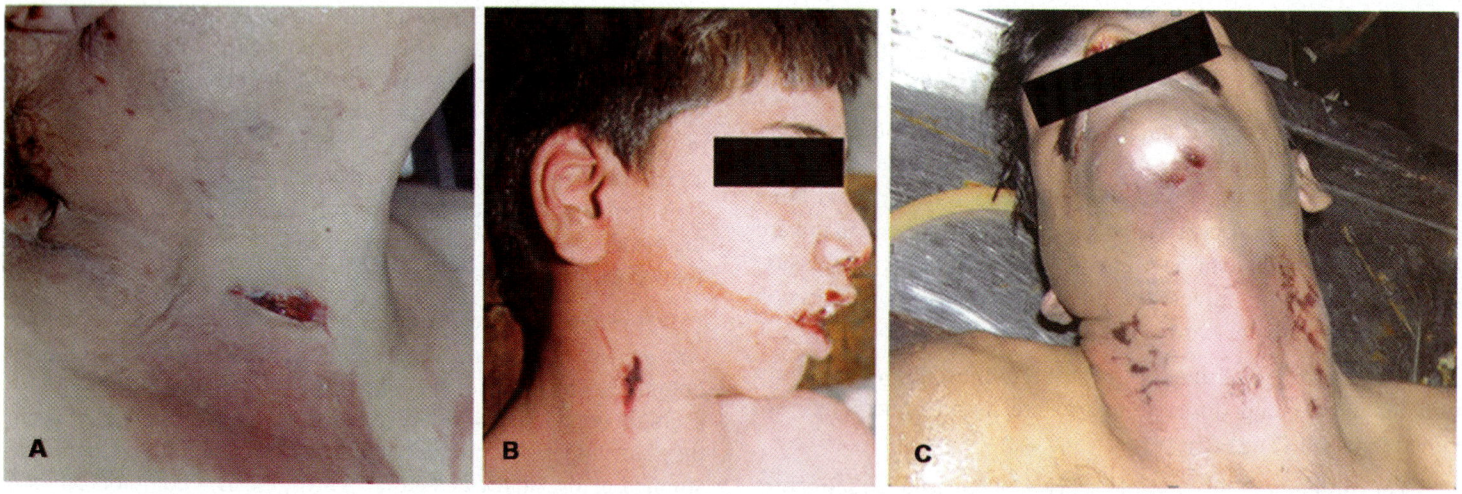

Figure 24.26A to C: Multiple bruises over neck in manual strangulation. Note crescentic scratch abrasions produced by nail

may go for the usual colour change. When fingertips are deeply pressed, nails produce crescentic marks on the skin. During grip thumb exerts more pressure than the other fingers. Two types of abrasions may be seen. When nails skid down the skin parallelly, linear lines for several centimeters may be seen. In other cases regularly curved, comma like, disk like or straight 1.5 cm in length and few mm in width. Many scratches are produced by the victim while trying to pull away from the assailant's hand. As most victims are females, usually having long nails, scratches are more severe than those of assailants. Parallel lines in vertical direction are seen in such cases. The nail marks are more marked when the skin is dry.

Internal findings: (i) Haemorrhages are found in the muscles of the neck (Figure 24.27). Carotid artery tear may be present. (ii) Fracture of hyoid bone is very common especially in the elderly. It is seen as inward compression, which can be bilateral. (iii) Thyroid cartilage may also be fractured in many cases.

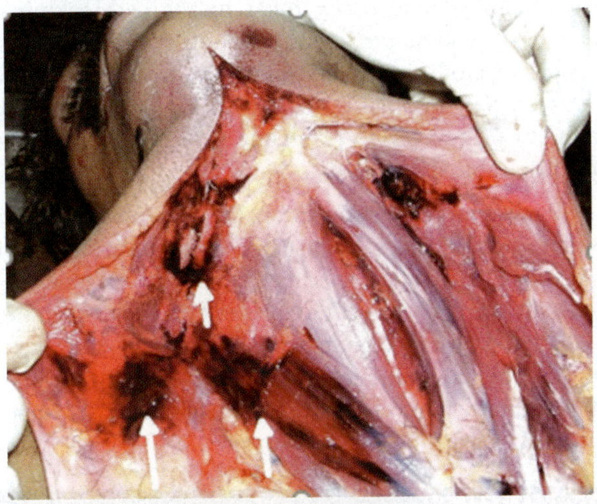

Figure 24.27: Internal findings in neck in manual strangulation, note effusion of blood in soft tissues of neck

BANSDOLA (Figure 24.28)

Strong bamboo or stick is put in front of neck and another one at the back of neck. Both ends are tied and squeezed, from front of chest and back to cause death. It interferes with respiration, and causes fracture of ribs etc.

GARROTING

In this the victim is attacked from behind without warning, the throat may either be grasped by hand or a ligature which is quickly tightened, by twisting it, with a lever causing sudden loss of consciousness and collapse leading to death. In one of the refined methods of garroting, a spike was used behind a clamp, which penetrated the spine and caused the death of the person. It was a mode of execution in Spain and Turkey. **Spanish Windlass** is an iron collar around the neck that is tightened by screw for strangulating the victim (Figure 24.29).

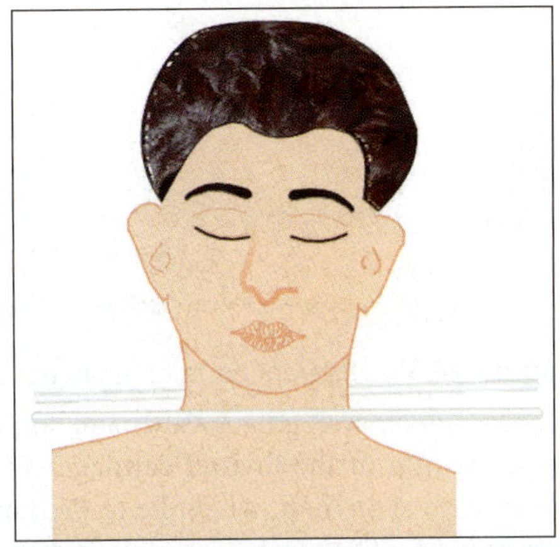

Figure 24.28: Bansdola with bamboo sticks over front and back of neck

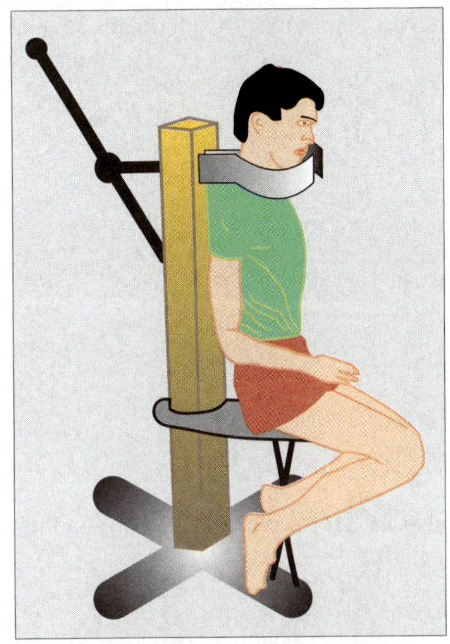

Figure 24.29: Garroting

MUGGING

Strangulation is caused by holding the neck of the victim in the bend of the elbow. Pressure is exerted either on the front of larynx or at the sides of neck by forearm or arm. Rarely, foot or knee is used to press the neck. In mugging, marks over the neck may be minimal. On autopsy, there are findings similar to ligature strangulation by a broad object. The friction of the forearm may produce a diffuse abrasion along the jaw margin. On opening the neck, bruising of strap muscles of neck and in the soft tissues behind the larynx is seen. Rarely, fracture of hyoid or superior horn of thyroid may be produced.

Fractures of Hyoid Bone in Asphyxial Deaths

Hyoid bone (Figure 24.30) lies at the root of the tongue and consists of a central horizontal body to which are attached two

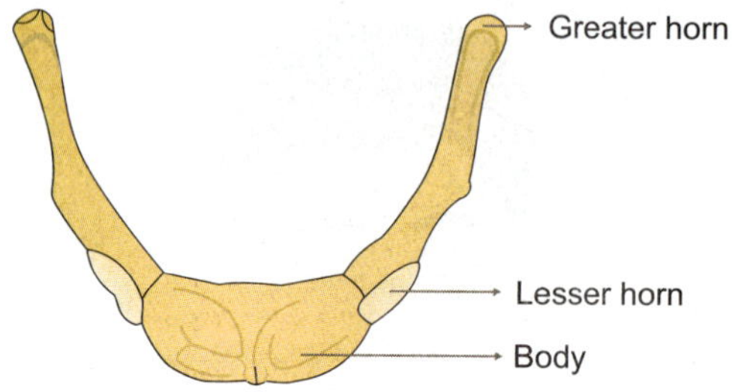

Figure 24.30: Different parts of hyoid bone

long greater horns which sweep backwards and slightly upwards above the upper margin of the thyroid cartilage (Figure 24.31). Sometimes even with synovium, which lie at the junction of the body with greater horns. The two lesser horns in the upper surface have no forensic significance. The horns of hyoid calcify during middle and later life. Various types of fractures (Figure 24.32) of hyoid bone may be seen in asphyxial deaths such as:

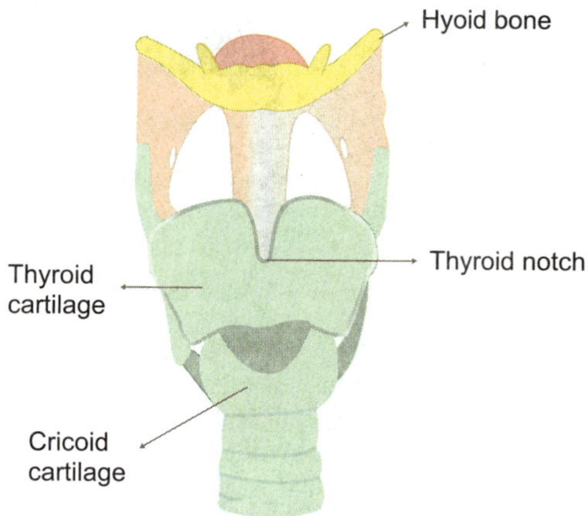

Figure 24.31: Larynx as viewed from the front

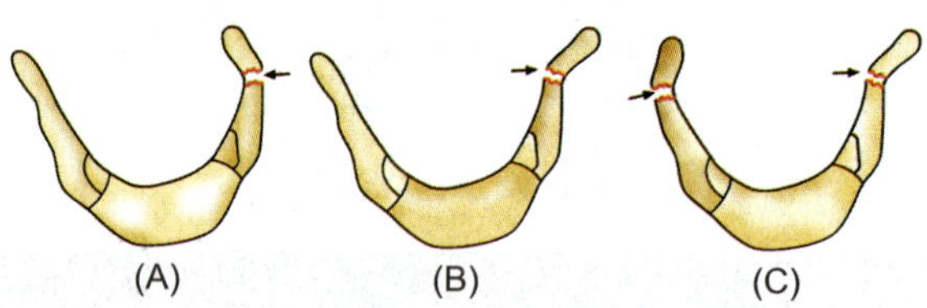

Figure 24.32A to C: Different types of hyoid bone fractures (A) Inward compression (B) Outward compression (C) Avulsion

1. **Inward compression fracture:** In this the greater horns of hyoid are compressed inwards causing fracture of the bone with tear of its periosteum on the outer side and not on inner side displacing the posterior fragment inwards. It is seen in manual strangulation. This type of fracture can occur on both the sides.
2. **Outward compression (anteroposterior compression) fracture:** In this hyoid bone is driven backwards, when divergence of greater horns is increased, causing fracture with outward displacement of posterior small fragment. As a result, the periosteum on inner side of fracture only is torn when the fragment can be easily moved outwards but inner movement is limited to normal position only. Either this type of fracture can occur in the greater horn at its junction with the body or it may be bilateral. This type of fracture is seen in hanging and ligature strangulation.
3. **Avulsion fracture:** This occurs due to muscular overactivity without there being direct injury to the hyoid bone. This type of fracture is also called traction 'tug' fracture. This occurs as a result of traction on thyrohyoid ligament either by downward or lateral movement of the thyroid cartilage from anteroposterior or lateral compression or when direct pressure is exerted between the hyoid and thyroid by the pressing fingers.

SUFFOCATION

The term suffocation is usually regarded as synonymous with asphyxia. However, the term is restricted to a group of circumstances except drowning in which asphyxia is produced by causes other than constriction of the neck by a ligature, hands, or a stranglehold. This includes closing the external respiratory orifices either by hand or by other means or blocking up the cavities of nose and mouth by introduction of a foreign substance, mud, paper or clothes etc. The following types of suffocation is usually seen: (i) Smothering (ii) Overlaying (iii) Burking (iv) Choking (v) Gagging (vi) Traumatic asphyxia (vii) Suffocation due to irrespirable gases.

In all these forms of suffocation, the asphyxial symptoms and signs are severe since death is usually the result of slow asphyxia, often taking 2-5 minutes to kill. Usually the external signs of asphyxia such as cyanosis of the face and petechial haemorrhages of the facial skin and conjunctiva is common. However, there may not be any external injury at all. Alternatively, these injuries may be slight and can escape the eyes of the most experienced examiner.

SMOTHERING

Smothering refers to the death resulting from mechanical occlusion of the mouth and nose that prevents breathing. The smothering agent is usually a fabric, an impervious sheet or a hand, though occasionally a mobile solid such as sand, mud, grain or flour may be responsible for blocking the air passages. In smothering, death may occur either by the occluding substance pressing down upon the facial orifices, or by the passive weight of the head pressing the nose and mouth into the occlusion. Deliberate homicide is seen usually in the old, the debilitated and in infants. It is extremely difficult to prove homicide from the objective findings. The smothering of babies whether intentional or accidental is not so rare in India compared to western world. However, in these cases, the findings are not significant as the classical signs of asphyxia such as congestion, cyanosis and facial and conjunctival petechiae are not commonly present. Since intrathoracic petechial haemorrhages are common in sudden infant death syndrome, these cannot be accepted in isolation as evidence of suffocation.

External findings: (i) No external signs are there when the obstruction is by some soft material such as bed-clothing, pillow, cushion, mother's breast or even assailant's hand that is gently applied. (ii) There are scratch abrasions, bruises, finger nail marks, laceration of soft parts of victim's face (Figures 24.33, 24.34). (iii) There may be bruising and laceration of lips, gums and tongue (Figure 24.35). (iv) Pressure marks on the face can rarely be distinguished from postmortem postural changes, where circumoral and circumnasal pallor is caused merely by passive pressure of the dependent head after death, preventing the gravitational hypostasis from entering these areas. Even when the head is found supine, variation in colour is still common on the face, with contrasting white and pink patches, which usually change as the postmortem interval lengthens. (v) Unless there are bruises or abrasions on the cheeks, around the mouth, lips or lesions within the lips or mouth, it is dangerous to overinterpret mere colour variations from alterations for blood in the facial capillary bed, which is usually a postmortem phenomenon.

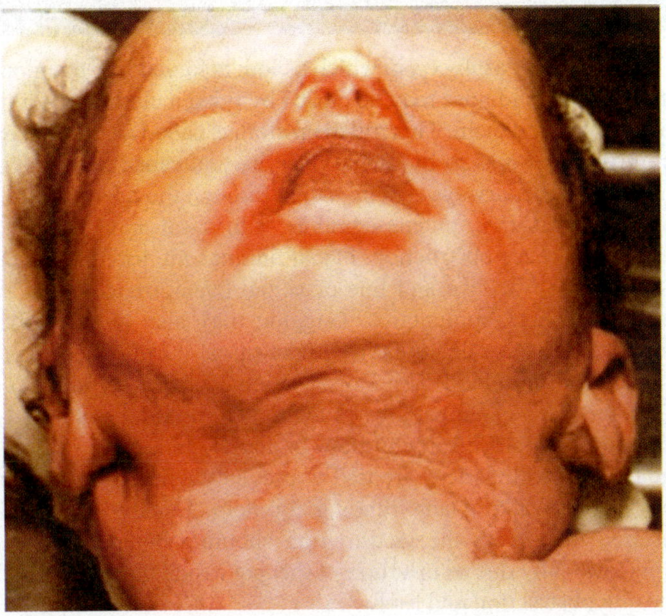

Figure 24.33: Contusion and abrasions in and around the lips in a newborn in case of smothering

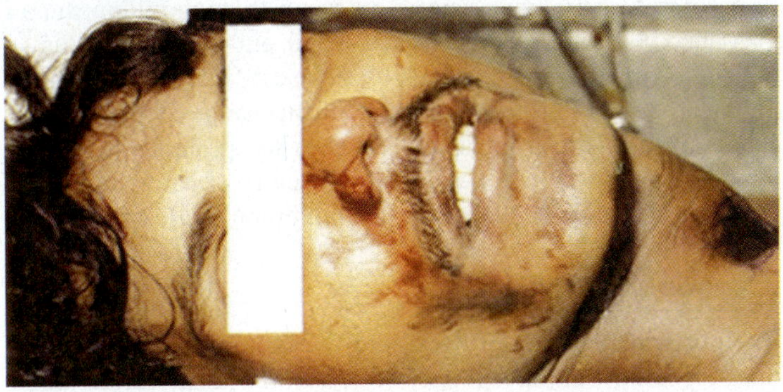

Figure 24.34: Abrasions and bruises over mouth and nostrils in a case of smothering

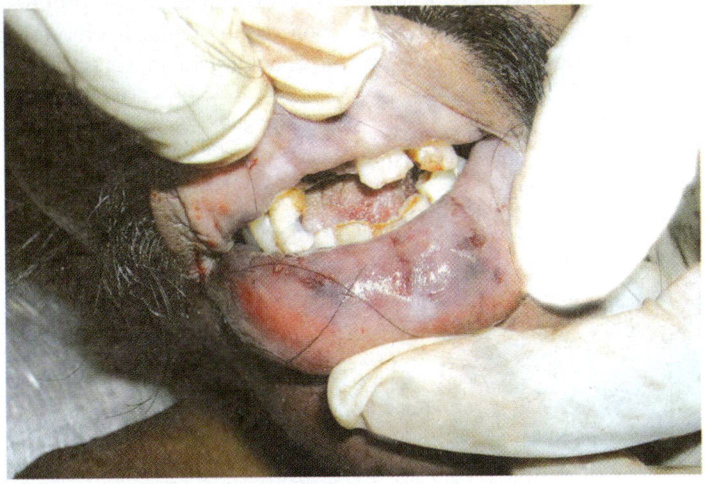

Figure 24.35: Contused lacerations over the inner sides of lips in a case of smothering

Medicolegal Aspects

Suicidal smothering: This can occur in mental patients or prisoners. Suicide is practicable merely by burying the face in a flock of mattress or even it would appear by lying against the bed clothing to obstruct the nose and mouth, especially when drunk. The death by cut throat may occasionally terminate by smothering. If the trachea is completely severed, the lower end is likely to be drawn down within the thorax by the weight of the heart and lungs. If the soft parts then close over the wound, they can obstruct the trachea and the victim is smothered.

Accidental smothering: The circumstances of accidental smothering vary according to the age of the victim. The bed clothes cover the nostrils and mouth of the infants during first month of life especially premature with resulting death. Suffocation of the infant is also possible when it turns on its face in its cot and buries his face in a soft pillow or mattress. Accidental smothering in children and young adults may be predisposed to by an epileptic fit. Another variety of accidental smothering likely to involve children in an airtight place or one in which ventilation is negligible such as in disused refrigerator. Accidental smothering of adults by precipitation into a quantity of finely divided, solid materials such as flour, sand, coal-dust, cinders, grain or feathers may occur in the course of their occupation. Besides, smothering may occur subject to epileptic or epileptiform fits. Accidental smothering may occur outdoors when the victim, in the course of an epileptic fit or under the influence of drinks or drugs, falls face down into mud, snow or thick grass.

Homicidal smothering: Homicide of an adult by smothering is possible when there is a gross disparity between the assailant and the victim or else when the victim is helpless by virtue of his age, ill health or incapacity from drink or drugs or when stunned by a blow. It is a common mode of infanticide. Usually infant's mouth and nostrils are closed by means of hand, or even a plaster. Usually the assailant uses far more force than is necessary to kill and consequently finger marks in the form of scratches and bruises are found over the victim's face.

GAGGING

This is a type of asphyxia in which a cloth is forced into the mouth or the mouth and nose may be closed by tying a cloth or a similar material around them. This rolled up cloth is called a **gag**. The gag is introduced so as to block the pharynx and cause asphyxia. In these cases the airways remain patent through the nostril initially but later on saliva, mucus combine with nasal and pharyngeal oedema to cause obstruction. Facial findings are prominent such as congestion of face and fine petechial haemorrhages over the face, sclera and conjunctiva. Gagging may also be caused by impaction of false dentures inside the throat during anaesthesia. In addition, the blood with clots may enter the throat and cause blockage. This is almost always homicidal mode of death and is commonly employed in children. In adults the hands are tied at the back as well as legs are tied to prevent them from removing the gag or walking and running for help. Usually the gag is inserted to prevent the victim from shouting but death occurs unintentionally due to insertion of the gag inside the pharynx and causing obstruction and asphyxia.

CHOKING (Figure 24.36)

It is a form of asphyxia caused by an obstruction within the air passage. It is almost always accidental and is usually due to inhalation of a foreign body, but it can be caused by the inhalation of the products of disease or by anatomical changes due to disease. The usual mechanism of asphyxia in choking is simple mechanical obstruction. However, occasionally the entry of foreign material may cause sudden death from vagal inhibition **(Café-coronary).**

Causes of Choking

(i) Inhalation of foreign body into the glottis such as bolus of meat, potato, button, coins, marbles, corns, fish, screws, pins or artificial dentures. (ii) Inhalation of vomited material in an unconscious, when intoxicated, during anaesthesia or epileptic fits. (iii) Belching out of milk by infants and young children may be aspirated into the air passages. (iv) Inhalation of products of disease or violence such as blood or pus while haemoptysis in Tuberculosis, rupture of an aortic aneurysm in air passages, or due to flooding of air passages with pus and necrotic debris in a lung abscess. (v) Anatomical changes due to disease such as a bronchial growth, laryngeal oedema, laryngeal tumours, pharyngeal abscess and angioneurotic oedema. (vi) In conditions such as poliomyelitis or bulbar palsy, accidental inhalation of food occurs due to disturbance in swallowing mechanism.

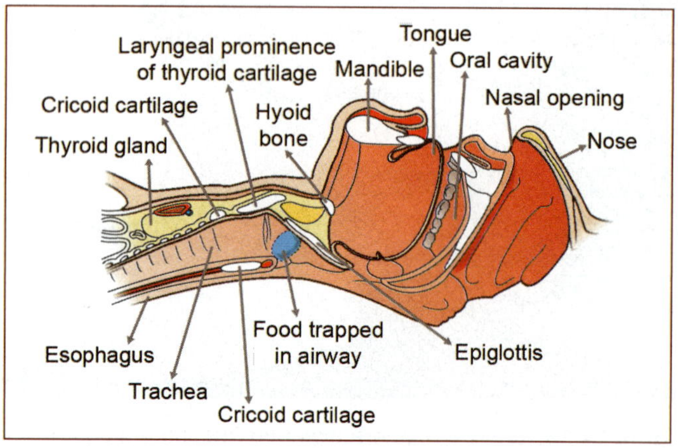

Figure 24.36: Choking

Mechanism

The usual mechanism of asphyxia in choking is mechanical obstruction but the entry of foreign body may cause sudden death from vagal inhibition.

Causes of Death

(i) *Asphyxia:* It is most common. (ii) *Vagal inhibition:* There are cases where the immediate result of choking is vagal inhibition and sudden death. The diagnosis is difficult due to absence of overt signs especially in an infant with small quantity of foreign material in the respiratory passages. The diagnosis is simple when a massive foreign body causes the obstruction but even when the foreign body is small, yet the cause of death seems to be vagal inhibition. Sudden death can occur when there is flooding of postnasal space with regurgitated food or even when minute particles are exposed to the vocal cords. The surgical procedures on larynx with light anaesthesia may cause sudden death from vagal inhibition. (iii) *Laryngeal spasm:* This occurs due to entry of an irritating foreign material in the air passages. This is likely if acid gastric juice alone suddenly enters the air passages.

Medicolegal Aspects

Death by choking is commonly an accident but occasionally it may be homicidal.

Accidental choking: It is very common and is seen in very young, elderly and psychiatric patients when the ability to chew or swallow is impaired. It may commonly occur during a meal when food is accidentally inhaled while the person is laughing or crying or even when someone unexpectedly slaps the person of the back.

Suicidal choking: Suicide by choking is quite rare but may be seen in mentally ill patients or prisoners who do not have access to other methods of committing suicide.

Homicidal choking: Choking is an uncommon and rare mode of committing homicide. However, the literature suggests that cases are on record where murders have been committed by choking the victim. Choking due to regurgitation of food may occur during rape or violent sexual intercourse.

Autopsy Findings

(i) Presence of impacted foreign body in the air passages. (ii) Regurgitated food particles such as vomitus, milk etc. may be found mixed with mucus in trachea, bronchi and lower bronchioles. (iii) All organs are congested. (iv) Other findings of asphyxia may be present.

CAFÉ-CORONARY

A condition where a healthy and grossly intoxicated person, suddenly turns blue, coughs violently, then collapses and dies. Death appears to be due to sudden heart attack. However, at autopsy one may find some food material or piece of meat obstructing the larynx. Clinical signs of choking are absent, as there is a high blood alcohol content, which anaesthetizes the gag reflex.

As the person vomits, the vomited matter may be inhaled leading to choking. Infants often regurgitate clotted milk after a meal into larynx and children may often place coins or small stones in the larynx. Rubber balloons may also be accidentally ingested by children and may get stuck in the pharynx or glottis. Suffocation may be caused by some diseases like diphtheria, infectious mononucleosis, haemoptysis in pulmonary tuberculosis. Larynx and bronchial growths may cause haemorrhage into trachea. Insect bites and drug reaction causes laryngeal oedema leading to death. Blow to the front of the neck may cause swelling of the mucosa, oedema and haemorrhage. Death may occur due to reflex vagal inhibition.

TRAUMATIC (CRUSH) ASPHYXIA

This is the name given to those kinds of asphyxia, which are caused due to mechanical fixation of the chest so that normal movements of chest wall are prevented. This occurs when a large weight falls onto or presses down on an individual's chest or upper abdomen. The most common form of traumatic asphyxia encountered is while repairing a car the jack slips and the vehicle falls on top of the individual. Great force is necessary to compress the chest and so this type of asphyxia is seen in cases like multiple deaths during stampede (chest is compressed and respiratory movements prevented by stampeding people piling on the top of each other causing **Riot crush or 'human pile' deaths),** hotel fire, and lane crowd in an enclosed place, building collapse and in coalmines. Traumatic asphyxia is usually accidental in manner. Individuals who survive an episode of traumatic asphyxia usually make an uneventful recovery, though occasionally there is some permanent visual impairment due to retinal haemorrhage.

Due to compression of chest, retrograde displacement of blood from superior vena cava into subclavian veins and veins of head and neck occurs leading to the cyanosis and congestion. Valves in the subclavian veins prevent spread of hydrostatic force to the veins of the upper limb and displacement of blood into the valveless veins of the head and neck causes the rupture of distal venules and capillaries. As a result, there is formation of numerous arterial haemorrhages into eyelid and conjunctiva with oedema of conjunctiva and bleeding from nose and ears. Internal organs are congested and petechial haemorrhages may be found in the pleura and pericardium.

Autopsy Findings

(i) There is deep red or purplish black discolouration of the skin of head, neck and upper trunk with numerous petechiae and ecchymoses in these areas (Figure 24.37). (ii) Petechiae of the sclera, conjunctiva and periorbital skin and retinal haemorrhages. (iii) There is intense cyanosis of deep purple or purple-red colour cyanosis above the level of compression usually to the level of third rib. If the patient recovers, the purple colour gradually disappears in 10-14 days without the usual colour changes. The abnormal purple red colour may persist for several days. (iv) Haemorrhage is seen in the tissues around the site of compression whereas below the level of compression, skin is pale and mild cyanosis may be seen. (v) Areas of pallor are seen at the level of collar of the shirt, folds or creases of garments. (vi) Internally, there is often no evidence of trauma in spite of the heavy weight on the chest. However, fracture of ribs may be present.

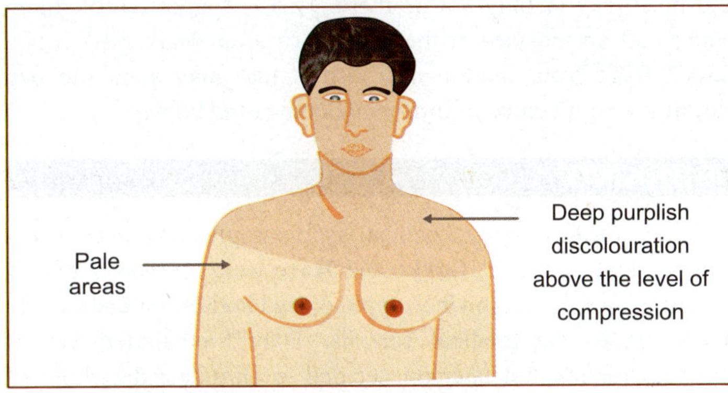

Figure 24.37: Findings in traumatic asphyxia

POSITIONAL ASPHYXIA

Positional asphyxia is virtually always an accident and is associated with alcohol or drug intoxication. An individual becomes intoxicated and falls into a restricted area, where because of position of his body, he cannot move out of that area or position and there is restriction on his ability to breathe. Positional asphyxia occurs if an individual falls down a well and is wedged between the walls. Every time he exhales, he slips farther and farther down the well preventing inhalation. There is usually marked congestion, cyanosis and petechiae at autopsy.

OVERLAYING

This form of asphyxia is a combination of mechanical asphyxia and smothering. It is seen most commonly when an infant is put to bed with one or more adults. During night, one of the adults inadvertently rolls on to or otherwise crushes and asphyxiates the infant by compressing the chest thus preventing respiratory movements and occluding the nose and mouth with bedding or the body of the adult. Later on the adult rolls off the child. The next morning the child is found dead without any evidence of trauma. These deaths are often thought to be due to SIDS. The autopsy findings are nonspecific with few fine petechiae over the face but not over the sclera or conjunctiva. The history of an adult sleeping with the child is important to differentiate such deaths from the 'cot deaths'. In England under the **Children and Young Persons Act, 1933**, it is a criminal offence to share bed by a person of the age of sixteen years or more with an infant in an intoxicated state. When individuals are buried in loose earth or sand (cave-ins) or in grain silos, they die as a result of occlusion of the nose and mouth along with immobilization of the chest and abdomen by external pressure sufficient to prevent respiratory movement.

Autopsy Findings

(i) Presence of petechial haemorrhages beneath the conjunctiva, epicardium and pleura. (ii) Evidence of contact flattening of face and nose may or may not be there. This is suggestive of infant being laid on the face at the time of or after death. (iii) Blood tinged froth from mouth and nostrils that may stain the bed clothing. (iv) Absence of injury marks over the body.

BURKING

Burking is a form of mechanical asphyxia plus smothering that is homicidal in nature. **Burke** and **Hare** were murderers during the 1820s in Edinburgh who supplied dead bodies for Anatomical dissection to the medical schools. They first started out as 'resurrectionists' but later on decided to eliminate the chore of digging up bodies. Instead, they would go straight to the source and would invite the individual to their house and intoxicate him. According to Hare, who turned King's evidence, Burke would kneel or sit on the chest, covering the mouth and nostrils with his hand thus producing a combination of traumatic asphyxia and smothering. External injury was absent and for Hare, the precise mechanism of asphyxia might not have been discovered. There was some bleeding into the tissues around the cervical spine but it was concluded that the injury occurred shortly after death. Burke later confessed to sixteen of such murders, which were committed for gain.

SUFFOCATION FROM IRRESPIRABLE GASES

Deaths from suffocating gases are due not to the toxic nature of the gases, but rather to displacement of oxygen from the atmosphere. Carbon dioxide and methane are two most commonly encountered suffocating gases. Both are essentially nontoxic and odourless and are found in sewers and mines. Methane is the principal constituent of the natural gas (94-96%). Reduction of atmospheric oxygen to less than 25% of normal displacement of oxygen by inert gases such as carbon dioxide and methane produces unconsciousness in seconds and death in a matter of minutes. The cause of death can be determined from the circumstantial evidences as there are no specific autopsy findings. If death is prolonged, the individuals appear cyanotic with petechial haemorrhages of the epicardium and visceral pleura. Petechiae are frequently absent in rapid anoxic deaths. Toxicological analysis for methane can be done. When it is detected in blood being nontoxic death cannot be attributed to it. However, it suggests that the individual was exposed to an atmosphere containing methane. As far as presence of carbon dioxide is concerned, it is a normal constituent of blood.

SEXUAL (AUTOEROTIC) ASPHYXIA

A subdivision of bondage includes those accidental deaths that occur during acts of sexual perversion practiced by one individual. Sexual asphyxia is used to describe deaths in which the fatal condition is self induced during the course of solitary erotic behaviour. Within this definition it follows that the death is asphyxial, but the classification excludes those deaths in other sexual cases where there is another person present and participating in the act.

These are asphyxial deaths principally due to hanging in which asphyxia is intentionally induced to enhance sexual arousal.

Typically, the deceased is found often tied up in a complicated fashion, in a secluded locality. Usually, the death scene is a lonely place, where the complicated preparation for the act cannot be discovered. The victim often goes through an elaborate ritual to enable to enjoy every stage. The attic, toilet or bedroom when other members are not present in the house or a secluded garden shed may be used.

Evidence of past use of the place for similar purpose can be observed by grooving of a wooden beam from which a rope has been suspended, the presence of concealed hook to suspend the rope and absence of paints in the pipes due to repeated use of rope etc. A mirror may be present to witness the procedure and to obtain self gratification. Pornographic books or pictures may be found thrown around the scene. Phallic shaped object, like broom handle or vibrator may be found near the body usually soiled with lubricants or fecal matter.

Sex and age distribution: The victim is usually exclusively male, rarely female in the age group of 12-25 years, with preponderance in 12-17 years; although cases at the extreme with children less than 12 years and old more than 60 years have been recorded.

Social class: No social class is exempt, but it is more commonly seen with professionals and artists.

Clothing: The deceased is almost naked, scantily dressed or dressed in a bizarre fashion. When wearing clothes, they are usually of the opposite sex. Quite often penis is covered in a handkerchief or a piece of cloth designed to prevent soiling of clothing during ejaculation.

Mode of Asphyxia

Death occurs as a result of asphyxia sustained during an attempt for sexual stimulation. The object is to produce a degree of hypoxia. Pressure over the neck is applied with some type of ligature with a pad in between for a soft feel on the neck. Sniffing of some noxious chemicals such as carbon tetrachloride, dichloroethane and other petroleum products (**Glue sniffing**) is also done at times to increase the effect. Pressure over chest may also be applied for a similar effect. Tying of whole body and limbs in a complicated manner is usually seen, which is meant to prevent voluntary relaxation of the ligature before achieving the required hypoxia. The pattern of binding and the use of apparatus often suggest that the act has been committed over a period of time. Careful examination of knots should be done to see if they can be self tied.

Mechanism

The object of this bizarre behaviour is to achieve sexual stimulation and to enhance orgasm by means of masturbation aided by hypoxia. Little evidence is present regarding the effect of hypoxia for sexual stimulation but women under effect of anaesthesia like nitrous oxide have often charged people with rape or indecent assault.

Cause of Death

Deaths result from the failure of "safety precautions" which are employed by the victim. The common causes are failure of slipknot to loosen, sudden collapse of stool, chain, extension weight. Plastic bags covering the face may cause suffocation. There is an absence of history of depression and no suicide notes are found. Death is most commonly accidental but not suicidal. Because of the absence of clinical cases involving living patients, no adequate understanding about the phenomenon is available.

The secret nature of the act is also a hindrance to the availability of full details regarding the incident. Even the closest relatives are unaware of them and moreover they are reluctant to seek medical advice. In married men, history from wife usually reveals a normal sexual life. These individuals are not dangerous to others, but at times sadistic murder may be committed.

Summary

(i) Evidence of abnormal sexual behaviour. (ii) Evidence of previous attempt. (iii) Evidence of padding between ligature and neck. (iv) No evidence of suicidal act such as absence of suicidal note. (v) Pornographic material should be collected from the scene, if present for corroboration of the evidence.

DROWNING

Drowning is a form of asphyxia due to aspiration of fluid into air passages caused by submersion in water or other fluid. Complete submersion is not necessary for drowning to occur. Our knowledge of the events that take place in the drowning victim is by no means complete. It is primarily derived from animal experiments and to some extent from the observations on human where drowning was witnessed and reported. Submersion is usually followed by a panicky struggle to reach the surface. When energy reserves are exhausted, the struggle subsides and actual drowning begins. When a person falls into water and sinks it is partly due to specific gravity of the body and partly due to force of fall. On sudden immersion into cold water, he may take a deep inhalation of water due to reflex from stimulation of the skin. The person may hold his breath for a varying period and then inhale carbon dioxide to stimulate the respiration center. As a result, inhalation of water may occur. He then cries to help that leads to inhalation of more water causing coughing and air is expelled out. If cerebral asphyxia will continue then death occurs in 3-10 minutes. The mechanism of struggle to breath before death in drowning is given in Figure 24.38.

Several phases are recognized in the drowning process: (i) Breath-holding lasts for a variable length of time until carbon dioxide accumulation in blood and tissues reaches a level at which stimulation of the respiratory center in brain leads to inevitable inhalation of large volumes of water. (ii) Swallowing of water, coughing, vomiting and progressive loss of consciousness follow in rapid succession. Escape of air remaining in the lungs, i.e., replaced by water leads to next phase. (iii) Profound unconsciousness and convulsions associated with gasping precede respiratory standstill, which is followed by failure of heart, irreversible changes in the brain and death supervene within a very short time.

Types of Drowning

Drowning is of following four types:

1. **Wet drowning:** In this type of drowning, more water goes to lungs.
2. **Dry drowning:** In this type of drowning, no water enters into the lungs and death occurs by laryngeal spasm.
3. **Secondary drowning:** It is post immersion syndrome and is also called **near drowning.** Death occurs after several episodes of resuscitation due to electrolytic disturbances such as metabolic acidosis. Lungs show haemorrhages and atelectasis. Myocardial anoxia may occur and may cause delayed heart failure.
4. **Immersion syndrome (Hydrocution):** Death in immersion syndrome is due to cardiac arrest as a result of vagal inhibition. It occurs in 1-2% cases of drowning. It is produced by: (i) Cold water stimulation by water striking the epigastrium. (ii) By cold water entering the ear drums, mucosa of pharynx or larynx. (iii) Cold water stimulating nerve endings of body surface.

   This can occur in circumstances of: (i) Falling or diving into the water with feet first; or (ii) 'Duck diving' by the inexperienced diver. (iii) Diving horizontally into water with blow to abdomen. This types of death occur in emotionally anxious those who intend to commit suicide with active nervous reflex. Alcohol increases such effects due to general vasodilatation.

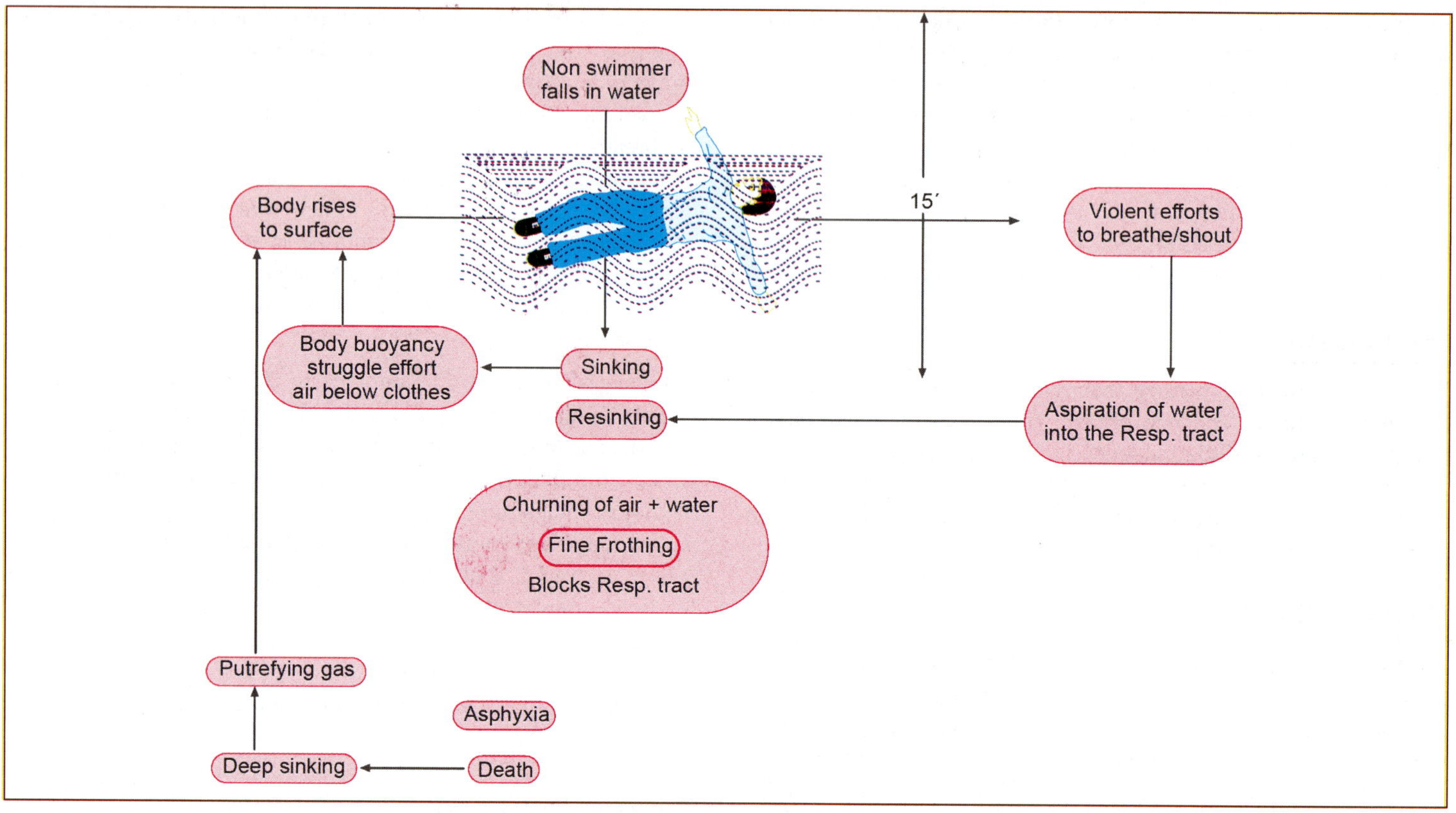

Figure 24.38: Mechanism of struggle to breathe before death in drowning

Pathophysiology of Drowning

Pulmonary alveolar lining is semipermeable and if water enters the alveoli, exchange of water takes place through the alveoli. The extent and direction depends upon the gradient between the osmotic pressure of blood and the water.

Drowning in fresh water or brackish water: In fresh water, water passes rapidly from the lungs to the blood, haemolysis and dilution of blood occurs thus increasing blood volume to 2.5 litres or more. Because of low salt content of these waters (brackish water has approximately 0.5% salinity), precipitous absorption into the circulation takes place. Fresh water alters or denatures the protective surfactant, which lines the alveolar wall. Loss of or inactivation of pulmonary surfactant and alveolar collapse decreases lung compliance causing severe ventilation perfusion mismatch up to 75% of the blood perfusing non-ventilated areas. When water is inhaled, vagal reflexes cause increased peripheral airway resistance with pulmonary vasoconstriction, pulmonary hypertension, decrease in lung compliance and fall of ventilation perfusion and increased Na^+ and K^+ concentration in serum leading to overburdening of heart causing pulmonary oedema. Pulmonary oedema occurs due to defective functioning of surfactant. Arrhythmias of heart beat, which culminate in ventricular fibrillation leading to death within 3-5 minutes from the start of submersion. Haemodilution leads to haemolysis causing haemoglobinemia and haemoglobinuria.

Drowning in Sea Water

In sea water (NaCl content is 3%) due to high concentration, water is drawn from the blood in the lung tissue causing severe pulmonary oedema, hypernatremia and haemoconcentration. At the same time, there is an attempt to reestablish osmotic balance, salts from sea water in the lungs pass to the blood stream with slow death from asphyxia. Death occurs in 4-8 minutes. Overall, death may occur from asphyxia, ventricular fibrillation, cerebral anoxia, injuries caused during drowning, vagal inhibition and laryngeal spasm. Salt water drowning usually lasts longer and hence is likely to be more amenable to resuscitation than drowning in fresh water.

Different mechanisms in fresh water versus salt water drowning has significant implications with respect to blood alcohol concentration of the victim. In fresh water drowning dilution of blood may be expected to cause a decrease in the alcohol level, whereas in salt water drowning a slight increase occurs.

Diagnosis of Drowning

Drowning is mostly accidental. In a relatively small number of cases, it is suicidal. In some cases, death in the water is due to natural causes, such as heart attack or cerebral haemorrhage during bathing or swimming. Disposal of victim of a homicide to simulate drowning is rare yet because of such possibility, distinction between changes due to drowning and those resulting from postmortem immersion of the body is of prime importance.

There is no reliable test permitting an equivocal diagnosis of drowning. Thus, the central question in the case of a body recovered from water is whether the individual was alive at the time he entered the water. The scene, the circumstances surrounding the incident with all available background information and deceased's clothing all play a significant role for example the finding of an alcoholic floating in water 20 ft below the cliff with his zip open suggests that he had been urinating before he fell. The rare instance of hand clutching weeds concludes that the deceased may have struggled to stay on surface. The presence of water in the lungs and stomach of a drowning victim is of no real significance. Water may well reach these organs after death. At autopsy, the lungs of a drowning victim commonly resemble those seen in cases of atherosclerotic heart disease.

Drowning in the bath tub occurs only if unconsciousness is brought down by disease (epilepsy, or heart disease) or after consumption of alcohol or drugs. Accidental drowning in the swimming pool sometimes results from jumping off the diving board. Impact of the forehead on the floor of pool may cause hyperextension of the head and loss of consciousness with subsequent inhalation of water. Common autopsy findings in these cases consist of haemorrhage in the deep neck muscles in the region of cervical 1 and 2 vertebra with or without vertebral fractures.

There are cases seen in which young healthy individuals while engaged in underwater swimming died by sudden drowning. A plausible explanation is that usually a diver hyperventilates before entering the water, the overbreathing followed by exercise under water causes fall in arterial oxygen tension to a level at which consciousness is lost and water is inhaled.

Autopsy Findings in Drowning Deaths

A body in water will sink unless air trapped among the clothes keeps it afloat. The body will resurface when gas is formed because of putrefaction. Putrefaction in water proceeds at a considerably slower rate than in the air but once the body is removed from water, postmortem changes progress far more rapidly than is usual under the same prevailing environmental conditions. Putrefaction is slower in sea water compared to fresh water because high salinity retards bacterial growth. The time until reappearance of the body depends on the temperature of water. It may take two to three days in summer and weeks or months in winter. While the body is underwater, it is subject to injuries by wildlife or by drifting along the ground. These injuries should be recognized and distinguished from injuries sustained during life. A victim of drowning tends to bleed more readily and more blood oozes from a wound of such an individual. Postmortem lividity is difficult to recognize in a body recovered from water due to swelling and loss of translucency of the upper layer of the skin, the skin becomes waterlogged if immersion is prolonged. Algae grow on the exposed part giving prolonged green or black colour to those areas. Adipocere formation is common in victims of submersion.

Caisson disease: It occurs in underwater diving when the diver remains underwater for prolonged period at great depths due to change of ambient pressure causing formation of bubbles in his blood and tissues if the ascent is too fast. At autopsy, the finding consistent of foci of ischemic necrosis especially in brain, lungs show haemorrhage, oedema, atelectasis and areas of emphysema.

Signs of Immersion

1. **Maceration of skin:** It begins within minutes in warm water, such as death in bath tub, but in cold water is visible after variable time; the minimum probably being 4-5 hours. The first sign tends to be on areas with an appreciable keratin layer such as fingertips, palms, back of hands and then soles where the surface becomes bleached, wrinkled, pale and sodden, the so called **washer women's skin** (Figure 24.39A). After some days in warmer water and up to several weeks in cold, the thick keratin of hands and feet becomes detached and eventually peels off in 'glove and stocking' fashion. The nails and hairs become loosened at the same time. It is not associated with the process of drowning but is due to prolonged immersion. It cannot be used to determine the length of time the body was in water. In cold water, several days may elapse, while in warm water several hours may suffice. The glove may be used for fingerprint for identification. In second degree burns and in decomposition, peeling of skin from hands and feet occurs in similar fashion. Soddening of the skin due to absorption of water occurs into its outer layer. This involves first the fingertips, then in 2-4 hours it spreads to palm and to back of the hand in 24 hours. Similar changes are seen in the foot. If shoes are there, it takes twice as long.
2. **Cutis anserina or goose flesh:** It is a common finding in immersed bodies but is related to cold water than warm water. The erector pilae muscles attached to each hair follicle can contract in any type of death and cause a generalized dimpling of skin. Skin has granular and puckered appearance due to spasm of erector fibers and the muscles attached to hair follicles. It can occur in those living in cold weather and it may occur in submersion of body in cold water after death during molecular death. Retraction of scrotum and penis occurs due to cutis anserina.
3. **Estimation of duration of immersion:** This is another difficult problem and one that is often too dogmatically answered by doctor with insufficient experience to appreciate the potential error. The overriding variable factor is water temperature that has most common effect on decomposition. When a body falls into water in average temperature climate the following is an approximate guide to timing: (i) If no wrinkling of finger pads is present, less than few hours have elapsed. (ii) Wrinkled fingers, palm and feet progressively

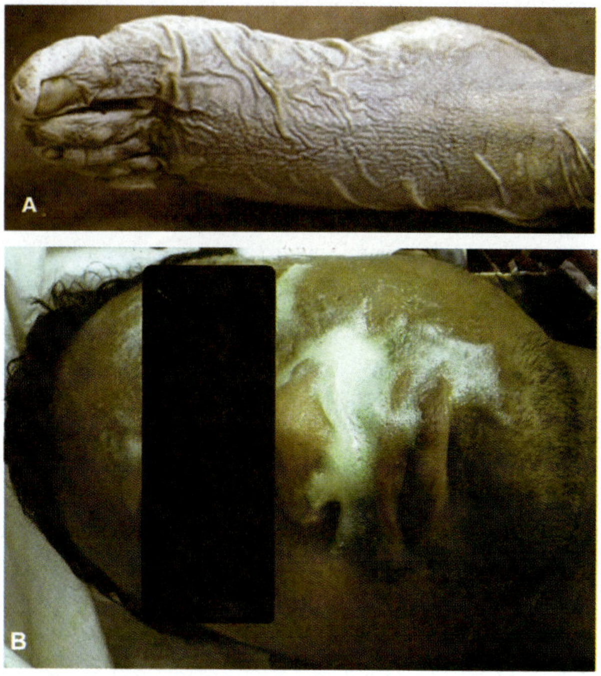

Figure 24.39A, B: Washer women's skin on foot (A) and froth (B) in drowning

occurs from ½-3 days. (iii) Early decomposition often first in the dependent head and neck, abdomen and thighs is 4-10 days. (iv) Bloating of face, abdomen with marbling of veins, peeling of epidermis on hands and feet is 2-4 weeks. (v) Gross skin shedding, muscle loss with skeletal exposure, partial liquefaction in 1-2 months.

This time may be reduced or exceeded by wide margin depending on animal predation, climatic changes, bodily built and type of water whether contaminated or not.

External

(i) Clothing is wet and skin is wet, cold clammy and pale due to vasoconstriction. (ii) ***Distribution and colour of postmortem hypostasis:*** It is usual for most corpses to float or hang in water in prone position and the head and limbs hang down. Head, neck and face, upper part of chest and upper arm show postmortem staining in such cases. However, water movement often roll the body constantly unless in a placid lake. Other corpses may float upon the back and gravitational staining of the skin may therefore be in any pattern if the body is subject to frequent change of posture. Postmortem staining is usually pink due to oxygenation but may be dusky and cyanotic. (iii) ***Haemorrhage in middle ear and mastoid air cells:*** These are occasionally encountered in persons recovered from water. However, this is not specific for drowning, as it can also be seen due to pressure change as in underwater diving or from extreme congestion as seen in other types of asphyxial deaths or heart failure. (iv) Cyanosis may or may not be there. (v) Conjunctiva is congested and petechial haemorrhages may be present. An occasional small haemorrhage may be seen in the conjunctiva but multiple pinpoint haemorrhages as seen in strangulation or hanging do not occur in drowning. (vi) Pupils may be dilated and the tongue is swollen and protruded. (vii) Rigor mortis appears early, when violent struggle takes place before death. (viii) ***Abundant foam:*** It is usually noted extruding from mouth and nostrils of a drowning victim (Figure 24.39B). The froth may extend to the trachea, bronchi and lower air passages. This foam may not be apparent when the body is recovered from water, but it appears when pressure is applied to the chest. The froth is fine, leathery, tenacious and white or mixed with blood present over mouth and nostrils. This results from inhalation of water that irritates the mucous membrane and stimulates the secretion of mucous. Air with mucous and water creates a churning effect and causes the froth. Thus, the foam is produced by mixture of air, mucous and water in presence of respiratory movements. There is formation of fine bubbles that do not easily collapse when touched with the points of a knife. It may project as a small balloon or mushroom like mass or a curved horn from the mouth and nostrils. The froth may not be there in dry drowning. Hence, the presence of foam in the airway indicates beyond doubt that the victim was alive at the time of submersion. Frequently the foam is bloodstained, not as a result of injury to the chest, but due to the tears of the lung tissue by increased pressure within the lungs, which is part of drowning process. When decomposition sets in foam is rapidly changed to a foul smelling, brown somewhat bubbly fluid. (ix) ***Cadaveric spasm*:** Presence of weeds, ground and grass in the hands that are clenched. It indicates the person was alive when drowned. Damaged nails and abraded fingers may be present due to struggle to survive.

Differential Diagnosis of Froth in Drowning

(i) Strangulation (ii) Acute pulmonary oedema (iii) Electrical shock (iv) Epilepsy (v) Opium poisoning (vi) Putrefaction.

Internal

Internally lungs show the main features suggestive of drowning. Macroscopically they are voluminous, completely covering the pericardial sac and bulge out of the chest when the sternum is removed. Passive collapse which usually occurs in death does not occur due to the fact that oedema fluid blocks the bronchi. The lungs show rib impressions on the surface and do not collapse when kept on a table. On cut section they may appear dry, but large amount of water, sometimes foamy, ooze from the surface on squeezing. If lungs are left alone, water will start to trickle from the surface and they will slowly collapse because of increased pressure during forced expirations.

1. **Paltauf's haemorrhages:** Alveolar walls rupture producing haemorrhages and when located subpleurally these are called Paultauf's haemorrhages. These are usually present in the lower lobes of the lungs. They may be seen on the anterior surface and interlobar surfaces of lungs. They may however be absent. These haemorrhages are shining, pale bluish and may be minute or 3-5 cm in diameter. Spot like **haemorrhages**

in the lungs especially under the pleura are often noted in drowning. These haemorrhages result from overdistension of the lungs by drowning liquid and hemolysis and dilution accounts for their pink appearance. This drowning lung is fairly characteristic but not pathognomic. This condition of the lung is called '**Emphysema aquosum**' and '**trockenes oedema**'. Active respiratory movements is a prerequisite for the drowning water to reach all the peripheral parts of lungs.

2. After death, water cannot reach the lungs by hydrostatic pressure when the body is submerged but the amount of water would be small and it would gravitate only to the lower parts of the lungs. Therefore, **hydrostatic lung** cannot simulate drowning lung. Muller, Reh and Eisele, using high pressure chamber or lowering the body in normal water showed that it is possible to develop hydrostatic lung that cannot be distinguished from drowning lung. Thus, drowning lung was developed by putting the body 3 meters deep for 65 hours (when death is due to hanging) and even a depth of 2 meters for 20 hours may produce drowning lung.

   Therefore, **Reh** was of the opinion that drowning lung is diagnostic for drowning only if the: (i) Body has remained floating on or very near the surface. (ii) Drowning lung with frothy fluid over mouth and nostrils should not leave any doubt about the diagnosis of drowning.

3. **Histological findings of drowning lung:** Much of the work has been done to confirm histologically the genuineness of 'emphysema aquosum' in both fresh and decayed bodies, but the dilation and rupture of the terminal air space can occur not only as a result of drowning but of passive immersion in water deeper than 4 meters. Dilatation of the alveoli, thinning of the walls and compression of the capillaries are easy to obscure but the significance is ambiguous. The number of macrophages in the alveoli adjusted to the size of the alveoli where distended was studied by **Betz**, who carried a diagnostic usefulness of the method as long as no autolytic changes are present. **Haffner** has used the weight of spleen as a diagnostic marker in drowning compared with other modes of asphyxia about an 18% reduction in weights and spleen-liver ratios were recorded. The skin changes in maceration are also well recorded.

   Drowning cases with relatively dry lungs are occasionally observed. Heart action continues in drowning after cessation of respiration. This is sufficient to absorb water from the lungs into the bloodstream and as no significant amount of water reaches the alveoli after inhalation is stopped and the same can be seen when resuscitative measures are started immediately.

   The microscopic findings after haematoxylin and eosin staining does not yield much about the diagnosis. Following stages are encountered:

   Stage 1: Thickness of the alveolar wall (normally 2-3 times the capillary width) is reduced to capillary width. Capillary appears round or oval like a chain. Partial fiber rupture may be observed.

   Stage 2: Alveoli are more distended and capillaries lie separately. Fiber rupture is more marked.

   Stage 3: Maximal distension of alveolar walls. Capillaries appear thread like and only occasional lumina are observed. Distinct intraseptal fiber rupture is there.

   Stage 4: This stage is seldom seen and may involve only scattered alveoli. There is complete rupture of alveolar walls and retraction of the fibers like a corkscrew.

   The microscopic findings in the lungs in drowning are not characteristic, yet they differ to some extent depending on whether drowning occurred in fresh water or in sea water.

   Differences in lungs in fresh water and sea water drowning: In fresh water drowning, the lungs are over-distended, alveolar walls are torn and structures in the way of the inundating fluid are disrupted. This picture is referred to as '**aqueous emphysema**' and the intraalveolar haemorrhage leading to pinkish or red staining of foam in the airway. In sea water drowning, the architecture of lungs is often better preserved and aqueous emphysema is less pronounced.

   Differential diagnoses of drowning lung: (i) Aspiration of blood (ii) Capillary bronchitis (iii) Fatal asthmatic attack (iv) Hypoxia from strangulation and throttling (v) Chronic emphysema.

   In hydrostatic lung, reticular fibers show different picture. The fibers do not withstand hydrostatic pressure. Therefore, the fibers show coarse rupture and fragmentation. No stage of 2 and 3 of drowning lung is seen.

4. **Water in stomach and duodenum:** Water is present in the stomach and duodenum. Much amount of water may be swallowed which passes into the duodenum. It does not enter into the stomach after death as a result of the hydrostatic pressure. If a body is kept at a depth of 15 meters for 65 hours then no water enters the stomach. Thus, it is very vital sign that the person entered the water when he was alive and also a significant sign of drowning. The fallacy is that the deceased might have drank water prior to death or taken beverages before drowning in water. Therefore, absence of water proves nothing. The stomach may contain even foreign materials from the water such as slit, weed or sand but this cannot be accepted as positive aid in the diagnosis.

5. **Over-inflation of lungs:** Apart from generalized water-logging, the lungs may be markedly over inflated, filling the thoracic cavity when the sternum is removed. The texture is rather pale and crepitant, superficially resembling that in

asthma. The older name for this condition is '***emphysema aquosum***'. In drowning on the lateral surfaces of the lungs impression of the ribs, leaving visible and palpable grooves after removal of the organs from the thorax.

6. **Other organs:** The heart and great veins have often been said to be 'dilated and engorged' with fluid blood especially the right side but this is a nonspecific finding.

Cause of Death in Drowning

During the autopsy at times it poses problems as findings are minimal, obscure or completely absent. In such cases, the cause of death may be given as: (i) Consistent with drowning; or as (ii) Cause cannot be given; or (iii) Death is due to drowning.

Laboratory Diagnosis of Drowning

There are considerable doubts about the reliability of these chemical tests.

1. **Carrara in 1902** established disproportionate dilution of left heart blood in fresh water versus salt water based on specific gravity, and freezing point. Also, there is difference in electrical activity between the two sides but no definite findings were given.
2. **In 1921, Gettler** published a test for drowning from right and left heart chambers, a **difference of 25 mg/100 ml between the chloride concentrations** of the two sides of the heart indicated that the death was due to drowning. In fresh water drowning the chloride level in the blood in the left side of the heart was lower than in the right side; the reverse situation was noted in salt water drowning. Positive is seen in sea water drowning due to hemoconcentration and negative in fresh water drowning due to hemodilution.
3. **In 1944, Mortiz** suggested magnesium as being reliable than chlorides particularly for sea water drowning. He proposed that plasma concentration of magnesium differed between the left and right side of heart due to absorption of the ion from the drowning water especially if it is sea water.
4. **In 1953, Durlacher *et al.*** suggested that the plasma specific gravity in the left and right sides of the heart could accurately diagnose a case of drowning death. They revealed that both in fresh water and salt water drowning death, the plasma specific gravity in the left heart is lower than the right heart. If it is higher in left than right heart, then the person died of some other cause.
5. **In 1955, Freimuth *et al.,*** using specific gravity of heart plasma, concluded that negative differences between the left and right side may be obtained either in drowning or non-drowning cases, while positive values usually indicate that the death was caused by means other than drowning.
6. Quantitative assays of peroxidase in animal lungs yielded value close to 800 units in fresh water drowning and 6400 units in salt water drowning.

Diatoms and Drowning

In 1941 **Incze** demonstrated that diatoms could enter the systemic circulation via the lungs during drowning. The portal of entry of diatoms into bloodstream was believed to be via lungs through microscopic tears of alveolar walls that occur in the process of forceful water inhalation. All waters, fresh or salt water contain microscopic plants, the algae. The algae do not grow or grow only in small numbers in heavily polluted waters. Such water may also contain particulate matter characteristic for local pollution and the algae.

In 1963, the value of this method was questioned by recovery of diatoms in the liver and in other organs of individuals who had died of causes other than drowning. These diatoms may have been absorbed through gastrointestinal tract when the water containing diatoms was drunk.

Revenstrof in 1904 was the first to attempt to use diatom as a test for drowning. The basic premise is that when a living person is drowned in water containing diatoms, many diatoms will penetrate the alveolar walls and be carried to distant organs such as brain, kidneys, liver and bone marrow. After autopsy, samples of these organs can be digested with strong acid to dissolve soft tissue, thus leaving the highly resistant diatom to be identified under microscope. When a dead body is deposited in water or when death in the water is not due to drowning then although diatom may reach lungs by passive percolation, the absence of beating heart prevents circulation of diatoms to distant organs. The great advantage of the diatom test, if it were reliable would be that a positive diagnosis of drowning could be made even in the frequently putrefied bodies that are removed.

There are two main types; green algae and diatoms that are supplied with a delicate and beautiful heat and acid resistant siliceous shell, which is unicellular. Cell wall is usually strongly impregnated with silica and contain chlorophyll and a brown pigment. Diatom secretes hard siliceous outer box like skeleton called **frustule**. They resist heat and acid and vary in size from 2 microns to 1 mm though most of them are 10-80 microns in size and 10 microns in width. Diatoms upto the size of 60 microns can enter the pulmonary circulation during drowning. They vary from place to place and there is seasonal variation in the same place. They occur in cultivated soils and surface of moist rocks. Large numbers of free-floating diatoms are found in sea water and fresh water. Their shape is circular, triangular, oval, linear or rectangular (Figure 24.40). They can be demonstrated by the following:

Direct microscopic examination: This is only used in the examination of the lungs. Water is squeezed out of the lungs and centrifuged and the sediment is examined.

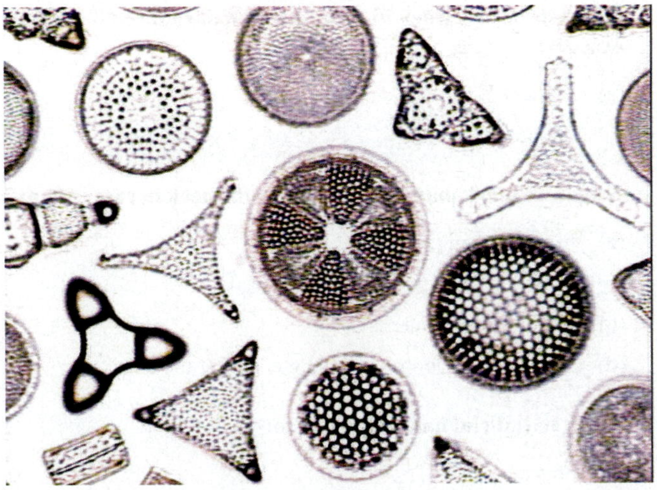

Figure 24.40: Different types of diatoms

Microscopic examination of tissue sections: Optically empty sections are prepared and quantitative analysis is done.

Chemical digestion: The tissue is prepared with acids whereby all organic matter is digested, but the siliceous shells of the diatoms are well preserved.

Incineration: Organic matter is destroyed with heat in an oven.

Principle of diatoms (Figure 24.41): The drowning fluid and the particles in it, i.e., diatoms and planktons pass from the ruptured alveolar wall into the lymph channels and pulmonary veins and left side of heart. Only in living body the diatoms are found in bone marrow, brain, liver and skeletal muscle etc. It is also found in bile and urine etc. Bone marrow is highly suitable and reliable. After cutting the bone the marrow is curetted from the gutter.

There can be situations where the diatoms may be absent even though the person is known to have drowned or they are present without drowning. These are: (i) *Seasonal variation:* A person may have drowned when the water is almost devoid of diatoms so no diatoms are recovered. (ii) A person may eat raw fruits or vegetables, which have been in contact with soil diatoms and shellfish, which feed on diatoms and show diatoms in the body. (iii) Large amounts of diatoms are found in materials used for manufacturing of buildings like cement, paint, paper, insulators etc. The atmosphere near the plants providing such material is highly polluted and the person might have inhaled and may have such diatoms in his body. (iv) Certain dusting powders contain diatoms, which may have been inhaled by the person and are found in his body. (v) Diatoms are ubiquitous, being present in soil, water supplies and in the air. (vi) They can also penetrate the intestinal lining and gain access to the bloodstream and hence any body tissues. (vii) Certain food, notably shellfish contains vast quantities of diatoms that may enter the circulation.

According to **Henday**, following two requirements to be fulfilled: (i) All the species recovered from the organs of the body must be present in the samples of water in the place of submersion. (ii) They must be present in approximately the same proportion in the organ as in the sample from the place of submersion.

LONG QUESTIONS

1. Define asphyxia. Discuss the various types of hanging and the autopsy findings in a case of hanging.
2. Define strangulation. What are the different postmortem findings and causes of death in strangulation.
3. Discuss the pathophysiology in drowning and role of diatoms in drowning cases.
4. Discuss the various types of drowning with the autopsy findings in fresh water drowning.
5. What is Gordon's classification of asphyxial deaths and discuss in detail pathophysiology in such deaths.
6. What is suffocation? Discuss the postmortem findings and medicolegal importance in such deaths.

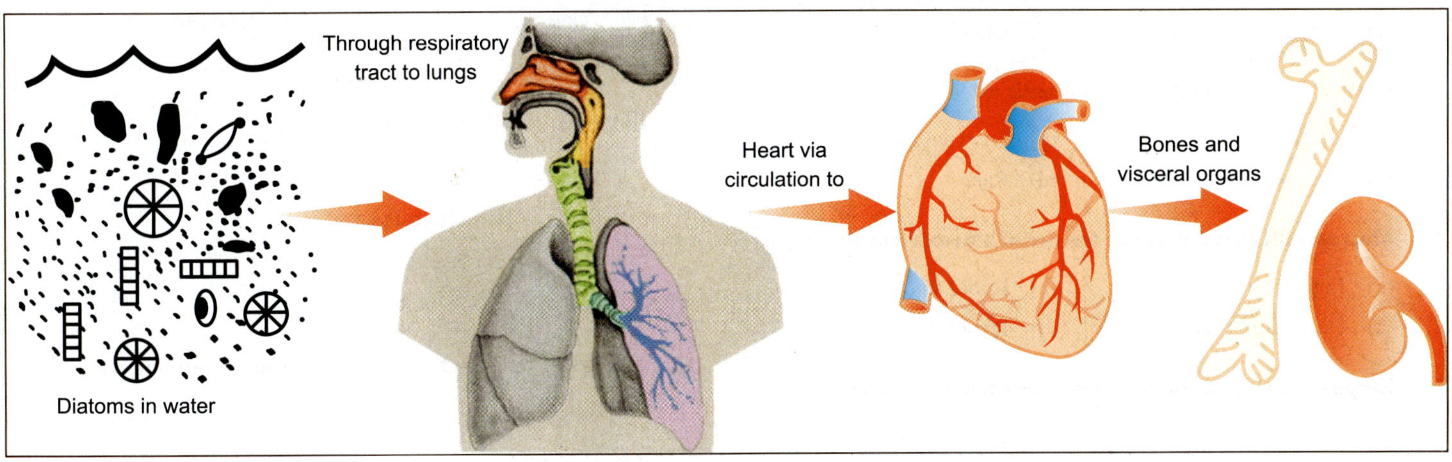

Figure 24.41: Transmission of diatoms

SHORT QUESTIONS

1. Hyoid bone and Asphyxial deaths.
2. Bansdola.
3. Judicial hanging.
4. Cafe coronary.
5. Gettler's test.
6. Suffocation.
7. Throttling.
8. Mugging.
9. Garroting.
10. Burking.
11. Paltauf's haemorrhages.
12. Differences between fresh water and sea water drowning.
13. Dry drowning.
14. Diatoms.
15. Sexual asphyxia.

MULTIPLE CHOICE QUESTIONS

1. Presence of diatoms in the bone marrow indicates the death due to:

(a) Choking (b) Drowning
(c) Strangulation (d) Hanging

2. Paltauf's haemorrhage found in:

(a) Arsenic poisoning (b) Strangulation
(c) Drowning (d) Hanging

3. Hyoid bone fracture is commonly found in:

(a) Manual strangulation (b) Ligature strangulation
(c) Hanging (d) Choking

4. Gettler's test is useful in the diagnosis of:

(a) Hanging (b) Drowning
(c) Strangulation (d) Rape

5. Most specific and diagnostic feature of antemortem hanging is:

(a) Ligature mark (b) Hyoid fracture
(c) Dribbling of saliva (d) Incontinence of urine

6. Emphysema aquosum and trockenes edema is seen in:

(a) Wet drowning (b) Dry drowning
(c) Immersion syndrome (d) Secondary drowning

7. Cyanosis occurs when in concentration of reduced haemoglobin exceeds:

(a) 3 grams % (b) 5 grams %
(c) 7 grams % (d) 9 grams %

8. A ligature mark may not be found in the neck in case of hanging:

(a) In partial hanging
(b) When the ligature is of soft material
(c) If a narrow ligature is used
(d) When a fixed loop with a single knot at the chin

9. Death in judicial hanging is due to:

(a) Shock
(b) Fracture dislocation of upper cervical vertebrate
(c) Rapid asphyxia
(d) Inhibition of heart

10. A 35-year-old male, healthy and grossly intoxicated, suddenly collapsed while eating at a dining table, the likely cause of death is:

(a) Choking (b) Myocardial infarction
(c) Acute asthmatic attack (d) Gagging

11. The cause of death in Cafe Coronary is:

(a) Asphyxia (b) Laryngeal spasm
(c) Sudden heart attack (d) Coronary thrombosis

12. Which one of the following asphyxia deaths is suggestive of homicide?

(a) Overlaying (b) Café coronary
(c) Gagging (d) Positional asphyxia

13. Most common method of suicide in India is:

(a) Hanging (b) Poisoning
(c) Fall from height (d) Consuming sleeping pills

14. In typical hanging, the knot is found:

(a) On mentum at anterior side of neck
(b) On right ear at lateral part of neck
(c) On left ear at lateral part of neck
(d) At nape of neck on the back

15. Amussat's sign can be seen in following conditions *except:*

(a) Hanging (b) Whiplash injuries
(c) Drowning (d) Blunt trauma to neck

16. During autopsy of a hanging death, stripe like haemorrhages on anterior aspect of the intervertebral disks of the lumbar part of the spinal column is observed. This feature is named as:

(a) Simon's bleeding

(b) Tua's bleeding

(c) Amussat's sign

(d) Hanging artefacts

ANSWER KEY

1. (b)	2. (c)	3. (a)	4. (b)	5. (c)	6. (a)	7. (b)	8. (b)	9. (b)	10. (a)
11. (a)	12. (c)	13. (a)	14. (d)	15. (c)	16. (a)				

25 CHAPTER

Infanticide

Infanticide: It is unlawful killing of a newborn below the age of one year. It was a recognized practice in many primitive communities. This problem persists throughout the world and took place for a variety of reasons in the past. It does not include death during labour by craniotomy or decapitation.

Foeticide: It is killing of the foetus at any time prior to birth.

Neonaticide: It is intentional killing of a child within 24 hours of its birth.

Fillicide: It is killing of a child by the parents.

Motives of Infanticide

Uncivilized societies: (i) The basic motive is survival of the fittest with destruction of those suffering from malformation and females being of less potential value to the community are killed. (ii) Some newborns are killed owing to tribal superstitions as some of them are considered unlucky such as twin births, those having teeth at birth and those with leg presentations. (iii) Due to the age long desire for strength and fertility some communities believe that destruction and eating the first newborn child added strength to those who devoured it.

Civilized societies: (i) To get rid of illegitimate children (ii) To get rid of child when mother is widow or unmarried (iii) When the parents belong to socially and economically weaker section of the society.

Laws in Relation to Infanticide

The infanticide laws differ in different countries but its evolution in England is of particular interest. Until 1922, the unlawful killing of newborn was murder, no matter by whom it is done. This made no allowance for the fact that the effects of delivery may temporarily disturb the balance of the mother's mind and she would then not be responsible if at that time her act or omission led to the destruction of her child.

1. **The Infanticide Act (1922):** This Act made provision of infanticide being committed by the mother with disturbed mental balance under the effects of delivery. This was applicable only to England (not applicable to Ireland or Scotland). This Act also did not take into account lactation and did not define any age limitation.

   In 1926, this Act was re enacted and defined the age limit of infanticide that is the child under 12 months. There are some points that should be stressed regarding the Infanticide Act: (i) It is only the mother who can be charged with the offence (ii) Child must be born alive (of course be viable) (iii) It must have been killed (iv) There must be evidence to establish that the mother is suffering from the disease of the mind for the reasons mentioned.

   The Act clearly states that it is applicable only to the mother and anyone else including the husband will be charged with *Murder or Manslaughter.*

2. **Infanticide Act 1938:** Section I enacts that "where a woman by any willful act or omission causes the death of her child being under the age of 12 months, but at the time of the act or omission the balance of her mind was disturbed by reason of her not having fully recovered from the effect of giving birth to the child or by reason of the effects of lactation consequent upon the birth of the child, then, notwithstanding

that the circumstance were such that but for this Act the offence would have amounted to murder." She is guilty of the felony of infanticide and may be dealt with and punished as if she had committed manslaughter. This Act talks of the 'balance of mind was disturbed at the time of the act'. This being a broader term needs to be proved by the doctor who is conducting her obstetrical checkup and by the psychiatrist.

In pursuance of **section 60 "Offence Against the Persons Act, 1861"** for which the child is deemed to have been recently born, if it has been born within 12 months before its death.

In every case of infanticide, legal presumption is that the child is born dead, and the onus of proving that the child was born alive rests on the crown. There is no need to produce the body and it is not necessary to prove that the child has been viable.

3. **Infant Life (Preservation) Act 1929:** The law was amended with regard to the destruction of children at or before labour. This Act defined the crime of child destruction as "Any person who, with intent to destroy the life of a child capable of being born alive, by any willful act causes a child to die before it has an existence independent of its mother, shall be guilty of felony, to wit of child destruction and shall be liable on conviction thereof on indictment to imprisonment for life". Thus, this offence cannot be committed during the earlier stages of pregnancy. The criteria to be fulfilled for the purpose of this Act are as follows: (i) Woman must be pregnant for a period of 28th weeks or more (ii) There shall be prima facie proof that she was at that time pregnant of a child capable of being born alive.

   This Act provides that if the person is not guilty of offence of murder, manslaughter or infanticide, he can be charged to be guilty of child destruction.

4. **Criminal Law of England:** According to this law, a child is considered to be born alive when it is completely born external to the mother irrespective of the attachment or severance of the cord. Hence, according to the English Law destruction of an infant before its complete birth has taken place is not homicide.

5. **Laws in India:** The definition held by Indian law is more correct and appropriate. It constitutes live birth even **if any part of child** has been brought forth external to the mother, though the child may not have breathed or completely born. The law in India draws no distinction between the murder of the newborn and that of any other individual and the provisions of the law that apply to homicide also apply to infanticide. Hence, according to Indian law, killing of an infant before any part of it is born is not homicide, but destruction of an infant after any part of it has been brought forth external to the mother, even before its complete birth constitutes homicide. Therefore, the definition of infanticide could be applied not only to the mother but also to the father. Legal bearing is same as culpable homicide except that the **law presumes that child is born dead**. It is for the prosecution to prove that the child is born alive and died from criminal violence. The crime is usually committed at the time or within few minutes or hours after the birth of the child.

Examination of the Woman

Signs consistent with a precipitate or difficult labour are impossible to find if more than 3 weeks have passed after delivery. However, immediately after delivery extragenital and genital signs can be discerned. In such cases, the Medical Officer is required to examine the woman. It should include: (i) Time interval between delivery and examination (ii) Mental status that is general demeanor and emotional state (iii) Signs of recent delivery.

Points in Relation to Infanticide

(i) Is the body of the child found that of a viable child? (ii) Is the body of the child belongs to the accused woman? (iii) Was the child still born or dead born? (iv) Was the child born alive? (v) If born alive, how long has the child survived? (vi) What was the cause of death?

Is the child viable? **Viability** means capability of having a separate existence after birth by virtue of certain degree of development. It should be explained that unless the child born has reached a stage of development, which is consistent with the possibility of a live birth, the charge of infanticide or child destruction would not be preferred against mother. In law, a foetus which has not attended a completion of 7th month of intrauterine life is said to be incapable of maintaining a separate existence and therefore nonviable. Where it can be shown that the child was premature, there is a strong presumption of stillbirth or death from prematurity shortly after live birth. If the child shows evidence of less than 7th month that failed to live by reason of immaturity. On the other hand, if there is any evidence that the foetus has lived after birth charge of infanticide will apply. Viability need not be proved, but in doubtful cases, it is improbable that the child had a separate existence. The Court sometimes requires to know whether the infant had attained the 28th week of gestation at the date on which it was killed. The opinion is based not only on a single criterion but upon several parameters. These are:

i. *General condition of the foetus:* Its plumpness that is fullness or fatness of the body and absence of apparent disease or malformation.

ii. *Weight of the foetus:* In multiple births, the weight of each of the infants is appreciably less than that of a single birth at the same stage of gestation. The female foetus is 100 gm less in weight than the male foetus.

iii. *Crown-heel length of the foetus:* It has been established that there is a close relationship between age and height of the foetus. To calculate age from height, crown-heel length is the best criteria (Table 25.1).

Table 25.1: Weight and length of the foetus in relation to age		
Age	Weight	Crown-heel length
28 weeks	2½-3lb (1.1-1.3 kg)	35 cm
32 weeks	3½-4lb (1.6-1.8 kg)	40 cm
36 weeks	5lb (2.2 kg)	45 cm
40 weeks	6-7lb (2.7-3.2 kg)	50 cm

Is the body of the child belongs to the accused woman? Proof on this point is most usually established for the evidence of persons with whom the suspected woman has more or less intimately associated in work or social life. At times careful examination by the police of the wrappings, which envelop the body of a child, may throw some light on the identity of the mother.

Was the child stillborn or dead born? A distinction must be drawn between still born and dead born:

Stillborn foetus: According to W.H.O. it is defined as one, which has issued forth from the mother after 28th week of pregnancy and did not at any time after being completely expelled, breathed or showed any other signs of life. This definition poses some problems in the English law. For example, the mother, whilst one foot of the child is still in the vagina, strangle it or kill it by some other means, even if it has cried since the delivery of the head, she is not guilty of offence, because the child by definition a still birth, not being completely expelled.

From practical point of view, it is highly unlikely that a woman who does not know the law would invent the story of incomplete expulsion, hence if she volunteers it in her original statement, it is difficult to refute. In cases of unidentified children, it is slightly impossible for the pathologist even if he finds evidence of breathing to say that the foetus had a separate existence.

Causes of still birth: (i) Anoxia of premature foetus (ii) Excessive moulding of head due to prolonged labour (iii) Toxaemia of pregnancy (iv) Rh incompatibility (v) Congenital defects in foetus/placenta.

To constitute still birth: (i) Period of pregnancy shall be ≥ 28 weeks (ii) The child was alive in uterus but had died during the process of birth and did not breath or show any signs of life or of separate existence after birth.

Dead born child: The foetus had died in the uterus itself and may show one of the following signs after it is completely born:

1. *Rigor mortis:* Rigor mortis present at birth suggests death *in utero* 2-3 hours before delivery.
2. *Maceration (Figure 25.1A to C):* Maceration is a process of aseptic autolysis and is the usual change if the foetus remains in the uterus for 3-4 days surrounded with liquor amnii, but exclusion of air and intact membranes. It is not seen if the foetus is born within 24 hours after death. If air enters, then putrefaction will set in. Macerated baby is soft, flaccid and flattens out when placed on a surface level. It has a sweetish, disagreeable odour; skin is red or purple. The signs of maceration are: (i) Earliest sign is slippage of skin that is seen within 12 hours of death of child inside the uterus (ii) If there is presence of gas in great vessels (Aorta), it indicates fetal death (iii) Large blebs filled with serous fluid are present (iv) Epidermis is easily peeled off leaving a moist and greasy area (v) Tissues are oedematous, abdomen is distended, and serous cavities are filled with serous turbid fluid (vi) Soft parts are readily detachable from the bone (vii) There is abnormal mobility of the joints and the small bones are separated (viii) All the viscera is softened except lungs and uterus which are unchanged for a long time. (ix) ***Spalding's sign***: Spalding sign is loss of alignment and overlapping of the bones of the cranial vault due to shrinkage of brain. It develops earlier in vertex presentation. It can be detected by X-ray examination within a few days of death of the foetus but often takes much longer time like 2-3 weeks. It is one of the surest signs of intrauterine death. (x) ***Robert' s sign:*** It is the presence of gas in the foetal vascular system of the dead foetus *in situ* uterus seen on X-ray. (xi) ***Deuel's halo sign:*** It is separation of the subcutaneous fat of the foetal scalp from the cranial bones in dead foetus in situ uterus observed on X-ray or ultrasound. (xii) ***Hyperflexion sign:*** Hyperflexion of the fetus may indicate intrauterine death; however, the feature more often indicates intrauterine growth retardation. ***Ball sign*** is the hyperflexion of the spine in IUD. (xiii) ***Helix sign:*** Gas in the umbilical arteries may be observed. (xiv) Crowding of ribs shadow can be seen.

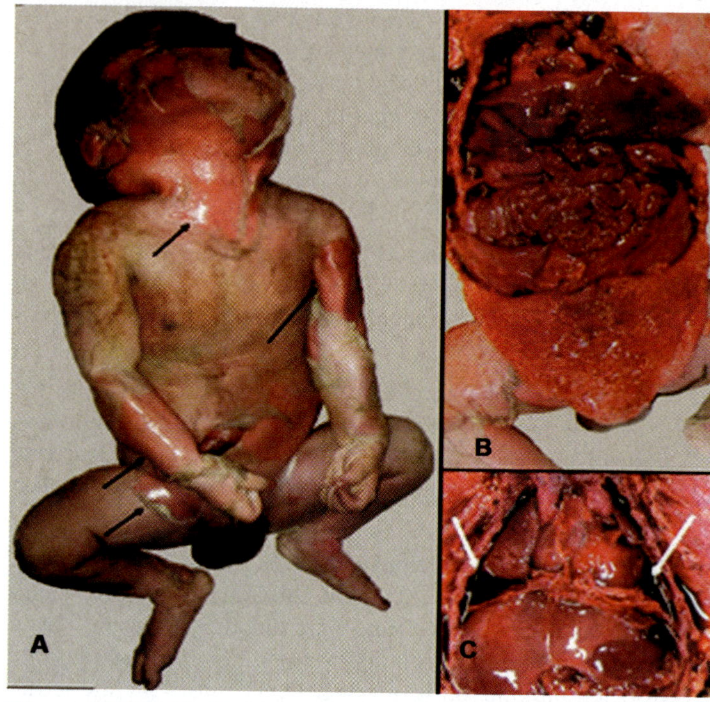

Figure 25.1A, B, C: Maceration of fetus showing skin slippage (A) and abdominal organs are softened, fluid in chest cavity (B, C)

3. *Mummification (Figure 25.2):* Mummification is dried up and shriveled appearance of foetus due to deficient blood supply and scanty liquor amnii when no air enters within the uterus.

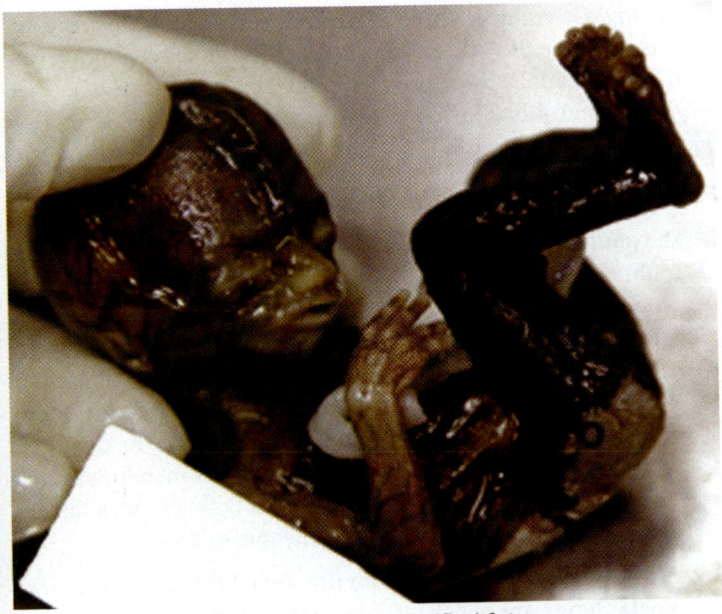

Figure 25.2: A mummified fetus

Was the child born alive? Separate existence and live birth are the two terms that are not synonymous with each other. The principal requirement of legal birth is that the child had or was capable of having a separate existence independent of its mother. In cases of child destruction, it is required to be proved that the child was capable of being born alive. The pregnancy must have reached 28th week or over and that the child was viable. Further, it must be proved that a willful act caused its death before it had an existence independent of its mother. Viability is the crux of matters of child destruction. Infanticide requires proof that the child had a separate existence and it had lived after complete extrusion of its body from that of his mother. The viability need not be proved. However, when the viability is doubtful, it is improbable that the child had a separate existence.

External examination: A separate existence requires complete extrusion of the foetus from the body of the mother but does not include the severance of the cord and detachment of the placenta. Umbilical cord should be examined for tears. In accidental tear of the umbilical cord, the break is usually close to one of its attachments, either near the placenta or the navel end of the infant. However, at the naval end of placenta little haemorrhage is unlikely to cause death. According to **Morris and Hunt (1966),** the cord can easily be broken by the hands and for this a force of 5 kg is required.

The ends of the cord should be examined at a low magnification by placing two portions in water or on a board and their ends are then gently spread out. Gross irregularities suggest tearing whereas a linear break with regular margin is indicative of separation by cutting. A blunt instrument can also produce a ragged line of separation. In addition, the tear can resemble superficially a clean-cut division of the cord. If the body has decomposed or there is severe drying, no opinion can be formed on the mode of severance of the cord.

Internal examination: Internal examination may provide for strong evidence of a separate existence. The evidences are: (i) If extraneous material, which could enter only after complete extrusion of the infant, is present either in the air passage or digestive tract. (ii) Extraneous material can enter the air passage for a limited distance after death but its entry into intrapulmonary bronchi is resisted by air in the lungs. Therefore, for material to be demonstrated in secondary bronchi or beyond, it must have been inhaled. It excludes contamination and milking of the material, downwards from trachea and bronchi by compression of the infant's body. During examination, such artefacts must be avoided and thoracic contents should be removed by 'no touch technique'. The thoracic viscera are placed on a clean slab or dish. The bronchial contents should be obtained by a clean pipette or syringe. Specimen obtained must be compared with the source of extraneous material such as soil or sand to obtain proof that the two samples are identical. (iii) Extraneous material may enter into the oesophagus, stomach and pass beyond even into small intestine during life but unlikely to reach up to the stomach after death. A sample of extraneous material must be compared with the probable source. The demonstration of food, e.g., milk in infant's stomach is suggestive of live birth.

Examination of Respiratory System

The aeration of lungs: This is based upon the expansion of the alveoli by postnatal breathing and is ascertained by inspection. However, it does not take into consideration the phenomenon of partial aeration or the fact that the child may cry in utero or breathe after expulsion of the head and before complete expulsion. Proof of breathing is not proof of live birth. There are illustrations of authentic cases in literature where breathing can occur before complete delivery. In addition, breathing is by no means rare while the head of the child is still in the vagina and in the uterus (**Clouston 1933**). Earliest cases of **Lebarius (1596)** alleges that the child's cry could be heard from a distance. **Ryder (1943)** reviewed the literature relating to vagitus uterinus. **Vagitus uterinus** and **vagitus vaginalis** is the hearing of the cry while the foetus is in the uterus or vagina respectively. This is due to rupture of the membranes resulting in entry of air in the lungs and the stimulation of the baby. Besides this other signs like movements of the limbs, muscle twitching etc. should also be taken into account.

Gross examination of lungs: Abdomen should be opened before the thorax and position of diaphragm is noted. In unexpanded lung it lies at the level of 4th-5th rib and after respiration at the level of 6th-7th rib. The position of the diaphragm is affected by decomposition. When the lungs are generally distended, soft and crepitant they have been aerated out. It is not true that the lungs are not expanded in the stillborn. Osborn (1953) disproved the belief that size of lungs has any relation to aeration. He has disproved the former belief that small solid lungs are indicative of stillbirth. The lungs fill the thorax in at least three quarters of all cases whether the child is born alive or not. The weight of the lung is recorded.

The weight of the lung is 1/70th of body weight that increases to 1/35th of the body weight after respiration (**Ploucquet's test**). Lungs are ligated across the hila and separated and then weight. The weight is 30-40 gm in unexpanded lungs that increases to 60-70 gm after respiration (**Fodere's test**). Both the tests result due to increased circulation though the weight of the lungs may not remain constant. Osborn also demonstrated that lungs may fail to expand due to bilateral pneumothorax with surgical emphysema, a result of artificial respiration. The presence of Tardieu's spots of asphyxia and evidence of bronchopneumonia are not evident of live birth as they may be seen in the stillborn. Occasionally subpleural interstitial emphysema may be seen and may represent attempted resuscitation by mouth-to-mouth respiration after birth. The consistency of the lung is noted and they are dense, firm, liver like and non-crepitant before respiration whereas they are soft, spongy, elastic and crepitant after respiration. The lungs are crepitant in artificial respiration and putrefaction also. In artificially inflated lungs, mottling is absent and on cut section little blood with no froth comes out. The differences in lungs before and after respiration are given under Table 25.2.

Hydrostatic (Raygat's) test: Scheyer first noted hydrostatic test in 1683. The basis of the test is that if the alveoli are compressed they will still contain some air if aerated at all. It is because on breathing the lung volume is increased. The specific gravity of lungs that is 1040 to 1050 diminishes to 940 after respiration. The test involves the determination of the buoyancy of lungs. The test depends upon the ratio of the specific gravity of the lungs to that of water as a lung containing air is lighter than water and therefore it floats. The lungs should be removed at autopsy with the bronchi, trachea and larynx intact. This 'pluck' is then placed in water, and if it floats, the test is positive. Finally, each lung is cut into 15-20 fragments which are again tested, and if they float the test is positive (this should exclude irregular and partial aeration). The pieces are then squeezed between thumb and index finger under the surface of water so that air bubbles comes out. If it still floats, then it is wrapped in a piece of cloth and squeezed by putting a weight. If these pieces are still floating that means there is presence of **residual air** that indicates that respiration has been established. Before performing this test, a piece of liver that serves as control is allowed to drop in water and if the liver also floats the test is of no use.

Fallacies of Hydrostatic Test

1. **Expanded lungs may sink due to:** (i) Diseases such as acute pulmonary oedema, pneumonia and congenital syphilis. (ii) Atelectasis (non expansion) (a) Air not reaching the alveoli due to feeble respiration (b) Complete absorption of air from the lungs by blood if circulation continued after respiration has been stopped or a state of asphyxia (c) More air being expelled from the lungs during expiration due to recoil of lung tissue (d) Obstruction by alveolar duct membrane. (iii) *Drowning:* When birth occurs in a toilet bowl or into a bucket containing water, the foetus may die due to drowning.
2. **Unexpanded lungs may float due to:** (i) *Putrefactive gases:* Foetal lungs are resistant to putrefaction due to less amount of blood. There is formation of soft, greenish air bubbles of different sizes that shift by pressure. (ii) *Artificial inflation:* In conditions of mouth-to-mouth respiration and blowing air by a tube, the lungs are inflated partially and stomach contains air. (iii) Alcoholic fixation.
3. **Hydrostatic test is not necessary, when:** (i) Foetus is <180 days (ii) Foetus is a monster (iii) Foetus is macerated or mummified (iv) Umbilical cord is separated or cicatrized (v) Stomach contains milk (vi) Whole of the thoracic contents float.

Applications of hydrostatic test: (i) When the body of the foetus is not putrefied and all portions of lung float after squeezing, it suggests that complete respiration has taken place. (ii) When some fragments of lung float it suggests that partial respiration has taken place. (iii) When all pieces of lungs sink, it suggests that the lungs are unexpanded and the infant has not breathed.

Table 25.2: Differences in findings in respiratory system before and after aeration

Features	Before respiration	After respiration
Shape of the chest	Flat, circumference is 1-2 cm less than the abdomen at the umbilical level	Expands, arch shaped or drum shaped
Position of the diaphragm	At the level of 4th-5th rib	At the level of 6th-7th rib
Lung volume	Normal or small	Larger
Margins	Sharp	Rounded
Consistency	Dense, firm, non-crepitant and liver like	Soft, spongy, elastic and crepitant
Colour and expansion of air sacs	Uniformly reddish brown, bluish or deep violet according to the degree of anoxia. On pressing little frothless blood oozes out	Mottled or marbled appearance, air sacs are distended and expanded, raised slightly above the surface with polygonal areas on the surface (mosaic appearance). On cut section, frothy blood comes out and blood is aerated
Blood in the lungs	The circulation is not increased	The circulation is twice after respiration
Weight of the lungs i. Fodere's (static) test ii. Ploucquet's test	 30-40 gm 1/70th of the body weight	 60-70 gm 1/35th of the body weight

In putrefied bodies, the problem is that whether such floating lungs were expanded before decomposition. The sinking portion of lung does not exclude the possibilities of having been expanded because putrefactive changes might have destroyed lung tissue, so that the respired air is squeezed out along with putrefactive gases.

Microscopic Examination of Lungs

1. **Preparation of the lungs:** Osborn (1953) stressed the importance of **"No touch" technique,** which aims at the elimination of artefacts produced by careless manipulation. Thoracic contents should be removed intact by cutting with a scalpel, the parts being controlled by holding the tongue or larynx with the forceps. After fixation for 48 hours, samples for microscopy are taken of whole lung in cross-section.
2. In the past, microscopical examination of the lungs was a secondary line of investigation and was confined almost exclusively to the condition of lining of the air sacs. If these retained a gland like appearance, it was concluded that the child has not breathed and therefore was still born. However, it is now known that the change in the kind of cell that lines the air sacs is not abrupt nor is it coincident with the onset of breathing. These gland like air sacs may be present in the lungs of liveborn infants also. This development occurs entirely during intrauterine existence before term. This gland like interpretation is indicative only of prematurity or of some diseased state in the mature foetus, e.g., hydrops foetalis that prevents normal differentiation. Microscopical findings are: (i) *4-5 months foetus*: Lung has a gland like appearance with thick walled ductules, lined by cubicle or columnar epithelial cells. Part of lung does not float in water. (ii) *In stillborn full term foetus,* the alveolar spaces have developed and lungs does not float. (iii) In typical stillbirths, the sections will show that alveoli and bronchi are collapsed. (iv) In the aerated lung, the alveoli and the bronchi are more or less expanded with increased degree of dilatation of vessels and existence of pathological change. (v) In live birth full term foetus, lungs float in water but microscopically findings are alike stillborn foetus. (vi) According to **Ham**, during 5th month, gland like structure is seen. Upto this stage alveoli appear as hollow round epithelial structure lined by cubical or columnar epithelial cells. (vii) After 5th month, alveoli separate from each other and capillaries in the alveolar walls bulge into the spaces. This development occurs inside the uterus, independent of extrauterine respiration. (viii) Alveoli undergoes expansion as fluid is displaced by air. Amniotic fluid is partly absorbed from the alveoli and partly drained through the upper respiratory tract.

Microscopical examination is nowadays the main line of investigation and only reliable means of solving problems related with aeration of lungs such as: (i) Some of the foetus are clearly stillborn, and show maceration on naked eye examination. These appearances are uncommon and unless seen soon after the delivery the interpretation is difficult once putrefaction has started. (ii) Another 1/3rd children have lung appearances simulating those who had breathed. (iii) Some children show signs of obstructive emphysema. (iv) Rest show signs of "struggle to breathe". Of these some may be still born and some die soon after delivery.

Signs of Struggle to Breathe

Sequence of changes in both still born and those who die soon after delivery include:

1. Dark fluid blood due to raised carbon dioxide haemo-concentration (**pseudo-clots**).
2. Cyanosed, expanded lungs, the expansion is due to: (i) Inhaled liquor amnii, vernix or vomitus (ii) Obstructive emphysema (iii) Oedema with or without air or liquor amnii.
3. Tardieu's spots on the pericardium, pleura, and thymus in both live born and still born foetus.
4. Liver swelling due to congestion of the whole organ.
5. Distension of the large bowel with meconium. This may be extruded into liquor amnii and later inhaled, a point of importance in the recognition of still birth because phagocytosis of meconium may be demonstrated in the lungs.
6. **Development of oedema of lungs:** It is a late change and not found always Osborn found that the newborns are prone to oedema. It can arise very rapidly, i.e., within 1-2 minutes. It is not a terminal event and acute neonatal oedema is a primary cause of death. The recognition of oedema may be difficult, if the fluid had been drained out during preparation of sections and cellular contents are very few. In the **Osborn** series the oedema was present in the ratio of live birth (17): still birth (1). The absence of oedema in still born is to be expected since a rise of blood pressure after delivery favours production of oedema. The haemorrhagic oedema may be found in some cases since increased capillary permeability permits escape of red cells in fluid in the air sacs.
7. **Other findings:** (i) On examination of the sections specially stained to demonstrate fat, it may be seen that the alveolar ducts, the passage leading to air sacs are lined by a membrane which is made prominent by the stain. This membrane may be a fatty material derived from the vernix **(Ahlstrom 1942)**. This was called **alveolar duct membrane by Osborn.** Nowadays it is well known as hyaline membrane disease which is associated with Respiratory Distress Syndrome **(Davis 1981).** (ii) *Desquamation of bronchial epithelium:* Specimen is obtained by 'No touch technique' and thoroughly fixed prior to sampling. Its occurrence is a probable indication of maceration of the lungs, uterine death and still birth. (iii) *Bronchopneumonia:* It is not an indication of live birth as it is also present alike in still births. (iv) *Phagocytosis of meconium:* By the cells that line the air sacs provided artefacts be excluded, is important evidence of inhalation of liquor amnii and thus of still birth. (v) *Contusion of the lungs*: This is subpleural bleeding that can be readily distinguished from Tardieu's spots as it is more extensive and bears the pattern of rib markings. These result from vigorous attempts at artificial

respiration. Osborn finds them in 1:4 live births but in none of the still borns. These are taken to be good evidence of live birth.

Summary: (i) *Still birth is permissible when there is:* (a) Maceration of the infant (b) Flooding of lungs with liquor amnii (c) Evidence of phagocytosis of meconium by cells lining air sacs (d) Desquamation of the bronchial epithelium (e) Lower bowel distended with meconium (f) Small solid lungs of uniformly dark colour do not necessarily indicate still birth (g) Gross oedema makes still birth doubtful and probably excludes it. (ii) *Live birth is probable when:* (a) All the lobes of the lung are fully expanded with or without obstructive emphysema (b) Gross pulmonary oedema is present (c) Alveolar duct membrane is present and is widely distributed in the lungs (d) Pulmonary atelectasis due to obstruction by an alveolar duct membrane is present (e) Pulmonary contusions (when haemorrhagic disease of the newborn has been excluded). (iii) A gland like appearance of alveoli does not exclude live birth but indicates prematurity. (iv) Tardieu's spots although indicate the struggle to breath are present in both live and still births. (v) Bronchopneumonia is also indicative of both live and still births. However, proper history of the case is important to diagnose whether still birth or live birth.

Other Important Findings Suggesting Live Birth

1. **Saliva in the stomach** is suggestive of live birth even though the child has survived a few hours after birth. If no saliva is found in stomach it indicates still birth.
2. **Air in the gastrointestinal tract (Breslau's second life test):** If the air has reached the duodenum, it is a strong evidence of separate existence. In still births, there is absence of air. In artificial respiration, air can enter the stomach. **Hajkis (1943)** believed the radiological demonstration of air in the stomach and intestine to be a confirmatory sign of respiration. If air has reached the duodenum, he considered this a strong evidence of a separate existence. Air was not shown in the stomach and intestine of the still born child.
3. **Unequivocal neonatal line in the enamel of unerupted teeth** is suggestive of separate existence (**Gustafson 1966**). This would be of considerable importance to establish whether the child really had been born alive and survived, provided off-course the child in this case had lived for longer then it would be possible to detect a neonatal incremental line in the enamel and dentine of all the deciduous teeth and perhaps the first permanent molar.

   According to **Stack 1960** assuming knowledge of the rate of growth of the hard tissues to know the length of time the child had lived after the birth, incremental lines have a uniform intensity and a regular periodicity. Developing teeth increase in tissue thickness, weight and volume. According to him, weight of dry mineralized tissue is the best criteria.

   According to **Euler 1955** by 7th month, dentine of central incisor is 2.9 mm in width and that of lateral incisor, canine and molars has 2.4 mm width.
4. **Changes in the middle ear (Wredin's test):** Before birth, middle ear contains gelatinous embryonic connective tissue. With respiration, sphincter at the pharyngeal end of eustachian tube relaxes and air replaces the gelatinous substance within few hours to 5 weeks. To demonstrate air in middle ear, it should be opened underwater and tegmen tympani to be removed, the test is positive if air comes out.
5. **Changes in kidney and bladder:** Brownish yellow crystals of uric acid in the pelvis of the kidney and bladder with absence of urine.

Other Signs of Live Birth Depending on the Time of Survival

1. **Blood:** By 24 hours, nucleated RBCs disappear and by 3rd month of life foetal haemoglobin (normal 70-80%) is reduced to 7-8% and disappears completely by 6th month.
2. **Meconium:** It is a green viscid substance consisting of inspissated bile and mucous. It is acid in reaction, stiffens and stains the cloth brownish green. It is completely expelled from the GIT within 24-48 hours. In anoxia and breech presentation, it is completely excreted before birth.
3. **Caput succedaneum (Figures 25.3A, B and 25.4):** It is a swelling due to edema formed in the scalp over the presenting part on the head during prolonged or ventouse (vacuum cup) delivery. It contains blood and serum. It occurs due to compression of tissues in the girdle of contact which results in interference of the venous return and lymphatic drainage from the unsupported area of the scalp. Caput can cross the suture line. It disappears in 1-7 days, usually without any complication.

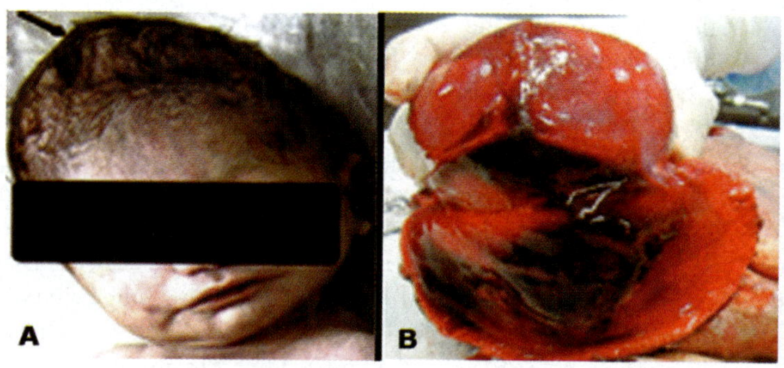

Figure 25.3A, B: Caput succedaneum

4. **Cephalhaematoma (Figure 25.4):** It is localized accumulation of blood deep to the scalp between periosteum and bone surface. It is limited by attachment of the periosteum to the fibrous tissue between the sutures. It never crosses suture line and is commonly limited to periosteal sheath of single bone usually right parietal bone. The bleeding occurs due to rupture of small vein from the skull due to friction between maternal pelvis and fetal skull as in cephalopelvic disproportion or precipitate labour. It can be seen also during forceps delivery which may be associated with fracture of skull bone. It occurs in only less than 1% of the newborn and varies in size from 1-5 cm. This swelling increases during the first two days after birth due to accumulation of more

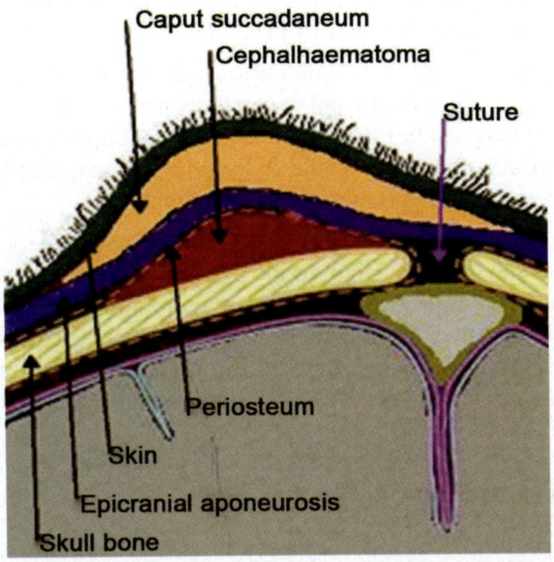

Figure 25.4: Caput succedaneum and cephalohematoma

blood but gradually decreases during the next weeks due to absorption of blood. Due to extra load of blood pigment neonatal jaundice may be increased.

5. **Skin changes:** (i) At first the skin is bright red and by 2-3 days it becomes darker then brick red then yellow and is normal by 7th day. (ii) Vernix caseosa covers the skin in the axilla, inguinal region and neck folds. It persists for 1-2 days. It may be absent at birth and can be removed by washing. (iii) Skin of the abdomen exfoliates for the first three days after birth.
6. **Findings in the gastrointestinal tract:** The air travels in the GIT at the same speed in full term infants as in premature infants. The air reaches the stomach after 15 minutes, small intestine after 1-2 hours, colon after 5-6 hours and rectum after 12 hours. The attempts at resuscitation and bacterial gas formation may cause an error.
7. **Changes in the umbilical cord:** If the cord is attached to placenta, it is suggestive of newborn. If the cord is clamped or tied and there is no evidence of reaction it is newborn. Both the site of severance and method of severance should be noted, but whether cut or torn may not always be easy to decide. It is best to remove the cord and examine microscopically in the laboratory. As far as finding of mummification of cord is concerned, it can also occur after death if exposed to air. The changes in umbilical cord with time are shown below:

Time	Changes in the umbilical cord
2 hours	Blood clots
12-24 hours	Cord shrinks and dries
36-48 hours	Inflammatory ring forms at the base
2-3rd day	Cord shrivels and mummifies
5-6th day	Cord falls off leaving a raw area
10-12 day	Heals and leaves the scar

8. **Changes in the umbilical vessels:**

Obliteration of umbilical vessels

	Starts	Closes
Umbilical artery	10 hours	3rd day
Umbilical vein Right Left	 — 3rd day	 6-7 months IUL 4-5th day
Ductus venosus (Left umbilical and common hepatic vein)	—	5th day
Ductus arteriosus	—	10th day
Foramen ovale	—	3rd month (rarely 2 years)

CAUSES OF DEATH

Natural Causes

Causes in the mother: (i) Diseases in the mother: (a) Syphilis (b) Smallpox (c) Plague (ii) Preeclamptic toxaemia: (a) Hypertension (b) Proteinuria (c) Fits (iii) Placenta praevia (iv) Abnormal gestation (Ectopic pregnancy).

Causes in the newborn: (i) Immaturity (ii) Debility (lack of general development) (iii) Congenital diseases of heart and lungs (iv) Malformations (v) Haemorrhage from umbilical cord, genital organs (vi) Postmaturity (vii) Neonatal infections (viii) Cerebral trauma (ix) Erythroblastosis foetalis: (a) Congenital hydrops foetalis (b) Icterus gravis neonatorum (c) Anaemia of the newborn.

Unnatural (Accidental) Causes

1. **During birth:**
   i. *Prolonged labor:* Intracranial haemorrhage and death with or without linear fracture of parietal bones of skull may result when the head is severely compressed against the contracted or deformed pelvis. Subdural haemorrhages are present bilaterally. Rarely extradural haemorrhage may occur. The cause of haemorrhage is rupture of bridging veins and internal or great cerebral veins and rarely tears of falx cerebri. The finding of moulding and caput succedaneum are usually seen. In addition, fracture dislocations of clavicles and limb bones may be present.

   ii. *Prolapse of cord:* This usually occurs in breech presentations when the cord gets compressed by head of foetus. The foetus dies as a result of asphyxia and on autopsy blood, meconium, liquor amnii, vernix caseosa is found in bronchial tubes.

   iii. *Twisting of the cord:* The twisting of the cord and knots in the cord can cause death by strangulating the foetus (Figure 25.5). The cord get compressed and there are no findings of abrasions or ecchymosis in the cord.

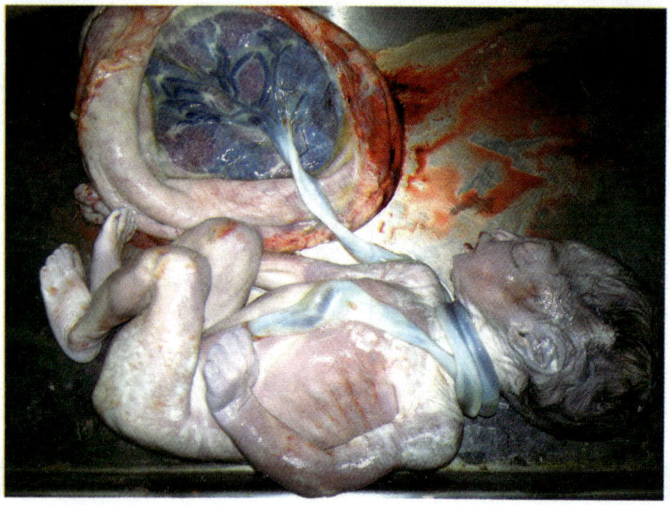

Figure 25.5: Strangulation of fetus by umbilical cord

iv. *Injury to the mother:* When the mother's abdomen is hit by heavy blows or kicks or fall from height, there may be fracture of skull or rupture of blood vessels and signs of concussion of brain.

v. *Death of the mother:* The child may die with death of the mother and can only be saved when delivered within 5-10 minutes of her death.

2. **After birth:**

i. *Suffocation:* The child may die when the foetal membranes cover the head during birth, face gets pressed accidentally on to the clothes. Also, when the foetus is submerged in the blood, liquor amnii or meconium discharges the child may die of suffocation. There are chances that the foetus may survive when covered by membranes only for 20-30 minutes.

ii. *Precipitate labour:* Precipitate labour terminating in a disproportionately shorter time than that taken on an average either by a primipara or multipara is called precipitate labor. All the stages of labor are merged into one and delivery occurs even without the knowledge of the mother. Foetus is normal or premature. It usually occurs in multiparous woman with large, roomy pelvis. A woman may deliver unconsciously because the contractile power of uterus is independent of volition. The child may die from: (a) Suffocation by falling into the lavatory pan (b) Head injury and fracture of skull occurs usually from a fall from 30" height but it can occur in a fall from a height of 18" (c) Haemorrhage from the torn ends of the cord.

If birth occurs in the toilet bowel, the infant may inhale the liquid, blood, meconium and vaginal mucus that may be found in the air passages. On microscopical examination of the lungs and examination of the cord on the slide under low magnification, the foreign particles can be seen in the drowning fluid.

In accidental fall usually bilateral subdural haemorrhage is present. The average length of the cord is 50 cm that is sufficient to protect the child from falling on the ground. It can withstand the weight of the infant. In these cases, caput succedaneum is not formed. Fissured fracture of skull is present that is limited to the parietal bone and may extend to frontal or squamous part of the temporal bone (Table 25.3).

Medicolegal Aspects

(i) The mother or her relative may be accused of infanticide, whilst the death of the foetus may be due to injury, asphyxia etc. (ii) In cases of infanticide, death may be attributed to precipitate labour.

Criminal Causes

These may be (i) Acts of commission (ii) Acts of omission.

Acts of commission: These are the acts done intentionally to cause death. The injuries may be found on the face, head and neck of the foetus when there are attempts at self-delivery. In such cases, on examination multiple circumscribed abrasions with scratch marks of finger nails may be found over the neck that may simulate homicide. Various acts of commission are:

1. *Suffocation:* The usual method employed is closing the infant's nose with two fingers and pushing the jaw upwards with palm in order to occlude airway. Other method can be placing pillow or towel over child's face or the face may be pushed down into bed clothing. Since the amount of force is less in these cases, at autopsy there may not be any evidence of trauma. Rarely overlaying, introducing mud, cotton-wool, rags into the mouth to kill the child may also be used.
2. *Strangulation (Figure 25.6A, B):* Manual or ligature strangulation are very commonly used. The umbilical cord may also be used as ligature at times.
3. *Drowning:* The body of foetus may be thrown into well, tank, drains.
4. *Burns:* This method is used for disposing the body but is not used for infanticide purposes.

Table 25.3: Differences in findings of head injury due to precipitate labour and blunt force

Features	Head injury due to precipitate labor	Head injury due to blunt force
Bruise	Present on the presenting part of scalp	Present anywhere on the scalp
Laceration	Not present	Usually present
Fracture	Fissured fracture, involves the parietal bones, runs downwards to the right angle of sagittal suture	Extensive comminuted fracture, sometimes depressed, affects all the bones of the vault
Brain	Usually not injured	Contusions, lacerations and haemorrhages present

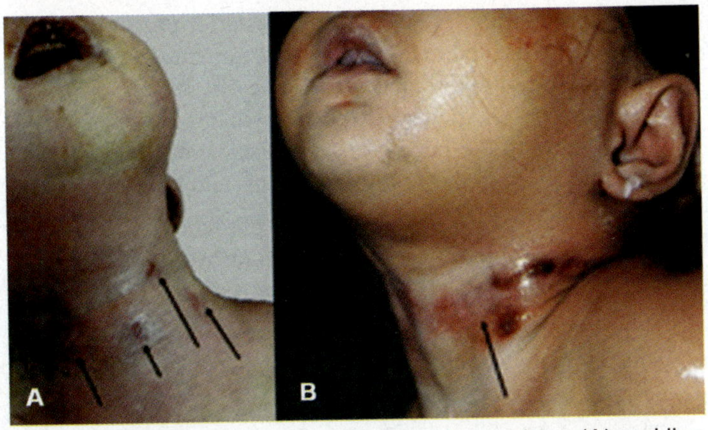

Figure 25.6A, B: Manual strangulation of a newborn (A) and ligature strangulation of an infant (B)

5. *Blunt force injury:* In cases of child battering, the head may be dashed against the wall or floor by holding feet. Findings of bruising over the ankles and feet at the site of gripping is seen. Besides this, there are findings of subdural and subarachnoid haemorrhages accompanied by fractures. Extradural haemorrhages in infants are usually limited to single bones since the dura adheres to the skull along the suture lines.
6. *Fracture and dislocation of cervical vertebra by twisting the neck:* This is seen in cases of child battering when there is twisting of neck.
7. *Wounds:* Occasionally the child may be killed by stabbing or by cut throat injuries.
8. Poisoning is a rare method of infanticide.

Acts of omission or neglect: The woman will be guilty of criminal negligence if she does not take ordinary precautions necessary to save her child after birth. These are acts of intentional neglect or care: (i) Failure to provide proper assistance during labour resulting in death by suffocation or head injury. (ii) Failure to tie the cord that results in death from haemorrhagic shock. (iii) Failure to protect the child from undue exposure to heat or cold. (iv) Failure to supply proper food. (v) Failure to clear respiratory passages of mucous or amniotic fluid that causes suffocation.

Concealment of Birth

It is an offence in England to conceal a birth and in Scotland to conceal pregnancy. The **Offences Against the Person Act 1861 (section 60)**, provides that "If any woman shall be delivered of a child, every person who shall, by any secret disposition of the dead body, whether such child died before, at, or after its birth, endeavour to conceal the birth thereof, shall be guilty of a misdemeanor."

This section makes it an offence for every person who has tried to conceal the birth of the child by any secret disposal of its dead body, at or after its birth. If the person tries for the murder of the child and acquitted, he may be convicted under concealment of birth, depending upon the evidence. There is no need to prove live birth. It is sufficient that there has been a birth and that the child was dead at the time of concealment.

In India, it is defined under **section 318 IPC (Concealment of birth by secret disposal of dead body):** Whoever by secretly burying or otherwise disposing the dead body of a child, whether dies before, during or after its birth, intentionally conceals the birth of such child shall be punished with imprisonment upto 2 years or with fine, or with both. This Act is similar to the section 60 of 'Offence Against Persons Act' 1861 of England.

Abandoning of Infants (S. 317 I.P.C.)

If the mother or father of a child under the age of twelve years, or anyone having care of such child, leaves such child in any place with the intention of abandoning the child, shall be punished with imprisonment up to seven years or with fine, or with both.

BATTERED CHILD SYNDROME

Definition: The term battered baby syndrome was coined by **Henry Kempe.** It is also known as the **Cafey's syndrome, Child abuse syndrome or the maltreatment syndrome.** The Brandel's University (Massachusetts) definition of child abuse is "Non accidental physical attack or physical injury including minimal as well as fatal injury, inflicted upon children by persons caring for them". Five classical features of the syndrome are obscure illness or unexplained injury in infants of up to four or five years–from six or eight weeks, due to repeated abuse, physical hurt over a period of weeks or months by either or both parents, guardian or baby sitter, who fail to report or delay reporting the incidents, and, who, when they do mislead, indeed deliberately deceive, the nurse, doctor over the cause.

Social history in relation to family and parents: These factors appear to be consistent as all social classes may batter their children but it is more common in lower socioeconomic groups. The age of the parents is in early twenties having marital discords and the family is usually isolated. Sometimes the father may not be the biological father and the child is unwanted usually as a result of failed contraception, failed abortion, and is undesired. The physical provision for the family is good, the standard of mothering is good and the nutrition and well being of the child is good. The intelligence of the parents is quite normal, usually a dominant aggressive father and a less intelligent dominated overstressed mother. The father may have criminal records.

There is lack of stability of family in geographical sense. The battering parents were themselves battered children. The act of the child like crying, refusal to be quiet and persistent soiling of napkins precipitates the violence of the parents. In the family of battered children, if one child is battered other will be battered too.

The perpetrator is a low income or low education bracket with mothers of low intelligence with increasing family and domestic strain. The parents are aggressive with demand for discipline and may be schizophrenic.

Incidence

Age: Most of the children are below the age of three years; about 70% are less than two years of age, about 55% are less than one year and less than 20% are more than five years of age. The mean age is fourteen months.

Sex: The incidence is seen slightly more in boys that is in about 55-63% cases.

Position in the family: Usually there is only one child in the family who may be youngest or eldest and is often unwanted who may be born before marriage, due to failure of contraception and is usually an illegitimate child.

Race: The incidence of battered baby syndrome is not related to any particular race.

Nature of injuries: The assault is usually carried out by unaided hands of the adult that is the injuries are **noninstrumental**, but sometimes objects such as feeding bottles, pokers may be used for hitting. The injuries produced are of the following types.

1. *Bruises, lacerations and abrasions:* Bruises, abrasions and lacerations are the commonly produced injuries and soft tissue injuries are almost universal with an incidence of 80-100%. The injuries are found in **different stages of healing** (Figure 25.7A to D). The areas most commonly affected are head, face and neck. Bruising of scalp and forehead and underlying skull and brain injuries are produced that is visible on autopsy. Bruising of external ear, cheeks and the lips especially the upper lip associated with laceration of frenulum is of diagnostic significance. The detachment of inner surface of the lip from the gum margin suggests punching or slapping of the mouth. Bruising of the neck and sides of the chest may reveal finger tip pressure marks. The neck may be held on each side in turn to immobilize the face while it is assaulted with the other hand, leaving symmetrical bruises beneath the angle of the jaw. The child may be gripped forcibly on each side of the chest and shaken violently to stop him from crying thus leaving the bruises on the skin of the armpits and lower ribs with multiple fractures of the posterior parts of the ribs. Bruising of the abdomen is most common after head injuries. The rupture of abdominal viscera may occur and externally the classical **six penny piece bruises** extending from the breast bone to the pubis are seen. The limbs show bilateral multiple bruising of the forearms, arms and legs.

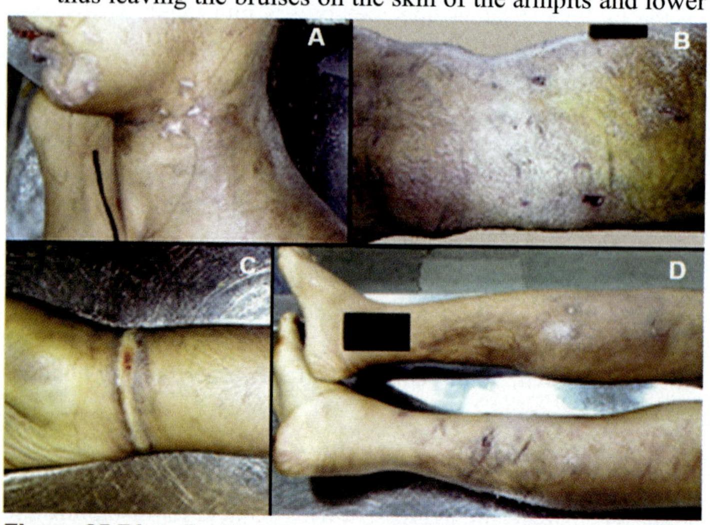

Figure 25.7A to D: Abrasions and contusions at different stages of healing over face, back of trunk, wrist and legs

2. *Bites:* The bites are very commonly produced by the mother that is to be differentiated from the bites by other children.
3. *Eye injuries:* The injuries to the eye that are found in battered baby syndrome are **retinal separation**, lens displacement, subconjunctival, subhyaloid and retinal haemorrhages.
4. *Head injuries:* Head injuries are common in a battered child. There may be presence of external scalp injuries. The fracture of skull along with the brain injuries are most frequent cause of death. The skull fractures are commonly fissured sometimes a segmental break in the parietal area caused by impact of head against a solid object rather than direct blow against a fixed head. There are cerebral contusions and scattered patches of bleeding in the meninges.
5. *Visceral injuries:* Rupture of liver, intestine and mesentery account for most of the fatalities due to blows over front of abdomen. The visceral injuries are the most common cause of death. The lacerations of the undersurface of liver with gross intraregional bleeding due to tears in mesentery of small intestine are falsely attributed by the parents to an accident.
6. *Skeletal lesions and radiologic appearances:* In all the cases of battered baby syndrome, radiography is most important. A whole-body X-ray must be performed before autopsy. It provides two kinds of useful information about general skeletal damage especially of different times of infliction and the characteristic bony lesions. The **formation of callous** is important in identifying and approximately dating old healing fractures. The characteristic radiographic lesions are the **separation of epiphysis** especially around the elbow and knee joint although any limb may be involved. There is shearing and elevation of periosteum which is not firmly attached in infants. The subperiosteal calcification in **periosteal haemorrhages** is a characteristic feature. There are multiple fractures of ribs that show a **beading effect**. The fracture of clavicle is also common. The **chipping of the corners of epiphysis at large joints** of limbs is again a characteristic feature due to shaking and rotating strains imposed upon limbs by forceful application of adult hands. The metaphyseal fragmentation is also common. The fractures of shaft of long bones from direct blows either from a fist or from the child hitting a fixed object can also occur. **Nobbing fracture** are the rib fractures observed on both sides close to spine due to holding the child with hands and shaking it violently or squeezing from side to side by the assailant.
7. *Burns:* **Punctate burns** often accompanied by older scars may indicate deliberate stubbing of cigarette ends upon child's skin. Child may be seated upon a stove or electric radiator and may be dipped in hot fluids.

Diagnosis of Child Battering

1. **Discrepancy between history and findings:** Variation and inconsistencies in explanation given by the parents; the story changes even after hours or days and different versions are given to different investigators. This is a characteristic finding. There is inconsistency of parent's explanation with the extent and chronology of injury. The bruises are multiple and there are multiple fractures in different stages of healing. The explanations of parents may change several times on repetition. In addition, there is tendency of the parents to take the child to different doctors or to a different accident center at each episode of injury.
2. **Delay in seeking advice:** There is delay in seeking medical advice or treatment. This is a highly significant feature that is seeking medical advice and injuries have a long interval.
3. **Classic lesions** such as torn upper lip frenulum, multiple bruises on the face, thorax or abdomen and around joints of the limbs, bite marks, unusual burns, fractures in different stages of healing and multiple bruises with different colours are typically present.
4. There are evidence of repeated visits to different doctors or different medical centers.
5. A general medical history as mentioned under definition given before exists.

SUDDEN INFANT DEATH SYNDROME

Sudden infant death syndrome is also known by the names of **Cot death** in Britain and **Crib death** in North America and is the most common cause of sudden death in infancy.

Definition

International conference in **Seattle in 1990** defined sudden infant death syndrome as "The sudden death of any infant or young child which is unexpected by history and in whom a thorough necropsy fails to demonstrate an adequate cause of death. It is not a recognized cause of death in India due to much higher level of infant mortality as the increased rate of death from causes like infections and malnourishment overshadows Cot death.

Historical Aspects

SIDS has been known for at least 3,000 years in Jewish Old Testament. It also occurs in animals such as pigs.

Incidence

UK (2/1000 live birth), USA (2.3/1000 live birth). The incidence decreased in Britain and other European countries as there were campaigns for sleeping babies on their backs and not on their face; avoiding overheating the baby and avoiding smoking near the baby. In India, no studies are available signifying incidence of SIDS.

Age: It is usually 1 month-1 year and is rare after 1 year. The official age is 2 weeks-2 years. Most of the deaths occur during 2-8 months. Peak is 4 months due to lowest level of infant's antibodies and decline of maternal antibodies.

Sex incidence: Male to female ratio is 1.3:1.

Incidence of twins: There is an increased risk that is five times more than in single babies. Prematurity and low birth weight increases the risk. Sometimes both the twins die on the same day.

Social class: There is a marked increase in lower socio-economic class in Western countries.

Seasonal variation: In temperate regions, it is more common in colder seasons. In Northern hemisphere it occurs in October to April and in Australasia it occurs in July to August.

Time of death: Most of the deaths occur before mid morning. The infants are usually found dead after night sleep or after their morning feeds. Minority of them dies in afternoon or in the evening.

Typical history: The typical history given is that the child was either quite well or had some upper respiratory tract infection or slight diarrhea the previous day and was found dead in the morning. Almost all deaths occur in the morning in their sleeping place. In 85% of the cases no postmortem findings are found whereas in 15% of the cases some chest infection, congenital anomalies and old birth injuries are demonstrable. Petechial haemorrhages in lungs, epicardium and thymus are usually seen and due to these findings the death was attributed to suffocation, called overlaying when the child was smothered by mother in the bed but even when the children slept in bed this continued to occur.

Various theories of causation of SIDS: (i) Cow's milk protein allergy (ii) House mite allergy (iii) Deliberate suffocation (iv) Botulism (v) Deficiency of selenium, vitamins E, C, D, thiamine, calcium, magnesium and biotin (vi) Staphylococcus aureus causes anaphylactic shock due to its growth in unabsorbed milk (vii) Hypoglycemia (viii) Hypothyroidism (ix) Carbon dioxide and carbon monoxide poisoning (x) Overlaying (xi) Pharyngeal hypotonia (xii) Nasal obstruction (xiii) Respiratory syncytial virus (xiv) Prolonged sleep apnea (xv) Deficient or abnormal pulmonary surfactant (xvi) Cardiac conduction anomalies (xvii) Narrow foramen magnum (xviii) Hypothermia or hyperthermia (xix) Immunodeficiency (xx) Hypogammaglobulinemia (xxi) Status lymphothymaticas (very enlarged thymus) (xxii) Cardiovascular system anomalies.

Prolonged sleep apnoea: In 1970s and early 1980s this theory gained favour. Some infants with poor respiratory drive suffered from exaggeration of normal periods of apnea that all infants have during sleep. Progressive hypoxia and failure to respond to hypercapnia and hypoxia in sleeping infant results in hypoxia resulting in apnea then hypoxia then bradycardia and finally cardiac arrest. Respiratory infection, sleep and nasal obstruction contributed to acute on chronic state hypoxia. For this apnea alarms were built but the theory was deflated after prospective studies.

To summarize SIDS is a final common pathway leading to death in infants compromised by a number of deleterious factors summating to final fatal outcome. It is multifactorial and the factors such as sleep depress the brainstem, virus infections of respiratory tract cause viremia, reduce oxygenation and narrow effective airway lumen by mucus and exudates. The constitutional factors like botulism, prematurity and low birth weight are contributory. Mode of death is respiratory failure due to brain stem dysfunction.

Role of pathologist in SIDS: (i) A meticulous autopsy examination should be undertaken (ii) Natural diseases and other injuries should be excluded (iii) Parents to be given sympathetic advice.

Autopsy Findings

External findings: Scene of death is rarely available and at autopsy following are the external findings but are not significant: (i) Gross findings are nil. (ii) Hands are clenched around the fibers from bed clothes as if there were spasmodic agonal grasping movements. (iii) Some children are found under bed clothes huddled upside down at the foot of the cot but this has no significance as some infants habitually sleep this way. (iv) Body is moist with sweat with raised body temperature and there is preventive advice in Britain to avoid infants from overwrapping and overheating. (v) Length, weight and physical measurements should be recorded carefully. (vi) Few infants will have significant pathological lesions in about 15% cases that may be some mild congenital heart lesion or some congenital anomaly such as Down's syndrome. (vii) Face is pale, slightly cyanosed and congested. (viii) If the infant has slept face down pallid area is seen around the mouth and nose where pressure prevents postmortem staining from settling. (ix) There is inconstant froth at lips and nostrils. (x) Slight oedema fluid that is blood tinged is exuding out of the mouth and nostrils. (xi) Stomach contents may be present on mouth, nostrils and face.

Internal findings: Internal findings are non-specific in a typical case of SIDS and for this no diagnosed criteria have been confirmed. The findings commonly are: (i) Petechial haemorrhages on visceral pleura, thymus glands and epicardial surface of heart especially posteriorly occur in 70% of true SIDS cases and are almost agonal in origin. The theory for this that is not substantiated is that they are the result of forced inspiratory efforts against a closed airway due to laryngeal spasm or collapsed pharynx in hypotonic infants. (ii) Thymic haemorrhages and large ecchymoses are found in SIDS as opposite to mechanical suffocation. These haemorrhages are in thymic cortex rather than the medulla but few pathologists accept this criterion. (iii) Presence of milk curd in air passage, is either an agonal regurgitation or a postmortem phenomenon. (iv) Respiratory infections in the form of inflamed laryngotracheal mucosa. If the infection is severe, it produces pus with obvious inflammatory changes in lung parenchyma. (v) Pulmonary oedema is moderate and the lung surface shows patchy sublobular partial collapse with areas of blue lung alternating with better-aerated pink zones. (vi) Other abnormalities such as Down's syndrome, congenital heart disease and chronic systemic disease are contributory causes of death in SIDS.

Histological findings in SIDS: (i) In the lungs, inflammatory changes and peribronchiolar cell infiltration is usually sparse or as small collections of leukocyte are found whereas in control infants, lymphocytes are found. (ii) Chronic hypoxia occurs due to thickened pulmonary artery walls, gliosis in brainstem, retention of brown fats in adrenals and abnormalities in the carotid body.

MUNCHAUNSEN SYNDROME BY PROXY

This is a **peculiar and dangerous type of child abuse usually involving the mother**, in which children are brought to doctors for induced signs and symptoms of illnesses with a fictitious history. The sex ratio is almost equal. It has been described in children of few weeks of age to 21 years. The child is admitted frequently in the hospital for medical evaluation for the nonexistent conditions. These patients appear to be compulsively driven to make their complaints. The person is aware that he is acting an illness, but he cannot stop the act. There is continuity, ranging from exaggerated claims of infirmity to actual self induced illness. At the extreme end, life-threatening injuries are masqueraded as being legitimately contracted. **Rosenberg (1989)** gave four diagnostic criteria (i) Illness produced or alleged, or both by a parent (ii) Repeated requests for medical care of a child, leading to multiple medical procedures (iii) Parenteral denial of knowledge of the cause of symptoms (iv) Regression of symptoms when the child is separated from the parents.

Methods of Production: (i) The mother pricks her finger and adds blood to the urine of the child and takes the sample to the doctor (ii) The child's nose is closed with two fingers and the lower jaw is pushed up with the palm to block the airway. (iii) A pillow or towel is put over the face of the child and the face is pushed down into bed clothing (iv) The mother gives insulin to the child and takes to hospital with hypoglycaemia (v) Allegation of vomiting by ipecacuanha (vi) *Diarrhoea:* Laxatives, salt poisoning (vii) *Convulsions:* Allegation or by theophylline, insulin, psychotropic drugs (viii) *Bleeding:* Anticoagulants, phenolphthalein poisoning, exogenous blood. (ix) *CNS depression:* Barbiturates, benzodiazepines (x) Alleged fever (xi) Scratching or intoxication rash.

LONG QUESTIONS

1. Define infanticide. What are the signs of live birth?
2. Describe the causes of death in case of infanticide.

SHORT QUESTIONS

1. Hydrostatic test.
2. Differentiate between respired and unrespired lung.
3. Differentiate between head injury due to blunt force and precipitate labour.
4. Munchaunsen syndrome by proxy.
5. Battered baby syndrome.
6. SIDS.

MULTIPLE CHOICE QUESTIONS

1. For "Infanticide" the age of the newborn should be below:

(a) 1 year (b) 2 years
(c) 3 years (d) 4 years

2. Hydrostatic test is done in case of :

(a) Hanging (b) Infanticide
(c) Drowning (d) HCN poisoning

3. Following is true regarding lungs in Ploucquet's Test:

(a) Smaller and constitute 1/50th of body weight
(b) Larger and constitute 1/40th of body weight
(c) Voluminous and constitute 1/35th of body weight
(d) Dark and heavy

4. Vagitus uterinus is:

(a) An infection of vagina
(b) An infection of uterus
(c) Infection of both vagina and uterus
(d) A cry of unborn baby from uterus

5. Concealment of birth by secret disposal of dead body is punished under section:

(a) 315 IPC (b) 316 IPC
(c) 317 IPC (d) 318 IPC

6. Abandoning an infant is punished under section:

(a) 315 IPC (b) 316 IPC
(c) 317 IPC (d) 318 IPC

7. The test that demonstrates air in the middle ear for diagnosis of live birth is:

(a) Wreden's test (b) Breslau's second life test
(c) Raygat's test (d) Fodere's test

8. Nobbing fractures are seen in cases of:

(a) Forceps delivery
(b) Battering of child
(c) Accidental fall of child
(d) Self-inflicted injuries by the child

9. All these features can be seen in case of a full-term dead born foetus at birth *except*:

(a) Rigor mortis (b) Maceration
(c) Mummification (d) Cadaveric spasm

ANSWER KEY ☞

1. (a)	2. (b)	3. (c)	4. (d)	5. (d)	6. (c)	7. (a)	8. (b)	9. (d)

26 CHAPTER

Impotence and Sterility

IMPOTENCE

Impotence is inability to have sexual intercourse. Presently, the term **"erectile dysfunction" (ED)** is used in male instead of impotence which is defined as the failure to achieve or maintain a rigid penile erection suitable for satisfactory sexual intercourse. Impotence is a ground for voidable marriages under S 12 Hindu Marriage Act. The question of impotence arises in both civil and criminal cases.

Civil cases: (i) Adoption (ii) Nullity of marriage (iii) Divorce (iv) Adultery (v) Disputed paternity and legitimacy (vi) Claims for compensation when loss of sexual functions is a result of accident.

Criminal cases: (i) Adultery (ii) Rape (iii) Unnatural offences. In these situations, the accused pleads impotence as a defence (iv) When an injured individual think that he has become impotent as a result of wounds or injuries inflicted by others.

STERILITY

Sterility is the inability of the male to beget children and in the female to conceive children. A person can be sterile without being impotent and can be impotent without being sterile.

Causes of Impotence and Sterility in Males

1. **Age:** Power of coitus starts earlier, then after 1-2 years power of procreation starts, i.e., at 14-15 years. A male is sexually potent at the age of puberty. As age advances, potency and power of procreation decreases. There is no definite age for this decrease but it occurs at the extremes of ages.
2. **Malformations and developmental anomalies:** (i) Absence or nondevelopment of penis (ii) Adhesion of penis to the scrotum (iii) Hypospadias associated with marked deformity and the person is also sterile as sperms cannot be deposited (Figure 26.1) (iv) Epispadias is rare; associated with rudimentary and stunted penis (Figure 26.2) (v) Loss

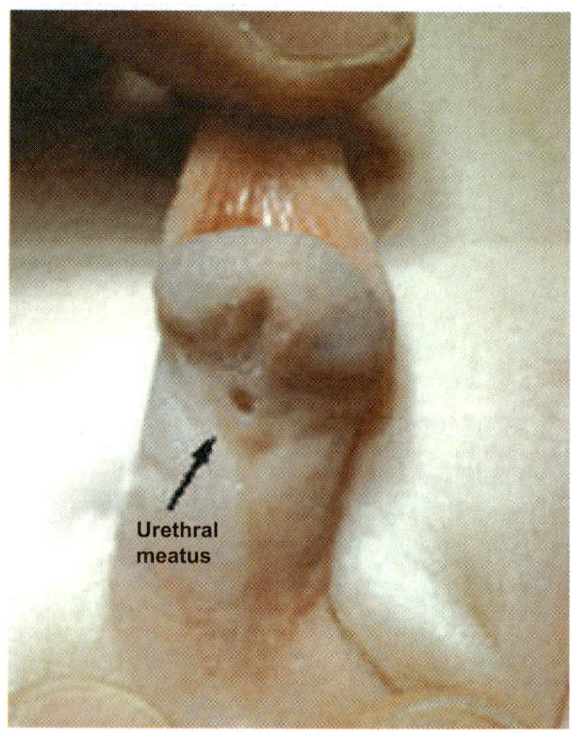

Figure 26.1: Hypospadias

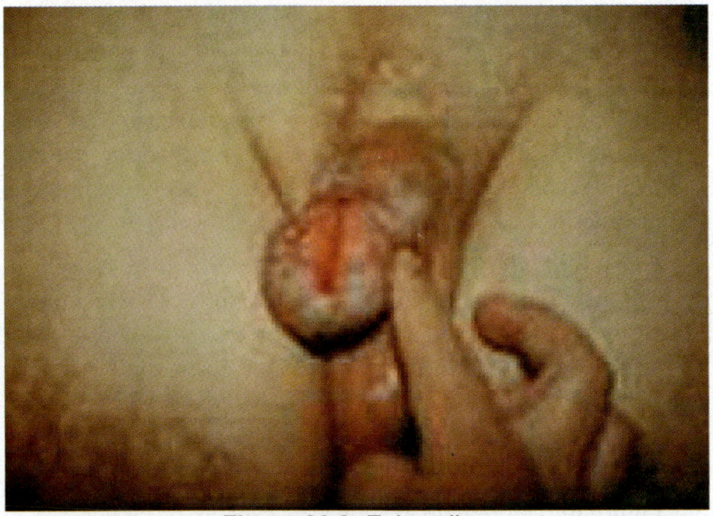

Figure 26.2: Epispadias

of both testicles or absence of them (vi) Cryptorchids are not necessarily sterile or impotent, but sterility is common due to azoospermia.

3. **Local diseases:** (i) Diseases causing temporary impotence that is cured by surgery: (a) Large hydrocoele (b) Scrotal hernia (c) Elephantiasis (Figure 26.3) (d) Phimosis (e) Paraphimosis (ii) Diseases of penis or scrotum causing impotence or sterility: (a) Syphilis (b) Cancer (c) Tuberculosis (iii) Gonococcal infection of the testis, epididymis, prostate etc. (iv) Atrophy of testicles (Mumps) (v) Surgical operations in Lithotomy position may result in the injury to ejaculatory duct and sterility.

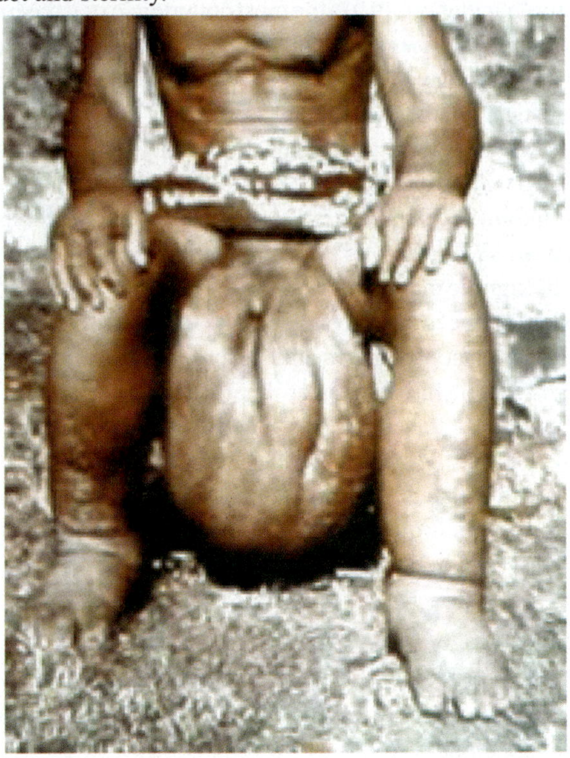

Figure 26.3: Elephantiasis

4. **General diseases:** (i) Endocrine disturbances like diabetes, pulmonary tuberculosis and chronic nephritis (ii) Injury to spinal cord resulting in paraplegia (iii) Tumour or injury to cauda equina (iv) General paralysis of insane (v) Blow on the head affecting brain or spinal cord (vi) Exposure to X-ray radiation leading to temporary azoospermia.
5. **Excessive and continued use of drugs:** Like opium, alcohol, cannabis, tobacco, cocaine may lead to impotency.
6. **Psychical influence:** Fear, anxiety, excessive passion, and sense of guilt, all lead to impotence.
7. **Quoad:** Quoad is also called selective impotence as in this condition the male is impotent with a particular woman. The phenomenon is known as **impotence quoad hoc.**
8. Earlier, psychogenic disorder was considered as the main cause of erectile dysfunction, however, current evidence suggests that more than 80% of cases have organic diseases.

Examination of the Male

The examination of the male person is carried out when asked by the Court or police in alleged rape cases. They are usually examined in casualty or by Forensic Medicine expert in their department of when specifically referred. They give opinion whether the person examined is capable of performing sexual intercourse or not.

Procedure for examination: (i) There should be written order from the Court/or request from investigating officer of the case. (ii) Informed consent of the accused, duly attested by the witness with time date and address should be obtained. (iii) Identification of the male is to be done by a close relative and at least two identifying marks to be mentioned. A recent photograph should also be attached duly signed by the doctor.

Medical Examination Proper

1. **History:** History of previous illness like mental illness or nervous system disorders and sexual history should be recorded.
2. **General examination:** It should include complete examination of all systems of the body in detail including the nervous system.
3. **Local examination:** It includes examination of: (i) Condition of testes, epididymis, spermatic cord, penis etc. They are to be tested for the presence of sensations. (ii) Prostate and seminal vesicle to be palpated per rectum. In addition, pressure to be applied over seminal vesicle, giving pressure by finger along the urethra thus the semen is brought to meatus and examined for spermatozoa.

Following tests may be required:

4. **Laboratory tests:** (i) Blood–Complete blood count (CBC), electrolytes, baseline renal and liver function tests, lipid

profile, TSH level, morning testosterone assay and fasting blood sugar and HbA1c for screening diabetes etc.

5. **Further testing:** (i) **Nocturnal Tumescence Testing (NPT):** It is helpful in differentiating psychogenic from organic erectile dysfunction. (ii) **Penile Duplex Doppler Ultrasound:** It is done to access the cavernosal vascular flow. Prostaglandin E1 or papaverine is injected intracavernosally and a doppler examination carried out. (iii) **Pudendal arteriography:** It is done to access the arterial vasculature of penis. (iv) **Penile Biothesiometry:** It is done to screen penile neuropathy using skin vibrational threshold sensitivity.

If there is no disease or abnormality, there is no reason to believe that the man is not capable of performing the sexual act. Existence of potency is a matter of inference to be drawn from negative findings. As **Casper** states that the possession of virility and the power of procreation neither requires to be, nor can be proved to exist by any physician but is rather like any other function to be supposed to exist within the usual limits of age.

Opinion: If there is no detectable finding or disease/deformity in a person, the opinion is given in a negative form, "There is no finding to suggest that the person examined is not capable of performing the sexual act." However, if there is any gross abnormality in the penis or scrotum, then the doctor can opine that "the person examined is not capable of performing the sexual act because of the disease".

Causes of Impotence and Sterility in Females

1. **Age:** Puberty starts at 13-14 years of age. **Catamenia** is the first menstrual flow. It lasts till menopause that is up to the age of 45-50 years. However, sexual instinct lasts till old age. There are cases in which 61-62 years old gave birth to a full-term child and 63 years old gave birth to her 22nd child.
2. **Congenital malformations:** (i) Total occlusion of vagina (ii) Adhesion of labia (iii) Imperforate hymen (iv) Congenital absence of vagina (v) Absence of uterus, ovaries and fallopian tubes (vi) Turner's syndrome.
3. **General diseases:** As women is the passive agent general diseases cannot cause impotence. The general disease and debility do not cause a barrier to sexual act or conception. A paraplegic can also become pregnant.
4. **Local diseases:** As a passive agent local diseases usually do not produce impotence but can produce sterility provided per vaginum examination is normal.
5. **Vaginismus** is a definite cramp like spasm of the adductor muscle and hysterical hyperasthenia coexists. The hyperasthenia is present all over the vulva, abdomen and thigh etc. Contraction is so severe that penile penetration is not possible. It occurs equally in virgin and in those who have children. The causes of vaginismus are as follows: (i) Sexual frustration secondary to husband's impotence (ii) Psychosexual inhibiting influence due to social, religious and orthodox practices (iii) Prior sexual trauma as a virgin at low age (iv) Dyspareunia (v) Personal repulsion to the idea of intercourse. Psychotherapy is essential to overcome this disorder.

Causes of sterility in females: Sterility is produced as a result of following conditions: (i) Gonorrheal infection of cervix, ovaries and fallopian tubes (ii) Removal of both ovaries due to disease (iii) Diseases of uterus (iv) Recto-vaginal fistula, leucorrhoea, menstrual disorders (v) *Psychological:* Fear, passion and neurotic temperament leads to hysterical fit during an attempt of coitus and leads to temporary sterility.

Opinion: The female examined is capable of taking part in sexual act (**Aptavira**) or she is not capable of taking part in sexual act (**Nonaptavira**).

Sexual Dysfunction

Sexual dysfunction is the problem with sexual function of a person at any stage of the sexual response cycle that includes sexual desire, sexual arousal, orgasm, and either sexual pain or lack of sexual pleasure, that leads to significant personal distress. It applies to people of different sexes and sexual orientations.

Premature Ejaculation

Premature ejaculation (PE) is the most common sexual dysfunction in men (upto 30% of male population is affected) who ejaculate prematurely during vaginal intercourse. As per DSM-5 (Diagnostic and Statistical Manual of Mental Disorders, fifth edition), there are four criterions for diagnosis of PE (i) The person consistently ejaculating within one minute or less of vaginal penetration. (ii) The symptom has persisted for at least 6 months and has been experienced 75%-100% of the time. (iii) The symptoms cause clinically significant distress, sexual frustration, dissatisfaction or tension between partners. (iv) The condition is not better explained by a nonsexual mental disorder or as a consequence of severe relationship distress or other significant stressors and is not attributable to the effects of a substance/medication or another medical condition. As per ICD-10 (International Classification of Diseases and Related Health Problems-10), the PE is defined as the inability to control ejaculation sufficiently for both partners to enjoy sexual interaction.

Frigidity

It is the inability to experience a sexual response of any kind, i.e., absence of desire, inability to experience of orgasm or sexual pleasure in a female.

LONG QUESTIONS

1. Define impotence. What are the causes of impotence and sterility in male? How you proceed to examine such cases and give your opinion?
2. Define sterility. What are the causes of impotence and sterility in females. How will examine such cases and give opinion?

SHORT QUESTIONS

1. Vaginismus.
2. Quoad.

MULTIPLE CHOICE QUESTIONS

1. The Quoad is impotent to:

(a) All the ladies
(b) To a particular woman
(c) To wife
(d) To elderly ladies

2. The most common cause of erectile dysfunction is:

(a) Psychogenic disorder (b) Organic diseases
(c) Drug abuse (d) None of the above

3. Impotence may be pleaded as a ground for defence in males in all *except:*

(a) Divorce
(b) Rape
(c) Adultery
(d) Unnatural sexual offence

4. 'Impotency' is defined as:

(a) Inability to conceive
(b) Inability to perform sexual act
(c) Premature ejaculation
(d) Inability to achieve an orgasm

ANSWER KEY ☞

1. (b)	2. (b)	3. (a)	4. (b)

27 CHAPTER

Virginity, Pregnancy, Delivery and Legitimacy

VIRGINITY

Virgin (Virgo intacta) is a female who has not experienced sexual intercourse whereas loss of virginity is known as **defloration.**

Marriage: It is a contract between man and woman which implies the sexual union.

The question of virginity arises in cases of nullity of marriage, divorce, rape, defamation etc.

1. **Nullity of marriage (S. 12 Hindu Marriage Act, 1955):** Marriage may be annulled that is never existed in the following conditions: (i) Either party being under age at the time of marriage (ii) Either party already validly married (iii) One party is of unsound mind (iv) Marriage has not been consummated due to impotence or willful refusal (v) When the woman was pregnant at the time of marriage.
2. **Divorce (S. 13 Hindu Marriage Act, 1955):** The following are the grounds for divorce. Dissolution of previously valid marriage will be granted in the following circumstances: (i) Adultery (ii) Husband is found guilty of rape, sodomy or bestiality (iii) Incurable insanity, leprosy, venereal disease (iv) Cruelty (v) Deserted the petitioner for two years continuously (vi) Ceased to be Hindu* (vii) Renounced the world by entering into religious worship* (viii) Not heard for 7 years* (ix) *Section 13 B of Hindu Marriage Act:* Divorce by mutual consent on the ground that they are living separately for the period of 1 year or more.
3. Defamation.
4. Rape.

In all such cases, the doctor is called upon to give the opinion after examining the female whether she is virgin or not.

Signs of Virginity

1. **Extragenital**
   - ***Breasts***: In a young adult female breasts are hemispherical, firm and rounded. Nipples are small and areola is pink or darker. Occasional act of coitus will not alter the character of breasts, hence little significance is given to findings of breasts as evidence of virginity. Breasts can be pendulous and large as a result of handling even though the woman had never been pregnant and is a virgin.
2. **Genital (Figure 27.1)**
   - ***Labia majora:*** Labia majora are two elongated folds of skin projecting downwards and backwards from Mons veneris. The point at which they meet centrally is known as **anterior commissure.** They meet posteriorly in front of anus is known as **posterior commissure.** In virgin they are thick, firm, elastic and rounded; lie in apposition to close the vaginal orifice. This is not seen in woman habituated to sexual intercourse.
   - ***Labia minora:*** These are soft, small, pink and sensitive. The labia minora meet anteriorly to form the clitoral hood that is small. The triangular area between clitoris as apex and anterior margin of hymen as base is known as **vestibule,** which is very narrow. The lower part of labia minora fuses posteriorly in midline and forms a fold called fourchette. **Fossa navicularis** is the concave area of vestibule bound anteriorly by vaginal opening,

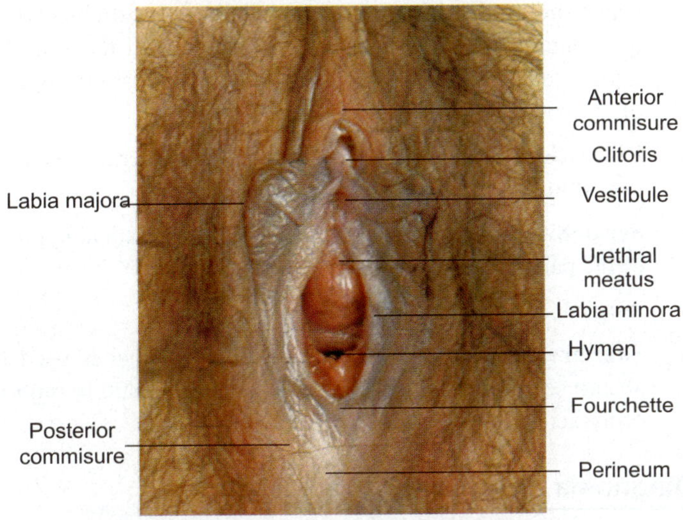

Figure 27.1: Anatomy of female external genitalia

posteriorly by fourchette and laterally by labia minora. The depression between fourchette and vaginal orifice remains closed in a virgin. The edges of labia minora project between labia majora.

- ***Vagina:*** Vaginal passage is a pocket, irregular in shape, about 7.5 cm long; 6 cm anterior wall, 9 cm posterior wall. It is collapsed to form a slit like opening crosswise of the body. It is pear (balloon) shaped when distended. Width of the upper end is 3-4 cm in nulliparous; 6-7 cm in multiparous. Vagina is narrow and tight, full of rugosity, reddish and sensitive to touch and its walls are approximated. Rugosity is removed only after childbirth but in some cases, it is absent in virgin with intact hymen. During sexual intercourse, the vagina expands to accommodate the male organ. A single intercourse does not alter the anatomy of genitalia apart from the rupture of hymen.
- ***Hymen:*** It is a fold of mucous membrane about 1 mm thick, situated at the vaginal outlet partially closing the vaginal orifice. The average adult hymen consists of folds of membrane having annular or crescentic shape. In children, it appears as a taut membrane when thighs are separated. During puberty, hymen enlarges and appears as a series of folds. Normal hymen may be rigid and fibrous. It is usually elastic and easily distensible. It is supplied by blood vessels that bleeds during rupture. In virgins it admits tip of little finger.

  According to some authors hymen is practically always present in a virgin though it may be congenitally absent. However, the latter view is quite erroneous. The hymen may remain intact even after repeated acts of coitus depending upon: (i) Force of penetration (ii) Size of male organ (iii) Type of structure (iv) Consistency (v) Nature of opening. In children during attempted sexual intercourse the hymen is usually not ruptured due to high up position.

  The term **Virgo intacta** is applied to such woman when the hymen is intact despite the fact that she had experienced sexual intercourse.

  When the hymen is intact, the woman may not necessarily be virgin. However, if hymen is ruptured the woman may still be a virgin because in such case the rupture had resulted due to causes other than the sexual act.

Types of Hymen (Figure 27.2)

1. **Semilunar or crescentic:** The hymenal opening is placed anteriorly present at the lateral and posterior margins of vaginal opening.
2. **Annular:** Hymenal opening is oval situated in the center and encircles the vaginal opening.
3. **Infantile:** There is small linear opening in the midline.
4. **Cribriform:** There are several hymenal openings.
5. **Vertical:** A vertical hymenal opening is seen.
6. **Septate:** There are two lateral openings side by side.

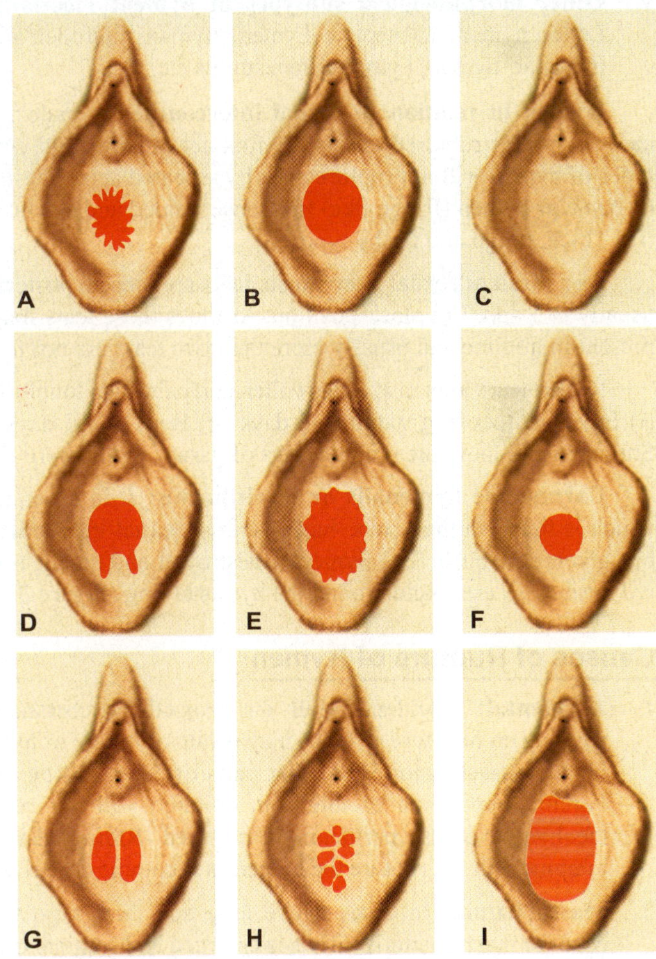

Figure 27.2: Different types of hymen (A) Fimbriated hymen (B) Semilunar hymen (C) Imperforate hymen (D) Hymenal tears (E) Carunculae mytiformes (F) Annular hymen (G) Septate hymen (H) Cribriform hymen (I) Parous introitus

7. **Imperforate:** No hymenal opening is there.
8. **Fimbriated or notched:** Free margin of hymen sometimes presents natural notches. This is to be differentiated from tears as a result of sexual intercourse. This type of hymen is also called **frilly edged**. The differences between fimbriated and ruptured hymen are as given below:

Features	Fimbriated hymen	Ruptured hymen
Situation of notches	Present anteriorly, doesn't extend to the base of hymen	Present posteriorly at one or both sides of median line; extend to the point of attachment of hymen to the edge of vagina
Shape and size of notches	Bilaterally symmetrical	Asymmetrical
Mucous membrane over notches	Intact	Not intact
Cause	Occurs naturally; making the edges of hymen notchy	Caused by sexual inter-course or by introduction of foreign bodies

9. **Other morphological subtypes of hymen:** Falciform or Lunar hymen, subseptate hymen, hymen microperforatus, irregular hymen, hymen trifenestratus etc.

Hymen in relation to sexual intercourse: In majority of cases hymen is ruptured during the first act of coitus but certain types of hymen will not rupture even by repeated acts. These are: (i) Annular hymen (fringe like) (ii) Loose, folded and elastic type (iii) Thick, tough and fleshy type.

As a result of sexual intercourse, tears are present posteriorly usually at 5 and 7'O clock position. At times these tears may be present in midline and usually more than two tears are not found.

Recent tears look raw, red, swollen and painful to touch. They (i) Bleed on touching within 1-2 days (ii) Heal in 5-6 days (iii) Shrunken and look like granular tags of tissues within 8-10 days.

Carunculae hymenalis or myritiformis: It is a condition which is found in those who have habitual sexual intercourse or has given childbirth. The hymen is destroyed and small, round, red fleshy tags are found around the hymenal ring (Figure 27.2).

Causes of Rupture of Hymen

1. **Accidental:** Accidental fall on projecting substance or slipping on furniture or fence may result in rupture of hymen. In these cases, injuries to other parts of body will be there. Forcible separation of thighs in children will not rupture the hymen unless perineum is ruptured. Riding, dancing, jumping will not rupture the hymen as is commonly believed.
2. **Masturbation:** In cases where long and thick objects are used for masturbation, clitoris is enlarged and vaginal orifice is dilated.
3. **Foreign body:** To render young girls fit for sexually intercourse, *Solapith* is introduced into the vagina. This soaks water and swells. This is done specially in prostitutes when the young girls are asked to sit in water with the *solapith* introduced into the vagina. The *solapith* swells and rupture of hymen occurs.
4. **Ulceration:** This could result from diphtheria, repeated fungal infection.
5. **Scratching:** Due to uncleanliness and poor personal hygiene of the part.
6. Surgical and gynecological operations.
7. **Sanitary tampons:** A plug of cotton wool that is used to absorb secretions and stop haemorrhage can result in rupture of hymen.

Diagnosis of Virginity

Usually, intact hymen indicates virginity but sometimes married woman and even prostitutes have intact hymen. Thus, an intact hymen does not automatically prove virginity. With an intact hymen there may be true virgin or false virgin. Hence due considerations should be given to accessory signs of virginity before giving the diagnosis of virginity.

If hymen is intact, labia majora is flabby and not in apposition and in addition, labia minora are not in apposition, vagina is roomy and admits two fingers then it is highly probable that the female is not a true virgin.

A virgin was once defined by judges as a ***rara avis*** and so far as the medical evidence is concerned, the definition is almost correct.

Signs of breasts and genitalia particularly intactness of hymen was always held to signify the physical virginity. However, hymen has limited value in defining virginity as sometimes repeated acts of coitus may not rupture the hymen. Intactness of hymen is not an absolute proof of virginity. With intact hymen there are true as well as false virgins.

Findings in true virgins: (i) Hymen is intact and is well stretched (ii) Edges are distinct and regular (iii) Vaginal orifice is of small dimension and allows admission of terminal phalanx of a finger. When all these findings are present, presumptions are in favour of the virginity or non-penetration of penis into the vagina.

Findings in false virgins: (i) Hymen is intact (ii) Hymenal orifice lets one, two or more fingers to pass easily (iii) Hymen is relaxed as to undulate and allow itself to be depressed in a virgin. However, the size of penis in erection can also penetrate without rupturing the hymen one or several times.

Accessory signs of virginity: In such cases suggestive of false virgin, accessory signs of virginity are to be reviewed and carefully weighed. These signs are: (i) Labia majora are separated and flabby (ii) Labia minora are thickened and separated (iii) Fourchette is torn (iv) Vagina is roomy and enlarged. Thus, with intact hymen there is little possibility of the female being a true virgin. If the above accessory signs are not present, there is greater possibility of female being a true virgin.

Thus, it is quite clear that in certain cases diagnosis of virginity is a delicate matter and there are cases when one cannot say for absolute in favour for or against it. However, unfortunately defloration without rupture of hymen is not the rule and at first coitus, hymen is torn in majority of cases.

To conclude there are no definite findings suggestive of a true or a false virgin and one cannot be certain of either nor can one express such certainty. Anyway, the diagnosis of virginity is a very delicate matter and undoubtedly difficult in some of the cases.

Virginity in relation to rape: On medical examination in a rape victim all the signs of virginity can be present. However, according to section 375 I.P.C., it is said that vaginal penetration to any extent, even if applying mouth to vagina is sufficient to constitute rape. The question of loss of virginity arises when the victim is a virgin prior to rape. Following points should be taken into consideration: (i) Laceration or tear of hymen is the principal evidence of defloration or loss of virginity. (ii) Other signs are not affected by a single act of coitus. (iii) Even at times repeated acts of coitus do not rupture the hymen. Thus, rupture of hymen should not be considered as principle evidence of loss of virginity due to rape. (iv) Age of rupture of hymen should be correlated with time of occurrence. (v) Other causes of rupture of hymen are to be considered while examining such a case.

Hymenoplasty: It is an operation for the repair of ruptured hymen and is more popular in Western countries when the unmarried girl gives gift to her husband. However, Indian women are also not lagging behind. The unmarried girls undergo hymenoplasty before marriage to avoid suspicion by their husbands. Even cases are on record that a lady on her 25th wedding anniversary underwent hymenoplasty to give a gift to her husband. The findings of hymenoplasty are narrow hymenal orifice that is unusual for the age group. There is congestion and scars at the site of united tears.

Differences between virginity and defloration

Features	Virginity	Defloration
Hymen	Intact, rigid, inelastic, edges are regular with a narrow opening allowing passage of tip of little finger	Torn or intact; loose elastic; two fingers pass easily
Labia majora	Fully developed, appose to each other; close the vaginal orifice completely	Not apposed, loose; vaginal opening may be seen at lower end
Labia minora	In contact and covered by labia majora	Exposed, separated from labia majora
Fossa navicularis	Intact	Disappears
Vagina	Narrow, rugae more folded; vault more conical	Grows in length; rugae less obvious, dilated

PREGNANCY

Pregnancy is a state that occurs in a female when an ovum is fertilized by spermatozoa. It occurs during the reproductive period of the female, the average being from 15-45 years. The question of pregnancy arises in the following cases:

Civil cases: (i) To avoid attendance in a Court of law as a witness. However, pregnancy is not a bar unless advanced state is reached as at that time delivery may be imminent and there may be risk to child (ii) Feigned pregnancy soon after death of her husband to claim succession to the estate (iii) To assess damage in a seduction or breach of promise of marriage (iv) When the woman blackmails a man and accuses him that she is pregnant by him (v) In cases of libel or slander of an unmarried woman, widow or wife having depart of from her husband and she is pregnant (vi) To secure greater compensation when her husband dies through negligence of the other (vii) A surgeon may terminate pregnancy by carrying out surgery for fictitious tumour (viii) To get more relief in cases of divorce.

Criminal cases: (i) To reduce the capital punishment, when convicted of capital crime (S. 416 Cr.P.C.). The High Court can postpone or commute it to life imprisonment (ii) Motive for suicide or murder of unmarried girls or widows (iii) In cases of alleged criminal abortion (iv) Alleged concealment of birth (S. 318 I.P.C.), pregnancy and infanticide.

To examine such cases a written order either from the police officer or court is obtained and informed written consent is taken. The lady must be examined by a female registered medical practitioner (S. 53 Cr.P.C.) or by a male doctor in the presence of a female attendant. In case the registered medical practitioner is encountering difficulty, the help of the specialist is taken.

Diagnosis of Pregnancy in the Living

1. **Presumptive signs**: (i) Amenorrhoea (ii) Morning sickness (iii) Breast changes (iv) Quickening (v) Pigmentation of the skin (vi) Changes in vagina (vii) Urinary disturbance (viii) Fatigue (ix) Sympathetic disturbances.
2. **Probable signs:** (i) Enlargement of abdomen (ii) Uterine changes (iii) Cervix changes (iv) Intermittent uterine contractions (Braxton Hick's sign) (v) Ballottement (vi) Foetal parts (vii) Uterine soufflé (viii) Biological tests (ix) Immunological tests (x) Pharmacological tests (xi) Radioimmunoassay for chorionic gonadotropins.
3. **Positive signs:** (i) Foetal movements (ii) Foetal heart sounds (iii) X-ray diagnosis (iv) Ultrasonography (v) Umbilical or Funic soufflé (vi) Foetal electrocardiogram.

Presumptive Signs

1. **Amenorrhoea:** It is the earliest and the most important symptom of pregnancy. There may be occasional spotting but full menstruation is not possible. Besides pregnancy,

amenorrhoea may occur due to anaemia, TB, disorders of thyroid and pituitary gland, mental stress, fear or nervousness of illicit relationship and when there is intense desire of pregnancy. Amenorrhoea may sometimes be feigned as a strong motive for deceit.

2. **Morning sickness:** It appears from the end of first month up to three months. Vomiting in the morning is not a reliable sign and may be due to migraine or some hormonal imbalance.
3. **Breast changes:** These changes are important in primigravida but are of less value in multipara. The breasts have increased growth and become physiologically more active. These changes are also found in ovarian or uterine tumours and in spurious pregnancy. The various breast changes are: (i) Tenderness (ii) Tingling sensation (iii) Size is increased due to hypertrophy of mammary gland. (iv) Superficial veins are engorged. (v) Nipple becomes deeply pigmented and erectile. (vi) Areola becomes deep darkly brown in 2nd month. (vii) Sebaceous glands are enlarged and tubercles are formed around the nipple ***(Montgomery's tubercles)*** by the end of 3rd month. (viii) Colostrum formation occurs during 3rd month, is thin yellowish fluid consisting of fat globules and large phagocytic cells filled with droplets of fat. (ix) After 6 months, silvery lines and striae are seen due to stretching of skin. (x) Rarely no appreciable breast changes occur and even the size may diminish.
4. **Quickening:** Quickening literally means "Coming to life". It is first perception of fetal movements by the mother that occurs during the 14-20th weeks. In a nonpregnant woman flatulence and peristaltic movement can be mistaken for quickening. In spurious pregnancy commonly seen in hysterical woman and those who are anxious to have children, false quickening can be felt.
5. **Pigmentation of skin:** The skin of vulva, abdomen and axilla become darker. There is formation of dark circles around eyes. The formation of **linea nigra** that are dark, pigmented lines starts from pubes, divides to encircle the umbilicus and continues upto xiphoid process is observed by 20th week.
6. **Changes in vagina:** The mucous membrane of vagina changes from pink to violet and finally blue as a result of venous obstruction. It is seen after 4th week and is known as ***Jackquemier's* sign** or ***Chadwick's sign.*** The tissue becomes softer, secretions are increased and the pulsations of vaginal artery can be felt at an early period.
7. **Urinary disturbance:** The enlarging uterus presses upon bladder and results in increased frequency of micturition. This symptom gradually passes off as the uterus comes into the abdomen and again reappears before term when head descends into pelvis.
8. **Fatigue:** It is very frequently present.
9. **Sympathetic disturbances:** These are salivation, perverted appetite and irritability.

Probable Signs

1. **Enlargement of abdomen:** It occurs due to enlargement of the uterus as:

Months	Enlargement of uterus
End of 3rd	Fills the pelvis
3rd-4th	Over the pelvic brim
5th	Midway between symphysis pubis and umbilicus
6th	At the level of the umbilicus
7th	Midway between umbilicus and ensiform cartilage
8th	At the level of ensiform cartilage
9th-10th	The uterus sinks into pelvis

Due to stretching of the abdominal wall, red coloured subcutaneous scars are seen on the abdomen.

2. **Changes in the uterus:** These are: (i) At 3rd month, angle between body and cervix is accentuated. On bimanual examination, uterus has a doughy or elastic feeling (ii) ***Hegar's sign*** is appreciable at **8-10 weeks** and can be elicited by putting one hand over the abdomen and two fingers inside the vagina. The cervix is felt as firm and hard whereas uterus is felt as elastic body. In between the two, the isthmus is felt as a soft compressible area. At about **6 weeks** of gestation, manual examination of uterus reveals softening at the midline of uterus anteriorly at the junction of uterus and cervix called ***Ladin's sign.*** At **7-8 weeks,** on clinical examination, a palpable lateral bulge or soft prominence can be observed at the junction where the uterine tube meets the utters is called ***Piskacek's sign.*** On bimanual examination, rhythmic contraction of uterus can be elicited as early as **4-8 weeks** which is called ***Palmer's sign.*** Increased pulsation can be felt through the lateral fornices at about **8th week** is called ***Osiander's sign.***
3. **Changes in the cervix:** The cervix softens from below upwards from the 2nd month onwards. This is well marked in the **4th month** and is known as ***Goodell's sign.*** There is softening of the cervix towards the last month of pregnancy. The cervical orifice becomes circular instead of transverse, admitting the tip of finger more readily.
4. **Intermittent uterine contractions (Braxton-Hick's sign):** These are intermittent, painless uterine contractions, are usually felt **after 3rd or 4th month**. These contractions last for one minute with relaxation for 2-3 minutes. The sign is elicitable even in cases of dead foetus, diseases like myomas, haemometra etc.
5. **Ballottement:** Ballottement means 'to toss up like a ball'. It is positive during **4th and 5th month** because the foetus is small in relation to liquor amnii. It is of two types: (i) **Internal**

ballottement: It can be elicited by inserting two fingers into the anterior fornix and the uterus is tapped upwards suddenly. The foetus moves upwards and after a while drops back on the finger tip like a ball. (ii) **External ballottement:** It can be obtained by sudden motion of the abdominal wall, in a few seconds the foetus rebounds back. These findings can be negative if there is less amniotic fluid.

6. **Foetal parts:** These can be felt by the **5th month** by palpating through the abdominal wall.
7. **Uterine soufflé:** It is a soft blowing murmur, heard by auscultation, which is synchronous with the mother's pulse. It is heard above the pubis at the end of **4th month** due to passage of blood through the uterine vessels.
   The uterine soufflé is also heard in enlarged ovaries and myomatous tumour of uterus.
8. **Biological tests:** These tests depend upon the presence of chorionic gonadotropins in the urine of a pregnant woman. The early morning sample of urine is taken for the test. The test depends on the hormones derived from the placenta. The diagnosis is made as early as **10-12 days** whereas other external signs of pregnancy prove not to be reliable. The test is false positive in hydatidiform mole, chorion epithelioma, ectopic gestation, pituitary tumours. **Galli Mainini test** has certain advantages as it is rapid there is easy availability of animals, has low cost and the accuracy is 94-96%. Various biological tests are given under Table 27.1.
9. **Immunological tests of pregnancy: Agglutination test:** Human Chorionic Gonadotropins has antigenic properties and when it is injected into animals, Anti Human Chorionic Gonadotrophic serum (Anti-HCG) is produced. The urine (suspected case of pregnancy-HCG) is mixed with anti HCG and incubated for one hour. If the patient is pregnant, HCG in urine will neutralize Anti-HCG in serum. Then RBC or latex particles coated with HCG are added and incubated for 2 hours. The mixture is then centrifuged and if the mixture remains turbid without deposit (No agglutination), it is taken as positive for pregnancy, because Anti-HCG has neutralized HCG in the urine of pregnant woman. Absence of agglutination indicates neutralization of the antiserum by gonadotropins in the urine.
10. **Pharmacological tests for pregnancy:** The sudden withdrawal of exogenously administered progesterone may precipitate endometrial bleeding in an amenorrhoeic patient. Thus, if no withdrawal bleeding occurs, pregnancy may be the likely explanation.
11. **Radioimmunoassay for chorionic gonadotropins:** This assay has been recently developed. The test detects minute amounts of HCG (0.003 international units per ml of serum) with accuracy concentration in 1 liter of plasma (mother)= 24 hours of urine concentration.

    HCG level starts rising after 2 weeks of missed period and the level is maintained upto 5th month. It gives 98% accuracy in the diagnosis of pregnancy. The test is false positive, due to luteinizing hormone (L.H.) of pituitary cross-reacting with antibody of HCG. It is false negative from more than 20 weeks to less than 10 days.

Positive Signs of Pregnancy

1. **Foetal movements:** Foetal movements are felt at **4th month** and the parts can be felt at **5th month** by placing the hand on the abdomen.
2. **Foetal heart sounds:** This is an important and definite sign of pregnancy. The foetal heart sounds become audible at **18-20 weeks** like tickling of a watch placed under a pillow. The heart rate is approximately 160/min at 5th month and 190/min at 9th month. The foetal heart sounds are not synchronous with mother's pulse and is not heard in a dead foetus or when there is excessive liquor amnii, fatty abdomen, or foetus < 18 weeks.

Table 27.1: Biological tests

Tests	Animals	Procedure	Time	Observations
Rapid Rat test	Two immature albino female rats	2 ml of morning sample of urine or 1 ml of serum is injected intraperitonially	4-24 hours later killed with chloroform asphyxia	Congested ovaries positive
Aschheim-Zondek test	Five immature white female mice; wt. 6-8 gm, 3-4 weeks old	0.2-0.3 ml of morning urine sample is injected subcutaneously BD for 3 days	Killed on 5th day	Haemorrhagic follicles or corpus luteum positive of ovary
Friedman's test	Adult female Rabbit; 12-12 week old, wt. 2 kg	5-10 ml of urine through ear vein for 2 days	24 hours after last injection	Haemorrhagic follicle or graffian follicle positive of ovary
Hogben (Female Toad) test	Mature female African Toads	5 ml of morning urine in dorsal lymphatic sac	Animal is isolated in a glass jar 1/3rd of water	After 12-18 hours Toad ovulates
Galli Mainini (Male frog) test	Rana tigrina	5-10 ml of morning urine in dorsal lymphatic sac of two male Toads	Cloacal urine is withdrawn ½-1 hour for 3 hours	Presence of sperms in the urine in 2-3 hours and latest within 24 hours, if pregnancy is present

3. **Umbilical or Funic soufflé:** It is a hissing sound synchronous with foetal heart rate due to movement of blood in the umbilical vessels. It is usually heard between **13 and 18 weeks.**
4. **X-ray diagnosis:** On radiological examination foetal parts can be detected from 16 weeks onwards and occasionally can be detected as early as **10-12 weeks**. On X-ray the foetus is seen as: (a) Annular shadow for skull (b) Small dots with linear arrangement for vertebral column (c) Series of parallel lines for ribs (d) Linear shadow of limbs. At a later stage, X-ray is of value in the diagnosis of twin pregnancy, foetal abnormalities, intrauterine death and hydatidiform mole.
5. **Ultrasonography (B-scan ultrasonography):** It is direct visualization of ultrasonic apparatus. **At 5-6 weeks** of gestational sac is large enough with uterus to be visualised by ultrasonography. Heart is the first functional organ and cardiac activity can be seen at 5-6 weeks of gestation.
6. **Foetal electrocardiogram:** It is more accurate at **after 17 weeks** of intrauterine life.

Determination of Period of Pregnancy

1. By counting the days since last menstrual period.
2. From quickening that occurs at 14-18th week.
3. Height of uterus above symphysis pubis.
4. ***Macdonald's Rule:***

$$\text{The no. of lunar months of pregnancy} = \frac{\text{Ht of fundus above the symphysis (cm)}}{3.5}$$

For example: If the height of uterus is 30 cm or 12 inches, then period of pregnancy = 30/3.5= 8½ lunar months = 34 weeks.

Pseudocyesis (spurious pregnancy): It is usually seen in women nearing menopause, in young woman who intensely desire a child or those with psychic or hormonal disorder. Such patients may present with all the subjective symptoms of pregnancy like: (i) Abdominal size is increased due to ascites, fat etc. (ii) Breast changes are sometimes present (iii) In many cases, women imagine fetal movements (iv) In some cases, pregnancy has gone to full term and even labour pains started when the patient was told that she is not pregnant. In these situations, the patient must be convinced about her condition and X-ray abdomen should be taken that will allay her doubts.

Diagnosis of Pregnancy in the Dead

An examination may help to retrieve or restore the reputation of a dead woman suspected of unchastity. The findings of pregnancy in the dead woman are: (i) ***Presence of an ovum:*** Presence of ovum for 7-10 days, presence of an embryo for 1-9 weeks or presence of foetus from 9 weeks onwards or presence of placental tissue and membranes or any other product of conception signifies that the woman is pregnant. A well formed corpus luteum in one of the ovary is very important feature. Even in an exhumed body foetal bones can be recovered. (ii) ***Corpus luteum:*** Corpus luteum continues to develop during pregnancy and maximum size is reached at 5th month forming a firm projection on the surface of the ovary. It then passes through a retrogressive change. However, it is well-marked at the time of delivery and may be evident up to 1-2 months thereafter. (iii) ***Uterine changes:*** Marks of placental attachment are found upto 8-9 weeks after delivery. Period of gestation is the possible period of pregnancy and is not the average period. (iv) In doubtful cases, microscopic examination will reveal products of conception, condition of endometrium and corpus luteum. (v) ***False positive pregnancy*** can be due to fibroid tumour, other pathologies of uterus and ovaries. Pregnancy can also occur without the formation of corpus luteum.

DELIVERY

The term delivery means expulsion or extraction of the child at birth. It means spontaneous delivery. The question of delivery may arise in situations such as: (i) Abortion before foetus is viable (ii) Infanticide (iii) Concealment of birth (S. 318 I.P.C.) (iv) Feigned delivery (v) Contested legitimacy (S. 112 I.E.A.) (vi) Blackmailing (vii) Defamation of character (viii) Nullity of marriage (ix) Divorce.

Signs of Recent Delivery in the Living

Recent delivery means 10-14 days after the date of delivery and is applicable to full term deliveries, rather than premature ones. In strong and healthy woman especially multiparous, the signs of recent delivery disappear within a week or so and sometimes earlier. The signs of recent delivery are:

1. **General appearance or indisposition:** (i) Woman has languished look with shrunken eyes for the initial 2-3 days (ii) There is dark coloured pigmentation over the lower eyelids (iii) Pulse and body temperature are slightly increased. These signs may be found in some other illness also and not specifically produced after delivery. These may not be produced in multiparous woman who resume work immediately.
2. **Intermittent contractions of uterus:** Intermittent contractions of uterus known as **after pains** are vigorous and painful and remain up to 4-5 days.
3. **Findings in the breasts:** Breasts are full and prominent and have a knotty feeling and are tender. Nipples are enlarged and surrounded by darkened areola. **Montgomery's tubercles** are present. Milk or colostrum corpuscles are present within few days. Veins over breasts are prominent.
4. **Abdominal findings:** Abdomen is lax, flabby with wrinkled skin. **Stria gravidarum and linea albicantes** are suggestive of past delivery in the absence of other possible causes. These are pink when recent and subsequently becomes white. These may not be present in previous prolonged distension of abdomen and if present, may disappear.

Linea nigra, a dark pigmented line in the midline of abdomen extending from symphysis pubis upwards is also seen.

5. **Uterine changes:** After delivery, uterus is contracted, retracted and feels like a hard cricket ball. Its height is three cm below the umbilicus. It diminishes in size at the rate of 1.5 cm/day. On 6th day, its height is midway between umbilicus and pubis.

   On 14th day, fundus is at the level of pubic symphysis and comes to normal position at about 9th week.
6. **Labia majora:** Labia majora are tender, swollen, bruised or lacerated.
7. **Vagina:** Vagina is smooth walled, relaxed and capacious. It shows recent tears, which heal by 7th day. The rugae start reappearing in 3rd week.
8. **Fourchette:** Fourchette is lacerated in primipara and perineum shows recent tears.
9. **Cervix:** After delivery, cervix is soft and patulous, edges are torn and lacerations are present transversely. By 24 hours the internal os closes, external os admits two fingers and is soft. At the end of 1st week, external os admits 1 finger with difficulty and by 2nd week it closes.
10. **Lochia:** Lochia is the discharge for 2-3 weeks after delivery and has a peculiar sour, disagreeable odour. The appearance of lochia after delivery varies with the passage of time as (i) For 4-5 days (**Lochia Rubra**): Bright red containing blood clots (ii) Next 4 days (**Lochia Serosa**): Serous and pale in colour (iii) After 9th day (**Lochia Alba**): Yellowish green or turbid (iv) It finally disappears.
11. **Biological tests:** They are positive upto 7-10 days after delivery and is strong corroborative evidence of recent delivery.

Signs of Recent Delivery in the Dead

1. **Uterine changes:** All the local signs of delivery may be present. Size of uterus will vary according to the period of gestation and time of survival. Immediately after the delivery, uterine wall is 4-5 cm thick and uterine cavity is obliterated by apposition of anterior and posterior walls. Total length of the uterine wall is 20 cm and length of the cavity is 15 cm. The weight and size of uterus varies according to the passage of time after the delivery as tabulated below. The thickness of uterus at six weeks is 5 cm.

Duration	Length of uterus	Breadth of uterus	Weight of uterus
2-3 days	17.5 cm	10 cm	1000 g
7 days	13-14 cm	5 cm	500 g
14 days	<12 cm	5 cm	350 g
6 weeks	7-8 cm	5 cm	100-120 g

2. **Changes in placental area:** Shortly after the delivery placental site appears as an irregular, nodular and elevated area 15 cm in diameter. By the end of 2nd week it is 3-4 cm in diameter and at 6th week it is 1-2 cm in diameter.
3. Ovaries and fallopian tubes are congested and normal within few days.
4. Corpus luteum is found in one of the ovaries for 1-2 months.
5. Peritoneum covering the lower part of the uterus is arranged in folds.
6. Bladder is hyperemic and submucosal haemorrhages are present.

Signs of Remote Delivery in the Living

(i) Abdomen is lax and flabby and linea albicantes is present (ii) Breasts are soft and pendulous with dark areola (iii) Labia are not in apposition, are more or less separated (iv) Vagina is capacious, dilated with relaxed walls (v) Fourchette and posterior commissure are lacerated (vi) Hymen shows carunculae myritiformes (vii) Perineum will show old tears (viii) Cervical cleft is transverse with ragged, irregular margins.

These signs may disappear in a woman who had delivered only once several years ago. Passage of uterine fibroid tumor through the vagina may produce some of the above mentioned signs.

Signs of Remote Delivery in the Dead

1. Abdomen lax and flabby and linea albicantes present.
2. Breasts are soft and pendulous.
3. Various uterine changes in parous and multiparous woman are:

Features	Multiparous uterus	Nulliparous uterus
Size	9 cm long; 6 cm wide; larger and thicker	7 cm long; 4.5 cm wide; smaller and thinner
Weight	80-120 gm	40-60 gm
Length	Body is twice the length of cervix	Body is of same length as cervix
Fundus	Top of fundus is convex and at higher level than the line of broad ligament	Not so
Cavity	Walls are concave from inside and with wider rounded cavity	Walls are convex with smaller triangular cavity
Cervix	Irregular, external os transverse, admits tip of finger; internal os not well defined	Regular with no scars. External os small, dimpled in the middle, internal os is well defined

LEGITIMACY

Legitimacy is defined under **Section 16 of Hindu Marriage Act** of children of void and voidable marriages. According to this section:

1. Any child of null and void marriage who would have been legitimate if the marriage had been valid, shall be legitimate whether such child is born before or after the commencement of the **Marriage laws (Amendment) Act, 1976** and whether or not a decree of nullity is granted in respect of that marriage under this Act and whether or not the marriage is held to be void otherwise than on a petition under this Act.
2. Where a decree of nullity is granted in respect of voidable marriage under **Section 12 of Hindu Marriage Act**, any child begotten or conceived before the decree, who would have been the legitimate child if at the date of decree marriage had been dissolved instead of been annulled, shall be their legitimate child.

According to **Section 112 Indian Evidence Act** a child is presumed to be legitimate if it was born during the continuance of a valid marriage between his mother by any man or within 280 days after its dissolution, the mother remaining unmarried. The presumption can be rebutted if it is shown by competent evidence that: (i) Parties to marriage had no access to either at any time when the child could have been begotten. (ii) It does not necessarily mean that the child is bastard because he is born beyond 280 days, as there is a wide variation.

Differences from English law: Presumption of legitimacy can be rebutted in England by proof of impotence and sterility of the husband, but no special point is given in the Indian law. In English law, illegitimate children become legitimate after subsequent marriage between parents and the child inherits the property.

Illegitimate children: Illegitimate children are: (i) Born out of wedlock between parents (ii) Within wedlock, if the husband is sterile, is under age or due to other causes (iii) Born out within competent period after cessation of relationship between husband and wife (iv) After blood tests paternity is excluded.

S. 5 of Hindu Marriage Act 1955: It defines the conditions of a Hindu marriage as: (i) Neither party has a spouse living at the time of marriage. (ii) At the time of marriage neither party: (a) Is incapable of giving valid consent as the result of unsoundness of mind (b) Though capable of giving a valid consent has been suffering from mental disorders to such an extent to be unfit for marriage and procreation of children (c) Suffering from recurrent attacks of insanity. (iii) The groom has completed 21 years of age and the bride 18 years of age at the time of marriage. (iv) The parties are not within the degrees of prohibited relationship unless the custom allows such a marriage. (v) Both the parties are not *sapindas* of each other unless customs or usage permits such a marriage.

S. 11 of Hindu Marriage Act: It defines **void marriages** as any marriage solemnised after the commencement of this Act shall be null and void and may be so declared by a decree of nullity if it contravenes any of the condition in clauses (i), (iv) and (v) of Section 5 of Hindu Marriage Act.

S. 12 of Hindu Marriage Act: It defines **voidable marriages** as:

1. Any marriage solemnised, whether before or after the commencement of this Act shall be voidable and may be annulled by a decree of nullity on any of the following grounds: (a) The marriage has not been consummated due to impotence of the respondent or (b) Marriage in contravention of condition specified in clause (ii) of section 5 or (c) Or the consent of the petitioner or guardian was obtained by force or fraud (d) That the respondent was at the time of marriage pregnant by some person other than petitioner.
2. No petition for annulling a marriage (a) On the ground specified in clause (c) of sub section (1) shall be entertained if (i) Petition is presented more than one year after the force had ceased to operate or fraud has been discovered. (ii) Petitioner with his/her full consent had lived with the other party after the force had ceased to operate or fraud has been discovered (b) Of the ground specified of clause (d) of subsection (1) shall be entertained unless (i) Petitioner at the time of marriage was ignorant of the alleged facts (ii) Proceedings have been instituted within one year of commencement of this Act and in case of marriages solemnized after the commencement of this Act, within one year from the date of marriage. (iii) Marital intercourse has not taken place with the consent of the petition since the discovery of the existence of impotence of respondent.

Until 1976, the children of legal marriage and voidable marriages were called legitimate and that of void marriage were called illegitimate. After 1976, Marriage Laws Amendment Act 1976 came into force and according to this, the children born of void or voidable marriage shall be legitimate as if the marriage between their parents were valid, irrespective of the fact whether or not the marriage has been declared null and void under this Act or whether or not the marriage is held to be void otherwise than in a petition under this Act.

Thus, it is quite encouraging policy by the legislature conferring legitimacy on all children, born of void and voidable marriages. The question is why the innocent children should suffer for the fault of their parents and why they should be deprived of their legitimacy as to their birth and be forced to carry the social stigma throughout their life, apart from being deprived of the rights in the properties and assets of their parents.

The only provision is that under provisions of the Hindu law of succession legitimate children have right to properties of their parents and also to the properties of relatives as reversionary. Children of void and voidable marriages are liable to the properties of parents only.

Posthumous child: Is the one who is born after the death of the father; begotten during the lifetime of his father, the mother being conceived by said father.

Medicolegal Aspects of Legitimacy

The question of legitimacy arises in connection of right to inherit property when disputed and affiliation cases etc. The following questions need to be discussed:

1. **Average duration of pregnancy between conception and delivery:** (i) ***Period between last menstrual period and delivery***: It cannot be relied upon because menstruation may cease from other causes and may continue after pregnancy has commenced. Impregnation may occur at any period during menstrual period. (ii) ***Observation of the period between a single coitus and delivery:*** It is not so precise as single coitus does not fix the date of conception, but only the date of insemination. Sperms retain their activity for 2-3 days in the vagina and 4-5 days in cervix, uterus or fallopian tube. Thus, the exact time of conception is not known. It is known that ovulation occurs 14 days prior to next period and the ovum probably persists for a day or two after it is shed unless fertilised. Therefore, fertilization occurs if sperm retains its power and unites with the egg cell in the fallopian tube. Thus, the exact period is not known but calculated from experience, i.e., 280 days or 40 weeks or 10 lunar months which is equivalent to 10 times of normal intermenstrual period.
2. **Maximum period of pregnancy:** No fixed limit is laid in India, England or USA. English Courts have accepted up to 349 days as maximum period, the child being legitimate. **Mckown and Gibson** in their extensive study stated that 354 days are not impossible.
3. **Minimum period and viability:** Legitimacy may be disputed when a child is born within a short time of the husband and wife living together after a long separation. Thus, important question is whether it is possible for a fully developed child to be born before usual period of gestation. Although, age of viability is 210 days but even at 180 days the fetus is viable and capable of separate existence.
4. **Superfecundation:** It is fertilization of two ova in the same cycle of ovulation by two separate acts of coitus, committed at short intervals. Here, incidence of twin pregnancies is 1.5%. It occurs in 70% of binovular twins, resulting from separate fertilization of two ova at the same period. Development of twins in the uterus is parallel, not equal depending upon placental blood supply. The two placentas are developed. One foetus may abort, die or may remain till the end. The other may press the dead foetus, so that it becomes one mass called **foetus compressus**. Spermatozoa causing fertilization may be from different man having different blood group. Cases are on record where one of the twins belonged to the one father by blood group (one father being B^+ and other being A^+).
5. **Superfoetation:** It is the fertilization of second ovum in a woman, who is already pregnant. Subsequently the two foetuses are born either at the same time showing different stages of development or two fully developed foetuses are born at different periods varying from 1-3 months. There are cases on record where 2nd child is delivered after a period of the 1st one, when twins are expected. Thus, after the delivery of 1st one second gets proper nourishment and as a result it gets delivered later on. However, nowadays, it is said that this condition is possible though quite rare because of: (i) Ovulation may take place during first three months of gestation until decidua vera and decidua reflexa come in contact and close the decidual cavity. (ii) There is possibility of double uterus.
6. **Inheritance:** Legitimate child inherits the property of the father; a monster not having the shape of the mankind is incapable of inheriting. No special points relating to this are mentioned in Indian law.
7. **Affiliation cases:** A woman who alleges a putative man to be father of her illegitimate child may file a case. By some suitable method like exclusion of blood group, DNA fingerprinting paternity is fixed.

   S. 125 CrPC Order for maintenance of wives, children and parents: If a person having sufficient means neglects or refuses to maintain his wife, his legitimate or illegitimate minor child, his legitimate or illegitimate child who has attained majority, his mother or father, all unable to maintain themselves; the magistrate of 1st class may order such a person to make a monthly allowances. In determining the amount of maintenance under the Hindu Maintenance Act 1956, the court has to consider following points: (i) The position and status of the party (ii) Reasonable wants of the claimant (iii) The value of the claimant's property and any income derived from them (iv) The number of persons entitled for the maintenance.
8. **Supposititious children:** Supposititious children are fictitious that is not real or imaginary. A woman may substitute a living male or female for dead child or may feign pregnancy and delivery and subsequently produce a living child as her own when she wants to extort or to gain the right to property. In such cases, it is to be decided whether the age of the child corresponds to the date of pretended delivery.
9. **Paternity:** The question of paternity arises in cases relating to legitimacy, posthumous child or supposititious children. It is decided from: (i) *Paternal likeliness*: The child may resemble the father in features and mannerism etc., but this is only corroborative. (ii) *Atavism:* The child does not resemble the parents, but resembles its grandparents due to inheritance of characteristics from remote rather than immediate ancestors. It is due to recombination of genes. In addition, mental, physical characteristics, tendencies, disease, and diathesis peculiar to remote ancestor may be inherited. (iii) *Developmental defects*: Disease or deformity may sometimes be transmitted

from parents to offspring. (iv) *Blood groups and mutations*: Mutation are changes seen between generations resulting in an altered character in the child in 1:30,000.

SHORT QUESTIONS

1. Types of hymen.
2. True and false virgin.
3. Vaginismus.
4. Frigidity.
5. Superfecundation.
6. Medicolegal aspects of pregnancy.
7. Precipitate labour.
8. Superfoetation.
9. Atavism.

MULTIPLE CHOICE QUESTIONS

1. The common site of rupture of hymen in a virgin is:

(a) Anterior (b) Posterior
(c) Anterolateral (d) Posterolateral

2. Atavism is resemblance of features to the:

(a) Mother (b) Father
(c) Neighbour (d) Grandfather

3. The positive sign of pregnancy is:

(a) Quickening (b) Amenorrhoea
(c) Foetal heart sounds (d) Hegar's sign

4. Presence of caruncula myrtiformes indicates:

(a) Previous childbirth (b) Defloration
(c) Rape (d) Virginity

5. Positive sign of pregnancy:

(a) Quickening (b) Ballottement
(c) HCG analysis (d) Foetal movement

6. Pregnancy can be diagnosed by X-ray at about:

(a) 10-12 weeks (b) 12-14 weeks
(c) 15-16 weeks (d) 19-20 weeks

7. Superfoetation means:

(a) Fertilization of two ova in same cycle by two separate acts of coitus
(b) Fertilization of a second ovum in a woman who is already pregnant
(c) Abortion of one fetus in twin pregnancy
(d) Retention of one macerated foetus

8. Superfecundation means:

(a) Fertilization of two ova in same cycle by two separate acts of coitus
(b) Fertilization of a second ovum in a woman who is already pregnant
(c) Abortion of one fetus in twin pregnancy
(d) Retention of one macerated foetus

9. A 22-year-old lady died. The postmortem appearance that will indicate that she has had delivered a child are all *except:*

(a) Walls of uterus are convex from inside
(b) Cervix is irregular and external os is patulous
(c) Body of uterus is twice the length of cervix
(d) Uterus is bulky, large and heavy than nullipara

10. Spot out the wrong statement about nullity of marriage as per Hindu Marriage Act:

(a) Either party is suffering from unsound of mind
(b) There is wilful refusal to consummate
(c) When wife was pregnant by any person other than the husband
(d) Same gotra marriage

11. Accessory signs of false virginity includes all the following, *except:*

(a) Labia minora are fully covered by labia majora
(b) Clitoris is enlarged
(c) Vestibule is gaping
(d) Vagina is roomy

12. In Nulliparous, cervical opening is:

(a) Longitudinal (b) Circular
(c) Transverse (d) Fimbriated

13. The following findings are present in genitals of a virgin girl, *except:*

(a) Fourchette and posterior commissure are intact
(b) Labia minora are covered by the labia majora
(c) Hymen is a narrow opening
(d) Vagina is rugose and separated apart

ANSWER KEY ☞

1. (d)	2. (d)	3. (c)	4. (a)	5. (d)	6. (a)	7. (a)	8. (b)	9. (a)	10. (d)
11. (a)	12. (c)	13. (d)							

28 CHAPTER

Abortion

Bleeding is one of the important abnormalities during early pregnancy that occurs due to spontaneous abortion (due to natural causes), ectopic gestation, tumors, cervical lesions and endometrial bleeding.

Medical definition of abortion: Abortion means spontaneous or induced expulsion of products of conception before viability (28 weeks) whereas premature labor is delivery of fetus after 28 weeks of pregnancy upto 40th week. In medical practice, the **abortion** occurs in 1st trimester, **miscarriage** in the 2nd trimester and **premature labor** in the 3rd trimester. Legally, all the above terms are synonymous.

Legal definition of abortion: Abortion means expulsion of products of conception from the uterus at any period prior to full term. Law makes no distinction between abortion, miscarriage and premature labor. The products of conception are termed by the terminologies such as **Ovum, Embryo** and **Foetus.**

Classification of Abortion

1. *Natural due to natural causes before 28 weeks*:

   (i) Spontaneous abortion (ii) Accidental abortion.

2. *Artificial (Induced) abortion*: (i) Justifiable abortion (ii) Criminal abortion.

3. *Clinically abortion can be*: (i) Inevitable abortion (ii) Incomplete abortion (iii) Threatened abortion (iv) Complete abortion (v) Septic abortion (may be due to incomplete abortion) (vi) Missed abortion in which there is formation of careous or blood mole with more than 8 weeks gestation (vii) Habitual or recurrent (When abortion occurs three consecutive times) (viii) Criminal abortion when the pregnancy is terminated unlawfully without any proper indication.

Threatened abortion: Threatened abortion usually occurs in the early weeks of pregnancy. The patient presents with moderate vaginal haemorrhage and mild pain. On examination, the opening of cervical os is closed.

Inevitable abortion: The patient presents with severe pain, increased uterine contractions and dilated cervix.

Incomplete abortion: There is continuous bleeding from the placental site and retention of placenta is one of the most common complications of incomplete abortion. The patient presents with severe anemia. These cases are to be evacuated by surgery and drugs like ergometrine is to be given to induce uterine contraction so that the placenta comes out.

Missed abortion: In this type of abortion, the foetus dies in utero and is retained for more than weeks in the uterus. The history is quite characteristic in such cases, as initially for 12 weeks, there are normal signs and symptoms of pregnancy. Thereafter slight bleeding occurs that stops suddenly and the patient develops amenorrhoea. The abdomen is not enlarged but brown discharge occurs per vaginum after several weeks or months. In this type of abortion, the products of conception are converted to ovoid, fleshy mass due to recurrent or slow haemorrhage into chorionic spaces.

Mechanism of Abortion

Abortion corresponds to the process of normal labor at term. The body of uterus contracts and retracts and cervix dilates. Any of the following mechanism may be followed: (i) *Expulsion of the whole ovum in one piece:* During early weeks of pregnancy, the vera and basalis layer of decidua separates, so that the entire decidua and ovum are expelled out together. (ii) *Expulsion of the whole ovum by inversion of the decidua vera or parietalis:* This common method of typical abortion is due to detachment of ovum by means of retro-placental clot, the ovum is pushed into the uterine cavity and is expelled. Then the inversion of decidua vera and parietalis occurs. (iii) Incomplete expulsion of ovum with the retention of the placenta and its membranes. (iv) In missed abortion, ovum is separated from its attachment to the uterus to a degree sufficient to kill the embryo, but the detached embryo is retained. Pregnancy tests previously positive becomes negative.

Types of abortion: It can be (1) Natural (2) Criminal. The difference between the two are tabulated under Table 28.1.

Table 28.1: Differences between natural and criminal abortion

Features	Natural abortion	Criminal abortion
Cause	Any woman with predisposing disease	Unmarried woman or widow
Infection	Rare	Frequent
Marks of violence on abdomen	Not present	May be present
Genital organs	No injuries	Injuries present
Toxic effect of drugs	Absent	Present
Foreign bodies in genital tract	Not present	Present
Foetal wounds	Absent	Present

NATURAL ABORTION

Natural abortion occurs before 28 weeks of pregnancy and the incidence being 5-20% of all pregnancies with an average of 10%.

Etiology

Abnormalities of the fetus: It accounts for 50% of all abortions. These are: (i) *Maldevelopment of the fetus:* The abortus in first two months shows errors of development of foetus like hydatidiform mole, degeneration of placenta and maldevelopment of the embryo. (ii) *Intrauterine death:* The death of the fetus *in utero* can occur from the following causes: (a) *Infections*: If mother contracts infections such as pneumonia, malaria, typhoid, dysentery, smallpox, syphilis etc, foetus is liable to die *in utero.* The infecting organism in syphilis, smallpox and rubella does not pass through the placental barrier. As a result, patient usually dies from the pyrexia and not the ill effect of the causative organism (b) *Poisons*: The most dangerous of the poisonous substances is lead and to some extent quinine. In such cases, the mother becomes gravely ill before there is any effect on the ovum (c) *Radiological effects*: Usually, the patient is being treated for malignant disease without the knowledge of status of pregnancy. When the patient gets sufficient exposure in the 1st trimester, the foetus dies in the uterus or else foetal abnormalities occur.

Abnormalities of the placenta and membranes: (i) *Acute hydramnios:* In acute hydramnios, the amount of amniotic fluid is more than 2000 ml (ii) Hydatidiform degeneration of placenta (iii) *Placenta praevia:* The placenta is attached in lower uterine segment resulting in severe bleeding after abortion. This usually occurs in second trimester.

General diseases of the mother: (i) *Acute infections:* The generalized infections can result from the diseases namely measles, scarlet fever, cholera, typhoid, diphtheria, malaria and smallpox. The localized infections resulting in abortion are pneumonia, pneumococcal peritonitis after evacuation, erysipelas and upper respiratory tract infections. (ii) *Chronic infections:* The chronic infection in mother that can cause abortion are syphilis (never causes an abortion before mid pregnancy), Tuberculosis (not a common cause but if the disease is widespread and rapidly progressive, abortion can occur), other chronic diseases such as hypertension and chronic nephritis. These diseases basically interferes with placental circulation and foetal blood supply.

Local abnormalities of the mother: (i) Local abnormalities of the genitalia such as genital hypoplasia, hypoplasia of uterus associated with gross ovarian deficiency, partial duplication of upper part of uterus, bicornuate uterus, septate uterus and subseptate uterus. (ii) *Displacement of uterus:* The attempts at correcting the position of retroverted uterus in second and third trimester causes abortion. As in fourth month, the uterus comes out of pelvis, there are no chances of abortion. (iii) *Fibromyoma of submucous or polypoid type:* This may also result in abortion. However, removal of tumour surgically results in normal pregnancy. (iv) *Cervical incompetence:* The cervix is patulous and abortion usually occurs in 2nd trimester due to premature rupture of membranes. (v) *Surgical operations:* Any operation on pregnant woman however trivial and anaesthesia involves risk of abortion. The risk increases nearer to the genital tract the operation is performed. Myomectomy carries the greatest risk of abortion and nervous women are liable to abort even after tooth extraction. (vi) *Drugs:* Drugs such as phosphorus, lead, quinine, ergot and mercury in poisonous quantities may lead to abortion from their toxic effects upon the mother. (vii) *Injuries:* The following injuries are liable to cause abortion: (a) Accidents and injuries to lower abdominal region and vulva results in formation of haematoma in the region of uterus with dislodgment of placenta (b) Trauma of coitus (c) Fatigue and jolting of a long vehicle journey (d) violent physical exercise, riding bicycle etc. (viii) *Immunologic causes:* The maternal lymphocytes invade the foetus and the women who reject skin graft of their husband are liable to abort more. (ix) *Disturbance of endocrine system:* Secretion of corpus luteum is essential for embedding of the fertilized ovum in the first few weeks of pregnancy. After 12-14 weeks, the functions of corpus luteum are replaced by placenta and even if both ovaries are removed, patient goes to term. In diabetes and thyrotoxicosis, there is tendency to abort because of the increase in prostaglandins E_2 and F_2 in amniotic fluid. (x) *Psychiatric causes:* The abortions result from fright, fear, acute mental tension and acute anxiety neurosis.

Abnormalities in the male: During investigations for infertility and repeated abortions the semen analysis is done. The analyses reveals large number of abnormal sperms that result in foetal abnormalities and abortion.

ARTIFICIAL ABORTION

Justifiable (Therapeutic) Abortion

Abortion is justified when done in good faith to save the mother's life if it is materially endangered by continuation of pregnancy. It is not done just to save family honour or for ethical or economical reasons. Abortion is justifiable if mother's health is likely to be permanently damaged by continuation of pregnancy. WHO defines **health** 'As a state of complete physical, mental and social well being and not merely the absence of illness and disease'.

Precautions to be taken by the doctor while performing therapeutic abortion: (i) It is always wise to consult another doctor preferably a specialist in the field of obstetrics and gynaecology. (ii) Written consent of woman and her husband is to be taken. (iii) Procedure should be undertaken in a government hospital. (iv) Doctor should wait for conducting abortion till the child attains viability. (v) While performing abortion, the presence of a witness preferably a nurse is must.

Indications for performing therapeutic abortion: (i) *Obstetrical indications:* (a) Severe eclampsia, hypertensive disorder (convulsion and coma) (b) Psychiatric conditions such as relative depression, suicidal tendencies and schizophrenic states (c) Unwanted pregnancy in a mentally subnormal woman. (ii) *Malignant conditions:* Invasive carcinoma of cervix, carcinoma of ovary and breast cancer with metastasis. (iii) *Cardiovascular conditions:* Valvular heart disease, cardiac failure, congenital heart disease, atrial fibrillation and hypertension. (iv) *Respiratory conditions:* Respiratory insufficiency in lung diseases, chronic bronchitis and asthma. (v) *Alimentary conditions:* Peptic ulcer, ulcerative colitis with perforation and bleeding, pancreatitis and acute hepatitis. (vi) *Renal conditions:* Nephrotic syndrome. (vii) *Endocrine and Metabolic conditions:* Diabetes mellitus, parathyroid tumour and osteomalacia. (viii) *Neurological conditions:* Spinal and cerebral tumours, recurrent epilepsy, hereditary spastic paraplegia and myasthenia gravis. (ix) *Psychological and emotional conditions:* (a) When the child is unwanted and is the result of incest and rape (b) When the patient is suffering from grave neurosis and suicidal tendencies. (x) *Conditions causing foetal abnormalities:* (a) Infective conditions (Rubella, Mumps) (b) Mother exposed to drugs (Thalidomide, androgens and oestrogens) (c) Rh incompatibility (d) Down's syndrome (Mongolism).

Methods of Termination of Pregnancy

Methods for first trimester MTP: These are (i) ***Menstrual regulation:*** This consists of aspiration of contents of uterine cavity by means of a plastic cannula (Karman's cannula), and a plastic 50 ml syringe capable of creating a vacuum of over 60 cm Hg. It is carried out effectively within 42 days of the beginning of last menstrual period. (ii) ***Dilatation and suction evacuation*:** This is most efficient method of terminating pregnancy up to 12 weeks of gestation. The gestation size and position of the uterus are carefully assessed. After administrating a paracervical block, the cervix is held with an Allis' forceps and dilated by means of specially designed dilators with a guard, or with sialistic dilators until adequate dilatation is achieved to permit introduction of suction cannula of appropriate size (diameter corresponding to the weeks of gestation) into the uterine cavity. A standard negative suction force of 650 mm (65 cm) of Hg is applied and the products are aspirated. (iii) ***Medical methods:*** Prostaglandin and more recently RU 486 have been extensively investigated as methods for MTP in early pregnancy but are unable the replace the more effective and safe surgical aspiration.

Methods of second trimester MTP: (i) ***Dilatation and evacuation*:** MTP up to 16 weeks is done by slow and deliberate dilatation of the cervix with laminaria tents, prostaglandin gel or pessary prior to evacuation of the uterine contents using either vaccum aspiration, aspirotomy ovum forceps or a blunt curette. (ii) ***Aspirotomy:*** This procedure involves suction aspiration of the liquor amnii, followed by evacuation of the fetal parts in pieces with the help of a specially designed instrument called the aspirotomy forceps. (iii) ***Hysterotomy:*** Once popular and used in combination with tubectomy is not advocated today, because safer medical procedures are available. (iv) (a) Intra-amniotic instillation of drugs such as hypertonic glucose and saline, mannitol, urea, hydrocortisone and prostaglandins (b) Extra-ovular instillation of drugs such as ethacridine lactate, hypertonic saline and prostaglandins.

MTP Act 1971

The Central Family Planning Board of Government of India, a policy making body, at a meeting held on 25th August 1964 expressed concern about problems of abortion and recommended to appoint a committee to examine the subject of abortion in its legal, medical, moral, and social aspects and to make suitable suggestions to alter the existing law. On 19th September 1964 Ministry of Health appointed, Mr. Shantilal Shah, Health Minister of Maharashtra as Chairman of the committee. In December 1966, the committee submitted its recommendations and the Bill was introduced in 1969. The Bill was passed in Rajya Sabha and Lok Sabha on 2nd August 1971. The Act was enforced on 1st April, 1972 in India except the state of Jammu and Kashmir. The Act lays down the: (i) Conditions under which a pregnancy can be terminated. (ii) Person/persons who can perform such terminations. (iii) Place where such terminations can be performed.

Conditions under which the pregnancy can be terminated: Section 3(2) provides the grounds on which MTP can be done.

These are:

1. **Therapeutic:** The continuance of pregnancy would involve

a risk to the life of the pregnant woman or grave injury to her **physical or mental health.**

2. **Eugenic:** There is a substantial risk that if the child were born, it would suffer from such **physical/mental abnormalities** as to be seriously handicapped.

Explanation 1: When pregnancy of the alleged woman has been caused by rape, which shall be presumed to constitute a grave injury to mental health of the woman.

Explanation 2: Where the pregnancy has occurred as a result of failure of contraceptive, which may be presumed to constitute grave injury to the mental health of the woman.

Person/persons who can perform the terminations: The Act provides safeguards to the mother by authorising only a registered medical practitioner having experience in obstetrics and gynaecology upto 12 weeks to perform such terminations. Two registered medical practitioners are necessary for termination after 12 weeks upto 20th week.

Place where terminations can be performed: The Act stipulates that MTP should be performed in the government, semi-government, or private hospitals approved for this purpose.

Consent: (i) Written consent of the guardian is required where age of woman is less than 18 years and in lunatics. (ii) In other cases only consent of the pregnant woman is necessary and that of the husband is not required. (iii) Professional secrecy should be maintained by the doctor. (iv) Sterilisation is not a criterion but the patient should be advised to use contraceptive methods.

Section 8 provides safeguards to the doctors that no legal action will be taken against any registered medical practitioner for any damage caused or likely to be caused which has been done in good faith.

MTP Rules 1975: MTP Rules were altered in October 1975 to eliminate time consuming procedure and to make MTP services more readily available. MTP rules include the following criteria:

1. **Approval by Board:** Chief Medical Officer of the district is empowered to certify that a doctor has the necessary training in Obstetrics and Gynaecology, to conduct the abortion. Under these rules, procedure of doctors applying for certification to Board was abolished.
2. **Qualification required to conduct abortion:** The new rules allows for the medical practitioners to qualify through on the spot training, if he has assisted in 25 cases of MTP in an approved institution. The doctor also qualifies if he has done: (i) 6 months housemanship in Obstetrics and Gynaecology. (ii) A postgraduate qualification in Obstetrics and Gynaecology. (iii) 3 years practice in Obstetrics and Gynaecology before 1971 Act. (iv) 1 year practice in Obstetrics and Gynaecology after 1971 Act.
3. **Place where abortion can be conducted:** Under new rules, non-governmental institutions may take up abortions provided they get a license from the Chief Medical Officer of the district, thus eliminating the requirement of private clinics obtaining a Board license.
4. It also provides emergency provisions when any registered medical practitioner can terminate the pregnancy to save the life of mother.

Medical Termination of Pregnancy Rules 2003: The Medical Termination of Pregnancy Rules 1975 stands repealed by Medical Termination of Pregnancy Rules 2003. It lays down the experience and training of the registered medical practitioners required for conduction of M.T.P. (i) Any medical practitioner having experience of 3 years in obstetrics and gynaecology or who has completed 6 months housmanship in obstetrics and gynaecology or worked in a hospital in department of obstetrics and gynaecology for at least one year can perform the MTP. (ii) Any registered medical practitioner who has assisted 25 cases out of which five cases he has performed independently in a hospital approved by the government can perform the MTP. The registered medical practitioner who have assisted in 25 cases can perform only first trimester terminations. (iii) Any medical practitioner having diploma or degree in obstetrics and gynaecology can perform MTP.

MTP Regulations 2003 define the conditions of maintaining records in the centres in which MTP can be done. All the forms filled for the procedure of conduction of the medical termination of pregnancy must be kept confidential and are not to be kept open to inspection. The consent form filled up by the patient together with the certified opinion of the doctor along with the intimation of termination of pregnancy should be kept in a sealed envelop and marked SECRET and then sent to the head of the hospital or the Chief Medical Officer of the state.

Other Aspects of the Act: Failure of contraceptive is quite rare and difficult to prove and sometimes there are circumstances where unmarried girls undergo voluntary intercourse.

THE MEDICAL TERMINATION OF PREGNANCY (AMENDMENT) ACT, 2021

The Act came into force from 25 March 2021. The key amendments are: (i) The Act extended the upper limit for abortions from 20 weeks to 24 weeks for special categories of women which includes survivors of rape (excluding marital rape), victims of incest and other vulnerable women like differently-abled women and minors. (ii) For termination of pregnancy of 20-24 weeks of gestation, the opinion of two registered medical practitioners is required. (iii) The opinion of one registered medical practitioner is needed for the termination of pregnancy upto 20 weeks of gestation (Earlier one RMP required for MTP upto 12 weeks gestation and two RMP required for MTP of 20-24 weeks of gestation). (iv) There is no upper gestation limit (beyond 24 weeks) for MTP in cases of substantial foetal abnormalities diagnosed by a Medical Board. The medical board consists of one gynaecologist, one radiologist or sonologist, one paediatrician, and other members prescribed by the State/UT government which will decide on such pregnancies. (v) ***Confidential clause, u/s Section 5A:*** No registered medical practitioner shall reveal the name and other particulars of a woman whose pregnancy has been terminated under this Act except to a person authorised by any law for the time being in force. Failure to protect the privacy and confidentiality of women shall be punishable with imprisonment which may **extend to one year, or with fine, or with both.** (vi) Under this Act, an unmarried woman can also terminate pregnancies under the failure of contraceptive clause within the gestational limits. As per previous law, a single woman could not cite contraceptive failure as a reason for seeking an abortion.

Criminal Abortion

Criminal abortion is the induced destruction or expulsion of the foetus from the womb of the mother unlawfully that is when there is no therapeutic indication. Criminal abortion is usually undertaken by the: (i) Widows for remarriage. (ii) Unmarried girls owing to rigid social customs and pregnancy resulting from illicit intercourse. (iii) Married woman of educated middle class to avoid addition to the family. Nowadays it is less due to widespread knowledge of contraceptives. (iv) Abortion may be undertaken solely for the purpose of sex determination to avoid female child. It is done in 2nd and 3rd month but rarely during 4th or 5th month. Cases of criminal abortion needs to be investigated when the woman dies or some one informs the police.

Types of Abortionists

The abortionists can be divided into three groups:

(i) Expert or medically qualified professionals (ii) Semiskilled abortionists such as midwives, nurse and chemists (iii) Unskilled abortions such as quacks or untrained dais.

Methods to Induce Criminal Abortion (Figure 28.1)

Mechanical Violence

(1) **General:** These methods may act directly on the uterus or act indirectly by promoting congestion of pelvic organs and causing haemorrhage between uterus and pelvic membranes. These methods are: (i) *Severe pressure over the abdomen* as caused by the blows, kicks, tight lacing and jumping. (ii) *Violent exercise:* Riding, cycling, jumping from height, jolting, driving on rough roads and lifting heavy weights. (iii) *Cupping:* Cupping is placing a lighted wick over the hypogastric area and turning a brass mug over the wick (Figure 28.2). The traction is applied over the mug that results in separation of placenta. The method is usually employed in advanced months of pregnancy. (iv) Application of Leaches to pudenda, perineum and inner surface of thigh. (v) Very hot and cold baths alternatively. (vi) Massaging the uterus through abdominal wall.

(2) **Local:** While correcting the retroverted uterus bimanually, the abortion may result.

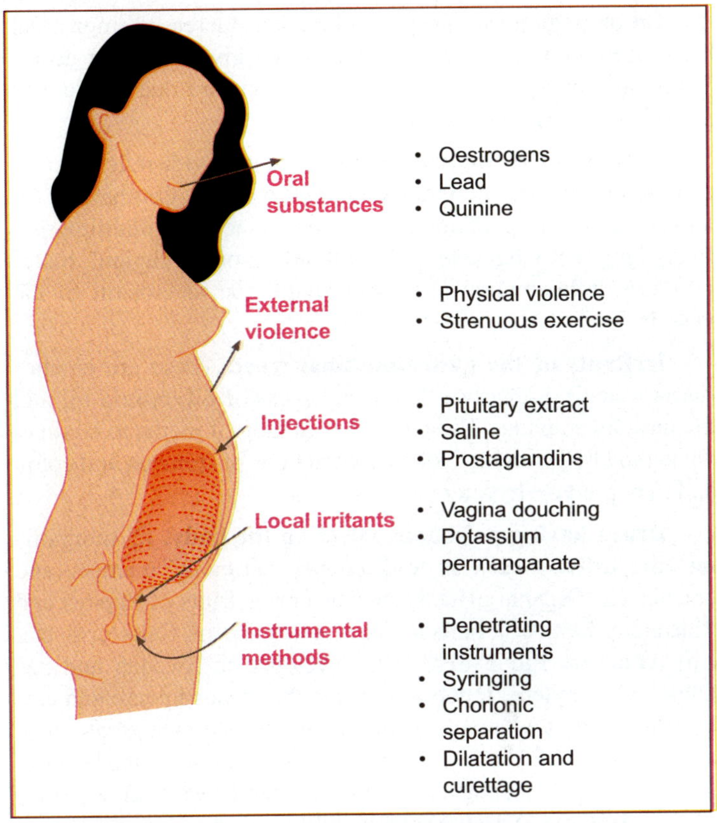

Figure 28.1: Various methods of criminal abortion

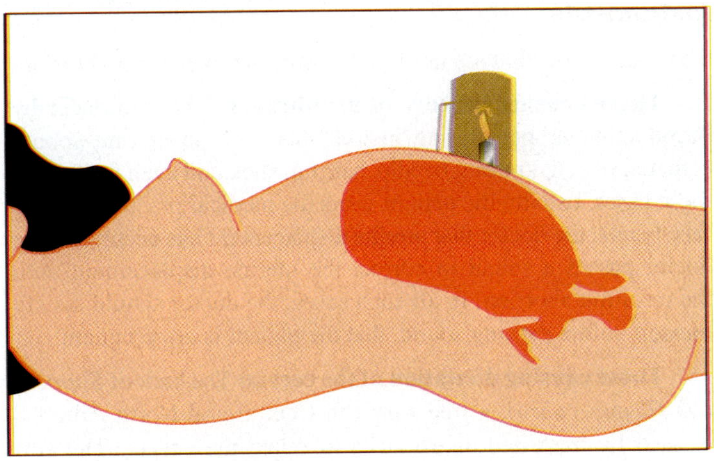

Figure 28.2: Cupping

Abortifacient Drugs

The abortifacient drugs are:

Ecbolics: They act directly on the uterus and increase the uterine contraction that causes abortion. These are Ergot (Ergometrine) that is used quite commonly, Quinine, Cotton root bark, posterior pituitary extract, potassium permanganate tablets (used locally in vagina and cause local ulceration and bleeding), Lead pills (lead oleate causes tonic contraction of uterus), Nitrobenzol and Strychnine.

Emmenogogues: They produce an increased menstrual blood flow and act as abortifacient when given in large doses. These are Savin, Borax, Apiol (toxic effects are due to tricresyl phosphate) and Prostaglandins.

Irritants of genitourinary tract: They provide reflex uterine contraction and are Oil of tansy, Oil of turpentine, Cantharides (in large doses produce inflammation of the kidney and albuminuria), Potassium permanganate (120-300 ml through vaginal route) produces inflammation and hemorrhage due to erosion of the vessels.

Irritants of the gastrointestinal tract: These are emetics (tartaric acid), purgatives (colocynth), castor oil, croton oil and magnesium sulphate. These cause excitation of uterus to contract "in sympathy" with the violent contractions of stomach and colon and may produce hyperemia.

Drugs having poisonous effect on the body: (i) Inorganic metallic irritants such as lead, copper, antimony, mercury and arsenic. (ii) Organic irritants such as unripe fruits of Papaya and Pineapple, bark of Plumago rosea and juice of Calotropis etc. (iii) **Abortion Pill F-6103** was developed in Sweden and has Diphenyl-Ephylene. It concentrates in the corpus luteum and acts by stimulating a woman's natural inclination to menstruate even after presence of fertilized ovum and causes incomplete abortion. The other forms of abortifacient pills are **Dr. Reed's extra strong female pills** and **Widow Welch's pills** etc.

Instruments

The instruments that are used for the purpose of causing abortion:

Those causing rupture of membranes: This can occur by introduction of penetrating instruments such as uterine sound, catheter, pencil, knitting needle, hairpin, stick and even fingers. In these cases, usually the patient visits the medical practitioner and falsely tells the doctor that uterine displacement has occurred. The doctor passes a sound to correct the uterine displacement with the resulting abortion. In all such cases, the doctor should satisfy himself before passing sound, that the patient is not pregnant.

Those causing dilatation of the cervix: The bark of *Slippery elm (Ulmus rubra)*, a tree found in Central and North America is used by unskilled abortionists to dilate the cervix. The soft flat pieces of wood of different size with the usual thickness of about 3 mm is passed into the cervical canal and left in situ. It absorbs moisture and vaginal secretions and swells up that dilates the cervical canal resulting in abortion. Even compressed sponge when left in situ in the cervical canal swells up to cause cervical dilatation and abortion. *Slippery elm* bark on each side bears a jelly like layer as thick as the bark itself. This property makes the bark self lubricating that swells on absorbing the vaginal secretions and causes cervical dilatation. The disadvantages are that the method is unhygienic and there are chances of infection. At times the stick may pass into urethra and gets lodged in bladder as foreign body.

Abortion stick: Abortion stick is a thin wood or bamboo stick, 12 to 18 cm (5-8 in) long and its one end is wrapped with cotton wool or a piece of rag whose greater part is soaked with juice of Marking nut, Calotropis or a paste made of Arsenic oxide, sulphide or red lead etc. Instead of stick, a twig of irritant plant such as calotropis, Nerium odorum or Plumago rosea can be used.

Air insufflation: The air is instilled into vagina by means of syringes or pumps.

Electricity: Negative pole is applied over the cervix and positive pole over sacrum or lumbar vessels and then the current is passed that results in uterine contractions and subsequent abortion.

Paste: The paste containing iodine, thymol or mercury (**utus paste**) is injected from a collapsible tube with uterine applicator into the uterus.

Syringing: Enema syringe with a hard bulb is commonly used to inject fluid into the uterus and the hard nozzle is inserted into cervix. Sometimes **Higginson's syringe** is used. The suction valve is placed in a bowl of fluid and pressure is applied on the bulb. A mixture of air and fluid is forced into uterine cavity at a higher pressure than uterine veins. The fluid detaches parts of amniotic sac and placenta from the uterine walls. The uterus contracts causing haemorrhage and thus abortion. The fluid comprises soap water, water containing inorganic and organic acids, lead, arsenic, lysol, cresol, formalin, $KMnO_4$ etc. The fluid can be administered by the patient or by an abortionist. *Major risks of syringing are:* (i) Due to the injection of cold or hot water death may result from vagal inhibition when injected into cervix. (ii) Air embolism due to stripping of the edge of placenta when air enters in the venous channels.

Complications of Criminal Abortion (Figure 28.3)

(i) *Toxaemic shock and death:* Due to absorption of substances through uterine and vaginal mucosa. (ii) *Sepsis*: Resulting from peritonitis, endometritis and salpingitis. (iii) *Fatal haemorrhage:* Resulting from retained products of conception and perforation of cervix, vaginal vault and fundus of uterus. (iv) *Necrosis of cervix:* Necrosis of cervical region can also result in death. (v) *Delayed air embolism:* The mechanism of delayed air embolism is yet to be explained. Air is held in the same fashion in the uterus till placental separation opens the vessels to allow it to pass into circulation. The mucus plug would possibly prevent escape of air via cervix. The lethal dose to cause air embolism and death is minimum 100 ml whereas in animal experiments it is 10-480 ml.

Medicolegal Aspects

Fabricated abortion: To have a false charge of abortion the females sometimes present animal foetus. In such cases, precipitin test is confirmatory as it is a species-specific test. In cases presenting with symptoms and signs of extrauterine pregnancy it may give rise to the suspicion of criminal interference.

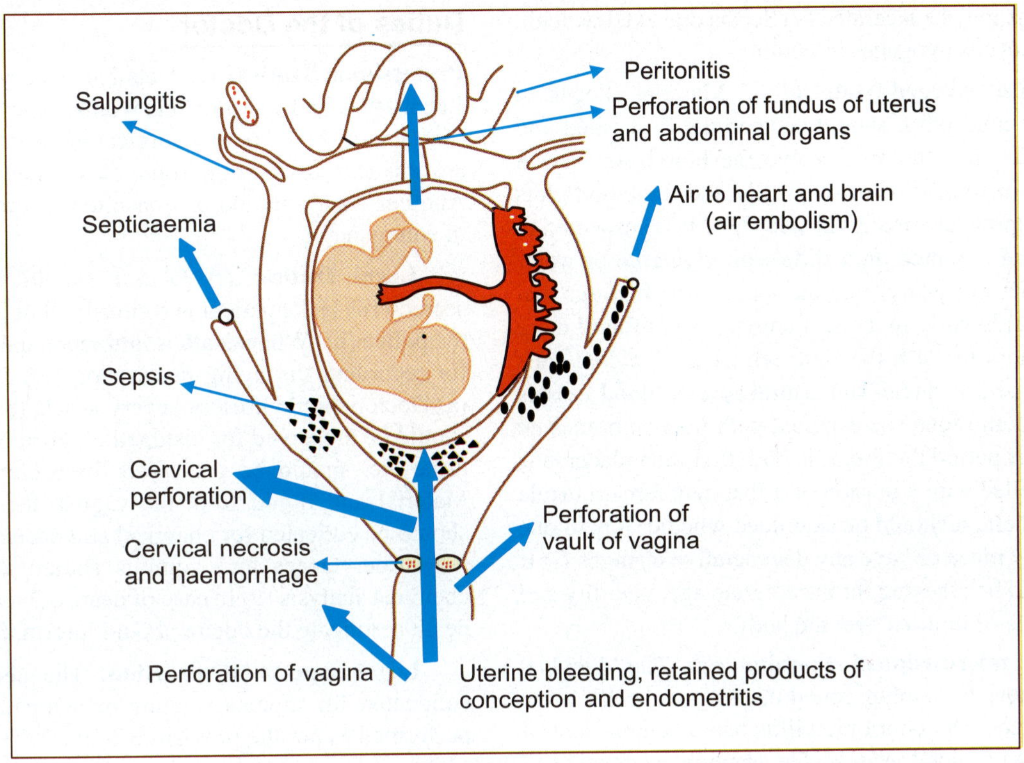

Figure 28.3: Various complications of procuring criminal abortion

Trauma and abortion: To establish causal relationship between trauma and abortion, following factors should be considered: (i) Traumatic event was followed within 24 hours by a process that ultimately lead to abortion. (ii) Foetus and placenta should be normal. (iii) Appearance of foetus and placenta should be compatible with the state of gestation when the traumatic event occurred. (iv) Factors known to cause abortion should be absent.

Rupture of membranes or separation of placenta may occur in some cases directly due to trauma. Following criteria suggests a causal relationship between trauma and abortion: (i) Normal progress of pregnancy (ii) There is absence of predisposing factors (iii) Signs and symptoms start within 48 hours of placental detachment (iv) There is adherent clot or depression of the placental surface.

Medicolegal questions that should be answered: (i) Was the deceased pregnant recently? (ii) Was there any evidence of abortion? (iii) Was there any evidence of criminal abortion? (iv) Was the cause of death related to abortion?

Causes of Death in Criminal Abortion

Immediate causes: (i) Shock *and haemorrhage:* Due to injury as a result of criminal interference uterine perforation and death results from haemorrhage. (ii) *Air embolism:* Entry of about 100 ml of air into the veins of uterus causes air embolism. When a soapy solution that is mixed with air is injected with pressure, the patient collapses within 10 minutes. (iii) *Reflex vagal inhibition:* Vagal reflex starts by touching the cervix, lower uterine segment by an instrument or irritant fluid and during anaesthesia prior to abortion. (iv) Fat embolism may result due to injection of soapy water and corrosives such as Lysol.

Delayed causes: (i) *Septicemia and pyaemia:* Sepsis may result from the dirty surroundings, dirty instruments and injury to uterus while performing abortion. The organisms commonly involved are Clostridium welchii and Clostridium tetani (ii) General peritonitis (iii) Toxaemia (iv) Tetanus.

Remote causes: (i) Jaundice and renal suppression (ii) Bacterial endocarditis (iii) Pulmonary embolism (iv) Pneumonia (v) Empyema and Meningitis (vi) Poisonous effects of the drug itself.

Diagnosis of Abortion in the Living

The cases of abortion come to the doctor for examination when: (i) Woman alleges abortion after a blow or quarrel in order to inflict penalty on assailant. (ii) Woman is charged with abortion but wishes to conceal it. The signs of recent abortion are essentially the signs of recent delivery. The findings depend upon the length of gestation and the time elapsed between abortion and examination. The signs of recent abortion are:

At 2-3 months: (i) Haemorrhage (ii) Slight softening of external os and maternal passage (iii) Slight enlargement of uterus (iv) Breast changes.

At 4-5 months: (i) Increased haemorrhage (ii) Internal os admits one finger (iii) Os is not injured if abortion is of less than

6 weeks (iv) Vagina may be lacerated (v) Sepsis due to Cl welchii, *E. coli* or Streptococcus pyogenes infection.

Examination of Alleged Material: (i) Material alleged to be the product of conception should be thoroughly washed and kept for sometimes in water to dissolve the blood clot. (ii) A portion should be examined microscopically and the blood clots submitted for grouping and precipitin test. (iii) Mass suspected to be foetus is cut and mounted on a slide with glycerine or water and then seen under low power microscope and the findings that will be seen are: (a) In early months, if embryo is not found there is formation of chorionic villi (b) Upto 9th week, decidual cells show cells with eccentric nuclei and central core of blood vessels (c) At 1st to 3rd month foetus is expelled with its membranes *en masse* (d) After this period the foetus is born first then placenta is detached and expelled with a portion of it that may remain inside (e) If placenta is there, it should be examined whether it is in one piece or torn at any place or have any degenerative changes (f) If it is foetus it should be assessed for intrauterine age, viability and presence or absence of injuries over the body.

Findings on microscopical examination: The decidual cells appear as fine, pale staining, round or polygonal cells, often with eccentric nuclei. The chorionic villus has a central core of connective tissue with blood vessels. The trophoblast consists of inner layer of cells of Langhans and the outer syncytial layer that is richly nucleated protoplasm without cell boundaries.

Postmortem Evidence of Criminal Abortion

The evidence of abortion should be obtained from:

(i) Medical history (ii) Clinical or autopsy examination (iii) Examination of aborted material (iv) In cases of sudden death of a woman of childbearing age when the: (a) Deceased is pregnant and deeply cyanosed (b) Instruments or drugs found at the scene of death (c) Underclothing is apparently disturbed (d) Fluid, soapy water or blood stained discharge coming out of vagina should always arouse suspicion of criminal abortion (v) To convict the abortionist it is important to ascertain that the: (a) Dead woman was pregnant (b) Accused was responsible for the act that resulted in the interruption of pregnancy (c) Accused acted in for the purpose of producing an illegal abortion (d) Death occurred as a result of abortion.

The autopsy findings depend upon the mode of abortion and time elapsed between death and examination. The pathologist should exclude causes of spontaneous abortion while conducting autopsy.

Special methods of dissection while performing autopsy: An incision is made just outside the labia majora that is carried backwards to include anus and forwards upto symphysis pubis that is then divided. Parietal peritoneum is cut around the brim of pelvis and by careful dissection the whole of pelvic viscera including uterus, vagina, anus, rectum, and bladder is removed and examined carefully in detail for the presence of any injuries.

Duties of the Doctor

Professional Duties: (i) Detailed history should be taken (ii) Record the condition and treat woman with best available facilities (iii) Doctor should not try surgical methods on the patient as there are chances of levying some false charge against the doctor. Another doctor should be consulted if some treatment is needed in emergency.

Legal Duties: (i) Doctor should maintain professional secrecy (ii) If the patient is seriously ill, it is mandatory to inform the police (iii) When death is imminent, the doctor should arrange for recording the dying declaration (iv) For chemical analysis: (a) Doctor should preserve every article (b) Uterus with contents should be preserved for histopathological examination (c) Blood, urine etc. should be preserved for bacteriological analysis (d) Material and liquid from the vagina, uterine cavity and blood should be collected for chemical and bacteriological examination (e) Urine, faeces and vomitus should also be preserved for chemical analysis (v) In case of death of woman instead of issuing death certificate the doctor should inform the police.

Legal aspects of abortion: The abortion should not be conducted for monetary gains or sympathy. It should only be performed as per the provisions of the MTP Act.

Provisions in Indian Law

Sections 312, 313, 314, 315 and 316 I.P.C. refers to the offences of criminal miscarriage and punishments awarded for these offences.

S. 312 I.P.C. Causing miscarriage: Whoever voluntarily causes a woman with child to miscarry, shall, if such miscarriage be not caused in good faith for the purpose of saving the life of the woman, be punished with imprisonment of either description for a term which may extend to three years, or with fine, or with both; and if the woman be quick with the child, shall be punished with imprisonment of either description for a term which may extend to seven years and shall also be liable to fine.

Explanation: The woman should be pregnant and miscarriage should be caused with her consent. Both are liable to punishment unless done in good faith to save the life of mother. The punishment is extended to seven years if the woman is quick with the child, i.e., above 16th week.

If the means used for causing miscarriage are not successful, is liable to be punished under S. 511 I.P.C. that is half of the punishment under section 312 will be awarded.

S. 313 I.P.C. Causing miscarriage without woman's consent: Whoever commits the offence defined in the last preceding section without the consent of the woman, whether the woman is quick with child is not, shall be punished with imprisonment for life or with imprisonment of either description for a term which may extend to ten years and shall also be liable to fine.

S. 314 I.P.C. Death caused by act done with the intend to cause miscarriage: Whoever, with the intent to cause miscarriage of a woman with the child, does any act which causes the death of such woman, shall be punished with imprisonment of either description for a term that may extend to ten years and shall also be liable to fine. If the act is done without the consent of the woman, shall be punished either with imprisonment for life or ten years.

Explanation: It is not essential to this offence that the offender should know that the act is likely to cause death.

S. 315 I.P.C.: Act done with intend to prevent child from being born alive or to cause it to die after birth: Whoever before the birth of any child does any act with the intention of thereby preventing that child from being born alive or causing it to die after birth, and does by such act prevent that child from being born alive, or causes it to die after its birth, shall, if such act be not caused in good faith for the purpose of saving the life of the mother, be punished with imprisonment of either description for a term which may extend to ten years, or with fine, or with both.

S. 316 I.P.C.: Causing death of the quick unborn child by act amounting to culpable homicide: Whoever does any act under such circumstance, that if he thereby caused death would be guilty of culpable homicide, and does by such act cause death of a quick unborn child, shall be punished with imprisonment of either description for a term, which may extend to ten years and shall also be liable to fine.

In cases of offences against children in uterus, where pregnancy has advanced beyond stage of quickening and where death is caused after the quickening and before the birth of the child, the person would be guilty of culpable homicide if he caused the death of the woman by an act which he knows is likely to cause her death and if his act causes the death of unborn child and injured the woman will be held guilty under section 316 I.P.C.

THE PRE-CONCEPTION AND PRENATAL DIAGNOSTIC TECHNIQUES (PROHIBITION OF SEX SELECTION) ACT

The Prenatal Diagnostic Techniques (Regulation and Prevention of Misuse) Act, 1994 was enacted by the Indian Parliament to provide for the regulation of the use of prenatal diagnostic techniques for the purpose of detecting generic or metabolic disorders or chromosomal abnormalities or certain congenital malformations or sex linked disorders and for the prevention of the misuse of such techniques for the purpose of prenatal sex determination leading to female feticide and for matters connected therewith or incidental thereto key milestones related to PNDT Act.

- Maharashtra was first State to enact Maharashtra regulation of use of PNDT Act in 1987.
- PNDT Act was passed in 1994.
- Hon. Supreme Court passed an Interim judgment in 2001 for more stricter implementation of Act based on PIL filed by CEHAT, MASUM and Adv Sabu George.
- PNDT Act amended in 2003 to Pre-conception and Prenatal Diagnostic Technique Act (PC-PNDT).
- Applicable to all Govt/NGO/Private/Corporate establishments.

Salient Features of the PC-PNDT Act

- The Act prohibits sex selection, before or after conception (Section 6).
- Use of Prenatal diagnostic techniques are allowed only on medical grounds for detecting abnormalities and anomalies such as: (i) Chromosomal abnormalities (ii) Genetic metabolic diseases (iii) Haemoglobinopathies (iv) Sex-lined genetic diseases (v) Congenital anomalies (vi) Any other abnormalities or diseases as may be specified by the Central Supervisory Board (Section 4(2)).
- The prenatal diagnostic techniques shall be conducted only by the qualified person if he/she is satisfied that any of the following conditions are fulfilled, namely: (i) Age of the pregnant woman is above 35 years. (ii) Pregnant woman has undergone two or more spontaneous abortions or foetal loss. (iii) Pregnant woman had been exposed to potentially teratogenic agents such as drugs, radiation, infection or chemicals. (iv) Pregnant woman has a family history of mental retardation or physical deformities such as spasticity or any other genetic disease. (v) Any other condition as may be specified by the Central Supervisory Board (Section 4(3)).
- No person conducting prenatal diagnostic procedures shall communicate to the pregnant woman concerned or her relatives the sex of the foetus by words, signs or in any other manner (Section 5).
- All clinics conducting ultrasound must be registered and certificate displayed. No. of machines, qualification of person conducting sonography and period of registration (Section19(4)).
- All clinics should display prominently disclosure of sex of the fetus is prohibited under the law in English as well as local language (Rule 17 (1)).
- All clinics should have available copy of Act (Rule 17 (2)).
- Doctors or clinics advertising sex determination test in any form are liable for punishment (Section 22).
- Every offence under this Act is cognizable, non-bailable and non-compoundable (Section 27).
- Implementing Authority under the Act is Appropriate Authority (Section 17).
- Under Act Appropriate Authority has power to search, seize and seal clinics (Section 30).
- Act has made it mandatory to maintain all records for a period 2 years or for a such period as may be prescribed (Section 29 and Rule 9) Section 5 and Rule 10 (1A).

Punishment Under the Act

- This Act provides for the punishment for contravention of any of the provision of the Act or rules by any medical geneticist, gynaecologist, registered medical practitioner or any person who owns or is employed at a Genetic Counselling Centre, a Genetic Laboratory or a Genetic Clinic with imprisonment for a term which may extend to 3 years and with fine which may extend to Rs. 10,000. For subsequent conviction the imprisonment will extend to 5 years with fine upto Rs. 50,000 (Section 23(1)).
- Name of the registered medical practitioner who has been convicted by the Court shall be removed from the register of the respective State Medical Council for a period of 5 years for the first offence and permanently for the subsequent offence (Section 23(2)).
- Any person who seeks the aid of a Genetic Counselling Centre, Genetic Laboratory or Genetic Clinic or of a medical geneticist, gynaecologist or registered medical practitioner for conducting prenatal diagnostic techniques on any pregnant woman (including such woman unless she was compelled to undergo such diagnostic techniques) for purposes other than those specified above, shall, be punishable with imprisonment for a term which may extend to three years and with fine which may extend to Rs. 10,000 and for subsequent conviction may extend to imprisonment upto 5 years and fine upto Rs. 50,000 (Section 23(3)).
- Woman who is compelled to undergo such diagnostic techniques or such selection is exempted from punishment–Presumption in case of conduct of prenatal diagnostic techniques (Section 24).

Methods of Contraception in the National Family Welfare Programme

The methods available currently in India may be broadly divided into two categories, spacing methods and permanent methods. The spacing methods include Oral Contraceptive Pills (OCPs), Condoms, Intrauterine Contraceptive Devices (IUCD) etc. The **permanent methods (Surgical methods)** are generally considered irreversible methods. For female tubectomy is used, where as in female vasectomy is used.

Tubectomy: In this method, the fallopian tubes are slightly cut and tied or artificial clips are placed so that the egg is unable to travel to the uterus for fertilization. Two techniques are used: (i) *Mini-laparotomy (Mini-lap)*: Under general or regional (mostly epidural) anaesthesia, a small incision is made in the abdomen and the fallopian tubes are cut or blocked. (ii) *Laparoscopic*: It is a sophisticated surgical procedure in which a long thin tube with a lens in it (fiber-optic device) is inserted through the abdominal wall through a keyhole incision. Then through this laparoscope, the doctor block or cut the fallopian tubes. It is a minimally invasive procedure which can be done by trained and certified MBBS doctor or specialist. It can often be performed on an outpatient basis.

Vasectomy: It is a simple, safe and effective method of contraception. It is usually performed under local anaesthesia. Two techniques are used in India: (i) *Conventional Vasectomy*: Small incisions are given on both sides of the scrotum and a section of tubes (vas deferens) are removed by cutting. The tubes are then sealed, tied, or cauterized using an electric current, and the cuts are closed with stitches. (ii) *Non-Scalpel Vasectomy*: In this technique, no incision is given and only performed by puncturing, hence, no stitches are required.

The procedure is performed by trained MBBS doctors. However, the couple needs to use an alternative method of contraception for first three months after sterilization till no sperms are detected in semen.

National Family Health Survey in India

The National Family Health Survey (NFHS) is a large-scale, multi-round survey conducted in a representative sample of households throughout India. The objectives of this survey are: (i) To provide essential data on health and family welfare needed by the Ministry of Health and Family Welfare (MOH and FW), Government of India and other agencies for policy and programme purposes; and (ii) To provide information on important emerging health and family welfare issues.

The survey provides state and national information for India on fertility, infant and child mortality, the practice of family planning, maternal and child health, reproductive health, nutrition, anaemia, utilization and quality of health and family planning services. Five rounds of NFHS (1992-93, 1998-99, 2005-06, 2015-16, 2019-2020 have been conducted by the International Institute for Population Sciences (IIPS), Mumbai, as the national nodal agency. The latest report (2019-2020) of the survey **(NHFS-5)** is available in the website of MOH and FW, Government of India.

Major Results of National Family Health Survey–5 (NHFS-5)

1. **Population:** (i) Use of family planning methods increased in most states/UTs. Contraceptive prevalence rate is highest in Himachal Pradesh and West Bengal. (ii) Total fertility rate (TFR) reduced in most states. The replacement level fertility (2.1) has been achieved in 19 out of 22 states except Manipur, Meghalaya and Bihar. (ii) Sex ratio at birth has remain unchanged in most states, however, it has declined in few states, the ratio is below 900 (Goa, Himachal Pradesh, Telangana, DNH and Delhi).
2. **Health and Nutrition:** (i) Proportion of institutional births across states increased. In Kerala, nearly 100% of the births were institutional births. Only 46% of the births in Nagaland were institutional births. (ii) There is increase in percentage of women receiving the recommended four or more ANC visits by health providers. (iii) Out of pocket expenditure on deliveries increased in 8 of the 17 states. (iv) Infant Mortality Rate (IMR) has declined across states. Assam has seen one of the largest drops in IMR, from 48 deaths (per 1,000 live

births) to 32 deaths. IMR remains high in Bihar (47 deaths per 1,000 live births). (v) Malnourishment among children (<5 years) is increasing in several states. The proportion of children who are underweight (low weight with respect to age) has increased in 11 of the 17 states. In Bihar and Gujarat, 40% or more of the children under the age of five years are underweight. (vi) Obesity is rising for both men and women across all states. (vii) Men are more likely to have slightly higher blood glucose levels in the range of high or very high compared to women. (viii) Prevalence of hypertension among men is somewhat higher than in women.

3. **Access to infrastructure:** (i) Access to electricity, improved source of drinking water and sanitation facility has increased across states. (ii) More women using mobile phones across all states; however, many of them do not have access to internet. (iii) More women using bank accounts; ownership of house/ land amongst women declines in several states.
4. **Gender related indicators:** (i) Use of hygienic methods of protection during menstrual period has increased across states (ii) Gender based violence still remains high, has increased in some states.

LONG QUESTIONS

1. What is abortion? Discuss various methods of medical termination of pregnancy.
2. Discuss the various methods used for criminal abortion and what are the findings in such cases?

SHORT QUESTIONS

1. Abortion Stick.
2. Cupping.
3. MTP Act 1971.
4. MTP Rules 2003.
5. PC-PNDT Act.
6. The Medical Termination of Pregnancy (Amendment) Act, 2021.

MULTIPLE CHOICE QUESTIONS

1. MTP Act was passed in the year:

(a) 1952 (b) 1961
(c) 1971 (d) 1981

2. Legally abortion means, pre-mature expulsion of the foetus from uterus:

(a) At any time before full term (b) Before 20th week
(c) Before 28th week (d) Before 210 days

3. Slippery elm bark (Ulmus rubra) is commonly used for:

(a) Causing fabricated injuries
(b) Aphrodisiac purposes
(c) Criminal abortion
(d) Treatment of arsenic poisoning

4. The minimum age of the women for MTP is:

(a) 16 years (b) 18 years
(c) 20 years (d) No age limits

5. All of the following methods are used for criminal abortion in India *except*:

(a) Cupping (b) Syringing
(c) Amniotic fluid replacement (d) Utus paste

6. Causing miscarriage without consent of woman is punishable under section:

(a) 31 IPC (b) 313 IPC
(c) 314 IPC (d) 315 IPC

7. As per recent amendment in MTP Act, how many doctors' opinion is required for termination of pregnancy upto 20 weeks of gestation?

(a) One (b) Two
(c) Three (d) Four

8. Causing death of the quick unborn child by act amounting to culpable homicide is punishable under section:

(a) 313 IPC (b) 314 IPC
(c) 315 IPC (d) 316 IPC

9. As per The MTP (Amendment) Act, 2021, the upper gestation limit for termination of pregnancy in cases of substantial foetal abnormalities diagnosed by a Medical Board is:

(a) 20 weeks (b) 24 weeks
(c) 28 weeks (d) No gestation limits

10. All are true statement for PC-PNDT Act, *except*:

(a) Prenatal diagnostic techniques are not allowed for sex determination
(b) All clinics conducting ultrasound must be registered and certificate displayed
(c) Doctors or clinics advertising sex determination test in any form are liable for punishment
(d) The pregnant woman is always liable for the punishment

ANSWER KEY

1. (c)	2. (a)	3. (c)	4. (d)	5. (c)	6. (b)	7. (a)	8. (d)	9. (d)	10. (d)

29 CHAPTER

Assisted Reproduction Techniques and Cloning

ASSISTED REPRODUCTIVE TECHNOLOGY (ART)

ART includes all techniques that attempt to obtain a pregnancy by handling the sperm or the oocyte outside the human body and transferring the gamete or the embryo into the reproductive system of a woman. There are many techniques used for ART like in vitro fertilization (IVF), and intracytoplasmic sperm injection (ICSI), embryo transfer techniques, ovarian stimulation, egg retrieval etc. IVF technique is the most common and effective type of ART. As per World Health Organisation (WHO), ART does not include assisted insemination (artificial insemination) using sperm from either a woman's partner or a sperm donor.

ARTIFICIAL INSEMINATION

Artificial insemination is a process when the sperms are deposited in the female genital tract artificially when the female cannot conceive through the sexual intercourse with her husband. The sperms may be introduced in the cervical canal **(intracervical)** or inside the uterus **(intrauterine).** There is higher success rate in intrauterine insemination (IUI), hence it is the most commonly used method. Less common techniques are **intrafallopian and intraperitoneal insemination** when the sperms are placed near the mouth of the fallopian tube and ovaries respectively. Rarely, a technique called **intravaginal insemination** is used, in which sperms are placed in the female partner's vagina.

History: Artificial insemination is commonly thought of as a modern technology but it has a long history. Thus, apparently artificial insemination was first attempted **on Juana, wife of King Henry IV of Castile** (1425-1474). The first artificial insemination in a dog was reported by the Italian scientist **Lazzaro Spallanzani** (1729-1799). The application of artificial insemination was first documented by John Hunter in the 1770s at London. Efforts to develop practical methods for artificial insemination were started in Russia in 1899. Papers on artificial insemination in horses had been published by 1922. By the mid 1940's artificial insemination had become an established industry. In 1949 improved methods of freezing and thawing sperm were developed. The idea for adding antibiotics to the sperm solution came in 1950 from Cornell. Improved methods of sperm collection were developed in the 1970's and 1980's. Research to improve methods of artificial insemination continues till today.

Indications for Artificial Insemination

Indications related to males: (i) Incurable defects in the husband's semen rendering him incapable of procreation. (ii) Premature or retrograde ejaculation. (iii) Hereditary disease in the husband as to contraindicate paternity. (iv) Rhesus incompatibility resulting in failure of children to survive because of erythroblastosis foetalis and husband being homozygous rhesus positive. (v) When the husband is impotent making sexual intercourse impossible. (vi) Abnormalities of penis such as epispadias or hypospadias etc. (vii) When the husband is being treated for cancer with radiotherapy or chemotherapy.

Indications related to females: (i) Cervical mucus may not be enough to allow sperm to move easily, or it may be too thick and sticky. Sometimes, cervical mucus is not compatible with the sperms. (ii) Women with mild uterine endometriosis thus preventing the passage of ovum. (iii) Anatomical defects of the uterus or cervix that prevents sperm from reaching the ovum.

Types of Artificial Insemination

Artificial Insemination Homologous (A.I.H.): In this type the semen of woman's husband is used. This is usually employed when the husband is oligospermic.

Artificial Insemination Donor (A.I.D.): The semen from some unrelated donor is used. This is usually undertaken when the husband is impotent, azoospermic, sterile or suffering from some genetic or hereditary abnormality.

Pooled Donor—Artificial Insemination Heterologous Donor (A.I.H.D.): In this to the husband's semen the semen of the donor is mixed.

Prerequisites for Artificial Insemination

(i) Consent of both the husband and wife as well as donor's wife should be taken. (ii) Identity of the donor should not be revealed and the donor should not know the recipient parents' identity and the results of the technique. (iii) Donor should be between **21 and 55 years** [As per ART (Regulation) Act, 2021], unrelated to the couple and should have his own children. (iv) Donor should be of sound physical, mental and emotional health as well as devoid of any hereditary or genetic disease. (v) Race and physical characteristics of donor should resemble as closely as possible to that of the husband. (vi) Procedure should be properly explained to the donor and his wife. (vii) Husband of the woman should be sterile or suffering from some genetic or hereditary disorder. (viii) Pooled semen should be preferably used as in that case there is a technical possibility of the husband being the father of the child. (ix) As per ART (Regulation) Act, 2021, **semen from two individuals should not be mixed** for the procedures. (x) Physician should select the donor after carrying out the semen analysis, chromosomal studies, testing for HIV status and other sexually transmitted diseases. (xi) Physician should maintain relevant records of the donor avoiding the possibility of single fecund donor and consanguineous marriages in future. (xii) While carrying out the procedure presence of a disinterested witness preferably a nurse is must.

Procedure for Artificial Insemination

Artificial insemination is carried out close to ovulation as the time of maximum fertility coincides with it. About one ml of semen is injected into the top of vagina, cervix or uterus through a small plastic tube. The procedures for the two most common forms of artificial insemination are:

Intracervical insemination: The male partner produces a semen sample by means of masturbation. The patient is advised to avoid coitus three days before the sample is taken to obtain good quality sperms. The sample can be collected at the hospital, or should be delivered from home within one to two hours. The semen is injected into the top of the vagina of the female. A plastic cap, to be taken out about 6 hours later, can sometimes be placed in the vagina to keep the sperm near the cervix. Intracervical insemination is used for couples in whom sperms cannot reach the cervix.

Intrauterine insemination (IUI): Intrauterine insemination has a higher success rate than other artificial insemination techniques, because in these sperms are placed near the fallopian tubes. It may also be combined with hormone treatment to encourage ovulation. Sperm from the male partner or donor is inserted into the uterus using a thin plastic tube that is passed through the cervix. The treatment can be repeated for a further three menstrual cycles, although these should not necessarily be consecutive for conception to occur.

Intrauterine insemination is often used when the cervical mucus is incompatible to sperms and many other unexplained infertility problems. Sperm washing prior to intrauterine infiltration removes most of the bacteria from the semen, but it is impossible to completely sterilize the sperm or the cervix. The sperm cells are washed to separate them from the plasma to avoid emergence of uterine infection and endometriosis (in less than 1% of the cases). The sperms are then incubated before being carefully placed in the uterus.

Success Rates with Artificial Insemination

Artificial insemination is successful in only 5%- 30% of cases. The success rate is increased when fertility drugs are used before carrying out artificial insemination. Semen analysis is to be carried out to know whether the sperms are suitable for the technique. Total sperm count, their morphology, motility, survival period and presence of anti-sperm antibodies should be assessed. Success rate increases to 70-75% pregnancies within 3-4 months of starting the treatment. For 90% of couples, if treatment is successful, it occurs within the first six cycles of treatment.

Successful treatment depends upon the following factors: (i) Cause of infertility (ii) Morphology and sperm count (iii) Conception is more likely to occur when the female has received hormonal treatment for ovulation (iv) Condition of the fallopian tube, ovaries, uterus and the regularity of menstrual cycle (v) Age of the woman as the fertility decreases after the age of 30 years.

Medicolegal and Ethical Issues Related to Artificial Insemination

There is no statutory law for artificial insemination in India. However, the present practice in India is as per the "National Guidelines for Accreditation and Regulation of ART Clinics in India" issued by ICMR, India. In Delhi, the practice is followed by the "The Delhi Artificial Insemination (Human) Act 1995".

The legal aspects in relation to A.I.H. applicable to India: (i) Artificial insemination with the semen of the husband (A.I.H.) is justifiable and unobjectionable since the child is actually the biological product of both husband and wife but does not constitute evidence of proper consummation of marriage. Hence nullity of marriage may still be granted to the wife on the ground of impotency of the husband or his wilful refusal to consummate the marriage. However, such a decree could be excluded on the grounds of approbation. (ii) Posthumous AIH through a sperm bank–Child born to a woman artificially inseminated with the stored sperms of her deceased husband must be considered to be a legitimate child notwithstanding the existing law of presumptions under our Evidence Act.

In case of A.I.D., there have been debates over the rights of sperm donors. When considering the ethics of sperm donation, several factors must be considered: (i) Rights of the sperm donor (ii) Rights of the clients (who are purchasing the sperm) (iii) Criteria by which sperm are collected (i.e., choosing a donor who has certain traits) (iv) Amount of sperm that a single man can donate.

These rights were developed through the principles of medical ethics and informed consent and are not mandated technically by law. However, sperm banks are approved by the authority as per the Assisted Reproductive Technology (Regulation) Act, 2021. If certain criteria are not met, the banks are not accredited. Sperm donor and client rights are usually established via an informed consent form that is signed by the client and verified by the client's doctor. This form ensures that the client understands his/her rights and the rights of the sperm donor.

Ethics of choosing sperm: Sperm banks differ in their selection of sperm donors. All are highly selective, but some are more selective than others. The disparity between ultra-selective sperm banks and ones that cater to a more "normal" population raise ethical questions. As of yet, these ethical issues have not been resolved.

How much sperm can be donated? If a donor desires too many kids, the risk of producing children who will eventually copulate increases. Although it sounds unbelievable, half brothers and sisters (from the same donor father) have actually married not knowing they were related. As per ART (Regulation) Act, 2021, semen bank shall **not supply the sperm of a single donor to more than one commissioning couple**. This limit prevents the problem mentioned above and is adhered to by all sperm banks.

The legal aspects in relation to A.I.D. as applicable to India are: (i) *Adultery:* The donor and recipient cannot be held guilty of adultery in India as section 497 I.P.C. requires sexual intercourse necessary for adultery. (ii) *Legitimacy:* The husband is not the actual father of the child thus; the child is illegitimate and cannot inherit property. (iii) *Nullity of marriage and divorce:* Mere artificial insemination is not a ground for nullity of marriage and divorce but if A.I. is due to impotence of the husband then it is a ground. If the procedure of artificial insemination has been carried without the husband's consent, he can sue his wife for divorce and doctor for damages. (iv) *Natural birth:* The child will remain the product of natural birth if the parents do not disclose the actual fact. The status of the child born by artificial means shall be presumed to be legitimate child of the couple, having been born through in wedlock and with consent of the both spouses. Sperm donor shall have no parenteral right. (v) *Unmarried woman/widow:* There is no legal bar on an unmarried woman/widow going for AID. The status of such a child born by artificial insemination would be legitimate. (vi) *Incest:* Risk of incest exists between children born by artificial insemination and child of donor but the offence is not punishable in India.

The Delhi Artificial Insemination (Human) Act 1995: This Act is applicable in the National Capital Territory of Delhi. The objectives of this Act are: (i) To allow issueless couple to have a child through artificial insemination and give it a legal status (ii) To control the spread of HIV 1 and 2 through artificial insemination (iii) To regulate donation, sale or supply of human semen/ovum for artificial insemination (iv) To make it obligatory on the part of the medical practitioner to: (a) Seek the written consent of the husband and the wife, seeking artificial insemination (A.I.). (b) Seek the written consent of the donor and the recipient and their spouse, in case of requests of semen/ovum from specified donor/recipient. (c) Test the recipient for HIV 1 and 2 and other sexually transmitted diseases before performing A.I. (d) Not to segregate the XX/XY chromosomes for A.I. (e) Not to disclose the identity of the donor or recipient to avoid disputes relating to succession as far as possible that are likely to arise due to artificial insemination. (f) Doctor should keep complete record of the biodata including marks of identification of the donor and the recipient of the semen and ovum. (v) To prohibit carrying on semen bank without registration and yearly renewal that is punishable with fine up to 5,000 rupees and in case of second or subsequent offence, imprisonment for a term up to 3 months or with fine up to 5,000 rupees. (vi) The semen bank before accepting the semen for artificial insemination shall test the donor for the presence of HIV 1 and 2, antibodies by highly sensitive ELISA kit and screen for Hepatitis B surface antigen and if found negative, only then, the donor shall be allowed to donate. (vii) Donated semen shall be stored either by cryo-preservation of liquid nitrogen freezing or any other safe method for a minimum period of three months in order to exclude window period of HIV 1 and 2 infections in the donor. Second ELISA test is performed on the donor after three months, and if negative, the semen shall be used. The doctor should seek the written consent of the recipient for using the semen on the basis of only one ELISA test, being negative, where facilities for cryo-preservation and liquid nitrogen for semen are not available.

Semen Banking

Semen banking is the preservation of human semen by adding glycerol and after slow cooling and rapid freezing it is stored below a temperature of -79°C. When the semen used is that of the husband after his death (Posthumous artificial Insemination) due to availability of semen banking, it may give rise to problems in connection with the inheritance rights of such a child born, which did not start its life when the genetic father was alive.

Amendment to Human Fertilization and Embryology Act (HFEA) has allowed posthumous artificial insemination using the semen of the deceased husband.

Egg Donation: It is a process in which a fertile woman donates an egg, or oocyte, to another woman to help her conceive. It is a part of implantation procedure such as IVF. The donor should be healthy and in the age group of **23-35 years. An oocyte donor shall donate oocytes only once in her life time and not more than 7 oocytes shall be retrieved from oocyte donor** [As per ART(Regulation) Act, 2021]. Oocytes are obtained mostly by surgical intervention. It is fertilized in a laboratory with husband's semen and the resultant embryo then transferred to the infertile female partner.

Controlled Ovarian Stimulation: It is used for (i) To retrieve multiple oocytes during a single IVF cycle for IVF treatments. (ii) To store oocytes (eggs) for future use. (iii) To induce ovulation in patients with ovulatory dysfunction to help them conceive. Many stimulations have been introduced for controlled ovarian hyperstimulation of patients undergoing in vitro fertilization treatment. However, commonly used protocols for ovarian stimulation are either Follicle-stimulating hormone (FSH) in combination with Gonadotropin releasing hormone (GnRH) agonist (GnRH agonist protocol) or GnRH antagonist (GnRH antagonist protocol). Human chorionic gonadotropin (hCG) is used for final maturation of the eggs and for the induction of ovulation.

Ovarian Hyperstimulation Syndrome (OHSS): It is an iatrogenic complication, which results from uncontrolled ovarian stimulation induced by exogenous methods. As per World Health Organization (WHO), the incidence of OHSS is 0.2-1% of all stimulation cycles in ART. The exact pathophysiology of OHSS is remained unexplained. The syndrome is characterized by an acute shift of protein-rich fluid from the vascular compartment into the third space leading to haemoconcentration, decreased renal perfusion, oliguria, thromboembolism, eventually renal shutdown, and death in the most extreme cases. The primary risk factors associated with the development of OHSS are young age, low body mass index, polycystic ovarian diseases (PCOD), and previous episodes of OHSS and the secondary risk factors are serum E2 level >3000-4000 pg/ml in IVF cycles and >1500-2000 pg/ml in COS cycles, follicle number >20-25 in both ovaries, large number of oocytes retrieval, stimulation procedure and agents, which are used, hCG administration for luteal support and pregnancy. Ovarian stimulation should be carried out with the utmost caution to avoid Ovarian Hyperstimulation Syndrome (OHSS).

SURROGATE BIRTH

The word 'surrogate' means 'substitute. Surrogacy means the situation in which a woman (the surrogate), bears a child for the benefit of others, commissioning parents. In a surrogate pregnancy, eggs from the surrogate mother or from an egg donor are fertilized with sperm from a sperm donor to make an embryo.

Full Surrogacy/Gestational Surrogacy: It is a situation where the embryo is provided by the commissioning couple or intending woman. The surrogate remains only the gestational mother.

Partial Surrogacy/Traditional Surrogacy: When the carrying woman (the surrogate) has her own egg fertilized. The surrogate mother is artificially inseminated with barren woman's husband's sperms or with sperms from a sperm donor. In this situation, the surrogate is both biological as well as gestational mother of the child.

Indications of Surrogate Birth/Motherhood: (i) Inability of the couple to produce the child as the wife is unable to conceive or carry the child to term. (ii) There are some eugenic reasons, genetic defects or inherited diseases. (iii) Wife does not wish to take time to carry the foetus through. (iv) Wife may suffer from anxiety or labour phobia. (v) Couple wishes to adopt the child but since the facilities are scarce and it takes long for adoption. (vi) Sometimes the adopted child is in emotional conflict when he/she discovers that they are not his biological parents.

Legal Scenario for Practice of Surrogacy in India

Before 2021, ICMR guidelines, Home Ministry's order was regulating surrogacy policy in India. Presently, the policy of surrogacy is guided by **the Surrogacy (Regulation) Act, 2021.** As per this Act single men, and gay couples are banned from opting for surrogacy. Single woman–either divorced and widowed between the age of 35-45 years and couple of Indian origin are allowed to avail surrogacy. Foreigners are banned from opting surrogacy. Only gestational/full surrogacy is allowed. No commercial surrogacy is allowed.

THE SURROGACY (REGULATION) ACT, 2021

This Act received the assent of the President on the 25th December, 2021. The purpose of the Act is to regulate the practice and process of surrogacy in India.

Some Major Features of the Act are:

1. **Definition** [S2(1)]:
   (i) ***"Surrogacy"*** means a practice whereby one woman bears and gives birth to a child for an intending couple with the intention of handing over such child to the intending couple after the birth.
   (ii) ***"Altruistic surrogacy"*** means the surrogacy in which no charges, expenses, fees, remuneration or monetary incentive of whatever nature, except the medical expenses and such other prescribed expenses incurred on surrogate mother and the insurance coverage for the surrogate mother, are given to the surrogate mother or her dependents or her representative.
   (iii) ***"Commercial surrogacy"*** means commercialisation of surrogacy services or procedures or its component services or component procedures including selling

or buying of human embryo or trading in the sale or purchase of human embryo or gametes or selling or buying or trading the services of surrogate motherhood by way of giving payment, reward, benefit, fees, remuneration or monetary incentive in cash or kind, to the surrogate mother or her dependents or her representative, except the medical expenses and such other prescribed expenses incurred on the surrogate mother and the insurance coverage for the surrogate mother.

(iv) ***"Surrogate mother"*** means a woman who agrees to bear a child (who is genetically related to the intending couple or intending woman) through surrogacy from the implantation of embryo in her womb and fulfils the conditions as provided in sub-clause (b) of clause (iii) of section 4.

(v) ***"Intending couple"*** means a couple who have a medical indication necessitating gestational surrogacy and who intend to become parents through surrogacy.

(vi) ***"Intending woman"*** means an Indian woman who is a widow or divorcee between the age of 35 and 45 years and who intends to avail the surrogacy.

(vii) ***"Surrogacy procedures"*** means all gynaecological, obstetrical or medical procedures, techniques, tests, practices or services involving handling of human gametes and human embryo in surrogacy.

(viii) ***"Surrogacy clinic"*** means surrogacy clinic, centre or laboratory, conducting assisted reproductive technology services, in vitro fertilisation services, genetic counselling centre, genetic laboratory, Assisted Reproductive Technology Banks conducting surrogacy procedure or any clinical establishment, by whatsoever name called, conducting surrogacy procedures in any form.

2. **Prohibition and Regulation of Surrogacy Clinic (S. 3):**

(i) No surrogacy clinic, unless registered under this Act, shall conduct or associate with, or help in any manner, in conducting activities relating to surrogacy and surrogacy procedures; or employ or cause to be employed or take services of any person, whether on honorary basis or on payment, who does not possess such qualifications as may be prescribed.

(ii) No surrogacy clinic, paediatrician, gynaecologist, embryologist, registered medical practitioner or any person shall conduct, offer, undertake, promote or associate with or avail of commercial surrogacy in any form; or store a human embryo or gamete for the purpose of surrogacy except storage for other legal purposes like sperm banks, IVF and medical research; or conduct or cause to be conducted sex selection for surrogacy.

3. **Regulation of Surrogacy and Surrogacy Procedures (S. 4):** (i) The Act only ***allows altruistic surrogacy and prohibits commercial surrogacy.*** (ii) Surrogacy is permitted for **intending couples** who suffer from proven infertility. (iii) It is permitted when an intending couple has a medical indication necessitating gestational surrogacy: provided that a **couple of Indian origin** or an **intending woman** who intends to avail surrogacy, **shall obtain a certificate of recommendation from the Board** on an application made by the said persons in such form and manner as may be prescribed. (iv) It is permitted for any other condition or disease as may be specified by regulations made by the Board. (v) It is not permitted for producing children for sale, prostitution, or other forms of exploitation.

A. **Eligibility Criteria for Intending Couple:** The intending couple should have a **'certificate of essentiality'** and a **'certificate of eligibility'** issued by the appropriate authority.

(a) ***The certificate of essentiality*** will be issued upon fulfilment of the following conditions: (i) A certificate of proven infertility of one or both members of the intending couple from a District Medical Board. (ii) An order of parentage and custody of the surrogate child passed by a Magistrate's court of the first class or above. (iii) Insurance coverage for a period of 36 months covering postpartum delivery complications for the surrogate mother.

(b) ***The certificate of eligibility*** to the intending couple is issued upon fulfilment of the following conditions: (i) The couple being **Indian citizens and married for at least 5 years.** (ii) **Between 23 and 50 years old (wife) and 26 and 55 years old (husband),** on the day of certification. (iii) They **do not have any surviving child** (biological, adopted or surrogate); this would not include a child who is mentally or physically challenged or suffers from life threatening disorder or fatal illness with no permanent cure; and (iv) Other conditions that may be specified by regulations.

B. **Eligibility Criteria for Surrogate Mother:** To obtain a **certificate of eligibility** from the appropriate authority, the surrogate mother has to be: (i) A **close relative** of the intending couple (ii) A **married woman** having a child of her own (iii) **25 to 35 years old** (iv) A **surrogate only once** in her lifetime (v) Possess a **certificate of medical and psychological fitness** for surrogacy (vi) The surrogate mother cannot provide her own gametes for the procedure (vii) No woman shall act as a surrogate mother more than once in her lifetime, provided that the number of attempts for surrogacy procedures on the surrogate mother shall be such as may be prescribed.

4. **Prohibition of Conducting Surrogacy (S. 5):** No person including a relative or husband of a surrogate mother or intending couple or intending woman shall seek or encourage to conduct any surrogacy or surrogacy procedures on her except for the purpose specified in clause (ii) of section 4.
5. **Written Informed Consent of Surrogate Mother (S. 6):** A written informed consent of the surrogate mother to undergo surrogacy procedures shall be taken. The information regarding all known side effects and after effects of such procedures shall be informed to the surrogate mother in the language she understands. There shall be an option for surrogate mother to withdraw her consent for surrogacy before the implantation of human embryo in her womb.
6. **Prohibition to Abandon Child Born Through Surrogacy (S. 7): The intending couple or intending woman shall not abandon the child,** born out of a surrogacy procedure, whether within India or outside, for any reason whatsoever, including but not restricted to, any genetic defect, birth defect, any other medical condition, the defects developing subsequently, sex of the child or conception of more than one baby and the like.
7. **Rights of Surrogate Child (S. 8):** A child born out of a surrogacy procedure shall be **deemed to be the biological child of the intending couple or intending woman** and the said child shall be entitled to all the rights and privileges available to a natural child under any law for time being in force.
8. **Number of Oocytes or Human Embryos to be Implanted (S.9):** The number of oocytes or human embryos to be implanted in the uterus of the surrogate mother for the purpose of surrogacy, shall be such as may be prescribed.
9. **Prohibition of Abortion (S. 10):** No person, organisation, surrogacy clinic, laboratory or clinical establishment of any kind shall force the surrogate mother to abort at any stage of surrogacy. An abortion of the surrogate child requires the **written consent** of the surrogate mother and the authorisation of the appropriate authority. This authorisation must be compliant with the **Medical Termination of Pregnancy Act, 1971.**
10. **Registration of Surrogacy Clinics:** Surrogacy clinics cannot undertake surrogacy related procedures unless they are registered by the appropriate authority. Clinics must apply for registration within a period of 60 days from the date of appointment of the appropriate authority (S.11). There shall be established a Registry to be called the **National Assisted Reproductive Technology and Surrogacy Registry** for the purposes of registration of surrogacy clinics under this Act (S. 15).
11. **Constitution of National Assisted Reproductive Technology and Surrogacy Board (S. 17):** The central and the state governments shall constitute the **National Assisted Reproductive Technology and Surrogacy Board and the State Assisted Reproductive Technology and Surrogacy Boards,** respectively.

    Functions of the National Board Include (S. 25): (i) Advising the Central Government on policy matters relating to surrogacy (ii) Laying down the code of conduct of surrogacy clinics (iii) Supervising the functioning of State Boards (iv) Reviewing and monitoring the implementation of the Act, and the rules and regulations made under the Act and recommend to the Central Government, changes therein (v) Setting the minimum standards of physical infrastructure, laboratory and diagnostic equipment and expert manpower to be employed by the surrogacy clinic (vi) Overseeing the performance of various bodies constituted under the Act and take appropriate steps to ensure their effective performance.
12. **Appointment of Appropriate Authority (S. 35):** The Central and the State Governments shall constitute one or more appropriate authority for each of the Union territories and whole or any part of the State respectively for the purposes of this Act and the Assisted Reproductive Technology.

    Functions of the Appropriate Authority include (S. 36): (i) Granting, suspending or cancelling registration of surrogacy clinics (ii) Enforcing standards for surrogacy clinics (iii) Investigating and acting against breach of the provisions of the Act (iv) Recommending modifications to the rules and regulations.
13. **Offences and Penalties:** The offences under the Act include [S. 38(1)]: (i) Undertaking or advertising commercial surrogacy (ii) Abandoning, exploiting or disowning a surrogate child (iii) Exploiting the surrogate mother (iv) Selling embryo or gametes for surrogacy (v) Running an agency, a racket or an organisation for selling, purchasing or trading of human embryos or gametes for the purpose of surrogacy. The penalty for such offences is imprisonment for a term which **may extend to 10 years and with fine which may extend to 10 lakh rupees** [S. 38(2)].

    The Act specifies a range of offences and penalties for other contraventions of the provisions of the Act (S. 39-42). Every offence under this Act shall be cognizable, non-bailable and non-compoundable (S. 43).

IN VITRO FERTILIZATION (IVF)

The term "**test tube baby**" is a non-medical term earlier used for IVF.

Historical perspectives: (i) World's first test tube baby was born in England on July 24, 1978 (ii) World's second test tube baby was born at Calcutta (iii) The first test tube baby clinic started operating in Norfolk Virginia since February 1980.

In IVF, the eggs are surgically removed from the women, fertilized with available sperms in a dish and embryo replaced into the womb of the woman who completes the carriage till delivery. Semen samples of husband are screened two or three times for Hepatitis B surface antigen and HIV I and HIV II.

Process of In Vitro Fertilization

Hormone like gonadotropin is injected into ovary, which induces superovulation. Approximately 30 hours later, the oocytes are removed from the ovary by laparoscope. The removed oocytes are placed in a petridish or test tube containing a growth medium simulating the environment of the woman's body. The medium is composed of the woman's fluids from her reproductive tract. A sperm held in vitro then fertilizes the oocytes. The resulting conceptus is kept in an environment at room temperature where it divides and grows for a few days until it reaches the **blastocyst stage**. The conceptus is then picked up with a small hollow tube injected through the vagina and cervix into the uterus where it is implanted at a proper time in the menstrual cycle. After successful transplantation the woman carries the blastocyst to term. The IVF may be performed in many contexts in which the presence or absence of the following four factors will emerge: (i) A genetic link between parents and child (ii) A gestational link between mother and child (iii) A marital relationship (iv) Necessity of the process to fulfill an individual procedure potential.

Possible hypothetical situations for I.V.F. are described in Table 29.1.

Table 29.1: Possible hypothetical situations for in vitro fertilization

Sperm	Ovum	Uterus (Blastocyst implantation)
Husband	Wife	Wife
Donor	Wife	Wife
Husband	Donor	Wife
Donor	Donor	Wife
Husband	Wife	Surrogate
Husband	Donor	Surrogate

Case I: In this I.V.F. may be necessary because wife may have a tubal occlusion which prevents her to conceive and in some cases voluntarily couple may desire to conceive through IVF to permit early screening of genetic defects, control the timing of pregnancy and select a blastocyst with certain characteristics. In this case the ovum of the wife is fertilized in vitro by sperm of the husband and then is transferred to wife's uterus.

Case II: In this case, the husband is sterile or he suffers from some genetic disorder that he does not want to transmit to the child or he is sterile. In this case the sperm of the donor are used for fertilizing the wife's ovum in vitro and then implanted in the uterus of the wife.

Case III: In this case the wife is either sterile or has some genetic defect that she does not want to transmit to the child. The sperm of the husband fertilizes the donor's ovum in vitro and then transferred to the wife's uterus.

Case IV: The couple employs this method when both the partners are sterile. The ovum from the donor is fertilized by the sperms of the donor in vitro and then transferred in the uterus of the wife.

Case V: This is employed when the wife is unable to carry the child to term then the uterus of the surrogate is used for the purpose.

Case VI: This might be used by a woman who wishes to have a child but cannot conceive naturally or through artificial insemination or does not wish to conceive by method. Then the husband's sperms fertilize donor woman's ovum in vitro and then it is transferred in the uterus of the surrogate.

Various Techniques for IVF

1. **Gamete Intrafallopian Transfer (GIFT):** The egg and sperm are put together in the fallopian tube for fertilization.
2. **Embryo Transfer (ET):** The embryo that is created from the egg and sperm is transferred into the carrier's womb, and the carrier may or may not be the originator of the egg.
3. **Zona Drilling (ZD):** In this the prepared semen is introduced through a partial opening of zona pellucida.
4. **Partial Zona Pellucida (PZD):** This method is employed if due to any reason it's not possible to penetrate zona pellucida. It is of two types: (i) *Sub zonal injection (SUZI):* The sperm is injected between the egg and the surrounding membranes with a sharp micropipette. (ii) *Intracytoplasmic sperm injection (ICSI):* The sperm is directly injected into inner cellular structure of the egg.

Ethical and Legal Aspects in Assisted Reproduction Techniques

The ethical and legal aspects involved with in vitro fertilization and allied procedure are many and most of them remain unresolved. The reason for this uncertainty is the rapid advancement of the technology thereby resulting in the lag in legal and ethical response. There are a number of ethical and religious issues regarding IVF of which some are unanswered and others remain the topic for debate. These are: (i) Issues relating to experimentation on human beings as this is important to define when life begins in IVF (ii) Moral issues relating to non-coital reproduction (iii) What are the rights of inheritance in case of ovum or sperm donation? (iv) Whether there should be any age limit? (v) Does surrogacy resemble baby selling as the ability to bear the child is being used commercially. (vi) What should be the fate of orphan embryos and what are the legal rights of embryos? (vii) Issues relating to embryo research and should genetic engineering be totally banned.

Besides these other areas that have generated public enquiries and legal debate are many such as: (i) What is the fate of excess and stored embryos and is selective breeding for male child being employed? (ii) Are there any practices where the use of drugs to trigger false positive pregnancy tests are undertaken and the falsification of test reports indicating pregnancy. (iii) In relation to donation of genetic material it is important whether the secrecy is maintained or not and the donors are properly screened or not. (iv) Financial gains related to the procedure and regularization of sperm banks are important issues. (v) Legitimacy of motherhood in relation to surrogacy is an important issue. (vi) There are chances of exploitation of surrogate mother and the effects of this practice on the offspring.

Many enquiry committees including Warnock Committee in England were established. All of them suggested continuation of assisted technology with proper control. In most of the developed countries like USA, UK, Australia and Singapore there is strict control of regulatory bodies. Recommendations of these committees are amended from time to time and binding on all centers.

Warnock Committee 1982: Political involvement started in U.K. and a commission of inquiry was appointed in 1982 with Mary Warnock as its chairman. The committee gave recommendations of statutory licensing authority and licensing of research and practice: (i) A statutory licensing authority should be formed to regulate infertility services and research (ii) AID, IVF, egg and embryo donation is to be regulated by law (iii) Cryopreservation was permitted (iv) Research on spare embryos was permitted 14 days after fertilization.

Human Fertilization and Embryology Act (HEFA) 1990: This Act was enforced in England. It is related to various research and clinical procedures of assisted reproduction. HEFA is a corporate authority, which can issue licenses for treatment, storage and research. Other European countries also enacted code of ethics within their own clause. They formulated more or less similar regulation based on Warnock's report keeping in mind local, social and political pressure.

Assisted Reproduction in United States: American College of Obstetricians, Gynecologists and American Fertility Society similar to British voluntary licensing authority formed a national advisory board on the ethics of reproduction.

Indian Scenario

In India, the Indian Council of Medical Research (ICMR) laid out guidelines for ART clinics as far back as 2005, however, these do not enjoy legislative backing. Since many ART clinics have been running in the country without regulation, a need was felt for regulation of such clinics as there are implications on the health of those who undertake the procedure. The Act allows **accessing ARTs for a married heterosexual couple and any woman between the age of 21 years to 55 years (single woman, unmarried, divorced, or widowed)** and **excludes single men, cohabiting heterosexual couples and LGBTQ+ individuals**.

THE ASSISTED REPRODUCTIVE TECHNOLOGY (REGULATION) ACT, 2021

This Act received the assent of the President on the 18th December, 2021. The purpose of the Act is to regulate and supervise the assisted reproductive technology clinics and the assisted reproductive technology banks, prevention of misuse, safe and ethical practice of assisted reproductive technology services.

Some Major Features of the Act are:

1. **Definition [S. 2(1)]:**
   (i) ***"Assisted reproductive technology"*** means all techniques that attempt to obtain a pregnancy by handling the sperm or the oocyte outside the human body and transferring the gamete or the embryo into the reproductive system of a woman.
   (ii) ***"Assisted reproductive technology clinic"*** means any premises equipped with requisite facilities and medical practitioners registered with the National Medical Commission for carrying out the procedures related to the assisted reproductive technology (ART).
   (iii) ***"Commissioning couple"*** means an infertile married couple who approach an assisted reproductive technology clinic or assisted reproductive technology bank for obtaining the services authorised of the said clinic or bank.
   (iv) ***"Infertility"*** means the inability to conceive after **one year** of unprotected coitus or other proven medical condition preventing a couple from conception.
   (v) ***"Woman"*** means any woman above the age of **21 years** who approaches an assisted reproductive technology clinic or assisted reproductive technology bank for obtaining the authorised services of the clinic or bank.
2. **Establishment of Assisted Reproductive Technology and Surrogacy Board:**

   The Central and the State Governments shall constitute the **National Assisted Reproductive Technology and Surrogacy Board and the State Assisted Reproductive Technology and Surrogacy Boards,** respectively (S. 3).

   A. ***Functions of the National Board include (S. 5)***: (i) Advising the Central Government on policy matters relating to the assisted reproductive technology. (ii) Reviewing and monitoring the implementation of the Act, rules and regulations made thereunder and recommending it to the Central Government, any suitable changes therein. (iii) Laying down the code of conduct to be observed by persons working at clinics and banks. (iv) **Setting the minimum standards** of physical infrastructure, laboratory and diagnostic equipment and expert manpower to be employed by clinics and banks. (v) Overseeing the performance of various bodies constituted under this Act and taking appropriate steps to ensure their effective performance. (vi) Supervising the functioning of the National Registry and liaison with the State Board.

   B. ***Functions of the State Board (S. 8):*** (i) It shall have the responsibility to follow the policies and plans laid by the National Board for clinics and banks in the State. (ii) It shall co-ordinate the enforcement and implement the policies and guidelines for assisted reproduction in the state.

3. **Establishment of National Registry of Clinics and Banks:** The Central Government may, within a period of 90 days from the date of commencement of this Act, by notification, establish for the purposes of this Act and Surrogacy Act, a Registry to be called the National Assisted Reproductive Technology and Surrogacy Registry (S. 9). The National Registry shall consist of such scientific, technical, administrative and supportive staff and the terms and conditions of their service under the Act (S. 10).
4. **Functions of National Registry include (S.11):** (a) It shall act as **a central database** in the country through which the details of all the clinics and banks of the country including nature and types of services provided by them, outcome of the services and other relevant information shall be obtained on regular basis. (b) It shall assist the National Board in its functioning by providing the data generated from the central database of the Registry. (c) The data generated from the National Registry shall be utilised by the National Board for making policies, guidelines and shall help in identifying new research areas and conducting research in the area of assisted reproduction and other related fields in the country. (d) Such other functions as may be prescribed.
5. **Appointment of Appropriate Authority (S. 12):** The Central and the State Governments shall appoint one or more appropriate assisted reproductive technology and surrogacy authorities for each of the Union territories and for the whole or any part of the State, respectively for the purposes of this Act.
6. **Functions of Appropriate Authority are (S. 13):** (a) To grant, suspend or cancel registration of a clinic or bank (b) To enforce the standards to be fulfilled by the clinic or bank (c) To investigate complaints of breach of the provisions of this Act, rules and regulations made thereunder and take legal action as per provisions of this Act (d) To take appropriate legal action against the misuse of assisted reproductive technology by any person and also to initiate independent investigations in such matter (e) To supervise the implementation of the provisions of this Act and the rules and regulations made thereunder (f) To recommend to the National Board and State Boards about the modifications required in the rules and regulations in accordance with changes in technology or social conditions (g) To take action after investigation of complaints received by it against the assisted reproductive technology clinics or banks (h) Such other functions as may be prescribed.
7. **Registration of Assisted Reproductive Technology Clinic or Assisted Reproductive Technology Bank (S. 15-18):** (i) All ART clinic and bank must be registered under the National Registry of Banks and Clinics of India. (ii) Clinics shall make an application to the Registration Authority within a period of 60 days from the date of establishment of the National Registry. (iii) The **Registry is meant to act as a central database** for all facilities providing ART services in India, with State Governments appointing relevant authorities in their respective states to facilitate the registration process. (iv) No clinics or banks shall be registered under this Act, unless the appropriate authority is satisfied that such clinics and banks are in a position to provide such facilities and maintain such equipment and standards including specialised manpower, physical infrastructure and diagnostic facilities as may be prescribed. (v) The appropriate authority shall grant registration within a period of 30 days of receipt of application. (vi) Registrations must be **renewed every 5 years** and may be cancelled or suspended if an entity contravenes the provisions of the Act.
8. **General Duties of Assisted Reproductive Technology Clinics and Banks (S. 21):** The clinics and banks shall perform the following duties, namely:
   (a) The clinics and banks shall ensure that commissioning couple, woman and donors of gametes are eligible to avail the assisted reproductive technology procedures subject to such criteria as may be prescribed.
   (b) The clinics shall obtain donor gametes from the banks and such banks shall **ensure that the donor has been medically tested** for such diseases as may be prescribed.
   (c) The clinic shall: (i) Provide professional counselling to commissioning couple and woman about all the implications and chances of success of assisted reproductive technology procedures in the clinic. (ii) Inform the commissioning couple and woman of the advantages, disadvantages and cost of the procedures, their medical side effects, risks including the risk of multiple pregnancy. (iii) Help the commissioning couple or woman to arrive at an **informed decision** on such matters that would most likely be the best for the commissioning couple.
   (d) The clinics shall make commissioning couple or woman, **aware of the rights of a child born through the use of ART.**
   (e) The clinics and banks shall ensure that information about the commissioning couple, woman and donor shall be kept **confidential and the information about treatment shall not be disclosed to anyone except to the database to be maintained by the National Registry, in a medical emergency** at the request of the commissioning couple to whom the information relates, or by an order of a court of competent jurisdiction.
   (f) Every clinic and every bank shall maintain **a grievance cell** in respect of matters relating to such clinics and banks and the manner of making a complaint before such grievance cell shall be such as may be prescribed.

(g) The clinics shall apply the assisted reproductive technology services: (i) **To a woman above the age of 21 years and below the age of 50 years;** (ii) **To a man above the age of 21 years and below the age of 55 years.**

(h) The clinics shall issue to the commissioning couple or woman **a discharge certificate** stating details of the assisted reproductive technology procedure performed on the commissioning couple or woman.

(i) All clinics and banks shall co-operate and make available their premises for physical inspection by the National Board, National Registry and State Boards.

All clinics and banks shall provide all information related to (i) Enrolment of the commissioning couple, woman and gamete donors (ii) The procedure being undertaken (iii) Outcome of the procedure, complications, if any, to the National Registry periodically, in such manner as may be prescribed.

9. **Written Informed Consent (S. 22):**

(1) The clinic shall not perform any treatment or procedure without—(a) The **written informed consent of all the parties** seeking assisted reproductive technology (b) An **insurance coverage** of such amount as may be prescribed **for a period of 12 months in favour of the oocyte donor** by the commissioning couple or woman from an insurance company or an agent recognised by the Insurance Regulatory and Development Authority.

(2) The clinics and banks **shall not cryo-preserve any human embryos or gamete, without specific instructions and consent in writing from all the parties seeking assisted reproductive technology, in case of death or incapacity of any of the parties**.

(3) The clinic shall not use any human reproductive material, except in accordance with the provisions of this Act to create a human embryo or use an in vitro human embryo for any purpose without the specific consent in writing of all the concerned persons to whom the assisted reproductive technology relates.

(4) **Any of the commissioning couple may withdraw his or her consent under sub-section (1), any time before the human embryos or the gametes are transferred to the concerned woman's uterus**.

10. **Duties of Assisted Reproductive Technology Clinics and Banks to Keep Accurate Records (S. 23):**

(a) All clinics and banks shall **maintain detailed records of all donor's oocytes, sperm or embryos used or unused**, the manner and technique of their use in such manner as may be prescribed.

(b) All clinics and banks shall, as and when the **National Registry is established, submit by online,**–(i) All information available with them in regard to progress of the commissioning couple or woman (ii) Information about number of donors (sperm and oocyte), screened, maintained and supplied and the like to the National Registry **within a period of one month from the date of receipt of such information**.

(c) The records maintained under clause (a) shall be maintained for **at least a period of ten years**, upon the expiry of which the clinic and bank shall transfer the records to a central database of the National Registry: provided that if any criminal or other proceedings are instituted against any clinics or banks, the records and all other documents of such clinics and banks shall be preserved till the final disposal of such proceedings.

(d) In the event of the closure of any clinic or bank before the expiry of the period of ten years under clause (c) such clinic or bank shall immediately transfer the records to the central database of the National Registry.

(e) All such records shall, at all reasonable times, be made available for inspection to the National Board or the National Registry or the State Board or to any other person authorised by the National Board in this behalf.

11. **Duties of Assisted Reproductive Technology Clinics Using Human Gametes and Embryos (S. 24):** While using human gametes and embryos, the duties to be performed by the clinics and banks shall be as under: (a) The clinics shall retrieve oocytes in such manner as may be specified by regulations. (b) **Not more than three oocytes or embryos may be placed in the uterus of a woman during the treatment cycle** in such manner as may be specified by regulations. (c) **A woman shall not be treated with gametes or embryos derived from more than one man or woman during any one treatment cycle**. (d) A clinic shall **never mix semen from two individuals** for the procedures specified under this Act. (e) **The embryos shall not be split and used for twinning to increase the number of available embryos**. (f) The **collection of gametes posthumously shall be done only if prior consent of the commissioning couple** is available in such manner as may be prescribed. (g) The clinic shall not use ovum that are derived from a foetus, in any process of in vitro fertilisation. (h) Such other duties as may be prescribed.

12. **Preimplantation Genetic Diagnosis (S. 25):**

(1) The Pre-implantation Genetic testing shall be used to **screen the human embryo for known, pre-existing, heritable or genetic diseases only**.

(2) The donation of an embryo after Pre-implantation Genetic Diagnosis to an approved research laboratory for research purposes shall be done only: (a) With the approval of the commissioning couple or woman; and (b) When the embryo suffers from pre-existing, heritable, life-threatening or genetic diseases.

(3) The National Board may lay down such other conditions as it deems fit in the interests of the Pre-implantation Genetic testing.

13. **Sex selection (S. 26):** (1) Subject to the provisions of the Pre-conception and Pre-natal Diagnostic Techniques (Prohibition of Sex Selection) Act, 1994, the **clinic shall not offer to provide a couple or woman with a child of a pre-determined sex**. (2) It is prohibited for anyone to do any act, at any stage, to determine the sex of the child to be born through the process of assisted reproductive technology to separate, or yield fractions enriched in sperm of X or Y variations. (3) A person shall not knowingly provide, prescribe or administer anything that shall ensure or increase the probability that an embryo shall be of a particular sex, or that shall identify the sex of an in vitro embryo, except to diagnose, prevent or treat a sex-linked disorder or disease.

14. **Sourcing of Gametes by Assisted Reproductive Technology Banks (S. 27):**

    (1) The screening of gamete donors, the collection, screening and storage of semen; and provision of oocyte donor, shall be done only by a bank registered as an independent entity under the provisions of this Act.

    (2) **The banks shall:** (a) **Obtain semen from males between 21 years of age and 55 years of age**, both inclusive; (b) **Obtain oocytes from females between 23 years of age and 35 years of age;** (c) Examine the donors for such diseases, as may be prescribed.

    (3) **A bank shall not supply the sperm or oocyte of a single donor to more than one commissioning couple.**

    (4) **An oocyte donor shall donate oocytes only once in her life and not more than seven oocytes shall be retrieved from the oocyte donor.**

    (5) All unused oocytes shall be preserved by the banks for use on the same recipient, or given for research to an organisation registered under this Act after seeking written consent from the commissioning couple.

    (6) **A bank shall obtain all necessary information in respect of a sperm or oocyte donor, including the name, Aadhaar number** as defined in clause (a) of section 2 of the Aadhaar (Targeted Delivery of Financial and other Subsidies, Benefits and Services) Act, 2016, address and any other details of such donor, in such manner as may be prescribed, and shall undertake in writing from such donor about the confidentiality of such information.

15. **Storage and Handling of Human Gametes and Embryos (S. 28):** (1) The standards for the storage and handling of gametes, gonadal tissues and human embryos in respect of their security, recording and identification shall be such as may be prescribed. (2) The gamete of a donor or embryo shall be **stored for a period of not more than ten years** and at the end of such period such gamete or embryo shall be allowed to perish or be donated to a research organisation registered under this Act for research purposes with the consent of the commissioning couple or individual, in such manner as may be prescribed.

16. **Restriction on Sale, Etc., of Human Gametes, Zygotes and Embryos (S. 29):** The sale, transfer or use of gametes, zygotes and embryos, or any part thereof or information related thereto, directly or indirectly to any party within or outside India shall be **prohibited except in the case of transfer of own gametes and embryos for personal use with the permission of the National Board**.

17. **Research on Human Gametes and Embryos (S. 30):** (1) The use of any human gametes and embryos or their **transfer to any country outside India for research shall be absolutely prohibited**. (2) The research on human gamete or embryo within India shall be performed in such manner as may be prescribed.

18. **Rights of Child Born Through Assisted Reproductive Technology (S. 31):** (1) **The child born through ART shall be deemed to be a biological child of the commissioning couple** and the said child shall be entitled to all the rights and privileges available to a natural child only from the commissioning couple under any law for the time being in force. (2) **A donor shall relinquish all parental rights over the child or children which may be born from his or her gamete**.

19. **Offences and Penalties:**

    A. **S. 32:** (1) The clinic, or bank or agent thereof, shall **not issue, publish, distribute, communicate** or cause to be issued, published, distributed or communicated any advertisement in any manner including internet, regarding facilities of **sex selective assisted reproductive technology** (2) Contravention of provisions under sub-section (1), shall be punishable with imprisonment for a term of **5 years, extendable to 10 years or with fine which shall not be less than 10 lakh rupees but may extend to 25 lakh rupees or with both**.

    B. **S. 33:** (1) Under the Act, any medical geneticist, gynaecologist, registered medical practitioner or any person shall not:

       (a) Abandon, disown or exploit or cause to be abandoned, disowned or exploited in any form the child or children born through ART.

       (b) Sell human embryos or gametes, run an agency, a racket or an organisation for selling, purchasing or trading in human embryos or gametes.

       (c) Import or help in getting imported in whatsoever manner, the human embryos or human gametes.

       (d) Exploit the commissioning couple, woman or the gamete donor in any form.

(e) Transfer human embryo into a male person or an animal.

(f) Sell any human embryo or gamete for the purpose of research.

(g) Use any intermediates to obtain gamete donors or purchase gamete donors.

(2) Any contravention of the provisions of clauses (a) to (g) shall be punishable with a fine which shall **not be less than 5 lakh rupees but may extend to 10 lakh rupees for the first contravention and for subsequent contravention, shall be punishable with imprisonment for a term which shall not be less than 3 years but may extend to 8 years and with fine which shall not be less than 10 lakh rupees but may extend to 20 lakh rupees**.

CLONING

Cloning: It is the technique of producing a genetically identical duplicate of an organism artificially.

Clone: It is an organism that has same genetic information as another organism or organisms. A clone is said to be all descendents derived asexually from a single individual, as by cutting, bulbs, by fissions by mitosis, or by parthenogenesis reproduction.

With the birth of cloned sheep, mice, and cloned cows soon to be borne in Japan, the art of carbon copying adult mammals is developing rapidly, but according to scientists, the prospect of humans is remote. Researchers predict that they will be able to rechannel the embryo's normal development to grow a new heart or any other organ of the body.

Nuclear Transfer: This is transferring of nucleus from the cell of one organism to an enucleated egg cell. This will produce an organism that has exact genetic material as that of the donor cell. Scientists are using current techniques exceedingly more and more with variety of species.

In nature and even in the lives of humans, clones are present. Cloning occurs with all plants, some insects, algae, unicellular organisms that conducts mitosis or binary fissions, and occasionally by all multicellular organisms, including humans.

Monozygotic twins (identical twins) are clones of each other. They have exactly the same genetic information due to the division of an embryo early in development that produces two identical embryos. About eight million human clones inhabit the world. In unicellular organisms, a cell will produce two daughter cells that have the same genetic material.

The first organisms that were cloned using nuclear transfer were frogs because they have large egg cells and scientists can obtain up to 2,000 of them from one ovulation.

Successful cloning has occurred with livestock. The drive towards success is not because livestock like cows and sheep are model organisms but farming industry has made and continues to make a big effort towards finding a way to implement the technique of nuclear transfer to livestock. Research in cloning is also occurring in primates, due to their similarities with humans. This leads to the most talked about aspects of cloning, the use of the techniques with human cell eggs.

Dr. Seed, physicist who researched fertility sciences in 1980's and now specializing in embryology, states that he has set up a fertility clinic that can conduct nuclear transfer and thus accomplish the task of human cloning. He successfully transferred human embryo from one human to another in the 1970s.

History of Cloning

(i) **Adolph Edward Driesch** could let the eggs of a sea Urchin develop into the two blastomere stage. Then he separated it by shaking it in a flask and allowing them to grow cells that developed into dwarf sea urchins. (ii) First implantation of a nucleus in to an egg cell occurred in 1952 by **Robert Briggs** and **Thomas J King** in Philadelphia. They had transferred the nuclei of Leopard Frog's eggs but the egg cells did not develop. (iii) **Dr. John Gurdin** accomplished the successful nuclear transfer of embryo cells later in 1970's but frogs did not develop beyond tadpoles. (iv) In 1984, **Dr. Steene Willadsen** announced that he had successfully transferred nuclei from embryo of sheep to produce clones. He was successful with cows and even monkeys. He began cloning embryos that were in 64-128 stages suggesting that perhaps nuclear transfer was possible with differentiated cells (v) In 1994, **Dr. Neal** first produced calves by nuclear transfer from fully develop embryos. (vi) In 1997, **Dr. Lan Wilmut** and **Dr. Keith Campbell** of the Roslin Institute in Edinburgh, Scotland produced Megan and Morag, the first cloned sheep from embryo cells. Their new technique starved the donor embryo of the nutrient serum they feed the cells. This would put the cell in the right moment in the cell cycle, thus allowing the genetic material to be accepted more easily by the egg cell. This was the integral step of nuclear transfer.

Dolly (First Clone Sheep): Dr. Wilmut and Dr. Campbell of the Roslin Institute in Edinburgh, Scotland produced the first cloned sheep from embryo cells on February 22, 1997. These scientists took a mammary cell from a sheep and put it into an egg. They let this egg to grow into an embryo and then transplanted this fused embryo and put it in a recipient Ewe, acting as a surrogate mother. This occurred late in January 1996 that was the day of fusion date for Dolly.

Methods Used for Cloning (Nuclear Transfer)

The method used is called nuclear transfer since nuclear information is transferred and involves following steps:

(i) First step is to find something to clone. Dr. Wilmut and Campbell grabbed some cells, which were growing in the lab from mammary cells of a six-year-old Finn Dorset Ewe.

(ii) Next step is to get an oocyte and take the DNA out so that the donor DNA can be added.

(iii) Donor cell and the oocyte without a nucleus are put together in a petridish and electric current is sent through it to fuse as a zygote.

(iv) This cell then grows and divides like a fertilized egg cell and then it becomes a blastocyst.

(v) For each clone Roslin researchers combined material from two sources: (a) Extracting immature oocytes from the ovaries of Ewes. (b) Removing the DNA from it to make enucleated egg cells and then take cells containing donor genetic material.

(vi) ***Cloning in dolly:*** Dolly's DNA came from a Finn Dorset sheep, she was developed from an oocyte donated from a Poll Dorset and her surrogate mother being Scottish Blackface Ewe. The variation in breeds was used to show that Dolly is not of the same breed as her surrogate mother or the egg cell she developed from. Dr. Wilmut and his colleagues fuse the empty oocyte with the donor cells by bringing them together and subjecting them to an electric current to fuse as one cell. After growing and dividing for a week or so in lab culture dish, the fused cell formed an early embryo called a blastocyst, which Wilmut's team implanted into a surrogate mother. Dolly was the only lamb born from 217 fusions of oocytes with udder cells after 5 months.

There are chances of failures because it is difficult to ensure that the empty oocytes and donor cells are at the same stage of the cell division cycle.

Aims and Objectives of Cloning

(i) Cloning could also directly offer means of curing diseases. As a technique that could extend means to acquiring a new data for the embryology and how organisms develop as a whole over time. (ii) Agricultural industry demands nuclear transfer to produce better livestock with ideal characteristics for the agricultural industry and to be able to manufacture biological products such as proteins for humans since many human diseases are caused by defects in the production of proteins. (iii) Cloning endangered species to increase their population. (iv) Livestock can produce biological proteins helping people having diseases like parkinson's, diabetes and cystic fibrosis. (v) Cloning provides better research capabilities for finding cures to many diseases. (vi) Provides benefit to those who would like to have children like in infertility or those with genetic disorders. (vii) Single women could have child using cloning instead of IVF or artificial insemination. (viii) Cloning also provides children to those who needs organ transplants to have a clone born to donate organs. (ix) Provides a copy of a child for a couple whose child had died. (x) Making copies of diseased to better the engineering of offspring in humans and animals thus producing animals of high genetic value. (xi) Cloning of pigs that will produce organs which will not be rejected by humans after a transplant.

Application for Cloning

Various applications for cloning can be: (i) Infertile couples that cannot conceive due to some genetic disorder can only seek cloning. (ii) Couples who are infertile as a result of gametic insufficiency might choose to clone one of the partners rather than the sperm, egg or embryo from some unknown donor. (iii) Couples, who are at the risk of having a child with some genetic disorder, may seek to clone one of them or some of their already present child. (iv) Obtaining tissues or organs for transplantation in case of a child lacking a suitable donor. (v) Therapeutic cloning aims to develop medical therapies for which the cloned embryos grown only upto fourteen days can harvest the stem cells that will be useful in treating certain diseases.

Ethical Issues of the Use of Cloning

(i) Decline in genetic diversity and even depriving a person of his uniqueness. (ii) If a population of organisms has the same genetic information then the disease would wipe out entire population. (iii) If we try to clone endangered species, we could possibly kill the last females integral to survival of species, e.g., it took 227 tries to produce Dolly. (iv) If everyone has the same genetic material, ability to clone will be lost and we have to resort to natural reproduction, causing it to inbreed, which may pose problems. (v) It is similar to taking nature in to our own hands by cloning animals and humans. (vi) Religious organizations consider nuclear transfer to cause men to be reproductively obsolete since cloning requires only oocyte, any cell and a woman to develop in. (vii) Rights to human beings will be defied since clones are not granted the birth of newness. (viii) Mental and emotional problems of a clone. (ix) Cloning would enable rich or powerful persons to clone themselves several times over and commercial entrepreneurs might hire women to bear clones of sports or entertainment celebrities. (x) Current reproductive techniques can be abused.

Medicolegal Aspects of Cloning

1. **Identification:** Problems would arise in identification of the person.
2. **Paternity and maternity testing:** In matter involving paternity and maternity, it would be difficult who is the biological father or social father or genetic father.
3. **Property and inheritance:** In matters related to inheritance of property, it would cause great problems.
4. **Religious problems:** There is no religious sanction.
5. **Ethical problem:** Believe in only the natural method of reproduction, it is like playing with nature and taking nature into their own hands.
6. In India, there is no specific law regarding cloning. The ICMR guidelines on cloning prohibits whole human cloning or reproductive cloning. However, it allows therapeutic cloning and the use of embryonic stem cells for research purpose.

Hormonal Replacement Therapy (HRT)

Hormone therapy (HT) is used to boost the hormone levels of the menopausal women. It relieves some of the symptoms of menopause like hot flashes, vaginal dryness, night sweats, dry itch skin, and mood swings etc. It also prevents osteoporosis, decreases tooth loss, lowered the risk of diabetes and colon cancer in menopausal women.

There are two main types of hormone therapy: (i) **Estrogen Therapy Alone:** Low doses of Estrogen as a pill or patch is given to the women every day. It can be prescribed as a cream, vaginal ring, gel or spray. (ii) **Estrogen Progesterone/Progestin Hormone Therapy (EPT) (Combination Therapy):** Combined doses of estrogen and progesterone (or progestin, a synthetic form of progesterone) is prescribed. The therapy usually continues about 2-5 years.

Health risks associated with HRT (estrogen alone or combination therapy) include increased risk of endometrial cancer, gall bladder/gallstone problems, urinary incontinence, dementia, stroke, blood clots and heart attack. The combination hormonal therapy may be resulted in more vaginal bleeding and breast cancer.

LONG QUESTIONS

1. Discuss artificial insemination, test tube baby, surrogate mother, hormonal replacement therapy with respect to appropriate national and state law.
2. Discuss the Assisted Reproductive Technology (Regulation) Act, 2021.

SHORT QUESTIONS

1. Artificial insemination.
2. Surrogate motherhood.
3. Cloning.
4. IVF.

MULTIPLE CHOICE QUESTIONS

1. Legal problems of adultery in artificial insemination are dealt under:

(a) Sec. 497 IPC (b) Sec. 420 IPC
(c) Sec. 32 IPC (d) Sec. 175 IPC

2. World's first test tube baby was born in:

(a) England (b) USA
(c) Germany (d) Israel

3. As per "The Surrogacy (Regulation) Act, 2021", in a life time, how many times a woman in India is allowed to act as surrogate?

(a) Not more than one
(b) Not more than two
(c) Not more than three
(d) Not more than four

4. A 23-year-old multiparous woman, an anonymous egg donor, who died a few hours after undergoing a procedure to donate eggs at an in vitro fertilization clinic. Autopsy revealed massive pulmonary oedema, intra-alveolar hemorrhage, ascites and pleural effusion. Both ovaries were enlarged and associated with the presence of multiple cysts. The most likely cause of death in this case is:

(a) Ovarian hyperstimulation syndrome
(b) Pulmonary thromboembolism
(c) Polycystic ovarian disorder
(d) Fat embolism

ANSWER KEY ☞

1. (a)	2. (a)	3. (c)	4. (a)

30 CHAPTER

Medicolegal Aspects of AIDS and Covid-19

Acquired immune deficiency syndrome is causing both health and legal problems. Much of the controversy about AIDS and its victims involve the legal rights of the public whose health should be protected; the risks and methods of transmission of AIDS; the right of those with the disease to receive full medical attention and to receive public services like schooling and the right of the victims to their privacy.

This is further complicated by the need of the AIDS victim for protection from communicable diseases that are life threatening to the victim but not to the general public. Health personnel are concerned because of greater chance of contact with patients with the disease.

According to estimates from the Joint United Nations Programme on HIV/AIDS (UNAIDS) 37 million adults and 2.5 million children were living with HIV at the end of 2003. This is more than 50 percent higher that the figures projected by WHO in 1991 on the basis of the data then available. The worst affected are the countries of Sub-Saharan Africa and South East Asia. During the period 2003, a total of 5.3 million people were affected in India, which increased to 5.7 million during the period 2005. During 2003, some 5 million people became infected with the Human Immunodeficiency Virus. The year also saw 3 million deaths from HIV/AIDS a high number despite retroviral therapy which saved AIDS and AIDS deaths in the richer countries.

AIDS is a viral disease involving the breakdown of the body's immune system. The full blown syndrome is believed to be both incurable and almost inevitably fatal, striking most frequently among certain high-risk groups, such as male homosexuals, intravenous drug users, recipients of blood transfusions and hemophiliacs.

AIDS represents a form of secondary immunological disorder that results in profound depression of cell mediated immunity. It is caused by a retrovirus known as Human T-lymphotropic virus type III/Lymphadenopathy-associated virus or HTLV III/LAV. The virus inhibits body's ability to resist diseases by infecting white blood cells called T-lymphocytes, which are an integral part of the human immune system. Specifically the disease selectively destroys and generates qualitative abnormalities in the patient's T-helper/inducer cells, which enable other components of the immune system to function and thus comprises T-lymphocyte subset primarily responsible for the generation of most specific human immune responses. As a result, the immune system of patients with AIDS is characterized by functional defects in virtually all limbs of the immune system. This suppression of the immune system exposes patients to a variety of 'opportunistic' infections and malignant conditions that generally do not afflict otherwise in individuals in similar situation without AIDS. It also possibly infects B-cells and causes macrophage dysfunction and thus an acquired immune deficiency state results.

Included under 'diseases at least moderately predictive of cellular immune deficiency' are two neoplasia-Kaposi's sarcoma and primary lymphoma of the brain, and a wide spectrum of opportunistic infections such as:

1. Protozoal and Helminthic infections caused by Pneumocystitis carinii, Toxoplasmosis, cryptosporidiosis and strongyloidosis.
2. **Bacterial infections:** Atypical myobacteriosis.
3. **Viral infections:** Cytomegalovirus; herpes virus I or II; and progressive multifocal leukoencephalopathy by papovavirus.

The signs and symptoms in the patient may be non-specific and are often due to infections or neoplastic complications rather than to the disease itself. There are no pathological lesions diagnostic of AIDS. The patients may present as: (i) Unexplained loss of weight (ii) Low grade fever (iii) Unexplained generalized lymphadenopathy (iv) Diarrhoea.

WHO Definition

The patient should present with at least one major and two minor signs to be diagnosed as a case of AIDS.

Major signs: (i) Weight loss more than 10% of body weight (ii) Chronic diarrhoea for more than one month (iii) Prolonged fever for more than one month.

Minor signs: (i) Cough for more than one month (ii) General pruritic dermatitis (iii) Recurrent herpers zoster infections (iv) Oropharyngeal candidiasis (v) Chronic progressive disseminated H. simplex.

Pathogenesis

The incubation period for AIDS varies from 4 months to 57 months. HIV attaches itself to the T_4 receptor molecule on T-helper lymphocytes in order to infect them. These T-helper lymphocytes are found in most fluids such as breast milk, semen, tears and saliva. HTLV-III/LAV has been isolated in a wide range of body fluids including blood, semen, saliva, tears, breast milk and urine. How much exposure is needed for the syndrome to develop is unknown. Random exposure is not sufficient and in the absence of contamination with blood products by direct passage and/or sexual contact AIDS is unlikely. Persons are not considered to have AIDS merely because tests show them to be generating antibodies to the AIDS virus that is to be 'seropositive'. Indeed, a person is not considered to have AIDS even if he or she is seropositive, displays a number of elements in the definition of AIDS used for reporting purposes by the Centers for Disease Control (CDC), and is afflicted with one or more of the opportunistic diseases that takes advantage of the patient's immune system.

The high risk groups in the community for acquiring AIDS are: (i) Recipients of blood transfusion (ii) Homosexuals (iii) Prostitutes and eunuchs (iv) Drug addicts and drug abusers (v) Groups with sexual interaction with foreign travellers.

Routes of Transmission

AIDS may be transmitted in any of the following ways: (i) By way of unprotected (vaginal, anal or oral) sexual intercourse both homosexual or heterosexual. (ii) By exchange of contaminated blood and blood products by way of sharing needles by drug abusers and through blood transfusions. (iii) Needle type exposure resulting from cuts by knife while carrying out surgeries in operation theatres and in the autopsy rooms. (iv) Perinatal transmission (From HIV positive mother to her unborn child).

Precautions to be Taken in Health Care Settings by the Health Care Personnel

(i) Medical officer while examining a homosexual male especially one with history or the external stigmata of drug abuse, should take precautions to avoid contamination himself with blood or seminal fluid especially from infected syringes and needles. (ii) In invasive procedures such as surgery, dental procedures in which bleeding might occur and vaginal or caesarean section deliveries gloves, masks, eye coverings and other barrier precautions should be routinely used. (iii) Extraordinary care should be taken to prevent injuries to hands caused by needles, scalpels and other sharp instruments or devices during procedures; when cleaning used instruments; during disposal of used needles and when handling sharp instruments following procedures:

Precautions to be taken while performing autopsies: High risk postmortems are those wherein lies the danger of infection to the mortuary staff and doctor performing autopsies. Precautions to be taken for autopsy in cases of deaths due to AIDS include: (i) Wiremess gloves should be used but since they are expensive, double gloves can be used. (ii) Facemasks and goggles must be used by the doctor and the assistants. (iii) A dead body should be well marked with a label as to 'HIV positive' before transfer from hospital to mortuary. (iv) Bleaching powder (Sodium hypochloride solution) should be used to cover areas wherever body fluids are spilled and instruments should be heat sterilized and then put in a solution of bleaching powder. (v) Re-capping of needles should be avoided. (vi) All open wounds should be properly covered. (vii) Body should be properly carried and cremated.

Medicolegal Problems Surrounding AIDS

Apart from the diagnostic and treatment problems, AIDS has thrown up many legal and social issues. It should be kept in mind that, AIDS patients, like all other patients are entitled to equality, confidentiality, right to information etc. At the same time the doctor has the social duty of making a privileged communication in the larger interest of the society. Recently, **Supreme Court of India** has ruled that the sexual partner of an AIDS/HIV positive patient is to be informed of the fact. The treating doctor also has the duty to inform the paramedical staff involved in the treatment of such patients, the mortuary staff, pathologist and the staff of the crematorium so that due precautions can be taken by these people who are likely to come in direct contact with the infected biological material. The hospital administrators as well as the nursing officers' in-charge of safe custody of medical documents should ensure that HIV positivity is not revealed to unauthorized persons.

Admission to hospital: Although people suffering from AIDS need medical care to prolong their lives, the law does not guarantee such care. When there is no emergency, the Hospital Superintendent may decide on admission of patients taking various factors such as urgency and availability of beds into account. His unreasonable denial to admission may lead to the decision being contested on administrative law grounds as prejudiced or with gross irregularity. Also, if the patient who is turned away dies and is proved in Court of Law that his life would have been saved or prolonged by timely admission, a civil action for damages may be instituted against the hospital.

Medical Practitioners and Their Freedom to Treat

A private medical practitioner is free to decide to whom he wants to accept as a patient. The relationship between patient and doctor is the result of an agreement which often comes about on an ad hoc and tacit basis. There are a number of exceptions to the patient's freedom of choice: (i) A doctor has to treat a patient in an emergency or when no other treatment facility is available. If other medical care is available, it would not be unreasonable for the doctor to refuse treatment in case he has open wounds and it is necessary to protect him and blood to blood contact is virtually certain. Danger to oneself may become the limit of responsibility to help others; and doctors cannot be expected to treat patients with a lethal transmissible disease, if they are virtually certain to contact the disease themselves. (ii) Where the likelihood of infection is minimal, as in case of normal health care setting and where necessary precautions can be taken, it would be unreasonable for a doctor to refuse emergency treatment to an AIDS patient. (iii) Doctor cannot commence treatment and then stop when he finds the patient to be HIV positive. He can escape liability if he can show that the patient made it impossible for him to continue the treatment or if he transferred the patient, with the latter's consent, to another doctor. (iv) A doctor may be under a statutory duty to treat. However, the regulations issued in terms of the Health Act only grants the power, but does not impose duty on medical officers to examine patients in order to prevent the spread of AIDS. The medical officer will be obliged to exercise his discretion. (v) Doctors in government employment are obliged to treat all patients who consult them or are referred to them in the course of their duties. Failure to treat could lead to disciplinary action and liability for damages vicariously for the hospital or personally for the doctor. (vi) **In India** it is considered unethical for a medical practitioner to deny treatment, investigation or operation to a person infected with HIV. An enquiry can be made by the State Medical Council or Medical Council of India (now National Medical Commission) and the practitioner may be held guilty of professional misconduct on this ground. (vii) Ethical and professional guidelines of the **South African Medical and Dental Council** states that although the South African medical practitioner or dentist is under no legal obligation to accept a particular patient in his private practice (other than circumstances mentioned above) and may terminate the relationship between them if his diagnostic ability is compromised by the patient's refusal to undergo a simple investigation; such as a blood test, he should show compassion and make every effort to avoid such an impasse. (viii) **Article I of the Spanish Law** provides for special measures in matters of public health and to prevent its loss or deterioration, the health authorities or the various public administrators may within the scope of their powers, adopt the measures laid down in this law whenever medical reasons of emergency or need may so require.

Informed consent: Any medical treatment (including the taking of a blood sample) constitutes an invasion of the patient's bodily integrity, for which consent is essential, if intervention may constitute assault. (i) **United Nations HIV/AIDS and Human Rights International Guidelines** express the requirement that apart from surveillance testing and other unlinked testing done for epidemiological purposes, public health legislation should ensure that HIV testing of individuals should only be performed with specific informed consent of that individual. Exceptions to voluntary testing would need specific judicial authorization, granted only after due evaluation of the important considerations involved in terms of privacy and liberty. (ii) Person administering the test has duty of care to avoid that risk of harm by ensuing that patient understands the risk before agreeing to be tested. (iii) 'Golden standard' for HIV testing requires both pre-test and post-test counselling. A failure to perform adequate pretest counselling would ordinarily imply a lack of informed consent to any HIV test subsequently administered. To that end, it is a practice for a consent form to be signed by the patient once they have agreed to submit to an HIV test, and for that form to be retained for the protection of the doctor or counsellor. (iv) Post-test counselling is the process by which ideally, it is ensured that the test result and its implications are understood, that the person being tested has a strategy for dealing with that information in relation both to her or himself and to others who might be affected such as a spouse, and has access to any resources needed. (v) Golden standard for HIV testing requires that patients be informed face to face about the test result and not over the telephone or by a third party. (vi) **United Nations HIV/AIDS and Human Rights International Guidelines** suggest "In view of the serious nature of HIV testing and in order to maximize prevention and care, public health legislation should ensure, whenever possible that pre and post test counselling be provided in all cases." The consent cannot be said to be implied when HIV testing is included in tests undertaken routinely in some medical or surgical treatment. (vii) According to provisions of **Australian State of Tasmania** it does not stipulate the consent need be "informed". The patient should also be informed about the treatment options. If the patient is under the age of 18 years, his parents or guardian normally give consent to treatment. The Tasmanian Act goes on to provide that a medical practitioner may undertake HIV test without the consent of a person, if: (a) Person is unconscious, unable to consent and (b) Medical practitioner believes that such test is clinically necessary. (viii) **Child Care Act of South Africa** provides that when parents refuse or are not able to give their consent, the minister may give his consent. In cases of emergency where the life of the child is endangered or lasting injuries may result, the Hospital Superintendent, where child is being treated or the principal of the institution can give consent. (viii) According to **Article 10.6 of Spanish General Law of Health**, written informed consent is needed for any intervention. (ix) **American Medical Association** and the National Academy of Science Institute of Medicine also advise against mandatory testing and recommend voluntary informed consent for testing of patients in the high risk groups undergoing surgery or invasive procedures.

Marriage and professional secrecy: The relationship between a doctor and patient being sacred, the physician is expected to maintain professional secrecy, with regard to the information about the patient's condition in order to avoid discrimination. (i) A World Health Organization consultative committee has suggested that the treating doctor can override the rule to maintain professional secrecy and inform the sex partner of the HIV positive patient about his/her HIV status in the larger interest of the society. (ii) In 1995, Supreme Court was approached by HIV positive doctor who tested HIV positive in 1995 and was supposed to marry in December 1995, had to call off his marriage as the hospital where blood tests were performed had disclosed the result. It was argued by the appellant that 'duty of care' in the medical profession includes confidentiality and since this was violated by the hospital, it was liable to damages. (iii) After going into the ethics of confidentiality based on the Hippocratic Oath, and the national and international codes of medical ethics, the **Supreme Court ruled that the duty to maintain secrecy is not absolute**. It said "The argument that the respondents were under a duty to maintain confidentiality formulated by the Indian Medical Council cannot be accepted as the proposed marriage carried with it the health risk to an identifiable person who had to be protected from being infected with the communicable disease from which the applicant suffered." The argument as regards to the right to privacy was also not accepted by the Court. In addition, the Court observed that had the appellant married the lady, he could have committed offences under section 269 and 170 I.P.C. (iv) In Spain, professional secrecy is protected by several legislative measures. The Spanish constitution (Article 18.1) states that 'The right to honour, personal and family privacy and one's own image is guaranteed'. (v) According to Spanish law, failure to disclose in the case of HIV infected patient does not constitute a criminal offence. If a doctor, who is treating a seropositive health care worker, considers that there is a risk of contagion to third parties, he or she may break the oath of professional secrecy, seeking judicial protection in article 8 of the Spanish Criminal Code. (vi) **Ethical guidelines of the South African Medical and Dental Council** state that where there is a serious and identifiable risk to a specific individual who, if not informed will be exposed to HIV infection, the doctor shall consider it a duty to seek to ensure that such person is informed. As regards the legal position, AIDS and HIV infection are not notifiable diseases in South Africa. Justification for disclosure should lie in overriding public interest, such as protection of interest of third parties. If the patient who has donated blood is HIV positive, doctor should inform blood bank, as this would be in public interest. The doctor would also have the right to inform the sexual partners of the HIV positive patient, if it is evident that the patient does not follow doctor's advice to inform them and take precautions. (vii) In United States, a doctor's ethical duty to keep medical information confidential is not absolute. He may have an overriding duty towards society, when the benefits of disclosure outweigh its harm. This duty to disclose confidential medical information in appropriate circumstances is not only an ethical duty, but a legal one under public health law in US. The partner of an HIV infected person may be considered to have a right to information that is directly relevant to his/her health.

Blood transfusion: AIDS has an enormous impact on blood transfusion services because of 'window period' that is the period between contracting the HIV virus and the HIV test becoming positive. This is generally taken to be about 2-4 weeks. During this period, the blood is infective and will transmit the disease to the recipient of the blood despite the test's being negative. The WHO in association with the League of Red Cross Societies and the Red Crescent Societies initiated a 'Global Blood Safety Initiative'. They published a consensus statement on the question of AIDS in blood transfusion in March 1989 as to "Accelerated plans to recruit safer donors should include to motivate and recruit donors from low risk community groups and components should be prepared only from blood of the safest donors." This is particularly important in areas of high HIV prevalence in which the possibility of false negative tests is increased. There is universal agreement that screening of all blood, plasma, blood byproducts, donated tissues, organs and semen for HIV is necessary.

Laws and Regulations Governing HIV Infected Persons

Rights of AIDS patients: (i) **Article 21 of the constitution of India** guarantees right to life and personal liberty to every HIV positive individual and it is the fundamental right of every AIDS patient to have access to adequate treatment provided by the government. (ii) The HIV infected person also has the right to privacy which is considered as part of the right of life with human dignity. The right to privacy of a person has been stated in Article 12 of the Universal Declaration of Human Rights, Article 17 of the International Covenant on Civil and Political Rights and Article 21 of the Constitution of India. (iii) WHO guidelines state that there is no public health rationale to justify isolation, quarantine or discrimination based on a person's HIV status or sexual behaviour. (iv) Strong laws have been enacted around the world to protect the confidentiality of people who undergo HIV testing. **The United Nations HIV/AIDS and Human Rights International Guidelines** recommend "Public health legislation should ensure HIV and AIDS cases are reported to public health authorities for epidemiological purposes are subject to strict rules of data protection and confidentiality."

Confidentiality: In the **Australian State of New South Wales**, the law states that:

(i) A medical practitioner must not state the name or address of the patient (a) In a certificate sent to the Director General in relation to HIV/AIDS, or (b) Except as may be prescribed, in a written or oral communication made by medical practitioner for the purposes of arranging a test to find out whether the patient suffers from HIV/AIDS. (ii) Information about a person required to be tested or infected with HIV may be disclosed (a) With the consent of the person, or (b) In connection with the administration of this Act or another Act, or (c) By order of Court or a person authorized by law to examine witness, or (d) To a person who is involved in the provision of care to or treatment or counselling of the other person if the information is required in connection with providing such care, treatment or counselling. (iii) A medical practitioner or other person who fails to comply with the requirement of this section is guilty of an offence. Maximum penalty is 50 penalty units.

Discrimination: Discrimination is defined as 'treatment of one person less favourably than the other in the same or comparable circumstances on the basis of a characteristic that is not immediately relevant to the situation'.

(1) **Article 14 and 16 of the Indian Constitution** guarantees equality and provide against discrimination in employment respectively. Article 16 prohibits discrimination in public employment on grounds of religion, caste, creed, sex, colour etc. However, these rights are available against the state and not against private employers. There is no specific employment law that provides protection from discrimination to people living with HIV/AIDS. (ii) Laws have been enacted in every **Australian State and territory** and nationally to protect people from unwarranted discrimination on the grounds of disability and perceived disability. It is unlawful to discriminate even on the ground of a belief that a person has HIV simply because they had a test for the virus. (iii) The U.S. Department of Justice's new AIDS policy states that a person infected with the HIV virus is only protected against discrimination if he or she is able to perform the duties of the job and does not constitute a direct threat to the health or safety of others. (iv) In countries like UK, France, Germany, Spain and Netherlands, it is standard procedure for life and disability insurers to demand an HIV test when insuring a certain amount of money. Below this amount the insurers sometimes demand an HIV test on medical grounds. (v) At present, AIDS and HIV seropositive patients are uninsurable except in case of health insurance programme in Netherlands. (vi) The joint declaration made by the **WHO and the International Labour organization** stated that a worker may not be dismissed because of HIV infection and that infected people must go on working as long as they are medically capable of performing their jobs satisfactorily. (vii) It is ethical and moral to treat patients regardless of disease. American Medical Association provides that a physician shall in the provision of appropriate patient care, except in emergencies, be free to choose whom to serve. (viii) Many countries have policies that require visitors and migrants to be tested for HIV and to leave country or be refused entry if found positive. In some countries, prisoners are also being tested for HIV sero-status. Armed forces establishment argue for mandatory testing of recruits and discharge of anyone found to be HIV positive irrespective of length of service, qualifications or duties.

Medicolegal Aspects in Relation to HIV/AIDS Patient

In India:

(i) A person with HIV infection can be prosecuted under **section 269 I.P.C.** Whoever unlawfully does any act which is, and which he knows or has reason to believe to be, likely to spread the infection of any disease dangerous to life, shall be punished with imprisonment for a term which **may extend to six months, or with fine, or with both if he** performs a negligent act likely to spread the infection of the disease. (ii) If the act is willful, he may be punished under **section 270 I.P.C.** whoever negligently does an act which he knows or has reason to believe to be likely to spread the infection of any disease dangerous to life shall be punished with imprisonment of either description for a term which may extend to two years, or with fine or, with both). (iii) A civil suit under the law of tort may be filed to claim compensation for violation of the fundamental rights to personal liberty.

Criminal liability for transmitting AIDS by sexual intercourse: (i) When a person knows that he is suffering from the virus and also knows how it is spread: (a) Intentionally have sexual intercourse in order to infect the other person from fatal disease (and the person dies) (b) Has sexual intercourse with another person/persons not caring whether or not they contract the disease and one or more of his sex partners contract disease and die, is held guilty of murder **(S. 302 I.P.C.).** (ii) Criminal liability of person in high risk AIDS group such as male homosexuals, prostitutes who (a) Knows AIDS and how it is spread (b) Is HIV positive or in fact has AIDS, but is genuinely unaware of the fact and (c) Has done nothing to ascertain whether or not he has AIDS, nor does he take any precaution in his sexual activity and who transmits AIDS to his sex partners who become infected and die, held guilty of manslaughter/culpable homicide **(S. 299 I.P.C.).** (iii) Accused can be prosecuted under S. 44 I.P.C., S. 440 I.P.C. (punished for fraud, deceit or mispresentation), 320 I.P.C. (The accused can be prosecuted under the 8th clause) S. 304-A I.P.C., even if the accused did not know that he has AIDS or that AIDS is incurable and fatal he may be charged under this section.

Civil liability for transmitting AIDS by sexual intercourse: The patient can be held liable for: (i) Negligence (ii) Battery (iii) Intentional infliction of physical harm or emotional distress (iv) Fraud.

Outside India:

(i) An accused in Lafayette, Indiana, US suffering from AIDS tried to commit suicide. Three risk workers stopped him but he beat and scratched the risk workers. He was found guilty of attempted murder (**Cape Times 15 Jan 1988).** (ii) **First criminal law in the World on AIDS:** According to Louisiana state legislation, "A person who intentionally exposes another to the AIDS virus through sexual contact without the knowledge or lawful consent of the victim is guilty of an offence and liable of conviction to a fine of not more than 5000 dollar and/or imprisonment with or without hard labour for not more than 10 years (**Louisiana Act, 663 of 1987**).

Important Case Discussions in Relation to AIDS

(i) Earliest civil case for transmitting a venereal disease was in 1878, the Irish case **Hegarty vs Shine**, Hegarty sued her lover for battery for having infected her with venereal disease. She lost the case. Court held that *exturpicausa non iritur actio* (from a base or immoral action no legal cause will be upheld by the court), the fact that defendant concealed the fact that he suffered from venereal disease did not affect the judgement. (ii) **RV Clarins 1888 22 QBD 23:** In the above case the man knowingly transmitted venereal disease to the wife but was not found guilty of assault. Court held that wife's ignorance for her husband's disease would not affect her consent for sexual intercourse. This is an old case and it is doubtful if the courts will still follow the same ruling. (iii) **Crowel vs Crowel** 1920, a US court held that a wife whose husband has wrongfully infected her with a venereal disease may obtain damages from her husband.

Defences Which the Accused May Raise

The following discussion is best on actual defences raised by the accused in the recent cases: (i) Defence constitutional right to privacy barring any investigation by the court. Many US courts have faced an objection by the defendants. The investigations into matters of marriage, etc. an invasion of the constitutional right of privacy. But the courts held that: (a) No duty on the part of the defendant to disclose the fact that he is infected with the disease can be held (b) No one acquires a right of action by his own wrong. This defence has not been sustained in the court. (ii) *Volenti non fit injuria:* In cases of AIDS a defence of consent may be sustained. (iii) Contributory negligence. (iv) *Defence taken by the husband:* That the wife had given unconditional consent for sexual intercourse at the time of marriage.

COVID-19

Introduction

Coronavirus disease 2019 (COVID-19) caused by severe acute respiratory syndrome coronavirus-2 (SARS-CoV-2). The first case was reported at Wuhan, China in a market worker who was admitted to hospital on 26 December 2019 with severe pneumonia and respiratory failure. On 31 December, 2019, the China health authority informed the World Health Organisation (WHO) regarding reports of several cases of pneumonia of unknown aetiology in the same city. Then it spread rapidly to the other part of China and other countries. The Ministry of Health and Family Welfare (MOHFW), Government of India reported first confirmed case of SARS-CoV-2 infection in India on 30 January, 2020 in Kerala's Thrissur district in a student who had returned home for a vacation from Wuhan University in China. On 30 January, the WHO declared COVID-19 to be a Public Health Emergency of International Concern. On 11 March, 2020, the WHO declared Covid-19 outbreak as a pandemic worldwide.

The SARS CoV-2 Virus

The SARS CoV-2 virus (initially known as 2019 novel coronavirus/2019-nCoV), belongs to corona virus group (genus-Beta coronavirus), single stranded RNA virus, with a crown due to the presence of spike glycoproteins on the envelope. It shares 79% genome sequence identity with SARS-CoV and 50% with MERS-CoV. There are many genetic variants of SARS CoV-2 virus identified, e.g., Alpha, Beta, Delta, Gamma, Eta, Theta, Kappa, Epsilon etc. According to WHO, the variants Alpha (B.1.1.7), Beta (B.1.351, B.1.351.2, B.1351.3), Gamma (P.1, P.1.1, P.1.2) and Delta (B.1.617.2, AY.1, AY.2**) Omicron (B.1.1.529) are designated as a 'variant of concern'.** Genetic evidence suggests that SARS-CoV-2 is a natural virus that likely originated in animals, However, there is no conclusion yet about when and where the virus first entered humans.

Modes of Transmission

It is a highly infectious virus which has the ability to establish sustained human-to-human transmission. The virus is primarily transmitted between people through respiratory droplets and contact routes (both direct and indirect). Its basic reproductive number (R0), i.e., the number of secondary infections generated from one infected individual, is estimated to be between 1.4 and 6.49, with a mean of 3.28.

Prevention of COVID-19 Transmission

Preventive measures for COVID-19 transmission via respiratory droplets include physical distancing, community use of well-fitting masks (e.g., barrier face coverings, procedure/surgical masks), adequate ventilation, and avoidance of crowded indoor spaces. Spread of virus through contact routes can be prevented by practicing good hand hygiene and environmental cleaning.

Pathogenesis

The SARS CoV-2 virus enters to the respiratory tract through inhalation. Early in the infection, it targets nasal and bronchial epithelial cells and pneumocytes, through the viral structural spike (S) protein that binds to the angiotensin-converting enzyme 2 (ACE2) receptor. The virus then enters the cell cytoplasm, where it releases RNA genome and replicates, resulting in the formation of new viral particles. The virus propagates and migrates down the respiratory tract along the conducting airways. SARS-CoV-2 infects pulmonary capillary endothelial cells, accentuating the inflammatory response and triggering an influx of monocytes and neutrophils. This presentation activates both innate and adaptive immunity causing the production of large amounts of pro-inflammatory cytokines and chemokines that aggravates interstitial pneumonia and acute respiratory distress syndrome (ARDS). In some patients, this activation becomes so massive that cytokine storm develops, resulting in thrombotic tendency and multi-organ failure, and eventually causing death.

Diagnosis

History: History of exposure to someone confirmed or suspected to have Covid -19.

Symptoms: The commonly reported symptoms include fever or chills, cough, shortness of breath or difficulty breathing, new loss of taste or smell, sore throat, myalgias, nasal congestion or runny nose, nausea, vomiting, diarrhoea, fatigue, headache.

Laboratory: There can be lymphopenia, thrombocytopenia, elevated liver enzymes, ↑ LDH, ↑ inflammatory markers (e.g., C-reactive protein, ferritin) and ↑ inflammatory cytokines (IL-6, TNF alpha), ↑ D-dimer (>1 mcg/ml), ↑ prothrombin time (PT), ↑ troponin, ↑ creatine phosphokinase (CPK).

Radiological: Chest X-Ray: Consolidation followed by ground glass opacity (GGO) are the most common findings. Pleural effusion can also be observed**. CT chest** may be considered as the first-line imaging test for detecting COVID-19 pneumonia. GGO in combination with reticular and/or interlobular septal thickening and consolidation are characterstic features observed in a CT chest.

Molecular Diagnosis: (i) **RT-PCR** is a highly sensitive and specific method which detects viral RNA. It is used as the gold standard for SARS CoV-2 diagnosis. The preferred samples for this test are nasopharyngeal and throat swabs as well as lower respiratory samples. However, the results are variable and there is scope of false negatives owing to either sampling errors or due to usage of different primers and reagents by different vendors. (ii) **Rapid antigen test** (sometimes known as a rapid diagnostic test – RDT) detects of viral antigens (spike protein and nucleocapsid being target antigens). The samples are collected from the nose and/or throat with a swab. It is a cheaper and quick method than RT-PCR, however less accurate than RT-PCR. (iii) **Viral isolation with culture:** Detection of the virus by its cytopathic effects on cell lines is highly limited, as the procedure requires bio-safety level-3 facility. (iv) **Antibody estimation** by immuno-chromatography and ELISA methods is helpful in determination of past infection. This test cannot be used for diagnosis of Covid-19 in the early stages of infection or disease. However, false positive report is due to cross reactive antibodies against other HCoVs. A false negative test does not rule out SARS CoV-2 infection.

Autopsy on Covid-19 Deaths

The pathobiology of the disease largely remains unknown. Hence, autopsy on suspected or confirmed COVID-19 infection particularly in the presence of several comorbidities, can ascertain the exact cause(s) of death, optimize clinical management, and assist clinicians in pointing out a timely and effective treatment to reduce mortality.

Precautions: SARS-CoV2 is a microorganism categorized as Hazard Group 3. Necessary safety measures should be taken during autopsy procedures, during specimen collection and handling, to prevent occupational transmission of this infectious pathogens. To exclude or confirm Covid-19, before postmortem nasal and oral swabs can be tested by RT-PCR. (i) An autopsy room conforming to BSL 3 standards would be ideal but is not mandatory. (ii) Adequate ventilation in autopsy room is required. (iii) The dead body should be handled by trained staff. (iv) The staffs should maintain high standard of personal hygiene and wear personal protective equipment (PPE). (v) Avoid direct contact with blood and body fluids. (vi) Any aerosol producing procedures should be avoided. (vii) Any electric bone saws used should have a vacuum that isolates aerosolised particles. (viii) In case, autopsy is essential medicolegally, it should be done under strict precautionary measures. (ix) Minimally invasive autopsy-by biopsy and partial autopsy can be done. (x) Embalming should be avoided in Covid-19 deaths.

Gross findings: (i) *Lungs:* Heavy and boggy, patchy as well as diffuse consolidation along with pleural fibrinous exudate and/or fibrosis, sometimes with purulent inflammation due to secondary bacterial infection with/without evidence of pericarditis (Hanley *et al.* 2020).

Microscopic findings: Maiese *et al.* (2021) systematically reviewed the autopsy findings in Covid-19 and found that the major histological feature in the lung is diffuse alveolar damage with hyaline membrane formation, alongside microthrombi in small pulmonary vessels. There is also a high incidence of deep vein thrombosis and pulmonary embolism, suggesting endothelial involvement, but more studies are needed.

Medicolegal Autopsy on Covid-19 Deaths

A. **Standard Guidelines for Medicolegal Autopsy in Covid-19 Deaths in India by ICMR:** (i) The deaths in hospital and under medical care due to Covid-19 are non-medicolegal cases. The certification for cause of death in these cases can be done by the treating doctor. Hence, no medicolegal postmortem is required. (ii) Some of the cases of suspected Covid-19 death which are brought dead to the hospital, labelled by emergency doctor as medicolegal case (MLC) and police is informed. These cases may need postmortem examination for clarity of the cause of death and to differentiate between MLC and Non-MLC case. The Forensic autopsy of these cases may be waived off. (iii) **Autopsy on MLC cases**: During autopsy of cases which are homicidal/accidental/suicidal with Covid-19 positive or suspected Covid-19 positive, invasive postmortem procedures should be avoided. In these cases, multiple photographs of the body should be taken and general examination, external examination, cloth examination, verbal autopsy (as depicted by WHO) should be done to find out cause of death.

B. **Covid-19: Guidelines on Dead Body Management by MOHFW, Government of India:** The guideline mentions how to disposed of dead body of a suspect or confirmed case of COVID-19 and standard and standard precautions to be followed by health care workers while handing dead bodies of Covid-19. Salient features are: (i) There is unlikely to be an increased risk of COVID infection from a dead body to health workers or family members who follow standard precautions while handling body. (ii) Only the lungs of dead COVID patients, if handled during an autopsy, can be infectious. (iii) Autopsies should be avoided. If autopsy is to be performed for special reasons like in MLC cases, the following infection prevention control practices should be adopted (a) The Team should be well trained in infection prevention control practices (b) The number of forensic experts and support staff in the autopsy room should be limited (c) The Team should use full complement of PPE (coveralls, head cover, shoe cover, N 95 mask, goggles / face shield) (d) Round ended scissors should be used (d) PM40 or any other heavy duty blades with blunt end points to be used to reduce prick injuries (e) Only one body cavity at a time should be dissected (f) Unfixed organs must be held firm on the table and sliced with a sponge–care should be taken to protect the hand (g) Negative pressure to be maintained in mortuary. An oscillator saw with suction extraction of the bone aerosol into a removable chamber should be used for sawing skull, otherwise a hand saw with a chain-mail glove may be used (h) Needles should not be re-sheathed after fluid sampling–needles and syringes should be placed in a sharps bucket (i) Reduce aerosol generation during autopsy using appropriate techniques especially while handling lung tissue (j) After the procedure, body should be disinfected with 1% Sodium hypochlorite and placed in a body bag, the exterior of which will again be decontaminated with 1% Sodium hypochlorite solution (k) The body thereafter can be handed over to the relatives (l) Autopsy table to be disinfected as per standard protocol.

Dead bodies should be stored in cold chambers maintained at approximately 4°C. Embalming of dead body should not be allowed.

Autopsy on Deaths Following Covid-19 Vaccination

Vaccines are not entirely without risk and adverse reactions including death may occur following vaccination. Few deaths have been reported following Covid-19 vaccination. In case of alleged deaths following vaccination, investigation should be done meticulously as per Adverse Events Following Immunization **(AEFI) guidelines** issued by the Ministry of Health and Family Welfare (MOHFW), Government of India. (i) Postmortem examination of such cases should be carried out at the nearest medical college or district hospital by a forensic expert and pathologist. (ii) The process of postmortem examination (external and internal) should be videographed. (iii) The tissues samples (viscera) should be sent for histopathogical examination in all cases and for toxicological analysis in specific cases to the designated medical college/forensic science laboratory for analysis and followed up for early submission of reports. (iv) The autopsy should be performed as soon as possible (within 72 hours) to avoid tissue damage, development of postmortem artefacts and lysis of the adrenal glands, which can alter diagnosis.

Other laboratory test: Femoral vein blood (serum) can be tested for tryptase, Anti-PEG antibodies, total immunoglobulin E (IgE), the inflammatory markers interleukin-6 and C-reactive protein (CRP) as well as complement activity C3/C5.

Apart from routine organs, histological examinations of the injection site, pharyngeal mucosa, the spleen, regionally draining lymph nodes, especially axillary, and the deltoid muscle should be performed.

Medicolegal Aspects of COVID-19 Pandemic in India

1. **The Epidemic Disease (Amendment) Ordinance, 2020**

   The ordinance amends the Epidemic Diseases Act, 1897 with aim to provide for the better prevention of the spread of Covid-19 in India. The act provides protections for health care personnel combatting epidemic diseases. **S. 3 (2,3)**, The Ordinance specifies that no person shall (i) commit or abet the commission of an act of violence against a health care service personnel, or (ii) Abet or cause damage or loss to any property during an epidemic. Contravention of this provision is punishable with imprisonment for a term which is not less than 3 months, but which may extend to 5 years and with fine between Rs 50,000 and two lakh rupees. If an act of violence against a health care service personnel causes grievous harm, the person committing the offence will be punishable with imprisonment between six months and seven years, and a fine between one lakh rupees and five lakh rupees. These offences are cognizable and non-bailable.

   The act expands the powers of the Central Government to prevent the spread of such diseases. Section 2 of the Epidemic Act empowers the State Government to take suitable temporary measures to prevent an outbreak or threatened outbreak or spread of an epidemic. Section 4 gives legal protection to every person who has acted under this Act or the directions issued under this Act subject to only one condition that the act must have been done in good faith.

   S. 144 Cr. P.C.: States may issue orders by invoking Section 144 of Cr.P.C., 1973 to restrict public gatherings and impose a curfew. Violation of orders under section 144 Cr.P.C. is also punishable under S. 188 I.P.C.

   S. 188 I.P.C. prescribes punishment of upto 6 months and fine of up to Rs. 1,000 for not following government orders.

   S. 269 I.P.C. prescribes punishment of upto 6 months, or with fine, or with both for negligent or unlawful act of a person which he knows or has reason to believe to be likely to spread the infection of any diseases dangerous to life.

   S. 270 I.P.C. prescribes punishment of upto two years, or with fine, or with both for malignant act of a person which

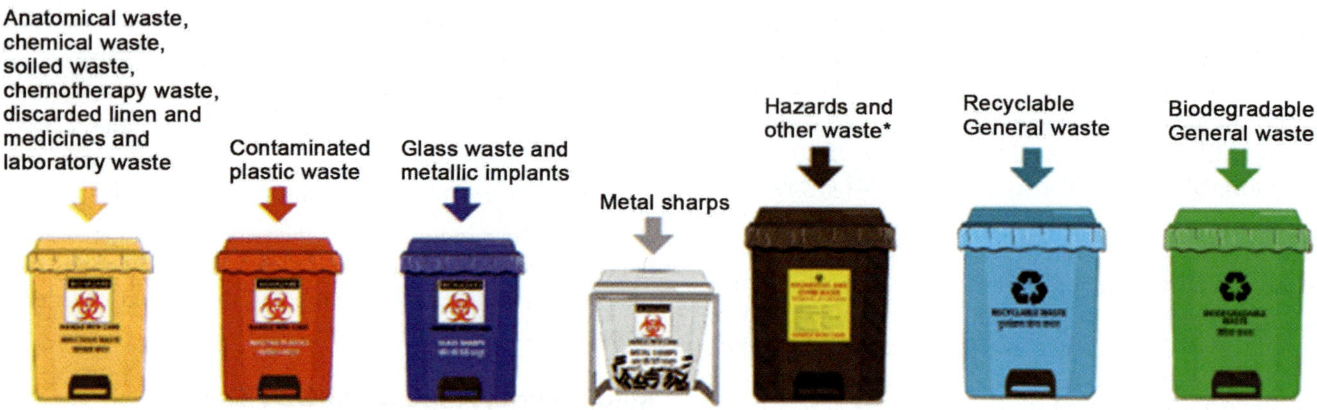

Figure 30.1: Colour coded containers for biomedical waste disposal

he knows or has reason to believe to be likely to spread the infection of any diseases dangerous to life.

S. 271 I.P.C. prescribes punishment upto 6 months, or with fine, or with both for disobedience to quarantine rule.

2. **The Disaster Management Act, 2005**

The Act provides power to Central Government and national disaster management authority (NDMA) for effective management of disaster. On March 14, the Central Government termed COVID-19 as a 'notified disaster' as a "critical medical condition or pandemic situation". The Act enables the Centre and States to enforce a lockdown and restrict public movement. It allows the Government to get access to the National Disaster Response Fund, the State Disaster Response Fund and the District Disaster Response Fund. The Act has provisions for allocation of resources for prevention, mitigation, capacity building etc. The Act also being used to control the circulation of fake news about the pandemic. There is provision of penalties for specific offences under sections 51 to 60 of the Act.

3. **Biomedical Waste Management Rules, 2016 (Amendment 2018, 2019)**

This rule provides the framework of the management and handling of disposal and scientific management of biomedical waste. In wake of the COVID-19 pandemic, the Centre Pollution Control Board (**CPCB**) and the Ministry of Health and Family Welfare (**MoHFW**) issued various guidelines for handling, treatment and safe disposal of BM Waste generated during treatment, diagnosis and quarantine of patients confirmed or suspected to have COVID-19. The biomedical waste should be discarded in colour coded containers (Figure 30.1)

4. **Practice of Telemedicine**

Before 25, March 2020, the practice of telemedicine was not legal India. Due to emergence of the COVID-19 pandemic, The Board of Governors of the Medical Council of India allowed telemedicine practice and issued guidelines for its use. On 9 August, 2020 the Government of India introduced its telemedicine service, *eSanjeevani*, as part of its 'Digital India' initiative.

LONG QUESTIONS

1. Discuss the medicolegal as well as ethical issues of AIDS.
2. Discuss pathogenesis, autopsy findings and medicolegal aspects of Covid-19.

MULTIPLE CHOICE QUESTIONS

1. **A person introduces HIV infected needle to another with intent to spread the disease. He may be charged under section:**
   (a) 269 I.P.C. (b) 270 I.P.C.
   (c) 279 I.P.C. (d) 302 I.P.C.

2. **A man suffering from AIDS knowingly transmits the infection to a woman, would be guilty under:**
   (a) 268 I.P.C. (b) 270 I.P.C.
   (c) 271 I.P.C. (d) 274 I.P.C.

3. **A person deliberately introduces COVID-19 virus infection to another with intent to spread the disease. He may be charged under section:**
   (a) 269 I.P.C. (b) 270 I.P.C.
   (c) 279 I.P.C. (d) 302 I.P.C.

4. **Disobedience to quarantine rule is punishable under section:**
   (a) 271 I.P.C. (b) 270 I.P.C.
   (c) 279 I.P.C. (d) 273 I.P.C.

ANSWER KEY

1. (b)	2. (b)	3. (b)	4. (a)

31 CHAPTER

Sexual Offences

Sexual Violence: The World Health Organization (WHO) defines Sexual Violence as "any sexual act, attempt to obtain a sexual act, unwanted sexual comments/advances and acts to traffic, or otherwise directed against a person's sexuality, using coercion, threats of harm, or physical force, by any person regardless of relationship to the victim in any setting, including but not limited to home and work".

Sexual Assault: A form of sexual violence, is a term **often used synonymously with rape**. However, sexual assault could include anything from touching another person's body in a sexual way without the person's consent to forced sexual intercourse–oral and anal sexual acts, child molestation, fondling and attempted rape.

Sexual Offences are the acts of sexual intercourse and/or sexual interference with a person or animal against the provisions of law. These can be classified as:

1. ***Natural offences:*** It includes those offences which are committed *in order of nature*, i.e., penis-vaginal sexual intercourse. (i) Rape (ii) Incest (iii) Adultery
2. ***Unnatural offences:*** It includes offences which are committed *against the order of nature*, i.e., sexual intercourse other than penis-vaginal. (i) Sodomy (ii) Buccal or oral coitus (iii) Tribadism/Lesbianism (iv) Bestiality.
3. ***Sexual perversions (Paraphilias)*** are conditions in which sexual excitement or orgasm is associated with acts or imagery that are considered unusual within the culture (i) Exhibitionism (ii) Frortteurism (iii) Pedophilia (iv)Voyeurism (v) Sexual Sadism (vi) Sexual Masochism (vii) Fetishism (viii) Transvestism (ix) Other specified paraphilias.
4. ***Other sex related crimes*:** (i) Indecent assault (iii) Sexual harassment (iii) Immoral trafficking such as kidnapping, prostitution, etc.

Earlier, rape was only considered as natural sexual offences. As per Criminal Law Amendment Act, 2013, the definition of rape widened to include all forms of forceful sexual violence–penetrative by penis (oral, anal, vaginal, urethral), by objects/weapons/fingers (vagina, urethra or anus) and non-penetrative (touching, fondling, etc.). Hence, sexual offences (natural/unnatural/perversions) fall under the definition of rape.

RAPE

The word 'rape' originates from the Latin word *"rapere"* that means to seize or take away by force. In Latin, the term for rape is **raptus**. Originally, the word rape was simulated with the words such as *rapine*, *rapture*, *rapacious* and *raptor* that were referred to the general violations. In antiquity the word rape was used for violence against some person. Rape is a crime where the victim is forced into sexual activity particularly sexual penetration without her will or consent. Article 21 of the Indian Constitution guarantees the right to life and liberty. In the common law of the United Kingdom, Australia and the United States, 'rape' traditionally describes the act of a man who forces a woman to have sexual intercourse with him. Until the late 20th century, forced sex by a husband against his wife was not considered 'rape', since a woman (for certain purposes) was not considered a separate legal person with the right of refusal, or sometimes was deemed to have given advanced consent to a lifelong sexual relationship through the wedding vows. However, most Western countries have now legislated against this exception. They now include spousal rape (vaginal intercourse), and acts of sexual violence, such as forced anal intercourse in their definitions of 'rape'.

In English law, the legal definition of rape relates to nonconsensual penile penetration of the mouth, anus, or vagina. A new offence of assault by penetration has been recently created to cover nonconsensual penetration of the anus or genitalia by an object or a body part; this new offence has the same maximum sentence as rape. In Scotland, nonconsensual penile-vaginal penetration is defined by common law, as "carnal knowledge of a female by a male against her will". The changes also made rape punishable with a maximum sentence of life imprisonment. Some American states define all penetrative acts as sexual assaults subcategorized by the degree of force and coercion used. The legal interpretation of 'vaginal penetration' refers to penetration of the labia and does not require that penis actually enter the vagina. The age at which a female can legally give consent for penile-vaginal intercourse in England is 16 years, whereas in California it is 18 years same as in India.

The statute in California also includes a new sexual crime, called "assault by penetration", which also has the same punishment as rape, and is committed when someone sexually penetrates the anus or vagina with a part of his or her body, or with an object, without that person's consent.

'Rape' as a clearly defined offence was first introduced in the Indian Penal Code in 1860. Prior to this, there were often diverse and conflicting laws prevailing across India. There have been several piecemeal amendments to the IPC, but it hasn't been reformed in any way. The brutal gang rape and murder of **Nirbhaya** in 2012 shook the nation's consciousness like no other. The Central Government constituted a judicial committee headed by Justice J.S. Verma, a former Chief Justice of India to suggest amendments to criminal law to sternly deal with sexual assault cases. Considering the justice Verma's committee report, the policy makers made amendments to criminal law and came up with stringent punishment in rape and sexual assault cases. On 3 February, 2013, **The Criminal Law (Amendment) Act, 2013 (Nirbhaya Act)** became effective which widened the scope and definition of rape. Subsequently, it was amended in 2018.

LAWS IN RELATION TO RAPE IN INDIA

S. 375 of the Indian Penal Code defines rape:

A man is said to commit '**rape**' if he:

(a) Penetrates his **penis**, to any extent, into **vagina**, **mouth**, **urethra** or **anus** of a woman or makes her to do so with him or any other person; or

(b) Inserts, to any extent, any **object** or a **part of body,** not being the penis, into the **vagina**, the **urethra** or **anus** of a woman or makes her to do so with him or any other person; or

(c) **Manipulates any part of the body** of a woman so as **to cause penetration** into the **vagina**, **urethra**, **anus**, or **any part of body of such woman**, or makes her to do so with him or any other person; or

(d) **Applies his mouth to vagina, anus, urethra** of a woman or makes her to do so with him or any other person.

Under the circumstances falling, under any of the following seven descriptions:

Firstly: Against her **will**.

Secondly: Without her **consen**t.

Thirdly: With her consent, when her consent has been obtained by putting her or any person in whom she is interested, in fear of death or hurt.

Fourthly: With her consent, when the man knows that he is not her husband and that her consent is given because she believes that he is another man to whom she is or believes herself to be lawfully married.

Fifthly: With her consent, when, at the time of giving such consent, by reason of unsoundness of mind or intoxication or the administration by him personally or through another of any stupefying or unwholesome substance, she is unable to understand the nature and consequences of that to which she gives consent.

Sixthly: **With or without her consent, when she is under 18 years of age**.

Seventhly: When she is unable to communicate consent.

Explanation 1: For purposes of this section, **vagina shall also include labia majora**.

Explanation 2: **Consent means** an unequivocal voluntary agreement when the woman by words, gestures or any form of non-verbal communication, communicates willingness to participate in the specific act.

Provided that a woman who does not physically resist to the act of penetration shall not by the reason only of that fact, be regarded as consenting to sexual activity.

*Exception 1: **A medical procedure or intervention shall not constitute rape**.*

Exception 2: **Sexual intercourse or sexual acts by a man with his own wife, the wife not being under 15 years of age, is not rape.**

Further Explanation: The "will" and "consent" are two different attributes. Every act done against the will of a person is done without consent also but an act done without consent is not necessarily against the will. For example, sexual intercourse with an unconscious woman is without her consent but cannot be said to be against her will. A girl under 18 years of age cannot give valid consent for sexual act, but it cannot be said to have occurred against her will. Submission does not necessarily mean consent but consent involves submission. The sexual intercourse should be against her will, wish or desire. Whether the alleged consent is merely a passive submission or willing consent depends upon the circumstances of each case.

Age of giving consent for sexual intercourse is 18 years in India. Consent must be obtained prior to the act. Consent after the act is no defence. Even a prostitute cannot be forced to have sexual intercourse. Consent is not valid if taken by fraud or force. Presumption and proof of consent can be presumed from the circumstances of each case. The only evidence of lack of consent is various signs of struggle found on the person of the victim. It is necessary to prove that maximum resistance was offered to prevent the act. Resistance depends upon the type of woman, built, age etc. **The burden of proof lies on the accused**. Prosecution has to prove all elements for the offence. In most of the cases no signs of injury or intoxication are there and the sexual act is based on fraud and fear.

Further explanation provided to the section states that slightest vulval penetration, even touching of penis with vulva constitute the offence of rape, whereas the exception leaves out marital rape altogether if the wife is not under 15 years of age. In **R vs. R, the House of Lords** widened the scope of criminal liability by declaring that the husband could be charged as a principal offender in the rape of his wife. This decision seems to have obliterated the protection of the husband from such prosecution under the doctrine of marital exemption. This exemption was based upon the belief under which the wife was regarded as the husbands' chattel. She was supposed to have given a general consent to her husband as a natural implication of the marriage. This has now become an outdated view of marriage in England.

However, the above decision of the House of Lords has not been followed in India where marital exemption to the husband still exists.

There is considerable debate as to what constitutes proper and complete consent in a sexual relationship. How explicit should consent be, how often should it be established, and what constitutes diminished capacity (usually due to drugs or alcohol) are all subjects of some disagreement. These debates take place both on moral and ethical grounds, and as a legal issue, since rape can only be convicted as a crime with intent in many jurisdictions, and the erroneous belief of consent is a common defence.

S. 376: Punishment for rape (Table 31.1)

(1) *Whoever, except in the cases* provided for by sub-section (2), commits rape, shall be punished with imprisonment of either

Table 31.1: Punishment for rape

I.P.C. section	Type of rape	Punishment
376(1)	Rape of a woman ≥ **18 years**	≥10 years imprisonment, but may extend to imprisonment for life, and shall also be liable to fine.
376(2)	Rape in custody, rape by relative or guardian or teacher or a person in a position of trust or authority, rape during communal or sectarian violence, rape of a pregnant woman or woman with mental/physical disability or woman incapable of giving consent, repeated rape of same woman, rape causing grievous bodily harm or maims or disfigures or endangers the life of a woman etc.	≥10 years imprisonment, but may extend to imprisonment for life which means remainder of person's natural life and shall also be liable to fine.
376(3)	Rape of a girl **<16 years**	≥ 20 years imprisonment, but may extend to imprisonment for life which means remainder of person's natural life and shall also be liable to fine.
376AB	Rape of a girl **<12 years**	≥ 20 years imprisonment, but may extend to imprisonment for life which means remainder of person's natural life and shall also be liable to fine or with **death**
376A	Rape resulted in persistent vegetative state or causing death	≥ 20 years imprisonment, but may extend to imprisonment for life which means remainder of person's natural life and shall also be liable to fine or with **death**
376B	Sexual intercourse by husband upon with his wife during separation without her consent	Imprisonment between 2 and 7 years and shall also be liable to fine.
376C	Sexual intercourse by person in authority (not amounting to the offence of rape)	Imprisonment between 5 and 10 years and shall also be liable to fine.
376D	Gang rape	≥ 20 years imprisonment, but may extend to imprisonment for life which means remainder of person's natural life and shall also be liable to fine.
376DA	Gang rape of a girl **<16 years**	Imprisonment for life which means imprisonment for remainder of person's natural life and shall also be liable to fine.
376DB	Gang rape of a girl **<12 years**	Imprisonment for life which means imprisonment for remainder of person's natural life and shall also be liable to fine or with **death**.
376E	Repeat offenders	Imprisonment for life which means imprisonment for remainder of person's natural life and shall also be liable to fine or with **death**.

description for a term which shall **not be less than 10 years but which may extend to imprisonment for life, and shall also be liable to fine.**

(2) *Whoever,*

(a) Being a **police officer**, commits rape:

(i) Within the limits of the police station to which such police officer is appointed; or

(ii) In the premises of any station house; or

(iii) On a woman in such police officer's custody or in the custody of a police officer subordinate to such police officer; or

(b) Being a public servant, commits rape on a woman in such public servants' custody or in the custody of a public servant subordinate to such public servant; or

(c) Being a **member of the armed forces** deployed in the area by the central or state government commits rape in such area; or

(d) Being on the **management or on the staff of a jail, remand home or other place of custody** established by or under any law for the time being in force or of a women's or children's institution, commits rape on any inmate of such jail, remand home, place or institution; or

(e) Being on the **management or the staff of a hospital,** commits rape on a woman in that hospital; or

(f) Being a **relative, guardian or teacher of, or a person in a position of trust or authority** towards the woman, commits rape on such a woman; or

(g) Commits rape **during communal or sectarian violence**; or

(h) Commits rape on a **woman knowing her to be pregnant**; or

*(i) -----------

(j) Commits rape, on a **woman incapable of giving consent**; or

(k) **Being in a position of control or dominance** over a woman, commits a rape on such a woman; or

(l) Commits rape on a **woman suffering from mental or physical disability**; or

(m) While committing **rape causes grievous bodily harm or maims or disfigures or endangers the life of a woman**; or

(n) Commits rape **repeatedly on the same woman**

shall be punished with rigorous imprisonment for a term which shall **not be less than 10 years** but **which may extend to imprisonment of life, which shall mean imprisonment for the reminder** of **that person's natural life and shall also be liable to fine.**

*Clause (i) omitted by Act 22 of 2018, before omission, clause (i) read as–Commits rape on a woman when she is under 16 years of age.

(3) *Whoever,* commits rape on a woman **under 16 years** of age shall be punished with rigorous imprisonment for a term which shall not be **less than 20 years, but which may extend to imprisonment for life, which shall mean imprisonment for remainder of that person's natural life, and also liable for fine.**

Provided that such fine shall be just and reasonable to meet the medical expenses and rehabilitation of the victim. Provided further that any fine imposed under this section shall be paid to the victim.

S. 376AB: Punishment for rape of woman under 12 years of age: Whoever, commits rape on a woman under **12 years** of age shall be punished with rigorous imprisonment for a term which shall not be **less than 20 years, but which may extend to imprisonment for life, which shall mean imprisonment for the remainder of that person's natural life, and with fine or with death:** Such fine shall be paid to the victim and shall be used for medical expenses and rehabilitation of the victim.

Provided that such fine shall be just and reasonable to meet the medical expenses and rehabilitation of the victim. Provided further that any fine imposed under this section shall be paid to the victim.

S. 376A: Punishment for causing death or resulting in persistent vegetative state of the victim: Whoever, commits an offence punishable under sub-section (1) or sub-section (2) of section 376 and in the course of such commission inflicts an injury which causes the death or causes the woman to be in a persistent vegetative state, shall be punishable with rigorous imprisonment for a term which **shall not be less than 20 years**, but which may extend to **imprisonment for life**, which shall mean **imprisonment for the remainder of that person's natural life, or with death.**

S. 376B: Sexual intercourse by husband upon with his wife during separation: Whoever has sexual intercourse with his own wife, who is living separately, whether under a decree of separation or otherwise, without her consent shall be punished with imprisonment of either description for a term which shall **not be less than 2 years** but which may **extend to 7 years** and shall also be liable to fine.

S. 376C: Sexual intercourse by person in authority: Whoever, being:

(a) In a position of authority or in a fiduciary relationship; or

(b) A public servant; or

(c) Superintendent or manager of a jail, remand home or other place of custody established by or under any law for the time being in force, or a women's or children's institution; or

(d) On the management of a hospital or being on the staff of a hospital.

Abuses such position or fiduciary relationship to induce or seduce any woman either in his custody or under his charge or present in the premises to have sexual intercourse with him, such **sexual intercourse not amounting to the offence of rape, shall be punished with rigorous imprisonment** of either description for a term which shall **not be less than 5 years**, but which may **extend to 10 years** and shall also be liable to fine.

S. 376D: Gang Rape: Where, a woman is raped by one or more persons constituting a group or acting in furtherance of a common intention, each of those persons shall be deemed to have committed the offence of rape being the superintendent or manager of a jail, remand home or other place of custody established by or under and shall be punished with rigorous imprisonment for a term which shall **not be less than 20 years**, but which **may extend to life**, which shall mean imprisonment for the remainder of that person's natural life and with fine.

Provided that such fine shall be just and reasonable to meet the medical expenses and rehabilitation of the victim. Provided further that any fine imposed under this section shall be paid to the victim.

S. 376DA: Punishment for gang rape on woman under 16 years of age: Where a woman under 16 years of age is raped by one or more persons constituting a group or acting in furtherance of a common intention, each of those persons shall be deemed to have committed the offence of rape and shall be punished with **imprisonment for life, which shall mean imprisonment for the remainder of that person's natural life, and with fine**.

Provided that such fine shall be just and reasonable to meet the medical expenses and rehabilitation of the victim. Provided further that any fine imposed under this section shall be paid to the victim.

S. 376DB: Punishment for gang rape on woman under 12 years of age: Where a woman under 12 years of age is raped by one or more persons constituting a group or acting in furtherance of a common intention, each of those persons shall be deemed to have committed the offence of rape and shall be punished with **imprisonment for life, which shall mean imprisonment for the remainder of that person's natural life, and with fine or with death**.

Provided that such fine shall be just and reasonable to meet the medical expenses and rehabilitation of the victim. Provided further that any fine imposed under this section shall be paid to the victim.

S. 376E: Punishment for repeated offenders: Whoever has been previously convicted for an offence punishable under sections 376 or 376A or 376AB or 376D or 376DA or 376DB and is subsequently convicted of an offence punishable under any of the said sections shall be punished with **imprisonment for life, which shall mean imprisonment for the remainder of that person's natural life**, or **with death**.

DEBATABLE POINTS IN LAW

There are a few points in the law, which are open to debate. Sexual intercourse by a man with his own wife, where the wife is over 15 years of age, where the age of marriage being 18 years is not rape. Sexual intercourse in a custodial situation is deemed an offence (policemen, public servants, managers of public hospitals and remand homes or wardens of jails), even if it is with the consent of the woman.

S. 54 I.E.A. states, "In criminal proceedings (including rape) the fact that the accused person has a bad character is irrelevant, unless evidence has been given (by him) that he has a good character, in which case it becomes relevant."

S. 21 (2) I.E.A.: An admission may be proved by or on behalf of the person making it, when it consists of statements of the existence of any state of mind or body, relevant or in issue, made at or about the time when such state of mind or body existed, and is accompanied by conduct rendering its falsehood improbable.

In cases where the accused sexually harasses or insults the modesty of a woman by way of either obscene acts or songs or by means of words, gesture, or acts intended to insult the modesty of a woman, he shall be punished under sections 294 and 509 I.P.C. respectively.

Under **S. 294 I.P.C.:** The obscene act or song must cause annoyance. Though annoyance is an important ingredient of this offence, it being associated with the mental condition, has often to be inferred from proved facts. However, another important ingredient of this offence is that the obscene acts or songs must be committed or sung in or near any public place with the imprisonment up to 3 months and/or with fine.

S. 509 I.P.C. comes into effect when there is an intention to insult the modesty of any woman by the offender by uttering any word, making any sound or gesture or by exhibiting any object, with the intention that such word or such sound be heard, or that such gesture or object be seen by such a woman, or by intruding upon the privacy of such a woman shall be punished with simple imprisonment that may extend to 3 years and fine.

The instances of indecent assault are: (i) In ***Rupan Deol Bajaj vs. K.P.S. Gill***, a IAS officer, the Supreme Court in January, 1998 fined Mr. K.P.S. Gill for slapping the posterior of Rupan Bajaj (a senior IAS Officer) Rs. 2.5 lakh in lieu of three months rigorous imprisonment under sections 294 and 509 of the I.P.C. (ii) In 1997 in ***Vishaka vs. State of Rajasthan and others*** on a writ petition filed by 'Vishaka'–a non-governmental organization, for the first time sexual harassment had been explicitly legally defined as an unwelcome sexual gesture or behaviour whether directly or indirectly as: (a) Sexually coloured remarks (b) Physical contact and advances (c) Showing pornography (d) A demand or request for sexual favours (e) Any other unwelcome physical, verbal/

nonverbal conducts being sexual in nature. It was in this landmark case that the sexual harassment was identified as a separate illegal behavior. (iii) ***A.K.Chopra's case,*** is the first case in which the Supreme Court applied the law laid down in Vishaka's case and upheld the dismissal of a superior officer of the Delhi based apparel export promotion council who was found guilty of sexual harassment of a subordinate female employee at the place of work on the ground that it violated her fundamental right guaranteed by Article 21 of the Constitution. (iv) ***The Mathura case:*** In case of Mathura, a 16-year-old tribal girl the judgment turned out to be in favour of the accused. Mathura was accused of being a "liar". It was stated that since she was "habituated to sexual intercourse", her consent was given.

As a whole, the process of law is biased against the victim. If the victim is a minor, the onus is on the accused to prove his innocence. But if the victim is a major, it is up to her to prove her charge. Therefore, the defence finds it worthwhile to prove that the victim is a major. Also, in rape cases, unless the woman is examined medically within 24 hours, it becomes difficult forensically to prove that rape has occurred.

OTHER LEGAL PROVISIONS FOR RAPE

1. **S. 114A I.E.A. Presumption as to absence of consent in certain prosecution for rape:** In a prosecution for rape under clause (a), (b), (c), (d), (e), (f), (g), (h), (j), (k), (m) or (n) of subsection (2) of section 376 I.P.C. where sexual intercourse by the accused is proved and the question is whether it was without the consent of the women alleged to have been raped and she states in her evidence before the court that she did not consent, the court shall presume that she did not consent.

   In a recent Supreme Court judgement (2006) it has been stated that the victim's testimony alone is sufficient to convict the accused, and it does not require any corroboration including that of a doctor.

2. **S. 228A I.P.C. Disclosure of identity of the victim of certain offences etc.** (1) **Whoever prints or publishes the name** or any matter which may make known the identity of any person against whom an offence under section 376, 376A, 376B, 376AB, 376C, 376D, 376DA, 376DB or 376E is alleged or found to have been committed shall be **punished with either term which may extend to two years and also fine.** (2) Printing and publication can be done with the permission in writing from the officer-in-charge of the police station or I.O. of the case acting in good faith for the purpose of investigation or with the authorization in writing of the victim or if the victim is dead or minor or of unsound mind with the authorization in writing of the next of the kin of the victim.

3. **S. 327(2) Cr.P.C.:** The inquiry into under the trial of rape or an offence under section 376, 376A, 376B, 376AB, 376C, 376D, 376DA, 376DB or 376E I.P.C. shall be conducted **in camera.** It means the presiding officer and staff along with both parties and their lawyers will be inside the court room.

   However, if the presiding judge thinks fit on an application made by either of the parties may allow a particular person to have access to, or be or remain in, the room or building used by the court.

4. According to **S. 13 Hindu Marriage Act 1955,** it is a ground for annulment of marriage when the husband is found guilty of rape.

What Constitutes Rape?

Slight penetration of the vulva by the penis is sufficient to constitute the sexual intercourse necessary for the offence of rape. Orgasm or emission of semen is not mandatory for establishing the crime. If there is no penetration by the penis, however partial, the charge of rape cannot be ruled out. All forms of forceful sexual violence–penetrative (oral, anal, vaginal, urethral), by objects/weapons/fingers (anal, vaginal, urethral) and non-penetrative (touching, fondling, etc.) constitutes the offence of rape. Absence of injury on the body of the victim or presence of intact hymen does not exclude rape. Hence, in the absence medical findings, the doctor should not opine that rape has not been committed.

Types of Rape

Gang rape: Where a woman is raped by more than one person acting in furtherance of their common intention, each of the person shall be deemed to have committed gang rape. It is also known as **group rape or pack rape**. It occurs when a group of people participate in the rape of a single victim. It is far more damaging to the victim, and in some jurisdictions, is punished more severely than rape by a single person. The term "group rape" is now often preferred to "gang rape", as the word "gang" can have racial connotations when used against minority defendants in western nations.

Violent rape: Violent rape occurs when violence beyond the rape itself is a part of the assault. This may include physical force, harm, threat of harm, including death threats, or threats against a family member.

Statutory rape: Any sexual contact with persons under the age of consent for sexual intercourse is defined as statutory rape, even if he or she agrees to the sexual activity. The offence is often based on a presumption that people under a certain age are unable to give informed consent. The age of consent is the age at which individuals are considered competent to give consent for sexual intercourse. The age is different for different countries. **In India it is 18 years** and ranges from 12 to 21 in various states internationally. The sex which violates age of consent law, but is neither violent nor physically coerced, is described as statutory rape.

Acquaintance (date) rape: The term, acquaintance or date rape refers to rape or nonconsensual sexual activity between people who are already acquainted, or who know each other socially such as friends, acquaintances, people on a date, or even people in an existing romantic relationship. In these cases, it is alleged that consent for sexual activity was not given, or was given under duress. In most jurisdictions, there is no legal distinction between rape committed by a stranger, or by an acquaintance, friend or lover. In general, evidence suggests that 80% of all rapists know their victims.

Spousal rape: Spousal rape is also called marital rape, wife rape, partner rape or **intimate partner sexual assault** (IPSA), because there is a widely held view that a woman surrenders consent upon entering a relationship. However, the law has been slow to criminalize this form of rape or sexual assault. It is now a crime in most parts of the West.

Rape of females by males: Every minute someone is sexually assaulted in the world. The rape of females by males is the most well-known and most well-reported form of rape. Young females are four times more likely than any other group to be the victims of sexual assault.

Rape of males by males; Although rape and sexual assault is usually known as a crime against women, men can also be raped. According to the US Bureau of Justice Statistics for 2003, 9.9% of rape and sexual assault victims in the United States of more than 12 years are male. Therefore, nearly 17 out of every 100,000 males are victims. According to the data for 2004, this number has fallen to 2.95%; therefore, slightly more than 5 out of every 100,000 males are victims. In India, males are not raped but this type of crime falls under sodomy, an unnatural offence.

Rape of males by females: It is widely, considered impossible because male erectile response is seen as voluntary. Female rapists are usually seen as much less culpable than male rapists by the courts. In many countries, male rape is legally classified under a different law or name. Under the Indian law, a man can only commit rape. Woman can only be charged with indecent assault.

Rape of females by females: Female-female rape is rape that can occur against heterosexual females, lesbians and within lesbian relationships. As in male-male rape, the victim of female-female rape is not necessarily homosexual simply because she is the target of assault by a woman. The attacker may not be necessarily homosexual.

Although a woman who forces a man to have sex cannot be prosecuted for rape under English law, if she helps a man commit rape she can be prosecuted for the crime but a woman can also be prosecuted for causing a man to engage in sexual activity without his consent, a crime which also carries a maximum life sentence if it involves penetration of the mouth, anus or vagina. In India Supreme Court recently held that a woman cannot be prosecuted for rape or gang rape but can be prosecuted for abetment of rape depending upon the merit of the case.

Custodial and prison rape: The prison rape is routine in India and also in US prisons. Women prisoners are especially vulnerable to assault by guards and other staff members.

Rape and drugs: Any drug that incapacitates another person and renders that person vulnerable to a sexual assault, including rape is called "**date rape drug**". The incidents of sexual assault and rape are not exclusively reported when two people are dating rather it can happen to anyone, in varied situations or settings. An attacker could be someone you just met or someone you've known for a while. That's why **Drug-facilitated sexual assault (DFSA)** is an appropriate terminology which can be defined as a non-consensual sexual act in which the victim is incapacitated or unconscious due to the effects of alcohol, a drug and/or other intoxicating substances. Alcohol is the most commonly detected substance in DFSA globally and co-occurrence with other drugs is common. Common drugs that have been used include "**club drug**" like Gamma-Hydroxybutyrate (GHB), flunitrazepam (Rohypnol), Ketamine and MDMA (ecstasy). Prescription medicine such as sleeping pills, anxiety medicines, muscle relaxers, tranquilizers, and street drugs are also used for DFSA.

GHB is a date rape drug also known as liquid ecstasy, G, or soap etc. It is clear, tastes salty, odourless liquid that looks like water and so can be added to a beverage such as sodas, liquor, or beer without the person knowing it. It is a designer drug which causes CNS depression. Euphoria, increased sex drive, and tranquillity are reported positive effects of GHB abuse and side effects include sweating, loss of consciousness, nausea, hallucinations, amnesia and coma.

Flunitrazepam (Rohypnol) commonly called Roofies can incapacitate victims and prevent them from resisting sexual assault. It is a colourless, odourless and tasteless drug. It causes CNS depression and can produce anterograde amnesia, which means that individuals may not remember events they experienced while under the effects of the drug. The sedative effects of Rohypnol begin to appear approximately 15–20 minutes after the drug is ingested. The effects typically last from 4-6 hours after administration of the drug, but some cases have been reported in which the effects were experienced 12 or more hours after administration.

It is imperative that any investigation into the suspected use of date rape drugs involve the immediate carrying out of a blood test, as waiting too long to test for the presence of drugs may cause false negatives.

Effects of Rape

A proportion of violent sexual assaults end with the death or serious injury of the victim. Other consequences can include pregnancy or sexually transmitted diseases. Because of the sexual nature of rape crimes, the most common effect of rape on victims, however, is serious psychological trauma. This is especially true in societies with strong sexual customs and taboos. For example, a woman (and especially a virgin) who is raped may be deemed by society to be "damaged": she may suffer isolation, be prohibited to marry, be divorced if she was married, or even killed. She may also feel "dirty", even though the crime was not her fault.

Rape trauma syndrome: In the past, survivors of rape and sexual assault were often diagnosed with Rape trauma syndrome (RTS), and then considered to be a psychological disorder. RTS is no longer considered a diagnosis, but rather a set of normal psychological and physiological reactions that a victim is likely to experience. These include, but are not limited to, feelings of guilt and shame, tension, anger, eating disturbances, and sometimes depression. The reactions are very similar to those that would be experienced by a survivor of any other traumatizing experience, and sometimes result in a diagnosis of post-traumatic stress disorder. These traumatic responses are often cited as one of the reasons why rape goes unreported.

The process to denounce and eventually convict an offender is often hindered by similar psychological effects. Victims frequently feel shame when describing what has happened. Also, the intimate questions and medical examinations required for prosecution can make the victim uncomfortable. In societies that do not provide equal civil rights to women and men, this process is even more difficult for female victims.

Secondary victimization is the re-traumatization of the sexual assault, abuse or rape victim. It is an indirect result of assault which occurs through the responses of individuals and institutions to the victim. The types of **secondary victimization** include victim blaming, inappropriate behaviour or language by medical personnel and by other organizations with access to the victim post assault.

In the United States, rape is unique in that it is the only crime in which there are statutory protections designed in favour of the victim (known as rape shield laws). These were enacted in response to the common defence tactic of "putting the victim on trial". Typical rape shield laws prohibit cross-examination of the victim with respect to issues, such as his or her prior sexual history, or the manner in which he or she was dressed at the time of the rape. Most states and the federal rules, including law in India, however, provide exceptions to the rape shield law where evidence of prior sexual history is used to provide an alternative explanation for physical evidence, where the defendant and the victim had a prior consensual sexual relationship, and where exclusion of evidence would violate the defendant's constitutional rights.

Types of Rapist

The rapists may be: (i) Normal well-adjusted men who behave abnormally under the influence of alcohol (ii) Sexually deviated but with no psychological disorder (iii) Psychologically deviated but sexually non-deviated (iv) Both psychologically as well as sexually deviated males.

Social Aspects of Rape

Rape is a worldwide crime that affects people of all ages, castes, religions and geographical locations. The perpetrator can be anyone, however, as per National Crime Record Bureau (NCRB), India, most rapes are committed by people known to the victims such as relatives, neighbours and employers etc. In India, social factors are primarily responsible for high incidence of rapes. There are rape myths (male sexuality–men cannot control their sexual urges, male pathology–rapists are mentally ill and female precipitation) present in our society and contribute to the high incidence of rapes in India. These myths have put the responsibility for prevention rape on the victim and exonerate the perpetrator. Other reasons for high incidence of rape cases in India are like social hierarchy, poverty, low literacy rate, greater sex imbalance (the lower the number of women to men), drug abuse, lack of public safety measures, lack of sex education etc.

Rape is associated stigma and the victim may be viewed by society as being 'damaged'. She is blamed for the incident. Following rape, interpersonal relationships of the victim with intimate partners, friends and family members can be affected. The victim and her family may suffer social isolation and many times the victim disowned by friends and family. She may be prohibited from marrying, be divorced if already married. This phenomenon is known as secondary victimization. The rape victim may be killed and burnt to conceal the crime. Rape victims experience devastating mental health problems like post-traumatic stress disorder, anxiety and depression. There can be difficulty in communication, intimacy, trust and sexual relations. Enjoyment of social activities can be also be adversely affected. They are vulnerable to repeated suicidal behaviour and incidences of suicide after rape are common.

Recording of statement of sexual assault victim by women police officer:

1. ***In S. 154 Cr.P.C. Sub-section (1):***

   If the information is given by the woman against whom an offence under sections 326A, 326B, 354, 354A, 354B, 354C, 354D, 376, 376A, 376B, 376AB, 376C, 376D, 376DA, 376DB, 376E or section 509 of the Indian Penal Code is alleged to have been committed or attempted, then such information **shall be recorded, by a woman police officer or any woman officer:**

   Provided further that:

   (a) In the event that the person against whom an offence under sections 354, 354A, 354B, 354C, 354D, 376, 376A, 376B, 376AB, 376C, 376D, 376DA, 376DB, 376E or S 509 of the Indian Penal Code is alleged to have been committed or attempted, is **temporarily or permanently mentally or physically disabled**, then such **information shall be recorded by a police officer, at the residence of the person seeking to report such offence** or **at a convenient place of such person's choice, in the presence of an interpreter or a special educator**, as the case may be;

   (b) The recording of such information **shall be video-graphed**;

   (c) The police officer shall get the statement of the person recorded by a Judicial Magistrate under clause (a) of sub-section (5A) of S 164 as soon as possible.

2. ***In S. 161 Cr.P.C. sub-section (3):***

   The statements of a woman against whom an offence under sections 354, 354A, 354B, 354C, 354D, 376, 376A, 376B, 376AB, 376C, 376D, 376DA, 376DB, 376E or S 509 of the Indian Penal Code is alleged to have been committed or attempted shall be **recorded by a woman police officer or any woman officer**.

   The responsibilities of the physician in the examination of the victim of sexual assault are: (i) Collection of physical evidence to corroborate the charges of the offence (ii)

Management of the injuries and other ailments (iii) Prevention and treatment of venereal diseases (iv) Psychological counseling and referral to the psychologist.

S. 164A Cr.P.C. Medical examination of the victim of rape–the victim should be medically examined **within 24 hours from the time of receiving the information** relating to the commission of the offence. The examination should be conducted by **a registered medical practitioner (RMP) employed in government hospital or a local authority and in the absence of such practitioners by any other medical practitioner** with the consent of such woman or of a person competent to give such consent on her behalf. The doctor shall examine without delay and prepare a report. The exact time of start and close of examination to be recorded. The RMP shall forward the report without delay to Investigating Officer (IO) and in turn IO to magistrate.

Punishment for Health Professionals

I. **If the physician fails to examine the victim properly or doesn't collect the required materials for evidence purpose, he/she may be punished under:**

S. 166A I.P.C.*: *Public servant disobeying direction under law: Whoever, being a public servant, (c) fails to record any information given to him under sub-section (1) of S. 154 Cr.P.C., in relation to cognizable offence punishable under IPC sections 326A, 326B, 354, 354B, 370, 370A, 376, 376A, 376B, 376AB, 376C, 376D, 376 DA, 376DB, S. 376E or S. 509, shall be punished with rigorous imprisonment for a term which shall **not be less than six months** but which may **extend to two years, and shall also be liable to fine**.

II. **For non-treatment of victims of sexual violence, may be punished under:**

S.166B I.P.C.: Whoever, being in charge of a hospital, public or private, whether run by the Central Government, the State Government, local bodies or any other person, **contravenes the provisions of S. 357C Cr.P.C.**, shall be punished with imprisonment for a term which **may extend to one year or with fine or with both**.

Ministry of Health and Family Welfare, Government of India, Guidelines and Protocols for Medicolegal Care for Victim/Survivor of Sexual Violence:

After the Nirbhaya case, to supplement the procedure laid in S. 164A Cr.P.C, the Ministry of Health and Family Welfare in 2014 gave certain guidelines and protocols for medicolegal care for the survivor/victims of sexual violence. Those are: (i) **Operationalise informed consent** and respect autonomy of survivors in making decisions about examination, treatment and police intimation. (ii) Specific guidance on dealing with persons from **marginalised groups** such persons with disabilities, sex workers, LGBT persons, children, persons facing caste, class or religion-based discrimination. (iii) Ensure **gender sensitivity** in the entire procedure by **disallowing any mention of past sexual practices** through comments on size of vaginal introitus, elasticity of vagina or anus. Further **it bars comments of built/height-weight/ nutrition or gait that perpetuate stereotypes about 'victims'**. (iv) Focus on history by recognising various forms and dynamics of sexual violence including activities that lead to loss of evidence. (v) **Evidence collection based on science and history**, with specific guidance for taking relevant samples and preservation of evidence. (vi) Lay down Standard Treatment protocols for managing health consequences of sexual violence. (vii) Lay down guidelines for provision of first line psychological support.

Survivor: The term survivor recognizes that the **person has agency** and she is capable of taking decisions despite being victimized, humiliated and traumatized due to the assault. This term is preferably used instead of victim.

Victims means a person suffering harm including those who are subjected to non-consensual sexual act which could be sexual assault, rape or sexual violence. The person **doesn't possess agency** and is not fully capable of comprehending situation at hand because of the victimhood faced.

MEDICAL EXAMINATION OF RAPE VICTIM/ SURVIVOR (Figure 31.1)

I. **General Procedure:** Medical examination of rape victims is a **"medicolegal emergency"**. A hospital may receive a victim of rape when victim voluntarily reports to the hospital, or on requisition by the police or by the court. A woman police officer not below the rank of sub inspector (SI) can request for examination of victim. The victim should be **medically examined within 24 hours** from the time of receiving the information relating to the commission of the offence. The examination should be conducted by a registered medical practitioner employed in government hospital or a local authority and in the absence of such practitioners by any other medical practitioner **(S. 164A Cr.P.C.)**. The victim should be examined **preferably by a female doctor**, however in case a female doctor is not available, a male doctor can conduct the medical examination in the presence of a female attendant. Police personnel should not be allowed in the examination room, however, if the victim requests, her relative may be present while the examination is done.

II. **Preliminary Data:** Name, age, sex, address, marital status, date and time of arrival in the hospital, date and time of commencement of examination and name of the person who brought the survivor and relationship to accompanying persons should be documented. Two identification marks of the victim should be noted. Left thumb impression of the victim should be taken.

III. **Initial Resuscitation/First Aid:** If the victim has sustained serious injury or in an unconsciousness state, necessary emergency treatment should be given.

IV. **Informed Consent:** First, nature and purpose of examination should be explained to the victim and in case of child to the

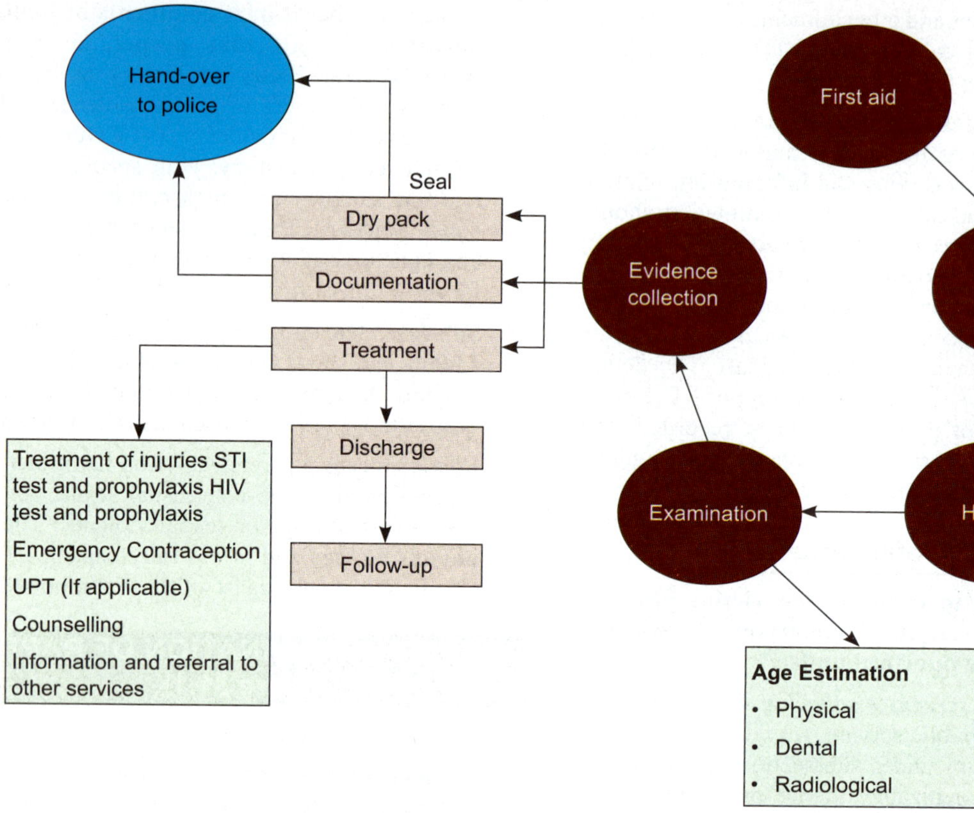

Figure 31.1: Steps for medical examination of rape victim

child's parent/guardian. A written consent must be obtained from the victim for medical examination and treatment. The medical examination includes the history, physical examination and collection of physical evidence and specimens for laboratory analysis. The consent form must be signed by the victim, a witness and the examining doctor. In case of minor, i.e., below 12 years and persons with mental disability, parental/guardian's consent must be obtained.

If a victim has come directly to the hospital without the police requisition, the hospital is bound to provide treatment and conduct a medical examination with consent of the victim/parent/guardian (depending on age). A police requisition is not required for this. If victim has come on her own without FIR, she may or may not want to lodge a complaint but requires a medical examination and treatment. Even in such cases **the doctor is bound to inform the police** as per law. However, neither court nor police can force the victim to undergo medical examination. It has to be with the informed consent of the victim/parent/guardian (depending on the age). In case the victim does not want to pursue a police case, a **Medicolegal Case (MLC) must** be made and she must be informed that she has the right to refuse to file FIR. An **informed refusal** must be documented in such cases.

V. **History:** A general medical history of injury or any illness should be documented. Any history of drug allergies should also be noted. Vaccination history is important with regard to tetanus and hepatitis B, so as to ascertain, if prophylaxis is required. History of the incident and post-incident events should be recorded in detail.

A history of menarche, date of last menstrual period and history of previous pregnancies should be recorded. If the victim is menstruating at the time of examination then a second examination is required on a later date. A history of previous consensual coitus should also be recorded. History regarding specific nature of sexual assault should be noted. The statement of the victim's words must be written down as much as possible **(word for word)**. If history is narrated by a person other than the victim herself, her name should be noted. Especially if the identity of assailants is revealed it is better to also have a counter signature of the informant. The history of the events should include statements regarding various aspects of the assault that may be further corroborated by physical or laboratory examination. The time and place at which the assault occurred should be recorded. This would help the physician to look for the dirt, grass or twigs of leaves and further corroborate with the allegation. The specific nature of the assault should be noted that is whether any body fluids through ejaculation, urination or defecation were left on the victim or if the vaginal, oral and anal penetration has occurred. If any history of oral sex by the assailant on the victim or sucking, licking, kissing of body parts is present, it should be noted. This would help in collecting proper samples. The history relating to the use of weapons or materials such as restraints should be noted and signs of application of restraints should be noted on the body of the victim. Information regarding use of condom during the assault is relevant because in such cases, vaginal swabs and smears would be negative for sperm/semen. Post incident events whether the victim has bathed, douched, defecated, urinated or has changed clothes should also be noted.

VI. **General Physical Examination:** The physician examining the victim of sexual assault should be gentle and empathic. In all the cases, examination should be performed in a private area of the hospital along with a nurse who can assist the physician, as **chaperon**. The physical examination must be complete enough to note any abnormalities that have occurred as a result of the assault. The physician should assess and record the patient's general appearance before she disrobes such as patient's demeanor, emotional distress or depression, which may manifest itself by inappropriate laughing, agitation or withdrawal. Vital signs such as blood pressure, pulse, temperature or respiratory distress should be taken and documented. Abnormalities such as elevated pulse may reflect emotional stress or major trauma.

The victim should be requested to stand on a white platform or paper and to undress herself one by one. The physical evidences that are lodged on the garments may fall on the white surface and will be easier to collect from there.

The whole body (top-to-toe) should be thoroughly inspected for stains such as dirt and blood, injuries, skin disease, and scars of old injuries including those that are self-inflicted. Foreign material such as blood or dried semen should be scraped and submitted for evidence.

All the injuries such as bruise, abrasion, and lacerated or incised wound should be described in terms of location, size, shape as well as color and whether it is scabbed, bleeding or swollen. Areas like scalp, face, neck, shoulders, breasts, wrists, forearms, medial aspect of upper arms, thighs and buttocks should be specially inspected for injuries. The tender areas on the body surfaces should be noted after palpation. The bruise undergoes color changes with the passage of time that is to be noted. All the injuries should be photographed. The injuries should be marked on body charts and numbered. Bite marks should be photographed (Figure 31.2A,B). A complete medical examination should be conducted to document injuries and also to note any diseases that may affect interpretation of medical findings.

VII. **Age Estimation:** It is required when there is no documentary proof of age, or documents or certificates are found to be fabricated or any dispute regarding age of the victim. If there is enough documentary proof (Birth Certificate, School Certificate etc.), medical age (Bone ossification test) determination is not required. The age estimation can be done on the basis of physical, radiological and dental examination.

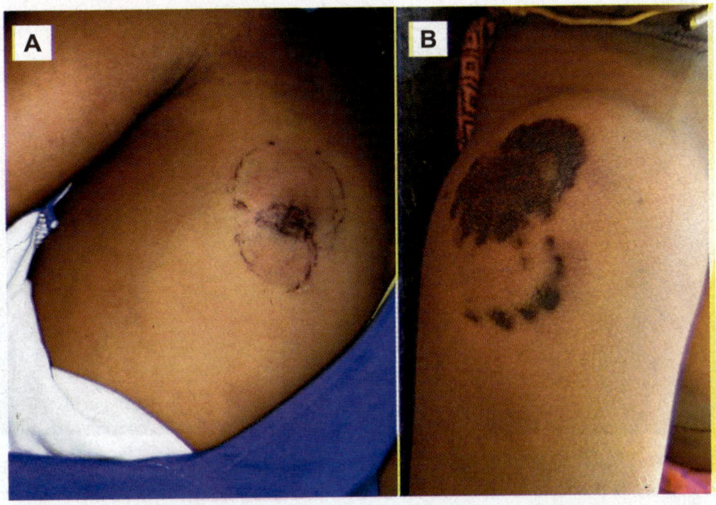

Figure 31.2A,B: Bite marks over breast (A), shoulder (B) in case of sexual assault of a 9-year-old girl (*Courtesy:* Dr Kiran Patnaik, Assoc. Prof. MKCG Medical College, Berhampur, Odisha)

VIII. **Anogenital Examination:** Anogenital examination is required in order to assess the degree of trauma and also to collect specimens for evidentiary purposes.

First, make the victim feel comfortable and as relaxed as possible. The victim should be explained each step of the examination procedure. Then, the victim is placed in the lithotomy position (legs drawn up and widely open) on the examination table with parts fully exposed. If the separation of the thighs causes too much pain, local anesthetic may be required. The examination should be done in good light.

Initially the external genitalia and perineum should be inspected carefully. Signs of trauma such as bruising on inner thighs may result from attempts to pull apart the legs should be searched. The pubic hairs should be examined for matting from seminal fluid or blood or lubricants etc. The portion of matted hairs must be cut off and preserved for examination. Invisible stains or foreign particles on the skin can be detected using **Wood's lamp**, which emits filtered UV light. Combing the pubic hair for specimens of free foreign hair and clippings of few (15-20 hairs) of the victim's pubic hair for comparison (control samples) should be done. If pubic hair is shaven, it is to be noted. If there is bleeding from the genital tract, the possible source of bleeding whether it is menstrual or resulting from the injuries should be noted.

Examination of Vulva: The vulva (external female sex organ) which includes labia majora, labia minora, clitoris, urethral meatus and vestibule, mons pubis, fourchette, vaginal opening and hymen should be inspected systematically. These parts should be inspected for any signs of recent injury such as bleeding, tears, bruises, abrasions, swelling, or discharge and infection (Figures 31.3 to 31.6). Tears are most frequently seen on posterior

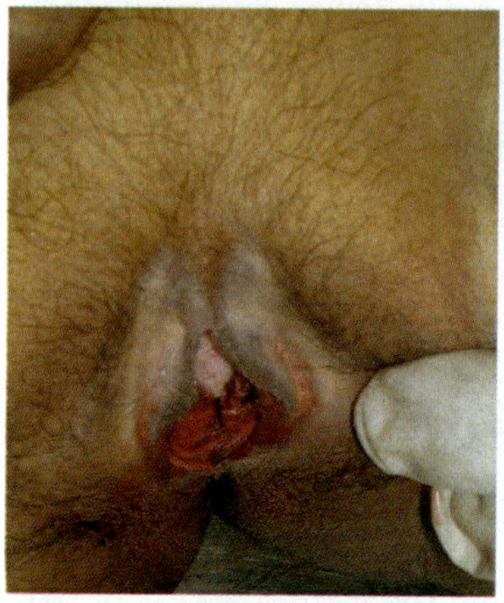

Figure 31.3: Bruising with tears over labia minora at 6 O'clock and 7 O'clock position in a rape victim

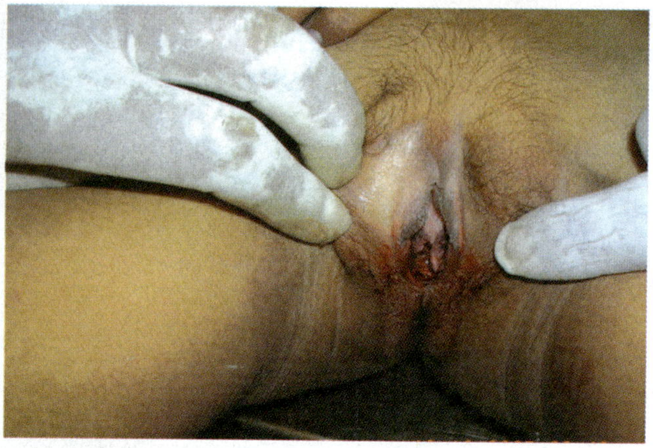

Figure 31.4: Findings of sexual assault in a minor girl, note bruising of the genitalia

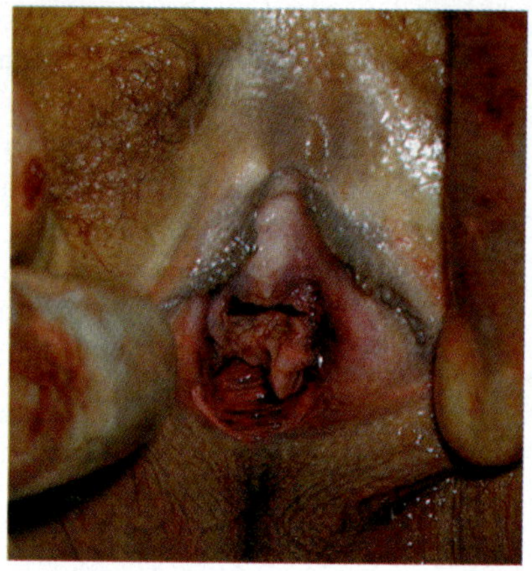

Figure 31.5: Hymenal and vaginal tear in a rape victim

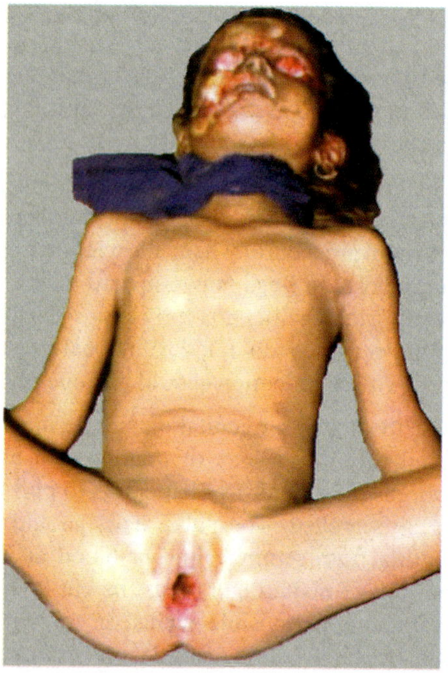

Figure 31.6: Mutilation of face and lacerations over genitalia and anus in a case of sexual assault

fourchette and fossa navicularis and abrasions are seen on labia minora frequently. The bruises are most commonly found on the hymen. The hematoma of the labia is also seen grossly in some of the cases. The injuries are commonly detected on one or more of the following sites; posterior fourchette, labia minora, hymen and fossa navicularis. Two vulval swabs (for semen examination and DNA testing) should be taken. Many times, microinjuries may not visible on **direct visual inspection**, hence, **a magnifying glass** or **colposcope** or **toluene blue contrast method** can be used.

Toluidine blue stains nuclei and it has been used on the posterior fourchette to identify injuries of the keratinized squamous epithelium that were not apparent grossly. Toluidine blue (1%) is sprayed on the posterior fourchette and excess is wiped out. The time parameters within which application of toluidine blue helps in highlighting injuries have not been identified. Lacerations, abrasions, bruising at the posterior fourchette are enhanced by the use of colposcope and toluidine blue.

A **colposcope** is a freestanding, binocular microscope on wheels particularly useful for external, internal genital and anal assessments in cases of sexual assault. It provides 5-30 times magnification and greater illumination, enabling detection of more abnormalities.

Examination of Hymen: When the hymen is fimbriated, a moistened swab can be used to visualize the hymenal edges. When the hymenal opening cannot be seen at all, application of a few drops of warm sterile water or saline on to the hymen will often reveal hymenal edges. **Foley's catheter** can also be used in post pubertal females. To visualize hymen, **Glaister keene rods or globes** that are glass or plastic rods about 6 mm diameter having a globe at one end can be used. They vary in size from 1-2½ cm. To visualize hymen, the rod is warmed to body temperature and then spherical head is first passed into hymenal orifice. The rod is then passed round the posterior surface of hymen that is stretched slightly by separating labia minora. The edges of the hymen are slightly everted this way. The sphere is slightly rotated around the edges of the hymen to differentiate natural notches from tears. To detect tears, a **hymenoscope** can be utilized, which provides good transillumination of the hymen. Hymenoscope is a refinement of Glaister knee rods with source of light within the ball. After the sexual act, lacerations with bruising may be seen at 3 O'clock and 9 O'clock positions of the hymen and are commonly seen at 5 O'clock and 7 O'clock positions (Posterolateral positions). The injuries to hymen can be an abrasion, bruise, laceration and swelling and also redness. Post pubertal females can experience penile vaginal penetration without sustaining any hymenal deficits due to the elasticity of hymen.

The presence of an intact hymen should be documented but does not rule out vaginal penetration. Evidence of the recent disruption of the hymenal ring, such as reddening, laceration or bleeding is rarely found but should nevertheless be sought. In practice, hymenal tissue is difficult to identify in a number of cases. The hymen can be torn due to several reasons such as cycling, riding or masturbation etc. Thus, the status of the hymen (intact or absent) is irrelevant. *The hymen should be regarded as any other part of the genital while documenting examination in cases of sexual violence.*

Examination of Vagina: Per Vaginum examination can only be done on adult women when medically indicated. The vaginal canal can be inspected with gentle retraction. In adult female, it can be done with the help of a sterile **speculum** lubricated with warm saline/sterile water. In young females, look for bruises, redness bleeding and tears that may be extended to the perineum. Lacerations as well as ruptures of the vagina are most commonly located in the right fornix or extending across the posterior fornix. Although most vaginal lacerations result from sexual intercourse but they can also result from vaginal instrumentation, use of plastic tampon inserters, and trauma after a fall or a sudden increase of intra-abdominal pressure. If injuries aren't apparent but are suspected, use good lighting and a **magnifying glass/ colposcope**, if one is available, to examine for tiny injuries. If **Toluidine blue** at 1% is available, it is sprayed and the surplus is wiped away. Micro-injuries will be highlighted in blue. All of these tests should be performed only after swabs for trace evidence have been collected. If there is vaginal discharge, take note of the texture, colour and odour.

When there is no history of penetration and no visible injuries, a per speculum examination is not required in the case of children/young girls. In case of minors and when injuries inflicted are severe, the examination and treatment as needed may have to be performed under general anesthesia.

*Per-Vaginum examination by inserting two fingers for determination of whether the hymen is broken or not and laxity of vagina, commonly referred to by lay persons as **'two-finger test', or "virginity test", must not be conducted** for establishing rape/sexual violence.* The Ministry of Health and Family Welfare, Government of India issued a guideline after the Supreme Court's judgement which held that the test is a violation of a woman's right to privacy. There should be no comments made about the size of the vaginal introitus, the elasticity of the vagina or the hymen, or past sexual experience or habituation to sexual intercourse because it has no bearing on a case of rape.

Examination of Cervix: Bruises and lacerations of the cervix have been described after nonconsensual sexual acts. Cervical abrasions are more common in digital penetration than in penile penetration. It's important to distinguish between abrasions and erosions. Cervical erosions do not occur during penetration. **Colposcopy** is commonly used to visualize cervix directly.

Examination of Anus and Anal Canal: Bleeding/swelling/ tears/discharge/stains/warts around the anus and anal orifice must be documented. A per-rectal examination is indicated if a history of rectal intercourse is elicited and similar to genital examination. This examination is done to detect tears/stains/ fissures/hemorrhoids in the anal canal. Signs of tenderness and trauma can be elicited by palpation with a gloved finger. A proctoscope can be used inspection for signs of trauma and foreign material. Relevant swabs from these sites should be collected. There should be no comments on the shape, size, and/or of the anal opening, as well as previous sexual experience or habituation to anal intercourse.

Examination of Oral Cavity: Oral cavity should also be examined for any evidence of bleeding, discharge, tear, edema, tenderness.

IX. **Recovery of Physical Evidence:** To prevent contamination of samples, the gloves should be worn and changed when collecting samples from different parts of the body. Recovery of certain physical evidence material in strict keeping with the proper medicolegal and forensic requirement can be done from the use of pre-assembled evidence collection kit **(Rape kit)**. It is also called sexual assault evidence collection kit **(SAFE kit)** or physical evidence recovery kit **(PERK)**. Normally, the SAFE kit consists of: (i) Instructions, authorisation and documentation forms (ii) Large sheet of paper to undress over (iii) Paper bags for collection of clothing of victim (iv) Equipment for collection of samples–Comb for pubic hair combing, nail cutter, wood stick for fingernail scrapping, small scissor (v) Container for sample preservation–urine sample container, Tubes/vials/vacutainers for blood samples (EDTA, Plain, Sodium fluoride) (v) Glass slides (vi) Disposable gloves, Syringes and needle (vii) For packaging and sealing forensic evidence–Envelopes or boxes for individual evidence samples, labels, lac (sealing wax) (vii) Clean clothing, shower/hygiene items for survivors use after the examination.

Forensic swabs should be placed in plastic sheaths without any transport media or in specially designed boxes that allow the swabs to air dry. Blood and urine samples for drug and alcohol analysis should be placed in containers with a preservative (such as sodium fluoride) that prevents decomposition and fermentation. Blood sample should contain potassium oxalate. Blood sample for DNA analysis should be placed in a container with appropriate preservative such as EDTA. Besides these samples, control samples such as an unopened swab should be retained for analysis. All the items should be packaged quickly to prevent accidental loss of material and also to minimize decomposition. Proper labeling and sealing of all the recovered items or material is mandatory. The clothing worn by the victim during or after the incident may be an invaluable source of information in terms of the nature of the assault that is evident from the damage to clothing and presence of body fluid stains as well as the identification of the assailant. Even stains on clothing that have been washed have been found to contain sufficient spermatozoa for DNA profiling. Clothing should be placed in paper bags and not in plastic that due to condensation cause decomposition. The clothing should be properly labeled and sealed. If clothing is to be held for forensic examination, replacement clothing needs to be provided by the hospital.

The various samples to be collected for analysis in a rape victim are:

Skin samples: All the areas of skin where there is deposition of saliva or semen and bearing injury marks should be swabbed using the surgical gauze pads to recover trace evidences. If the skin is moist, dry swabs should be used to retrieve the stain that are then packed without transport medium and sealed. For dried stains, a cotton swab whose tip is moistened with the sterile water is used. The tip of the swab is rolled over the skin using circular motions while rotating the swab on its long axis to ensure maximum contact between the skin and the swab. A second dried swab is then rolled over in the same area to absorb the water left on the skin by the initial swab and collect any remaining cells. Minimal pressure should be applied to prevent exfoliation of the patient's own epithelial cells. Two swabs are sufficient when no stains are visible but in a stained area any number of swabs will suffice. Ultraviolet light causes fluorescence of semen and saliva and can be used in determining the areas of skin to be swabbed. But detergents, lubricants containing petroleum jelly and milk also fluoresce. The only means of confirming the presence of saliva on the skin is by detecting the enzyme amylase. From the salivary sample it is possible to determine the ABO secretor status.

Hairs: Hair is most commonly sampled to detect body fluids or retrieve foreign hair or particles. Hair should be cut if they are matted due to deposition of semen or saliva. About twenty-five hairs should be cut. For drug analysis at least 50 strands of hair should be cut. The ideal site for sampling is the crown of the head. The sampled hairs are then wrapped in aluminum foil. Any foreign particles or hairs identified on the head or pubic hair should be collected with forceps and submitted for analysis. Pubic hair may be transferred between individuals during sexual intercourse. The loose pubic hair on the victim that is grossly different from her own hair should be routinely combed onto an uncontaminated paper, with the victim in semi-lithotomy position. Similarly, the loose pubic hairs from the suspect are also collected. Then the paper along with the comb is folded inwards and submitted for forensic analysis. When it is not possible to obtain buccal cells or a blood sample, then 10-25 strands of head hair with attached roots can be plucked individually. Hair is most commonly sampled to detect body fluids or retrieve foreign hairs or particles. Hair may be used as reference sample for DNA analysis. Various drugs such as benzodiazepines, amphetamines, cannabis, cocaine, opiates and barbiturates are deposited in the hair and are accessible to analysis for longer periods in hair compared to blood and urine.

Nails: During the course of sexual assault, trace material such as skin, body fluids, hairs, fibers and soil can collect under the fingernails of both the victim and assailant. Clippings of the whole fingernail are taken but when short, samples from the fingernails should be obtained by scrapping. Scrapping of the material under the nail should be taken using a **tapered stick** or both sides of the fingernails should be swabbed. Each hand should be sampled separately and specimens packaged along with the stick.

Samples from oral cavity: To look for the presence of spermatozoa and for DNA analysis, the oral cavity should be sampled by collecting 10 ml of saliva, application of gauze pads, swabs, filter paper and mouth rinses using 10 ml of distilled water. Firstly, the saliva sample is obtained, then swabs are rubbed over the inner and outer gum margins with particular attention to margins around the teeth, over the hard palate, if tolerated over the soft palate, on the inside of the cheeks and lips and over both surfaces of the tongue. The mouth is then rinsed with 10 ml of sterile water which is retained in a bottle as the final sample. Buccal cells are the preferred DNA reference sample for both suspect and complainant. The buccal cells are obtained by firmly rubbing a swab over the inside of the cheek. The sample of saliva can also be used for the secretor status. It is important that forensic samples should be rapidly retrieved from the oral cavity. Even though the maximum persistence of spermatozoa in the oral cavity is recorded as 28-31 hours, only a few spermatozoa are detected unless the sample is taken within a few hours of ejaculation. Although rinsing of the mouth, drinking and brushing of teeth do not necessarily remove all traces of spermatozoa, such activities should be discouraged until the samples have been obtained.

Samples from female genital area: The following samples should be collected to maximize the recovery of spermatozoa: (i) Any external sanitary napkins or internal tampons is collected and submitted for analysis. (ii) Two swabs are then used to sample the vulva that is inner aspects of labia majora, the labia minora and the vestibule. The interlabial folds should be properly swabbed. These should be labelled as vulval swabs. The moist stains should be recovered on dry swabs. (iii) Two dry swabs are then used to swab the lower vagina after separating the labia, are labeled low vaginal swabs. (iv) A transparent speculum of proper size lubricated with sterile water is passed gently about 2/3rds into the vagina and then opened and any foreign bodies such as tampons or condoms are removed and submitted for analysis. Two dry swabs are then used to swab the vagina beyond the end of the speculum, particularly the posterior fornix and these are labeled as high vaginal swabs. Two cervical and two urethral swabs are then taken and sampled for sexually transmitted diseases. The used speculum should also be retained and packaged separately for analysis of spermatozoa. (v) Aspiration of any pools of fluid in the high vagina can be undertaken. Also 2-10 ml of normal saline or sterile water can be placed in vagina and the vaginal washings can be aspirated and submitted for analysis.

Complete spermatozoa are found in the vagina for 24 hours and are likely to be found up to 3 days later and occasionally up to 7 days later. The quantity of semen in the vagina will diminish with time. The posture and activity of the victim and washing, bathing, douching accelerates loss of semen. The spermatozoa can be isolated for longer periods of up to 17 days in the endocervix. The spermatozoa may remain motile in the vagina up to 24 hours and longer in the cervical mucosa. The morphology of the spermatozoa shows consistent changes. The presence of large number of spermatozoa with tails is indicative of recent sexual intercourse. The longest time after intercourse the spermatozoa with tails have been found on external vaginal swabs is 33 hours and 122 hours on internal vaginal swabs.

Rectal and anal swabs: If the skin is moist, the swabs should be taken using dry swabs and when dry after moistening with normal saline. Two swabs should be taken from the perianal area that is within 3 cm around the anus. These are labeled as external anal swabs and placed in sheaths with no transport medium. The anal canal is then sampled by passing a wet swab and then a dry swab up to 3 cm into the anus. The proctoscope lubricated with sterile water is then passed 2-3 cm into the anal canal and the lower rectum is sampled using a dry swab. As the proctoscope is withdrawn, the anal canal can be sampled again with a dry swab.

Oral swabs: Oral swabs should be taken from the posterior parts of the buccal cavity, behind the last molars where there is the best likelihood of discovering evidence.

X. **Laboratory Evaluation:** Specimens collected from the sexual assault victim have medicolegal significance. All the specimens should be properly labelled with patient's name, age and sex, date and time of collection, police station to establish written documentation of the custody of evidentiary material to **maintain chain of evidence**. Specimens collected routinely include any clothing that is torn, bloody or soiled in the course of the assault, any foreign debris such as hairs or dried secretions adhering to the patient's body and fingernail scrapping. Blood and saliva samples obtained from the victim are used to determine her blood type in other body fluids. By comparing blood group substances found in various specimens to the patient's blood group, a secretion (semen) may be identified as foreign.

Seminal Fluid Analysis

Examination of seminal fluid and stains has both civil and criminal importance.

Civil importance: (i) Compensation on ground of acquired sterility (ii) Disputed paternity (iii) Legitimacy (iv) Artificial insemination (v) Compensation on the ground of failure of vasectomy cases leading to pregnancy of wife.

Criminal importance: (i) Concerning commission of sexual offences (ii) Identification of offender of sexual offence cases.

Composition of seminal fluid: *Physical appearance:* Seminal fluid is pale or grayish white thick, viscid and has a characteristic smell. The seminal stain fluoresces under ultraviolet light. It comprises seminal plasma and spermatozoa. ***Seminal plasma:*** It contains large amount of fructose, inositol, spermine, sorbitol, citric acid glycerylphosphorylcholine, ergothioneine, proteases, alkaline and acid phosphatases, prostaglandins, etc. ***Spermatozoa contains:*** (i) Deoxyribonucleoprotein in the nucleus (ii) Lipoglycoprotein and other lysosomal enzymes (iii) Dehydrogenases, glycosidases, glycolysing enzymes and other enzymes, in the middle piece (iv) Contractile protein system in the tail (v) Hyaluronidase (vi) Plasmalogen (aldehydrogenic lipid).

Routine studies performed on these include analysis for the presence and concentrations of acid phosphatase, an enzyme present in the ejaculate. The presence of this enzyme in a specimen serves as an indirect verification of the presence of semen. Specimens are also tested for the identification of blood group substances. Immediate microscopic examination of the wet mount of the material obtained from the vaginal fornices to identify motile spermatozoa can be carried out. Other routine studies are performed to detect sperm, either live sperm in a wet mount or dead sperm or sperm products on a dry slide. It is possible to estimate the length of time the sperms were present in their current state at the site of examination. If no spermatozoa are detected, an attempt is made to corroborate the allegation by the microscopic identification of seminal choline crystals. Seminal choline is present in high concentrations in seminal fluid and choline crystals can be precipitated by the addition of reagents. The seminal fluid can also be identified by electrophoretic techniques. If the assailant is secretor, his seminal fluid will contain his ABO blood group.

Morphology and motility of human spermatozoa: The length of the sperm varies from 52-55 microns in length. It has got a head, neck and tail (Figure 31.7). The head consists of the nuclear matter, which is covered with acrosome.

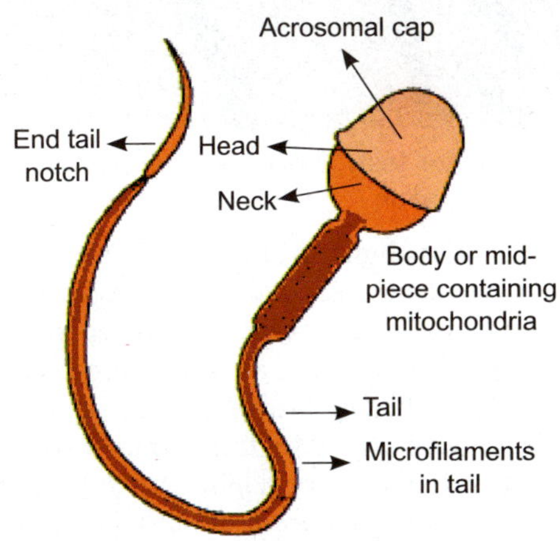

Figure 31.7: Morphological appearance of spermatozoa

The body consists of the head and the neck, it contains the mitochondria which are the energy providers to the tail for its motion to propel the sperm forwards.

The sperms retain full (90-100%) motility for about 3 hours at the room temperature, which decreases to about 50% in eight hours and further to 10% in about 24 hours. At body temperature the full motility persists for about 6-8 hours in vagina. Later the sperms disintegrate and separate into head and tails which may be recovered from the vagina upto 7-10 days in the vagina and 12 to 14 days in the cervix and uterus respectively. Some literature reports presence of sperm head in the vagina even upto 17 days. Oral cavity may show sperms upto about 9 hours and anus upto 2 days.

Tests for Seminal Fluid

Various tests can be done to confirm the nature of a stain or wet material collected as evidence.

1. ***Physical examination:*** When seminal stains are dry they have a greyish white or yellowish grey colour with irregular map like outline. A fresh stain is translucent whereas it becomes yellowish brown after the passage of a month. The stain when examined under filtered UV light, it fluoresces giving bluish white colour. The fluorescence is given by other albuminous materials such as nasal mucous, vaginal discharge and detergents.

2. ***Chemical examination***

   Florence test (Figure 31.8): The stain is extracted using 10% solution of hydrochloric acid and a drop of this is kept on a glass light and then dried. Now, a coverslip is placed over it and a drop of florence solution (containing potassium, iodine and water) is allowed to run under the coverslip. This is now examined microscopically and if semen is present dark brown rhombic crystals of choline iodide (choline originates from seminal vesicles) appear immediately. These crystals resemble haemin but their arrangement is in the form of clusters, rosettes, crosses etc. This test is proof of presence of some vegetables and animals' substance. However, a negative reaction proves that the stain is not seminal.

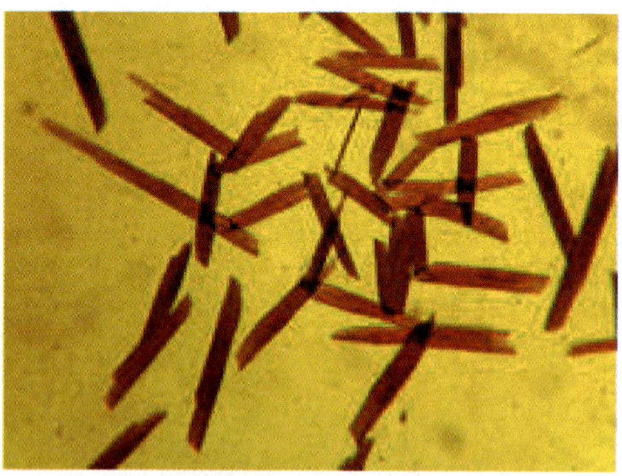

Figure 31.8: Florence test, choline iodide crystals as seen on microscopical examination

   Barberio's test: In this test a saturated aqueous or alcoholic solution of picric acid is added to seminal fluid. Yellowish needle shade rhombic crystals of spermine picrate are produced. The reaction depends on presence of spermine from prostatic secretions.

   Acid phosphatase test: The main bulk of seminal fluid is composed of prostatic fluid that has high concentration of acid phosphatase, i.e., 20 to 400 times more than any other body fluid. Undiluted semen has acid phosphatase activity of 340-360 Bodanksy units. The concentration of acid phosphatase gradually falls with time in vaginal secretions. Positive reactions are seen for 36 hours that disappear in 72 hours. The test is conducted using alpha naphthyl phosphatase and fast black K dye. Positive reaction is indicated by purple colour appearing very rapidly (within ½ minute) in comparison with acid phosphatase of other origin. Detection of more than 100 Bodansky units/ml is indicative of semen and it is detectable from vagina for about 36 hours. Dried unputrefied stains give a positive reaction though the enzymatic activity decreases with time and is destroyed in about 5 minutes at 60° C. The test is more of negative value and can establish conclusively that a given stain is not semen.

   Creatine phosphokinase test: The concentration of creatine phosphokinase in the spermatozoa is nearly double than in any other body fluid. Also, the enzyme is quite stable and the test gives a positive result in stains as old as about 6 months. The normal concentration of creatine phosphokinase in seminal fluid is 385-14000 units/ml. Levels above 400 units/ml are considered conclusive of seminal stains.

   Ammonium molybdate test: All these chemical tests are screening tests; many other body fluids also give positive reactions for these tests. If these tests are negative then presence of seminal fluids in the stain is excluded. Rapidly positive acid phosphatase test is a more dependable one.

   Semen specific glycoprotein (P 30): This glycoprotein is of prostatic origin and is present in the seminal fluid independent of the spermatozoa. It can be found in the vagina up to a maximum of about 2 days. This is a more dependable test than the previous ones and has replaced them.

   Gel electrophoresis test: Gives almost diagnostic result for presence or absence of seminal fluids.

3. ***Microscopic examination*:** This is the most definitive test to ascertain the presence of spermatozoa (Figure 31.9). It can be done for both wet specimen as well as dry stains. Wet specimen recovered from the vagina is placed on a slide, diluted with a drop of normal saline and examined for motile spermatozoa.

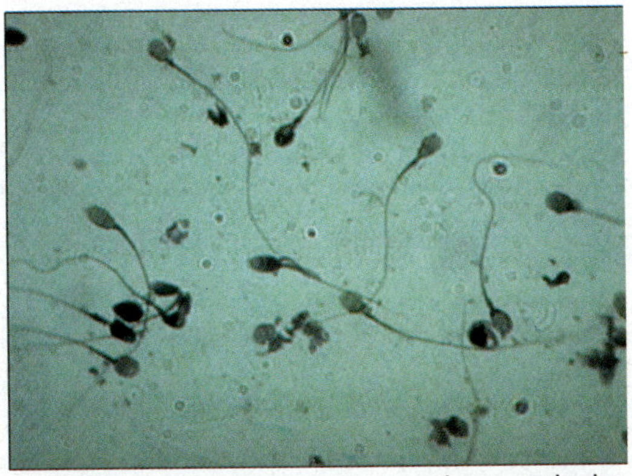

Figure 31.9: Spermatozoa as seen on microscopical examination

In case of dry seminal stains, it is first moistened with 1% hydrochloric acid or 3% acetic acid for a few hours. The material is then transferred to a glass slide, stained with Methylene blue and counterstained with Eosin. The posterior half of the head is stained with eosin while the anterior half stains lightly if at all with methylene blue. The tail is stained pink. Complete sperms have been found in specimens as old as about 5 years. The finding of even a single unbroken sperm is an absolute proof of presence of semen.

Tests for venereal diseases: Studies performed for the detection of venereal disease include gram staining and culture of secretions for gonorrhea and baseline serology for syphilis. It should be noted that it takes about a month from the time of infection before the blood test becomes positive for syphilis, so that the blood test is not always negative after successful treatment or prior syphilis infection. The test thus serves only as a baseline in recent assaults.

Blood and urine analysis: About 10 ml of blood sample with potassium oxalate for DNA analysis and another 2 ml sample with sodium fluoride for drug and alcohol analysis is collected. 20 ml of urine with sodium fluoride is collected. Pregnancy tests may be required in the post-menarche female if the history or physical examination indicates the presence of a preexisting pregnancy.

Corroborative Signs of Rape: (i) Marks of violence on body and genitalia of the victim (ii) Presence of seminal stains on the body and genitalia of the victim (iii) Detection of spermatozoa in the seminal stains or fluid on laboratory analysis (iv) Finding of spermatozoa in vagina on wet smear and hematoxylin eosin preparations (v) Findings suggestive of existence of syphilis, gonorrhea and other sexually transmitted diseases.

XI. **Opinion:** The issue of whether an incident of **rape occurred is a legal issue and not a medical diagnosis**. The doctors should not, on the basis of the medical examination conclude whether rape had occurred or not. Only findings in relation to medical findings should be recorded in the medical report. A provisional opinion should be immediately given after examination of the victim on the basis of history and findings of detailed clinical examination of the victim (Table 31.2). The final opinion can be given after receipt of the forensic analysis of the samples sent to forensic science laboratory (FSL) (Tables 31.3 and 31.4). **The opinion can be furnished as per the guidelines issued by the Ministry of Health and Family Welfare, Government of India**.

Table 31.2: Provisional opinion in case of alleged sexual assault

Physical injuries	Genital injuries	Provisional opinion
Present	Absent	There are signs suggestive of recent use of force/forceful penetration of vagina/anus. Sexual violence cannot be ruled out
Present	Absent	There are signs suggestive of recent forceful penetration of vagina/anus
Absent	Present	There are signs of use of force, however vaginal/anal/oral penetration cannot be ruled out
Absent	Absent	There are no signs of use of force; however, final opinion is kept pending till availability of FSL reports. Sexual violence cannot be ruled out

Table 31.3: Final opinion in case of alleged sexual assault

Physical injuries	Genital injuries	FSL report: Presence of semen/ drugs/other forensic evidence	Final opinion
FOR PENILE PENETRATION			
Present	Present	Positive for presence of semen	There are signs suggestive of forceful vaginal/anal sexual intercourse
Present	Absent	Positive for presence of semen	There are signs suggestive of forceful vaginal/anal sexual intercourse
Absent	Present	Positive for presence of semen	There are signs suggestive of forceful vaginal/anal sexual intercourse
Absent	Absent	Positive for presence of semen	There are signs suggestive of forceful vaginal/anal sexual intercourse
Absent	Absent	Positive for presence of semen, drugs or alcohol	There are signs suggestive of forceful vaginal/anal sexual intercourse under the influence of drugs/alcohol

Contd.

Contd.

FOR NON-PENILE PENETRTION			
Present	Present	Negative for presence of semen/ drugs/alcohol/lubricant	There are no signs of vaginal/anal intercourse, but there is evidence of physical and genital assault
Present	Absent	Negative for presence of semen/ drugs/alcohol/lubricant	There are no signs of vaginal/anal intercourse, but there is evidence of genital assault
Absent	Present	Negative for presence of semen/ drugs/alcohol/lubricant	There are no signs of vaginal/anal intercourse, but there is evidence of physical assault
Absent	Absent	Negative for presence of semen/ drugs/alcohol/lubricant	There are no signs suggestive of penetration of vaginal/anus
Absent	Absent	Positive for presence of lubricant only	There is possibility of vaginal/anal penetration by lubricated object

Table 31.4: Opnion for non-penetrative assault

History, physical and forensic evidence from FSL	Opinion
Bite marks present and/or FSL detects salivary stains	There are signs suggestive of evidence of bite mark/s on ___________ site (time the injury)
Sucking marks (discoid, subcutaneous extravasation of blood, with or without bite marks) present and/or FSL detects salivary stains	There are signs suggestive of sucking mark/s on ___________ site (time the injury)
Forceful fondling, with presence of bruises or contusions with or without fingernail marks	There are signs suggestive of forceful physical injuries on ___________ site (time the injury) (which may be due to fondling)
Only forceful kissing and FSL detects salivary stains	There are signs suggestive of salivary contact (which may be due to kissing)
If the history suggests forced masturbation of the assailant by the survivor and if there is evidence of seminal stains detected on the hands	There are signs suggestive of the survivor of seminal fluid contact (which may be due to masturbation)
In case there are no signs of sucking, licking___________detected, but the history suggests some such form of assault	It is still important to document a good history because the survivor may have had a bath or washed him/herself

Medical and Psychological Treatment

Medical therapy requires attention to life threatening conditions first. In the absence of such conditions, prophylactic treatment for venereal disease and pregnancy should be addressed. **Rape trauma syndrome** is of concern. The appropriate management of the patient may minimize additional stress. The victim should receive all services completely free of cost. Privacy after assault is a sensitive issue and questioning must be approached carefully. Despite the need for sensitivity, it is important to ask about specific acts that the rapist performed, since the patient's embarrassment may lead to minimal response.

Concept of 'One Stop Centre'

Ministry of Women and Child Development (MWCD), has formulated a Centrally Sponsored Scheme for setting up One Stop Centres (OSC) across India. This is a sub-scheme of Umbrella Scheme for National Mission for Empowerment of Women including Indira Gandhi Mattritav Sahayog Yojana, popularly known as Sakhi. The scheme is being implemented since 1st April 2015 and is funded through Nirbhaya fund. The objectives of establishment of OSC are: (i) To provide integrated support and assistance to women affected by violence, both in private and public spaces under one roof. (ii) To facilitate immediate, emergency and non-emergency access to a range of services including medical, legal, psychological and counselling support under one roof to fight against any forms of violence against women.

Causes of Death in Rape Victims

(i) ***Shock*** due to fright and emotion can be overwhelming and may lead to death without any bodily injury. It's more common in young women especially teenagers and in virgins who are very much frightened by the first encounter. (ii) ***Hemorrhage*** can occur in cases of violent rape when the victim is forcibly raped and massive hemorrhage occurs from tears in the vagina. Also, in cases of the assailant having a sadist tendency, excessive bites on the body can lead to hemorrhage and death. (iii) ***Suffocation or asphyxia*** is one of the very common causes of death. The assailant at times tries to close the mouth of the victim to prevent her from shouting and calling for help. The assailant may either suffocate the victim or strangulate her.

Medicolegal Aspects of Rape

(i) ***Rape and Resistance:*** It is important to differentiate between the false allegations and true rape. Resistance by the victim is an important indicator of rape. Any injuries present on the body of the victim which correlate with the description of the circumstances provided should be given due importance to differentiate true and false allegations. (ii) ***Rape under narcotics or sleep:*** If the victim is incapacitated by narcotic drugs or alcoholic intoxication then there are no injuries on the body. In such cases even if the victim has consented it's considered invalid and sexual intercourse is considered as rape. Partial penetration can rarely occur during sleep in a virgin female though complete penetration is highly improbable. (iii) ***Rape by impersonation of the husband:*** This is a very rare occurrence, the only possibility occurs when the person alleged is and identical twin of the husband, who is away for a long time and the woman is unable to identify the person as different from her husband. (iv) ***Rape during unconsciousness:*** Rape can be committed on a woman during syncope, epileptic coma, hypnosis and unconsciousness resulting from administration of narcotics, anaesthetic agents and intoxicating substances. However, when she regains consciousness a virgin female would feel pain, tenderness and moistening of her genitalia. In these cases, she is bound to complain immediately but suspicion may arise when she complains after a lapse of long time.

Examination of the Accused (S. 54 Cr.P.C.)

The procedure of examination is same as that of the victim and it is preferable to examine the accused after the victim has been examined. For examination of the accused following methods are to be adopted: (i) A written request from the investigating officer/court to be obtained. (ii) Consent of the accused is taken after explaining him the detailed procedure and outcome of the examination preferably in the presence of a third party whose signature is obtained. (iii) He should be identified by the police officials who accompanies and also two identifying marks to be written in the report. Recent photograph of the accused to be pasted on the report with a signature of the doctor examining him as it is very convenient to identify him in the court of law. (iv) Exact time and date and place of examination to be noted. (v) Examination must be carried as soon as possible as there is chances of loss of trace evidence and other vital points. (vi) General development including the genital development to be noted. (vii) Detailed history of the case is obtained from the accused which is to be corroborated with the history given by the investigating officer. (viii) Mental status and general behaviour should be observed and noted down in the report. If at all any suspicion of any drugs or alcohol is present it should be noted. (ix) Clothes are to be examined for the presence of soil, mud, blood and seminal stains etc. and if at all there is any loss of button or a tear it should be noted down. (x) Evidence of cosmetics like lipstick, face powder, perfume etc. to be searched for. (xi) Nails scrapping should be examined for the presence of fibers, hair, blood, epithelial cells etc. (xii) Marks of struggle on the body to be looked for and the detailed examination of the injuries such as teeth bite, scratch especially over the inner side of thigh or genitalia to be looked for.

Local examination: (i) Development of the genital organs and are there is any scratch abrasions and bruising of the genitalia caused by the victim during struggle for prevention of intercourse to be noted down. (ii) Forceful penetration against the resistance may produce tears or bruising of the frenulum of the prepuce in the uncircumcised penis, but rupture of the frenulum is very rare. (iii) There may be abrasion of the glans penis in both circumcised and uncircumcised penis. The above injuries are more common in connection with children because of the disproportionate sizes of female and male genitalia. (iv)There may be bloodstain over the glans or shaft of the penis. (v) Groove behind the glans to be examined for the presence of smegma. Absence of smegma may indicate that the intercourse might have been performed. However, presence of smegma rules out the possibility of complete penetration because smegma is rubbed off during intercourse. The smegma is nothing but a mixture of the shed off epithelial cells and secretions from the Tyson's glands over the glans. It takes about 24 hours to be deposited again.

Specimens to be collected: (i) Swabs from the coronal sulcus, shaft, urethral orifice and adjacent areas. They may reveal the presence of semen or vaginal cells. (ii) Blood for grouping, drugs, alcohol and DNA analysis etc. (iii) Pubic hair combing may reveal female pubic hair and at least 10-20 pubic hair should be collected by closely shaving them for future comparison. (iv) Stained areas on the clothing should be marked and the clothing sealed and handed over to the police.

***Opinion*:** The opinion in cases of accused can be expressed as: (i) There is nothing to suggest that the person is incapable of performing the act. (ii) Person is not capable of performing the act because of gross abnormalities in the genital organs. (iii) Findings are suggestive of recent sexual act.

Tests to be Carried Out in An Accused

(i) ***Lugol's iodine test:*** This is done by cleaning the organ with a filter paper and subsequently exposing the paper with a vapor of Lugol's iodine. The filter paper becomes brown if the vaginal epithelial cells are present because of their content of glycogen. This indicates that the penetration has occurred. (ii) Genital organ to be washed with saline and the material is stained with **Papanicolaou's stain.** It reveals the vaginal and cervical cells and Barr body identification that is suggestive of recent intercourse. (iii) Shaft of the **penis is squeezed** to see if there is any discharge of semen at the meatus that indicates the recent emission.

Tests to Detect Truth

The following methods can be used to ascertain the truth behind the statement given by the accused. These tests can be done for any other type of crimes and are not specific to the accused of sexual offences.

1. **Narcoanalysis test:** The subject's imagination is neutralized by making him semiconscious. In this state, it becomes difficult for him to lie. His answers are restricted to facts he is aware of and becomes incapable of resistance to questioning as well as incapable of inventing falsehood that he is using to conceal the guilt. The drugs used for the purpose are: (a) Scopolamine hydrobromide ½ mg S.C. followed by ¼ mg every 20 minutes for an average 3-6 injections till the subject reaches proper stage for questioning (b) Sodium amytal or sodium pentothal (**truth serum**) is given intravenously as 2.5-5% solution at a rate not to exceed 1 ml till proper stage is induced (c) Sodium seconal 0.1 gm is given 1½ hours before induction. Then 15 mg morphine sulphate and ½ mg

scopolamine hydrobromide are given subcutaneously after 45 minutes. All three drugs may also be given intravenously to save time. These drugs make the person more talkative and he loses inhibitions. These drugs depress the actions of CNS and causes hypotension and bradycardia. In a relaxed state the person reveals repressed feelings or memories and is susceptible to suggestions. However, there are chances of larger number of false negatives.

2. **P 300 test:** Sensors are attached to the head and the subject is seated before a computer monitor. He is then shown certain images or made to hear certain sounds. Waves are generated only if the subject has some connection with the pictures or sounds. The subject is not asked any questions.
3. **Lie detector test (Polygraph):** A polygraph is an instrument that simultaneously records changes in physiological processes such as heartbeat, blood pressure, respiration and electrical resistance (galvanic skin response or GSR). The polygraph is used as a lie detector by police departments, the FBI, the CIA, Federal and state governments, and numerous private agencies. The underlying theory of the polygraph is that when people lie they also get measurably nervous about lying. The heartbeat increases, blood pressure goes up, breathing rhythms change, perspiration increases, etc. A baseline for these physiological characteristics is established by asking the subject questions whose answers the investigator knows. Deviation from the baseline for truthfulness is taken as sign of lying. There are three basic approaches to the polygraph test: (i) ***Control question test (CQT):*** This test compares the physiological response to relevant questions about the crime with the response to questions relating to possible prior misdeeds. (ii) ***Directed lie test (DLT):*** This test tries to detect lying by comparing physiological responses when the subject is told to deliberately lie to responses when they tell the truth. (iii) ***Guilty knowledge test (GKT):*** This test compares physiological responses to multiple choice type questions about the crime, one choice of which contains information only the crime investigators and the criminal would know about.
4. **Brain fingerprinting:** It is a technique that measures recognition of familiar stimuli by measuring electrical brain wave responses to words, phrases, or pictures that are presented on a computer screen. Brain fingerprinting was invented by Dr. Lawrence Farwell. The theory is that the suspect's reaction to the details of an event or activity will reflect if the suspect had prior knowledge of the event or activity. This test uses the memory and encoding related multifaceted electroencephalographic response to detect familiarity reaction. The person to be tested wears a special headband with electronic sensors that measure the EEG from several locations on the scalp. In order to calibrate the brain fingerprinting system, the testee is presented with a series of irrelevant stimuli, words, and pictures, and a series of relevant stimuli, words, and pictures. The test subject's brain response to these two different types of stimuli allow the testor to determine if the measured brain responses to test stimuli, called probes, are more similar to the relevant or irrelevant responses.

The technique uses the fact that an electrical signal known as P300 is emitted from an individual's brain approximately 300 milliseconds after it is confronted with a stimulus that has special significance to that individual (e.g., a murder weapon or a victim's face). Because it is based on EEG signals, the system does not require the testee to issue verbal responses to questions or stimuli.

Brain fingerprinting uses electrical brain responses to detect the presence or absence of information stored in the brain. Because it depends only on information stored in the brain and cognitive brain responses, brain fingerprinting does not depend on the emotions of the subject, nor is it affected by emotional responses. Brain fingerprinting is fundamentally different from the polygraph, which measures emotion-based physiological signals such as heart rate, sweating, and blood pressure. Also, unlike polygraph testing it does not attempt to determine whether or not the subject is lying or telling the truth. Rather, it measures the subject's brain response to relevant words, phrases, or pictures to detect whether or not the relevant information is stored in the subject's brain.

Incest

Incest is sexual intercourse by a man with a woman closely related either socially or genetically and law forbids them to marry. Although incest is taboo or forbidden in the majority of cultures, the precise meaning of the word varies widely because different cultures have differing notions of sexual activity. Some jurisdictions consider only those related by birth and others for those related by adoption or marriage. Various types of incest are: (i) **Oedipus complex** (son and mother) (ii) **Electra complex** (daughter and father) (iii) **Pharoan complex** (brother and sister). Parental incest including opposite sex and same sex forms committed by both fathers and mothers is the most common incestuous relationship. It often occurs in situations where one parent is either absent from the household or emotionally or sexually unavailable. The other parent may use the child as a substitute for their missing partner. Parental incest has tremendous potential for causing psychological harm to the child. Also such a relationship can be established by an adult who are in some responsible roles such as teachers, religious authorities, caretakers of prisons, juvenile reformatories. Incest between siblings is fairly common part of sexual exploration by children especially in families with children who are close in age. Consensual incest between adults occurs where there is no dependence on the adults as parent-child or sibling-sibling dependence precludes independent consent such as that between mother and son. Examples of incest in mythology are rampant. In Greek mythology Zeus and Hera were brother and sister as well as husband and wife. The Bible also contains a number of references to incest. Incestuous relationships were widespread during part of Egyptian history. Incestuous unions were frowned upon and considered as a violation of natural and social order in Roman times. In India, incest as such is not an offence but the accused can be penalized for rape whereas in Western countries it is a cognizable offence.

Adultery

S. 497 I.P.C. describes adultery as: "Whoever has sexual intercourse with a person who is and who he knows or has reason to believe to be the wife of another man without the consent or connivance of that man, such sexual intercourse not amounting to the offence of rape is guilty of the offence of adultery". The woman must be married while the man may or may not be married. In India, the wife is not punishable as an abettor.

In September 2018, the Supreme Court of India had declared Section 497 of the Indian Penal Code–that makes adultery a punishable offence for men–unconstitutional and struck it down. Adultery is no longer offence in India, however, it still can be a valid ground for divorce and nullity of marriage. **Fornication** refers to consensual sexual intercourse between two people not married to each other.

THE PROTECTION OF CHILDREN FROM SEXUAL OFFENCES ACT, 2012 (AMENDMENT 2019, 2020)

The Protection of Children from Sexual Offences (POCSO) Act became effective from 9th March, 2012. For the first time, a special law has been passed to provide for the protection of children from the offences of sexual assault, sexual harassment and pornography while safeguarding the interests of the child at every stage of the judicial process by incorporating child-friendly mechanisms for reporting, recording of evidence, investigation and speedy trial of offences through designated Special Courts. It was amended in 2019 and the Act has enhanced punishment under various sections of the Act including punishment for aggravated penetrative sexual assault. The Act has also tightened the provisions to counter child pornography. The Act is gender neutral and recognizes that boy can be victims of sexual violence as well. It defines a child as any person below the age of 18 years.

A. **Definitions of the Offences Mentioned in the Act are:**

(i) ***Penetrative Sexual Assault* (S. 3):** A person is said to commit "penetrative sexual assault", If (a) He penetrates his penis, to any extent, into the vagina, mouth, urethra or anus of a child or makes the child to do so with him or any other person; or (b) He inserts, to any extent, any object or a part of the body, not being the penis, into the vagina, the urethra or anus of the child or makes the child to do so with him or any other person; or (c) He manipulates any part of the body of the child so as to cause penetration into the vagina, the urethra or anus of the child or makes the child to do so with him or any other person; or (d) He applies his mouth to the penis, vagina, anus, urethra of the child or makes the child to do so to such person or any other person.

(ii) ***Aggravated Penetrative Sexual Assault* (S. 5)**: Whoever, being a police officer, or a member of the armed forces or security forces or being a public servant or being on the management or on the staff of a jail, remand home, protection home, observation home, or other place of custody or care and protection or being on the management or staff of a hospital, whether government or private, or being on the management or staff of an educational institution or religious institution commits penetrative sexual assault on a child or commits such assault in gang or by using deadly weapons, fire, heated substance or corrosive substance; or causes grievous hurt or bodily injury or injury to the sexual organs of the child is said to commit aggravated penetrative sexual assault.

Amendment 2019: These include: (i) Assault resulting in death of child; and (ii) Assault committed during communal or sectarian violence/a natural calamity, or in any similar situations of violence.

(iii) ***Sexual Assault (S. 7):*** (a) Any Act namely touching with sexual intent vagina, penis, anus or breast of the child or makes the child touch the vagina; (b) Causing the child to touch such parts of the body of the offender or any other person; (c) Any other act with sexual intent involving physical touch **except penetration**.

(iv) ***Aggravated Sexual Assault (S. 9):*** Similar to aggravating circumstances mentioned in S. 5. Amendment 2019 includes: (i) Assault committed during communal or sectarian violence or a natural calamity; and (ii) Administrating or help in administering any hormone or any chemical substance, to a child for the purpose of attaining early sexual maturity.

(v) ***Sexual Harassment of the Child (S. 11):*** Acts done by one with sexual intent, namely: (a) Utters any word, sound, makes any gesture, exhibits any object or part of body with the intention that such word shall be heard, or such gesture shall be seen by the child; or (b) Makes a child exhibit his body or any part of his body so as it is seen by such person or any other person; or (c) Shows any object to a child in any form or media for pornographic purposes; or (d) Repeatedly or constantly follows or watches or contacts a child either directly or through electronic, digital or any other means; or (e) Threatens to use, in any form of media, a real or fabricated depiction through electronic, film or digital or any other mode, of any part of the body of the child or the involvement of the child in a sexual act; or (f) Entices a child for pornographic purposes or gives gratification there for. *Explanation:* Any question which involves sexual intent shall be a question of fact.

(vi) ***Use of Child for Pornographic Purposes (S.13):*** Whoever uses child in any form of media (including programs/advertisements telecast by television channels or internet or any electronic/print form, whether or not such programme or advertisement is intended for personal use or for distribution) for purposes of sexual gratification, which includes: (a) Representing sexual organs of child (b) Using child in real/simulated sexual acts (with or without penetration) (c) Indecent/obscene representation of child.

[S. 2(1da)], defines "child pornography" as any visual depiction of sexually explicit conduct involving a child which include photograph, video, digital or computer-generated image indistinguishable from an actual child, and image created, adapted, or modified, but appear to depict a child.

[S.15(1-3)], offences for storage of pornographic material involving children: These include: (i) Failing to destroy, or delete, or report pornographic material involving a child, and (ii) Transmitting, displaying, distributing such material except for the purpose of reporting it. It also enhances the punishments for such offences.

B. **Procedures for Reporting, Recording of Evidence, Investigation and Trial of Offences:** The Act incorporates a **child friendly procedure** for all stages. These include: (i) Recording the statement of the child at the residence of the child or at the place of his choice, preferably by a woman police officer not below the rank of sub-inspector. (ii) Police officer not to be in uniform while recording the statement of the child. (iii) The statement of the child to be recorded as spoken by the child. (iv) Assistance of an interpreter or translator or an expert as per the need of the child. (v) Assistance of special educator or any person familiar with the manner of communication of the child in case child is disabled. (vi) History seeking should be facilitated by use of dolls and body charts. (vii) No child to be detained in the police station in the night for any reason. (viii) Medical examination of the child to be conducted in the presence of the parent of the child or any other person in whom the child has trust or confidence. If not available, hospital has to provide a female who will be present at time of examination (S.27). (viii) In case the victim is a girl child, the medical examination shall be conducted by a woman doctor. (ix) Genital and anal examination should not be conducted mechanically or routinely. (x) Collection of evidence after a thorough medical examination. (xi) Conduct age assessment of the victim (if required). (xii) Treatment for the physical and genital injuries. (xiii) Offer prophylaxis for sexually transmitted diseases including HIV. (xiv) Discuss emergency contraceptives with the pubertal child and her parent. (xv) Do baseline evaluation for mental health issues. (xvi) Monthly follow-up at least for six months to look for development of psychiatric disorders. (xvii) Establishment of **Special Courts** for trial of offences. (xviii) Frequent breaks for the child during trial. (xix) Child not to be called repeatedly to testify. (xx) No aggressive questioning or character assassination of the child. (xxi) Do family counselling. (xxii) **In-camera trial** of cases. (xxiii) For speedy trial, the Act provides for the evidence of the child to be recorded within a period of 30 days. And Special Court is to complete the trial within a period of one year.

C. **Relief and Rehabilitation of the Child:** Soon after the complaint is made to the Special Juvenile Police Unit (SJPU) or local police, these will make immediate arrangements to give the child, care and protection such as admitting the child into shelter home or to the nearest hospital within twenty-four hours of the complaint and report the matter to the Child Welfare Committee within 24 hours of recording the complaint, for long-term rehabilitation of the child.

The Act casts a duty on the Central and State Governments to spread awareness through media including the television, radio and the print media at regular intervals to make the general public, children as well as their parents and guardians aware of the provisions of this Act.

The National Commission for the Protection of Child Rights (NCPCR) and State Commissions for the Protection of Child Rights (SCPCRs) have been made the designated authority to monitor the implementation of the Act.

D. **Punishments for Offences Covered in the Act are:**

Offence	Minimum	Maximum	Fine
Penetrative Sexual Assault (S. 3)	10 years (Child <16 years: 20 years) (S.4)	Life imprisonment–means remainder of natural life	Yes (for medical expenses and rehabilitation)
Aggravated Penetrative Sexual Assault (S. 5)	20 years (rigorous) (S. 6)	Life imprisonment–means remainder of natural life or death penalty	Yes (for medical expenses and rehabilitation)
Sexual Assault (S. 7)	3 years (S. 8)	5 years	Yes
Aggravated Sexual Assault (S. 9)	5 years (S.10)	7 years	Yes
Sexual Harassment (S. 11)	–	Up to 3 years (S. 12)	Yes
Use of child for pornographic purposes	5 years	7 years	Yes
Use of child for pornographic purposes resulting in penetrative sexual assault	10 years (Child <16 years: 20 years)	Life imprisonment	Yes
Use of child for pornographic purposes resulting in aggravated penetrative sexual assault	20 years	life imprisonment or death	Yes
Use of child for pornographic purposes resulting in sexual assault	3 years	5 years	Yes
Use of child for pornographic purposes resulting in aggravated sexual assault	5 years	7 years	Yes

For the more heinous offences of Penetrative Sexual Assault, Aggravated Penetrative Sexual Assault, Sexual Assault and Aggravated Sexual Assault, the **burden of proof is shifted on the accused**. To prevent misuse of the law, punishment has been provided for making false complaint or proving false information with malicious intent. Such punishment has been kept relatively light (6 months) to encourage reporting. If false complaint is made against a child, punishment is higher (one year). The **attempt to commit an offence** under the Act has been made liable for punishment up to half the punishment prescribed for the commission of the offence. Punishment for **abetment of the offence** is the same as for the commission of the offence. The media has been barred from disclosing the identity of the child without the permission of the Special Court. The punishment for breaching this provision by media may be from six months to one year.

- **S. 19 POCSO Act and S. 357C Cr.P.C.** both instruct the doctor/hospital to mandatorily inform the police when they are examining a case of sexual violence.
- **S. 21 POCSO Act and S. 166B I.P.C.** prescribe punishment for not following the directions of S. 19 POCSO Act and S. 357 Cr.P.C.

E. **Protection of Children from Sexual Offences Rules, 2020**

The Ministry of Women and Child Development of Central Government on 9th March 2020 notified Protection of Children from Sexual Offences Rules, 2020. Significant additions in the new rule include: (i) Provision of mandatory police verification of staffs in school (ii) Zero tolerance to child pornography (iii) Reporting of pornographic material involving a child (iv) Imparting age-appropriate child rights education (iv) Provision for compensation within 30 days (v) Provides definition of the "District Child Protection Unit", "expert", "special educator", and "Person familiar with the manner of communication of the child" "support person".

F. **The Juvenile Justice (Care and Protection of Children) Amendment Act, 2021**

The amendment Act empowers the District Magistrate to issue adoption orders to ensure speedy disposal of cases and enhance accountability. The Amendment Act also re-defines the category of 'serious offences'. Serious offences, will also include offences for which maximum punishment is imprisonment of more than seven years, and minimum punishment is not prescribed or is less than seven years.

UNNATURAL SEXUAL OFFENCES

S. 377 I.P.C. Unnatural offences: Whoever voluntarily has carnal intercourse against the order of nature with any man, woman, or animal, shall be punished with imprisonment for life, or with imprisonment of either description for a term which may extend to ten years and shall also be liable to fine.

Explanation: Penetration is sufficient to constitute the carnal intercourse necessary to the offence described in this section.

The unnatural sexual offences are classified as sodomy, buccal coitus and bestiality.

Current Legal Status of S. 377 I.P.C.

On 2 July, 2009, in *Naz Foundation v. Government of NCT of Delhi* case, two-judge benches of the Delhi High Court partially struck down the provision of S. 377 I.P.C. which criminalised consensual unnatural sexual acts between adults in private, holding that it violated the fundamental right of life and liberty and the right to equality as guaranteed in the Constitution. However, S. 377 I.P.C. will continue to govern non-consensual penile non-vaginal sex and penile non-vaginal sex involving minors. It is a landmark case in legal history of India. It de-criminalised consensual sex between gay adults.

On 11 December, 2013 while hearing in *Suresh Kumar Koushal v. Naz Foundation*, a two-judge panel of the Supreme Court overturned the Delhi High Court decision and reinstated S. 377 I.P.C., ruling that amending the law was the responsibility of the legislature.

On 24 August 2017, in case *Justice K.S. Puttaswamy (Retd.) and Anr. v. Union of India and Ors.*, the Supreme Court of India held that the Right to Privacy is a fundamental right protected under Article 21 and Part III of the Indian Constitution.

On 6 September, 2018, a five-judge Constitution bench of Supreme Court of India in case *Navtej Singh Johar v. Union of India*, **decriminalized part of S. 377 I.P.C**. It ruled that all consensual unnatural sexual acts between adults in private are not violative of S. 377 I.P.C. However, the court clarified that the provisions of S. 377 I.P.C. will continue to govern for bestiality, non-consensual penile non-vaginal sex and penile non-vaginal sex involving minors.

I. **Sodomy or Buggery or Greek Love**

Sodomy is a term of religious origin to characterize certain sexual acts. It is most commonly used to describe the specific act of anal sex between two males, between a woman and a machine, between a male and a female, human and animals. The term sodomy also includes the non-coital sexual act such as oral sex in the natural orifices like nose, ear, umbilicus and sometimes between the toes. The term sodomy is derived from the name of the ancient city of *Sodom*, which according to the Bible was destroyed by God for its misdeeds. The epistle of Jude in the New Testament, however, echoes the Genesis narrative and recalls mainly the sexually immoral aspects of Sodom's sins just as Sodom and Gomorrah and the surrounding cities, which likewise indulged in sexual immortality and pursued unnatural desire; serve as an example by undergoing a punishment of eternal fire. The first known use of the term sodomy used in a more general sense to mean 'crime against hookers' is found in the writings of Jewish historian Josephus. In today's common language it identifies the practices of anal or oral intercourse. From the earliest times in the United States, sodomy was prohibited and in the 1950s, all the states had some form of law criminalizing sodomy. In 2003, only 10 states had laws prohibiting sodomy with penalties ranging from 1 to 15 years imprisonment. Additionally, four other states had laws that specifically prohibited same-sex sodomy. In 2003, the USA Supreme Court in *Lawrence v. Texas* case, ruled that Texas' sodomy law was unconstitutional. The verdict made sexual activity between homosexuals legal in every state in America. In UK, sodomy is legal for consenting adults, if it is done in private.

In India, sodomy implies an anal intercourse. It can be heterosexual or homosexual depending on whether two men or a man and a woman are involved. If the passive agent is an adult, its known as **gerentophilia** and if the passive agent is a young boy it is known as **pederasty** and the habitual passive agent is called a **catamite.** A **pedophile** is an adult who repeatedly engages in sexual activities with children. When sodomy is practiced between two men they alternately act as active and passive agents.

Sodomy is commonly seen in prisoners, sailors and persons staying in military barracks, hostels etc. If the male organ is inserted or thrust between the thighs it implies penetration necessary to constitute unnatural offence.

In India, male prostitutes called **eunuchs** act as passive agents in sodomy. They dress up like females and also adopt their tastes and habits. Of these **Hijrahs** are those who have been castrated mostly before puberty. After the wounds heal the male organ resembles female genitalia. In addition, some hormonal imbalance may cause some feminine characters in them. **Zenanas** are those in whom the genitalia are intact.

In India, consensual sodomy between two adults is legal. In case of nonconsensual sodomy or sodomy with a minor is a criminal offence under S. 377 I.P.C. Offence for nonconsensual sodomy by a man with an adult woman shall be considered under S. 375 I.P.C. However, offence of nonconsensual sodomy by a man with his wife is considered as cruelty, which is a ground for divorce and the husband can also be punished under S. 377 I.P.C. According to *S.13 Hindu Marriage Act, 1955* it is annulment of marriage when the husband is found guilty of sodomy. Any degree of penetration or any attempt for penetration is punishable and proof of emission is not necessary. It is a cognizable, non-bailable offence to be tried by a 1st class magistrate and the accused is punishable with life imprisonment or imprisonment up to 10 years and also liable for fine.

Medical examination in a case of sodomy: A medical examination of the accused (active agent) as well as victim (passive agent) is necessary.

Preliminaries: A written request must be obtained from the police authorities for the purposes. A written informed consent for examination of the victim should be obtained. If minor (<18 years), consent of parent/guardian is required for examination. In case of female victim, there should be a female chaperone. The victim can also request for an examination but the doctor should inform the police. A detailed medical history should be taken before commencing the examination and it must be enquired whether the accused (active agent) has obtained the other party's consent by means of force or fraud and also if the active agent was under influence of drugs, or by reason of his disease or age incapable of committing the offence. The name, date, place, time along with identification marks should be noted.

Examination of the victim (non-habitual passive agent): The examination should be carried in proper light in the knee elbow position. In case of a young child, the examination should be done on left lateral position. The findings are: (i) Anal muscle are dilated with loss of elasticity and tone on digital examination. (ii) There is pain and tenderness during the examination. (iii) Diffuse swelling of anal margins with obliteration of normal anal skin folds. (iv) Linear abrasions on the perianal area are more marked in children due to disproportion in the size of the penis of the active agent and the anal canal of the passive agent. (v) Sudden force may produce anal lacerations with bruising that are sometimes triangular with base at the anus and sides vertically inwards into the rectum (Figures 31.10 and 31.11). (vi) Anal fissures may also be present. (vii) Blood and seminal stains may be found sticking to the clothes of the passive agent and in and around the anus and perineum. (viii) Swabs from inside and around the anus should be preserved for microscopic examination. (ix) Any loose pubic hair or lubricant found on the undergarments and around the anus also suggests the evidence of the crime.

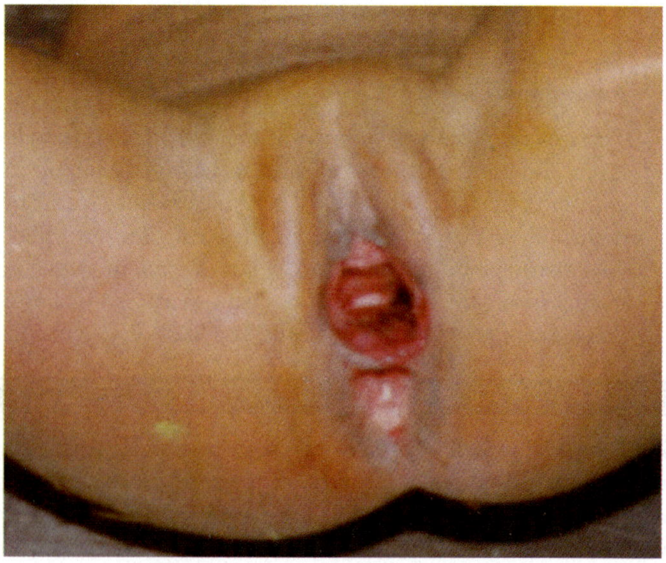

Figure 31.10: Anal tear in sodomy

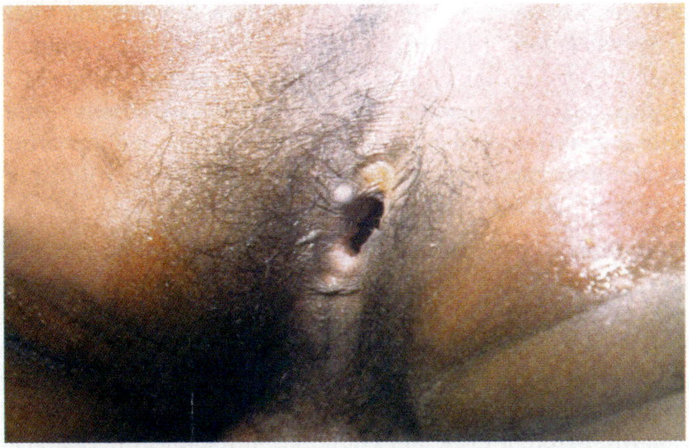

Figure 31.11: Anal tear at 3 O'clock position in sodomy

Examination of the victim (habitual passive agent): (i) There is shaving of perianal skin. (ii) Victim does not experience pain or tenderness on examination. (iii) Skin around the anus is smooth and thickened. (iv) These are loss of anal tone and disappearance of radial folds. (v) Funnel shaped depression of buttocks towards anus due to absorption of fat is more demarcated in old, thin victims than the fatty adult. (vi) Anus is dilated and patulous with loss of rugosity. (vii) Anal fissure, piles and scars of old lacerations are seen. (viii) Evidence of venereal diseases such as gonorrhea and syphilis may be present.

***Examination of accused (active agent)*:** The person should be examined soon after the commission of the crime, in which case following findings are evident: (i) Peculiar smell of anal glands transferred to the penis persists for sometime after the act unless washed thoroughly. (ii) Traces of fecal matter and lubricant on the organ. (iii) There are abrasions on the prepuce and glans penis and tearing of frenulum. (iv) Presence of blood and seminal stains is corroborative. (v) Presence of sexually transmitted diseases such as gonorrhoea and syphilis. (vi) Marks of violence on the body of the active agent in the non-consenting act. (vii) Penis may be elongated with constriction of glans and twisting of urethra. (viii) Clothing may have seminal stains.

II. **Tribadism**

This is female homosexuality and also known as **lesbianism or sapphism**. Women of the **Isle of lesbos** practiced this perversion. Sexual gratification is obtained by kissing, general body contact or manual manipulation of breast and genitalia. Clitoris may be elongated or an artificial penis or phallus may be used. The active partner is known as **butch or dyke** and the passive partner is called **femme**. A lesbian who did not identify as either butch or femme is called **kiki**. Lesbians who are morbidly jealous of one another when rejected can commit crimes like homicide and suicide. In India, lesbianism is not punishable under S. 377 as it criminalizes only non-consensual 'penile non-vaginal sex'.

III. **Bestiality**

Sexual intercourse by a human being with lower animals like calves, sheep, she-ass, goats and larger birds like chicken, duck etc. at times. Vaginal intercourse is very common though it may be done through anus or any other natural orifice. Persons who go out with animals usually indulge in such practice and are commonly mentally deranged. There is a false belief that sexually transmitted diseases are cured by sexual intercourse with a she-ass. Females use dogs and cats to manipulate their genitalia. Actual coitus is rare. Both the human and the alleged animal have to be examined. Presence of human spermatozoa in the vagina or anus of the animal, presence of animal hairs on the body or the clothing of the accused and presence of abrasions on the genitals can confirm the commission of the crime. Bestiality is punishable under section 377 I.P.C. According to *S.13 Hindu Marriage Act, 1955* it is annulment of marriage when the husband is found guilty of bestiality.

IV. **Buccal Coitus (Sin of Gomorrah)**

According to Bible it was prevalent in the town called **Gomorrah**. Male organ is inserted into the mouth of a young child. Faint teeth marks and abrasions may be seen on the penis. Aspiration of semen can result in accidental deaths and seminal fluid is found in respiratory tree that should be examined microscopically. Buccal swabs are useful up to 9 hours to demonstrate the sperm. In India, consensual buccal coitus between adults in private is legal in India, however buccal coitus without consent and with minor is a criminal offence. It is punishable under S. 377 I.P.C. with punishment up to 10 years. Offence for nonconsensual buccal coitus by a man with an adult woman shall be considered under S. 375 I.P.C.

SEXUAL PERVERSIONS OR PARAPHILIAS

Sexual perversions are persistently indulged sexual acts in which complete satisfaction is sought and obtained without sexual intercourse. **Uranism** is the general term for perversions of the sexual instinct. Sexual perversions are conditions in which sexual excitement or orgasm is associated with acts or imagery that are considered unusual with problems associated with the stigmatization of labels. The neutral term paraphilia derived from the Greek roots meaning "alongside off" and "love" is used to describe what used to be called sexual perversions. Paraphilia is defined in DSM-V as "any intense and persistent sexual interest other than the sexual interest in genital stimulation or preparatory fondling with phenotypically normal, physiologically mature, consenting human partners. The aetiology of paraphilia is not known. Paraphilias often result from a variety of associated problems such as guilt, depression, shame, isolation and impairment in the capacity for normal social and sexual relationships. Psychoanalysts generally theorize that paraphilias represent a regression to or fixation at an earlier level of psychosexual development resulting in a repetitive pattern of sexual behaviour that is not mature in its application and expression. Another psychoanalytic theory holds that these conditions are all expressions of hostility in which sexual fantasies or unusual sexual acts become a means of obtaining revenge for a childhood trauma. The persistent, repetitive nature of the paraphilia is caused by an inability to erase the underlying trauma completely. A history of child abuse is sometimes seen in individuals with paraphilias. This condition may result from fear of sexual performance or intimacy, excessive alcohol intake, some physiological problems or psychosocial trauma. The nature of a paraphilia is generally specific and unchanging and is more common in males than females (Except for masochism, paraphilias are almost exclusively diagnosed in men).

Paraphilias causing distress or impairment of person's own life or the paraphilic need which has to be satisfied with involvement of personal harm or risk of harm to the community, are considered as paraphilic disorders. According to DSM-V, **Paraphilic disorder** is defined as "persistent and intense atypical sexual arousal patterns that are accompanied by clinically significant distress or impairment". For diagnosis of paraphilic disorder two criterion should be fulfilled. (i) Criteria A is the paraphilia component of the disorder, which requires an atypical focus of sexual arousal and an arousal pattern that is recurrent, intense, and persists for at least six months. (ii) Criterion B is the harm component, which requires the presence of distress, impairment in functioning, or involvement of nonconsenting victims. For diagnosis of voyeuristic disorder, a new Criterion C is added, i.e., the person should be an adult (a minimum age of 18).

There are eight specific relatively common paraphilic disorder which can be sub grouped as **criminal and noncriminal type**. In criminal Paraphilic Disorders (Exhibitionistic, Frotteuristic, Paedophilic and Voyeuristic Disorders), a nonconsenting victim is involved, and individuals acting on these sexual urges would constitute a crime. In noncriminal Paraphilic Disorders (Sexual Sadism, Sexual Masochism, Fetishistic and Transvestic Disorders) usually a consenting partner is involved, and acting on these sexual urges would not constitute a crime necessarily.

Exhibitionism

Exhibitionism means exposure of genitalia in public to obtain sexual pleasure with or without masturbatory acts, mostly by males to the persons of opposite sex. It is one of the most common type of paraphilia. The lifetime prevalence of exhibitionism by male is 2-4%, peaking in late adolescence. In some cases, the act is impulsive and spontaneous. It may be premeditated. Occasionally the women may expose themselves in public. Majority of them are psychopathic or suffer from compulsive neurosis. It is an obscene act punishable under section 294 I.P.C. with 3 months imprisonment or fine or both. The exhibitionists are divided into: (i) ***Typical male exhibitionist:*** They exhibit sometimes only with erection and never make any gesture towards his victim. (ii) ***Masturbators:*** Masturbation is the deliberate self-stimulation which effects sexual arousal. Mild masturbation exercises are common both to men and women. Techniques are largely manual, urethral insertions and anal stimulations are rare. Hollow articles like, bottles, candles, test tubes, devices made of rubber and plastic are used to stimulate female genitalia.

In females, finger is gently and rhythmically moved over the clitoris or labia minora or steady pressure is applied over these parts. Genitalia may be rubbed against pillow or bed. Women may insert fingers, glass, tubes and bananas etc. Artificial masculine genitalia parts are also used. Masturbation is an offence if done openly in public places. The masturbators may or may not be primarily exhibitionists, but enjoy masturbation in public. Their fantasies are more active and related to that a woman has come over and perhaps performed fellatio or even got into intercourse with them. They are not violent or assaultive.

The aggressive group aim at producing maximum amount of shock and terror. They will hide in the hallways or a dormitories and jump out when women come by or they will expose to single women in dark place. They make menacing and threatening gestures. After therapy they have admitted that they had assaultive and homicidal fantasies but never carried them out. Basic motive behind the act is aggressive rather than sexual.

Frotteurism

The term Frottage is derived from the French word "*frotter*", which means "to rub". Frotteurism is the contact with another person to obtain sexual gratification by rubbing against non-consenting persons in the crowd and so on (fair, buses etc.). The person who practices this act is called frotteur. When these persons attempt intercourse, they have premature ejaculation or they are impotent. It is a very common perversion and it rarely occurs alone. It is mostly reported in young adolescent males and rarely in females. The victim is usually a female. It is a criminal offence under S. 354 I.P.C. (assault or criminal force to woman with outrage her modesty) punishable with imprisonment not less than 1 year, can be extended up to 5 years along with fine.

Pedophilia

It is defined as a persistent sexual interest in prepubescent children, as reflected by one's sexual fantasies, urges, thoughts, arousal, or behaviour. The pedophile is an adult or older adolescent (at least 16 years age) and minimum 5 years older than the child. This sexual deviation is often linked to personal distress, to a significant alteration of personal, family, professional and social life. It is the only paraphilic disorder without an 'in remission'and an 'in controlled environment' specifier. Pedophilia is a sexual orientation and it does not refer people who abuse children sexually. Pedophilia is not an offence in India, however, when a pedophile involved in sexual abuse with a child, it is a punishable offence under POCSO Act. **Infantophilia** is term used for erotic preference for infants or toddlers. The term **hebephilia (ephebophila)** means the erotic preference for pubertal adolescents.

Voyeurism

Voyeurism is a disorder of sexual arousal involving the act of observing unsuspecting individuals, usually strangers, who may be naked in the process of disrobing or engaged in sexual activity. Masturbation usually occurs during or shortly after voyeuristic activity. A variation of voyeurism entails listening to erotic conversations. Voyeurism may occur with exhibitionism. It is a sociopathic personality disorder. Onset is before the age of fifteen years. Childhood trauma of sexual abuse or significant childhood experience manifests itself in voyeuristic behaviour. Voyeurs do not commit major sex crimes, but at times they may assault the victim or commit murder. It is rare in females.

Voyeurism is now regarded as a serious offence and punishment for it is defined in **Section 354C I.P.C.**: Any man who watches, or captures the image of a woman engaging in a private act in circumstances where she would usually have the expectation of not being observed either by the perpetrator or by any other person at the behest of the perpetrator or disseminates such image shall be punished on **first conviction** with imprisonment of either description for a term which shall not be less than one year, but which may extend to three years, and shall also be liable to fine, and be punished on a **second or subsequent conviction**, with imprisonment of either description for a term which shall not be less than three years, but which may extend to seven years, and shall also be liable to fine.

For the purpose of this act, "private act" includes an act of watching carried out in a place which, in the circumstances, would reasonably be expected to provide privacy and where the victim's genitals, posterior or breasts are exposed or covered only in underwear; or the victim is using a lavatory; or the victims doing a sexual act that is not of a kind ordinarily done in public.

Bogging: It is a special form of voyeurism taking place on railways. It consists of leaning out of the carriage windows and observing love-making in the adjacent carriage.

Sadism

Sadism is the sexual pleasure or gratification in the infliction of pain and suffering upon another person. The term is derived from the name of a French writer, **Donatien Alphonse Francois de Sade (1740-1819)**. He was very infamous for his crimes and writings. Many of these stories were about sexualities, cruelty and torture. Sexual gratification is obtained or enhanced from the acts of physical cruelty or infliction of pain upon one's partner. It is commonly seen in males. The sadist brands his sexual partner, bites her severely, flogs with whips, beats with stick, inflicts cuts with knife and also ill treats her in many ways. There are 4 grades or levels of sadism. In extreme cases, the sadist may commit murder on a female child usually inflicting serious injuries on her genital that is called lust murder.

Lust murder: In extreme cases murder serves as stimuli for the sexual act and becomes equivalent of coitus, accompanies by erection, ejaculation and orgasm. The condition has periodic outbreaks due to patient's recurring compulsion to paroxysmal sexual desire. There are multiple injuries on the body with incised or stabbing of breast and genitalia accompanied by sucking, licking and biting. There is a desire to drink blood and to eat flesh. Erection and ejaculation may be followed by sexual intercourse with dying or injured victim. His behaviour is usually normal until next paroxysm. Every murder during sexual act is not a lust murder.

Necrophilia: Necrophilia involves the desire for and use of a dead body for sexual purpose. *First category:* Necrophilia may take the form of a fetish where the portions of the dead body like breasts of a female are removed and either worn by the male offender in a female fashion or retained in his possession for observation or physical contact. *Second category:* In this category, the individuals exhibit a far greater degree of sadistic tendency with the desire to mutilate body of the dead women stolen from funeral parlours or removed from graves in a cemetery. Extensive mutilation may be present with removal of portions of body, most often breast, genitalia etc. for later fetish. *Third category:* It involves either utilization of a dead body for sexual satisfaction by cunnilingus or vaginal intercourse or the murder of and individual in order to have sexual contact after he or she is dead. This is very rare in practice. *Fourth category:* In this lust murder is committed. Most instances involve destruction of a dead body rather than homicide.

Masochism

Masochism is the sexual pleasure or gratification of having pain or suffering inflicted upon self, often consisting of sexual fantasies or urges for being beaten, humiliated, abused, tortured, or otherwise made to suffer, either as an enhancement to or a substitute for sexual pleasure. The name is derived from the name of the 19th century author **Leopold von Sacher-Masoch**, an Australian novalist known for his novel **Venus in Furs** that dealt with highly masochistic themes.

Sadism and masochism often go together that is one person obtaining sadistic pleasure by inflicting pain or suffering on another person who thereby obtains masochistic pleasure, so collectively known as sadomasochism. The words are now commonly used to describe personality traits in an emotional rather than sexual sense. There is quite frequently a strong emotional aspect to the sexual desires, taking the form of a need for domination or submission, the desire to be controlled, or control another, as opposed to a simple desire for pain submission. Many sadomasochistic activities involve only mild pain or discomfort. The terms sadism and masochism were first used consistently to describe these behaviours by the **German psychiatrist Richard Freiherr von Krafft Ebing** in his 1886 compilation of case studies 'Psychopathia Sexualis', a famous study of sexual perversity. **Sigmund Freud**, a psychoanalyst noted that both were often found in the same individuals and combined the two into a single dichotomous entity known as **sadomasochism**. There are a number of reasons for sadomasochistic practices. For some, taking on a role of compliance or helplessness offers a form of therapeutic escape from the stresses of life, from responsibility or from guilt. For others, being under the power of a strong controlling presence may evoke the feelings of safety and protection associated with childhood. A sadist may enjoy the feelings of power and authority that comes from playing the dominant role, or receive pleasure vicariously through the suffering of the masochist.

Fetishism

Fetishism is a form of sexual deviation, is found only in males. The fetishist experiences sexual excitement leading to orgasm from seeing some part of the body of a woman (partialism) or some article belonging to her, e.g., shoe, undergarments or some other wearing apparel. These individuals may often be arrested for burglary and also for stealing the objects of his fetishistic desire. **Diaper fetishism** also known as diaperism or nappy fetishism denotes a condition of having sexual preferences for diapers.

Transvestism or Eonism

Magnus Hirschfeld coined the term 'transvestism' in 1915 in Berlin. In Latin, *trans* means across, over and *vestere* means to dress or to wear. He used it to describe a group of people who habitually and voluntarily wore clothes of opposite sex. Hirschfeld noticed that sexual arousal was often associated with transvestite behaviour and he also clearly distinguished between transvestism as an expression of a person's contrasexual (**transgender**) feelings and fetishistic behaviour, even if the latter involved wearing clothes of the opposite sex. The term **cross-dresser** was coined for heterosexual male who wear traditional feminine clothing. This group of cross-dressers is not transvestite or transsexual. Transvestism is a deviant desire to wear clothes of opposite sex. These are homosexuals with no genital abnormality. They have strong desire to become members of the opposite sex and also seek surgery for anatomical alteration. In Indian law no recognition for a changed sex exists. **Autogynephilia** is a subtype of transvestism that refers specifically to men who become aroused by thinking or visualizing himself as a woman.

Other important paraphilias: (i) ***Somnophilia:*** It is rare paraphilia of the marauding/predatory type in which there is interest in having sex with a sleeping person. It is more commonly referred to as **Sleeping Beauty Syndrome,** however, in this case the sleeping person waking up during the sexual contact. Griffiths (2014) opined that Somnophilia is not restricted to sleeping individuals only but there is an interest in sexual activity with an unconscious person. He suggests that the definitional shift to unconsciousness may be a response to the rise in drug-facilitated sexual offences. (ii) ***Sexual oralism:*** It is application of mouth to sexual organs. It is a very common perversion, both heterosexual and homosexual. It is of two types: (a) *Fellatio:* It is oral stimulation or manipulation of penis, either by male or female. (b) *Cunnilingus:* It is oral stimulation of female genitalia. (iii) ***Undinism:*** In this paraphilia, sexual pleasure is obtained by witnessing the act of urination by someone of the same or opposite sex. In some cases, pleasure is obtained by being urinated upon by the loved one or urinating on him or her, but this is rare. (iv) ***Pyromania:*** In most cases of pyromania, there is an underlying psychosexual disorder. Some people have latent form of sadism while others obtain sexual stimulation while viewing the flames and destruction of a building. Another form of pyromania is exhibited among homosexuals where there has been infidelity among the sexual partners. The feeling of jealousy and desire to obtain revenge can be exhibited by setting afire within the apartment or house of the transgressing partner. If the latter is trapped in the fire, severe injury and even death can occur. (v) ***Myxoscopia:*** In this the person gets sexual gratification by observing another couple performing the sexual intercourse. The individuals get sexual gratification by hearing sounds of sexual intercourse or lovemaking (**Ecoutage**). (vi) ***Triolism or Trolism:*** It is an extreme form of sexual perversion within the man who obtains gratification when he either shares his own wife or girlfriend with another man or exchanges wives or compel his wife to cohabit with another man. (vii) ***Bobbit Syndrome:*** In this type of perversion, the female partner amputates the penis of her male partner with a sharp cutting weapon. (viii) ***Scatalogia:*** It is associated with obscene telephone calls. (ix) ***Caprolalia:*** The sexual excitement is obtained by using obscene language. (x) ***Caprolangnia:*** The sexual excitement is associated with the sight or smell of faeces or defaecation. (xi) ***Urolangia/Urophilia:*** The sexual excitement is associated with the sight or thought of urine or urination. (xii) ***Pygmalionism:*** Falling in love with a self-made object. (xiii) ***Klismaphilia:*** Sexual arousal by receiving or administering enema. (xiv) ***Dippoldism:*** Sexual gratification by beating children.

OTHER SEX RELATED CRIMES

Indecent Assault and Attempt to Rape

In cases where an indecent assault is made upon the person of a woman, but where rape is not committed, the culprit is charged with section 354 of I.P.C.

S. 354 I.P.C. prescribes punishment for anyone who assaults or uses criminal force to any woman with an **intent to outrage her modesty. Indecent assault** cannot be complete unless there is intention or knowledge that the woman's modesty will be outraged. Indecent assault upon a woman does not amount to an attempt to commit rape, unless the court is satisfied that there was a determination in the accused to gratify his passion at all events and in spite of all resistance. The difference between 'mere preparation' and 'an attempt' to commit an offence consists chiefly in the greater degree of determination. For attempt to commit rape, the prosecution must prove that it has gone beyond preparation. For example, the accused, a medical man, asked a woman to lie down in the bedroom for injection. When she lied down he tried to proceed for criminal intention of rape. She raised an alarm and ran out of the room. The court held this to be an attempt to commit rape. In another example the accused caught hold of a girl, stripped her, sat over her and then people came. Court held that there was attempt to commit rape. An indecent assault upon a woman is punishable under this section. The offence under this section is of less gravity than rape.

An indecent assault is an assault which right minded persons would consider as 'indecent'. Accordingly, any evidence explaining the defendants conduct, or whether any admission by him or otherwise is admissible to establish whether he intended to commit an indecent assault, as is stated under section 21 subclause (2) of the I.E.A., which reads:

S. 354A (I.P.C.) sexual harassment and punishment for sexual harassment a man committing any of the following acts:

i. Physical contact and involving unwelcome and explicitly sexual overtures; or
ii. A demand or request for sexual favour; or
iii. Showing pornographic against the will of a woman; or
iv. Making sexually coloured remarks.

Shall be guilty of the offence and shall be punished with rigorous imprisonment for a term which may extend to three years or with fine or with both, but offence committed in clause (iv) shall be punished with **imprisonment for one year or fine or both**.

S. 354B (I.P.C.) Assault or use of criminal force to woman with intent to disrobe the punishment being minimum **three years may extent to seven years and fine**.

S. 354D (I.P.C.) Stalking

1. Any man who–(i) Follows a woman and contact, or attempts to contact to foster personal interaction repeatedly despite a clear indication of disinterest by such woman; or (ii) to monitor and used by a woman of the internet, email or any other form of electronics communication, commits the offence of stalking.
2. Who commits the offence shall be punished with **imprisonment up to 3 years** and **fine for the 1st conviction** and will be punished 2nd subsequent conviction, the imprisonment may **extend to 5 years and fine.**

Prostitution

Section 2 of Immoral Trafficking Prevention Act, 1956 defined prostitution as "the sexual exploitation or abuse of persons for commercial purposes". The practice of prostitution frequently involves sadomasochistic tendencies on the part of both the participating partners. Both male and female prostitutes fall into this category. Male prostitutes engaging in homosexual acts can express a conscious or subconscious desire for self-humiliation or they may receive partial or complete sexual gratification from the humiliation of their male partners. Others allow themselves to be participants in normal or sexual practices with masochistic overtones. In most cases there are call girls who are specialists in the acts of bondage. Even massage parlours maintain private rooms completely equipped with the practice of bondage and even call girls who will make house calls on demand.

In India, prostitutes can practice their trade privately, however, few activities related to prostitution such as prostitution within 200 yards of a public place, living on the earnings of the prostitution, running brothels, soliciting, trafficking and pimping are all punishable offence.

If a person engages in sex acts with a sex worker within 200 yards of a public place or "notified area", he will be punished with imprisonment up to 3 months. If the offence is committed against the will of the person, punishment shall imprisonment for a term for 7 years and can extend to 14 years. The client may also be punished if the sex worker is below 18 years of age (From 7 to 10 years of imprisonment).

Punishment for those who visit the brothel for the purpose of sexual exploitation of any victim of trafficking:1st visit–up to 3 months/fine up to 2000, 2nd and subsequent visits–up to 6 months and fine up to 50,000.

Long Questions

1. Define rape. How will you examine an alleged rape victim? Discuss the significant legal provisions in rape.
2. How will you examine a person who is accused of rape?
3. Discuss in detail the sexual perversions.
4. Discuss the role of seminal fluid in sexual offences cases.

Short Questions

1. Section 376 I.P.C.
2. Voyeurism.
3. Tribadism.
4. Sadism.
5. Smegma.
6. Paraphilias.
7. Unnatural sexual offences.
8. Incest.
9. Seminal fluid.
10. Truth serum.
11. Narcoanalysis.
12. Brain fingerprinting.

MULTIPLE CHOICE QUESTIONS

1. **A 28 years old man has intercourse with his wife aged 14 years. This constitute rape if:**
   (a) No consent is taken
   (b) He had extramarital relations
   (c) Age of wife is less than 16 years
   (d) Age of wife is less than 15 years

2. **The following tests are done to detect the seminal stains *except:***
   (a) Florence test (b) Luminal test
   (c) Barberio's test (d) Acid phosphatase test

3. **Florence test is useful in detection of:**
   (a) Blood (b) Semen
   (c) Urine (d) Saliva

4. **Presence of vaginal epithelium on the glans can be demonstrated by :**
   (a) Osmic acid (b) Potassium iodide
   (c) Lugol's iodine (d) Nitric acid

5. **All the drugs can be used for narcoanalysis *except:***
   (a) Sodium pentothal
   (b) Barbiturates
   (c) Sodium amytal
   (d) Scopolamine hydrobromide

6. **The term 'butch or dyke' is used in reference of:**
   (a) Sin of Gomorrah (b) Active lesbian
   (c) Catamite (d) Bestiality

7. **'Greek love' refers to:**
   (a) Sodomy (b) Coitus per os
   (c) Bestiality (d) Female homosexuality

8. **Non-treatment of victim of sexual offence by hospital is punishable offence under following section of Indian Penal Code:**
   (a) 164A (b) 164B
   (c) 166A (d) 166B

9. **Section 354C I.P.C. deals with:**
   (a) Compelling women to be naked
   (b) Voyeurism
   (c) Demand of sexual favours
   (d) Making sexually coloured remarks

10. **Section 354D I.P.C. deals with:**
    (a) Stalking (b) Voyeurism
    (c) Acid attack (d) Adultery

11. **Disclosure of the name of rape victim is punishable under I.P.C. section:**
    (a) 166A (b) 166B
    (c) 228A (d) 304A

12. **Lesbianism is synonyms with:**
    (a) Tribadism (b) Eonism
    (c) Undinism (d) Trolism

13. **Sexual excitement obtained by using obscene language is called:**
    (a) Sexual oralism (b) Scatalogia
    (c) Caprolalia (d) Myxoscopia

14. **A 21 years old male intentionally exposed his genitalia in a public place in front of females to obtain sexual pleasure. A police complaint is made by the females. He will be punished under section:**
    (a) 294 I.P.C. (b) 295 I.P.C.
    (c) 354 I.P.C. (d) 354C I.P.C.

15. **All are unnatural sexual offences *except:***
    (a) Tribadism (b) Bestiality
    (c) Incest (d) Sodomy

16. **Troilism refers to:**
    (a) Sexual gratification by hearing sounds of sexual intercourse
    (b) Sexual gratification by observing wife having sex with another person
    (c) Sexual focus on genital rubbing
    (d) Intercourse with lower animals

17. **Age limit for statutory rape as per current 375 I.P.C. is:**
    (a) 18 years (b) 16 years
    (c) 15 years (d) 12 years

18. **Adultery is laid down under section:**
    (a) 497 I.P.C. (b) 498 I.P.C.
    (c) 498A I.P.C. (d) 499 I.P.C.

ANSWER KEY

1. (d)	2. (b)	3. (b)	4. (c)	5. (b)	6. (b)	7. (a)	8. (d)	9. (b)	10. (a)
11. (c)	12. (a)	13. (c)	14. (a)	15. (c)	16. (b)	17. (a)	18. (a)		

32 CHAPTER

Forensic Serology and Trace Evidence

In the time that has elapsed since the discovery of the ABO system by Landsteiner, knowledge in forensic serology has expanded tremendously. Excluding hormones and some temporary pathological factors, more than 160 antigens, 150 serum proteins and 250 cellular enzymes have been found in human blood. Three classes of blood constituents have been chosen by serologists for analysis of blood samples; group specific antigens, cellular enzymes and serum enzymes and proteins.

Medicolegal Aspects of Blood

Blood in itself is very important entity in medicolegal practices which alone or along with other trace evidences plays a key role to unfold different problems. Estimation of blood and bloodstains has importance in both civil and criminal fields of investigation concerning identification of an individual on one side and many other medicolegal issues on the other side. No other body fluids or tissues have such divergent medicolegal importance as blood has.

Civil Importance: (i) Paternity or maternity issues (Table 32.1). (ii) Divorce and nullity of marriage cases, for example question of intersex and some forbidden diseases. (iii) Compensation cases related to workmen's welfare, e.g., industrial and commercial workers. (iv) Civil negligence cases arising in hospital or medical practices, e.g., transfusion cases, chemotherapeutic practices etc.

Criminal Importance: (i) Identification of victim or offenders of crime like homicide, sex offences or where death has occurred due to rash or negligent acts. (ii) Cause of death, e.g., detection of poison or some other pathology responsible for the death. (iii) Time of death by use of different chemical or biochemical tests. (iv) In cases of criminal abortion and investigation of sexual offence cases, e.g., examination of vaginal or seminal fluids on the person or undergarments of victim and the accused. (v) To establish the relationship between the offence, offender, offended (victim) and offending agent (Application of Locard principle). (vi) Cases of malingering.

Table 32.1: Paternity exclusion chances with different blood group systems

Group systems	Cumulative exclusion rate
• ABO	18%
• ABO + MNS	60%
• ABO + MNS + red cell antigens + serum proteins	82%
• ABO + MNS + red cell antigens + serum proteins + red cell enzymes	94%
• ABO + MNS + red cell antigens + serum proteins + red cell enzymes + HLA	98.5%
• DNA typing	100%

Examination of Blood Stains

Collection of blood stains: (i) A clean piece of white filter paper may be used, allowing blood to soak onto it, and then it is dried at room temperature. A control filter paper should also be sent for examination. (ii) If the object is porous, a portion of unstained area should also be taken. (iii) If the object is nonporous and particularly, if it is metallic, stains can be recovered by scrapping and placed in small glass containers. They should not be placed in envelop as may be reduced to powder. (iv) Stains on clothing may be scrapped of or a fragment of the material cut. (v) The solvents for bloodstains are the following: (a) 10% solution of potassium cyanide (b) 10% solution of glycerine in distilled water (c) Weak solution of ammonia.

A coloured solution is obtained immediately with any of the above solvents. Otherwise the material must be covered and left for 12-24 hours at room temperature.

Stains on clothing: In the case of clothing, type of garment, its colour and consistency should be noted and if the garments are torn, position of the tears should be noted. Whether the clothes were dried, damp or wet when received should be noted. Examine both the outer and inner surfaces of the garments. The position of all the stains should be given correctly by a description of the stains in its relation to the manner in which a garment is actually worn, i.e., a stain on the trouser should be described as being above, behind, or on the inner side of the knee. Stains may also be described in relation to the pocket, the button, or the seams of garments. The size and the shape of the stains should be noted. Bloodstains are extremely resistance to washing by water. Dried blood on a dead body or article is very resistance to water. The dried blood will remain intact for quite a long time, even though the body has been submerged.

Medicolegal Questions in Relation to Blood Stains

1. **Whether the stain is due to blood or other stain?** Different stain that resembles blood stains are: (i) *Rust stain:* Instrument and weapons made of iron are rusted and the rust may resemble blood stain but on heating opposite side of the weapon they don't fall up in scales. They do not have a dark and a glazed appearance. Rust stain do not stiffen the cloth and are soluble in dilute hydrochloric acid. Moreover, they give positive test for iron. (ii) *Vegetable stain:* Fruits like mulberry, currants and *jamuns* produce tan that look like blood stain. In these cases vegetable debris and cells are found when visualized under microscope. On the other hand, *pan juice*, tobacco, fruit and leaves of some of the trees produce red stains resembling blood stain. By addition of a drop of ferric chloride these stains become black due to presence of tannin. (iii) *Synthetic dye:* The colour changes to yellow by addition of nitric acid and the original colour is restored by again adding a strong solution of alkali, if the stain is due to synthetic dye. (iv) *Mineral stains:* Compounds of iron, red lead, and red sulfide of mercury give red colouration that looks like blood stain. These metals can easily be differentiated from blood stain by appropriate tests. (v) *Miscellaneous group:* Spots of resin, grease and coaltar on fabric looks like an old blood stain but gives negative test for the blood.

   That the stain is due to blood can be known from simple microscopic tests, different colour tests and crystal tests.

2. **Whether the blood stain is of human origin or not?** This question can be answered by performing the precipitin test that is an immunological test and is species specific. When it is established that the stain is due to human blood, the following questions are to be answered.

3. **What is the source of bleeding?** (i) *Menstrual blood:* Usually found in female undergarments during the menstrual cycles. It is dark, fluid, has disagreeable smell and acid in reaction. On microscopy it shows endometrial cells, vaginal epithelium and number of bacilli and cocci. At times Trichomonas vaginalis or moniliasis may be present. Menstural blood contains fibrinolysins that prevents clotting. (ii) *Haemoptysis*: It is bright red and is mixed with froth and is alkaline in reaction. (iii) *Vomitus:* The vomited blood is chocolate brown in colour and acid in reaction due to presence of gastric contents. (iv) *Blood in cases of rape:* This is usually mixed with semen and pubic hair may be present at times. (v) *Blood stain due to boils and sores:* A mixed appearance of blood and a pus is found and one can find pus cells and bacteria under microscope.

4. **What is the age of the blood stain?** The age is usually determined by the colour changes which is quite unreliable:

   - *Fresh stain:* Bright red.
   - *24 hours:* Reddish brown.
   - *Within a few days:* Brown.
   - *After a long time:* Black.

   Fresh stains are moist, sticky and stiffen the cloth on drying due to presence of proteins. A drop of blood dries of in one to two hours in normal conditions. However, in cases of pool of blood it takes 24 to 36 hours to dry depending upon the amount of blood, surface of collection and temperature etc. The solubility gradually decreases with the age. Fluorescence decreases as the stain becomes older. On the whole at least this can be ascertained whether the stain is fresh, recent, a weeks duration or old.

5. **What is the sex of the person?** The sex can be ascertained from the presence of sex chromatin.

6. **What is blood group of the person?** Grouping can be known from the different blood group tests.

7. **Whether it is arterial or venous in origin?** The bleeding from the arteries has a sprouting effect and is bright red in colour when fresh. On the other hand, bleeding from a vein occurs passively and dark in colour even when it is fresh.

8. **Whether it belongs to the accused or victim?** The blood stains on the inner side of the garment definitely belongs to the victims whereas stains on the outer side may belong to the accused or the victim.

9. **Whether the blood stain is derived from a living person or dead one?** The blood which has shed during life can be removed in scales on drying due to presence of fibrin whereas, the postmortem blood breaks off into powder on drying.

Physical Tests for Blood

Naked eye examination: On naked eye examination, the non coagulated blood is thick, viscid and bright red or bluish depending on the source or region. Antemortem bleeding causes coagulation that separates the serum. The clot can be taken out *en masse* from the spot but leaves an impression over there due to the fibrinous network that results in the clot formation. The postmortem clot cannot be taken *en masse* and it leaves no impression on the spot. Roughly three layers are detected in the mass; one by the platelets, second by the RBC and third by WBC.

Microscopic examination: This can establish whether the sample is blood or not and can differentiate between the blood of various species. The human RBC is biconcave, spherical, nonnucleated disc (Figure 32.1) and the average diameter is 7.3

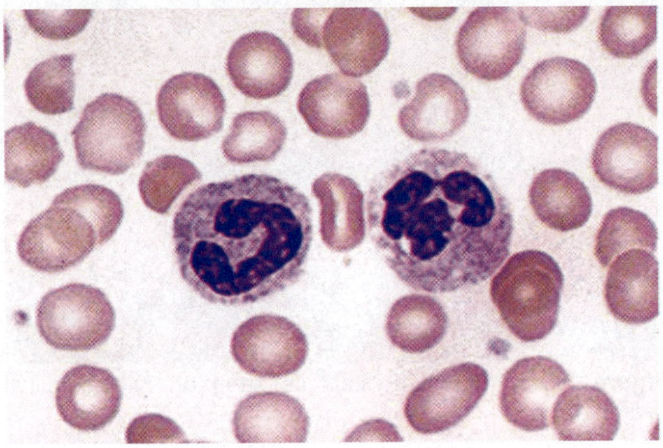

Figure 32.1: Red blood cells

microns, the maximum breadth is 2.5 microns and the minimum is 1 micron. The average volume of red cells is 90-95 cubic micrometers, whereas in other mammalians it is biconvex, nucleated and the size varies with the species.

Spectroscopic examination (Figure 32.2): This is one of the most definitive tests for establishing the presence of blood. It is based on the absorption spectrum of various types of haemoglobin in the blood. Even less than 0.1 mg of blood sample is sufficient for conducting this test. The bloodstain is dissolved in water, salt solution, or dilute ammonia and is placed in a glass tube and examined through a spectroscope. The absorption spectrum is characteristic for each type of haemoglobin. This definitely establishes that the sample is blood.

Colour Tests for Blood

Principle: The colour tests detect the presence of haemoglobin, the colouring matter of blood and enzyme peroxidase which in the presence of hydrogen peroxide oxidises the colourless bases to coloured salt. It is also possible to utilize the same peroxidase reaction at a much higher sensitivity by using luminal reagent. It shows bright fluorescence in the presence of blood. Various colour tests are:

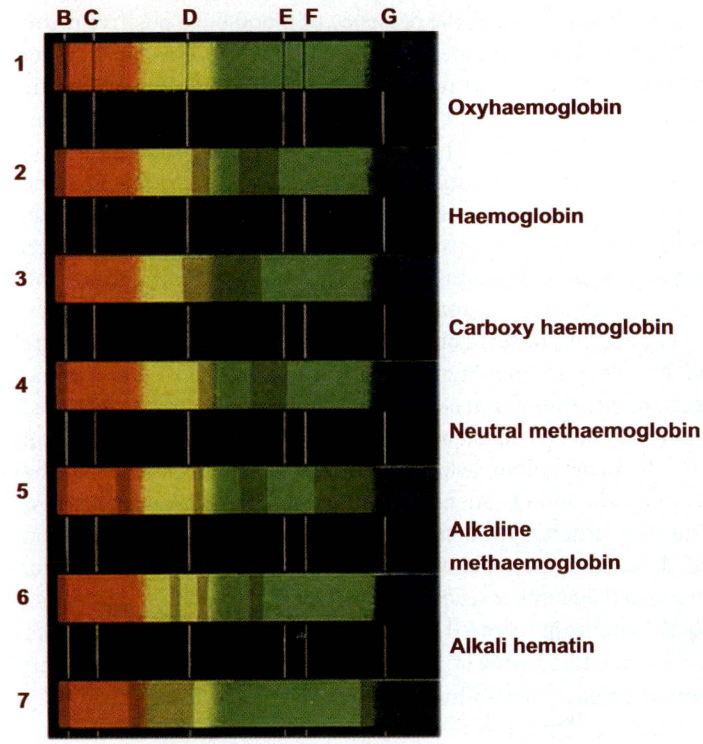

Figure 32.2: Spectroscopic examination of blood

Benzidine test: It uses 10% solution of benzidine in glacial acetic acid. When the stain extract is mixed with it, it produces an intense **blue colour** on addition of hydrogen peroxide, if blood is present. The test is positive in dilution of one part of blood in 500,000 parts and was commonly used in medicolegal practice. This test can detect blood from washed fabrics and old stains. Nevertheless, nowadays it is of limited use because of its carcinogenic properties.

Phenolphthalein test (Kastle Mayer tests): The reagent for this test is obtained by mixing a 2% solution in 20% aqueous solution of potassium hydroxide till the solution becomes colourless. The phenolphthalein is reduced by zinc dust in a strong alkaline medium. If the reduced phenolphthalein is oxidized by nascent oxygen liberated by the action of peroxidase on hydrogen peroxide this gives a **pink or purple colour** with blood stains.

Leucomalachite green test: It uses a 1% solution in 40% aqueous solution of acetic acid and produces a **bluish green** colour with blood stains. It is the most suitable presumptive test.

Orthotoulidine test (Kohn and Kelly test): This utilizes 1% solution in 40% alcohol and gives a **bluish green colour** with blood stains.

Luminal test: This utilizes a solution of 3- Amino pthalic acid hydrazide, sodium carbonate and hydrogen peroxide and produces a bright luminescence in presence of blood.

Interpretation of colour tests for bloodstains: These are presumptive tests for blood used at the scene and at laboratory. A negative result excludes the presence of blood but a positive result may indicate that the suspected stain could be blood as lots of other material gives false positive test. False positive coloured catalytic test reaction can be given by following substances: (i) ***Chemical oxidants and catalysts:*** This includes copper and nickel salts, rust, formalin, potassium permanganate, potassium dichromate, some bleaches, hypochlorite, iodine and lead oxides and vitamin C etc. Phenolphthalein gives positive results with oxidizing compounds such as copper, potassium ferricyanide, nickel, cobalt nitrates and some sulfocyanides. Luminol reacts with cupric ions and some compounds of copper, cobalt and iron. Potassium permanganate and hydrated sodium hypochlorite also gives positive luminal reaction. (ii) ***Plant sources:*** Vegetable peroxidases are the most important class of substances which show false positive reaction with chemical colour tests. The following plant tissues may be mistaken for blood such as Apple, Apricot, Bean, Blackberry, Jerusalem artichoke, horseradish, potato, turnip, cabbage, onion and dandelion root. Plant materials such as beetle leaf, garlic, tomato and cucumber react positively with tetramethyl benzidine. **Higaki and pulp** reported that plant peroxides does not contribute to false positive result in a three-stage phenolphthalein test. (iii) ***Animal origin:*** The following substances of animal origin may give false positive reaction with benzidine reagent such as pus, bone marrow, leukocytes, brain tissue, spinal fluid, intestine, lung, saliva and mucous.

Microchemical Tests

Takayama reagent test: This test is also known as the **Haemochromogen crystal test**. Takayama reagent is used in this test which is prepared from sodium hydroxide, pyridine and glucose. The sample material is placed on a glass slide and Takayama reagent is added to it and it is examined under microscope. Pink feathery crystals of hemochromogen are formed which are arranged in clusters, sheaves etc. (Figure 32.3). The test is considered negative if no crystals are formed in 30 minutes. ***Teichmann's test:*** This test is also known as **Haemin crystal test**. In this to the blood stain a crystal of sodium chloride is added along with a few drops of glacial acetic acid and it is heated with a coverslip in place. After cooling faint yellowish-red to brownish black rhombic crystals are seen if blood is present in the sample (Figure 32.4). The test gives a negative reaction if the stains are old, washed or treated by chemicals.

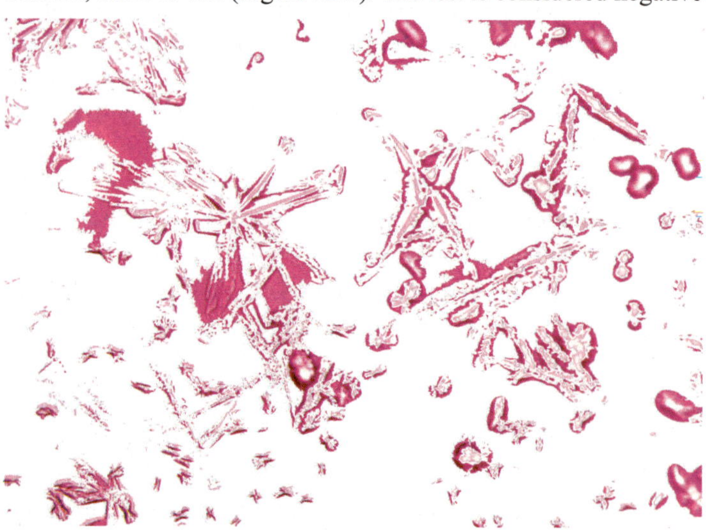

Figure 32.3: Haemochromogen crystals on microscopical examination

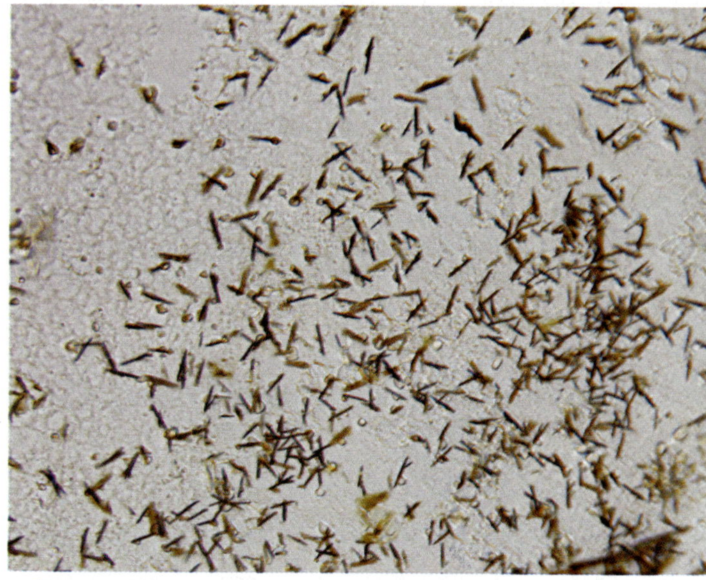

Figure 32.4: Haemin crystals as seen on microscopical examination

Interpretation of crystal tests: The sensitivity and specificity of the Takayama test is essentially the same as that of the Teichman's test. Takayama test is positive with as little as 0.001 ml of blood or 0.01 mg haemoglobin. It is superior to the Teichmann test in that it can often give positive results with blood removed from wood or leather surfaces. The drawback of the Takayama test is that a complete crystallization is difficult to obtain with old blood sample and there may be formation of different types of crystals. The failure to obtain a positive Takayama test does not necessarily indicate the absence of blood.

Immunoserological Tests

Principle: The serum of the blood stain contains protein. If antihuman serum is treated with blood stain from human source then there will be antigen antibody reaction which can be demonstrated by various serological tests mentioned above. It is to be remembered that many animal serum proteins may be agglutinated by or may be reacted upon by antihuman sera. The serum proteins preferred for these tests are globulin and antihuman globulin that is prepared by injecting human serum in rabbits. The antisera to be used should be first made free from reactivity with the animal blood proteins by treating the antisera with the similarly available animal protein or sera. Various immunological tests are:

Ring test: It is a precipitation test performed with antihuman serum and stain extract. 0.2 ml of stain extract of different dilutions are taken in round bottomed glass tubes of 5 cm length and 5.5 mm diameter. Equal volume of antihuman serum is added in the tube by running down along the wall of each tube. A precipitation ring is formed at the interface of the two fluids, with 1: 1000 dilution of the stain extract, if the stain is of human blood. Control tests are necessary with normal saline, human serum and sera of other animals.

Gel electrophoresis test: In this test the extracts of different stains are placed in separate holes on the side of a gel strip and antihuman globulin and antisera for other common animals are placed in separate holes on the other side of the gel strip. The set is then subjected to electrophoresis in such a way that albumin and non gamma globulins from the stain extract side travels to the antisera side and reacts with the gamma globulins there. A line of precipitate forms at the meeting point of proteins travelling from the stain extract side with the specific antisera, which denotes the species origin of the stain extract that underwent precipitation reaction with the antisera of a particular animal or human origin.

Mixed antiglobulin test: In this test antihuman globulin rabbit serum is prepared and treated with A, B, O blood group cells and sera of other species of common animals to avoid error in record of study, due to possible reaction with antihuman globulin sera and these agents. The red cells chosen are used after washing, for at least ten times, in normal saline solution. The antihuman globulin thus treated and obtained is suitable for use in the test. O Rh+ red cells are used as the indicator cells for the positive reaction in the test. Sensitized red cells are prepared by mixing 1 ml of 2% suspension of O group of Rh+ red cells with 1 ml of 10% incomplete anti D sera and the mixture is incubated for 1 hour at 37°C. These cells are washed and made to 1% suspension with rabbit protein which then becomes agglutinable by antihuman globulin serum.

Passive haemagglutination test: The RBCs, when treated with tannic acid becomes capable of binding proteins on their surface. If the extract contains protein due to the presence of human blood, then tanned human RBCs can bind the protein in the stain and hence the RBCs thereafter will be agglutinated when further treated with antihuman globulin. For the test a cell suspension is prepared and a drop of it is mixed with one drop of antihuman globulin serum. Clumping indicates the presence of human protein in the extract. Control tests are to be performed alongwith the main test.

Points to be remembered in relation to serological tests for extracting stains: All reasonable control tests are to be performed along with the tests. Ageing of the stain, heat and washing with soap or detergents may give false negative results. However, if the stain is otherwise protected from decomposition or contamination from the dirt or chemical then ageing alone does not damage the reacting capacity of the stain serologically. Once it is established that the stain is due to blood and that it belongs to human being then the next series of serological tests is involved. For detection of group factors in the blood to help to relate the stain extract with a particular individual further, various blood groups and types of tests are available such as:

Primary Blood Group Systems

The primary blood group systems are well known and defined blood group systems. These are ABO, MNS, P, PH, Diego, Donbrock, Duffy, Kell, Kidd, Lewis, Lutheran, XG and YT.

Secondary Blood Group Systems

The secondary blood group systems are antigens that are either foreigners to new systems or products of rare mutant genes in existing ones. They also include high incident antigens which have not been related to major systems. They include the following Auberger, August, Batley, Beaker, Bils, Bishop, Bga, Bgl, Box, Cavatiere and Chido.

Some of the red cell antigens such as A, B and I have been shown to be present on both leukocytes and platelets. Nevertheless, the antigens representing the majority of blood group systems such as Rh, Duffy, MN and so forth seem to be unique antigens characteristic to leukocytes and platelets. According to the present state of knowledge, there are four established leukocyte group antigen systems namely HLA-A, HLA-B, HLA-C and HLA-D.

Red blood cells like any other cells shrink in solutions with an osmotic pressure greater than that of normal plasma. NaCl solution is isosmotic with plasma. In solution with lower osmotic pressure, the cell becomes spherical rather than disk shaped.

The hemolysed red cells release their contents into the solution. More than 250 proteins and enzymes have been found in the red cells. The predominant erythrocyte protein is haemoglobin, whose more than 100 variants have been described. Many red blood cell enzymes show genetic polymorphism as do a significant number of proteins found in blood serum and other body secretions. Many of these persist in their biological activity even after blood has dried. Therefore, blood can potentially distinguish one person from the other.

ABO Grouping

The most well known and medically important blood types are the ABO group. All humans can be typed for the ABO blood group. The ABO typing of a person depends upon the presence or absence of two genes, A and B. These genes determine the configuration of the red blood cell surface. A person can be A, B, AB, or O. If a person has two A genes, their red blood cells are type A. If a person has two B genes, their red cells are type B. If the person has one A and one B gene, their red cells are type AB. If the person has neither the A nor B gene, they are type O.

The possible permutations of antigens and antibodies with the corresponding ABO type are given underneath ("yes" indicates the presence of a component and "no" indicates its absence in the blood of an individual).

ABO blood type	Antigen A	Antigen B	Antibody anti-A	Antibody anti-B
A	Yes	No	No	Yes
B	No	Yes	Yes	No
O	No	No	Yes	Yes
AB	Yes	Yes	No	No

Genetic inheritance patterns: ABO blood types are inherited through genes on chromosomes, and they do not change as a result of environmental influences during life. An individual's ABO type is determined by the inheritance of the 3 alleles (A, B or O) from each parent. The possible outcomes are shown below:

Parent alleles	A	B	O
A	AA (A)	AB (AB)	AO (A)
B	AB (AB)	BB (B)	BO (B)
O	AO (A)	BO (B)	OO (O)

Both A and B alleles are dominant over O. As a result, individuals who have an AO genotype will have an A phenotype. People who are type O have OO genotypes. In other words, they inherited a recessive O allele from both parents. The A and B alleles are codominant. Therefore, if an A is inherited from one parent and a B from the other, the phenotype will be AB.

Tests for Determining ABO Grouping

(i) ***Tube method:*** In this method a drop of washed suspension of red cells is added to equal volumes of each of the antisera of A, B and O in separate tubes. When agglutination is seen by naked eye or microscope in the tubes the blood group can be identified. (ii) ***Tile method:*** In this method, a porcelain tile rather than a tube is used and the results are similar to tube test. (iii) ***Absorption-inhibition method*:** In this technique the sample and antisera are allowed to react with each other for a longer period. This test is useful in cases where the cell membrane is damaged and agglutination test cannot be done. (iv) ***Mixed agglutination tests:*** In this test the sample piece of stained cloth is cut into pieces of 2-3 mm and the fibers are separated. Then they are added to tubes along with antisera of A, B, O types. Clumps of red cells seen adherent to the fibres is a positive reaction and the group can be known by the antisera which clumped to the cloth fibres. (v) ***Absorption-elution technique*:** This test is similar to mixed agglutination test but the clumps are noticed on the walls of the test tube rather than the sample cloth fibres. This technique can be used to find the blood group form body tissues also.

MN System

The MNSs system was discovered by Landsteiner and Levin in 1928. Two antibodies called anti-M and anti-N were identified. These two antigens are shown to be derived from a single pair of genes which are allelomorphic and codominant. The frequency for these groups in human population is: (i) Group M (20%). (ii) Group N (22%). (iii) Group MN (50%). These two antigens can be paired as: (i) M pairing with M—genotype MM and phenotype or group M. (ii) N pairing with N—genotype NN and phenotype or group N. (iii) M pairing with N producing genotype MN and phenotype or group MN. The possible groups of children under MN system are given below:

Groups of parents	Possible groups of children	Groups not possible
M × M	M	N, MN
M × N	M N	M, N
M × MN	M, MN	N
N × N	N	M, MN
N × MN	N, MN	M
MN × MN	M, N, MN	—

Ss System

This system was discovered in 1947 by Walsh and Montogomery. They discovered an antigen (S) and antibody (anti-S). The proportion of blood samples agglutinated by anti-S is about 55% and those not agglutinated are about 45% (in English and American white population). Of the M samples about 73% are agglutinated. The S occurs more often with M than with N suggesting an association between MN groups and S. Anti-S has been used for paternity testing but anti-S is too rare.

Rh System

Landsteiner and Wiener in 1940 discovered human blood factor called 'Rhesus' or 'Rh'. The guinea pigs and rabbits were immunized with blood from *Macacus rhesus* monkey. They obtained an antiserum that after suitable absorption agglutinated not only the red cells of rhesus monkey but also about 85% of blood samples from whites of New York. Those whose red cells were agglutinated by the new antibody were designated by **Rh-positive** and those whose red cell were not so agglutinated were designated **Rh-negative**. Antisera giving similar reaction to animal anti-Rh sera were found to occur in humans. The individuals who lack Rh antigen may in certain circumstances form Rh antibodies. This could be due to receiving a blood transfusion of Rh-positive blood or carrying of an Rh-positive fetus.

Kell System

Rarely there is presence of anti-K and this is sometimes helpful in paternity cases. The finding of a K-positive child with a K-negative mother and putative father would constitute an exclusion of paternity.

Duffy System

This system employs the use of two sera anti-Fy^a and anti-Fy^b. Anti-Fy^a provides evidence of nonpaternity when the putative father and mother are Fy^a and the child $Fy^{a}+$. Anti-Fy^b is a rare serum but is obtainable in sufficient quantity and strength could be used with anti-Fy^a in the testing of white races. In doubtful paternity cases involving Negroes it must be remembered that the phenotype Fy (a–b–) is common.

Kidd System

This system is defined by anti-Jk^a and anti-Jk^b sera. Both at present are rare, particularly anti-Jk^b. At the moment insufficient family studies have been made for this system to be used except with caution and as additional evidence in special cases.

Lutheran System

The finding of Lu (a+) child with Lu (a–) mother and putative father can be regarded as evidence for an exclusion based on another blood-group system. Anti-Lu^b is too rare for regular use and furthermore is of small value as it reacts with over 99% of samples.

Other Antigenic Factors Inherited in Serum

Haptoglobulins: Haptoglobulins are haemoglobin binding proteins that are found in human serum. They are observed as characteristics bands during electrophoresis. The differentiation of three different pattern of these proteins depends on superior resolving power of the starch-gel method. It is possible to classify most people into three consistently inherited haptoglobin (Hp): (i) Haptoglobulins 1-1 (Hp^1Hp^1). (ii) Haptoglobulins 2-2 (Hp^2Hp^2). (iii) Haptoglobulins 2-1 (Hp^2Hp^1). Haptoglobulins are only occasionally present at birth and 97% of infants can be typed by six months of age.

Gamma factors in blood serum: The gamma globulins are transmitted from mother through the placenta to the newborn. These are helpful in solving problems related to exchange of babies in hospital. GM factors in blood serum are GM1 antigen to GM 25 antigen.

Red cell enzyme systems: A large number of enzymes that catalyses various biochemical reaction are also present in blood plasma. Phosphoglucomutase (PGM) and adenylatekinase (AK) have an established value in paternity testing. Besides this Red cell acid phosphatase, Adenosine deaminase (ADA), 6-phosphogluconate dehydrogenase (G-6PD), glutamate pyruvate transaminase (GPT) and esterase D (Es D) may also be used. These enzymes are demonstrated by starch gel electrophoresis technique and do not persist for more than one month in stain material.

HLA typing: HLA system consists of protein substances present on the surface of tissues, organs, tumours, white cells and platelets. These are present on spermatozoa but not on ovum or trophoblast. They are also present on placental surface at term and fetal tissues at 6 weeks. Major human leukocytes antigens HLA-A, B, C, D and DR are determined by a single chromosomal segment, major histocompatibility complex (MHC). This is situated on the short arm of human chromosome 6. There are 68 antigenic factors present in white cells and each parent contributes to a child one of the two chromosomes containing the HLA region. Only fresh blood samples are examined for solving paternity or maternity. Presence of these antigens may be detected by using white cells and a suitable antiserum that either agglutinates white cells or damages them so that they can be stained with suitable dyes that do not affect damaged cells.

Abnormal haemoglobins: There are three varieties of normal haemoglobin: (i) ***Haemoglobin A:*** It consists of Alpha + Beta chains. (ii) ***Haemoglobin A2:*** It consists of 2 Alpha polypeptide chain + Delta chain. It is present in 2% of total haemoglobin. (iii) ***Haemoglobin F:*** It is present in newborn foetus upto extent of 80% maximum and consists of alpha type and gamma type. By two years of age blood will not have any foetal haemoglobin. (iv) ***Haemoglobin H:*** All four chains are Beta chains. (v) ***Haemoglobin barts:*** All four chains are gamma chains, the normal polypeptide chain is abnormally conjugated. (vi) Haemoglobin S. (vii) Haemoglobin C. (viii) Haemoglobin E. (ix) Haemoglobin D Punjab.

There are substitutions of some amino acids at some points by some other amino acid that are not present in normal haemoglobin. These abnormal haemoglobins can be detected with paper electrophoresis. Foetal haemoglobin can be differentiated by its property of alkali resistance and ultraviolet absorption curve.

Medicolegal aspects of abnormal haemoglobins: Haemoglobin A1 and A2 are normal varieties in adults and children above two years of age. Haemoglobin F is normal in the newborn and decreases upto the age of 2 years and by this time it is totally removed. This point may be helpful to determine the age of infants and young children. Inheritance of abnormal haemoglobin has importance in deciding the paternity and maternity disputes. Abnormal haemoglobin can be used to identify a person.

Group specific substances: In the body tissues, agglutinogens of ABO system are present. In the tissues they appear in lipoidal form and in about 80% people they appear in water soluble form that can be demonstrated in all body fluids except CSF. These substances are not found in nerve tissue, epithelium, appendages of skin, bones and cartilage. **Nonsecretors** are persons who possess only lipoidal form whereas secretors are the one who possess a water soluble form. A pair of allelic genes Se (dominant) and se (recessive) are responsible for capacity to secrete these antigens in body fluids. **Secretors** possess genotype Se Se, and Se se whereas nonsecretors possess genotype se se. Secretors also possess H antigen on the red cells irrespective of the ABO system. The amount of H antigen is highest on RBC of persons with O blood group.

Examination of Nails

From the nails, poisons (heavy metals like Arsenic) can be detected. Debris on the nail bed may show presence of foreign tissue and blood, which can give sex and blood group of the person.

Examination of Skin and Dandruff

The mixed agglutination principle is used for ABO grouping of skin and dandruff as described by **Swine burne.** Cell suspension of skin scrapping or dandruff flakes is used in this method. Positive result is shown by firm adherence of indicator cells to the skin or dandruff cells under tests.

Differences from fibers: These mixed agglutination clumps will be circular in appearance rather than elongated as in the grouping of fibers.

Examination of skin may help to know the sex and blood group of the person. Also, poisons can be detected. From dandruff blood group of the person can be known.

Examination of Vaginal Fluids

This is done for the purpose of: (i) Detection of semen in vaginal fluid (ii) Detection of blood in seminal fluid (iii) Detection of blood group specific substances in vaginal fluid, if the person is a secretor. Examination of vaginal epithelial cells is a good way to know the actual sex in gonadal dysgenesis cases. Presence of vaginal epithelium on the glans penis of the accused supports sexual intercourse. The glans is rubbed with a moist blotter and subjected to the vapour of iodine. The blotter becomes partly brown if vaginal epithelial cells are present as they contain glycogen that turns brown due to iodine. Vaginal stain extract should also be examined for poisons of a suspected case of criminal abortion.

Examination of Urinary Stains

The presence of urine is ascertained by the use of urease tablets, testing for creatinine and detection of an odour of urine in the concentrated extract. Blood group substances, anti A and anti B agglutinins are also detected. Species identification of urine can also be undertaken. A method of concentrating urinary proteins is based on a technique used by mejbaum-Katzenellenbogen. The concentrated urine proteins are subjected to precipitin test by the agar diffusion method against the antiglobulin of various relevant species, including humans. It is suggested that the method might apply to urine stains both for species identification and for the detection of isoagglutinin.

Medicolegal Aspects: Stain due to urine may be known by using urease test and also testing the stains for different constituents of urine. Examination of urine may also give blood group of the person if he is a secretor. Many poisons are extracted through urine and can be detected in the urine.

Examination of Salivary Stains

Saliva is a thin fluid secreted by salivary glands. It contains enzymes like ptyalin (alpha amylase, glucose 6 phosphate dehydrogenase, various proteins, lipids, chloride and thiocyanate ions etc.). Dried stains of saliva are not found on the crime related articles as often as the stains of blood and semen. In very peculiar context, their significance is high. Unburned portions of cigars, cigarettes or bidies are such example. Saliva stain grouping on such articles from the scene of crime is very helpful in the identification of the criminal. The presence of saliva can be confirmed by the presence of buccal squamous cells microscopically. Amylase can be detected if stains are due to saliva. In that case, there will not be any bluish discolouration because amylase digests starch partly to dextrose and then to maltose. α-Amylase in salivary stain can be detected by fluorescent spectroscopy in which usually UV light is used.

The sex of the person can be determined by the Barr bodies present in buccal mucosal cells present in the saliva. Blood group of the person can be known by mixed agglutination test with the buccal squamous cells or the fibers from the stained parts of the clothes.

LONG QUESTIONS

1. Discuss the medicolegal aspects of blood stains.
2. What are the different blood groups? How they help in solving the disputed paternity cases?

SHORT QUESTIONS

1. Trace evidences.
2. ABO grouping.
3. Colour tests for blood stain.
4. Haemin crystal test.
5. Haemochromogen test.
6. Precipitin test.
7. HLA typing.
8. Group specific substances.

MULTIPLE CHOICE QUESTIONS

1. If the father has blood group 'B', mother has blood group 'AB', the children are not likely to have blood group:

(a) O (b) A
(c) B (d) AB

2. An old blood stain in a cotton fibre can be best identified by:

(a) Haemin test (b) Precipitin test
(c) Benzidine test (d) Leucomalachite test

3. Benzidine test for blood is:

(a) Confirmatory test (b) Specific test
(c) Presumptive test (d) Double confirmatory test

4. Following are the confirmatory test for identification of blood in a suspected stain, *except:*

(a) Haemin crystal test
(b) Spectrophotometry
(c) Electrophoresis
(d) Benzidine test

5. Takayama test is used to detect:

(a) Seminal stain
(b) Urine stain
(c) Saliva stain
(d) Blood stain

6. The following are confirmatory tests for the blood, *except:*

(a) Takayama test
(b) Electrophoresis
(c) Teichmann's test
(d) Kastle Meyer test

7. Which test of blood is species specific:

(a) Phenolphthalein test
(b) Benzidine test
(c) Spectroscopy
(d) Precipitin test

8. HLA system is situated on:

(a) Chromosome X
(b) Chromosome 5
(c) Chromosome 6
(d) Chromosome 7

9. One of the following is absent in menstrual blood:

(a) Platelets
(b) White blood cells
(c) Fibrin
(d) Haemoglobin

10. Salivary stains on various substrates can be detected by:

(a) Infra-red rays
(b) X-rays
(c) UV light
(d) Gamma rays

11. Most specific test to detect blood stains is:

(a) Benzidine test
(b) Teichmann's test
(c) Orthotoluidine test
(d) Spectroscopic test

12. In Teichmann's test microscopy shows:

(a) Rhombic crystals
(b) Light pink feathery crystals
(c) Dark pink feathery structures
(d) Due to haemochromogen

13. Which of the following sign will indicate the menstrual blood was antemortem?

(a) Alkaline
(b) Light pink
(c) Does not clot
(d) Shows endometrial and vaginal cells

14. The test used to differentiate blood of humans from those of lower animals is:

(a) Benzidine test
(b) Teichmann's test
(c) Takayama test
(d) Precipitin test

ANSWER KEY

1. (a)	2. (c)	3. (c)	4. (d)	5. (d)	6. (d)	7. (d)	8. (c)	9. (c)	10. (c)
11. (d)	12. (a)	13. (c)	14. (d)						

33 CHAPTER

DNA Fingerprinting

DNA or Deoxyribonucleic Acid exists in the form of twisted double helix and governs various inheritance traits of human as well as animals. The characteristics of all living organisms, including humans are essentially determined by information contained within DNA that they inherit from their parents. Each person has a unique DNA fingerprint similar to the conventional fingerprints. Unlike a conventional fingerprint that occurs only on the fingertips and can be altered by surgery, a DNA fingerprint is the same for every cell, tissue, and organ of a person. It cannot be altered by any known treatment. Consequently, DNA fingerprinting is rapidly becoming the primary method for identifying and distinguishing among individual human beings. Any type of organism can be identified by examination of DNA sequence unique to that species.

Genetic fingerprinting exploits highly variable repeat sequences called **microsatellites**. Two unrelated humans are likely to have different numbers of microsatellites at a given locus. By using PCR to detect the number of repeats at several loci, it is possible to establish a match that is extremely unlikely to have arisen by coincidence, except in case of identical twins, who will have identical genetic profiles.

To identify individuals, forensic scientists scan 13 DNA regions that vary from person to person and use the data to create a DNA profile of that individual called **DNA fingerprint** (also called **DNA typing or DNA profiling**). Living organisms that look different or have different characteristics also have different DNA sequences. The more varied the organisms, the more varied the DNA sequences. DNA fingerprinting is a very quick way to compare the DNA sequences of any two living organisms. Only one-tenth of a single percent of DNA (about 3 million bases) differs from one person to the next.

History of Forensic DNA Typing

- 1980—Ray White described first polymorphic RFLP marker.
- 1985—Alec Jeffreys discovered multilocus VNTR probes at University of Leicester.
- 1985—First paper was reported on PCR.
- 1988—FBI starts DNA case work.
- 1991—First paper reported on STR.
- 1995—FSS launched UK DNA database.
- 1998—FBI launches CODIS database.

Structure of DNA

The length of DNA in a cell is about 180 cm. Each chromosome consists of two long linear DNA molecules, the polymers being hydrogen bonded via specific nucleotide pairing and coiled as a double helix, which is spiral in nature and looks like a spiral staircase. Nuclear proteins called histones, the complex of DNA and histones being referred to as chromatin structurally stabilize the helix. Each nucleotide is composed of phosphate, deoxyribose sugar, and organic nitrogenous bases. The bases are adenine (A), guanine (G), cytosine (C) and thymine (T). The bases of one strand are connected to the bases of the other strand by hydrogen bonds with adjacent nucleotides linked to each other by covalent bonds. Adenine combines only with thymine and guanine combines only with cytosine. The DNA molecule resembles a twisted rope ladder with four kinds of stair-steps, e.g., A-T, T-A, C-G or G-C. There are three hydrogen bonds between G and C, and two bonds between A and T.

The sequence of bases can code for many properties of the cells of the body as the cells can read this code. The **'coding DNA'** can encode the information contained in DNA that is determined primarily by the sequence of letters along the zipper. For example, the sequence ACGCT represents different information than the sequence AGTCC, in the same way that the word "POST" has a different meaning from "STOP" or "POTS", even though they use the same letters. The traits of a human being are the result of information contained in the DNA code. Our cells also contain much DNA that does not encode anything and is called the **non-coding or 'junk DNA'**. The DNA code or genetic code is passed by the sperm and egg to the offspring. A single sperm and egg contains about three billion bases consisting of A, T, G and C that follow each other in a well-defined sequence along the strand of DNA. The base sequence of sperms and eggs is quite different from each other. The appearance of double helical arrangement of DNA in the cell is shown in Figure 33.1.

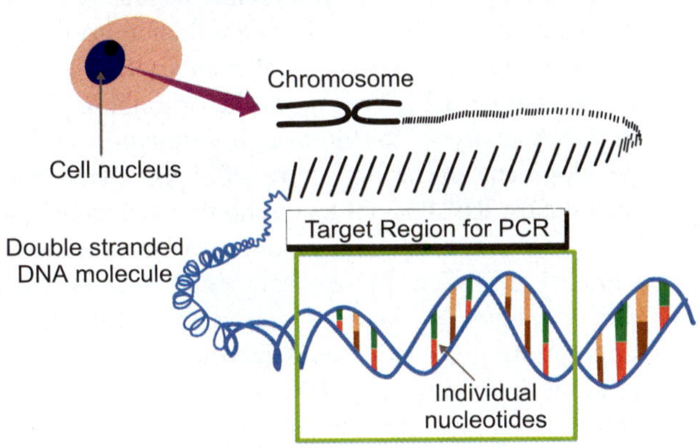

Figure 33.1: DNA in the cell

DNA Typing

DNA fingerprinting begins by extracting DNA from the cells in samples such as blood, bone, hair and other appropriate body tissues and products from the crime scene or the individual. The DNA is analyzed for the presence of a set of specific DNA markers. A series of probes bound to a DNA sample creates a distinctive pattern for an individual. Forensic scientists compare these DNA profiles to determine whether the suspect's sample matches the evidence sample. A marker by itself usually is not unique to an individual, if however, two DNA samples are alike at four or five regions, odds are great that the samples are from the same person. The portions of the DNA sequence that vary the most among humans is used.

The fresher the tissue the better and much putrefied material was formerly of little use, as the nuclear chromatin was degraded. DNA profiling has employed two main techniques for comparing a 'test' with the 'control' sample. The original Jeffrey's method was to use restriction enzymes, which split the DNA into a large number of fragments which when visualized by autoradiography, produced a series of bands in a 'bar code'. This obviously offered a more discriminative means of comparison, as multiple reference points were provided in the same test. As the chance of two random persons having the same band is about 25%, a profile with 11 bands has a chance of identity of only one in 3 million. Though **multilocus probes** are excellent in paternity work and any genetic investigations where high-quality fresh live material is available, the quality of many forensically obtained samples leaves much to be desired. When using poor material in multilocus tests, many of the bands are faint or absent due to degradation of the DNA. Here different restriction enzymes produce **single-locus probes**, which can be used to advantage, as although only two bands appear (one derived from each parent), the sensitivity, quality and discrimination is better than multilocus methods on poor samples. By using a series of single-locus probes in different tests, a battery of good-quality profiles can be built up, even on degraded material. Recent advances in identifying mitochondrial DNA, however, offer new scope for using tiny samples.

Samples and Controls Needed for DNA Profiling

The essence of DNA profiling in forensic work is comparison between two samples. One is the "test" sample from the living or dead subject (or objects with which he or she has been in contact, such as clothing) and the other the control.

Blood: As red cells have no nuclear DNA, sufficient blood must be obtained to extract DNA from the much sparser leukocytes (i) At least 1 ml and preferably 5 ml is taken into an EDTA tube, which extracts metallic ions and not only prevents clotting, but also inhibits enzymes in blood or microorganisms, which may break down DNA during storage. (ii) Blood sample should be taken in plastic tube and frozen solid in a deep freeze or ice making compartments of an ordinary refrigerator before transit to the lab. (iii) Blood stains should be either sent intact on surfaces, kept as cool as possible before and during transit to the lab. (iv) Blood stains may be rubbed with the cotton wool swab moistened with water. This swab is then air-dried without heat and then frozen. (v) Control samples for conventional blood grouping, including swabs rubbed on an area of fabric away from obvious stains as well as an unused swab should be provided to the lab. (vi) Dried blood stains on hard surfaces can be scraped off with a scalpel in a small plastic container and sent as they are and kept as cool as possible.

Seminal and vaginal fluids: (i) Swabs from vagina, rectum, mouth etc. should be air-dried as quickly as possible but not heated. They should be stored in deep-freeze before transit to lab. (ii) Liquid semen found in the vagina or elsewhere should be recovered with the fine pipette, placed in a small plain tube and frozen solid. (iii) Seminal stains on small items of fabric or any other small objects may be frozen or kept as cool as possible before and during transit. (iv) Clothing should be stored in paper bags and kept as cool as possible. (v) Damp swabs may be taken of suspect stains, which are then air-dried and frozen. (vi) Suspect's dried seminal stains on hard surfaces may be scraped off and transmitted dry to the laboratory. (vii) Mouth swabs at least 3-4 must be obtained by rubbing hard inside the cheek or the mouth lining scraped with an instrument and then smeared onto a swab.

Hairs: Whatever the source of the hairs–head, pubic, eyebrow, axillary they are of no use for DNA profiling unless nucleated root or follicle cells are present in sufficient numbers. The keratinized shaft contains no DNA-extractable material. The hairs shed naturally, as in "moulting", often from combs and hairbrushes, may have little or no root material and it is essential to have plucked hairs, from the living or dead. At least 10-20 hairs are the minimum required; these should be placed in a small plastic bag and frozen if there is to be a delay in arriving at the laboratory.

Autopsy tissue samples: (i) **At least 2 g of tissue** should be taken from the parenchyma of an organ and placed in a small plastic tube with no fixative or preservative. It should be frozen solid. (ii) **Spleen is the best organ for the DNA** recovery, though liver, muscle, kidney and brain may also be used. (iii) Dried bone such as femur, sternum or humerus can be used to detect DNA sample from the bone marrow in cases of decomposed, skeletonized bodies.

Levels of DNA in biological materials

Type of sample	Amount of DNA
Blood stain (1cm^2)	20-40 µg/100 ml
Blood stain (1mm^2)	200 µg
Semen	2 µg
Vaginal swab	150-300 µg/ml
Hair (plucked)	1-750 µg/hair
Hair (blood smeared)	0-12 µg/hair
Saliva (buccal cells)	0.5-19 µg/ml
Urine (urinary tract cells)	1-20 µg/ml

DNA Fingerprinting Process

1. Extraction of DNA

The principals involved in all those methods of DNA isolation can be categorized into four basic steps: (i) Cell lysis via disruption of cellular membranes. (ii) Denaturation and hydrolysis of proteins. (iii) Removal of denatured proteins and other cell debris. (iv) Purification of DNA. The commonly used DNA isolation procedure are organic isolation method, non-organic isolation method, column-based isolation and magnetic bid-based isolation of DNA.

2. Quantification of DNA

Quantification of DNA in a forensic sample is of major importance for proper DNA amplification and STR profiling. Several methods have been developed for quantification of DNA like yield gel method, absorption spectrophotometry and recently by Real Time PCR.

3. Making DNA Fingerprints

There have been two main types of forensic DNA testing called the RFLP and PCR based testing. The DNA can be analysed by using the restriction fragment length polymorphism (RFLP) technique in which the multiple repeating fragments are used to match with the sample. If the sample is too small then the available DNA can be amplified using the polymerase chain reaction process (PCR). Also in case of decomposed bodies, PCR technique has to be utilized for analyzing the available DNA.

A. Restriction Fragment Length Polymorphism (RFLP)

RFLP has been almost entirely replaced by the PCR based testing for DNA samples. RFLP is a technique for analyzing the variable lengths of DNA fragments that result from digesting a DNA sample with an enzyme called restriction endonuclease. This enzyme cuts DNA at a specific sequence pattern known as a **'restriction endonuclease recognition site'.** The presence or absence of certain recognition sites in a DNA sample generates variable lengths of DNA fragments, which are separated using gel electrophoresis. They are then hybridized with DNA probes that bind to complementary DNA sequence in the sample. RFLP is one of the original applications of DNA analysis to forensic investigation. With the development of newer, more efficient DNA analysis techniques, RFLP is not a commonly used technique, as it requires relatively large amounts of DNA. In addition, samples degraded by environmental factors such as dirt or fungus do not work well with RFLP. The DNA fingerprinting by RFLP is a laboratory procedure that requires following steps (Figure 33.2): (i) ***Isolation of DNA:*** DNA must be recovered from the cells or tissues of the body. Only a small amount of tissue like blood, hair, or skin is needed. For example, the amount of DNA found at the root of one hair is usually sufficient. (ii) ***Cutting, sizing and sorting:*** Restriction endonucleases are used to cut the DNA into fragments at specific places. For example, an enzyme called EcoR1, found in bacteria, will cut DNA only when the sequence GAATTC occurs. The DNA fragments are sorted according to size into bands by agarose gel electrophoresis. (iii) ***Transfer of DNA to nylon membrane:*** The bands of DNA are transferred via a technique called Southern blotting from the agarose gel to a nylon membrane. (iv) ***Probing:*** The Nylon membrane is then treated with a radioactively labeled DNA probe which binds to certain specific DNA sequence on the membrane. This produces a pattern called the DNA fingerprint. Each probe typically sticks into only one or two specific places on the Southern blot. The final DNA fingerprint is built by using multiple probes (5-10 or more) simultaneously. (v) ***DNA fingerprints:*** Excess of DNA probe is then washed off. An X-ray film placed next to the nylon membrane

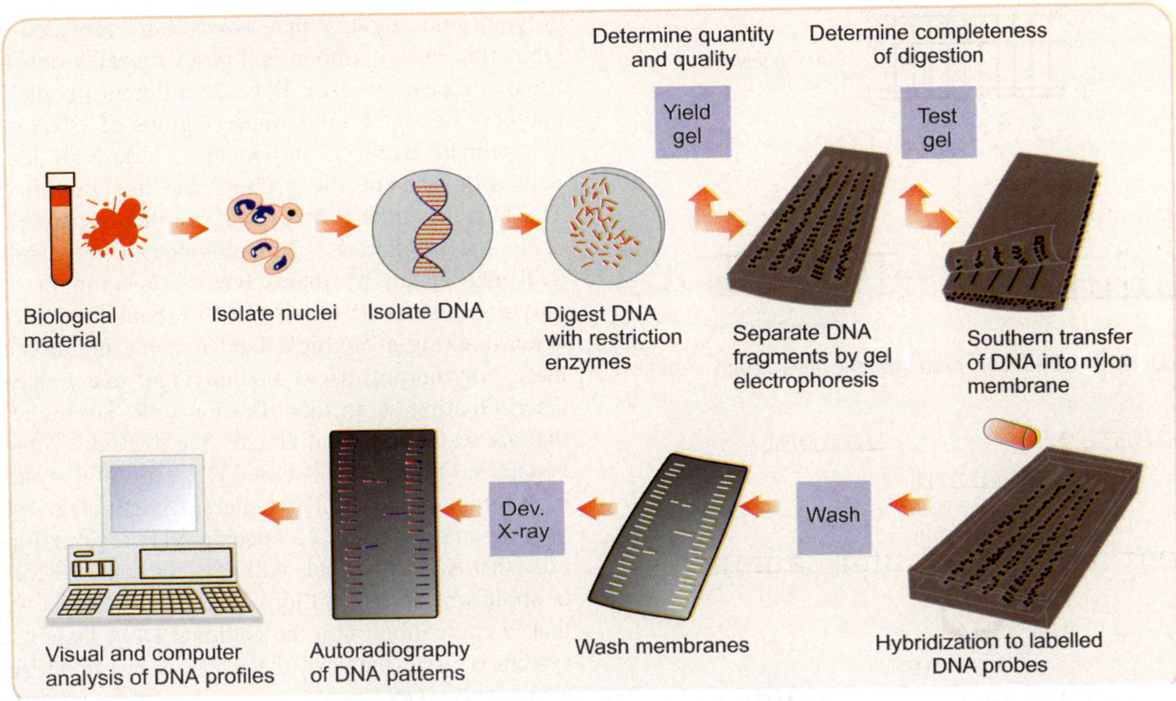

Figure 33.2: Procedure of DNA profiling

detects the radioactive pattern of bands. Development of this film (autoradiography) reveals visible pattern of bands **(DNA fingerprint)** indicating the sizes of alleles for the locus within each sample (Figure 33.3). These prints are called **'autorad'.** The band sizes are measured by comparing them with the bands of known DNA samples. By using multiple probes targeting various polymorphism in successive X-ray images, a fairly high degree of discrimination is possible.

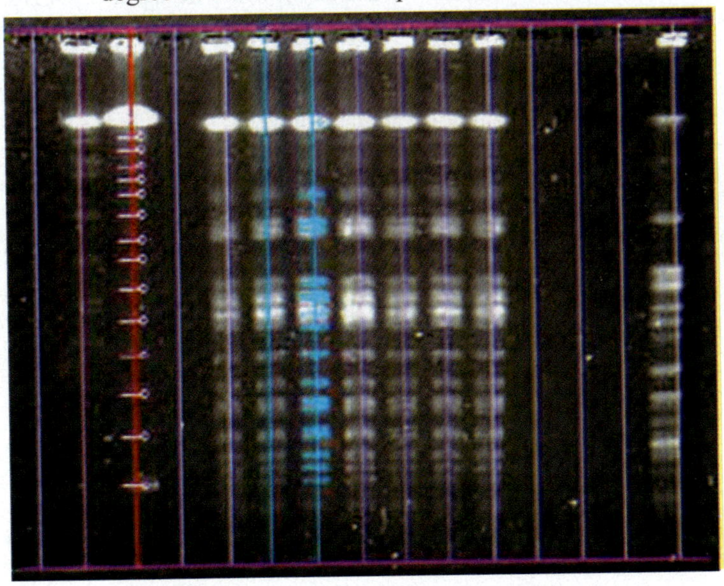

Figure 33.3: DNA pattern from blood on knife

The primary drawback of RFLP is that the exact sizes of bands are unknown and comparison to a molecular weight ladder is done in a purely qualitative manner. RFLP is a very time consuming method that required relatively high quantity of good quality DNA to be used.

B. Polymerase Chain Reaction (PCR)

With the invention of polymerase chain reaction, DNA fingerprinting took huge strides forward in both discrimination power and ability to recover information from the very small starting samples. PCR involves amplification of specific regions of DNA using a cycling of temperature and a thermostable polymerase enzyme along with sequence specific primers of DNA (Figures 33.4 and 33.5). PCR analysis is used to make millions of exact copies of DNA from a biological sample. PCR itself does not accomplish DNA typing but increases the amount of DNA available for typing. DNA amplification with PCR allows DNA analysis on biological samples in tiny quantities of DNA and enables even highly degraded samples to be analyzed. Commercial kits such as Profiler PlusTM, CofilerTM and PowerPlexTM that used single nucleotide polymorphisms for discrimination. These kits use PCR to amplify specific regions with known variations and hybridize them to probes anchored on cards, which results in a coloured spot corresponding to the particular sequence variation. However, in PCR analysis great care should be taken to prevent contamination with other biological materials during identifying, collecting and preserving of a sample. PCR uses primers that serve as starting points for copying of a region of DNA. Using multiplex PCR, over 10 markers can be copied at once. The sensitivities are to levels less than 1 ng of DNA and there is an increased ability to handle mixtures and degraded samples (Table 33.1).

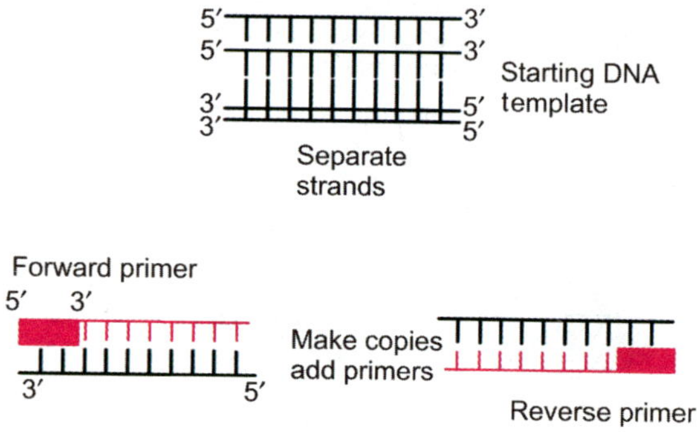

Figure 33.4: DNA amplification with polymerase chain reaction (PCR)

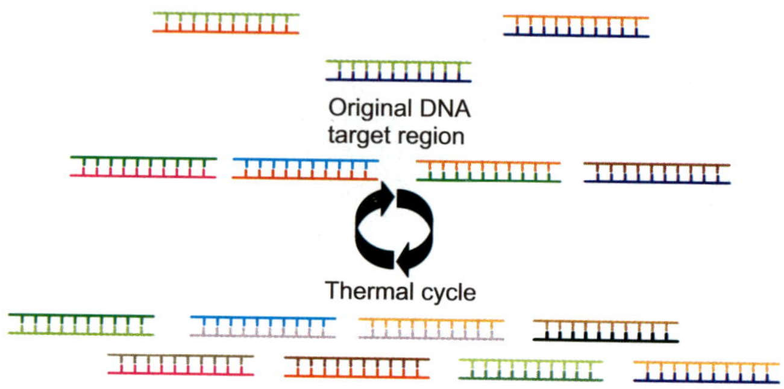

Figure 33.5: PCR copies of DNA exponentially through multiple thermal cycles

Table 33.1: Differences between the RFLP and PCR based testing

Properties	RFLP	PCR
Amount of sample	Requires large amount of DNA sample	Requires small amount of DNA sample
Moist and warm conditions	Sample degradation is accelerated in warm moist conditions	The chances of degradation in such conditions are less
Sensitivity	Tests are less sensitive	Tests are faster and extremely sensitive
Decomposed samples	Not useful	Useful
Contamination with other samples	Less sensitive to contamination	More sensitive to contamination

Short Tandem Repeats (STR) Analysis: STR technology is used to evaluate specific regions (loci) within nuclear DNA. STR is a term that describes any short, repeating DNA sequence (Figure 33.6). This technique is the most prevalent. It uses highly

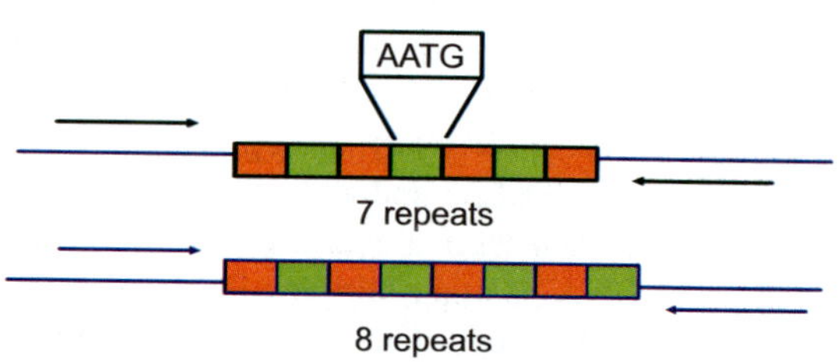

Figure 33.6: Short tandem repeats (STRs)

polymorphic regions that have short repeated sequences of DNA (the most common is 4 bases repeated but there are 3 and 5 bases repeats in use). Because different people have different numbers of repeat units, these regions of DNA can be used to discriminate between individuals. These STR loci are targeted with sequence-specific primers and are amplified using PCR. The DNA fragments that result are then separated and detected using electrophoresis. The polymorphisms displayed at each STR region are by themselves very common, typically each polymorphism will be shared by about 5-20% of individuals. When looking at multiple loci, it is the unique combination of these polymorphisms to an individual that makes this method discriminating as an identification tool. The more STR regions that are tested in an individual, the more discriminating the test becomes. Different STR based DNA profiling systems are in use in different countries. The Federal Bureau of Investigation (FBI) uses a standard set of 13 specific STR regions for CODIS. The odds that two individuals will have the same 13-loci DNA profile is about one in one billion. In U.K. the SGM+ system is used that is compatible with the National DNA Database. Whichever system is used, many of the STR regions under the test are the same. These DNA profiling systems are based around multiplex regions, whereby many STR regions will be under test at the same time. Compared to PCR based systems, multiplex STRs are more simple and direct at the allele detection stage and are slightly more vulnerable to missing alleles.

Amplified Fragment Length Polymorphism (AmpFLP): This technique was put into practice in the early 1900's and used PCR to amplify DNA samples. This technique relied on **'variable number tandem repeats'** (VNTR) polymorphism to distinguish various alleles, which were separated on a polyacrylamide gel using an allelic ladder. Bands could be visualized by silver staining gel. As the analysis is done on a gel, very high number repeats may bunch together at the top of the gel, making it difficult to resolve. Due to its low cost and ease of set up and operation, AmpFLP is popular in low income countries.

Lineage Markers in Forensic Analysis

1. **Mitochondrial DNA analysis (mtDNA) for maternal lineage:** For highly degraded samples, it is sometimes impossible to get a complete profile of the 13 CODIS STRs. In these situations, mitochondrial DNA (mtDNA) is sometimes typed as there are many copies of mtDNA in the cell, while there are only 1-2 copies of the nuclear DNA. Mitochondrial DNA analysis can be used to examine the DNA from samples that cannot be analyzed by RFLP or STR. While older biological samples that lack nucleated cellular material such as hair, bones and teeth cannot be analyzed with STR and RFLP, it can be analyzed with mtDNA. In the investigation of cases that have gone unsolved for many years, mtDNA is extremely valuable. All mothers have the same mitochondrial DNA as their daughters. This is because the mitochondrion of each new embryo comes from the mother's egg cell. The

father's sperm contributes only nuclear DNA. Comparing the mtDNA profile of unidentified remains with the profile of a potential maternal relative can be important technique in missing person investigations.

2. **Y-Chromosome analysis (Y Chromosome DNA test or Y-DNA test) for paternal lineage:** The Y-chromosome is passed directly from father to son, so the analysis of genetic markers on the Y chromosome is especially useful for tracing relationships among males or for analyzing biological evidence involving multiple male contributors.

Medicolegal and Ethical Aspects of DNA Fingerprinting

DNA fingerprints are useful in several applications in the legal setup: (i) *Paternity and Maternity:* Because a person inherits his or her variable number of tandem repeats (VNTRs) from his or her parents, VNTR patterns can be used to establish paternity and maternity. The patterns are so specific that a parental VNTR pattern can be reconstructed even if only the children's VNTR patterns are known (the more children produced, the more reliable the reconstruction). Parent-child VNTR pattern analysis has been used to solve standard father-identification cases as well as more complicated cases of confirming legal nationality and, in instances of adoption and biological parenthood. DNA paternity testing is because the child inherits the DNA from his mother and father. If the paternal alleles are not found in the child then it's called **exclusion.** The probability of exclusion (PE) is a statistical evaluation of the DNA tests being used. The PE is important, as it has to be at least 99% for the laboratory to provide a satisfactory report. Any series of tests has a probability of detecting at least one exclusion, if the man truly is not the father of the child. This is essentially the "probability of exclusion" for the series of tests. A probability of exclusion of 99% means that if 100 cases involving non-fathers are analysed, approximately 99 of them should show at least one exclusionary result. (ii) *Criminal Identification and Forensics:* DNA isolated from blood, hair, skin cells, or other genetic evidence left at the scene of a crime can be compared, through VNTR patterns, with the DNA of a criminal suspect to determine guilt or innocence. VNTR patterns are also useful in establishing the identity of a homicide victim, either from DNA found as evidence or from the body itself. (iii) *Personal Identification:* The notion of using DNA fingerprints as a sort of genetic bar code to identify individuals has been discussed, but this is not likely to happen anytime in the near future. The technology required to isolate, keep on file, and then analyze billions of much specified VNTR patterns is both expensive and impractical. Social security numbers, picture ID, and other more mundane methods are much more likely to remain the prevalent ways to establish personal identification. (iv) To identify endangered and protected species as an aid to wildlife officials. (v) To match organ donors with recipients in transplant programs. (vi) To detect bacteria and other organisms that may pollute air, water, soil and food. (vii) To determine pedigree for seeds or livestock breeds.

Ethical Issues: (i) *Privacy:* As DNA can provide insights into many aspects of an individual such as susceptibility to certain diseases, legitimacy etc. This could increase the potential for genetic discrimination by government, insurers, banks, schools and colleges etc. As the DNA samples and records are not discarded, there are chances of a person's entire genome being available that can be used to reveal personal information. (ii) *Individuals chosen for sampling:* In U.K, all suspects and arrestee can be forced to provide a DNA sample. In U.S., arresting people on less than probable cause to obtain DNA evidence raises the question of Fourth Amendment violations against unreasonable search and seizure. In India, the DNA profiling is limited to the forensic case work and it is not mandatory for all suspects and arrestee to provide the sample. (iii) *Practicality*: Since there is an enormous backlog of over half a million DNA samples to be entered into the CODIS system where the evidence would have been useful for conviction.

National DNA Databank (CODIS)

Combined DNA Index System (CODIS) is used for linking serial crimes and unsolved cases with repeat offenders. All 50 states have laws requiring that DNA profiles of certain offenders be sent to CODIS. The Convicted Offender Index contains DNA profiles of individuals convicted of sexual offences and other violent crimes. All DNA profiles stored in CODIS are generated using STR analysis. CODIS utilizes computer software to automatically search its two indexes for matching DNA profiles. It requires more than 4 RFLP markers and/or 13 core STR markers (CODIS core). In year 2017, seven additional STR markers were added.

DNA Database in India (UMID)

The Department of Forensic Medicine, AIIMS, New Delhi, has developed the first DNA database and identification portal for identification of unidentified bodies in India. It is named as UMID (Unidentified dead bodies, Missing person, Identification portal and DNA database) which is developed by Behera *et al.*, as part of Task Force Project funded by Indian Council of Medical Research (ICMR). It caters the identification of unidentified bodies reported from the south and south-east district of Delhi.

LONG QUESTION

1. Discuss the medicolegal aspects of DNA fingerprinting.

SHORT QUESTIONS

1. DNA fingerprinting.
2. RFLP.
3. PCR.
4. STR segments.

MULTIPLE CHOICE QUESTIONS

1. **DNA fingerprinting is done by:**
   (a) Sequence in nuclear DNA
   (b) Sequence in nuclear RNA
   (c) Non-sequence in nuclear DNA
   (d) Non-sequence in nuclear RNA

2. **Which of the following is the best method to determine paternity?**
   (a) Fingerprinting
   (b) DNA fingerprinting
   (c) Blood group
   (d) HLA

3. **Which one of the following will be the best sample preserved for DNA test?**
   (a) Hair (b) Skin swab
   (c) Blood (d) Nails clipping

4. **For DNA test, postmortem liquid blood is preserved in vial containing:**
   (a) Calcium oxalate (b) Potassium oxalate
   (c) EDTA (d) Sodium fluoride

5. **Alternate forms of genes known as:**
   (a) Alleles (b) Locus
   (c) Probes (d) Primers

6. **Three basic steps in DNA extraction are all *except:***
   (a) Lysis (b) Precipitation
   (c) Purification (d) PCR

7. **The DNA fingerprinting relies on:**
   (a) Difference in patterns of genes between individuals
   (b) Difference in junk DNA patterns between individuals
   (c) Difference in order of genes between individuals
   (d) None of the above

8. **Paternal lineage can be best established by:**
   (a) Autosomal DNA typing
   (b) Mitochondrial DNA typing
   (c) Y-STR
   (d) HLA typing

9. **Maternal lineage can be best established by:**
   (a) Autosomal DNA typing (b) Mitochondrial DNA typing
   (c) Y-STR (d) HLA Typing

ANSWER KEY ☞

1. (a)	2. (b)	3. (c)	4. (c)	5. (a)	6. (d)	7. (b)	8. (c)	9. (b)

34 CHAPTER

Forensic Psychiatry

Psychiatry: The study of etiology, diagnosis and treatment of mental disorders is called psychiatry.

Forensic Psychiatry: It is the application of psychiatry in the administration of justice. The attitude of the society towards persons afflicted with mental illness has changed considerably and it is now realized that no stigma should be attached to such illness as it is curable, particularly, when diagnosed at an early stage. Thus, the mentally ill persons are to be treated like any other sick persons and the environment around them should be made as normal as possible.

The experience of the working of the Indian Lunacy Act, 1912 has revealed that it has become outmoded. With the rapid advance of medical science and the understanding of the nature of the malady, it has become necessary to have fresh legislation with provisions for treatment of mentally ill persons in accordance with the new approach. Accordingly, the Mental Health Bill was passed in both the houses of Parliament on 22nd May 1987 and came into force on 1st April 1993.

INSANITY

The word insanity has no technical meaning in law or in medicine. It does not connote any definite medical entity but is solely a legal and sociological concept used to designate those members of society who are unable on account of mental disease to adapt themselves to ordinary social requirements, so that the community compulsorily segregates them and takes away their rights as citizens. Insanity is thus seen as a social inadequacy and medically it is a form of mental disease. Insanity is a degree of mental disturbance. The person may be considered from legal point of view to be immune from certain responsibilities. He may be disallowed certain privileges that may require a degree of competence for example to marry, to make contracts, to manage property etc.

The word unsoundness of mind, which finds a place in Indian penal code and is used as a synonym with other terms like insanity, lunacy, madness or mental derangement or disordered state of mind, due to which the individual loses the power of regulating his actions and conduct according to the rules of the society to which it belongs.

Binet-Simon Test for Intelligence Quotient: It is a measure of intelligence, based on psychological tests that is calculated as: IQ = mental age/chronological age × 100. When the mental age increases, the IQ provides an index of relative brightness that can be used to compare children of different ages. In adults, the concept of mental age becomes less relevant. There are separate age norms in various age groups upto age 65. The IQ as measured by most intelligence tests is an interpretation or classification of a total test score in relation to the norms. It can be misleading since it is an average of different abilities or levels of ability that themselves may show great variability. The IQ is a measure of present functioning ability and not necessarily of future potential.

Oligophrenia (Mental Subnormalities): In oligophrenia, there is retarded or incomplete and abnormal mental development. In these cases, the I.Q. is below 70 and it mostly results from environmental, genetic and endocrinal abnormalities. Even at times birth trauma can be a cause. The following three categories of oligophrenia are encountered: (i) ***Idiot:*** These are persons with an I.Q. between 0 to 20. There is defective mental development since birth or early childhood. It may be associated with physical abnormalities like microcephaly or mongolism and at times there is defective development of other organs of the body. (ii) ***Imbecile:*** These are persons with the I.Q. between 20 to 50. These persons also have the defective development of the brain from birth or early childhood and are not capable of being taught. (iii) ***Moron:*** These persons have an I.Q. ranging from 50 to 75 and have the mental development of a child of the age of 6-11 years. They require constant care and supervision for their protection.

Wechsler Adult Intelligence Scale (WAIS): WAIS is a general test of intelligence, which Wechsler defined as, "Global capacity of the individual to act purposefully, to think rationally, and to deal effectively with his environment." In keeping with this definition of intelligence as an aggregate of mental aptitudes or abilities, the WAIS-R consists of 11 subtests divided into two parts, verbal and performance. It is further divided into six verbal subtests and five performance subtests. Verbal tests are: (i) Information (ii) Comprehension (iii) Arithmetic (iv) Digit span (v) Similarities (vi) Vocabulary. Performance subtests are: (i) Picture arrangement (ii) Picture completion (iii) Block design (iv) Object assembly (v) Digit symbol. The scores derived from this test are: (i) Verbal IQ (VIQ), (ii) Performance IQ (PIQ), and (iii) Full Scale IQ (FSIQ). The FSIQ is a standard score with a mean of 100 and a standard deviation of approximately 15.

Causes of Insanity: (i) Hereditary conditions: (a) Huntington's chorea (b) Amaurotic familial idiocy (ii) Environment factors: (a) Faulty parental attitude (b) Lack of mental hygiene (iii) Psychogenic causes: Repression of mental conflicts (iv) Organic diseases: (a) Head injury (b) Senile degeneration (c) Atherosclerosis (d) Myxedema (v) Insanity due to drugs: These are alcohol, cocaine, hashish and opium (vi) Insanity of pregnancy and childbirth: It is quite commonly encountered.

Precipitating Factors for Insanity: (i) Financial and business worries (ii) Frustration and disappointment in love affairs (iii) Death of near and dear ones.

Alcoholic Insanity: It includes delirium tremens and Korsakoff 's psychosis.

Delirium Tremens: This is a type of delirium seen in chronic alcoholics. It occurs 1-2 days after sudden withdrawal of alcohol due to heavy bout of drink. Injuries, infections and shock may precipitate it. Patient becomes sleepless, restless, and irritable and there are disorders of perception. There are coarse muscular tremors of face, tongue and hands. Also, there is disorientation and hallucination and the person may commit suicide, homicide etc.

Medicolegal Aspects: Alcoholic insanity is considered as unsoundness of mind and the person is not responsible for the crimes committed during this delirium.

Korsakoff's Disease: In Korsakoff's psychosis, there is loss of memory for recent events, extreme dissociation. The crimes related to sexual jealousy which are homicidal in nature are committed.

Insanity Due to Drugs: Addiction of drugs such as cocaine, hashish, opium may lead to insanity.

Insanity of Pregnancy and Childbirth: During pregnancy and child birth attacks of mania, melancholia, dementia etc. are precipitated.

MENTAL AND BEHAVIOURAL DISORDERS CLASSIFICATION (ICD-10)

F00-F09 Organic, Including Symptomatic, Mental Disorders: Mental and behavioural disorders due to demonstrable cerebral disease or disorder, either primary (primary brain pathology) or secondary (brain dysfunction due to systemic diseases). Term organic here does not mean that other psychiatric disorders are 'non-organic' in nature. It simply means that the disorders listed in this section have a demonstrable and diagnosable cerebral disease or disorder, e.g., delirium, dementia, organic amnestic syndrome, and other organic mental disorders.

F10-F19 Mental and Behavioural Disorders due to Psychoactive Substance Use: This group includes mental and behavioural disorders due to the use of one or more psychoactive substances, e.g., acute intoxication, harmful use, dependence syndrome, withdrawal state, amnestic syndrome and psychotic disorders due to psychoactive substance use.

F20-F29 Schizophrenia, Schizotypal and Delusional Disorders: This group includes mental and behavioural disorders characterized by prominent disturbances of thought, perception, affect, and/or behaviour, e.g., schizophrenia, schizotypal disorder, persistent delusional disorders, acute and transient psychotic disorders, induced delusional disorder and schizo-affective disorders.

F31-F39 Mood (Affective) Disorders: This group includes mental and behavioural disorders with prominent disturbance of mood, e.g., manic episode, depressive episode, bipolar affective disorder, recurrent depressive disorder and persistent mood disorder.

F40-F48 Neurotic, Stress-related and Somatoform Disorders: (There is no category with code number F49) includes mental and behavioural disorders that were earlier labeled as neurotic disorders, with an emphasis on psychological causation, e.g., anxiety disorders, phobic anxiety disorders, obsessive-compulsive disorder, dissociative (conversion) disorders, somatoform disorders, reaction to stress, and adjustment disorders, and other neurotic disorders.

Post-Traumatic Stress Disorder (PTSD)

It is an anxiety disorder that develops in reaction to physical injury or severe mental or emotional distress, such as military combat, violent assault, natural disaster, or other life-threatening events. As per proposed ICD-11, Classical symptom clusters of PTSD include: (i) **Intrusion symptoms:** Recurrent unwanted distressing memories of the traumatic events, flashbacks, or nightmares, typically accompanied by strong and overwhelming emotions such as fear or horror, and strong physical sensations. (ii) **Avoidance:** Avoidance of thoughts and memories of the event or events, avoidance of activities, situations, or people reminiscent of the event or events. (iii) **Alteration in arousal and reactivity:** Persistent perceptions of heightened current threat–for example, as indicated by hyper vigilance or an enhanced startle reaction to stimuli such as unexpected noises. (iv) **Additional criteria for complex PTSD:** Severe and pervasive problems in affect regulation, persistent beliefs about oneself as diminished, defeated, or worthless, accompanied by deep and pervasive feelings of shame, guilt, or failure related to the stressor, persistent difficulties in sustaining relationships and in feeling close to others.

For diagnosis of PTSD, the duration of the symptoms must be more than one month. It is more common in women. Early diagnosis and intervention are necessary for effective management.

F50-F59 Behavioural Syndromes Associated with Physiological Disturbances and Physical Factors: Includes disorders that were earlier called psychosomatic disorders. The term psychosomatic is no longer used because its use implied that the association between the psychological factors and physical disorder is etiological, e.g., eating disorders, non-organic sleep disorders, sexual dysfunctions (not caused by organic disorder or disease), mental and behavioural disorders associated with puerperium, and abuse of non-dependence producing substances.

F60-F69 Disorders of Adult Personality and Behaviour: E.g., personality disorders, habit and impulse disorders, gender-identity disorders, disorders of sexual preference and psychological and behavioural disorders associated with sexual development and orientation.

F70-F79 Mental Retardation: Includes disorders with arrested/incomplete development of the intellectual abilities, which may or may not be associated with other mental disorder, e.g., mental retardation (mild/moderate/profound).

F80-F89 Disorders of Psychological Development: Mental and behavioural I disorders with an onset during infancy or childhood, e.g., specific developmental disorders of speech and language, specific developmental disorders of Scholastic skills, specific developmental disorders of motor function, mixed specific developmental disorders, and pervasive developmental disorders.

F90-F98 Behavioral and Emotional Disorders I with Onset Usually Occurring in Childhood I and Adolescence: Miscellaneous mental and I behavioral disorders that have an onset in I childhood and adolescence, e.g. hyperkinetic disorders, conduct disorders, mixed disorders of conduct and emotions, tic disorders.

F99 UNSPECIFIED MENTAL DISORDER

Psychosis

A major mental disorder of organic or emotional origin characterized by extreme derangements of the personality often accompanied by severe depression, agitation, aggressive behaviour, illusions, hallucinations, delirium etc. In these the person loses touch with reality and shows psychotic symptoms.

Neurosis

This is a mental disorder or a disease of the nerves. Any faulty or inefficient way of coping with anxiety or inner conflict, usually involving the use of an unconscious defence mechanism, that may ultimately lead to a neurotic disorder. Ability to function is markedly impaired but behaviour generally remains within acceptable social norms. Perception of reality can be affected. Usually no proof of organic cause can be found.

Delirium

Delirium is a syndrome generally produced by a transient disturbance of brain tissue function. It is a disturbance of consciousness in which: (i) Orientation is impaired (ii) Critical faculty is blunted or lost (iii) Thought content is irrelevant or incoherent. In the early stage, the patient becomes restless, uneasy and sleepless, loses self-control, and becomes excited. Although, the level of consciousness is altered, the patient is generally awake, and able to answer questions. However, his thinking, memory, perception and attention are disturbed. Delirium may be followed by complete recovery in an acute brain syndrome. It may also progress to an irreversible amaurotic syndrome, which may be defined as chronic brain syndrome leading to coma and death in which case the matter of deliberation seems irrelevant. It is found in cases of: (i) Trauma (ii) Anoxia (iii) Vascular infarction (iv) Toxic metabolic disorders (v) Drug abuse (vi) Inflammatory conditions (vii) Psychological disturbances (viii) Mental stress (ix) Overload of work.

Medicolegal Aspects: Delirium is less often associated with hallucinations and delusions and if the person commits crime then he is not responsible for his act.

Delusion

It is a false belief that arises without appropriate external stimulation in something, which is not a fact, and which persists even after its falsity has been clearly demonstrated. The belief held is not ordinarily shared by other members of the patient's sociocultural and educational group. Delusions are pathognomonic of the psychoses. They occur in schizophrenia. They can be observed in all psychotic states including that of organic origin. A normal person can have delusion but he corrects himself by his reasoning capacity.

Types of Delusion: (i) ***Of grandeur or exaltation (Megalomania):*** A man imagines himself to be very rich, though in reality he is a pauper. He thinks himself to be a king or a great personality, but actually he is a common man. (ii) ***Of persecution:*** He imagines that attempts have been made to kill him by his nearest relatives. (iii) ***Of references:*** He thinks that people, things and events etc. refer to him in a special way. People are talking about him and newspapers are writing about him. (iv) ***Of influence or of control:*** He complains that his actions, thoughts are being influenced and controlled by some outside agency, like radio, hypnotism or telepathy etc. This type of delusion is seen in schizophrenia. (v) ***Of infidelity:*** A man imagines that his wife is unfaithful to him while in reality she is chaste. (vi) ***Of self-reproach (self-accusation):*** The person reproaches himself for the past failure and misdeeds which are often of a trivial nature. (vii) ***Of nihilistic:*** The man declares that he does not exist or that there is no world. (viii) ***Hypochondria:*** A person has a firm belief in his mind that there is something wrong in his body, though he is quite healthy. (ix) ***Paranoid delusions:*** Over suspiciousness leading to persecutory delusions.

Medicolegal Aspects: Delusions often affect the conduct and actions of the sufferer. There is the tendency to commit suicide and homicide etc. Delusion is often taken as defence in Court of law. The person cannot be held fully responsible for the act.

During the examination of the mental condition of the person, the medical man should make a careful note as to which law he gives much importance. In the beginning of a disease delusion may not be evident. As person can conceal it, hence the doctor should examine or watch the person for days together.

Erotomania: It is a type of delusion in which the person believes that someone is deeply in love with him or her. So, it develops in those persons who has some obsession for a particular person and starts to believe that other person is reciprocating. The person is of higher status, famous or superior at work or business. the erotomaniacs tries to get close with the person through telephone, letters, emails, gifts or by frequent visits, otherwise the person is normal.

Empathy: The degree to which the observer is able to enter the thoughts and the feelings of the patient.

Fugue: It is a state of altered awareness during which the individual forgets the part or a whole of his life. He leaves home and wanders. It may occur in hysteria, schizophrenia, epilepsy.

Hallucination

Hallucination is a false sense of perception without any external object or stimulus to produce it. It is the apparent perception of an external object when no corresponding real object exists. A dream is a simple example of hallucination in everyday experience. It occurs in a number of conditions such as: (i) Schizophrenia (ii) Under the influence of drugs (L.S.D., Mescaline) (iii) Temporal lobe lesions (iv) Generalized organic brain diseases (v) Small doses of alcohol and cannabis (vi) Brain tumor, subarachnoid hemorrhage, uremia etc. (vii) High fever.

Types of Hallucinations: (i) ***Visual:*** In this type of hallucination, the person may see himself being followed by a lion though no lion exists. (ii) ***Auditory:*** In this the person listens to the voice and imagines that someone is talking to him, when nobody is there. (iii) ***Olfactory:*** In this the person smells pleasant or unpleasant when no smell is there. (iv) ***Gustatory:*** The person tastes sweet, sour or salt etc. when there is no food in mouth. (v) ***Tactile:*** The person imagines that mice or rats are crawling over him when practically no mice or rats are present, for example cocaine bugs as seen in cocaine poisoning. (vi) ***Kinesthetic/Psychomotor:*** There is feeling of movement of some parts of the body when they are stationary. (vii) ***Lilliputation or micro tic:*** Small size objects may appear very large or vice versa. (viii) ***Hypnagogic:*** False sensory perception occurring midway between falling asleep and being awake that is during drowsy state after deep sleep and before awakening.

Medicolegal Aspects: Hallucination may be pleasant or unpleasant. Delusions arising from unpleasant hallucinations may cause the person to commit suicide or homicide. The person is not held responsible for the deeds committed during the hallucinations.

Illusion

Illusion is a false interpretation by the senses of external object which has a real existence. Some of the examples are that the person feels a dog as a lion, rope as a snake or tree as a ghost. A sane person also has illusion, but he is able to correct the illusion but an insane person cannot correct his falsity. Illusions of sight and hearing are very common but those involving other senses also occur. Illusions can occur in insanity and other toxic states.

Medicolegal Aspects: The person is not responsible for his acts.

Obsession

In this a single idea or emotion is constantly entertained by a person in spite of all efforts of the sufferer to drive it away from his mind. It is a disorder of thought and attempts to resist makes them more strongly insistent.

Examples of Obsession: (i) Closing the door and checking for the locks repeatedly at bedtime. (ii) Counting the money again and again before going to the market. (iii) A wife may continuously believe her husband to be unfaithful to her or vice versa. (iv) Washing hands again and again.

Medicolegal Aspects: (i) Obsession is a disorder of mind that is borderline between sanity and insanity. (ii) Sane person also have obsession but he can correct it. (iii) It is usually seen in nervous people.

Impulse

Sudden and irresistible force compelling a person to the conscious performance of some actions without notice or forethought. A sane person has sufficient faculties to control the impulse. However, an insane person cannot control his impulses. It is usually seen in imbecility, dementia, acute mania etc.

Types of Impulse: (i) ***Kleptomania:*** There is tendency to steal small articles. (ii) ***Pyromania:*** An impulse to set fire to things. (iii) ***Multinomania:*** A desire to maim animals. (iv) ***Dipsomania:*** An excessive desire to drink alcohol. (v) ***Sexual impulses:*** It is a form of sexual perversions by abnormal means to obtain gratification. (vi) ***Suicidal or homicidal impulse:*** It is an impulse to commit suicide or homicide.

Lucid Interval

This is period occurring during insanity when all the symptoms completely disappear and the person becomes normal. It appears in melancholia and mania. The differences between lucid interval of head injury and insanity is given in Table 34.1.

Table 34.1: Differences between lucid interval of head injury and insanity

Features	Head injury	Insanity
History of	Injury	Mental disease
Preceded by	Phase of concussion	Phase of symptoms of insanity
Followed by	Phase of cerebral irritation and compression of brain	Phase recurrence of symptoms of insanity
Episodes	Only once	More than once

Medicolegal Aspects: The person is not legally responsible for the crimes done during lucid interval but it is very difficult to prove the same.

MENTAL HEALTH ACT, 1987

(i) This Act defines the criteria for admission and restraint of the mentally ill persons. (ii) As per this Act the words lunacy, insanity and unsoundness of mind have been **replaced by the word mentally ill that has been defined as** "a person who is in need of treatment by reason of mental disorder other than mental retardation". (iii) It provides the guidelines for establishment and maintenance of psychiatric hospitals and nursing homes. (iv) It describes the procedure for admission and detention of mentally ill persons, in psychiatric hospitals and nursing homes. (v) It describes the provisions for inspection, discharge, leave of absence and removal of mentally ill persons from psychiatric hospitals or nursing homes. (vi) It provides for judicial inquisition regarding possession of property by alleged mentally ill person, custody of the person, and management of his property. (vii) It provides for the liability to meet cost of maintenance of a mentally ill person detained in psychiatric hospital or psychiatric nursing home. (viii) It provides for protection of human rights of mentally ill persons. (ix) It provides for penalties and procedure for awarding the same, for violation of the provisions of the Act. (x) It also provides for certain other miscellaneous aspects regarding lunacy and the lunatics.

Admission of Lunatics or Insane Persons into Mental Hospitals or Psychiatric Nursing Homes

Part I: Admission As Voluntary Patient

S. 15: Request by major for admission as voluntary patient: Any person who considers himself to be mentally ill and desirous of getting admitted for treatment, he can request medical officer in-charge of a psychiatric hospital/nursing home and can get admitted in the same as a voluntary patient.

S.16: Request by guardian for admission of a ward (minor less than 18 years as voluntary patient) whom he considers to be mentally ill. He may request medical officer in-charge of the hospital/nursing home for the admission.

S. 17: Procedure to be followed: (i) On receipt of request under S.15 or S.16, the medical officer in-charge shall make such inquiry as he may deem fit within a period not exceeding 24 hours and if he is satisfied that the applicant (major or minor) requires treatment as inpatient, he may admit such him as a voluntary patient. (ii) Every voluntary patient admitted to a psychiatric nursing home/hospital will abide by the rules and regulations made by the medical officer in-charge or the licensee of such hospital/nursing home.

S.18: Discharge of voluntary patients: (i) Medical officer in-charge of the psychiatric nursing home/hospital after receiving the request for the discharge by the voluntary patient or his guardian, shall discharge him within 24 hours. (ii) When minor voluntary patient who is admitted in the hospital/nursing home as inpatient attains majority he should be informed about his attainment of majority by medical officer and unless a fresh request is made by him for continuation as inpatient, within one month of such intimation he shall be discharged. (iii) When the medical officer is satisfied that the discharge will not be in the interest of the patient, a medical board is constituted consisting of two medical officers within 72 hours of receipt of request period of expiry (under subsection (i) and (ii) above) and their opinion is sought as to whether the patient needs further treatment and if the board feels that the patient needs further treatment, the medical officer will not discharge the patient but instead will continue the treatment for the period not exceeding ninety days at a time.

Part II: Admission Under Special Circumstances

S. 19: Admission under special circumstances: (i) Mentally ill persons who does not or are unable to express willingness for admission as a voluntary patient may be admitted as an inpatient on an application made by relative or friends. The medical officer can admit such patient if he is satisfied that the admission is necessary for the benefit of the patient but he will be kept only for 90 days. (ii) For application, a prescribed medical form along with two medical certificates from two medical practitioners (one of these should be in government service) in the support of the mental illness of the person that requires him to be kept under observation and treatment as inpatient should be enclosed. If the application is not accompanied by medical certificates then the medical officer in-charge of the hospital may arrange examination of the person by two medical officers of the mental hospital/nursing home and if findings of the two medical officers are supportive of mental illness of the person then he may be admitted in the hospital. (iii) For the discharge of such patient, the relative or friend may apply to the magistrate. The magistrate after making inquiry and after giving notice to the person as he deems fit, may either allow or dismiss the application. (iv) Provisions of the section shall be without prejudice to the persons exercisable by a magistrate.

Part III: Reception Order

S. 20: Application for reception and detention order: (i) An application of reception order may be made by: (a) Medical officer in-charge of psychiatric hospital/nursing home (b) Husband, wife or any other relative. (ii) Medical officer in-charge of the hospital where the ill person is undergoing treatment under a temporary order is satisfied that (a) Treatment of mentally ill person is required to be continued for more than 6 months or (b) It is necessary in the interests and personal safety of the ill person or for the protection of others, that such person shall be detained in psychiatric hospital/nursing home. He may make an application to the magistrate with local unit of whose jurisdiction the hospital situated for the detention of the ill person under a reception order. (iii) Husband, wife or any other relative can make an application for detention under a reception order. (iv) Where the husband and wife are not available and relatives make an application, the request must be accompanied by reason of their absence. (v) No persons (a) Who is a minor or (b) Who has not seen the alleged mentally ill person within 14 days before the date of application shall make an application. (vi) Application must be made with the prescribed form alongwith two medical certificates out of which one should be of the Government Medical practitioner.

S. 21: Form and contents of medical certificates: The medical certificate shall contain a statement that (i) Each medical practitioners has examined the ill person independently and the opinion is given on the basis of his own observation. (ii) Ill person is suffering from mental disorder of such a nature and degree that he requires detention in a psychiatric hospital/nursing home. That such detention is needed in the interests of health and safety of the mentally ill person and for the protection of others.

S. 22: Procedure upon application for detention: (i) On receipt of application the magistrate may make a reception order, if he is satisfied that: (a) Mentally ill person is suffering from such a nature and degree that he requires detention in a psychiatric nursing home/hospital for treatment (b) It is in the interest of the health of mentally ill person or for the protection of others that he should be detained and a temporary treatment order would not be adequate in the circumstances, and it is necessary to make a reception order. (ii) On receipt of application, magistrate will consider the statement of the certificate and form. (iii) If the magistrate considers that there are sufficient grounds to proceed further he shall personally examine the ill person unless for reasons to be recorded, he thinks that it is not necessary. (iv) If he is not satisfied with the application he may fix a date for further consideration of the application and may make such inquiries concerning the alleged mentally ill person as he thinks fit. (v) The notice of the date fixed should be given to the applicant and any other person whom he thinks fit of receiving notice. (vi) During this period of pending disposal of the application, the magistrate may make an order for the proper care and custody of the alleged mentally ill person. (vii) The magistrate shall consider the application in camera in the presence of the (a) Applicant (b) Alleged mentally ill person (c) Person who may be appointed by the alleged mentally ill person (d) Any other person as the magistrate thinks fit. (viii) If magistrate is satisfied that the alleged mentally ill person is so mentally ill that in the interests of the health and personal safety of the person or for the protection of others his detention is necessary, he may pass a reception order and if not satisfied he may dismiss the application with reasons recorded and one copy is given to applicant.

S. 23: Powers and duties of police officer in respect of the mentally ill persons: (i) Every officer in-charge of police station may take: (a) Into protection any person found wandering within his jurisdiction whom he has reason to believe that he is so mentally ill that he cannot take care of himself and (b) Whom he has reason to believe to be dangerous by reason of mental illness. (ii) The police officer cannot detain the mentally ill person taken into protection without being informed of the grounds of such protection to the person himself or to his relatives or friends if the mentally ill person cannot understand those grounds. (iii) Police officer must produce the mentally ill person within 24 hours before the nearest magistrate excluding the time necessary for the journey from the place where he was taken into such protection of the Court of the magistrate and he cannot detain beyond the said period without the authority of the magistrate.

S. 24: Procedure on production of mentally ill person: When a person is produced before the magistrate by the police and in the opinion of the magistrate, there are sufficient grounds for proceeding further, the magistrate shall: (i) Examine the person to access his capacity to understand. (ii) Cause him to be examined by a medical officer. (iii) May make necessary inquiries. After completion of proceedings magistrate may pass a reception order authorizing the detention of the said person as an inpatient in a psychiatric hospital/nursing home (a) If the medical officer certifies that person to be mentally ill (b) Magistrate himself is satisfied the said person is mentally ill and that for his care and for the protection of others such order is necessary: Provided that (a) If the relative or friend of the mentally ill person desires of sending the mentally ill person to a particular licensed psychiatric hospital/nursing home and undertakes in writing a bond to pay the expenses of maintenance and if the medical officer in-charge of such hospital/nursing home also consents, the magistrate may pass a reception order for admission there (b) If any relative or friend enters into bond with or without sureties for such amount as the magistrate may determine undertaking that he will properly take care of the mentally ill person so that he longer remains dangerous to himself or to others, then instead of making a reception order the mentally ill person is handed over to the relative or friend.

S. 25: Order in case of mentally ill person cruelly treated or not under proper care and control: (i) Police officer who has reason to believe that any person within the limits of his station is mentally ill and is not under proper care and control, or is ill-treated or neglected by any relative or other person having his charge, can report the facts to the magistrate. (ii) Any private person who has reason to believe the above facts may report to the magistrate. (iii) Magistrate may cause the mentally ill person to be produced before him, and summons such relatives or other persons who ought to be in-charge of that person when it appears to the magistrate, on the report of police officer/private person that any mentally ill person is not under proper care and control, is ill treated or neglected. (iv) If such relative/person is legally bound to maintain the mentally ill person, the magistrate may pass an order to require them to take proper care of such person. In cases of non-compliance of the order, fine up to Rs. 2000 may be imposed. (v) If there is no person who is legally bound to take care of the mentally ill person or if such legally bound person refuses or neglects to maintain the ill person, or if magistrate thinks fit to do so, he may cause the mentally ill person to be produced before him and without prejudice to any action proceed in the manner provided under S. 24 and pass a reception order.

S. 26: Admission as in patient after inquisition: Any district court holding an inquisition under chapter VI is of the opinion that it is in the interest of mentally ill person, he may by order direct the admission of such person into hospital as in patient. Every such order may vary from time to time or revoked by the District Court.

S. 27: Admission and detention of mentally ill prisoners: An order under S.30 of the Prisoners Act, S.144 of the Air Force Act, S.145 of the Army Act, S.143 or S.144 of the Navy Act or S.330 or S.335 Cr.P.C. directing the reception of the mentally ill prisoner into any psychiatric hospital/nursing home, he may be lawfully transferred for detention therein.

S. 28: Detention of alleged mentally ill person, pending report by medical officer: This section provides for detention of the alleged mentally ill person brought before a magistrate under S. 23 or S. 25, the magistrate may by order in writing, authorize the detention of such person under proper medical custody in an observation ward of a general/psychiatric hospital/nursing or any other suitable place for such period not exceeding 10 days as the magistrate may consider necessary for enabling any medical officer to determine whether a medical certificate in respect of the alleged mentally ill person may properly be given under clause (a) of subsection (ii) of S. 24. Such further detention will be by order in writing by the magistrate for periods not exceeding 10 days provided that no person shall be authorized to be detained under this subsection for a continuous period exceeding 30 days in aggregates.

S. 40: Order of discharge by medical officer in-charge: (i) Notwithstanding anything in chapter IV the medical officer in-charge, on the recommendations of two medical practitioners, one of whom must be a psychiatrist, by order in writing, direct the discharge of any person, other than a voluntary patient detained or undergoing treatment therein as an inpatient, and such person shall thereupon be discharged from the psychiatric hospital/nursing home. (ii) Where any order of discharge is made, a copy of such order shall be forwarded to that authority by medical officer in-charge.

S. 41: Discharge of mentally ill persons on application: When any application is received to discharge to the medical officer in-charge by the person on whose application the admission was made, he may be discharged provided the medical officer in-charge certifies in writing that the person is not dangerous and is fit to be discharged.

S. 42: Order of discharge on the undertaking of relatives or friends for due care: (i) Where such person shall be delivered over to his care and custody, he may make an application to the medical officer in-charge who forwards it to the authority with remarks thereon. (ii) Friend/relative will furnish a bond with or without sureties for amount specified by the authority to take care of such person and that he will not cause injuries to himself or others.

S. 43: Discharge of person on his request: Any mentally ill person who feels that he has recovered except prisoners will (i) Make an application to the magistrate. (ii) It should be supported by a certificate from a medical officer in-charge of the hospital or psychiatrist. The magistrate after inquiry if deems fit can pass an order for discharging the person.

S. 44: Discharge of person subsequently found on inquisition to be of sound mind: If subsequently the ill person is found to be of sound mind or capable of taking care of him or managing his affairs, medical officer in-charge on production of a copy of such findings duly certified by district court discharge such person from the psychiatric nursing home/hospital.

MENTAL HEALTH CARE ACT, 2017

This Act came into existence on April 7, 2018 which superseded the previously existing Mental Health Act, 1987. The Act seeks to fulfil India's international obligation pursuant to the Convention on Rights of Persons with Disabilities and its Optional Protocol which was adopted by the United Nations (UN) on December 13, 2006 and came into force on May 3, 2008. This Act aims to provide for mental health care and services for persons with mental illness and to protect, promote and fulfil the rights of such persons during delivery of mental health care and services and for matters connected therewith or incidental thereto.

Highlights of the Act

1. **New Definition of Mental Illness: S. 2 (1s),** the new Act defines "mental illness" as a substantial disorder of thinking, mood, perception, orientation, or memory that grossly impairs judgment or ability to meet the ordinary demands of life, mental conditions associated with the abuse of alcohol and drugs.
2. **Rights of Persons with Mental Illness:** (i) **S. 18,** (a) All mentally ill persons have the right to access good quality, convenient, affordable, and accessible mental health care services run or funded by the appropriate government. There shall be free treatment for mentally ill persons if they are homeless or belong to Below Poverty Line (BPL), even if they do not possess a BPL card. (b) There shall be no discrimination on any basis including gender, sex, sexual orientation, religion, culture, caste, social or political beliefs, class or disability. (ii) **S. 23,** The mental ill persons have the right to confidentiality in respect of their mental health, mental health care, treatment and physical health care. (iii) **S. 24,** The photographs and other information pertaining to the mentally ill person cannot be released to the media without the consent of that person. (iv) **S. 25,** The persons have the right to access their medical records. (v) **S. 27,** The persons shall be entitled for free legal services. (vi) **S. 28,** The persons have the right to complain in the event of deficiencies in provisions.
3. **Advance Directive: S. 5-13,** A mentally ill person (who is not a minor) has the right to make an advance directive towards the way she/he wants to be treated for the requisite illness and who her/his nominated representative shall be. Advance directives have no place in the care of a capacitous individual or at times of emergency treatment. This directive has to be vetted by a medical practitioner.
4. **Prohibited Procedures:** (i) **S. 95,** Few procedures which seems barbarian and clearly against human rights shall not be performed on any person with mental illness (a) Electro-convulsive therapy without the use of muscle relaxants and anaesthesia (b) Electro-convulsive therapy for minors (c) Sterilization of men or women, when such sterilization is intended as a treatment for mental illness (d) Chained in any manner or form whatsoever. (ii) **S. 96,** No psychosurgery shall be performed until (a) The informed consent of the patient on whom surgery is being performed (b) Approval from the concerned board to perform the surgery. (iii) **S. 97,** (a) No seclusion or solitary confinement (b) Physical restraint may be used, if it is the only means available to prevent imminent and immediate harm to person concerned or to other.
5. **Admission of Persons with Mental Illness:** The admission of the mental ill person to a health establishment can be independent or supported. (i) **S. 85-86, Independent admissions** are voluntarily requested by capacitous patients, with freedom (and responsibility) to make decisions and care plans. There is no limit to the time period for independent admissions. (ii) **S. 89-90, Supported admissions** (replacing involuntary admission of mental health Act 1985), can take place with minimal or no agreement from the patient. The maximum duration for an initial supported admission is 30 days. It can be renewed further upto maximum 180 days.
6. **Decriminalisation of Attempt to Suicide: S. 115(1),** The Act decriminalized suicide attempt which was earlier punishable under section 309 I.P.C. A person who attempts suicide shall be presumed to be suffering from mental illness at that time and the government hall have a duty to provide care, treatment and rehabilitation of the person so that risk of recurrence suicide attempt does not occur.
7. **Mental Health Establishments:** (i) **S. 33, S. 45,** The government has to set up the **Central Mental Health Authority** at national level and **State Mental Health Authority** in every state. (ii) **S. 44,** All mental health practitioners (clinical psychologists, mental health nurses, and psychiatric social workers) and every mental health institute will have to be registered with this authority. These bodies will (a) Register, supervise and maintain a register of all mental health establishments (b) Develop quality and service provision norms for such establishments (c) Maintain a register of mental health professionals (d) Train law enforcement officials and mental health professionals on the provisions of the Act (e) Receive complaints about deficiencies in provision of services (f) Advise the government on matters relating to mental health.
8. **Responsibility of Certain Other Agencies:** (i) **S. 101,** A police officer in charge of a police station shall report to the Magistrate if he has reason to believe that a mentally ill person is being ill-treated or neglected. (ii) **S. 100,** There is a duty on the police officer in the charge of a police station to take under protection any wandering person; such person will be subject to examination by a medical officer and based on such examination will be either admitted to a mental health establishment or be taken to her residence or to an establishment for homeless persons.
9. **Offence and Penalties: S. 108,** Any persons violating the provisions under this Act will be punished with imprisonment upto 6 months or Rs. 10,000 one or both. Repeat offenders can face upto 2 years in jail or a fine of Rs. 50,000–5 lakh or both.

CRIMINAL RESPONSIBILITIES OF INSANE

Responsibility means liability of the person for his acts or omissions and also the liability to punishment for any illegal action. The law presumes that every person is mentally sound unless it is proved to the contrary.

S. 338 and 339 Cr.P.C. relates to provisions of accused persons of unsound mind including fitness to stand trial and subsequent procedures.

S. 328 Cr.P.C. provides for procedure in case of accused being lunatic: According to this when a magistrate holding an inquiry against person of unsound mind and incapable of making his defence, such persons will be examined by civil surgeon/ medical officer and after examination of such surgeon/officer as witness will reduce the examination to writing. If the person is of unsound mind, further proceeding in the case shall be postponed.

S. 329 Cr.P.C. provides for procedure in case of person of unsound mind before court: The court shall postpone further proceeding if at the trial of the person he is of unsound mind as proved by the medical and other evidence. **S. 338 Cr.P.C.** provides for procedure where lunatic detained declare fit to be released. **S. 339 Cr.P.C.** provides for delivery of lunatic in care of relative or friend.

The plea of insanity is taken: (i) In **bar of trial** when the accused is insane and cannot plead. (ii) In **bar of conviction** of the accused who was insane when the crime was committed. (iii) In bar of **infliction of capital punishment** when a condemned prisoner is insane. If insanity is established, the accused person is found "not guilty" and is kept in an asylum. The law presumes that every person is sane and responsible for his action, the proof that it is not so has to be produced by the person who sets up a defence. The law also presumes that for every criminal act there must be a Mensrea (Mens = mind, rea = criminal) that is criminal intent of mind.

Examination of Mentally Ill Person: The doctor examines the person and gives opinion as to whether the person is sane or insane. The doctor conducts the examination when insanity is taken as a defence in homicidal cases. Important points may be taken into consideration during the examination such as: (i) ***Family history:*** Of the disease, CNS disorders, chorea, epilepsy etc. is to be recorded. (ii) ***Personal history:*** History of intake of drugs or alcohol should be noted. In addition, sexual history and history of occupation and habits should be recorded. Whether any psychogenic factors like emotional conflict, repression and anxiety states are present, should also be recorded. (iii) ***Physical examination:*** Way of dressing, walking, cleanliness should be recorded. Vitals such as pulse, BP (raised in insane), condition of tongue (furred and coated) and skin (is dry and wrinkled) should be recorded. (iv) ***Mental condition:*** The general appearance has to be noted. Whether the person appears dirty, improperly dressed or naked. His behaviour, cooperation, abnormal conduct, memory, power of recovery and judgment should be noted. Sleep disturbances, walking and gait, attitude and posture, altered sexual behaviour incoherent speech etc. should be detailed. (v) ***Handwriting analysis:*** Misspellings and omission of letters shows mental confusion. (vi) Following features should be taken into account when an act is the result of insanity: (a) History whether melancholic, schizophrenic etc. (b) Absence of motive (c) Absence of secrecy (d) Multiple murders (e) Want of prearrangement (f) Want of accomplices.

The differences between true and feigned insanity are given in Table 34.2.

Table 34.2: Differences between real insanity and feigned insanity

Features	Real insanity	Feigned insanity
Onset	Gradual	Sudden
Motive	Nil	Presence of crime
Predisposing factors	Present	Absent
Signs and symptoms	Uniform	Present only when being observed and conscious
Facial expression	Peculiar vacant look	No peculiarity, frequently changing
Insomnia	Present	Absent
Exertion	Can stand exertion	Cannot stand exertion and fatigue
Habits	Dirty	Not so
Skin and lips	Dry	Not dry, normal
Frequent examination	Does not mind	Resists for fear of detection

McNaughten's Rule (Legal Test or Right or Wrong Test)

English courts dealing with responsibilities of mentally ill persons in criminal cases follow McNaughten's rule laid down in 1843. Daniel McNaughton a 29-year-old Scotsman and a paranoid schizophrenic believed that the Prime Minister of England Robert Peel was conspiring against him. He believed that the spies sent by the catholic priests with the support of the Tories Prime Minister were constantly following him, harassing him and hatching a conspiracy against him. He decided to kill the Prime Minister of England and made elaborate preparations for executing his plan. He heard voices accusing him of crimes which he claimed he never committed. But he shot Edward Drummond the private secretary to Prime Minister, by mistake. McNaghtan was acquitted as a result of medical evidence. Public reaction to this was most unfavourable. The debate took place in the House of Lords, and a number of questions were put to a bench of 14 judges but it was established that he was insane and acquitted. He was later sent to Bethlem Mental Hospital for the rest of his life.

The essence of McNaughtan's rule is to establish the defence on the ground of insanity. It must be clearly proved that "at the time of committing the act, the accused was labouring under such a defect of reason from disease of mind that he did not know the nature and quality of the act he was doing or he did not know that what he was doing was wrong".

In India the same law has been incorporated in **section 84 I.P.C.** which reads as: "Nothing is an offence which is done by a person, who at the time of doing it by reason of unsoundness of mind is incapable of knowing the nature of the act or that he is doing what is either wrong or contrary to the law".

Comments: It must be clearly proved that: (i) Offence is directly related to the insanity. (ii) Offence could not have occurred if there was no mental abnormality. (iii) Insanity subsequent to the act is not a defence.

Now, the terms 'defects of reason' and 'wrong' needs explanation.

Defect of reason: It must be clearly established that the reasoning powers of the accused were not functioning normally due to defect in intellectual and cognitive faculties. The nature and quality of act should be judged from the physical characters of the act but not from the moral aspects.

Wrong: Wrong means that the act is punishable by law. It concerns with the defendant's ability to distinguish between right and wrong. If he had the capacity to know that his act was wrong he will be fully responsible even if he was mentally ill and unable to refrain himself from doing the act.

Examples: (i) When a man thinks that another man is going to kill him and he kills that man in self-defence then this act is not punishable by law. (ii) If a person thinks another man to be a wild animal and kills him as a result, no responsibility is held for this act. (iii) If the man thinks of himself as a state executioner and executes someone then he is not held responsible for the act. (iv) When a man thinks himself a king and that it is his perogative to execute others as a criminal, he is not held responsible when he executes someone. (v) If under insane delusion a man thinks that another person has inflicted serious injury to his character and kills that person, he is held responsible as an insane person cannot take revenge.

Defects: For deciding that a person is insane only intellectual factors (reason) are taken into consideration but the: (i) Emotional factors (ii) Delusional beliefs (iii) Ability of the individual to control the impulse (resistible impulse) are not considered.

Charles Freeman was the heroin pusher and the Court found him guilty. The defence was that Freeman might have known that what he was doing was wrong. However, neither he had the capacity nor the will to be responsible for his acts and thus the Court of appeal reversed the decision (Justice Irving Kannan).

Durham Rule 1954

Monte Durham a 23-year-old who had been in and out of prison and mental institutions since he was 17 years old. He was convicted for housebreaking in 1953, and his attorney appealed. Although the district court judge had ruled that Durham's attorneys had failed to prove that he didn't know the difference between right and wrong, the federal appellate judge chose to use the case to reform the McNaughtan rule.

Citing leading psychiatrists and jurists of the day, the appellate judge stated that the McNaghtan rule was based on "an entirely obsolete and misleading conception of the nature of insanity". He overturned Durham's conviction and established a new rule. The Durham rule states "that an accused is not criminally responsible if his unlawful act was the product of mental disease or mental defect".

The Durham rule was eventually rejected by the federal courts, because it casted too broad a net as alcoholics, compulsive gamblers, and drug addicts had successfully used the rule as defence to defeat a wide variety of crimes. It was abolished in 1972.

Advantages: The rule was broader than McNaughten's rule and was widely acknowledged by the psychiatrists.

Disadvantages: (i) Deciding whether the act was the product of mental disease or defect is very difficult, and almost impossible at times as no definitions were given for these terms in the court. (ii) It gave the psychiatric a blank cheque and hardly granted any opportunity to the Court to render a judgment, i.e., rendering an independent social and legal judgment.

The Federal Rule

In 1984, Congress passed, and President Ronald Reagan signed, the Comprehensive Crime Control Act. The federal insanity defence now requires the defendant to prove, by "clear and convincing evidence", that "at the time of the commission of the acts constituting the offence, the defendant, as a result of a severe mental disease or defect, was unable to appreciate the nature and quality or the wrongfulness of his acts". This is generally viewed as a return to the "knowing right from wrong" standard. The Act also contained the Insanity Defence Reform Act of 1984 which, sets out sentencing and other provisions for dealing with offenders who are or have been suffering from a mental disease or defect.

Curren's Rule 1961

An accused person is not criminally responsible if at the time of committing the act he did not have the capacity to regulate his conduct to the requirements of law, as a result of mental disease or defect.

Irresistible Impulse Test

An accused person is criminally not responsible even if he knows the nature and quality of his act and is aware that it is wrong, if he is incapable of restraining himself from committing the act; because of the controlling agency or capacity has been destroyed by the disease. It is never used as a sole test for insanity.

American Law Institute Test 1970 (ALI)

Criminal responsibility as defined in ALI's model penal code 1970: "A man is not responsible for criminal conduct if at the time of such criminal conduct, as a result of mental disease or defect he lacks substantial capacity either to appreciate the wrongfulness of his conduct to the requirements of law." However, repeated criminal conduct does not alone prove such abnormality. This accepts the theory of combined McNaughten and irresistible impulse test. It takes account of the impairment of volitional capacity and impairment of cognitions. (i) It is broader than both McNaughten and irresistible impulse test. (ii) It demands that impairment be complete. (iii) Instead of knowing the difference between 'right and wrong' the defendant is subject to the subtler requirement of appreciating it. (iv) Instead of proving the act like "product of disease it has to be only shown that disease resulted in a loss of substantial capacity to obey the law.

Doctrine of Partial Responsibility

There are certain types of mental diseases like psychopathic personalities and paranoia in which criminal acts are committed. From the legal point of view, they are responsible for the act. At the same time from medical or psychiatric angle, such a person is of unsound mind. Thus, according to this doctrine, if these persons commit any crime, they should be considered partially responsible for the act. In England and in some states of USA it is not accepted as defence. However, in Illinois (USA) psychopaths may be declared insane and are treated in the hospital. In Scotland, it is taken as a defence and the charge of murder is reduced to manslaughter.

Homicide Act 1957 (England)

This Act brings the conception of diminished responsibility in a psychopath. The Mental Health Act 1959 defines the "psychopathic personality" as a persistent mental disorder or disability of mind which results in abnormally aggressive or seriously irresponsible conduct on the part of the patient requires or susceptible to treatment, for which he may be compulsorily detained in the hospital. The defence took the plea of diminished responsibility in the ground of sexual psychopath, who was unable to control the desire. The appeal was allowed and the charge for murder was converted into manslaughter that is diminished responsibility.

Somnambulism

Somnambulism means **walking during sleep**. A person leaves his bed and walks in the house or out of his house without any awareness of his actions. Nevertheless, he rarely injures himself. He is not asleep, but in a state of dissociated consciousness, a hallucinatory state unrelated to his immediate environment, similar to automatism. Such persons are well adjusted in life and are socially well behaved and not aggressive. Immediate stress and strain and mental conflicts etc. are present prior to walk. During this period, crimes are not willful or premeditated. Mental faculties are partially active and concentrated on a particular idea. Thus, a sleep walker may commit a crime and even solve a difficult problem but he has no recollection of the events. In some cases, the events of one fit are remembered in a subsequent fit. Such persons when commit a crime are not held criminally responsible for the act done during this period.

Somnolentia

Somnolentia is often called **sleep drunkenness.** It is a state that is midway between sleep and walking. If such a person is suddenly aroused from deep sleep, he may commit some crime due to confusion of mind as if he is having a dream at that time. He is not criminally responsible for the crimes committed during this period.

Drunkenness: The laws relating to drunkenness are laid down in section 85 and 86 I.P.C. Drunkenness caused by voluntary use of alcohol or some other intoxicating drugs is no excuse for the commission of a crime but insanity produced by drunkenness, voluntary or otherwise, absolves one of criminal responsibility, if it can stand the usual legal tests applied in other forms of insanity. In cases where the intention of a person committing an ingredient of the crime itself is present then simply being drunk is no defence. In King Emperor Vs Bishan Singh, the accused was charged with having murdered three persons by firing a gun in a state of intoxication. The court held that the accused was not in such an advanced state of intoxication as not to be fully aware of the act and held him responsible.

CIVIL RESPONSIBILITIES OF THE INSANE

Management of Property: On application by advocate general or a relative, court may direct to have an inquiry whether the person is suffering from unsoundness of mind and incapable of managing himself and his property. The court has to know: (i) Nature of his property (ii) Period of insanity (iii) Name of relatives or friends (iv) Any other relevant information. Then court fixes a date for medical examination and the medical officer/psychiatrist certifies that: (a) Person is insane but the insanity is of such a degree to render him incapable of managing the property and affairs (b) He is insane but capable of managing the property and affairs (c) In doubtful cases, opinion is given in favour of sanity.

If on inquiry by the court, the person is found incapable of managing his property/affairs but is not dangerous to him/other, the court appoints a manager to look after his property, granting him necessary power. The manager has to immaterial whether the vendor knew or not, but it is not responsible if the order is very much extravagant or if the vender has taken the advantages of his insanity. (i) Give the account of the whole property (ii) Submit the annual account within 3 months (iii) Removal/fine upto Rs. 500.

The court grants certain powers to the manager. He will not sell mortgages or gift any immovable property exceeding 5 years without prior permission of the court. The court may order to sell or raise money for the following purpose: (i) To pay lunatic's debts (ii) Discharge of encumbrance on his property (iii) Payment of debt or expenditure for the lunatics maintenance (iv) Provision for future maintenance and members who are dependent upon him (v) Payment of cost of judicial inquisition and other court expenditure.

If it is subsequently reported that the lunacy has ceased then second inquiry is held and necessary orders are passed to cease all proceedings in the lunacy.

Contracts: Under section 12 of Indian Contract Act, a contract is invalid if one of the parties was insane at the time of making the contract, or was unable to understand the nature of the contract. Lunatic is however responsible to pay for simple necessities he has purchased in accordance with his social position and status. A sane person, who occasionally becomes insane can make a contract when he is sane but not vice versa. When such person became insane after making the contract the Court orders for the fulfillment. The mental disorder of partner does not itself dissolve the partnership, unless steps bc taken for dissolution.

Marriage: Marriage is declared null and void if at the time of marriage, either party (i) Was incapable of giving consent to marriage owing to insanity; or (ii) Though either party was capable of giving valid consent but was suffering from such a kind or degree of mental disorder as to be unfit for marriage and procreation. (iii) Either party has been suffering from recurrent attacks of insanity or epilepsy. However, in cases when the insanity has developed subsequently it is not a ground for divorce. Mere weakness of mind or eccentricity are not sufficient to avoid marriage contract.

Evidence: According to **S. 118 IEA** a lunatic is not incompetent to testify, unless he is prevented by his lunacy from understanding the questions put to him and giving rational answers to them. It is for the Court to decide whether he is competent of giving evidence or not.

Consent: Section 90 I.P.C. provides that consent of an insane to certain acts is not valid:

1. *Consent for sex:* Although an insane woman had consented to sex it would amount to charge of rape, abetment of suicide or grievous hurt.
2. According to section 305 I.P.C., abetment of suicide of insane person, any delirious person, any idiot, any intoxicated person is punishable with death or life imprisonment or for a term not more than 10 years and also fine.

Testamentary Capacity: Testamentary capacity is the mental ability to made a valid will. (Testament = will; according to section 31 I.P.C., "will is any testamentary document"). For a valid will, the following conditions are to be fulfilled: (i) An understanding regarding nature of will. (ii) Knowledge of the property to be disposed of. (iii) Ability to recognize those who may have normal claims of the testator's bounty.

For a valid will following requirements should be fulfilled (i) There must be a written and properly signed and witnessed document. (ii) The testator must be more than 18 years of age, with sound disposing mind (a sound disposing mind is the one which has capacity of recollecting, judging and feeling the relations with connections and obligations of his family and blood relations). (iii) The will should not be made under any force, undue influence or dishonest representation of facts.

(i) A civil court may invalidate the will if the party was not of sound and disposing mind at the time of making the will. (ii) It is not a valid will if made under the influence of somebody. (iii) During lucid interval if he makes the 'will' it is valid. (iv) During fit of drunkenness it is valid if he understands the nature of will. (v) In extreme ages, the mental condition is seldom normal and the person is most of the time suspicious. They can make a valid will unless their mind has become so impaired that they are unable to understand its nature and consequences. (vi) Will is valid if the person commits suicide after making it and no other abnormalities are present. (vii) If a person is suffering from motor or sensory aphasia, agraphia or alexia or blind he can make a valid will if he knows what he does by it, if he can make clear by gestures that he wishes to make a will and also he is able to understand the meaning of questions put to him.

Holograph Will: It is a will which is written by the testator in his own handwriting.

At times doctor may be called upon to witness execution of will in case of a sick person. The doctor should examine in detail including the physical examination, mental examination with intelligence testing and laboratory investigations. To find out whether the testator is of sound and disposing mind following tests should be carried out. (i) Preliminary questions relating to his age, hobbies, number of relatives and degree of social contact with them. Besides this, his opinion on family, friends and partners etc. should be recorded. (ii) Questions pertaining to awareness of time, place and person should be asked. (iii) Nature, extent and value of his property and how he wants to distribute it should be asked. If any unjust or unusual distribution is noted, it should be asked whether it is intentional. (iv) If medical officer thinks that he is under the influence of somebody, he should be encouraged to tell the truth. (v) Testator's power of concentration is tested by asking simple arithmetic questions. (vi) On examination, the doctor should exclude any disease, pain, infirmity, strain and influence of drug or drink. The most common symptom of absence of legal capacity is impairment of memory. Dislike towards relatives without reason is not proof of want of capacity. (vii) It is to be determined whether at the time of making will the testator understood the business in which he was engaged and knew how he wanted to dispose his property.

LONG QUESTIONS

1. Discuss the civil and criminal responsibilities of insane.
2. Discuss the ways to restrain an insane person.

SHORT QUESTIONS

1. Delirium.
2. Delusion.
3. Illusion.
4. Hallucination.
5. Obsession.

6. Lucid interval.
7. Mental Health Care Act 2017.
8. True and feigned insanity.
9. McNaughtan's rule.
10. Impulse.

MULTIPLE CHOICE QUESTIONS

1. Lucid interval is seen in case of:

(a) Intracerebral haemorrhage
(b) Insanity
(c) Opium poisoning
(d) Chronic alcohol poisoning

2. McNaughten's rule is for:

(a) Civil responsibility of insane
(b) Testamentary capacity
(c) Criminal responsibility of insane
(d) Mental capacity of the witness

3. The capacity to make a will is determined by:

(a) McNaughten's rule
(b) Testamentary capacity
(c) Curren's rule
(d) Durham's rule

4. Kleptomania is a type of:

(a) Obsession (b) Delusion
(c) Illusion (d) Impulse

5. Delusion is a disorder of:

(a) Belief (b) Perception
(c) Interpretation (d) Memory

6. Obsession is a disorder of:

(a) Mood (b) Perception
(c) Intellect (d) Thought

7. Fluctuating level of consciousness is seen in:

(a) Hysteria (b) Delirium
(c) Dementia (d) Mania

8. Disturbances of consciousness, impaired orientation and blunting of critical faculty are the features of:

(a) Hallucinations (b) Delusion
(c) Hallucination (d) Delirium

9. Testamentary capacity refers to mental ability of a person to:

(a) Make a valid will (b) Testify in the court of law
(c) Sell the property (d) Be a legal guardian

10. In India, the present law on the defence of insanity is contained in section:

(a) 81 I.P.C. (b) 82 I.P.C.
(c) 83 I.P.C. (d) 84 I.P.C.

11. Abetment of suicide of insane person is related to:

(a) S. 304 I.P.C. (b) S. 305 I.P.C.
(c) S. 306 I.P.C. (d) S. 308 I.P.C.

12. As per Mental Health Care Act, 2017, all the following statements are true, *except:*

(a) All mentally ill persons have the right to access mental health care services
(b) The act decriminalizes suicide attempt
(c) There is time limit for independent admissions of a mentally ill person
(d) The mentally ill person cannot be chained in any manner or form whatsoever

ANSWER KEY ☞

1. (b)	2. (c)	3. (b)	4. (d)	5. (a)	6. (d)	7. (b)	8. (d)	9. (a)	10. (d)
11. (b)	12. (c)								

35 CHAPTER

Starvation Deaths

Starvation is a state that occurs from withholding the food or administration of unbalanced food. Starvation can be acute or chronic. The acute starvation occurs from the sudden and complete stoppage of food but chronic starvation occurs from the gradual intake of deficient food. The starvation deaths may be intentional or accidental and even homicidal. The usual causes are famine, neglect on the part of the guardians or parents, willful refusal to take food like in case of hunger strike, the passengers during shipwreck or landslides if they are stranded and when there is deficient supply of food.

Clinical Features

Acute Starvation

The sign and symptoms usually appear after 12-16 hours of stoppage of food. There is a hungry feeling followed by epigastric pain, which is relieved by pressure. The absorption of subcutaneous fat starts after 5-6 days resulting in general emaciation. Therefore, the eyes are sunken, pupils are mildly dilated, the cheeks sink and the bony prominences become more visible. The lips are dry and cracking is present, the tongue is coated and the person feels thirsty. There is salivation, voice becomes weak, the skin is dry becomes rough and pigmented at places. After a week, the muscles become weak. On physical examination the pulse becomes slow, the temperature is subnormal and constipation is the usual feature. The urine becomes scanty and evidences of acidosis are found. As time passes the body is reduced to a skeleton and the thoracic cage becomes more prominent. The loss of 40-45% of body weight is fatal. In these cases, the intellect remains clear. But in some cases, the person experiences delusions and at times hallucinations.

Chronic Starvation

The features of chronic starvation are: (i) The patient complains of hunger pains relieved by pressure, he becomes lethargic and disoriented. (ii) There is oliguria (iii) Evidence of pigmentation and the patient becomes anemic (iv) Subnormal temperature leading to hypothermia (v) Edema of the feet and limbs (vi) There is risk of infection like diarrhea, dysentery (vii) The death occurs due to exertion, cardiac failure and chronic absorption.

Fatal Period

When food is completely withdrawn then death occurs in 7-10 days. If the food alone is withdrawn death may prolong for 8-10 weeks or even more. If there is complete starvation without intake of both food and water then death occurs in 10-12 days. If water is continued then death may occur in 6-8 weeks or more. 80-90% body fat along with loss of 20-25% body weight should occur for death. However, the following factors may modify the fatal period:

1. The young and the old die earlier than the adults.
2. The females may tolerate starvation for a longer period than the males.
3. Fatty and healthy people tolerate better than the weak.
4. Persons with active physical exertion die earlier.

Cause of Death

Death occurs from exhaustion, circulatory failure due to brown atrophy of the heart or intercurrent infection.

Autopsy Findings

All organs and tissues show changes similar to premature senility. There is extreme emaciation and a reduction in the size and weight of all organs except brain. The brain become soft and pale. Muscles get atrophied and become dark in colour as the muscle fibers loose the striations due to granular degenerations. The fat of orbits and female breast is the last to go. Fat is absent from the subcutaneous tissues and almost completely lost from the mesenteries. Subepicardial fat is replaced by a gelatinous material. In acute starvation subcutaneous body fat is not lost completely. In children, the skeleton shows spinal curve, rickets and dental defects. In adults progressive demineralization and osteomalacia are seen. Stress fractures may be present and the skin is lusterless and looses its elasticity. The face becomes pale. Ascites may be present in some cases. Hairs are also dry and lusterless and the nails are dry and brittle. The lungs are pale and collapsed and exude very little blood on cutting. The stomach and intestine are atrophied and are stained with bile. The spleen is shrunken and the gallbladder is distended with bile. The kidneys show atrophy of the nephron. Blood volume is reduced, and there is severe anemia. The urinary bladder is also empty. In wasting diseases the gall-bladder is empty in contrast to death due to starvation.

Medicolegal Aspects

The diagnosis of starvation is done on the basis of history and other general findings. But at the same time one has to exclude the wasting diseases like malignant diseases: Addison's disease, diabetes mellitus, tuberculosis, even pernicious anemia and sometimes chronic diarrhea. Thus in the absence of above diseases diagnosis is usually made in favour of starvation.

Suicidal: Some persons have to voluntarily starve for the purpose of fulfillment of their grievances. At times the lunatics and hysterical women may refuse to take food. Rarely fasting is undertaken to attract the public attention. Right to life is guaranteed under Article 21 of the Constitution of India, which does not include the right to die. Thus, forcible feeding of these persons are lawful.

Homicidal: The victim is usually an infant or an aged person. At times the lunatics or mentally deranged persons also deprived of their food resulting in chronic starvation and finally death.

Accidental: Accidental starvation may occur during famine or being trapped in landslides or shipwreck. There is failure to provide food due to ignorance of the people. Certain diseases produces stricture of the esophagus resulting in intake of insufficient food.

LONG QUESTION

1. Define starvation. What are the postmortem findings in a death due to starvation?

MULTIPLE CHOICE QUESTIONS

1. In starvation death, the gallbladder is:

(a) Empty (b) Shrunken
(c) Full with bile (d) Filled with stones

2. All organs show atrophy in starvation deaths *except:*

(a) Liver (b) Mesentery
(c) Kidney (d) Brain

ANSWER KEY

1. (c)	2. (d)

Part 2: Forensic Toxicology

36 CHAPTER

General Toxicology

HISTORICAL PERSPECTIVES

The use of poisons dates back as far as spiritual and mythological beliefs have been recorded. Perhaps the first accounts deciphered are from the Sumerians of Mesopotamia, the modern day Iraq. Here there are associations of poisons with 'Gula' who was regarded as a spirit or 'the mistress of charms and spells'. This dates back to around 4500 BC and tabulated accounts of her have been found from about 1400 BC. Even in Greek mythology there is reference to poison, although no apparent citation to specific poisons used exists.

Records of Egyptian knowledge can be dated to about 300 BC. Menes, the earliest recorded Egyptian king studied the properties of poisonous plants. There is sufficient evidence from various papyri that the Egyptians were conversant with antimony, arsenic, copper, lead, opium and mandrake etc. Also, the Egyptians were probably the first to master distillation and discovered how to extract a powerful poison from peach kernels. A translation by Duteuil on a payrus in Louvre shows the earliest recording of a preparation of a substance for lethal purposes. Today this extract is known as prussic acid (cyanide). Also peach kernels contain 'cyanogenic glycosides' that release toxic substances in the presence of water. The ancient Greeks knew of arsenic in the form of realgar and orpiment, metals such as lead, mercury, copper, silver and gold and some of their properties. Amongst vegetable poisons, the Greeks chiefly employed Hemlock, for suicidal purposes and as State poison as a form of capital punishment. Socrates was found guilty of corrupting the youth of Athens with his philosophical teachings and in 402 BC was made to drink the State poison that is Hemlock.

Poisons and their effects were being studied predominantly to create a more virulent effect by the 14th and 15th centuries. Italian alchemists realized that combinations of known poisons could create a more potent effect. By the 17th century, poisoning had become such an art that there were schools in both Venice and Rome. During the late 18th century, an important case of poisoning in Britain was that of Sir Theodosius Boughton, whose body was exhumed and found to be impregnated with what appeared to be arsenic. Mathieu Orfila is considered to be the father of toxicology, having given the subject its first formal treatment in 1813 in his *Trait des poisons,* also called *Toxicologie generate.* The late 19th century is often associated with poisoning epidemic. To try to improve the way in which poisoners were caught and convicted the science of toxicology became increasingly important in the field of forensic medicine. However, as science progressed throughout the 19th century, so did poison detection tests for arsenic; Marsh test in 1836 and the Riensch test in 1841 and the science of toxicology grew in importance and reliability.

During the 20th century, the source, preparation and administration of poisons were stripped down; each process became cleaner, more attenuated and intellectually mastered. Due to toxicological studies, many formerly hazardous occupations are now controlled and present minimal risk. For example, exposure to substances such as lead, mercury and aniline is now strictly controlled. Pharmacological disasters such as the use of thalidomide as a sedative during pregnancy in the 1960s, led to the development of teratology and a greater understanding of potential *in utero* poisons. Arsenic remained a favourite for homicides in early part of the century. Cyanide too was popular around the middle of the century. The poison found a niche during the Second World War, and was used in liquid form as a suicidal tool for tortured agents of the resistance. Homicidally, cyanide enjoyed a resurgence of popularity in the latter half of the 20th century, with most of the poison secreted in food, drink and pharmaceutical products. Ricin, called the political poison of the 20th century became famous in the UK as a result of the **Umbrella assassination** of Georgi Markov in 1978, who died several days after he was stabbed by the point of the umbrella. At autopsy it was found that at the site of injury a device containing Ricin was implanted. Thallium, a true 20th century poison is found in pest control substances. It kills by disrupting the sodium potassium ATPase pump and thus causing cell depolarization.

In ancient India, women to get rid of their oppressive husbands used aconite, arsenic and opium. When we have a look at the history of ancient India, the literature describes various instances of poisoning. These include the description in Mahabharata of Bhim Sen being poisoned by Duryodhana.

In India, poisonous substances are used to commit suicide, or homicide. It can also be accidental more commonly in the children who may ingest the poison in lieu of the sweets. However, suicidal and homicidal poisoning is quite common in this country compared to the west.

These days the use of the chemicals for domestic and industrial purposes accounts for an increase in number of accidental poisonings. The use of quack remedies for a quick relief and the injudicious use of Ayurvedic and *desi* medicines also result in accidental poisoning very often. Poisoning is the fourth most common cause of accidents in children. Children less than 5 years of age and adolescent are prone to poisoning. Accidental ingestion are most common in children less than 5 years old. The pattern of misuse of substances is changing these days with increase in number of intake of pesticides and insecticides that is easily available. In India the most common agents for poisoning are the pesticides such as the organophosphates, carbamates and pyrethroids etc. Besides the pesticides, sedatives, corrosives and alcohol are also commonly used. Also plant toxins are rarely used in the rural India. In the North India, aluminium phosphide is most commonly used to commit suicide as it does not have any antidote and is highly fatal. The problem of illnesses and deaths is getting worse with the emergence of new drugs and chemicals. The properties, mechanism of action, lethal dose, detection and management of various poisonings will be discussed in the next few chapters.

Toxicology

Toxicology is the science dealing with the toxicity of substances. The word *toxicology* is derived from the Greek word *'toxon'* that refers to a bow used for shooting arrows. The word *'toxeuma'* meant an arrow, and *'toxicos'* is consigned to such a poison that in ancient times was often used on tips of arrows to produce a more lethal weapon. The substance inflicting toxic effect can be any drug, or any organic or chemical substance in the environment. Toxicology deals with the properties, actions, toxicity, lethal dose, symptoms, mechanisms, diagnosis, estimation and treatment of the poisonous substances.

Toxinology

Toxinology is the specialized area of toxicology that deals specifically with biological toxins, such as venoms or poisonous plants.

Forensic Toxicology

Forensic toxicology deals with medicolegal aspects of the harmful effects of the chemicals on the human beings. It combines the basics of toxicological principles with analytical chemistry.

Clinical Toxicology

It is a discipline within toxicology dealing with the bedside management of poisoned patients, including definitive toxicological diagnosis, assessment of immediate severity and long-term prognosis, and selection of treatments including antidotes.

Toxicokinetics: It is the study of absorption, distribution, metabolism and excretion (ADME) of toxicants/xenobiotics in relation to time. It the toxicological counterpart of pharmacokinetics.

Toxicodynetics: Baud *et al.* (2016) suggested this new discipline of learning within clinical toxicology which aims at describing the kinetics of clinically relevant toxic effects.

Toxicodymics: It is the study of dynamic interactions of a toxicant or their metabolites with a biological target and its biological effects. It is the toxicological counterpart of pharmacodynamics.

Poison

A poison is a solid, liquid or gaseous substance, which if introduced into the living body, or brought in contact with any part produces ill effects or death by its local, systemic or both types of action. This definition is unsatisfactory as a substance in particular dose causes beneficial effects to some whereas in the same dose it can cause the toxic effects to others. Drugs that are used for the treatment of diseases in higher doses will produce toxicity. As **Paracelsus,** the father of modern toxicology said, "All things are poison and nothing is without poison. It is the dose that determines the poison." Thus, every drug is potentially a poison when used erratically. **Paracelsus**, the 16th century toxicologist was the first person to explain the dose response relationship of toxic substances. In Indian law, there is no definition of 'poison' and there are various expressions for it. In biology, poisons are substances that cause injury, illness or death of organisms usually by a chemical reaction or other activity on the molecular scale. Some poisons are also toxins, usually referring to naturally produced substances that kill rapidly in small quantities such as bacterial proteins that cause botulism and tetanus. Animal toxins that are delivered subcutaneously (e.g., by sting or bite) are called **venom**. A poisonous organism is one that is harmful to consume but a venomous organism uses poison to defend itself while still alive. A single organism can be both venomous and poisonous. Deliberate application of poison has throughout the ages been used as a method of homicide, suicide and execution. As a method of execution, the poison can be administered as ingested, as the ancient Athenians did, breathed, such as carbon monoxide or hydrogen cyanide or taken intravenously. Many substances are regarded as poisons are toxic only indirectly such as methyl alcohol, which is not poisonous itself, but is chemically converted to toxic compound formaldehyde in the liver. Many drugs are made toxic in the liver, and the genetic variability of certain liver enzymes makes the toxicity of certain compounds differ between one individual and the next. Exposure to radioactive substances can produce radiation poisoning.

LD 50: It is the dose of a toxic substance that kills 50% of a test population (typically rats or other surrogates when the test concerns human toxicity).

Types of Poisoning

The poisoning can be acute, subacute or chronic.

Acute poisoning: In acute poisoning, whatever amount of poison is taken the toxicity is manifested immediately.

Chronic poisoning: Small amount of poison are repeatedly administered for a long period producing the toxic effects. The substances commonly causing chronic poisoning are metallic poisons, opium, antimony etc.

Subacute poisoning: In this the poisoning manifests between the acute and the chronic types of toxicity.

Mechanism of Action of Various Poisons

Some of the poisons on contact cause absorption and rapid death or impairment of function. The compounds acting on nervous system paralyze within seconds or less, include both biologically derived neurotoxins and so-called nerve gases, which may be synthesized for warfare or industry. Inhaled or ingested cyanide is used as method of execution on US. Gas chambers almost instantly starves the body of energy by poisoning mitochondria and synthesis of ATP. Intravenous injection of an unnaturally high concentration of potassium chloride, such as in the execution of prisoners in parts of the United States, quickly stops the heart by eliminating the cell potential necessary for muscle contraction. Such rapid reactions are often called **acute poisoning**. A poison may also act slowly known as **chronic poisoning** and is most common for poisons that accumulate such as lead, mercury, copper etc.

Factors Modifying the Actions of Poisons

There are a number of factors that modify the actions of poisons:

Quantity: The toxic effects of a poison vary with its quantity. Every drug is a poison when taken in a large quantity. But sometimes when a drug is ingested in a large quantity, it may induce vomiting and is rapidly eliminated leading to reduced toxicity. This occurs in alcohol and copper sulphate poisoning.

Route of administration: The severity and rapidity of action depends on the route of administration or intake of the poison. Inhaled poisons are rapidly fatal compared to the parenteral poisons whereas ingested poisons are less severe and act slowly compared to that taken subcutaneously or intramuscularly. The poisons are more effective when taken on an empty stomach.

Age and state of the body: Children, old, weak and diseased are more susceptible to the effect of the poison compared to the adults, healthy and stout persons.

Idiosyncrasy: Idiosyncrasy is allergic or anaphylactic response to a substance in which even a drug that is otherwise safe produces toxic effect. This effect can be produced by a large number of substances. A substance that is being used therapeutically may produce toxic effects. This can be due to anaphylaxis, idiosyncrasy or from the overdosage of the drug.

Tolerance: When a person uses some substance continuously, he is liable to tolerate larger than normal dose of that substance. This commonly occurs in an alcoholic who can tolerate larger than normal amount of morphine and related drugs.

Cumulative action: When a poison that is excreted may accumulate and produce toxicity when given in repeated doses for a long time.

Manner of Poisoning

Homicidal poisoning: It is the administration of poisonous substance by a person to kill another.

Suicidal poisoning: It is the intake of some poisonous substance by the individual himself for self-killing.

Accidental poisoning: It generally takes place due to the storage of poisonous and nonpoisonous substances at the same place. The injudicious use of the magic remedies and love-philters can also result in accidental poisoning.

The characteristics of ideal suicidal and homicidal poison are described under Table 36.1

Table 36.1: Differences between suicidal and homicidal poisoning

Characteristics	Suicidal	Homicidal
Availability	Easy and free	Not so
Cost	Low in cost	Not so
Colour, taste and odour	Tasteless or with pleasant taste	Colourless, tasteless and odourless
Solubility with food and drink	Present	Present
Signs and symptoms	Should not be there or very few	Resemble some natural disease
Onset of action	Quick onset	Slow onset

Contd.

Contd.

Antidote	Should not be available	Should not be available
Toxicity	Highly toxic	Highly toxic
Diagnosis from chemical tests	Difficult	Difficult
Death	Painless	Definite
Postmortem changes	May be produced	Nil
Common compounds used for the purpose	Aluminium phosphide, pesticides such as organophosphates and carbamates, barbiturates, potassium cyanide and copper sulphate and oxalic acid	Arsenic, antimony, aconite, thallium, organophosphorus compounds, strychnine, potassium cyanide

CLASSIFICATION OF POISONS

I. Corrosives

A. *Strong acids:* (i) Inorganic or mineral acids: (a) Sulphuric acid (b) Nitric acid (c) Hydrochloric acid (ii) *Organic acids*: (a) Carbolic acid (b) Oxalic acid (c) Acetic acid (d) Acetyl salicylic acid.

B. *Strong alkalis:* (i) Sodium hydroxide (ii) Potassium hydroxide (iii) Sodium carbonate (iv) Potassium carbonate (v) Ammonia.

C. *Acid like corrosives:* (i) Dimethyl sulphate (ii) Diethyl sulphate (iii) Ozone and atmospheric oxidants (iv) Sulphur dioxide.

D. *Metallic salts:* (i) Zinc chloride (ii) Potassium chloride (iii) Ferric chloride.

E. Phosphates such as polyphosphates.

II. Irritants

A. *Inorganic:* (i) Metallic: Arsenic, lead, mercury, copper, zinc, thallium etc. (ii) Non-metallic: Phosphorus, chlorine, bromine, iodine.

B. *Organic:* (i) Vegetable poisons: *Ricinus communis, croton tiglium, madar, semicarpus anacardium, calotropis,* capsicum, aloes, Abrus precatorius (ii) *Animal*: Cantharides, snake venom, insects, scorpion, spiders etc.

C. *Mechanical:* Powdered glass, diamond dust, chopped hair etc.

III. Neurotoxic

A. *Cerebral:* (i) *Somniferous:* Opium, barbiturates (ii) *Inebriant:* Alcohol, Ether and chloroform (iii) *Deliriant:* Datura, Belladonna, Cannabis, Hyoscyamus, Cocaine.

B. *Spinal:* Nux vomica and gelsemium.

C. *Peripheral:* Curare and Conium.

IV. Cardiotoxic

Aconite, quinine, digitalis, oleander, nicotine and hydrocyanic acid.

V. Asphyxiants

These are poisonous irrespirable gases such as carbon dioxide, carbon monoxide, hydrogen sulphide and coal gas. This category also includes the cyanides.

VI. Miscellaneous

A. *Food poisons* (Food borne botulism etc.).

B. *Agrochemicals:*

   i. Pesticides and insecticides (Organophosphates, Carbamates and Organochlorine compounds).

   ii. Bipyridal herbicides (Paraquats and diquat).

   iii. Chlorophenoxy herbicides (Bromoxynil, Ioxynil).

   iv. Rodenticides (Zinc phosphide, Strychnine sulphate, Sodium monofluoroacetate, Floroacetamide).

   v. Fumigants (Aluminium phosphide, Ethylene dibromide).

C. *Domestic and commercial poisons:*

   i. Petroleum distillates (Kerosene, Petrol mineral oil).

   ii. Disinfectants, detergents and cleansing agents.

D. *Drugs of abuse:* Alcohol, tobacco, cannabis, cocaine and opium derivatives, sedatives and hypnotics.

E. Chemical and biological warfare agents.

Common Household Poisons and Their Treatment

The common household poisons along with the symptoms and signs of their poisoning (Table 36.2).

DUTIES OF MEDICAL PRACTITIONER IN A CASE OF POISONING

The duties of medical practitioner are both legal and professional. Professional duties have priority over legal duties. **Pt. Parmanand Katara, Petitioner vs. Union of India and Ors., Respondents AIR 1989 S.C. 2039** held that every injured citizens brought for medical treatment should instantaneously be given medical aid to preserve life and thereafter the procedural criminal law should be allowed to operate in order to avoid negligent death.

PROFESSIONAL DUTIES (TREATMENT IN POISONING CASES)

A. Stabilise the Patient

It is very important to stabilise the patient first of all and to treat the most imminent danger to life immediately.

B. Removal of the Poisoning Material from the System (Decontamination)

Table 36.2: Various household poisons

Preparation	Poisonous substance	Symptoms and signs	Management
Moth balls	Naphthalene	Nausea, vomiting, pain abdomen albuminuria and hematuria, pulmonary oedema and coma	Stomach wash, soda bicarbonate, I.V. fluids. oxygen and artificial respiration
Baby powder	Boric acid	Nausea, vomiting, diarrhoea, convulsions, respiratory depression	Stomach wash, oxygen and artificial respiration
Insecticide spray	DDT/organophosphorus compounds	Nausea, vomiting, tremors, convulsions, coma	Stomach wash, paraldehyde, oxygen and artificial respiration
Chalk	Arsenic, copper and lead in coloured chalks	Nausea, vomiting, pain abdomen, symptoms of metallic poisoning	Stomach wash and treatment of metallic poisoning
Fireworks	Arsenic, mercury, lead and phosphorus	Burns	Burns to be treated
Cosmetics (nail enamel and thinners)	Potassium hydroxide, barium sulphate, acetone, methyl salicylates and denatured spirit	Nausea, vomiting, burning in stomach	Stomach wash
Baking powder neutralize	Tartaric acid	Nausea, vomiting, burning pain abdomen	Immediate soda bicarbonate to the acid
Baking soda	Sodium carbonate	Nausea, vomiting, abdominal distension	Vinegar
Crockery washing substance	Sodium and sodium polyphosphates	Variable symptoms depending on the substance	Symptomatic treatment
Match box and sticks	Silicates, antimony, hosphorus and potassium chlorate	Antimony and phosphorus poisoning	Symptomatic poisoning
Rat poison	Zinc phosphide	Nausea, hematuria	Stomach wash, Inj. vitamin K I.M.
Grain preservative	Aluminium phosphide	Bleeding	Oxygen and artificial respiration

(i) In cases of inhaled poisons, the individual should be shifted to fresh air and artificial ventilation should be started. (ii) In cases of injected poisons from bite or an injection, a ligature should be tied to prevent it from further reaching the circulation. The ligature is loosened for one minute after every ten minutes to prevent gangrene formation. (iii) In contact poisons affecting the skin, mucous membrane, any wound or when introduced in the uterus or vagina they should be irrigated with water and neutralized by application of suitable chemical.

The poisons are most commonly ingested orally. Depending on the time lapsed after ingestion; much of the poison lying unabsorbed in the stomach should be removed. In all ingested poisons the guidelines to treatment are: (i) Stomach should be emptied by gastric lavage or emesis but emetics are avoided in corrosive intake. (ii) Appropriate antidote should be given to neutralize the poisonous compound even despite gastric lavage and emesis as some poisons are secreted again in stomach after having been absorbed. (iii) Aid elimination of poison by the intestines and kidneys of what has been absorbed. (iv) Symptomatic treatment. (v) Egg whites are useful in most poisonings and tannin is antidotal to all alkaloids.

In ingested poisons, the methods of decontamination are: (i) Gastric lavage (ii) Emesis (iii) Catharsis (iv) Administration of activated charcoal (v) Whole bowel irrigation.

Stomach Wash (Gastric Lavage)

Gastric lavage is indicated in patients who present within three hours of ingestion of poison. The stomach wash can also be carried in the presence of gastric secretions, delayed gastric emptying or in case of ingestion of sustained release medications. Gastric lavage beyond 6-12 hours is recommended in ingestion of salicylates, tricylics, carbamazepine and barbiturates.

Gastric lavage tube: For gastric lavage, a soft rubber tube with a funnel at its one end known as **Ewald or Boas tube** is most commonly used (Figure 36.1A and B). In adults an ordinary, soft, non-collapsible tube with 36-40 French size having one cm diameter and 1½ mts length is used. In children with 22-28 French size (Ryle's tube) diameters should be used. The tube should have an attached glass funnel at one end and the other end should be rounded with lateral openings. There is a mark at a distance of 50 cm from its rounded end. A suction bulb is placed at the mid of the tube to pump out stomach contents.

Procedure for stomach wash: Before performing stomach wash, the patient should be lying in a left lateral position (Figure 36.2) or in a prone position with head hanging over the edge of the bed and the face is positioned downwards so the mouth is at a lower level than the larynx and chances of aspiration of fluid is eliminated.

The gastric lavage tube is gently passed into the stomach through the mouth by lubricating with glycerin or Vaseline jelly upto a distance of 50 cm in adults and 25 cm in children.

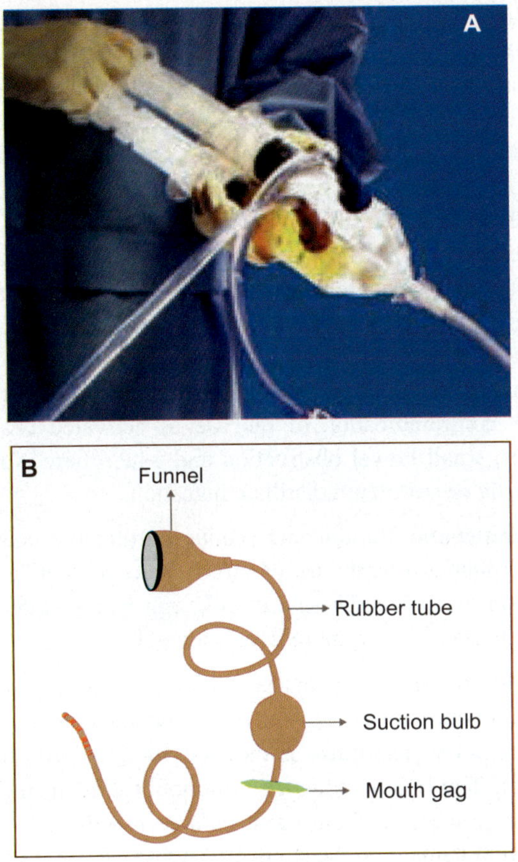

Figure 36.1: Ewald or Boas tube for gastric lavage

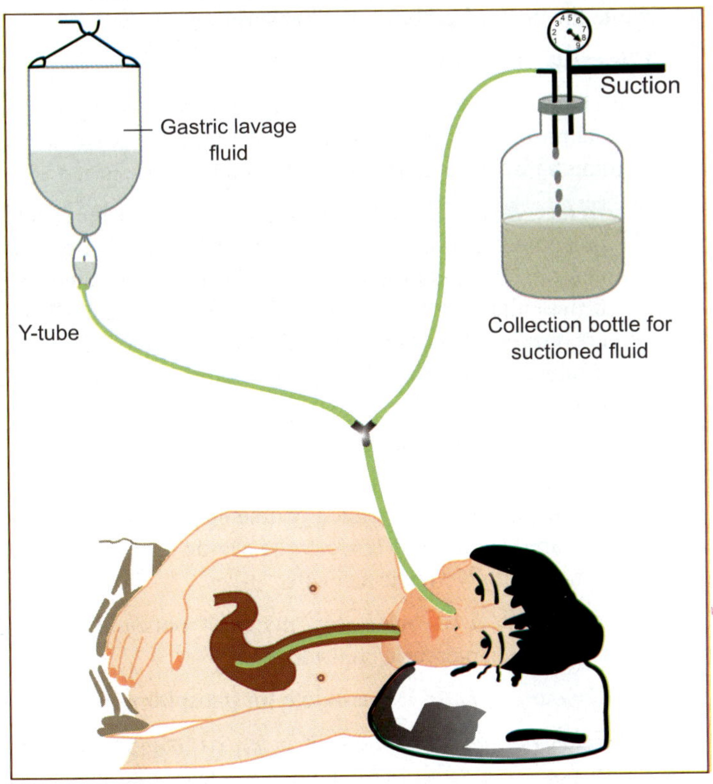

Figure 36.2: Position of patient for gastric lavage

The position of the tube in stomach can be checked by stethoscope or putting the upper end in a cup of water, if the lower end in the trachea, air bubbles will come out. For carrying out stomach wash, initially 250-300 ml of warm (35ºC) saline or plain water is passed through the funnel held high up. In children, instead of water 10-15 ml/kg body weight of warm saline is used as in them there are chances of inducing hyponatremia and water intoxication. The stomach contents can be siphoned by the use of suction bulb. The first sample of stomach wash should be preserved for chemical analysis. Then stomach wash is carried out with chemical agents specific to the poisons. In certain specific poisonings, instead of plain water or normal saline, other solutions can be used that are specific for particular poisons. These solutions are: (i) Potassium permanganate (1:5000 or 1:10,000) is used as gastric lavage fluid in various oxidizable poisons, e.g., alkaloids, salicylates (ii) Sodium bicarbonate (5%) (iii) Tannic acid (4%) (iv) Sodium thiosulfate (25%) can be used in cyanides (v) Calcium gluconate is used for oxalates (vi) 1:2 Castor oil and warm water solution is to be used for carbolic acid and phenolic group of poisons (vii) Desferrioxamine (2 gm in 1 liter of water) is used for iron poisoning.

In cases where potassium permanganate (a powerful oxidising agent) is used as gastric lavage fluid, the gastric lavage is continued till the colour of lavage fluid is colourless, odourless and no particulate matter is visible. At this time, a small quantity of fluid containing specific antidote or 1 gm/kg body weight of the suspension of activated charcoal and/or an ionic cathartic is left in the stomach.

Complications of gastric lavage: (i) Laryngeal spasm (ii) Aspiration pneumonitis (iii) Perforation of stomach or oesophagus (iv) Sinus bradycardia and ST elevation on ECG.

Contraindications of gastric lavage: The contraindication for stomach wash are absolute and relative.

Absolute contraindications: (i) Corrosive poisoning except carbolic acid as there is danger of perforation (ii) Convalescent poisons (iii) Comatose patient as there is risk of aspiration (iv) Volatile poisons due to the risk of inhalation (v) If the patient is hypothermic.

Relative contraindications: (i) If the patient is suffering from alimentary tract diseases like oesophageal varices (ii) Ingestion of alkali (iii) Advanced pregnancy (iv) Any haemorrhagic diathesis (v) Any history of recent surgical operation.

Emesis

The emesis should be avoided as there is danger of aspiration of stomach contents in an unconscious patient. The easiest way to induce vomiting is by tickling the fauces. Also vomiting can be produced by the use of emetics of which ipecac is the most effective whereas mustard powder and warm saline can give rise to complications. Also Apomorphine and zinc sulphate are no longer used. The emetics are: (i) Warm saline water comprising 2 tsf salt in 200 ml of water. (ii) Mustard powder 15 gms in 200 ml of water. (iii) Zinc sulphate 1-2 gms in 200 ml of water. (iv) Apomorphine 3-6 mg I.M. is the most potent and immediately acting emetic as it produces copious vomiting within 3-4 minutes. Apomorphine causes severe narcosis that is why it should not be used in comatose patients. If it is used, Naloxone hydrochloride, 5-10 mg I.M. should be administered that will counteract narcosis. (v) Ipecacuanha powder 1-2 gm or 30 ml (15 ml in children) of ipecac syrup causes vomiting with satisfactory results in a poisoned patient. It is derived from the root of *Cephalis ipecacuanha* and *C. acuminata*. The active principles are **cephalinc**, **emetine** and traces of **psychotropine** and it causes activation of peripheral sensory receptors in the GIT and also stimulates the chemoreceptor trigger zone and vomiting center in the medulla thus causing vomiting. The contraindications of emesis are:

Absolute contraindications: (i) Pregnancy (ii) Heart disease (iii) Haemorrhagic diathesis (iv) Cardiotoxic poison ingestion (v) In infants and old patients.

Relative contraindications: (i) During convulsions (ii) Ingestion of convalescent poison such as strychnine (iii) Ingestion of strong acids and alkalis due to the chances of perforation (iv) Ingestion of kerosene oil as there are chances of aspiration pneumonitis (v) Comatose or unconscious patients (vi) Foreign body ingestion (vii) Impaired gag reflex (viii) Poison that causes emesis (ix) Ingestion of petroleum distillates or drugs causing altered mental status.

Complications of emesis: (i) Features of cardiotoxicity such as bradycardia, atrial fibrillation and myocarditis (ii) Aspiration pneumonitis (iii) Oesophageal tears may be caused due to protracted vomiting.

C. Administration of Antidotes

An antidote is defined as a remedy to counteract or neutralize the effects of a poison. In various poisonings antidotes are used to counteract the pathophysiology produced by a toxin. According to the mode of action antidotes are classified as:

Mechanical or Physical Antidotes

The mechanical antidotes counteract the effect of poison mechanically preventing their absorption without inactivating the damaging action of the poisons. These are of the following types:

Adsorbent like activated charcoal: Activated charcoal is a fine, black, odourless and tasteless type of amorphous carbon prepared by destructive distillation of materials such as burning wood, coconut shell, bone, sucrose, or rice starch that have much higher surface area than charcoal followed by treatment with an activating agent such as steam, carbon dioxide etc. The large surface area of activated charcoal confers a great adsorptive capacity to this material. Each gram of activated charcoal works out to a surface area of 1000 m^2. Activated charcoal strongly adsorbs aromatic substances such as acetaminophen, salicylates, barbiturates and tricyclic anti-depressants thus reducing their absorption from the gastrointestinal tract. Most inorganic substances are poorly absorbed by activated charcoal. The dose is 1gm/kg body weight (50-100 gm in adults and 10-30 gm in children) after making a suspension in 4-8 times the water. 4-8 gms of activated charcoal acts mechanically by absorbing and also retains in its pores organic poisons and mineral poisons to a less degree. The side effects are vomiting, diarrhoea, constipation, pulmonary aspiration and intestinal obstruction. The contraindication of the use of activated charcoal are ileus, small bowel obstruction and when there is history of caustic or petroleum distillate ingestion.

Demulcents: Demulcents produce protective coating over the mucous membrane of stomach to protect it from the action of poison. These are milk, egg white, starch, milk of magnesia and aluminum hydroxide gel.

Bulky foods like bananas, boiled rice or potatoes allow smaller amount of poison to be available to the stomach mucosa for absorption as they are admixed with the poison itself. The bulky foods are commonly used in ingestion of glass powder as these particles are embedded in them and prevent damage to the stomach mucosa.

Diluents such as water, milk or other similar drinks that dilute the poison and delay their absorption.

Chemical Antidotes

The chemical antidotes disintegrate and inactivate poisons by undergoing chemical reactions along with the poisons and forming harmless or insoluble compounds. These are:

i. *Weak non-carbonate alkalis:* In corrosive acid poisonings, weak non-carbonate alkalis act as neutralizers. Strong alkalis are avoided as they can cause further damage to the stomach. Non-carbonate alkalis are preferred as carbonate alkalis react with acids to produce carbon dioxide gas that inflates the stomach and may get ruptured.

ii. *Weak vegetable acids:* In corrosive alkali poisoning, weak vegetable acids like citric acid, and acetic acid (vinegar, lemon juice) may be used. For arsenic poisoning, freshly prepared solution of ferric oxide can be used as it forms non-absorbable ferric arsenate.

iii. *Albumen:* It is used for mercury poisoning as it precipitates mercuric chloride.

iv. *Copper sulphate:* It is antidote for phosphorus.

v. *Potassium permanganate:* It is an oxidizing agent used in poisoning with oxidizable substances like cyanides, phosphorus, atropine and other alkaloids. A dilute

1:5,000 or 1:10,000 solution of potassium permanganate is used in any poisonings such as aluminium phosphide, opium derivatives, insecticides, nicotine, cyanides, hydrocyanic acid, atropine and strychnine etc.

vi. *Tincture iodine or Lugol's iodine:* In a solution of 15 drops in half a glass of water precipitates lead, mercury, silver, alkaloids and strychnine.

vii. *Tannic acid (4%) or strong tea or 1 tsf of tannic acid:* These are dissolved in water and used to precipitate metals like lead, mercury, nickel, zinc, copper, aluminium, cobalt, silver; strychnine, nicotine, cocaine etc.

Physiological Antidote

The physiological antidote acts on the tissues and various systems of the body and produces signs and symptoms opposite to the signs and symptoms produced by the poison. They are basically of use when some of the poison has already been absorbed into the circulation. They antagonize the effects produced by the poisonous substance. These are like atropine for organophosphorus compounds, physostigmine and neostigmine for dhatura and barbiturate for strychnine. The different types of antidotes for various poisons are listed below in Table 36.3.

Table 36.3: Poisons and antidotes

Poisons	Antidotes
Acetaminophen	N-acetylcysteine
Anticholinergics (Datura fastuosa)	Physostigmine
Carbon monoxide	Oxygen
Anticholinesterase (Organophosphorus compounds)	Atropine sulphate, Pralidoxime chloride (2-PAM)
Cyanide	Amyl nitrite, sodium nitrite and thiosulphate
Ethylene glycol	Ethanol
Heavy metal poisoning	Chelators, calcium disodium edentate (EDTA), dimercaprol (BAL), penicillamine and 2,3-dimer-captosuccinic acid (DMSA)
Iron	Desferroxamine
Methanol	Ethanol
Opioid	Naloxone hydrochloride
Arsenic compounds	Ferric oxide
Copper compounds	Potassium ferrocyanide

Universal antidote: When there is ingestion of an unknown poison or two or more poisons, universal antidote can be used. It comprises three antidotes: (i) **Activated powdered charcoal (2** parts by weight) (ii) **Magnesium oxide (1** part by weight) (iii) **Tannic acid (1** part by weight).

The powdered charcoal adsorbs alkaloid, magnesium oxide neutralizes acids, whereas tannic acid precipitates alkaloids glycosides and metals.15 gms of this powdered mixture should be added to half a glass of warm water before consumption. The activated charcoal alone is more effective as compared to universal antidote which contains equivalent amount of activated charcoal. This is due to interference of tannic acid and/or the magnesium oxide component with the adsorptive activity of activated charcoal. The use of universal antidote is **obsolete nowadays** but this can definitely as used as a first-aid measure at home before arrival at hospital.

Chelating Agents

Chelating agents inactivate a metallic ion with the formation of an inner ring structure in the molecule, when the metallic ion becomes the member of the ring. The chelating agents will form non-toxic stable soluble compounds with calcium and other heavy metals like arsenic, lead, mercury, copper, zinc, nickel, cobalt, manganese etc.

British Anti-Lewisite

B.A.L. (Dimercaptopropanol) was originally used as an antidote for Lewisite, a vesicant containing arsenic that was used as war gas. This compound is used in heavy metal poisoning especially arsenic, mercury, lead, antimony, gold and thallium and also to some extent against copper, bismuth etc.

Mechanism of Action

Heavy metal ions have a great affinity for sulphydryl (SH) radicals in the cells and tissue enzymes and they combine with them by displacing hydrogen, thereby depriving the body of certain tissue enzymes whose activity depend upon the SH groups. The thiol (SH) group of B.A.L. will combine with the heavy metals in the system and will dislodge them from their combination with the sulphydryl radicals in the tissue enzymes and thus sparing the tissue from its toxic effects. Dimercaprol forms a rather stable compound with the heavy metals and gets excreted out of the body mainly in urine without causing any damage to the liver, kidneys etc.

Dose: 3-4 mg/kg body weight that is to be administered deep intramuscularly within first 4 hours of poisoning. The ampoule of B.A.L. (100 mg/ml) contains 2 ml of 10% compound in Arachis or peanut oil with 20% benzyl benzoate solution. The injection must be given 4 hourly for first 2 days and then thrice daily for 10 days.

Contraindications: Administration of Dimercaprol is absolutely contraindicated in cadmium poisoning (forms a nephrotoxic compound with cadmium) and any preexisting liver disease. Also, it is relatively contraindicated in any kidney disease.

Side effects: The side effects of administration of Dimercaprol appear when it is administered in a dose more than 3.5 mg/kg body weight. These are: (i) Anorexia, nausea and vomiting (ii) Excessive salivation or lachrymation (iii) Generalized aches and pains (iv) Hyperthermia (v) Feeling of constriction of chest (vi) Burning of eyes and throat (vii) Fall of blood pressure.

Precaution: B.A.L. should not be used intravenously as death can result from fat embolism.

E.D.T.A.

E.D.T.A. (Ethylene diamine tetra-acetic acid) forms readily soluble, practically non-ionized and non-toxic compound with heavy metals. It is a useful antidote for those heavy metals that have an affinity for calcium.

Mechanism of Action

When lead, zinc, manganese, cadmium, iron and copper form compounds with edetate, calcium cannot displace them. Calcium disodium EDTA chelates extracellular lead in soft tissues as well as in bones. In practice, edetate is given in the form of calcium disodium versenate to prevent rapid removal of calcium from the body. In the presence of lead, this chelating agent readily exchanges calcium for lead and thus detoxification and excretion of lead is done. The chelating agent renders lead water soluble, nontoxic, non-ionized and non-metabolized to get excreted intact in the urine. Edetate does not get metabolized in the body like dimercaprol and is poorly absorbed by the gut. Calcium disodium versenate is the best known chelating agent against inorganic lead intoxication but not so effective in tetraethyl lead poisoning. It is used principally against lead intoxication but can also be used in copper, zinc and nickel poisoning. It is less effective in manganese, iron, cadmium and radioactive elements poisoning. It is superior to both BAL in the treatment of both arsenic and mercury.

Dose: 5 ml ampoule of 20% calcium edetate is dissolved in normal saline or 5% saline dextrose (250-500 ml) solution. It is administered by slow I.V. drip. The concentration should not exceed 3% and the drip should not take less than two hours to complete. The usual dosage is 50-70 mg/kg per day and in adults 1 gm can be given I.V. twice daily for five days. This should be repeated again after a gap of three days. E.D.T.A. should not be given orally as lead will get chelated in the G.I.T. and more of it will be absorbed.

Side effects: (i) Thrombophlebitis from administration of strong solution (ii) Lower-nephron nephrosis (iii) Hypersensitivity to the agent (iv) Fever, headache, generalized malaise and fatigability (v) Nausea, vertigo and vomiting (vi) Hypotension.

Contraindications: The only contraindication is raised intracranial pressure when fluids are to be restricted.

Penicillamine (Cuprimine)

Penicillamine is the product of hydrolysis of penicillin. It acts as a chelating agent because of possessing stable SH groups. It is advantageous to use this compound against poisoning due to lead, copper, mercury and zinc preparations, as it can be used orally and continuously for a long time without producing any major toxicity. It is also useful in treating Wilson's disease (hepatolenticular degeneration) resulting from disorders of copper metabolism and cystinuria.

Dose: It is given 0.5 gm orally half an hour before meals four times a day for a period of 8-10 days. Pyridoxine 25-50 mg/day can be given to counteract symptoms of pyridoxine deficiency.

Side effects: The side effects of penicillamine therapy are rare and are more pronounced when the patient is suffering from copper storage disease, cystinuria or scleroderma for a long period. These are: (i) Hypersensitivity reactions in the form of skin rashes and nephrotoxicity (ii) Optic neuritis resulting from pyridoxine deficiency (iii) Leucopenia, thrombocytopenia and agranulocytosis.

Desferrioxamine Mesylate or Deferoxamine

Desferrioxamine is a water soluble compound that has a great affinity for ferric ion. This acts as chelating agent against iron intoxication especially in case of acute poisoning through its role in accelerating removal of iron from the body in case of haemochromatosis cannot be challenged. It removes iron from ferritin, hemosiderin, a little from transferrin but not from haemoglobin and cytochromes.

Dose: It can be given orally, intramuscularly as well as intravenously:

- *Orally:* 8-10 gms dissolved in 80-100 ml of distilled water.
- *Intramuscularly:* 1 gm initially to be followed by 0.5 gms twice or thrice daily.
- *Intravenously:* 1-2 gm in 5% of 500 ml of dextrose saline solution; not more than 15 mg/kg body weight per hour or 80 mg/kg in 24 hours should be administered.

D. Elimination of Poison by Excretion

When more than 6-8 hours have elapsed after ingestion of the poison, the absorbed poison should be eliminated by excretory channels that are kidneys. In barbiturate and salicylates poisoning, this is the only treatment. Diuretics like chlorothiazide, mannitol or furosemide are commonly used drugs. Fluid balance is to be maintained by IV fluid infusion. Peritoneal dialysis and exchange transfusion is done in small children in poisonings due to barbiturates, salicylates and iron. Hemodialysis is employed for removing barbiturates, salicylates, bromides, boric acid and thiocyanates. The methods employed for the purpose are:

Catharsis

Cathartics reduce the transit time of the poisonous substance in the G.I.T. but their efficacy in reducing the mortality or morbidity is not established. The cathartics are:

Saline cathartics: These cathartics alter the physicochemical forces within the intestinal lumen leading to osmotic retention of fluid which activates motility reflexes and enhances expulsion. The dose of recommended cathartics is:

- *Magnesium citrate:* 4 ml/kg.
- *Magnesium sulphate:* 30 gm (250 mg/kg in children).
- *Sodium sulphate:* 30 gm (250 mg/kg in children) in copious amount of water.

The high dosage magnesium cathartics can result in hypermagnesemia.

Saccharide cathartics: Sorbitol (D-glucitol), 50 ml of 70% solution is the cathartic of choice in adults because of better efficacy than saline cathartics but in children there is risk of hypernatremia.

E. Symptomatic Treatment

The patient should be treated for the symptoms accompanied with good nursing care under constant supervision of the physician. Respiratory tract infection is commonly encountered more common in older patients who have been unconscious for hours and in whom gastric lavage was done. In such cases, routine antibiotic prophylaxis should be given. Dehydration, anuria, convulsions, circulatory collapse, hepatic and renal failure should be taken care of. Fluid balance to be maintained by I.V. fluid infusion and I.V. mannitol should be administered to combat renal failure. BP and pulse rate should be maintained continuously. The airways should be protected and artificial respiration with oxygen inhalation is to be given.

LEGAL DUTIES OF THE DOCTOR

(i) In all cases of suspected or confirmed poisonings the attending doctor should record all the findings and prepare a medicolegal case report and inform the nearest police station. (ii) If the homicidal poisoning is suspected by the doctor, the police officer should be informed **(S. 39 Cr.P.C.)**. If the doctor fails to report the matter to the police, he will be held culpable under **section 176 I.P.C**. (iii) Attending physician should collect, preserve and seal the evidence related to the case of poisoning such as the gastric lavage fluid, vomitus, faeces and urine etc. for onward transmission to the Forensic Science Laboratory for chemical analysis. If the doctor deliberately fails to do so he is liable to be punished under **section 201 I.P.C.** (iv) In all the cases of poisoning, it is the duty of the attending physician to divulge to the police whatever information he has. Withholding the information or providing wrong information makes the doctor liable to be punished under **section 202 and 193 I.P.C**. (v) In case of poisoned patient on the verge of dying it is the duty of the attending doctor to arrange for recording of dying declaration. Prior to declaration he should examine the patient and certify that he/she is mentally fit in regards to his consciousness and whether faculty of thought and judgment is clear *(compos mentis)* to give the declaration. Ideally the magistrate should record the declaration but, in his absence, the doctor can record it. (vi) In cases that are brought dead to the hospital or the patient has died during the course of treatment, the doctor should not issue death certificate but instead send the body for autopsy examination. (vii) In cases of food poisoning, the doctor should collect the contaminated food and sent it to the forensic science lab for chemical analysis. It is the duty of the doctor to report such cases to public health officials.

Diagnosis of Poisoning in the Living

(i) Symptoms appearing suddenly in a healthy person (ii) Symptoms appear uniformly and rapidly increase in severity (iii) When several persons are affected at the same time, e.g., food poisoning (iv) Detection of poison in the food.

In such cases the following material should be collected: (i) Stomach wash fluid (ii) Blood with sodium fluoride as preservative (iii) Urine with sodium fluoride as preservative (iv) Faeces.

Diagnosis of Poisoning in the Dead

1. **Postmortem appearances:** Clothes and external surface of the body should be looked for stains of poison, vomitus and faeces etc. The dark brownish or black stains of lips and cheeks occurs in sulphuric acid poisoning, yellowish brown stains appear in nitric acid poisoning and grayish white stains in carbolic acid poisoning.
2. **Colour of postmortem staining:** The colour of postmortem staining depends on the poison ingested; yellow or dark brownish coloured hypostasis develops in phosphorus, copper and cherry red discolouration occurs in CO poisoning.
3. **Odour from the body cavity:** Many poisons have a characteristic smell that is peculiar to that particular poison (Table 36.4).

Table 36.4: Poisons with their characteristic smell

Type of poison	Characteristic smell
Cyanides	Bitter almonds
Carbolic acid	Hospital disinfectant (soap like)
Alcohol	Acetone-apple like
Chloral hydrate and paraldehyde	Acrid-pear like
Aluminium phosphide, zinc phosphide	Fishy, phosphene like
Carbon monoxide	Coal gas
Organophosphates	Garlicky
Hydrogen sulphide and N-acetyl cysteine	Rotten eggs
Ethanol, Chloroform and Nitrites	Sweet or fruity

4. **Natural orifices:** The discharges from natural orifices are characteristic of some of the poisons.
5. Injection marks over the body should be noted in some injectable poisons.
6. Evidence of marks of violence may be seen in homicidal deaths. The bodies that are poisoned are not readily decomposed.

Postmortem Examination in a Case of Poisoning

Aims: (i) To identify the type of poison (ii) To find out time since death (iii) To find out cause of death (iv) To find out the manner of death whether suicide, accident or homicide (v) In infants to find out whether it is a live birth and its viability.

Diagnosis

The diagnosis in a case of poisoning should be made from postmortem appearances. The autopsy surgeon should read the inquest papers and the information relating to the poisoning should be gathered from the relatives about: (i) Quantity and quality of poison consumed (ii) Time of onset of symptoms after taking the poison (iii) Duration of illness (iv) Treatment given.

Very often the information is inadequate so it is quite a difficult task when the bodies are decomposed or has ingested corrosive or irritant poisons. For this a thorough examination is to be carried out along with the histopathological examination and chemical analysis of viscera.

External Examination

1. **Postmortem staining:** Normal colour of postmortem staining is coppery red or purple. It is:
   - Pink or cherry red in CO poisoning, hydrocyanic acid poisoning and in burns.
   - Purple or violet in asphyxial deaths.
   - Coffee brown in potassium chlorate poisoning.
   - Dark brown or yellow in phosphorus poisoning.
2. **Odour from the body:** No disinfectants should be used as they may mask the smell. On opening the body the characteristic smell of poisons like HCN, Carbolic acid, alcohol, ether, chloroform and opium can be felt.
3. **Examination of the natural orifices:** In the natural orifices the evidence of corrosive changes over the mouth, lips and tongue can be seen. They may be discoloured yellow in HCN poisoning.
4. **Injection marks:** This is particularly important in injectable poisons.
5. **Colour of the skin:** The skin may be discoloured yellow or jaundiced in phosphorus or acute copper poisoning.

Internal Findings

(i) All the organs must be examined and contents preserved for chemical analysis. (ii) Any peculiar smell should be noted. (iii) Mouth and throat should be examined for erosions or staining. (iv) Upper respiratory tract should be particularly examined in cases of poisoning with volatile irritants or there may be presence of inhaled poisonous matter. (v) Mucous membrane of the stomach and gastrointestinal tract should thoroughly be examined for the following signs of corrosive and irritant poisoning:

Colour of the mucous membrane of stomach: The normal mucous membrane of the stomach is pale and white. Irritant poisons cause patchy redness of the mucous membrane at the cardiac end and greater curvature of the stomach but rarely of the pyloric end. Due to the irritant action of the poison, there may be small haemorrhagic areas along with mucous secretion. Redness of the mucosa of the posterior wall may also be found after death. In a case, gastric redness was detected after nineteen months of arsenic poisoning and in another case twenty-one months after exhumation. The mucous membrane is velvety in appearance in arsenic poisoning and is covered with viscid secretion that is blood stained.

Redness of mucous membrane of stomach encountered in asphyxial deaths is due to generalized venous congestion. The hyperemia of stomach occurring in some of the diseased states is uniform in distribution. The colour of stomach walls may be discoloured due to the bile, fruit juice or food ingested that is uniform in distribution with no signs of inflammation. The mucous membrane may be red or hyperemic: (a) When the deceased had died during the process of digestion (b) Asphyxial deaths when there is generalized venous congestion (c) When the mucous membrane is exposed to oxygen (d) In diseased states like chronic gastritis or gastric ulcer, the redness is uniformly spread and the ridges are usually not involved (e) In deaths from poisoning, the redness is patchy; more marked at the cardiac end and greater curvature and also involves the mucosal ridges. The colour of stomach walls may be discoloured due to the bile, fruit juice or food ingested that is uniform in distribution with no signs of inflammation. The colour of the walls of the stomach in various poisonings are given in Table 36.5.

Table 36.5: Colour of stomach walls in various poisonings

Type of poisoning	Colour of stomach walls
Ferrous sulphate	Green
Amytal	Blue
Soneryl	Pink
Mercury	Slate
Oxalic acid	Black
Nitric acid	Yellow
Copper sulphate	Bluish green

Softening: Corrosive acids, alkalis and irritants cause softening of greater curvature and cardiac end of stomach as they damage the superficial epithelium. In diseased states such as peptic ulcer or malignancy this softening is uniform and limited to stomach whereas in putrefaction, the softening starts at the dependent parts and involves all the layers of stomach wall and inflammatory signs are absent. Carbolic acid causes hardening and shrinkage of mucous membrane.

Ulcers: Ulcers due to corrosives or irritant poisons are present on the greater curvature, have thin, friable margins and surrounded by signs of inflammation. The mucosa is soft and hyperaemic. The ulcers due to disease or malignancy are seen on the lesser curvature with their well-defined punched out margins that are thickened and indurated. Gastric ulcer involves the lesser curvature, has sharply defined, thickened and indurated edges and redness in the neighbourhood of the ulcer. But the redness in the irritant poisoning is diffuse and extends to duodenum and small intestine. In chronic ulcer due to disease, aperture is oval or rounded and the margins are punched out. There is no charring and chronic adhesions to other organs are present. Rarely both the ulcers will look similar. After death, autodigestion by gastric juices occurs that appears near cardiac end, is large, irregular with rough edges and no inflammation or charring is there.

Perforation: The perforation of stomach may be found in strong acids such as sulphuric acid poisoning. The stomach is usually black in colour with extensively damaged mucosa. The aperture is large with irregular edge and all the layers are lacerated through which acid escapes into the peritoneal cavity causing acute peritonitis. In a chronic gastric ulcer when perforation occurs, it looks either oval or round with a punched out appearance with indurated margin. In rare instances it may cause autolysis at the cardiac end of stomach without any peritonitis.

Stomach contents: The contents of the stomach should be thoroughly examined for presence of any identifiable food material and its consistency, traces of poison and also for any distinguishable odour.

All the organs of the body should be thoroughly examined for the signs of diseases to rule out diseased states leading to the death of the patient. Sometimes abortifacient drugs are introduced through the vaginal route for which the vagina and whole of the female genital tract should be examined.

Chemical Analysis in Poisoning

An important proof of poisoning is the detection of poisons in the faeces, blood and viscera. The finding of the poison in the food, medicines act as a corroborative but not a conclusive proof. The medical practitioner must preserve all the viscera and get it sealed in his presence for onward transmission to the police officer who will forward it to the Forensic science laboratory for chemical analysis.

Defence lawyer's argument: If the poison is present in the stomach, it might have been introduced after death. The argument is useless if the poison is found in the viscera and preserved in a clean container to avoid contamination. It is not necessary to lay stress on the amount of poison in the analysis, except that: (i) Poison might have been taken as a medicine (ii) Poison is used on a regular basis habitually (iii) It is a natural constituent of the body (iv) It is a normal constituent of food (v) It is produced during decomposition.

It is possible that a person may die from the effects of the poison but none is found after death. When the poison has not been detected, the judge should go by the symptoms, signs, postmortem report and oral evidence.

The viscera along with certain body fluids should be collected, preserved and sent to the Forensic Science laboratory for chemical analysis by the forensic pathologist. The presence of poisons should be demonstrated by standardized analytical methods. The preservative for the viscera is rectified spirit or saturated saline solution. The blood can be preserved in potassium oxalate or sodium fluoride and urine should also be preserved with sodium fluoride. The viscera that is preserved routinely should include the following (Table 36.6):

Table 36.6: Viscera preserved for chemical analysis

Viscera	Quantity	Preservative
Stomach with its contents	Whole of the stomach with entire contents	Saturated saline or rectified spirit
Small intestine with contents	Upto 30 cm with 100 gm of contents	–do–
Liver with gall-bladder	500 gm	–do–
Kidney	One half of each or whole	–do–
Spleen	Whole	–do–
Blood	10-20 ml	Potassium oxalate or sodium fluoride
Urine	30-50 ml	Sodium fluoride

About 10-20 ml of blood should be taken in a glass bottle from the femoral vein and should not be taken from the abdominal or pleural cavity, with potassium fluoride or sodium fluoride as preservative in suspected alcohol poisoning. About 30-50 ml of urine should be kept with sodium fluoride as preservative.

Most of the poisons are ingested, so stomach and intestines are preserved. As the poison passes through the liver, it is preserved. Kidneys being the organ of excretion are preserved and finally as poisonous substance are excreted in urine, it is also kept for analysis.

Methods of Preservation of Various Samples

Blood: After death the serous membrane of the stomach and intestine break down allowing the substance to migrate to the organs of the chest and abdomen as there is a false rise of the substance in the blood level. Ideally before autopsy about 50 ml of sterile blood should be collected from the peripheral (femoral, inguinal or subclavian) veins. After removal of the viscera again 10-15 ml of blood should be collected from these areas. No blood to be collected from the pleural and the peritoneal cavities. If the heart blood is clotted, the vena cava or the aorta should be punctured. If peripheral blood cannot be obtained samples from the right and left sides of the heart should be collected separately. In cases of drowning 10 ml of blood is removed from each side of the heart for separate sodium, chloride or magnesium determinations. In barbiturate and ethanol poisoning, toxicological examination of portal vein blood may be of interest. Any anticoagulant other than heparin may be used. Usually, the blood should be preserved by adding 10 mg of sodium or potassium fluoride and 3 mg of potassium oxalate.

CSF: It is usually collected by lumbar puncture or from the cisterna magna by inserting a long needle. This is to be done during internal examination. More than one blood free sample may be needed. Direct aspiration can be done from the lateral or third ventricle.

Vitreous: Vitreous humour can be used for determination of alcohol and for other toxicological studies, particularly when other body fluids are not readily available. It can be withdrawn using fine needles through the outer canthus of the eye. 1-2 ml can be taken from either eye. The tip of the needle should lie near the centre of the eyeball. Forceful aspiration must be avoided because it may detach retinal cells, which cloud the specimen and give spuriously high potassium values. The vitreous humour may be stored in a refrigerator at 4°C for upto 48 hours.

Bile: Bile is best removed by puncturing the gallbladder in situ.

Gastrointestinal tract: The stomach can be saved with its contents by placing ligatures around the lower end of esophagus and the upper end of duodenum. The organ is then opened to inspect the contents of the stomach and its walls. In poisoning with yellow phosphorus, the stomach has to be opened under nitrogen just before analysis. Several portions of the small and large intestine each about 60 cm long are tied by double ligatures. The separate portions are labelled and submitted unopened for toxicological examination.

Hair: Hair should be pulled from the scalp, not cut. A large sample of about 10 gm should be collected and tied in locks with cotton. This should be done in a manner that identifies the ends where the hair roots are.

Skin: In suspected injections of poisonous substances the skin around the suspected site is excised at a radius of 2-4 cm from the injection site. If a poisonous substance might have been taken up by absorption, the skin is excised in an area where the absorption is thought to have occurred, and a distant preferably a contralateral area. Control skin sample should be preserved from the opposite side.

Bone: In cases of subacute or chronic poisoning by heavy metals mostly arsenic, antimony and thallium about 10 cm of the shaft of femur is to be preserved for analysis.

Urine: Urine is best collected in a sterile needle and a syringe through the dome of the diaphragm. The sterilized wall is stretched between two hemostats and then punctured. Urine is of utmost importance for toxicological analysis. Every effort must be made to collect it. The urethra should be tied or clamped and the dome of bladder widely incised between hemostats, which then are used to hold the bladder open. Urine should be preserved in 50 ml bottles.

Uterus: In deaths due to criminal abortion, uterus and appendages along with upper part of vagina are preserved with any chemicals or poisonous substance. Foreign bodies found in the genital tract to be preserved separately.

Heart: Heart should be preserved in cases of poisoning by cardiac poisons like strychnine and digitalis.

Brain: Brain has to be preserved in poisoning from alkaloids, organophosphorus compounds and volatile organic poisons. Spinal cord should be preserved in strychnine poisoning.

Poisonings where special viscera is to be preserved

Special viscera	Poisonings
Strychnine	Heart, Brain, Spinal cord
Organophosphorus	Brain
Gaseous, Alcohol and Chloroform	Lungs
Skin with subcutaneous tissue	Injectable poisons, drugs of abuse and snakebite*

*In all these types of poisonings, control site should also be preserved.

Points to be followed while preserving the viscera: (i) Viscera are preserved in saturated solution of common salt or rectified spirit. Rectified spirit is not to be used in poisonings due to alcohol, acetic acid, phenol, phosphorus and paraldehyde where saturated solution of sodium chloride is used. Formaldehyde should not be used as a preservative because it makes extraction of poisons difficult. (ii) Stomach and intestine are kept together in a glass jar and in another jar pieces of liver, kidney and spleen are preserved. Blood and urine are preserved separately in two glass bottles. Rubber inserts should not be used as it extracts some poisons like chloroform and phenols. (iii) Quantity of preservative should be equal to the bulk of the organ. (iv) Only two-thirds of the bottle should be filled allowing space for decomposition gases. (v) Bottles should be properly sealed. (vi) Bottles should be well labelled bearing the name of the deceased, Postmortem No., date and name of the police station. (vii) Sample of the preservative used that is 100 ml of spirit or 25 gm of sodium chloride should be sent to the lab to rule out contamination. (viii) A copy of the postmortem report should also be sent along with the viscera. (ix) A sample of seal should be sent along with the viscera. (x) Viscera along with the sample of preservative and sample of seal should be handed over to the police for onward transmission to the laboratory. (xi) Polyethylene bags or containers can be used but the volatile poisons may diffuse through it. In cases where lungs have to be preserved for analysis like that of volatile poisons, nylon bags should be used and the blood should be kept in plastic capped tubes.

Failure to Detect Poison on Chemical Analysis of the Viscera

Failure to detect poison occurs many a times in forensic practice in an alleged case of poisoning, in spite of circumstantial evidences being pointing towards the poisoning. The poisonous substance may not be detectable due to some of the following reasons: (i) Some individuals may be unusually susceptible to the deleterious effect of the poisonous substance. (ii) Whole of the poison has already been eliminated from the stomach and intestines by vomiting or other means such as purging and if absorption had occurred it got detoxified, neutralized, conjugated and finally eliminated by the kidneys etc. (iii) Chemical analysis may be faulty due to submission of wrong, insufficient or decomposed material for analysis whereas sometimes faulty techniques are occasionally used in the laboratory or inexperienced technical staff result in improper evaluation of the results. (iv) Quantity of poison is below detection limits. (v) Some of the alkaloids, toxins of *Clostridium* and *Salmonella* and chemicals like LSD-25 cannot be detected by chemical analysis. (vi) There may be uneven distribution of absorbed poison in various organs depending on the type of poison and mode of administration, e.g., when a poison is injected intravenously the blood levels are higher than liver levels.

Bedside Tests for Detection of Poisons/Drugs

Bedside tests for detection of poison or drugs are important 'point of care tests' in emergency setting. These tests can be done anywhere outside the centralized laboratory and the results of these tests are obtained quickly. The test can be possible by using samples from urine, serum/blood, breath, sweat, or saliva. These tests are qualitative test used for screening of poisons/drugs (Table 36.7) and have limitations in sensitivity and specificity. Further testing may be needed to determine exact amount of a particular poison/drug (Quantitative test) in the sample and to confirm the results.

Table 36.7: Bedside test to detect some common poisons/drugs

Bedside test/Spot test	Poisons/Drugs
Ammonium molybdate test, Potassium hydroxide test	Organophosphorus
Dichromate test, Iodoform test, Ester test	Ethyl alcohol
Dille-Koppayani test	Barbiturate
Feigl's test, Benzoinoxime test	Cupper
Fujiwara test	Chloroform, Chloral hydrate
Fuchsine test	Sulphites
Gerrard's test	Hyocine, atropine
Gunzberg's test	HCL
Gutzeit test	Arsenic
Kappanyi-Zwikker test	Barbiturate
Keller's test	Oleander
Legal's test, Idoform test	Acetone
Prussian blue test	Cyanide
Marquis test	Opiates, Amphetamines, Aspirin, Ergot, Thebaine, Abrus precatorious
Marsh's test	Arsenic
Mayer's test	Nicotine
Mandelin's test	Strychnine
Mayers's test, Dragendorff's test	Nicotine
McNally's test	Salicylates
Nitric acid test	Argemone mexicana
Vitalis's test	Atropine, Brucine, Datura fastuosa
O-Cresol test, ammonium molybdate test	Parathion
Palets reaction test, Alverex reaction test	Aconite
Reinsch's test	Mercury, Arsenic, Antimony, Bismuth, Selenium, Thallium
Schiff's reagent test	Formaldehyde, Acetaldehyde
Scott test	Cocaine

Analytical Techniques in Medical Toxicology

The analytical techniques for the detection of poisons, drugs and various chemicals are more dependable and satisfactory than the usual chemical and biochemical methods. The common analytical techniques employed in toxicological analysis are:

1. ***Spectrophotometric:*** It is based on the absorbance or transmission of light from a colour reaction at a specific wavelength. It includes the following techniques: (i) Calorimetric (ii) Fluorimetric (iii) Automation.
2. ***Chromatographic:*** It is based on the migration of compound on adsorbent (solid phase) by a mobile phase. It includes: (i) Thin layer chromatography (TLC) (ii) Gas liquid chromatography (GLC) (iii) High pressure liquid chromatography (HPLC) (iv) Gas liquid mass spectrometry (GL-MS).
3. ***Competitive binding assay or immunoreactive assay:*** (i) Radioimmunoassay (RIA) (ii) Enzyme Immunoassay (EIA) (iii) Fluorescent Polarization Immunoassay (FPIA) (iv) Immunotubidimetric assay.

Samples to be collected for various analytical procedures: (i) Blood for recently used drugs (ii) Serum or plasma sample for protein bound drugs (iii) 24 hours urine sample for free drug analysis (iv) Random urine sample for drugs with a longer half life.

Important points to be remembered: (i) Sensitivity and specificity of the technique determines its utility. (ii) Target of drug testing is either the parent drug or its metabolite. (iii) Urine and blood are analyzed usually but urine contains 1000 times more drug than the blood so it is the preferred sample. (iv) Blood is useful to identify recently used drugs. (v) Cut off value is also critical in determining if a drug test is to be reported as positive or negative. (vi) False negatives are far more common than false positives.

Comprehensive drug testing is very important mainly for psychiatrists in arriving at precise evaluation and appropriate treatment plan for a drug addict. Diagnosis of polydrug abuse is not possible of which the psychiatrists and forensic toxicologists are now more aware of and are therefore interested in laboratory testing of body fluids for various drugs of abuse.

Atomic Absorption Spectroscopy (AAS): It is a spectro-analytical techniques used for quantitation of metals in different variety of samples. It works on the principle that the atoms of different elements absorb characteristic wavelength of light. The sample is first atomised (i.e., converted into ground state free atoms in the vapor state) and a beam of electromagnetic radiation emitted from excited lead atoms passed through the vaporised sample. The analyte concentration is determined from the amount of absorption. It is used for determination of gun powder residues analysis in firearm cases and one of the most popular methods for the determination of heavy metals in forensic as well as clinical samples.

Thin layer chromatography (TLC): Thin layer chromatography is used as a broad spectrum screen for detection of drugs of abuse. It is most inexpensive technique and does not require any sophisticated instruments. The results of this technique are only qualitative and cannot be quantified. Its major drawback is that it has a low sensitivity (1000-2000 mg/ml) and low specificity. TLC relies on a reproducible migration pattern by the drug on a thin layer adsorbent such as silica gel coated glass plates. The characterization of a particular drug is achieved by colour reactions produced by spraying the plates with colour complexing reagents. The patient's sample is spotted along with other known drugs on a TLC plate which is put in a solvent chamber. The solvent is dried and sprayed with various complexing reagents. The coloured spots of various known drugs are compared with unknown patient's sample. The location of spot is identified by an:

$$\text{Rf number} = \frac{\text{Distance travelled by a drug}}{\text{Distance travelled by solvent from the origin, where sample was spotted}}$$

The spots in the TLC plates can be visualized by UV or fluorescent light. TLC method was designed to detect high dose of a drug, recent drug abuse and toxic levels of drugs. It is a good test for an emergency where drugs taken are not known and presence or absence of a drug is necessary to start the specific treatment. TLC results are not generally admissible as forensic evidence. In this technique, it must be understood that whether the sample is positive or negative depends upon the concentration of drug in a sample or the sensitivity of cutoff value of the assay. Often the cutoff value is set high to avoid false positives especially for legal purposes. False positive results are quite unusual by TLC but they can be confirmed with a more specific test. The low level of substances is not easily determined by this method.

Gas liquid chromatography (GLC): Gas liquid chromatography separates molecules by the use of a glass or metal tube that is packed with material of a particular polarity. The sample of drug is vaporized at the injection site and carried through the column by a steady flow of gas. The column terminates at detector that permits recording and quantification. The time from injection till a response is observed at the recorder or integrator is referred to as **Retention time (RT)**. Identical compounds travel through column at the same speed because their interaction with packing material is same. The drug of abuse in patient's sample (urine/ blood) is extracted and purified before it is injected on to the column. Retention time of patient's sample is compared with RT of known drugs of abuse, processed under similar conditions. If the two are identical, the sample is confirmed with that particular drug of abuse. GLC is significantly more specific and sensitive than TLC and some drugs are detected better with GLC.

High pressure liquid chromatography (HPLC): High pressure liquid chromatography is similar to GLC but it uses liquid rather than gas to propel the sample through the column in HPLC. Some drugs are better chromatographed on HPLC, e.g., tricyclic antidepressants and benzodiazepines. HPLC is more specific and sensitive than TLC.

Gas chromatography–Mass spectrometry (GC-MS): Gas chromatography-mass spectrometry analyzes a drug according to its fragmentation pattern. Weaker bonds of molecules are broken under stress to produce a fragmentation pattern. A perfect match with a fragmentation pattern in a computer library is considered an absolute confirmation of the drug and is referred to as 'fingerprinting' of molecules. GC-MS is 100-1000 times more sensitive, specific, more reliable and most definitive forensic quality procedure than the TLC system. Being expensive, it is impractical for screening but vital for confirmation of drug presence and identity which is specific for medicolegal cases. GC-MS is generally used for analysis of volatile and heat stabile compounds.

Liquid chromatography–Mass spectrometry (LCMS): LC-MS is a chemistry technique that combines the physical separation capabilities of liquid chromatography (or HPLC) with the mass analysis capabilities of mass spectrometry (MS). The individual components in a mixture are first separated followed by ionization and separation of the ions on the basis of their mass/charge ratio. The separated ions are then directed to a photo or electron multiplier tube detector, which identifies and quantifies each ion. The major advantages of this technology include sensitivity, specificity and precision as analysis is done at molecular level. This technique is suitable for analysis of non-volatile and heat labile compounds.

Other more sophisticated methods used in modern toxicology laboratories include: Inductively coupled plasma ionization (ICP) is another ionization method used for elemental analysis, inductively coupled plasma ionization MS (ICP-MS) usually used for metal detection, tandem mass spectrophotometry (MS/MS) and multi-stage/sequential mass spectrometry (MS^n) etc.

Radioimmunoassay and enzyme immunoassay (RIA and EIA): They operate on the principle of antigen antibody interactions. The drugs of interest are compelled to large molecules and then injected into rabbits or sheep to produce antibodies against the drug. The immunologic methods used for detection employ antibodies against specific drug and competing drug molecules that are tagged enzymatically or that possess radioactivity. Immunoassay reliability depends on how specific and sensitive the antibodies are to a given compound. This is important because cross reacting compounds can result in false positives or falsely elevated results. That is why competitive binding assays are deemed to have much lower specificity than chromatographic techniques. **Enzyme Multiplied Immunoassay Technique (EMIT)** is the most widely used EIA methodology. It utilizes the enzyme glucose-6 phosphate dehydrogenase (G_6-PDH) as the active tag. The assay is based on the catalytic reduction of NAD to NADH, which is measured spectrometrically at 340 nm. EMIT procedures are less sensitive and specific in cannabinoids than the RIA but EMIT is quite popular and commonly used because no extraction or centrifugation is required and system levels itself to easy automation. EIA screens yielding positives should always be confirmed by alternative methods GC-MS.

Prevention of Poisoning

The poisonings usually result due to lack of proper storage places in the house. Various accidental poisonings can be avoided when the following precautions are taken: (i) Medicines and chemicals should be stored out of reach and site of children and at a considerable height and preferably locked and separately from other household products. (ii) Medicines, chemicals and household products should not be transferred and be kept in their original, labelled containers. (iii) Medicines should be stored in child resistant packs and all the medicines and chemicals etc. should be properly labeled. (iv) Before consuming the medicine, the label with its directions for use should be properly read. (v) Empty containers of liquid medications, chemicals and household products should be rinsed with water before throwing. (vi) Always protect skin and eyes while spraying insecticides with maintenance of adequate ventilation.

POISON INFORMATION CENTRES

The incidence of poisoning has increased markedly during the last decade but has received attention of public professionals and authorities quite recently. Poison information centre is a specialized unit that provides information on poisoning to the community. The main functions of such a centre are: (i) Provision of toxicological information (ii) Advice on the management of poisoning cases (iii) Training to the professional and paraprofessionals on first-aid, management and prevention of poisoning (iv) It also provides toxicological laboratory services (v) In developing contingency plans for chemical disaster with other responsible bodies (vi) Centre responds to chemical disasters (vii) Centre carries out epidemiological and experimental studies to find out the toxic risks and mechanisms.

National Poison Information Centre, Delhi: In India, National poisons information centre was established in 1995 at Department of Pharmacology, All India Institute of Medical Sciences, New Delhi. The centre provides information on poisoning management. It holds teaching and training program on poisoning prevention and management. It also plays an important role in developing contingency plans for chemical disasters and conducts research related to antidotes, environmental and biological monitoring of the chemicals and toxicokinetics. The centre provides information on management and treatment protocols of various poisonings all over the country. The centre provides round the clock service all 365 days of the year. Besides this, the center has the backup of latest literature on poisoning. The Poison Information consultant after taking an exact history and the relevant details about the product consumed provides the precise and concise information on the product involved, likely signs and symptoms, pre-hospital treatment, supportive and symptomatic care, antidotal therapy including dosage and availability. Also, the entire information is recorded in a specific performa for evaluation of data and further follow-up. The Poison Information Centre also conducts studies on the pattern of poisoning in a particular area and developing a prevention programme. National Poison Information Centre has readymade information cards covering the signs and symptoms, prehospital and hospital management protocols including therapeutic drugs and antidote dosing schedule on Organophosphates, Carbamates, Organochlorines, Aluminium phosphide, Ethylene dibromide, Pyrethroid, Rodenticides, Corrosives, Tricyclic antidepressants, Benzodiazepines, Phenytoin, Methyl alcohol, Carbon monoxide, Paracetamol, Opioids, Datura, Yellow Oleander, Scorpion sting, Copper sulphate and Cyanide. Various poisoning manuals and books are available at the centre. The centre is also in the process of setting up a National Antidote Bank that will stock all essential antidotes.

In India, besides this centre, there are poison information centres at Ahmedabad, Cochin and Chennai.

Western Australian Poisons Information Centre: This centre serves more than half of the area of Australia including Western Australia, South Australia, the Northern Territory, the Australian Capital Territory and a small region of western New South Wales. The centre provides telephonic consultation to medical professionals and the general public in cases of acute and chronic poisonings. The centre provides toxicological advice on the management of exposures to prescription and non-prescription pharmaceuticals, household and industrial chemicals, plants, animals, pesticides and other agricultural products. The centre also conducts formal training in clinical toxicology and toxinology for all its staff members. The centre also undergoes many research activities.

The American Association of Poison Control Centres: It is a nationwide organization of poison centres and interested individuals with the objectives: (i) To provide a forum for poison centres and interested individuals to promote the reduction of morbidity and mortality from poisonings through public and professional education and scientific research. (ii) To set voluntary standards for poison center operations. The activities of this centre include: (i) Certification of regional poison centres and poison centre personnel (ii) Interaction with private and governmental agencies whose activities influence poisoning and poison centres (iii) Development of public and professional education programs and materials (iv) Collection and analysis of national poisoning data.

Victorian Poisons Information Centre: This centre is located at the Royal Children's Hospital, Melbourne. The centre provides timely and safe information in cases of poisonings and suspected poisonings. Telephonic advice is provided on first-aid treatment of poisonings or suspected poisonings with or without referral to the hospital. To the health professionals information is given about formulations of products and management of poisoned patients.

National Poisons Information Service, UK: This centre also responds to queries relating to toxic exposures to drugs and chemicals. The queries from doctors and other health care professionals are answered. The NPIS online database, **Toxbase** is available for consultation.

LAWS IN RELATION TO THE POISON

Indian Statutes on Drugs

Many legal acts controlling and regulating the manufacture, sale, distribution and possession of drugs and poisons are passed in India. These include the following:

The Opium Act, 1857: This Act was the earliest enactment concerned with the issue of licenses for cultivation of poppy, the delivery of opium produced to the officers of the central government at the established rates, fixing the limits of issuing licenses from time to time within which licenses can be issued and fixation from time to time of prices to be paid for the opium produced in respect of which it ensured.

The Opium Act, 1858: This Act was enacted to regulate the possession, transport, export, import and sale of opium. The primary aim was protection of public welfare by preserving health, eliminating undesirable moral and social effects, commonly associated with the indiscriminate use of this drug.

The Poisons Act, 1919: The Poisons Act was passed in 1919 and it prohibits the import of any specified poison except when it is according to the conditions of license and regulates the grant of licenses. It also regulates the possession for sale and the sale of any specified poison. The Act was amended in 1958. The Act followed the Opium Act, 1878 as an important drug legislation touching dangerous drugs.

The Dangerous Drugs Act, 1930: This Act was enacted in pursuance of the obligation undertaken by the Government of India to ratify the Geneva Dangerous Drugs Convention 1925, for the suppression of illegal traffic in and abuse of dangerous drugs, especially cocaine and morphine. With that object it provided for the exercise of control by the Central government over the cultivation of dangerous drugs; production and supply of opium and opium derivatives; manufacture of or manufactured drugs like cocaine, methadone, morphine and other narcotic substances, medicinal opium; export, import and transhipment of dangerous drug. It deals mainly with opium, Indian hemp and coca leaves.

The Drugs and Cosmetics Act, 1940: The Drugs and Cosmetics Act deals with the import, manufacture, sell, stock or exhibit for sale, and distribution of proprietary medicine. Every patent or proprietary medicine should display on the label of the container either the true formula or list of ingredients contained. The Act was amended by the Drugs Act 1964 to include Ayurvedic, Siddha and Unani Drugs.

The Drugs Act, 1940: The Drugs Act 1940 regulates the import, manufacture, distribution and sale of the following drugs in India: (i) Patent or proprietary medicines (ii) Vaccines and sera, toxins, toxoids, antitoxins, antigens and other biological products of such nature (iii) Vitamins, hormones and analogous products (iv) The drugs meant for use of humans and animals and those used in the treatment, mitigation or prevention of a disease. This Act was amended by the Drugs Act 1955.

The Drugs (Control) Act, 1950: This Act seeks to control the sale, supply and distribution of drugs. It provides for the fixation of maximum prices chargeable, the maximum quantity which may at any time be possessed by the dealer or producer, the maximum quantity which may in any one transaction be sold to any person. It also includes the issue of cash memo for sale, markings of prices and exhibiting list of prices and stocks, etc.

The Drugs and Magic Remedies Act, 1954: This Act prohibits the advertisements of magic remedies for: (i) Procurement of miscarriage or prevention of conception in women (ii) Improvement and maintenance of the capacity of sexual pleasure (iii) To correct menstrual disorders (iv) For the diagnosis, cure, mitigation, treatment or prevention of any disease, disorder or condition specified in the Schedule to the Act or the rules. The Act also specifies the exceptions to these advertisements.

THE NARCOTIC DRUGS AND PSYCHOTROPIC SUBSTANCES ACT 1985

This Act repeals the Opium Act 1857, The Opium Act 1878 and the Dangerous Drugs Act 1930. The Act was amended in 1988, 2011, 2014 and 2021. The Act shall extend to whole of India. The object of the Act is to consolidate and amend the law relating to narcotic drugs, make stringent provisions for the control and regulation of operations relating to narcotic drugs and psychotropic substances and make provisions for matters connected therewith. The Act defines narcotic drug, psychotropic substance, medicinal cannabis, opium, opium derivatives, opium poppy, poppy straw, poppy straw concentrate, cannabis (hemp), cannabis plant, coca derivative, coca leaf, manufacture, production, preparation and addict etc.

Narcotic drug: It means coca leaf, cannabis (hemp), opium, poppy straw and includes all manufactured goods.

Manufactured drug: It means: (i) All coca derivatives, medicinal cannabis, opium derivatives and poppy straw concentrate. (ii) Any other narcotic substance or preparation that the Central government declares to be a manufactured drug.

Psychotropic substance: It means any substance, natural or synthetic, or any natural material or any salt or preparation of such substance or material included in the list of psychotropic substances specified in the schedule.

Addict: It means a person addicted to any narcotic drug or psychotropic substance.

Small quantity: It means such quantity as may be specified by the Central government in the official Gazette. The burden of proving that it was intended for personal consumption shall lie on the person found in possession of the drug or psychotropic substance. The small quantities as specified in the Central government in the official gazette given in the table below:

Drug	Quantity
Heroin	5 grams
Cocaine	2 grams
Hashish/Charas	100 grams
Opium	25 grams
Ganja	1 kg

Offences and penalties: Chapter IV of the Act defines offences and penalties under the Act. The **Section 27A** of the Act provides punishment for financing illicit traffic and harbouring offenders–Whoever indulges in financing, directly or indirectly, any of the activities specified in sub-clauses (i) to (v) of clause (viiia) of section 2 or harbours any person engaged in any of the aforementioned activities, shall be punishable with rigorous imprisonment which shall not be less than 10 years but which may extend to 20 years with fine which shall not be less than one lakh rupees but which may extend to two lakh rupees for the following contravention. The Court may for the reasons recorded in the judgement impose a fine exceeding two lakh rupees. The contraventions for which such punishment is contemplated, may be of any rule or order made or condition of a licence granted there under relating to poppy straw, coca plant and coca leaves, prepared opium, opium poppy and opium, cannabis plant and cannabis, manufacture dugs and preparations, psychotropic substances, embezzlement of opium by cultivator, illegal import or export or transshipment of narcotic drugs and psychotropic substances, external dealings in narcotic drugs and psychotropic substances in contravention of **S. 12 (S. 24),** allowing premises etc. to be used for the commission of an offence punishable under the **Act (S. 26). S. 31A gives Death penalty for certain offences after previous conviction.** (l) Notwithstanding anything contained in section 31, if any person who has been convicted of the commission of, or attempt to commit, or abetment of, or criminal conspiracy to commit, any of the offences punishable under **S.19, 24 and 27A.**

THE NARCOTIC DRUGS AND PSYCHOTROPIC SUBSTANCES (AMENDMENT) ACT, 2021

This amended Act, 2021, was notified vide the Gazette Notification dated 30th December, 2021.

Salient Features

Correction of the drafting error of 2014 amendment to the Act: Before the 2014 amendment, **clause (viiia) of Section 2 contained sub-clauses (i) to (v),** which defined the term **"illicit traffic".** In 2014, the Act was amended and the clause number of the **definition for such illicit activities was changed** and was catalogued under **Section 2 clause (viiib).** However, the **section (27A) which deals with penalty for financing these illicit activities was not amended** and continued to refer to the earlier clause number of the definition. The 2021 ordinance (Ord. 8 of 2021) on 30th September, 2021, **amended the section on penalty** to change the reference to the new clause number.

(a) **In NDPS (Amendment) Act, 2021: 'clause (viiib)' is substituted in place of 'clause (viiia)'** of **section 27A of the NDPS Act.** This Act replaced the 2021 amendment ordinance.

(b) This amendment will **retrospectively effective from May 1, 2014** (i.e., when the 2014 amendments came into effect).

LAWS IN RELATION TO POISONING IN THE INDIAN PENAL CODE

Section 272 I.P.C.: Adulteration of food or drink intended for sale: Whoever adulterates any article of food or drink, so as to make such article noxious as food or drink, intending to sell such article as food or drink shall be punished with imprisonment of either description for a term which may extend to six months, or with fine which may extend to one thousand rupees, or with both.

Section 273 I.P.C.: Sale of noxious food or drink: The person shall be punished with imprisonment of either description for a term which may extend to six months, or with fine which may extend to one thousand rupees, or with both.

Section 274 I.P.C.: Adulteration of drugs: The person shall be punished with imprisonment of either description for a term which may extend to six months, or with fine which may extend to one thousand rupees, or with both.

Section 275 I.P.C.: Sale of adulterated drugs: The person shall be punished with imprisonment of either description for a term which may extend to six months, or with fine which may extend to one thousand rupees, or with both.

Section 276 I.P.C.: Sale of drug as different drug or preparation: The person shall be punished with imprisonment of either description for a term which may extend to six months, or with fine which may extend to one thousand rupees, or with both.

Section 277 I.P.C.: Fouling water of public spring or reservoir: The person shall be punished with imprisonment of either description for a term which may extend to three months, or with fine which may extend to five hundred rupees, or with both.

Section 278 I.P.C.: Making atmosphere noxious to health: The person shall be punished with fine which may extend to five hundred rupees.

Section 284 I.P.C.: Negligent conduct with respect to poisonous substance: Whoever does, with any poisonous substance, any act in a manner so rash or negligent as to endanger human life, or to be likely to cause hurt or injury to any person, or knowingly or negligently omits to take such order with any poisonous substance in his possession as is sufficient to guard against any probable danger to human life from such poisonous substance, shall be punished with imprisonment of either description for a term which may extend to six months, or with fine which may extend to one thousand rupees, or with both.

Section 299 I.P.C.: Culpable homicide: Whoever causes death by doing an act with the intention of causing death, or with the intention of causing such bodily injury as is likely to cause death, or with the knowledge that he is likely by such an act to cause death, commits the offence of culpable homicide.

Hence if A administers a substance to B with such intent or knowledge and thereby causes B's death, A may be convicted under this section of the offence of committing culpable homicide, irrespective of whether the substance administered may or may not strictly be called a poison. For it is the intent which suffices to constitute a crime, irrespective of the dose or even the nature of substance.

Section 304A I.P.C.: Causing death by negligence: Whoever causes the death of any person by doing any rash or negligent act not amounting to culpable homicide, shall be punished with imprisonment of either description for a term which may extend to two years, or with fine, or with both.

Section 326 I.P.C.: Voluntarily causing grievous hurt by dangerous weapons or means: Whoever, except in the case provided for by the Section 335, voluntarily causes grievous hurt by means of any instrument for shooting, stabbing, or cutting, or any instrument which used as a weapon of offence, is likely to cause death, or by means of fire or any heated substance, or by means of any poison or any corrosive substance, or by means of any explosive substance, or by means of any substance, which is deleterious to the human body to inhale, to swallow or to receive into the blood, or by means of any animal, shall be punished with imprisonment of either description for a term which may extend to ten years and shall also be liable to fine.

Section 326A I.P.C.: Voluntarily causing grievous hurt by use of acid etc. Whoever causes permanent or partial damage or deformity to, or burns or maims or disfigures or disables, any part or parts of the body of a person or causes grievous hurt by throwing acid on or by administering acid to that person, or by using any other means with the intention of causing or with the knowledge that he is likely to cause such injury or hurt, shall be punished with imprisonment of either description for a term which shall not be less than ten years but which may extend to imprisonment for life and with fine which may extend to ten lakh rupees.

Section 326B I.P.C.: Voluntarily throwing or attempting to throw acid: Whoever throws or attempts to throw acid on any person or attempts to administer acid to any person, or attempts to use any other means, with the intention of causing permanent or partial damage or deformity or burns or maiming or disfigurement or disability or grievous hurt to that person, shall be punished with imprisonment of either description for a term which shall not be less than five years but which may extend to seven years, and shall also be liable for fine.

Section 328 I.P.C.: Causing hurt by means of poison, etc., with intent to commit an offence: Whoever administers to or causes to be taken by any person any poison or any stupefying, intoxicating or unwholesome drug, or other thing with intent to cause hurt to such person, or with intent to commit or to facilitate the commission of an offence or knowing it to be likely that he will thereby cause hurt, shall be punished with imprisonment of either description for a term which may extend to ten years, and shall also be liable to fine.

LONG QUESTIONS

1. Classify poisons and describe in detail the management of a case of unknown poisoning brought to casualty.
2. Write in detail the medicolegal duties of a doctor in a case of suspected poisoning.
3. What is antidote? Discuss different of antidote with suitable examples as their indications.
4. Describe simple bedside clinic tests to detect poison/drug in a patient's body fluids.

SHORT NOTES

1. Contraindications of stomach wash.
2. Ideal homicidal poison.
3. B.A.L.
4. Universal antidote.
5. Activated charcoal.
6. Chelating agents.

MULTIPLE CHOICE QUESTIONS

1. The poison administered to Socrates, the Greek philosopher as a form of execution is:

(a) Arsenic (b) Curare
(c) Hemlock (d) Aconite

2. Emetics are contraindicated in poisoning by:

(a) Arsenic
(b) Organophosphorus compounds
(c) Kerosene
(d) Barbiturates

3. **Gastric lavage is contraindicated in the following poisoning *except:***

(a) Sulphuric acid (b) Hydrochloric acid
(c) Nitric acid (d) Carbolic acid

4. **BAL is used in the treatment of poisoning by:**

(a) Mercury (b) Phenol
(c) Aconite (d) Morphine

5. **For gastric lavage in adult, stomach tube to be passed upto:**

(a) 25 cm (b) 30 cm
(c) 50 cm (d) 55 cm

6. **Universal antidote consists of the following *except:***

(a) Potassium permanganate (b) Animal charcoal
(c) Magnesium oxide (d) Tannic acid

7. **E.D.T.A. (Calcium Disodium Versenate) is useful in the treatment of:**

(a) Hypercalcaemia (b) Dhatura poisoning
(c) Opium poisoning (d) Lead poisoning

8. **Substance commonly used for preservation of viscera for toxicological purpose is:**

(a) 10% formalin
(b) Saturated solution of common salt
(c) 40% formalin
(d) Alcohol

9. **Deferoxamine is used in the treatment of poisoning by:**

(a) Iron (b) Mercury
(c) Lead (d) Arsenic

10. **Bluish discoloration of stomach wall at autopsy is found in all poisoning *except:***

(a) Copper sulphate (b) Copper subacetate
(c) Methylene blue (d) Lead subacetate

11. **All of following drugs are included under the 'NDPS Act' *except:***

(a) Opium (b) Hashish
(c) Amphetamine (d) Alcohol

12. **A dead body is having bluish green colour postmortem hypostasis. The most likely cause of death by poisoning in this case is due to:**

(a) Hydrocyanic acid (b) H_2S
(c) Dhatura (d) Sodium nitrite

13. **The proportion of tannic acid, magnesium oxide and activated charcoal in universal antidote is:**

(a) 2:1:1 (b) 1:1:2
(c) 1:2:1 (d) 2:2:1

14. **If the homicidal poisoning is suspected by the doctor and he/she fails to report the matter to the police, the doctor will be held culpable under section:**

(a) 176 I.P.C. (b) 270 I.P.C.
(c) 279 I.P.C. (d) 302 I.P.C.

15. **B.A.L. (Dimercaptopropanolol) is absolutely contraindicated in poisoning due to:**

(a) Cadmium (b) Arsenic
(c) Mercury (d) Thallium

16. **Section 274 I.P.C. deals with:**

(a) Administration of poisons (b) Adulteration of drugs
(c) Injury caused by corrosives (d) Negligence

17. **A recently married girl has consumed organophosphorus poison and admitted to an emergency of a government hospital. The attending physician withhold the information and willfully provided wrong information to investigating authority. He should be punished under section:**

(a) 201 I.P.C. (b) 304 I.P.C.
(c) 304A I.P.C. (d) 279 I.P.C.

18. **Which poison smells like rotten egg?**

(a) Nitrobenzene (b) Naphthalene
(c) Camphor (d) N-acetylcysteine

19. **A person having negligent conduct with respect to poisonous substance is punished under following Indian Penal Code:**

(a) 304A (b) 284
(c) 319 (d) 323

20. **If a private practitioner is convinced that the patient he is treating is a victim of homicidal poisoning, under which section of Cr.P.C. he is bound to inform the police or magistrate:**

(a) S. 37 (b) S. 39
(c) S. 174 (d) S. 176

21. **Dimercaprol is given in:**

(a) Intravenous route in cubital vein
(b) Deep intramuscular route
(c) Intraarterial route in femoral artery
(d) Subcutaneous route

ANSWER KEY

1. (c)	2. (c)	3. (d)	4. (a)	5. (c)	6. (a)	7. (d)	8. (b)	9. (a)	10. (d)
11. (d)	12. (b)	13. (b)	14. (a)	15. (a)	16. (b)	17. (a)	18. (d)	19. (b)	20. (b)
21. (b)									

37 CHAPTER

Corrosive Poisons

Corrosives are the poison that fixes, destroys and causes erosion of the surface coming in its contact. Some organic acids like oxalic and carbolic acid act as corrosives in concentrated form as do carbonates of sodium and potassium. Certain metallic salts, e.g., sodium chloride, potassium cyanide, ferric chloride, chromates and bichromates of alkalis also act as corrosives. Severity and extent of damage of tissues by corrosive depends upon (i) pH of the agent (ii) Amount, concentration and physical form (solid or liquid) of the agent (iii) Duration of contact. More severe injury occurs when corrosive substance with pH < 2 or pH > 12 is ingested.

Mode of Action

The mode of action of inorganic or mineral acids like sulphuric acid, hydrochloric acid and the nitric acid are: (i) Causes only local action but no remote effects on the system. (ii) In concentrated form, they cause corrosion and destruction of the tissue. (iii) Extracts the water from the tissues. (iv) Fixes, destroys and erodes the tissues. (v) Converts haemoglobin into hematin. (vi) Causes coagulation necrosis by precipitation of proteins forms an eschar, which is thought to prevent the acid from reaching deeper tissues. (vii) Mucosa of the esophagus is relatively resistant to the acids because of rapid transit of acids due to less viscosity and the resistance of squamous epithelium of oesophagus to acid. (viii) In acid ingestion, mucous membrane of stomach especially pyloric region is very susceptible and in this region necrosis commonly occurs. (ix) Acids "lick oesophagus and bite the pyloric antrum" whereas the opposite results from alkaline ingestion. (x) Complications develop from 3 weeks to 3 months of ingestion of the substance. (xi) Corrosives act as irritant and when well diluted act as stimulant.

General Principles of Management

A. **Initial Resuscitation**

For corrosive ingestion:

(i) Initial resuscitation with the maintenance of airway, breathing and circulation (ABC) should be followed. Tracheostomy with mechanical ventilation might be required in patients with laryngeal injuries. (ii) The supine position, gastric lavage, and induced emesis are contraindicated as this result in additional oesophageal injury secondary to reexposure of the oesophagus to the corrosive agent and risk of perforation of already thinned out stomach and oesophagus. (iii) Avoid giving neutralizing agents as heat generated by exothermic chemical reaction may increase tissue damage. (iv) Dilution of the corrosive with milk or water has a little role, as the extent of the injury is usually determined within minutes after ingestion of corrosive agent. (v) Gastric acid suppression with proton pump inhibitors (PPI) and H_2 blockers usually given to minimize oesophageal injury by suppressing acid reflux, however their efficacy is not proven. (vi) Corticosteroids may not prevent the development of strictures following corrosive ingestion and its use should be reserved for patients with airways involvement. (vii) Broad spectrum antibiotics should be given for patients with high grade caustic injury or those receiving systemic steroids or high suspicion for oesophageal perforation. (viii) Adequate pain relief with intravenous narcotics. (ix) Supportive care, rather than specific antidotes, is the mainstay of acute-phase treatment. (x) Do not feed orally until endoscopy.

For other exposure:

(i) In case of skin burns, wash with large quantities of water or apply paste of sodium bicarbonate. (ii) Eye burns are treated symptomatically after irrigating with water for 10-15 minutes. (iii) In case of corrosive inhalation, the person should be removed from exposure and supplemental oxygen should be given.

B. **Investigations for Severity of Injury**

Early upper GI endoscopy (not later than 24 hours) has role for diagnosis and management of corrosive injuries. It is the gold standard for determination of extent of injury which is performed in hemodynamically stable patients with no signs of perforation. However, the major drawback of endoscopy is its inability to accurately determine the depth of necrosis. To overcome the limitations of endoscopy contrast-enhanced computed tomography (CECT) can be used. Plain chest radiography may show gas shadow in the mediastinum or below the diaphragm suggesting oesophageal or gastric perforation, respectively.

C. **Surgery**

Emergency surgery is indicated in patients in whom initial evaluation suggests transmural necrosis/perforation of the GI tract. Long-term complications like strictures need endoscopic dilatation using either bougie like Savary-Gilliard dilators or balloon dilators in patients with short dilatable strictures. Topical mitomycin-C and intralesional triamcinolone can be administered during dilation procedures to reduce post-dilation recurrence of esophageal strictures. If endoscopic dilatation is not feasible, then definitive surgical treatment is performed.

Causes of Death

Time	Causes
Within few hours	Shock/glottic oedema
Within 24 hours	Perforation of stomach→peritonitis→shock
Within 1st few weeks	Septic absorption
After months or years	Exhaustion, malnutrition due to strictures, incurable dyspepsia

SULPHURIC ACID (OIL OF VITRIOL)

Properties

(i) Pure sulphuric acid is colourless with no fumes and it chars, and blackens the skin. (ii) Commercial sulphuric acid is dark or brown in colour due to the addition of impurities like lead sulphate, arsenic or nitric acid. (iii) Nordhausen acid or $H_2S_2O_7$ (pyrosulphuric acid) is stronger, brown, oily and fuming liquid used in the manufacture of indigo. (iv) Sulphate of indigo is 1 : 10 ($H_2S_2O_7$). (v) Sulphuric acid is chiefly used for preparing chlorine, battery (battery acid), for dissolving metal, for cleansing drains and toilets (toilet cleaners), for medicinal purposes, and to remove fur from kettles.

Signs and Symptoms of Sulphuric Acid Poisoning

Immediately after swallowing: (i) Intense burning pain in mouth, throat, oesophagus and upto the stomach. (ii) Dribbling of acid mixed with saliva on the angles of mouth and chin causing corrosion and brownish discolouration of skin over angles of mouth, chin and over the chest. (iii) Frothy eructation, retching and vomiting; vomited matter is acid, contains blood, mucous and shreds of mucous membrane. (iv) *Oral cavity:* Mucosa of mouth and lips are softened, excoriated, corrugated and covered with dirty white necrotic membrane that assumes brownish black discolouration. The oral cavity is full of secretions consisting of saliva, blood, mucous making speech and swallowing difficult and may even result in death from asphyxia. (v) Tongue is swollen, excoriated and discoloured with white coating that becomes dark later on. It may get disorganized into a shapeless, pulpy mass. (vi) Teeth are dead chalky white deprived of polish. (vii) Lips are swollen, excoriated with brown or black streaks resulting from the action of acid running from the angle of mouth to the chin and chest. (viii) Intense thirst and an attempt to drink water brings vomiting that leads to dehydration. Along with vomiting, there is extreme dysphagia. (ix) Voice is hoarse and husky and speech is painful and difficult due to the inflammation of epiglottis, uvula etc. (x) Breathing is difficult and noisy due to swollen and inflamed fauces and tender abdomen. (xi) Asphyxia may result from glottic oedema or aspiration of regurgitated acid contents (xii) Bowels are constipated with marked tenesmus and straining. during defecation. (xiii) Urine is scanty or suppressed with pain during micturition. (xiv) General condition of collapse like cold clammy skin, decreased BP and increased pulse may be there. (xv) Mind remains calm until the end. (xvi) Feeble pulse and difficult respiration, convulsions and death in 12-24 hours. (xvii) Complications in the form of mediastinitis or peritonitis from perforation of oesophagus or stomach and stricture of oesophagus may develop within a few weeks.

Fatal Dose: 5-10 ml.

Fatal Period: 12-18 hours.

Acid burns: The acid burns are full thickness burns with well defined edges and tend to heal slowly with scar formation.

Autopsy Findings

Postmortem findings depend upon the quantity and strength of acid and the time of survival.

A. **External Findings**

(i) Evidence of acid corrosion and chemical burns with brownish black parchment like and corroded spots are seen over chin, cheek, neck and chest resulting from trickling of the acid. (ii) Excoriation of lips, corrosion of mucosa of mouth and tongue, **chalky-white teeth** are characteristic.

(iii) Mucous membrane of mouth, tongue and lips shows brown or brownish black corroded spots with necrosis that are grayish white initially that changes to brownish black and leathery later on. (iv) When taken by spoon, lips and mouth escape injury.

B. **Internal Findings**

(i) Changes produced from corrosive poisoning are limited to the upper digestive tract and respiratory system. (ii) Mucous membrane of oesophagus is inflamed, swollen by oedema and severe interstitial haemorrhage is present even when corrosion is absent. The perforation is rare. (iii) Mucous membrane of stomach is inflamed, oedematous, **blackened and peppery feel** (Figure 37.1). (iv) Peritoneal cavity is filled with black grumous acidic liquid containing mostly altered blood from escape of the acidic stomach contents into peritoneal cavity following perforation of stomach. (v) Greater part of the stomach is converted into **soft, boggy, black mass** that readily disintegrates on touching. The mucosal ridges are more damaged than intervening furrows. The mucosa on stripping shows intense congestion and inflammation underneath. The perforated stomach has softened walls and edges of rupture looking black and irregular. (vi) Small intestine especially duodenum shows evidence of irritation. (vii) As a result of perforation of oesophagus or stomach, the thoracic and abdominal viscera is blackened and corroded by acid with features of chemical peritonitis. (viii) Corrosion and severe inflammation of larynx and trachea may be found. (ix) In delayed deaths formation of oesophageal strictures. (x) If patient survives longer fatty degeneration and toxic swelling of liver and kidney may be seen.

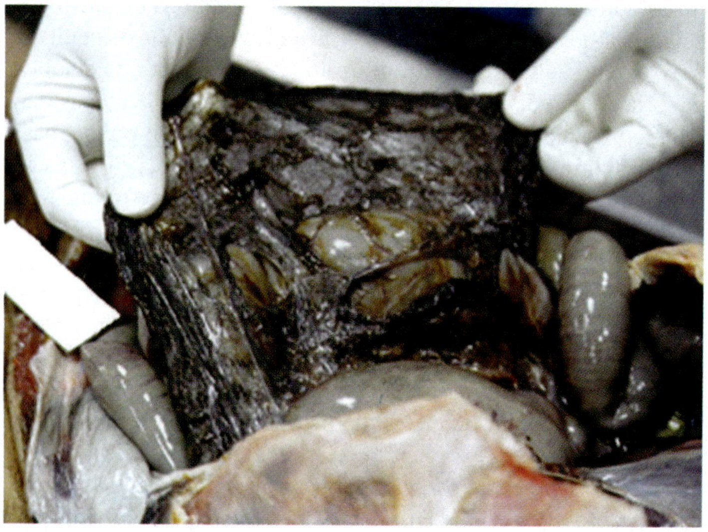

Figure 37.1: Blackened and peppery mucosa of stomach as seen in sulphuric acid poisoning

Diagnosis

(i) Haemoconcentration in red blood cells is noticed. (ii) Diffuse mottling of lung fields on X-ray when there is inhalation of acid vapour. (iii) *Chemical tests*: (a) When sulphuric acid is mixed with barium nitrate or chloride, white precipitate of barium sulphate is produced (b) Strong sulphuric acid chars organic matter.

Medicolegal Aspects

(i) Accidental poisoning occurs as it is mistaken for glycerine or castor oil. (ii) Mostly it is employed for suicidal purposes due to its easy availability. (iii) Homicidal ingestion is unusual. (iv) Cases of homicide by throwing acid on body are reported (Figure 37.2). (v) It acts as an abortifacient when injected into vagina. (vi) Employed for the purposes of vitriolage causing grievous hurt. (vii) Acid is sometimes thrown on the private parts, and face out of jealousy in cases of extramarital affairs. (viii) Acid bath murderer–John Haigh, a serial killer used to kill the victim and disposed their bodies using sulphuric acid.

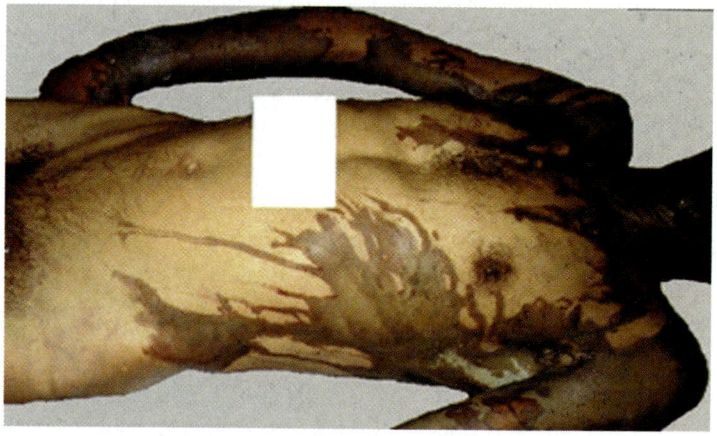

Figure 37.2: A victim of fatal corrosive attack at autopsy

Vitriolage or Vitriol Throwing

Vitriolage is throwing of strong sulphuric acid, concentrated mineral acid, corrosive alkalis, carbolic acid, or the juice of marking nut over the face or body of the victim for the purpose of disfiguring the face, destroying the vision for causing injury on the body or even destroying the clothing of the victim. Malicious persons do this when they have a hatred or enmity to the victim. Some people use old electric bulb filled with acid to carry out their motive.

Effects produced are: (i) There is severe burning pain and corrosion of the tissues with formation of brownish black burned areas that later on leave a permanent scar. (ii) Stains on skin and cloth are yellowish when nitric acid is used but blackish when sulphuric acid is used. (iii) Blindness may result if eyes are involved. (iv) Extensive disfiguring injuries are caused on the face. (v) Death may occur from shock, toxaemia or infection from severe chemical burns inflicted on the skin. The burns are penetrating, painless and the acid devitalizes the tissues and predisposes to infection. Slow repair and formation of scar tissue with contracture occurs.

Treatment

(i) Wash with plenty of water or soap solution. (ii) Apply magnesium oxide or carbonate as thick paste. (iii) Cover the raw surface with tannic acid jelly or soframycin or penicillin tulle gauze dressing. (iv) Wash the eyes with plenty of water and irrigate with 5 gm of sodium bicarbonate and one ounce of water. (v) Subsequently few drops of castor or olive oil are to be dropped into eye. (vi) Corneal ulcers are treated with atropine ointment, hydrocortisone and antibiotics.

Medicolegal Aspects

(i) Permanent loss of vision amounts to grievous injury (S. 320 I.P.C., clause 2). (ii) Permanent disfiguration of head or face due to scar tissue formation also amounts to grievous injury (S. 320 I.P.C., clause 6). (iii) Vitriolage amounts to dangerous injury either due to severe extensive burn or subsequent infection. (iv) **S. 326A I.P.C.** deals with voluntarily causing grievous hurt by use of acid etc. (v) **S. 326B I.P.C.** deals with voluntarily throwing or attempting to throw acid.

NITRIC ACID—HNO_3 (AQUA FORTIS)

Pure nitric acid is colourless, clear liquid gives fumes when exposed to air. It has a peculiar choking odour. A powerful oxidizing agent dissolves all metals except gold and platinum. It destroys organic matters with formation of xanthoproteic acid that imparts **deep yellow colour** to the affected tissues.

Signs and Symptoms

The signs and symptoms produced by ingestion of concentrated nitric acid are similar to those of sulphuric acid but since it has tendency to char the tissues, **perforation of stomach does not occur** (i) Lips, tongue and mucous membrane of mouth are soft. Initially it is white then yellow due to formation of **xanthoproteic acid.** (ii) Clothing is also stained yellow due to xanthoproteic reaction. (iii) Teeth and clothes are yellow stained. (iv) Abdomen is more distended and tender due to formation of large quantities of gas by direct action of acids on the organic matter of stomach. (v) Violent vomiting occurs and the vomitus is yellowish brown containing altered blood. (vi) Gaseous eructations are more frequent and distressing. (vii) Oliguria and anuria occurs and albumin and casts are seen in the urine. As nitric acid like hydrochloric acid but unlike sulphuric acid is volatile and gives fumes at room temperatures, the effects produced by the inhalation of fumes are: (a) Irritation of the eyes with lachrymation and sneezing (b) Photophobia (c) Burning in the throat (d) Cough (e) Feeling of constriction in the chest (f) *Dyspnea:* Death may occur immediately from suffocation due to oedema of glottis or later on from pulmonary oedema or bronchopneumonia.

Fatal Dose: 10-15 ml.

Fatal Period: 12-24 hours.

Tests for Nitric Acid

(i) When ammonia water is added to the yellow stains, it turns to yellow. (ii) When iodide and ammonia is added to the yellow stains, the stains disappear. (iii) When bile and ammonia is added to the yellow stains, there is no change. (iv) If strong solution of ferrous sulphate and sulphuric acid is added to a solution containing nitric acid, a brown ring is formed at the junction between the two. The test is for the presence of nitrates.

Autopsy Findings

(i) Postmortem appearances are similar to those of sulphuric acid but tissues are stained yellow. (ii) Oesophagus and stomach are not stained yellow but is brown or brownish black due to the formation of **acid haematin.** (iii) Perforation is not so common. (iv) If the death is from inhalation of fumes then the respiratory passages are congested; lungs are congested and oedematous and the lining membrane of right auricle may show inflammatory changes.

Medicolegal Aspects

(i) Poisoning is mostly accidental or suicidal. (ii) Rarely it is homicidal.

HYDROCHLORIC ACID (HCL)

Pure hydrochloric acid is colourless and fuming liquid with strong pungent irritating odour. The strong solution gives fumes even at ordinary temperature and air. When the solution is ingested, its liberated gas is also inhaled. It is a natural constituent of the fluids of stomach and bowel. It is used for preparing chlorine, for dissolving metal, for cleaning drains, to remove fur from kettles and as medicine.

Muriatic acid is the solution of hydrochloric acid gas in water having yellow colour and fumes strongly in damp air. It is used commercially and is less destructive than sulphuric and nitric acids. HCL does not stain skin and mucous membrane but stains dark clothes reddish brown. Since it is volatile, it readily affects the respiratory tract mucosa.

Signs and Symptoms

(i) Hydrochloric acid is less active than the other two acids hence symptoms are much milder. (ii) It does not corrode or damage the skin. (iii) It readily destroys the mucous membrane. (iv) Mucous membrane is gray or gray white changing to brown or black. (v) Inhalation of fumes causes: (a) Irritation of the air passages (b) Spasm of glottis (c) Symptoms of suffocation (d) Cough, dyspnea and cyanosis.

Chronic Poisoning

Constant exposure to fumes produces chronic poisoning. The

symptoms and signs of chronic poisoning are: (i) Coryza (ii) Conjunctivitis (iii) Corneal ulcer (iv) Pharyngitis (v) Bronchitis (vi) Inflammation of gums (vii) Loosening of teeth.

Fatal Dose: 15-20 ml.

Fatal Period: 18-24 hours.

Autopsy Findings

(i) Findings are same as that of sulphuric acid poisoning but there is less tendency to charring and tissue destruction. (ii) Oral cavity and oesophageal mucous membrane is ashy grey in colour but may get blackened, swollen and hardened if the acid is concentrated. (iii) Stomach contains brownish acidic fluid and mucosa is corroded and grayish white in colour. (iv) Perforation is rare.

Chemical tests: On addition of silver nitrate to a solution of hydrochloric acid, a white precipitate of silver chloride is formed.

Medicolegal Aspects

(i) Suicidal poisoning is common (ii) There are a few cases of accidental poisoning (iii) It is very rarely homicidal (iv) It is rarely injected into the vagina to produce abortion and it causes atresia of the vagina (v) It is used for erasing writing; attempts for forgery may be there.

CARBOLIC ACID

This is hydroxy benzene obtained from coal tar oil by fractional distillation. Pure carbolic acid has colourless, prismatic needle shaped crystals with burning sweetish taste. It turns pink and liquefies when exposed to air. It has carbolic smell, is slightly soluble in water and freely soluble in glycerine, ether and alcohol. It is used as an antiseptic and disinfectant agent.

Commercial carbolic acid is dark brown liquid containing several impurities chiefly cresol. Carbolic acid and its derivatives are commonly used as disinfectants, antiseptics, germicides, caustics and preservatives kept in cupboards and almirahs. Lysol is as dangerous as phenol, which is used in the manufacture of explosives, fertilizers, textile, rubber, plastics, dyes, drugs and in preservations of vaccines etc.

Significance of change in colour: It serves as a warning of toxic properties of acid when used as an antiseptic on the wounds.

Poisoning by carbolic acid is known as **Carbolism.**

Absorption: It is readily absorbed from gastrointestinal tract, respiratory tract, rectum, vagina, serous cavities, wounds and skin.

Elimination: Phenol is converted into hydroquinone and pyrocatechol in the body before it is eliminated in the urine. Only traces are excreted in lungs and it is partly detoxified in the liver. Complete elimination occurs by 36-48 hours.

Fatal Dose: 1-2 gm of pure phenol, or 25-50 ml of household phenol.

Fatal Period: 3-4 hours.

Mode of Action

(i) Carbolic acid acts locally as a corrosive and systemically as **narcotic, induces sleep and drowsiness.** (ii) Carbolic acid has a great penetrating power as it coagulates protein but does not occur in chemical combination with them. (iii) When applied to the skin, it produces burning sensation, numbness, and **anaesthesia** due to its action on the nerve endings. (iv) It produces a white opaque eschar, which falls off in a few days and leaves a brown stain that may persist for several weeks. (v) It causes irritation and necrosis of the mucous membrane that may slough and get inflamed. (vi) There may be gangrene of the tissue. (vii) In small doses, it stimulates respiratory centre. (viii) In severe cases, hemolysis and methemoglobinemia are characteristic features that can occur following poisoning with hydroquinone.

Signs and Symptoms

Following signs and symptoms arise immediately after swallowing the acid that are: (i) Burning sensation in the mouth and throat. (ii) Mucous membrane of the mouth and lips is hard and white. (iii) Rapid absorption of acid into the blood stream is soon followed by giddiness insensibility and coma. (iv) Face is pale and cyanosed. (v) Pupils are constricted. (vi) Temperature is decreased. (vii) Pulse is increased, feeble and thready. (viii) Respiration is slow and laboured. (ix) Smell of carbolic acid is present in the breath. (x) Convulsions and lockjaw may be present. (xi) ***Carboluria:*** Urine is scanty and suppressed, when passed there is normal or greenish hue that becomes dark or olive green on exposure to air due to oxidation of pyrocatechol and hydroquinone in air that are the oxidation products of carbolic acid. Phenol is partly oxidized; partly unchanged that is excreted in the urine; partly free and partly unstable in combination with sulphuric acid and glucoronic acid. Carboluria is diagnostic of carbolic acid poisoning. (xii) ***Oochronosis:*** The hydroquinone and pyrocatechol may cause pigmentation in the cornea and venous complexes and various cartilages, it is seen in chronic poisoning. It is normally associated with alkaptonuria and gets deposited in cartilage. It can be occasionally seen from exposure to other substances such as trinitrophenol, resorcinol, mercury, picric acid, benzene, hydroquinone and anti-malarials.

Causes of death: (i) Syncope (ii) Asphyxia due to respiratory failure, oedema of glottis and complications such as pneumonia.

Treatment

In case of ingestion: (i) Avoid emesis as emetics at times fail due to anaesthetic effect. (ii) Gastric lavage is usually not recommended. ***Stomach:*** For gastric lavage, a small bore nasogastric tube is passed carefully and the wash is done with plenty of warm water along with charcoal, olive oil, castor oil, magnesium or sodium sulphate. The combination with phenol of these substances forms a harmless compound. The soap solution or 10% glycerine can also be used, until the washings are clear and odourless. Then 2 ounce of castor oil or liquid paraffin is left in the stomach. (iii)

Demulcents such as milk and white of an egg are given. (iv) To combat circulatory collapse and metabolic acidosis, I.V. saline containing 7 gm/litre of sodium bicarbonate is administered. Sodium bicarbonate also helps to dilute carbolic acid content of blood and it promotes excretion by promoting the flow of urine. (v) Methemoglobinemia should be treated if greater than 30%, or in cases of respiratory distress, with methylene blue 1 to 2 mg/kg of 1% solution, slowly I.V. (vi) Oxygen inhalation and artificial respiration when needed. (vii) Haemodialysis, if there is renal failure.

In case of contact exposure: (i) Contaminated clothings should be removed. (ii) Wash skin with water if it is the only available liquid, but preferably wash with polyethylene glycol molecular weight 300 (Macrogol 300), isopropyl alcohol, industrial methylated spirits or Golytely for at least 30 minutes. (iii) Eyes should be immediately flushed with water (preferably tepid) for at least 15 minutes.

In case of inhalation: (i) Remove patient from the area of exposure to fresh air. (ii) Maintain a clear airway and adequate ventilation. (iii) Give oxygen, if required.

Autopsy Findings

External Findings: (i) Dark brown excoriations may be seen at the angle of mouth and chin (ii) Signs of splashing may be present on the other body parts (iii) Tongue is white or swollen (iv) Smell of phenol comes from the mouth (v) Mucous membrane of mouth is corrugated, sodden and white or ash gray small submucosal haemorrhages may be seen.

Internal Findings: (i) Oesophageal mucosa is tough, white gray, corrugated and arranged in longitudinal folds. (ii) Stomach mucosal folds are swollen and covered with opaque gray or brown mucous membrane with a leathery feel (Figure 37.3). The intervening furrows are less damaged and the mucosa is often dark red, partly separated and necrotic with severe congestion of underlying mucosa. The stomach may contain reddish fluid mixed with mucus and shreds of epithelium emitting odour of phenol. (iii) Duodenum and upper part of small intestine shows changes similar to the stomach. (iv) Liver and spleen are in the form of white, hardened patch when in contact with stomach. (v) Kidney is inflamed and shows haemorrhagic spots. (vi) Lungs are congested and oedematous. (vii) Brain is congested and at times oedematous.

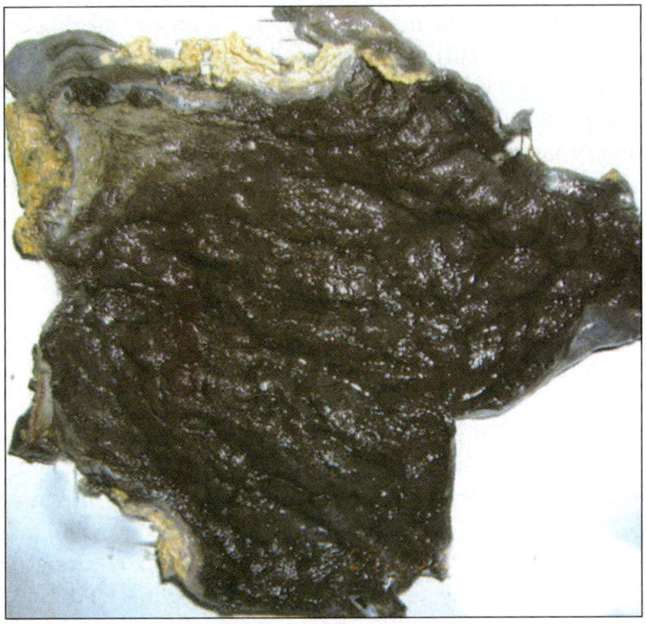

Figure 37.3: Opaque, gray brown and leathery mucosa of stomach as seen in carbolic acid poisoning

Medicolegal Aspects

(i) Used for suicidal purposes. (ii) Accidental poisoning results from its medicinal use and when it is introduced into vagina for abortion. Application of phenol preparations on wounds, ulcers, abraded skin, injections into abscess cavity, rectum, vagina or uterus can also result in accidental poisoning. (iii) Due to its peculiar phenolic odour and taste, it is rarely used for homicidal purposes.

OXALIC ACID (ACID OF SUGAR AND SALT OF SORREL)

Oxalic acid is colourless, transparent and prismatic crystals resembling magnesium sulphate. It is an organic corrosive acid. It is prepared from sugar by oxidation with nitric acid or by heating sodium or potassium formate. The differences between oxalic acid and magnesium sulphate are summarized below (Table 37.1):

Table 37.1: Differences in oxalic acid and magnesium sulphate

Features	Oxalic acid	Magnesium sulphate
Taste	Sour and acid	Nauseating and bitter
Reaction	Strongly acid, pH<7	Neutral, pH 7
On heating	Sublimes	Fixed
With sodium carbonate	No precipitate	Precipitates
Stains of ink or iron-moulds	Disappears	No action

Commercial use of oxalic acid: (i) Calico-printing (ii) Manufacture of straw hats (iii) Cleaning brass and copper articles, wooden surface and leather (iv) Photography (vi) Used by book binders.

Domestic use of oxalic acid: Oxalic acid is a common household remedy used for removing stains of ink and marks from clothing.

Illegal uses of oxalic acid: It is used for removing writing and signature from the paper.

Mode of Action

Oxalic acid has local as well as remote or systemic action:

Local action: (i) In solid or concentrated form or in large quantities, it acts as a corrosive. (ii) In weaker solutions, it acts as an irritant and this is more evident in the nervous system. (iii) When applied to the wound, it acts as a poison.

Remote action: (i) It precipitates ionized calcium and produces symptoms of **hypocalcaemia** (ii) Large doses cause rapid death from shock (iii) Causes tubular necrosis, uremia and death within 2-14 days.

Fatal Dose: 15-20 gm.

Fatal Period: 1-1½ hours.

Signs and Symptoms

The signs and symptoms produced vary with the amount taken and the concentration of the solution.

Fulminating poisoning: Large doses about 15 gm or more produces immediate symptoms and death within minutes. The following symptoms are produced: (i) Burning, sour and bitter taste in the mouth (ii) Throat constriction (iii) Burning pain in the mouth and upto the stomach; pain starts in the epigastrium and radiates to the whole abdomen (iv) Tenderness (v) Nausea, vomiting and eructation; vomitus contains blood and mucous (coffee ground colour) (vi) Thirst may be there (vii) Death usually occurs before the bowel is affected but if the life is prolonged, diarrhoea may occur.

Acute poisoning: (i) In a large dose when patient survives for hours, the symptoms are more of hypocalcaemia and less of digestive upset (ii) Muscle irritability and tenderness is there (iii) Convulsions occurs and there is numbness and tingling of fingertips and legs (iv) Cardiovascular collapse (v) Stupor and coma can occur at times.

Delayed poisoning: Symptoms of uraemia such as scanty or suppressed urine containing traces of blood, aluminium or calcium oxalate crystals are found.

Treatment

(i) Stomach wash by calcium lactate or gluconate (ii) Antidote is calcium lactate or gluconate, it converts oxalate to calcium oxalate that is insoluble; 10 ml of 10% calcium gluconate is administered intravenously at regular intervals (iii) Parathyroid extract 100 units I.M. is given in severe cases (iv) Demulcent drinks (v) Bowels may be relieved by enema (vi) Symptomatic treatment to be given (vii) Dialysis or exchange transfusion may be done.

Autopsy Findings

(i) Skin is rarely burned (ii) Strong solution may cause white as if bleached appearance of mucous membrane of mouth, tongue and lips. It may be red due to irritation (iii) Outer coat of stomach is inflamed and reddened with patchy softening, perforation is rare. The contents of the stomach are brownish due to acid haematin. At times the whole stomach is corroded and perforated. If death is immediate, stomach is pale and not corroded (iv) Kidneys are swollen and congested, tubules show oxalate crystals (v) All other organs are congested.

Medicolegal Aspects

(i) Accidental poisoning commonly as it is mistaken for magnesium sulphate (ii) Rarely it is found as suicidal poison (iii) Very rarely it is used for homicidal poisoning owing to its bitter taste (iv) It is used as an abortifacient rarely.

CORROSIVE ALKALIES

The strong solutions of alkalis act as corrosives but in dilute form, they act as irritants. Concentrated corrosive alkalis are more dangerous than acids. The chief alkaline corrosives with their fatal doses are the following:

1. Potassium hydroxide (Caustic potash): 5 gm.
2. Sodium hydroxide: 5 gm.
3. Potassium carbonate (Caustic soda): 18 gm.
4. Sodium carbonate (Washing soda): 30 gm.
5. **Ammonia:** 30 gm; gaseous ammonia dissolved in water forms strong solution of ammonia that is strongly alkaline, pungent liquid.
6. Ammonium carbonate.

Lye is a mixture of caustic soda and sodium bicarbonate that is used for cleaning purposes.

Uses of corrosive alkalies: (i) Caustic potash and caustic soda is extensively used for commercial purposes as cleansing agents in washing powders and pipe-cleaners. (ii) Used as liniments in medicines.

Actions produced: (i) Caustic action results from the absorption of water from the tissues. (ii) Alkalis combines with proteins to form proteinases and with fats to form soaps (saponification), resulting in liquefactive necrosis, which leads to deeper penetration into tissues with a greater likelihood of transmural injury. (iii) It causes blood vessel thrombosis of blood vessels during the injury. (iv) It produces more severe damage to esophagus because the alkalis are often more viscous that permit a longer contact time with esophageal tissues. (v) Alkali produces less severe injury to gastric tissue because the acidic contents in the stomach that act to neutralize gastric injury.

Signs and Symptoms

Signs and symptoms produced are similar to that of corrosives: (i) Soft, oedematous, translucent, swollen, red brownish scar formation is there (ii) Charring is not present (iii) Vomited matter is alkaline (iv) Purging is frequent; mucous and blood is present in the stools (v) When a strong solution of alkali is ingested, the mucosa of mouth and lips is discoloured and blister formation is there. ***Inhalation of Ammonia Vapours:*** Following symptoms are produced, when the ammonia vapours are inhaled: (i) Congestion and watering of the eyes (ii) Sneezing, coughing and choking (iii) Sudden collapse and death may occur (iv) Death is due to suffocation and oedema of glottis.

Treatment

(i) Immediate dilution with drinking of glass of water is recommended, when alkali is ingested. (ii) Ingestion of potentially neutralizing substances such as vinegar should be avoided. (iii) Induced emesis is contraindicated. (iv) Gastric lavage are generally ineffective and should be done carefully. (v) Further management should be done on the basis of clinical condition and extent of injury on the basis of radiological examination. (vi) Oxygen inhalation, when ammonia vapour is inhaled. (vii) Symptomatic treatment should be given.

Autopsy Findings

The findings are similar to corrosives.

Medicolegal Aspects

(i) Accidental poisoning is common as it is mistaken for medicines (ii) Homicidal poisoning is rare (iii) Poisoning by inhalation of ammonia vapour is common (iv) Sometimes caustic soda is thrown over the face and body producing chemical burns.

LONG QUESTIONS

1. Classify corrosive poisons. Describe signs, symptoms, management and autopsy findings a case of acute sulfuric acid poisoning.
2. Discuss signs, symptoms, management and postmortem findings in case of carbolic acid poisoning.

SHORT NOTES

1. Vitriolage.
2. Carboluria.

MULTIPLE CHOICE QUESTIONS

1. The actions of mineral acids include the following *except*:

(a) Extraction of water from the tissues
(b) Coagulation necrosis of the tissues
(c) Saponification of tissues
(d) Conversion of haemoglobin into acid haematin

2. Xanthoproteic reaction is observed in the following poison:

(a) Nitric acid (b) Sulphuric acid
(c) Carbolic acid (d) Oxalic acid

3. Green urine is passed in the poisoning due to:

(a) Oxalic acid
(b) Carbolic acid
(c) Iodine
(d) Copper sulphate

4. All the following are features of phenol poisoning *except*:

(a) Decreased body temperature
(b) Carbolic odour in the breath
(c) Dilated pupil
(d) Mucous membrane of mouth and lips are hard and white

5. A person attempts to throw acid on the face of his wife with intention to disfigure her. He will be punished under Section:

(a) 326 I.P.C. (b) 326-A I.P.C.
(c) 326-B I.P.C. (d) 354-A I.P.C.

6. A 23-year-old girl intentionally consumed some liquid kept in the toilet. She was brought dead to a hospital. Autopsy revealed excoriation of lips, chalky white teeth and the stomach is blackened and peppery feel. The most likely poison is:

(a) Nitric acid (b) Sulphuric acid
(c) Carbolic acid (d) Oxalic acid

7. Symptoms of hypocalcaemia are produced by poisoning with:

(a) Nitric acid
(b) Sulphuric acid
(c) Carbolic acid
(d) Oxalic acid

ANSWER KEY

1. (c)	2. (a)	3. (b)	4. (c)	5. (c)	6. (b)	7. (d)

38 CHAPTER

Metallic Poisons

LEAD

Lead was known to man as early as 4,000 BC. However, lead's toxicity was only recognized and recorded as early as 2000 BC. In 370 BC, Hippocrates was probably the first to describe lead colic, however without recognizing its aetiology. in 250 BC, the Greek philosopher Nikander of Colophon first described the clinical manifestations of lead poisoning. In ancient Rome, lead poisoning was a disease of the wealthy who used lead for preparing utensils, cosmetics, medicines and wines. It is believed that lead poisoning is primarily responsible for the collapse of the Roman Empire. Some researchers propose that Julius Cesar and Octavio had clinical manifestations associated with lead poisoning. In ancient times, it was regarded as father of all metals.

Lead is one of the truly toxic elements present in the human body. The compounds of lead are more dangerous than the lead itself, except when lead is in volatile state. Lead when inhaled acts 10 times more dangerously than when ingested.

Uses of Lead

(i) Lead is a major constituent of the lead-acid battery used extensively in car batteries. (ii) Lead was used as a white pigment in lead paint. (iii) Lead is used as a coloring element in ceramic glazes. (iv) Lead was used for plumbing in Ancient Rome. (v) Lead sticks were used as pencils but has been replaced by graphite for the last 450 years. (vi) Lead is used as projectiles for firearms and fishing sinkers because of its density, low cost verse alternative products and ease of use due to relatively low melting point. (vii) Lead is used in some candles to treat the wick to ensure a longer, more even burn. However, because of the dangers, European and North American manufacturers use more expensive alternatives such as zinc. (viii) Lead is used as shielding from radiation. (ix) Lead glass is comprised 12-28% lead. It changes the optical characteristics of the glass and reduces the transmission of radiation. (x) Tetraethyl lead has been used in leaded fuels to reduce engine knocking. However, this is no longer a common practice in the Western World due to health concerns. (xi) Lead is used as electrodes in the process of electrolysis.

Mechanism of Action

Most lead poisoning symptoms are thought to occur by interfering with an essential enzyme Delta-aminolevulinic acid dehydrase (ALA). ALA is a zinc-binding protein which is important in the biosynthesis of heme, the cofactor found in hemoglobin. It combines with sulphydryl groups and inhibits tissue enzyme systems. Lead also directly causes haemolysis of mature red cells. It affects erythropoiesis, and myelopoieis by depressing the bone marrow, resulting in anemia, basophilic stippling of RBCs, anisopoikilocytosis and thrombocytopenia.

Absorption of Lead

Lead is absorbed into the system by: (i) Inhalation (ii) Gastrointestinal tract by ingestion (iii) From abraded skin. Absorption of lead occurs at the rate of 1-2 mg/hour for a prolonged period. 0.01-0.1 m diameters are readily absorbed. Plumbism is caused ten times more by inhalation as fine dust or fumes. Lead is deposited in bones as tribasic lead phosphate that is an insoluble form. The lead is eliminated mainly in faeces and to a less extent in urine, bile, saliva, milk and sweat. Absorption of lead occurs within 3-6 minutes. Lead has blastophoric effect on the spermatozoa.

Idiosyncrasy: Some persons are not affected by the effects of lead compounds whereas persons addicted to alcohol are more prone to the effects. In addition, individuals with gout are affected soon.

Daily Intake of Lead

Daily intake of lead is 0.45 mg (i) 0.2-0.4 mg is taken along with the food (ii) 0.02 mg is ingested along with water (iii) 0.03 mg is taken by inhalation (iv) 0.04 mg is inhaled while smoking.

Salts of Lead that are Poisonous

(i) *Lead acetate* or sugar of lead; tastes sweet (ii) *Lead sub-acetate* (iii) *Lead carbonate* or white lead; used in oil painting. Commonly responsible for lead poisoning in children who suck and bite toys (iv) *Lead nitrate*; used in calico printing (v) *Lead sulphate*; is supposed to be non-toxic (vi) *Lead chromate* (yellow chrome); poisoning occurs from ingestion of sweets coloured with the salt (vii) *Lead chloride* is pigment, yellow oxychloride (viii) *Lead iodide* is bright yellow powder (ix) *Lead sulphide* (galena); in powder form as *soorma* (in place of Antimony sulphide) used to colour the eyes (x) *Lead monoxide* (Litharge, *Mudrasang,* Massicot); is pale brick red, used by the painters. Hair dyes also contain it (xi) *Lead tetroxide* (Read lead or *sindur*) is used as a pigment (Figure 38.1) (xii) *Lead tetraethyl:* It is an organometal compound, highly toxic, heavy, oily liquid and volatile at ordinary temperatures. It is added to the petrol to prevent it from knocking. This mixture is known as ethyl petrol or ethyl gasoline, used as a fuel for motor cars. Lead tetraethyl is absorbed by inhalation or through the intact skin. Poisoning occurs in persons engaged in the manufacturing of lead tetraethyl.

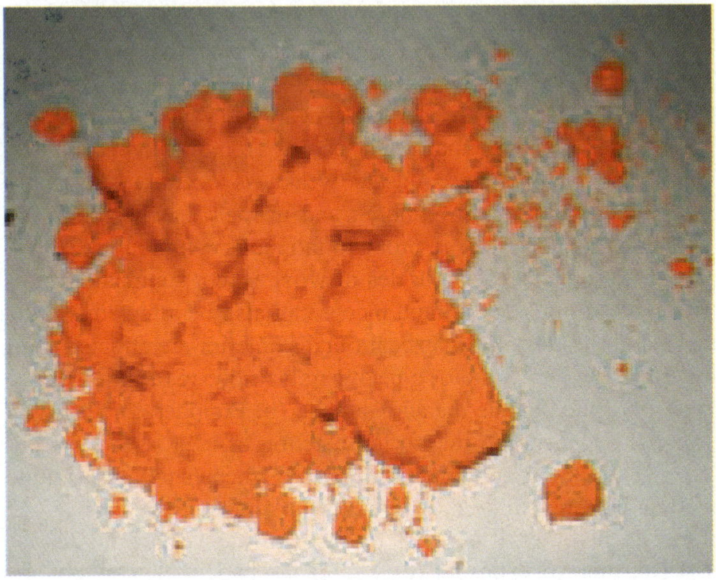

Figure 38.1: Lead tetraoxide (red lead)

The main compounds that produce poisonous symptoms are acetate, carbonate, chromate and oxides of lead.

Acute Lead Poisoning

Normally, blood contains 0.03 mg/100 ml of lead. In poisoning, the concentration of lead is usually between 0.1-0.6 mg/100 ml.

Acute poisoning is very rare and usually terminates in recovery hence it has little toxicological significance.

Acute poisoning occurs mainly *due to lead acetate*. The symptoms start immediately: (i) Metallic taste (ii) Burning sensation (iii) Dryness of throat and intense thirst (iv) Tongue is coated (v) Vomiting within half hour; vomitus is mixed with blood (vi) Nausea and colicky pain coming at intervals but relieved by pressure (vii) Constipation is a constant feature (viii) Poor appetite and weight loss (ix) Urine is scanty (x) Foul offensive breath (xi) Irritability, insomnia and excess lethargy (xii) Hyperactivity and headache (xiii) Neurological problems, such as drowsiness, insomnia, headache, vertigo, muscle cramps, convulsions and paralysis of lower limbs (xiv) In extreme cases, seizure, coma and death.

In acute poisoning by lead tetraethyl central nervous system is usually affected resulting in the signs and symptoms like irritability, convulsions, headache, delirium, low blood pressure, bradycardia and hypothermia. Sometimes nausea, vomiting, and loss of appetite occurs.

Acute lead encephalopathy: It is rare in the adults but many cases are reported in children. The clinical features include: (i) Anaemia (ii) Mild colic (iii) Vomiting (iv) Apathy (v) Drowsiness (vi) Stupor (vii) Ataxia; and (viii) Hyperactivity.

SUBACUTE POISONING

Intake of repeated small doses of a soluble salt like lead acetate results in subacute poisoning. Subacute poisoning resents as: (i) A blue line on the gums (ii) Gastrointestinal symptoms such as nausea and vomiting (iii) Face is livid and shrunken and bears an anxious look (iv) CNS symptoms are more prominent (v) Death is due to coma and convulsions within 3 days.

Fatal Dose:

- Lead acetate→20 gm.
- Lead tetraethyl→1.8-2.0 gm; usually uncertain.
- Lead carbonate→40 gm.
- Absorption of more than 0.5 mg/day.

Fatal Period:

Uncertain, usually 2-3 days.

Management

(i) Stomach wash by 1% Magnesium sulphate or Sodium sulphate or warm water and simple emetics should be administered. (ii) Whole bowel irrigation with polyethylene glycol. (iii) One ounce of magnesium sulphate to remove lead from the gastrointestinal tract. (iv) Demulcents such as milk, egg white etc. can be given. (v) Calcium gluconate 15 grain (1 grain= 0.0648 gm) I.V. for the abdominal colic. (vi) Injections of morphine should be given for severe pain. (vii) Mannitol for cerebral edema and diazepam, if patients having convulsions. (viii) Choice of chelation therapy depends upon the blood lead concentration (BLL) and clinical conditions. BAL or Calcium Disodium edetate (CaNa2EDTA) or both can be given. (ix) In case of renal failure, peritoneal or haemodialysis. (x) Symptomatic treatment.

Autopsy Findings

Findings of gastrointestinal tract irritation are usually found. (i) Intestines are contracted and thickened (ii) Stomach mucous membrane is thickened, softened and eroded at places (iii) A blue line may be visible on the gums (iv) The liver and kidneys are also contracted (v) Brain is pale and swollen (vi) Heart is hypertrophied with atheroma of aorta (vii) In the bone marrow, hyperplasia of leucoblast and erythroblasts are seen.

Chronic Lead Poisoning (Plumbism/Saturnism)

Chronic poisoning occurs with a daily intake of 1-2 mg of lead.

Sources of chronic lead poisoning: (i) Inhalation of lead dust and fumes among persons employed in factories and industries such as painters, compositors, plumbers, enamel workers, glass blowers, electric light workers and lead smelters. (ii) Drinking water stored in laden cisterns. (iii) Eating tinned food contaminated with lead. (iv) From use of ghee stored in brown or copper vessel lined inside with tin. Ghee becomes impregnated with lead derived from tin that contains it as an impurity and forms a poisonous salt (Oleate of lead). (v) Taking food cooked in lead vessels. (vi) *Absorption of lead through raw and intact skin*: Hindu married females apply *Vermillion* on the parting of scalp hair. *Vermillion* contains red lead mixed with red synthetic dye that is absorbed through the scalp. The use of hair oil helps to hold the lead in contact with scalp by forming lead soap with fatty acids of oil that favours absorption.

Signs and Symptoms

(i) **Facial pallor:** It is usually present around the mouth. It is one of the earliest and consistent signs and is independent of the degree of anaemia, seems to be due to vasospasm. (ii) **Anaemia:** Anaemia occurs at the lead level of 70-80 mg/100 ml of blood. In the early stages, polycythemia, polychromatophilia occurs and in late stages, microcytic or normocytic anaemia but not the macrocytic anaemia results. There is reticulocytosis, poikilocytosis, anisocytosis, cabot's ring and nucleated red cells are seen. The number of polymorphs and platelets is also decreased. **Punctate basophilia or basophilic stippling** is the number of discrete dark blue granules of pinhead size observed in the cytoplasm of red blood cells due to abnormal aggregated ribosomes. In lead poisoning, coarse basophilic stippling is observed as a result of precipitation of RNA secondary to pyrimidine-5′-nucleotidase inhibition. It cannot be used as a pathognomonic of lead poisoning, but provides a clue to the underlying diagnosis and an understanding of the underlying pathogenesis. It can also be seen in clinical conditions such as anemia, thalassemia, myelodysplasia, pyrimidine 5′-nucleotidase deficiency, post-chemotherapy, covid 19 patients and other heavy metal poisoning like arsenic etc. In chronic lead poisoning anaemia occurs due to: (a) Decreased life span of red cells as they are mechanically more fragile (b) Synthesis of hemoglobin is inhibited that further inhibits the action of Delta-amino-levulenic-acid dehydrogenase. (iii) **Lead line (Burtonian line/Burton's line/Burton's sign):** This clinical sign was described by Henry Burton in year 1840. It is a bluish/blue-purplish line, 1 to 2 mm wide, collar like seen at the junction of the gums and teeth due to subepithelial deposits of lead sulphide granules in chronic lead poisoning. The formation of lead sulphide (PbS) is due to the action of H_2S ($Pb_2^{+}+H_2S \rightarrow PbS+2H^{+}$), which is produced by bacterial degradation of organic material of food debris in the mouth. It is deposited in the dirty or carious teeth within a week of exposure usually in the upper jaw. It is observed only in 50-70% of patients. It is a reliable sign, but poor oral hygiene can produce a similar picture. A lead line may not be present even in severe lead poisoning if good oral hygiene is practiced. In edentulous patients a lead line is absent. There is sweetish, metallic taste in the mouth. (iv) **Colic and constipation (Dry bellyache):** It is usually a late symptom. Colic of intestine, ureter, uterus etc., occurs in 85% of the cases. It is very severe usually occurring at the night. During colic, the abdominal wall is rigid and contracted and heavy pressure results in some relief. The attack of colic lasts for few minutes **(lead colic/devonshire colic/painter's colic/saturnine colic/colica pictonum/colic of poitou).** The exact pathogenic mechanism of lead-induced abdominal colic is not known. However, three possible mechanism have been proposed (a) Changes in the visceral smooth muscle tone due to action of lead on the visceral autonomic nervous system (b) Changes in sodium transport in the small intestinal mucosa (c) Lead-induced interstitial pancreatitis. Constipation is usually present but diarrhoea and vomiting may also occur. (v) **Lead palsy:** Lead palsy is a late feature, seen usually in less than 10% cases. Tremors, hyperesthesia, numbness, cramps and muscle weakness occurs. It is more common in adults than children and in men than women. The muscle group that is more prone to fatigue is commonly affected. These are the extensor muscles of wrist except supinator longus **(wrist drop)** but deltoid and biceps can also be affected. All the extensor muscles of foot except tibialis anterior are affected **(foot drop)**. It is a purely motor type of paralysis due to (a) Interference with phosphocreatine metabolism and (b) Peripheral neuropathy (axonal degeneration due to toxic action of lead in the anterior horn cells). (vi) **Lead encephalopathy:** Encephalopathy is quite common in the children. It is present in almost every case in one form or the other. It depends on the: (a) Intensity of the disease (b) Duration of exposure (c) Age of the patient. The symptoms of lead encephalopathy are insomnia, headache, vomiting, restlessness, delirium, hallucinations, convulsions and coma develops after the nervous symptoms and finally the death. (vii) **Cardiovascular and renal symptoms:** Lead causes vascular constriction that results in hypertension, arteriolar degeneration, chronic arteriosclerotic nephritis, interstitial nephritis. (viii) **Coproporphyrin III:** In non-exposed individuals coporphyrin is less than 150 mg/l in urine. It is detected as reddish fluorescence when seen under U-V lamp; when a mixture of small quantity of urine, few drops of glacial acetic acid and equal quantities of ether are taken. (ix) **Reproductive system:** Menstrual derangements, sterility, abortion at 3-6 months and foetal abnormalities may occur. (x) **Visual system:** Lead pigments deposited in the retina **(retinal stippling)** which is an early sign of lead intoxication. Lead can cause optic neuropathy. (xi) **Other symptoms:** Other symptoms like anorexia, emaciation, alopecia, vertigo etc. may develop.

Diagnosis

1. Careful and detailed history regarding the nature of work to be taken.
2. **Blood levels:** Blood lead level (BLL) is measured in micrograms of lead per deciliter of venous blood (μg/dl). BLL is used to guide management and treatment decisions. Nearly everyone has a measurable BLL.

   Adult: Elevated BLL for an adult is now defined as ≥ 5 μg/dl by the National Institute for Occupational Safety and Health (NIOSH)/CDC's Adult Blood Lead Epidemiology and Surveillance (ABLES) program. The reference BLL was lowered from the previous level of >10 μg/dl. BLL between 40 and 79 μg/dl should be referred for prompt medical evaluation. When BLL is more than 80 μg/dl, urgent medical evaluation for probable chelating therapy is indicated. For BLL ≥ 100 μg/dl, chelating therapy is always necessary. The US Department of Health and Human Services recommends that BLL among all adults be reduced to <10 μg/dl.

   Children: In children, BLL ≥ 5 μg/dl is considered as elevated which requires further testing and monitoring. The CDC subcommittee on lead poisoning prevention has recently recommended to CDC that the reference value for blood lead in children be revised to 3.5 μg/dl. Chelation therapy may be considered with a level as low as 20 μg/dl. However, in case of BLL ≥ 45 μg/dl, chelation treatment should always be considered. Children should be hospitalized for parenteral treatment if BLL ≥ 70 μg/dl.
3. **Urine levels:** (i) In a 24-hour urine sample, an excretion of more than 0.08 mg/l is significant. On examination of urine: (a) Coproporphyrin level more than 0.15 mg/24 hrs are suggestive of lead exposure (b) δ-Amino-levulenic acid > 6 mg/l has some lead effects (c) δ-Amino-levulenic acid > 19 mg/l leads to lead poisoning (ii) Glycosuria, haematuria, proteinuria occurs. (iii) Urinary excretion of more than 1 μg of lead/mg of calcium edetate occurs after I.M. administration of calcium edetate at 25 mg/kg but not exceeding a total of 1 gm.
4. **Spinal fluid:** Spinal fluid analysis should be avoided unless it is quite essential. The pressure is raised with increased proteins and pleocytosis.
5. **X-ray findings:** Radiological examination shows transverse bands of increased density at the growing, i.e., metaphyseal ends of the bones in the children 2-5 years old mainly **(lead lines).** Multiple bands suggest repeated episodes of exposure. Abdominal X-ray shows opaque particles at the rectosigmoid area.

Tests for Lead

(i) *Qualitative test:* These are the color test which can be used (a) **Hydrochloric Acid Test:** One ml of dilute HCL is added to 1ml of test solution. A white precipitate is obtained which dissolves on boiling and reappears on cooling indicates the presence of lead. (b) **Potassium Iodide Test** (c) **Bicarbonate Test** (d) **Dithizone Test** (ii) *Quantitative test:* These techniques can be used for quantitative estimation of lead. (a) **ICP-MS** (Inductively Coupled Plasma-Mass Spectrometry) (b) Laser-induced breakdown spectroscopy **(LIBS).**

Treatment

(i) Remove the individual from the source of exposure.

(ii) Potassium or sodium iodide 1-2 gm thrice daily for 5-7 days to assist in the elimination of lead by the kidneys.

(iii) Sodium bicarbonate 20-30 G/day for 4-5 doses leads to transformation of tribasic lead phosphate to soluble dibasic phosphate and carbonic acid is liberated.

(iv) Magnesium sulfate or sodium sulfate 8-12 gm orally.

(v) **De-leading:** Body lead is stored in bones as triple phosphates and poisoning does not occur so long as the metal is immobilized and blood content of lead remains low. Therefore, in first two days: (a) High calorie diet including 3 pints of milk daily and calcium gluconate are administered. All these lead to alkalosis that lead is fixed in the bones and the symptoms are relieved then de-leading is done. (b) Low calorie diet like potato, rice and bread (no milk, egg or vegetables) are added. (c) Mild acidosis is induced with: (1) Ammonium chloride 8-12 gm/day and (2) Dilute phosphoric acid 4 ml, 6 times/day.

The de-leading is carried by: (a) *Correction of acidosis*: They become soluble, flow into blood stream and excreted in normal manner but an attack of plumbism may occur. (b) *Correction of alkalosis*: They tend to fix the lead in the bones so formerly the principle was to correct acidosis, thus lead is immobilized.

This method is replaced by chelating agents.

(vi) Chelating agents:

B.A.L.: The recommended dose for B.A.L. is 4 mg/kg body weight to be injected deep IM, every 4 hours for at least

3 days. It chelates lead both extracellularly and intracellularly. Two molecules of B.A.L. combine with one atom of lead to form a complex that is excreted in the bile and urine. B.A.L. is the chelator of choice in conditions of impaired renal function. It is only indicated when BLL ≥ 70 μg/dl. It is recommended as an agent of first choice for patients with lead encephalopathy. It is given in combination with CaNa2 EDTA for the treatment of lead encephalopathy. B.A.L. should be given at least 4 hours before CaNa2 EDTA as the latter mobilizes lead from tissue stores and aggravates symptoms of lead poisoning.

Derivatives of EDTA: Ethylene-diamine-tetra-acetic acid (Edetic Acid), Calcium or sodium edetate are used. For therapeutic use, calcium disodium versenate is used. Lead is one of the metal for which calcium disodium edetate has a great affinity. Calcium disodium versenate acts as an ion exchanger in which the calcium is exchanged for the heavy metal ion and a soluble, stable and unionized chelate of lead is formed that is excreted in the urine as lead ethylene-diamine-tetra-acetate. The complex is stable and is a less toxic molecule. The rate of excretion of lead as the EDTA complex in the urine increases fifty times above the normal untreated excretion rate. Therefore, chelation therapy serves to detoxify lead, withdraws it from effector sites and promotes excretion. Calcium disodium Edetate (CaNa2EDTA) only removes extracellular lead, and its effectiveness increases when used in combination with BAL. It should not be used alone in patients manifesting with lead encephalopathy, because it does not cross the blood-brain barrier and can potentially lead to exacerbation of lead encephalopathy. It is the preferred chelating agent in pregnancy but is a second line therapy for BLL ≤ 70 μg/dl.

Dose: EDTA 5 ml of 20% solution (15 grains) is diluted with 250-500 ml of normal saline or 500 ml of 5% glucose; the concentration should not exceed 3% and is given by I.V. drip over a period of 2 hours twice daily for 5 days. Then after a gap of 3-5 days, repeat the course for 5 days or calcium EDTA can be given 50 mg/kg/24 hours I.M. or I.V. for 5 days.

Side effects: The daily dose should not exceed 220 mg/kg in 12 hours and 75 mg/kg every 6-12 hours. The side effects that are produced are lacrymation, nasal congestion, sneezing, muscle pain, hypotension and chronic renal damage.

Penicillamine: It is another chelating agent that is effective in the excretion of lead by oral administration and is also useful in children. It is a degradation product excreted in the urine when patients with liver damage receive injections of penicillin. Commercially it is obtained by controlled decomposition of penicillin. It is at present very expensive. It is given orally in the doses of 0.6 to 1.5 gm daily in two equal doses for 7 days. It can be administered intravenously as 1-3 gm solutions in normal saline drip for 2-4 days. This increases the urinary excretion of lead. However, it is a third line chelating agent for lead poisoning, however, it is not approved by the US Food and Drug Administration (FDA).

DMSA/Succimer: It is an analogue of BAL approved by US Food and Drug Administration for oral use. It is the first choice for the treatment of children with mild and asymptomatic lead poisoning who have BLL ≥ 45 μg/dl. 100 mg capsules of DMSA are administered at 10 mg/kg (350 mg/m^2) every 8 hours for 5 days followed by same dose every 12 hours for 14 days.

(vi) N-acetylcysteine (NAC) is also considered as an antioxidant chelator.

(vii) **Dietary management:** Vitamin C, B_1 and B_6 has proved to be effective against lead toxicity. Essential metals such as zinc, calcium or iron can provide protective effects against lead intoxication. However, iron supplementation needs to be withdrawn during chelation therapy. Alpha-lipoic acid, methionine, homocysteine are other sulfur-containing compounds can reduce oxidative stress in lead poisoning.

(viii) Necessary measures are taken to prevent deposition of lead in the skeleton. This includes administration of diets such as plenty of milk or calcium chloride. Besides this, alkalosis is to be induced.

(ix) Mannitol is given to reduce cerebral edema and diazepam is given for the seizures in lead encephalopathy

Prophylactic treatment in chronic poisoning: (i) Adequate exhaust ventilation in factories (ii) Personal cleaniness should be employed (iii) The workers should take a diet rich in calories and plenty of milk (iv) Water containing minute quantities of sulphuric acid (v) Saline purgatives should be given (vi) Periodical medical examination of the staff working in lead factories.

Autopsy Findings

(i) Blue line on the gums at their junction with the teeth (ii) Fatty degeneration of paralysed limbs (iii) Stomach and intestine show ulceration and haemorrhages and the walls are contracted (iv) Liver and kidneys are contracted and show granular degeneration (v) Heart is hypertrophied and shows atheromatous changes.

Medicolegal Aspects

(i) Metallic forms are not poisonous, but when acted upon by secretions of the intestine and may act as a poison after being absorbed into the system as a salt that are poisonous. (ii) Compounds of lead are poisonous provided they are in a condition fit for absorption. In the absence of air, pure water has no action on lead, but in the presence of air, it is slightly soluble and lead hydroxide is formed. (iii) Chronic lead poisoning is regarded as one of the industrial diseases. (iv) Acute lead poisoning is very rare, when it occurs, recovery usually occurs. (v) In chronic poisoning, workers are referred to medical practitioners under 'Workman's Compensation Act 1923 so that next of kin gets compensation, if death occurs. (vi) Homicide by lead is rare as very few cases are reported when lead acetate is mixed with beer. (vii) Accidental poisoning occurs by use of *Litharge (Mudrasang)* (lead monoxide) as a remedy for syphilis by quacks. (viii) Used criminally as abortifacient, the paste used on abortion stick contains red lead or lead tetra oxide. (ix) Red lead alone or when mixed with Arsenic is used as a cattle poison. (x) It is used as to adulterate *snuff* to improve its colour. (xi) Lead is normally present in all human tissue, deposited in the bones, nail, tooth and hair. No lead is found in ovary but is present in the testes. It has got no affinity for fetal tissues. (xii) Accidental poisoning occurs in children by eating pica, old paint, plaster; feeding bottles made of glass contain lead, lead nipple shields, toys and street dirt. (xiii) Cosmetics like face powders, hair dyes used by the mothers secreted in the milk can cause accidental poisoning in the children.

ARSENIC

Arsenic is a metallic poison known since ancient times. The Greeks knew it as early as 500 B.C. and Hippocrates used it as an external remedy for ulcers, although there is no record of it being used as a poison this early. An eight-century Arab alchemist **Jabir ibn Hayyen** was the first to obtain white arsenic by heating realgar. It is thought that it was around this time when criminals first employed arsenic as a poison. Before white arsenic was known, most of the poisons used had a distinguishing taste, smell or colour but arsenic has very little smell or taste so it is undetectable by the victim. Arsenic often referred as the **"Poison of Kings" or "King of poisons"** because of its potency and the discreteness, by which it could be administered, particularly with the intent of removing members of the ruling class. It is believed that Napoleon Bonaparte was poisoned with arsenic as a part of political assassination It is the common environmental toxicant and is found in soil, water and air. It ranks 20th in elemental abundance in earth's crust and 12th in the human body.

PROPERTIES OF ARSENIC

Arsenic is element 33 in the periodic table and is classically considered a heavy metal. It exists in 3 allotropic forms and in several ionic forms. Environmental arsenic exists mainly as sulphide complexes realgar (As_2S_2), Orpiment (As_2S_3) and iron pyrites. On heating of these ores, arsenic sublimes and oxidizes to form arsenic trioxide (As_2O_3) a fine granular white powder also known as white arsenic. Arsine gas (AsH_3) is another arsenic compound, formed by the hydrolysis of metal arsenides and by the reduction of metals of arsenic compounds in acidic solutions. The main source of Arsenic is Arsenopyrites, realgar (Arsenic di-sulphide, As_2S_2) orpiment (Arsenic trisulphide, As_2S_3) and Arsenolite (Arsenic trioxide, As_2O_3). It is usually obtained as a byproduct from smelting of copper, lead, zinc and ether.

Natural sources of arsenic: The average daily intake of arsenic in adults is 0.5-0.1 mg. Arsenic is a widely distributed element and is found in: (i) Rocks and soil in concentrations of less than 1 ppm. (ii) Hot spring mineral waters. (iii) Drinking water supply. (iv) Seawater contains 2-5 mg/l. (v) Plant and plant products. (vi) Vegetables, fruits and grains. (vii) Seafood (Fish, Shellfish, crabs and Dover-sole) and meats. Marine organisms particularly shellfish may contain large amounts of well-absorbed trimethylated organoarsenic, arsenobentaine that exerts no known toxic effects when ingested by mammals and is excreted unchanged in the urine. (viii) Arsenilic acid has been used as a food additive for poultry and other livestock to promote growth and weight gain. The poisoning may result from regular consumption of such products but at times accidental poisoning of livestock has occurred. There are instances of Beef or cattle being poisoned by ingestion of field grass that has been previously sprayed by herbicides. The interaction of Arsenicals with bacteria is thought to account for the changes in the oxidation state and chemical form of arsenic.

Industrial sources of arsenic: Arsenic is used primarily in the production of glass and semiconductors, in wood and hide preservation, as an additive to metal alloys to increase hardening and heat resistance. In the past Arsenic was used as weed killer, rodenticide, in chemical warfare and in the production of pigments and enamels.

Arsenic may be introduced into the environment through (i) Industrial process such as smelting of other metals (ii) Application of arsenical pesticides and herbicides (iii) Generation of power from coal (iv) Geothermal sources (v) Coal and combustion of coal.

In the metallic form Arsenic is not poisonous as it is insoluble in water and cannot be absorbed from alimentary tract, but when it is oxidized by exposure to air it becomes poisonous. But some workers believe that the metallic form may undergo oxidation in the GIT producing symptoms.

Compounds of arsenic (Figure 38.2): The compounds of arsenic are organic as well as inorganic. The inorganic compounds are Arsenate (AS^{5+}) and Arsenite (AS^{3+}): (i) *Arsenious oxide or* **Arsenious trioxide (As_2O_3):** It is a heavy metal with a specific gravity 3.669. Its curious property is that it floats in water as a white film and is soluble in spirit. It is found as impurity in iron ores and mineral acids. It is also found in soils, mineral water and coal smoke. It is widely used in: (a) Calico-printing (b) Taxidermy (preparing, mounting skin of animals) (c) Preparation

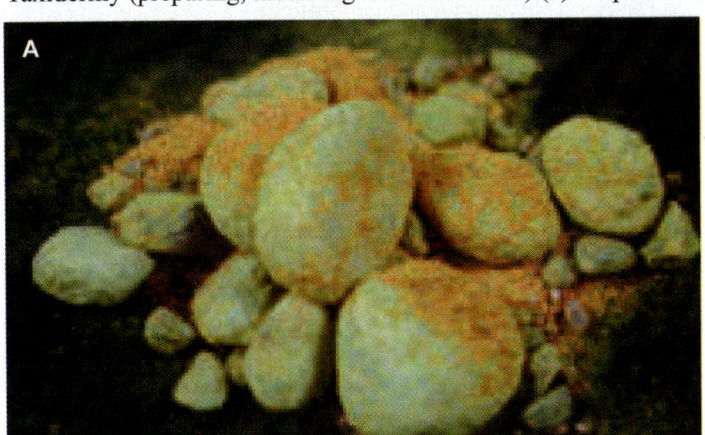

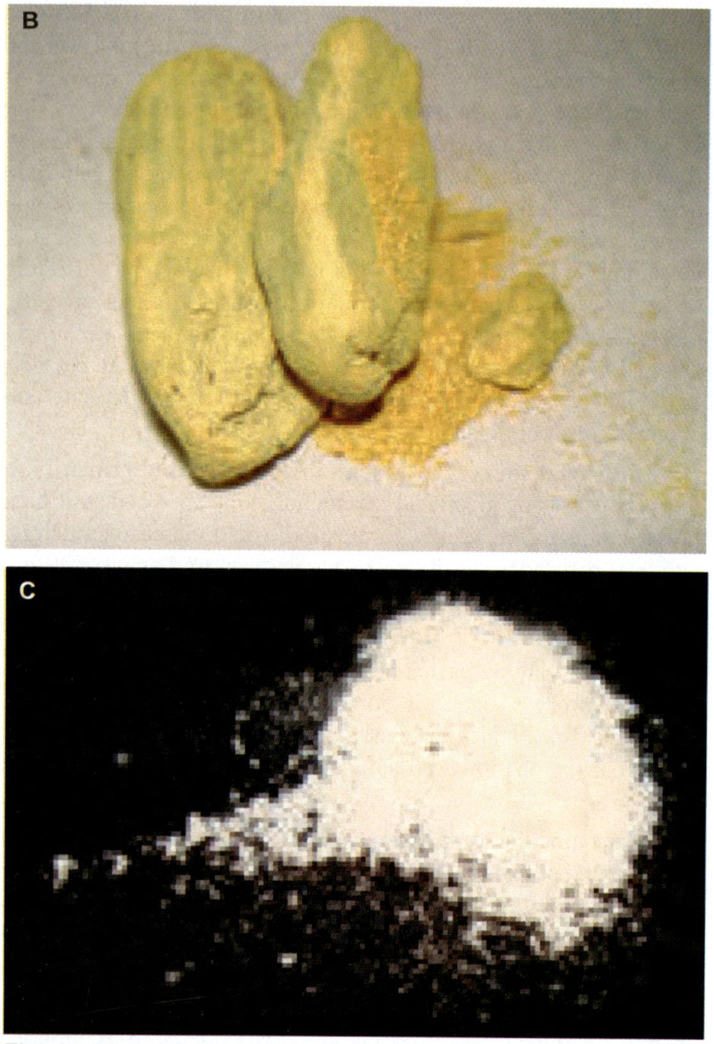

Figure 38.2: Compounds of Arsenic (A) Arsenic disulphide (B) Arsenic trisulphide (C) Arsenious oxide

of artificial flowers (d) Wall papers preparation (e) Preservation of timber and skin against ants (f) By *Hakims* and *Vaidhs* to treat rheumatism, skin diseases, syphilis and impotence. (ii) Copper Arsenite (Scheel's green, Paris green). (iii) Red Arsenic (Arsenic disulphide). (iv) Yellow Arsenic (Arsenic trisulphide). (v) Arsine gas (AsH_3) (is hemolytic and nephrotoxic).

Organo-chemicals: Many organo-chemicals ranging in toxicity from the war gas Lewisite to lead additives such as Arsenilic acid. In general their toxicity is similar to that of inorganic ones. These are: (i) Cacodylic acid (ii) Sodium cacodylate (iii) Atoxyl (iv) Salvarsan (v) Neo salvarsan.

Pharmacokinetics and general toxicity of Arsenicals: Arsenic can be inhaled and absorbed through the skin or through GI tract after ingestion. After a very small dose of arsenic (like that experienced daily by most people) most of the absorbed inorganic arsenic undergoes methylation, mainly in liver to monomethylarsonic acid and dimethylarsinic acid, which are excreted along with residual inorganic arsenic in the urine. However, if the dose of arsenic is very large, the elimination half-life is prolonged. Once absorbed, arsenic rapidly combines with the globin portion of haemoglobin and therefore localizes in the blood. There is minimal penetration of the blood-brain barrier and within 24 hours arsenic redistributes itself to the liver, kidney, spleen, lung and GI tract, with lesser accumulation in muscle and nervous tissue. Once in the tissues, arsenic exerts its toxic effect through several mechanisms, the most significant of which is the reversible combination with sulphydryl groups. Arsenic **blocks the Krebs cycle** and interrupts oxidative phosphorylation thus resulting in a marked depletion of cellular ATP and eventually death of the metabolizing cell. Arsenic also inhibits transformation of thiamine into acetyl CoA and succinyl-CoA resulting in the features of thiamine deficiency. **Arsenolysis** is a major form of toxicity in which the arsenic anions can substitute for phosphate in many reactions. Arsenic is capable of inhibiting oxidative phosphorylation through two different mechanisms. 2-4 weeks after ingestion, arsenic is incorporated into hair, nails and skin as it binds to the sulphydryl groups of keratin. Four weeks after ingestion, arsenic begins to localize in the bone where it substitutes for phosphate.

The toxicity is related to: (i) *How fast it is excreted from the system:* The inorganic forms are more toxic than the organic forms and the trivalent forms are more toxic than the pentavalent forms depending on their rapidity of excretion as organic arsenicals are more rapidly excreted than the inorganic form and pentavalent forms are cleared faster than trivalent form. (ii) *To what degree it may accumulate in the tissues:* Pentavalent forms are accumulated more rapidly than the trivalent forms which is approximately in the reverse order of excretion.

Arsine gas (AsH_3) causes rapid haemolysis and renal damage may persist for years following single acute poisoning. Arsenite is absorbed from GIT and retained in high levels in the tissues.

MECHANISM OF ACTION

The mechanism of toxicity of all arsenic compounds is the same. Once in the tissues, arsenic exerts its toxic effect through several mechanisms such as: (i) Reversible combination with sulphydryl groups (ii) Reacts with SH group in tissue proteins (iii) Interferes with number of enzyme system essential for cellular metabolism (iv) It is a capillary poison, dilates capillary (v) Fatty degeneration of liver (vi) Hyperemia and haemorrhages in the intestine (vii) Renal tubular necrosis (viii) Peripheral nerves show disintegration of axis cylinder (axonal neuropathy) with fragmentation and resorption of myelin.

Fatal Dose: The fatal dose of arsenic trioxide is 180 mg but the dose depends on the compound ingested, its physical form and the inherent tolerance of the patient to arsenic. A pinch weighing 20 grams can kill 8-10 persons.

Fatal Period: Fatal period for arsenic poisoning is 12-48 hours but can be fatal even within 2-3 hours.

The poisoning due to arsenic compounds can be acute, subacute and chronic.

Signs and Symptoms of Acute Poisoning

The acute arsenic poisoning results from the: (i) Oral ingestion (ii) Inhalation of arsenic gas (iii) Rubbing into the skin (iv) Introduction into rectum or vagina. Arsenic poisoning is usually the result of accidental or suicidal ingestion of insecticides; (Paris green) that is copper arsenite or calcium or lead arsenate. Pesticides containing arsenic are freshest source of poisoning.

The toxic symptoms of acute arsenic poisoning depends upon individual susceptibility. **Orchardists** can ingest 6.8 mg/day without any signs and symptoms but arsenic trioxide as low as 30 mg has been found fatal. This extraordinary degree of tolerance to ingestion of arsenic could be due to blockage of absorption, alteration in its distribution to tissues, enhanced or accelerated transformation of arsenite to less toxic arsenate, and decreased reduction of arsenate to arsenite by peripheral tissues.

The signs and symptoms start within half an hour but may be delayed for several hours when it is given in rectum, vagina or skin. The dilatation of capillaries is responsible for most of the symptom: (i) Initially the patient experiences a metallic taste in the mouth and slight garlicky odour in the breath along with xerostomia and dysphagia. (ii) Stomach pain which may increase on pressure. (iii) Increased salivation and intense thirst. (iv) This is followed abruptly by severe nausea and vomiting, colicky abdominal pain and profuse diarrhoea. The stools are dark coloured and bloody and later on are colourless, odourless and watery which changes to rice watery due to vasodilation with transudation of fluid into the bowel lumen in addition to mucosal vesicle formation and sloughing leading to increased peristalsis. Vomiting is projectile, dark brown or yellow in colour and contains stomach contents, blood and mucus due to capillary transudation of plasma following rupture of vesicles under intestinal mucosa. (v) Purging, tenesmus, pain and irritation around anus. (vi) Generalised vasodilation caused by capillary damage results in transudation of plasma and severe hypovolemia. (vii) If the ingested dose is smaller, the patient will have severe headache, vertigo, periorbital oedema, skeletal muscle cramping and evidence of renal damage manifested as oliguria, proteinuria, and haematuria. (viii) If the dose of arsenic ingested is large, cyanosis, cold clammy extremities, hypoxic encephalopathy, convulsions and acute tubular necrosis may occur following shock. (ix) Hyperpyrexia and acute haemolysis may also occur. (x) Face is pale and anxious. (xi) Eyes are shrunken. (xii) Pulse is irregular and quick. (xiii) Respiration is laboured. (xiv) Hypoxia, convulsions and coma precede death. (xv) If death does not occur in the first few hours from shock, patient may die a few days later from acute hepatic or renal failure. (xvi) Cirrhosis and ascites results from the therapeutic doses of Flower's solution (1% Arsenious trioxide). (xvii) The cardiac symptoms are due to decreased cardiac output due to hypovolaemia and direct toxic effect on the cardiac muscle. Cardiac manifestations include acute cardiomyopathy, subendocardial haemorrhages, and ECG changes (T-wave inversion and persistent prolongation of QT interval). (xviii) Arsenic has a predilection for keratin that is why the concentration is higher in hair and nails. The signs and symptoms of acute arsenic poisoning should be differentiated from Cholera (Table 38.1).

Table 38.1: Differential diagnosis of acute arsenic poisoning

Findings	Arsenic poisoning	Cholera
Pain in throat	Present before vomiting	Present after vomiting
Purging	Follows vomiting	Precedes vomiting
Vomitus	Consists of mucous bile and blood	Watery
Stools	High coloured, discharged with straining and tenesmus	Rice water and involuntary
Voice	Not affected	Peculiar and rough
Conjunctiva	Inflamed	Not inflamed

Narcotic form: It produces mainly CNS symptoms such as: (i) Giddiness (ii) Precordial distress (iii) Tenderness of muscles (iv) Delirium (v) Dilated pupils and complete paralysis of muscles at times. Unusual symptoms such as (i) Convulsions (ii) Lockjaw (iii) Raised temperature (iv) Loss of speech and memory (v) Joint pains can also be produced.

Arsine gas: Arsine gas acts as a poison to haemoglobin and causes haemolysis. It most commonly produces hemoglobinuria and anaemia. The other symptoms produced as a result of poisoning are jaundice, dark red urine, heart failure, delirium and coma.

Arsine dust: When arsine dust is inhaled, it causes cough with frothy sputum, pulmonary oedema, cyanosis, breathlessness, corneal ulcer and conjunctivitis.

SUBACUTE POISONING

Subacute poisoning results when the compounds of arsenic are given in small doses at repeated intervals. The signs and symptoms that are produced are dysphagia, cough, foul smelling tongue that is dry and congested and the motions are bloody.

Laboratory Findings

Diagnosis: Definitive diagnosis of arsenic poisoning is difficult because of the natural presence of trace amounts of arsenic in the body and because, due to the multi systemic toxicity of arsenic, the clinical manifestations vary widely so both acute and chronic poisoning simulate many other diseases and be overlooked in the differential diagnosis. Diagnosis is often particularly difficult in homicidal poisoning attempts because the patient will not usually know that he/she has ingested arsenic. As arsenic is widely distributed in nature, their presence may not always indicate the poisoning. (i) **Urine:** Normal value of arsenic is 0.01-0.06 mg/litre of urine and it may be even upto 0.2 mg/litre. Most patients with exposure have more than 0.1 mg/litre (upto 1 mg/litre) of urine. Proteinuria, casts and albuminuria are there. Arsenic poisoning is usually diagnosed with a urine test for arsenic since monomethylarsine and dimethylarsine are present in the urine 24 hours after ingestion and arsenic ions are present very shortly after ingestion (useful for diagnosis of acute poisoning). A urinary excretion of arsenic >200 mg/24 hr is regarded as indicative of exposure to a potentially toxic amount of arsenic. (ii) **Blood:** The normal blood level is 100 mg/litre. There is moderate anaemia and leucopenia (2000-5000 mm^3) except. Arsine poisoning that causes leukocytosis and mild eosinophilia. (iii) **Liver function tests:** There is failure to excrete bilirubin, decreased metabolism of protein. Serum alkaline phosphatase and bilirubin is raised and there is excretion of urobilinogen in the urine. (iv) **Gastric contents** can also be screened for arsenic and, if it is very soon after ingestion a blood test will also reveal arsenic. (v) **Hair and nails:** Analysis of body tissues, nails and hair is important in diagnosis of chronic arsenic ingestion. Colorimetry, polarography, atomic absorption spectroscopy and neutron activation analysis are effective methods for arsenic detection. Hair and nail samples containing >3 ppm or 100 mg of arsenic per 100 g of specimen are diagnostic of arsenic poisoning. In normal persons, average concentration is 0.05/100 gm of hair but more than 1 mg/100 gm indicates poisoning. Analysis of hair is often used many years after death to determine the cause of death. This is how the true cause of death (chronic arsenic poisoning) of Napoleon Bonaparte was determined 140 years after he died **(Weider, 1999).** (vi) **CSF analysis** is normal. (vii) **Reinsch test:** This test was developed by Hugo Reinsch. This test is done for the metals like arsenic, mercury, antimony and bismuth. 20 ml of stomach contents (vomitus or urine or dissolved powder of suspected material) is taken. It is placed in a conical flask alongwith 4 ml hydrochloric acid. A small strip or coil of copper is added. This strip or coil is then removed and examined for the colour of the deposit as silvery (mercury) or black (arsenic, antimony or bismuth). The last three metals can be distinguished by placing copper in 2 ml of 10% potassium cyanide and observe for dissolving of the deposit. If it dissolves, it is arsenic and remains undissolved in antimony or bismuth. (viii) **Gutzeit test.** (ix) **Marsh Berzelus test:** This test was developed by James Marsh in 1836 and was later modified by Berzedius. Hydrogen is generated in a hydrogen generator by zinc (free of traces of arsenic) and dilute sulphuric acid. The sample that is suspected to contain arsenic is introduced in this generator. If arsenic is present, arseniuretted hydrogen or arsine gas is produced as: $2As + 3H_2 \rightarrow 2AsH_3$. This gas is made to eject through a narrow tube that is heated. As it comes out in a jet, it is ignited. The flame is then cooled by placing a piece of cold porcelain in this flame. Arsine is decomposed back to arsenic and hydrogen, forming a brownish-black film of arsenic in a cold zone. The reaction being $2AsH_3 \rightarrow 2As + 3H_2$.

Treatment

(i) Empty stomach by emetics (tartar emetics should not be used). Copper sulphate also should not be used as it leads to the formation of copper arsenite. (ii) Stomach wash should be done with freshly prepared solution of ferric oxide in tablespoonful doses suspended in water; with arsenious acid it forms ferric arsenite that is a harmless and insoluble salt. Ferric chloride (45 ml) and sodium carbonate or magnesium oxide (15 gm) in half glass of water, strained through muslin is used for the lavage. Following reaction occurs: $FeCl3 + MgO \rightarrow Fe_2O_3 + MgCl_2$. (iii) For gastric lavage, 1% sodium thiosulphate in water is helpful. (iv) Dialysed iron may be used as a substitute. (v) 10% solution of sodium thiosulphate as 7½ gm I.V. injection is given but it is of doubtful value. (vi) British Anti Lewsite (B.A.L.) is administered 4 hourly for 2 days, 6 hourly for 1 day and total dose 12 hourly afterwards; total dose is 2.5-3 mg/kg body weight. The duration of B.A.L. depends upon clinical state response of the patient. B.A.L. is to be stopped if side effects like nausea, vomiting, burning sensation in the mouth, tachycardia, hypotension, constriction in the throat appear. (vii) DMPS 3 to 5 mg/kg, given IM every 4 hours administered as 5% solution for 2 days followed by Succimer or 3 to 5mg/kg IM every 6 to 12 hours. (viii) Oral Succimer given 10 mg/kg every 8 hours for 5 days followed by 10 mg/kg every 12 hours. (ix) To know when the chelation is to be stopped, 24 hours urine sample is to be collected and if Arsenic levels fall below 50 mg/24 hours, it should be stopped for 5 days and then started again so that the tissue arsenic is mobilized and ready for chelation. (x) Oral Penicillamine 100 mg/kg body weight in four divided doses is given in 24 hours for 4-8 days after initial 12-48 hours of B.A.L. therapy. (xi) Demulcents such as ghee and barley water are given. (xii) Castor oil or magnesium sulphate is administered to diminish intestinal absorption of arsenic. (xiii) Morphine is given to relieve pain. (xiv) Saline is administered intravenously for dehydration and enuresis. (xv) To relieve cramps, massage is employed. (xvi) Body temperature is to be maintained.

Treatment of poisoning by arsine gas: (i) Patient to be taken to fresh air (ii) Oxygen inhalation to be started (iii) Exchange transfusion should be undertaken (iv) Haemodialysis is ensued (v) Alkaline drinks are given. All of the above methods help to eliminate arsine from the blood. B.A.L. is not effective in arsenic gas poisoning.

Autopsy Findings

(i) Rigor mortis lasts longer. (ii) General shrunken appearance due to dehydration. (iii) Eyeballs are shrunken. (iv) Cyanosis of hands and feet is there. (v) Jaundice is also present. (vi) Mucous membrane of mouth and pharynx is inflamed and ulcerated. (vii) Stomach is the main organ to be inflamed; food particles are mixed with arsenic embedded in the mucous. The inner wall of the stomach is swollen, congested and tinged with streaks of blood and arsenic. On scraping the mucous membrane is congested inflamed and is brownish red or scarlet in color. The inflammation is more marked in the greater curvature and the cardiac end. Petechial hemorrhages are seen over the mucosa. Sub serosal haemorrhage also seen which may be extended into muscular and submucosal layer. The gross appearance of stomach mucosa is described as that of **red velvet like.** Ulceration, gangrene and perforation have been rarely reported. (viii) Small intestine is flabby and contains large flakes of mucous with little faecal matter, submucosal haemorrhages are present and the epithelium is flabby and oedematous. (ix) Large intestine contains seromucous and the intestinal glands are swollen and enlarged. (x) Lungs are congested, oedematous and show subpleural ecchymosis. (xi) Caecum and rectum are inflamed and the mucous membrane is flabby. (xii) Liver, spleen and kidney is enlarged and congested and shows fatty infiltration and degeneration. (xiii) Heart contains coagulated blood and ecchymosis of the endocardium and muscles of the left ventricle is there. (xiv) Brain is congested and ventricles are full of serum.

Autopsy findings in arsine gas poisoning: (i) Skin is dirty yellow in colour. (ii) Mucous membrane of stomach and intestine is yellow and inflamed. (iii) Liver is small or enlarged and shows fatty degeneration. (iv) Spleen shows evidence of destruction of blood and deposition of blood pigment throughout the organ. (v) Kidney is enlarged, congested and shows tubular necrosis. (vi) Lungs are congested and oedematous.

CHRONIC ARSENIC POISONING

This is much more insidious and the diagnosis is often difficult to establish. Chronic arsenic poisoning results from chronic repetitive inhalation of arsine gas or chronic repetitive ingestion by (i) Persons engaged in the occupation of: (a) Smeltering that is extraction of metals from ore by melting (b) Refining of ores (c) Manufacture of weed killers, insecticides, paints, dyes and cosmetics. (ii) Persons who ingest it as medicine for long periods. (iii) May follow the acute poisoning after recovery.

When the dose is not large enough to kill the patient, a number of secondary effects can be seen 2-4 weeks after ingestion of the poison. Patients who recover from the acute form of poisoning develop (i) Skin and mucosal changes. (ii) Peripheral neuropathy. (iii) Linear pigmentation in the fingers. (iv) Cutaneous manifestations appear within 1-4 weeks and consist of dry, diffuse and scaly desquamation with hyperpigmentation over the trunk and extremities and hyperkeratosis of palm and soles. (v) Mucosal surfaces also show signs of irritation like conjunctivitis, photophobia and pharyngitis. (vi) After 5 weeks, transverse white streaks 1-2 mm width appears above base of each fingernail called **Aldrich-Mee's line.** Those who have more than one exposure may show double line, several millimeters apart. (vii) After 1-3 weeks, features of peripheral neuropathy like decreased sensations of touch, pain and temperature appear in a symmetrical fashion. There is 'glove and stocking' distribution. There is distal weakness resulting in wrist drop, inability to walk, decreased distal reflexes and atrophy of muscles. Chronic poisoning consists of the following stages:

First stage: The following symptoms are produced in the first stage: (i) Loss of weight (ii) Loss of appetite and salivation (iii) Colicky pain and constipation (iv) Vomiting and diarrhoea (v) Gums are red and soft (vi) Tongue is coated, is thin white silvery and furred (vii) Oedema of eyelids and ankles (viii) Temperature and pulse is raised.

Second stage: In the second stage of chronic poisoning following symptoms are produced: (i) Catarrh of larynx and bronchial tube (ii) Dryness and itching of skin (iii) Voice is hoarse and husky (iv) Photophobia and conjunctivitis (v) Running nose and coryza (vi) Cough with bloody expectoration (vii) Liver is enlarged and cirrhotic (viii) Kidneys are damaged (ix) Prominent changes are produced in the skin: (a) Earliest cutaneous manifestation is persistent erythematous flushing caused by cutaneous capillary dilation (**"milk and roses" appearance of skin**) (b) Generalized or localized, **rain drop type of pigmentation** of the skin involving the covered parts of the body such as flexors, nipples, lower abdomen, temples and eyelids. This can be differentiated from Addison's disease as mucous membrane of the mouth is spared (c) Epithelial hyperplasia, discrete multiple wart like keratosis on the palm, soles, head and trunk (Basal cell carcinoma—Bowen's disease) (d) Hyperkeratosis then occurs with desquamation of the palms and soles (e) Epitheliomata are present in 20% of the cases (f) Nails are brittle with linear pigmentation. These include hair loss, **Aldrich-Mee's lines** (white transverse lines seen on the nail plate up to a year after arsenic intoxication) (g) Hairs are dry and there is patchy or diffuse alopecia (h) Painless perforation of the nasal septum.

Third stage: (i) Sensory symptoms are predominantly present such as headache, tingling, numbness and hyperaesthesia of the skin. (ii) Tenderness and muscle cramps. (iii) Oedema of the face, periorbital region, or ankles from localised transudation of intravascular fluid. (iv) Knee jerk is usually lost. (v) Impotence is commonly present. (vi) There is evidence of bone marrow depression and aplastic oedema. Haematologic abnormalities include normochromic and normocytic anaemia caused partly by haemolysis, leukopenia, thrombocytopenia and mild eosinophilia. Karyorrhexis is normally seen and manifested by bizarre nuclear forms seen on bone marrow examination. Interference with folate metabolism may lead to a megaloblastic picture.

Fourth stage: (i) Peripheral neuritis with glove and stocking type of anaesthesia. Neuropathy is the hallmark of arsenic poisoning. It is usually a symmetrical sensorimotor polyneuropathy, often resembling **Guillain-Barré syndrome**. The predominant clinical features of neuropathy are paresthesia, numbness and pain, particularly of the soles of the feet. Eventually, muscular atrophy (possibly even paralysis) and ataxia are seen. Encephalopathy may be seen in some cases, presenting as severe headache, personality disturbance, convulsions or coma. Peripheral neuropathy (may develop within a few hours of ingestion but usually seen 2-8 weeks after exposure). (ii) Muscular atrophy of extensor muscles resulting in **wrist drop** and **foot drop.** (iii) Muscular weakness (iv) Ataxia (v) Cramps (vi) Tremors and general emaciation (vii) Anaemia and dysuria (viii) Death is due to failure of heart muscles.

Differential Diagnosis

Chronic arsenic poisoning is to be differentiated from alcoholic neuritis. In the former the symptoms and signs are produced more rapidly, are widespread and there is no glycosuria whereas in alcoholic neuritis glycosuria is positive.

Treatment

(i) Remove the patient from source of poison (ii) B.A.L. is to be given 6 hourly for 2-3 days and then once daily (iii) Vitamin B_1 injection for peripheral neuritis (iv) Improve general health.

Medicolegal Aspects

(i) It is an **ideal homicidal poisoning** that is used frequently in India. It can be mixed with sweets, bread, cooked vegetable, drinks, milk, pan and cigarettes. Mass homicidal poisoning simulates cholera. It is tasteless, odourless, easily available and small doses are required for homicide. In western countries, small doses are given for a prolonged period that simulates gastroenteritis to conceal the crime. The **disadvantages** of being used as a homicidal poison are: (a) Can be detected even in the charred bodies (b) It delays putrefaction (c) Can be detected in decomposed bodies (d) Can be found in bones, hair even years after the poisoning. (ii) It is used on abortion sticks as paste or ointment. (iii) It is used as a cattle poison, is mixed with water in the well. (iv) Is used for suicidal purposes. (v) Poisoning can result accidentally due to its improper medicinal use when it is applied locally as a cure for impotence, poisoning can result from its application on the abraded skin, when it is accidentally mixed with food or drinks, when used as vaginal pessaries, and when it is mistaken for baking powder or soda. Beer drinkers in Lanceshire country in 1900 developed chronic arsenic poisoning and peripheral neuritis was produced. (vi) **Arsenophagists** use the drug as a habit as aphrodisiac and can acquire tolerance upto 0.3 gm or more in one dose. (vii) By dividing hair in small successive lengths from the root upwards and analyzing them separately, one may get the information regarding the time that has elapsed since the administration of arsenic. Arsenic starts depositing in the hair after 15 days. In about 25 days the arsenic is deposited in hair with the length of 1 cm. By neutron activation analysis, the relation between ingested arsenic and arsenic content of the hair can be known. (viii) Arsenic is excreted in the stomach and intestine after absorption, even when administered by routes other than mouth. (ix) It has the power of retarding decomposition and it does not disappear with decomposition.

Postmortem imbibition of arsenic: When there is a criminal charge of arsenic poisoning, the defence may take the plea that arsenic was introduced after death and postmortem imbibition has occurred in the tissues. The doctor can defend it by replying that signs of inflammation and ulceration of stomach will be absent in case of postmortem imbibition of arsenic.

Exhumed body: Arsenic cannot percolate in the cadaver from the soil, as it is an insoluble form, generally in combination with either lime or iron. To make soil arsenic soluble, hydrochloric acid is required. The nails and hair will have a higher concentration from the soil. The soil is to be kept for chemical analysis in exhumation.

MERCURY

Mercury is known as quick silver, a liquid metal with bright silvery luster that is volatile at room temperature. Some amount of mercury is ingested along with our diet and 5-20 mg is taken along with the foodstuffs daily.

The tolerable weekly intake of mercury per person is 300 mg out of which not more than 200 mg should be methyl mercury. It is not a normal constituent of the human body. Normal levels in unexposed individuals is: (i) 0-8 mg/100 ml of blood (ii) 0.6-1.6 mg per 100 ml of urine (iii) 5-150 mg per 100 gm may be found in liver and kidney.

Deadening of mercury: Mercury is converted into a dull gray powder (contains 33% of mercury): (i) When it is shaken with oil (ii) Triturated with sugar and chalk and is called deadening of mercury. It is used for the purpose of ointment.

Uses of Compounds of Mercury

1. *Inorganic salts:* (i) Calomel cathartic (Mercurous chloride, used as purgative) (ii) Mercurial ointment (iii) Vaginal creams (iv) Fingerprint powders (v) Amalgam (dental filling) (vi) Vermilion (Mercury sulphate).
2. *Organic salts* (Methyl and ethyl mercury: compounds) are an industrial waste and are used in manufacture of: (i) Thermometer (ii) Barometer (iii) Electrical industry (iv) Drug manufacturing (v) Mercury mining, hatters and furriers (vi) In agriculture as fungicide.

Compounds of Mercury

(i) Mercuric oxide, HgO (Sipichand) (ii) Mercuric chloride (corrosive sublimate); has (a) Antiseptic properties (b) Is largely used as medicine, taxidermy (c) Is deadly poison (iii) Mercuric iodide (Red iodide of mercury) (Figure 38.3) (iv) Mercuric cyanide, is poisonous (v) Mercuric nitrate (vi) Mercuric sulphide (Vermilion) (vii) Mercuric sulphate (viii) Mercurochrome contains 25-28% of mercury, discolours readily in water and toxic effects develop after prolonged use (ix) Mercury thiocyanate (Pharaoh' serpent) (x) Organic compounds are: (a) Ethyl and methyl mercury (b) Thiomerin sodium (c) Neptal.

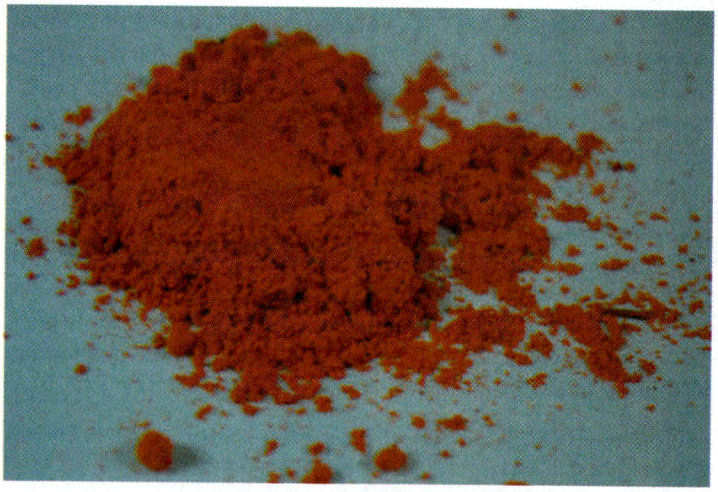

Figure 38.3: Mercuric iodide

Poisoning results from both organic and inorganic salts. The organic compounds produce irreversible effects and both the compounds affect CNS. Methyl mercury is more poisonous than the inorganic salts.

Fatal Dose: Mercuric chloride: 0.5-1 gm.

Mercurous chloride: 1.5-2 gm.

Fatal Period: 3-5 days.

Acute Mercury Poisoning

This poisoning is mostly due to corrosive sublimate, mercuric chloride. The signs and symptoms start immediately after swallowing the poison, and rarely they are delayed for half an hour (i) Acrid metallic taste in the mouth (ii) Feeling of constriction or choking sensation (iii) Hoarseness of voice (iv) There is difficulty in breathing (v) Mouth and tongue are corroded and swollen with gray-white coating (vi) Hot, burning pain in the mouth, stomach and abdomen (vii) Stools are blood stained (viii) Urine is suppressed and scanty, contains blood and albumin; is accompanied by necrosis of renal tubules and damage to glomeruli (ix) Pulse is quick, small and irregular; there is circulatory collapse (x) Thrombocytopenia and bone marrow depression (xi) When vapours are inhaled, following signs and symptoms are produced: (a) Salivation (b) Gingivitis (c) Loosening of teeth (xii) When injected intravenously, it produces: dyspnea, cyanosis, hypotension and convulsions (xiii) Death may be due to anaphylactic shock or ventricular fibrillation.

Diagnosis

Acute mercury poisoning is to be differentiated from arsenic poisoning from the following features: (i) The symptoms are produced quicker (ii) Acrid taste in the mouth (iii) Constriction of the throat is more marked (iv) Vomitus is more and often contains blood and mucous (v) Kidneys are more affected (vi) **Laboratory diagnosis:** (a) Urinary concentration is a good indicator of poisoning of elemental and inorganic mercury, but organic mercury (e.g., methyl mercury) can be detected easily in feces (b) Normal urinary concentration of mercury is <20 µg/l and 24 hours. urine excretion of mercury is <50 µg (c) Normal level of mercury in blood is <10 µg/l. (d) Blood mercury level is a useful test especially for acute exposure and the level of exposure is high (e) The 24-hour urine mercury level is the best biomarker for chronic long-term exposure (f) Hair analysis can help in diagnosis of chronic exposure (vii) **Nano technology:** It is a is high-sensitivity methods for analyzing ultra-trace amounts of heavy metals in biological samples. Gold nanoparticles (AuNPs) are used for detection of thymine bound mercuric ions. Silver nanoparticles are used as a sensitive detector of low concentration Hg^{2+} ions in homogeneous aqueous solutions.

Treatment

(i) Removal of the individual from the source of exposure. (ii) In case of vapor exposure, supplemental oxygen or endotracheal intubation and mechanical ventilation are recommended. (iii) In case of direct contact with mercury, the skin should be washed with soap and water. (iv) Correction of fluid and electrolyte. imbalance. (v) Whole bowel irrigation with polyethene glycol. (vi) Activated charcoal may be used but its efficacy is controversial. (vii) **Chelation therapy**: (a) **B.A.L.** is given in the dose of 5 mg/kg IM once, 2.5 mg/kg IM every 8 to12 hours for 1 day, and then 2.5 mg/kg IM every 12 to 24 hours for 7 days. It is indicated in elemental and inorganic mercury salts poisoning cases, however ineffective and it may even increase mercury levels in the brain and aggravate CNS symptoms in case of organic mercury poisoning (b) **DMSA or Succimer** is given orally or IV in the dose of 10 mg/kg every 8 hours for 5 days then 12 hourly for 14 days. If necessary, can be repeated with a 2 weeks interval. It is preferred for treatment of inorganic mercury poisoning (c) **DMPS** is given in the dose of 250 mg IV every 4 hours for the first 48 hours, then 250 mg IV every 6 hours for the second 48 hours and next 250 mg IV every 8 hours. After IV administration, oral therapy may be started with 300 mg tid for 7 weeks. It can remove mercury deposits in all human tissues except brain (d) **New DMSA analogues:** Mono isoamyl ester of DMSA (MiADMSA), Monomethyl DMSA (MmDMSA) and Monocyclohexyl DMSA (MchDMSA) can remove mercury from both intra and extra cellular sites, however, more studies are required to evaluate their efficacy. Combination of DMSA with MiADMSA has been found more effective (e) **N-acetyl DL:** Penicillamine an analogue of D-penicillamine which is more stable can be given. (viii) Hemodialysis, if renal failure occurs. (ix) Symptomatic treatment.

CHRONIC MERCURY POISONING (HYDRARGYRISM)

(i) Workers may get poisoned due to the vapours or dust (ii) When small doses are taken for prolonged period (iii) When used for external application as an ointment.

The signs and symptoms of chronic mercury poisoning start at a blood level of 100 mg/ml. The daily urinary excretion is more than 300 mg. The following signs and symptoms are produced: (i) Nausea, vomiting and diarrhoea (ii) Indigestion, dyspepsia and colicky abdominal pain (iii) Excessive salivation with swollen and painful salivary glands (iv) Foul smelling breathing (v) Inflamed and ulcerated gums with **brownish blue line** (vi) Loosening of teeth (vii) **Necrosis of jaw** that should be differentiated from phosphorus poisoning.

Mercuria lentis: A brownish reflex from the anterior lens capsule of both the eyes is seen when observed in slit lamp in persons exposed to mercury vapours for some years. It is bilateral and has no effect on the visual acuity.

Acrodynia (Pink disease): There is generalised rashes over the body. This results from chronic exposure to mercury in any form. Erythematous, eczematous (watery and weeping) papular type of skin lesions mostly in the hands and feet accompanied with thickening of skin are produced.

Mercurial tremors (Hatter's shake or glass blower's shake): In chronic mercury poisoning, moderately coarse tremors starting from hands then to lips and tongue and finally arms and legs occur **(Danbury tremors)**. These are detected early by writing. These are excited by voluntary movements and are absent during sleep. These are interspersed with jerky movements. There is incoordination of movements, increased deep reflexes, paresis of limbs and peripheral neuritis. The tremors should be differentiated from thyrotoxicosis in which there is presence of fine tremors, exophthalmos, raised pulse and goiter.

Mental symptoms (Erethism): Erethism develops in the persons working in mirror-manufacturing firms. Features of insanity such as shyness, timidity, irritability, loss of confidence, mental depression, loss of memory, insomnia, hallucinations and delusions develop in the workers. Sometimes suicidal melancholia or maniac depressive psychosis **(Mad hatter)** develops.

Minamata disease (Hunter Russell Syndrome): It is a chronic methylmercury poisoning that occurred in the Japanese inhabitants of Minamata and Niigata Bays due to consumption of fish and shellfish contaminated with toxic chemicals. The disease is characterized by peripheral sensory loss, tremors, ataxia, dysarthria and both visual and hearing loss.

Treatment

(i) Removal of the individual from the source of exposure. (ii) Plenty of milk should be given. (iii) Mouth wash by borax. (iv) Saline purgative to be given. (v) Sodium thiosulphate I.V. to be used. (vi) Chelation therapy–same as mentioned for acute poisoning. (vii) Prophylactic treatment including proper ventilation and periodic medical checkup of the workers.

Autopsy Findings

(i) If taken in concentrated form, appearances similar to corrosive poisoning will be present. (ii) Signs of irritant poisoning will be there. (iii) Mucous membrane of lips, mouth, pharynx and oesophagus will be grayish white. (iv) Stomach contents are coagulated, albuminous with mucous and blood. (v) Mucous membrane is eroded, inflamed and covered with grayish deposit of mercury or black deposits of mercury sulphide. (vi) There is great softening of the walls so great care must be taken during postmortem examination to remove it. However, perforation is rare. (vii) Caecum, colon and rectum are inflamed, ulcerated and gangrenous, if patient remains alive for sometime. (viii) Liver is congested with cloudy swelling. (ix) Spleen is congested. (x) Kidneys will be *enlarged, swollen and soft*; minute haemorrhagic spots scattered on its surface and the capsule will strip off easily; evidence of acute tubular and glomerular degeneration or *haemorrhagic glomerular nephritis*, in contradistinction to the *pale cortex* are characterstic. (xi) Heart shows fatty degeneration. (xii) Lesions are found in the alimentary canal even when applied on the skin or absorbed from the vagina or uterus.

Medicolegal Aspects

(i) Pure metallic mercury is not considered poisonous, as it is not absorbed by the gastric juice. 1-2 pounds of liquid metal is taken to cure constipation but has no harmful effects. In exceptional cases, mercury may undergo chemical change and acts as a poison. (ii) Few cases of mercury embolism are reported while the blood is collected from arteritis under the mercury seal. (iii) When injected subcutaneously, local abscess formation occurs. (iv) The mercurial vapours cause poisoning (0.5 mg/m^3 causes poisoning). (v) When it is rubbed on to the skin, is absorbed and poisoning occurs. There is a reported incidence of the death of three persons when they applied mercury ointment for itching. (vi) Amalgams that are used for filling carious tooth sometimes cause poisoning. (vii) Mercuric salts are more poisonous than mercurous salts. Trivalent salts are more poisonous than the bivalent salts. (viii) Mercuric chloride causes accidental poisoning when it is widely used as (a) Disinfectant and antiseptic (b) Contraceptive vaginal tablets (c) For antisyphilitic treatment. (ix) Phenyl mercuric acetate jelly leads to poisoning when used as a contraceptive. (x) Mercuric chloride *(Calomel)* is poorly absorbed and has a low solubility; used in teething powders, causes pink disease in infants. (xi) Mercuric sulphide *(vermilion)* is not absorbed through the skin and is nonpoisonous. (xii) It is eliminated through the saliva, urine, faeces, milk and perspiration. (xiii) By neutron activation analysis, it is found that the maximum amount of mercury in the human tissues is in the kidney, nails, scalp hair and skin. (xiv) Mercury may be detected in the bone in acute poisoning. (xv) Mercury is often used as a medicine; hence detection in small quantity in the viscera does not contraindicate death from other causes. (xvi) Mercury is not a constituent of human body; hence its presence indicates that it must have been introduced into the system. 5-150 mg/100 gm is normally present in the tissues like liver and kidney.

Test for Mercury: To a solution of mercury a piece of copper wire is introduced and few drops of HCl are added, a silver coating of mercury will be formed on the wire.

COPPER

Copper is also known as 'Tamba'. Metallic copper is not poisonous but some of its salts have a medicolegal importance. All salts of copper are poisonous. Copper alloyed with other metals when given in fine powdered state acts as a poison (i) Copper is a normal constituent of the body and is found in traces in urine, faeces, blood, tissue fluids and liver. It is also detectable in minute amount in various food materials such as potatoes, beans, spinach, fruits and mineral water. The normal dietary intake of copper is about 3 mg/day. In **Wilson's disease** there is increased absorption of copper in the system due to congenital defect in ceruloplasmin formation. All copper salts are powerful inhibitors of various enzyme systems. (ii) *Elimination*: Copper is eliminated more through faeces and bile than through urine. It is also excreted in saliva, milk and *in utero* from the mother to the foetus.

Copper sulphate (Figure 38.4) (Blue vitriol, $CuSO_4$, $5H_2O$, Nila tutiya): It occurs as large blue crystals, freely soluble in water having metallic taste. On heating upto 100°C, it loses its water of crystallization and becomes white with a blue tint and at 220°C it becomes completely white. On standing, it draws moisture and again becomes blue, as it is hygroscopic. Copper sulphate is used as astringent in small doses; as an emetic in slightly large doses and an irritant in larger doses.

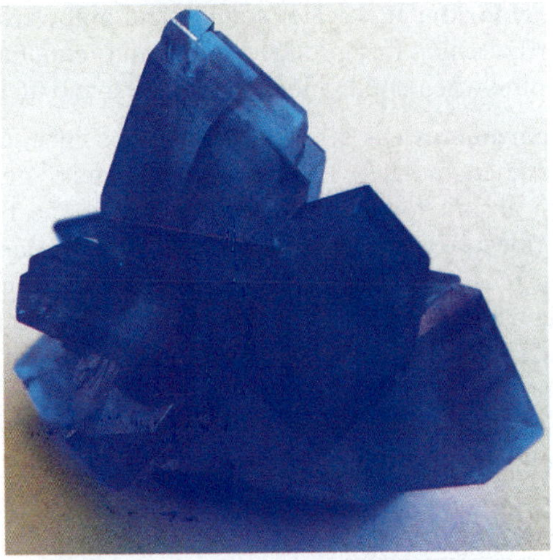

Figure 38.4: Copper sulphate crystals

Uses of copper sulphate: (i) It is used as an algaecide. (ii) It is also used by bookbinders and straw-hat makers. (iii) It is a constituent of Fehling's solution I. (iv) It was used for removal of excess granulation tissue in wounds. (v) To impart rich green colour and for preservation of fruits and vegetables but their dose should not exceed 15 mg/kg. However, the toxic effects does not result from their use as copper salts are converted into albuminate of copper, which is a harmless substance. (vi) In bakeries for fermentation of dough to make breads in winters. (vii) It is commonly used as an emetic in various poisonings except arsenic where it will form cupric arsenite or acetoarsenite of copper and produce toxicity. (viii) It is used as an antidote in phosphorus poisoning where it forms cupric phosphide (A nontoxic substance).

Copper subacetate (Verdigris or Zangal): Copper sulphate is a bluish green salt formed by the action of vegetable acids on improperly tinned copper cooking vessels. It is used as medicine for external use and is used in arts and industry. The signs and symptoms of verdigris poisoning are similar to that of copper sulphate poisoning.

Fatal Dose: 15-30 gms but small repeated doses are more fatal compared to single large dose.

Fatal Period: 1-3 days.

Signs and Symptoms of Acute Poisoning

Signs and symptoms appear within 15-30 minutes of the ingestion of the poisonous substance: (i) Metallic taste in mouth and sense of constriction in throat. (ii) Burning pain in the mouth, throat, oesophagus and up to the stomach. (iii) Repeated, violent and profuse vomiting; the vomitus is bluish or greenish blue in colour that becomes bluer on addition of ammonium hydroxide. The colour of vomitus will not change if it is bilious. (iv) Intense thirst, salivation, nausea and gaseous eructations. (v) Gums and tongue are stained bluish. (vi) Repeated diarrhoea with liquid, brown motions that is accompanied with tenesmus and colicky abdominal pain. (vii) Oliguria, anuria and albuminuria leads to uremia. (viii) Hemolytic tendencies due to increased concentration of copper in the erythrocytes, resulting in hemetemesis and malena. (ix) Jaundice may develop. (x) Muscular cramps, paralysis of limbs, convulsions, dyspnoea, quick, weak and feeble pulse, fall of blood pressure, cold clammy skin and coma. Death occurs in 1-3 days. (xi) Liver biopsy shows centrilobular necrosis and biliary stasis.

Chemical test: Ammonium hydroxide gives a greenish blue precipitate with substances containing copper salts; this precipitate is soluble in excess of ammonium hydroxide solution giving a deep blue colouration.

Treatment

(i) No emetics as copper sulphate itself causes emesis. (ii) Gastric lavage using 1% freshly prepared potassium ferrocyanide that acts as an antidote. It changes copper sulphate into insoluble cupric ferrocyanide. (iii) Demulcents like milk and egg albumen convert copper sulphate into insoluble cupric albuminate. (iv) To maintain fluid and electrolyte imbalance infuse 5% intravenous dextrose saline with vitamin C and amino acids. (v) Morphine is given to allay pain. (vi) Chelating agent, **penicillamine** 2 gm in divided doses is given orally for 5-7 days or parenterally 30 mg/kg body weight or B.A.L. as 300 mg I.M. stat and then 150 mg 4 hourly for next 6-7 days or until recovery. (vii) Calcium E.D.T.A. is also given as an antidote. (viii) D-penicillamine is the drug of choice for the treatment of Wilson's disease.

Autopsy Findings

(i) The skin is yellow due to jaundice. (ii) Greenish blue froth comes out of the mouth and nostrils. (iii) Mucous membrane of mouth, oesophagus, stomach and intestines will be inflamed, congested, swollen and excoriated and bluish green or bluish stained. (iv) Stomach contents are stained greenish blue or blue. (v) There is rectal perforation sometimes. (vi) Liver is enlarged, congested, soft and greasy showing features of fatty infiltration and degeneration. (vii) Kidneys are congested and features of tubular degeneration with deposition of copper is seen.

CHRONIC COPPER SULPHATE POISONING

Chronic copper sulphate poisoning results from: (i) Preservation and cooking of food in unclean copper utensils may result in poisoning as it is contaminated with verdigris. (ii) Chronic consumption of fruits and vegetables preserved and coloured with copper sulphate. (iii) Inhalation of copper dust or absorption through skin by workers in copper industry. (iv) ***Brass-founder's***

lung (Metal fumes fever): Inhalation of fumes of copper and zinc in workers engaged in smelting grass–an alloy of copper and zinc results in this condition. (v) ***Vineyard Sprayer's lung:*** Inhalation of Bordeaux mixture (1-2% aqueous solution of copper sulfate, neutralized with hydrated lime) observed in Portuguese vineyard workers.

Signs and Symptoms

(i) Styptic metallic copper taste in tongue and mouth. (ii) Bluish-green or purple line on the gums at its junction with the teeth called **Clapton's Line.** (iii) Lassitude, giddiness and headache. (iv) Nausea, vomiting, indigestion and dyspepsia. (v) Occasional diarrhoea with colicky abdominal pain. (vi) Laryngitis and bronchitis. (vii) Peripheral neuritis. (viii) Anemia and slight jaundice. (ix) Muscular weakness with atrophy may lead to paralysis. (x) Hair may be brownish golden in colour. (xi) Features of renal and hepatic damage are prominent. (xii) Conjunctivitis and corneal ulceration occur due to contact with copper dust. (xiii) Dermatitis due to skin contamination with copper salts. (xiv) **Chalcosis lentis:** It is the deposit of copper just below the anterior capsule of the lens in eye (characteristic **'sunflower'** appearance) after penetrating injury with copper containing metal.

Treatment

(i) Patient should be removed to fresh air. (ii) Correction of dyspepsia. (iii) Copper utensils used for cooking should be very clean and well-tinned. (iv) Chelating agents such as E.D.T.A, Penicillamine should be given. (v) Nutritious diet with multivitamins and intravenous fluids to be given.

Autopsy Findings

(i) Fatty degeneration, necrosis of liver cells and haemato-chromatosis. (ii) Degeneration and cloudy swelling of kidney.

Medicolegal Aspects

(i) Copper salts especially copper sulphate are not commonly used for suicidal purposes due to its blue or bluish-green colour, being self-emetic, strong metallic taste and big lethal dose. (ii) Compound is used for homicidal purposes. (iii) Rarely used for cattle poisoning. (iv) Accidental poisoning can occur from contamination of food stored or cooked in copper utensils due to formation of verdigris and eating fruits and vegetables preserved in copper sulphate. (v) Used on the abortion sticks to procure abortion.

IRON

Iron is a normal constituent of the body and is eliminated in faeces and urine. It is present in the food we take and in various multivitamin syrups, tablets, tonics and capsules. The salts of ferrous such as ferrous sulphate and ferrous carbonate are easily absorbed whereas ferric salts are not absorbed. The poisoning may result from ingestion of iron preparation available in the market by children in lieu of sweets. Teenagers and young females can also suffer from iron poisoning after a long period of treatment for anemia, in pregnancy or during postpartum period with these preparations. All iron preparations are dangerous except for ferrous gluconate.

Ferrous sulphate: It occurs as greenish crystals soluble in water and is used in industry for making blue black ink and dyes.

Ferric chloride: It is water soluble and a powerful irritant, forms triferriperchlor that produces sloughing endometritis and even peritonitis when applied locally in vagina and uterus.

Hemochromatosis is a relatively common inherited genetic condition due to mutated HFE gene. The faulty gene causes the body to absorb too much iron from food. The body lacks an efficient means of excreting the excess iron it takes in. Over time, this excess iron deposited in liver and pancreas. The pancreas damage can lead to secondary diabetes. This type of diabetes is called **Bronze Diabetes** due to the greyish colour of skin developed from deposition of excess iron. The trio signs for hemochromatosis are irreversible liver damage (cirrhosis), diabetes mellitus and a bronze discoloration of the skin.

Mechanism of Action

In dilute forms, the iron preparations act as astringent and corrosive in concentrated form leading to corrosion or perforation of gastric mucosa. It causes increased capillary permeability and inhibition of mitochondrial function. They may cause stricture formation.

Fatal Dose: 20-30 gm.

Fatal Period: Variable (24-48 hours).

Signs and Symptoms

The signs and symptoms are described in three stages:

Stage I: 30 min-6 hrs: (i) Metallic taste in mouth. (ii) Nausea, vomiting and epigastric pain. (iii) Hematemesis, diarrhea with black stools. (iv) Severe gastrointestinal hemorrhage results in shock followed by convulsions and coma, peripheral circulatory failure and death. (v) Iron released from the tablet or solution will exert its necrotizing effects on gastrointestinal tract mucosa and the unbound iron will soon get absorbed to produce systemic manifestations. (vi) Vomiting is most sensitive indicator of serious ingestions. Most patients resolve within 6 to 8 hours.

Stage II: 6 hrs-24 hrs: This phase is also referred as latent or quiescent period and is characterized by a transient resolution of gastrointestinal symptoms and cardiovascular instability. This phase is transient or not appears at all in with severe iron ingestions.

Stage III: 12 hrs-48 hrs: Life threatening symptoms predominate during this stage. Some patients may present with multiorgan failure. Recurrence of gastrointestinal hemorrhage, hematemesis, melena, and bowel perforation may be seen. Acute circulatory shock characterized by tachycardia, tachypnoea, pallor, hypotension and cyanosis may recur. Metabolic acidosis and coagulopathy present. The hallmark of this phase is progressive pulmonary dysfunction with a radiologic appearance of adult type respiratory distress syndrome or shock lung. Hepatic, renal and neurologic dysfunction all may occur during this time.

Stage IV: 4 wks-6 wks: Patients with severe poisoning who survive as well as those who do not develop systemic toxicity may go on to have gastric outlet obstruction or pyloric stenosis as result of gastric scarring. Vomiting is the presenting symptom of these late sequelae. Recurrence of shock and development of hepatic failure and features of acute hepatic necrosis with jaundice progresses to hepatic coma and death (This result from release of iron from reticuloendothelial system).

Diagnosis

(i) Iron levels in blood and gastric aspirate. (ii) Urine for bilirubin, bile salts and urobilinogen. (iii) Liver function tests and tests for rise in aminotransferases and prothrombin time should be carried out.

Chemical Test

Ammonium sulphide when mixed with ferric or ferrous salts gives black precipitate that is soluble in dilute hydrochloric acid.

Treatment

(i) Gastric lavage with water or normal saline by a large-bore orogastric tube is only indicated, if abdominal X-ray demonstrates a large number of visible pills in the stomach. (ii) Whole-bowel irrigation with polyethylene glycol solution is indicated, if abdominal X-ray demonstrates visible pills beyond the pylorus or throughout GI tract. (iii) **Desferrioxamine** (1 gm of Desferrioxamine chelates 85 mg of iron) is the most active antidote against iron poisoning. It is introduced in stomach in the dose of 5 gm dissolved in 100 ml of distilled water through stomach tube and be left out. Desferrioxamine 1 gm in 5 ml of distilled water can be given I.M. and further 500 mg in 12-24 hours depending upon the serum iron estimation. Intravenously maximum of 60-80 mg/kg in 24 hours can be infused. (iv) Shock and acidosis to be treated. (v) Correction of coagulopathy with Vit K. (vi) Symptomatic and supportive treatment.

Autopsy Findings

(i) Evidence of congestion, inflammation and corrosion of gastrointestinal tract. (ii) Liver will show hepatic necrotic changes. (iii) Kidney will show renal tubular necrosis.

Medicolegal Aspects

(i) Ferric chloride is rarely given to intoxicated persons for homicidal purposes. (ii) Accidental poisoning occurs in children commonly who ingest it in lieu of sweets. (iii) It is introduced locally in the genital tract to procure abortion.

THALLIUM

It is a soft white heavy metal that changes on exposure of air to formation of black Thallous oxide. The metal itself and its salts, e.g., thallium acetate and thallium sulphate are highly toxic, metal and its salts are chiefly used in dye and glass industries for preparation of optical lenses, imitation jewellery etc. thallium sulphate may be used rodenticide.

Fatal Dose: 200 mg to 1 gm; for children approx. 50 mg.

Fatal Period: 24 hours to 36 hours.

Mode of Action

Being highly poisonous it acts as strong gastrointestinal irritant; causes fatty degeneration of heart and liver and tubular necrosis of the kidney. It is accumulative in the skin and hair.

Sign and Symptoms

Acute Poisoning: The features include pain in abdomen, nausea, vomiting, diarrhea, followed by constipation, pain in legs and feet, conjunctivitis, rhinitis, bilateral ptosis with peripheral neuritis (sensory and motor), impaired vision, retrobulbar neuritis, optic atrophy, nail changes (Mees' lines), oliguria, albuminuria, pulmonary edema, followed by collapse and death from respiratory failure.

Chronic Poisoning: The features include painful peripheral neuropathy, alopecia, insomnia, erythematous skin rashes, mental confusion with lethargy.

The triad of gastroenteritis, polyneuropathy and alopecia is regarded as the classic syndrome of thallium poisoning (**Thallium triad**). The most characteristic sign of thallium toxicity is alopecia.

Thallium levels are usually examined in urine, blood and hair samples.

Treatment Symptoms

1. Give stomach wash with 1% potassium iodide to form insoluble salts of thallium iodide to be followed by activated charcoal and saline purgative,
2. Prussian blue 25 mg/kg body weight with 15% mannitol by duodenal drip may act as helpful chelating agent against thallium.
3. B.A.L. should be given in recommended doses as early as possible.

4. Potassium iodide and diuretics by mouth may help in excretion of thallium.

Postmortem Appearances

Congestion of gastric mucosa with submucus haemorrhagic spots, fatty degeneration of liver and heart, cloudy swelling and necrosis of cells of convoluted tubules of kidneys and congestion of all other organs, are characterstic. Externally, loss of large bunches of hair from scalp and outer 2/3 of eyebrows which are diagnostic.

Medicolegal Aspects

(i) It is considered as one of the better homicidal poisons. In India, cases of homicidal thallium poisoning have been reported in the recent past. (ii) Rarely used for suicide.

CADMIUM

Cadmium is a soft, silvery white with bluish color, odorless, tasteless and toxic heavy metal. It forms soluble salts of carbonates, arsenates, phosphates, and ferrocyanide compounds. It is commonly used in industries and present everywhere in the environment. Poisoning in humans occurs mainly through inhalation and ingestion.

Uses of Cadmium

(i) It is used as alloys in electroplating (auto industries). (ii) For production of pigments (cadmium sulfate, cadmium selenide. (iii) Used as a stabilizer for polyvinyl plastic. (iv) Used in batteries (rechargeable Ni-Cd batteries). (v) A cigarette contains cadmium and cigarette smoking is considered to be the most significant source of human cadmium exposure.

Mechanism of Toxicity

It binds to a sulfhydryl group–containing protein like metallothionein. It interferes with DNA repair mechanism, generates reactive oxygen species and induces apoptosis.

Mode of Action

It can cause severe pulmonary and gastrointestinal irritation, when inhaled or ingested. Absorbed cadmium predominantly accumulates in kidney and liver, but it can be found in other tissues such as bone and placenta. It impairs the Vitamin D metabolism in the kidney, gut absorption of calcium and disarranged collagen metabolism which leads osteomalacia and/or osteoporosis.

Fatal Dose: 100 mg soluble salt of cadmium.

Fatal Period: 5 to 7 days.

Signs and Symptoms

Acute Poisoning: Inhalation of cadmium causes flu like signs and symptoms such as fever with chills, muscle pain, chest pain, cough, shortness of breath and cyanosis (**Cadmium blues**). The features are similar to those seen in **metal fume fever**. In severe cases, pneumonitis, tracheobronchitis and pulmonary edema occurs which may lead to death.

Ingestion of cadmium causes nausea, vomiting, diarrhoea, abdominal cramps, headache, swelling of throat and tingling of hands. Flue like symptoms may occur. Large dose of cadmium causes damage to kidney, liver and heart resulted in death.

Chronic Poisoning: Inhalation of cadmium dust and fumes over a period of time leads to signs and symptoms of COPD. Both inhalation and ingest of cadmium cause kidney damage and affects skeletal system. **Itai-Itai (it hurts–it hurts disease/ ouch-ouch disease)**, is a severe form chronic cadmium poisoning characterized by osteomalacia with severe bone pain associated with renal tubular dysfunction. The disease was first noticed among the inhabitants of the Jinzu River basin of Japan. Chronic exposure to cadmium can lead cancers.

Diagnosis

(i) Blood cadmium levels reflect acute cadmium exposure. (ii) Urine levels appear to provide a better measure of chronic exposure. (iii) Hair, nail and saliva samples can be analyzed for diagnosis of chronic exposure. (iv) **Nano technology:** Nanoparticles quantum dots (QDS) can be used for detection of cadmium poisoning.

Treatment

(i) Removal of the individual from the source of exposure. (ii) Gastric lavage can be done. (iii) Activated charcoal cannot effectively absorb the metal. (iv) **Chelation therapy:** (a) **BAL and their analogues DMSA, DMPS** can be used (b) **New DMSA analogues:** Monoisoamyl DMSA (MiADMSA), Monomethyl DMSA (MmDMSA) and Monocyclohexyl DMSA (MchDMSA) can be used. Combination of DMSA with MiADMSA has been found more effective (c) **Dithiocarbonates:** Reduces general symptoms and enhances the urinary and biliary excretion of cadmium. (v) **NAC (N-acetyl cysteine)** can reduce cadmium-induced hepatic and renal metallothionein. (vi) **Nanoparticle:** Cadmium can be adsorbed by Al_2O_3 nanoparticles from solution/ sorbent systems.

Postmortem Appearances

Congestion of gastric mucosa, fatty degeneration of liver and heart, pulmonary edema, proximal tubular necrosis, interstitial nephritis in chronic cases and congestion of all other organs can be present.

Medicolegal Aspects

(i) It is an uncommon poisoning. (ii) Mostly cases are due to occupational exposure.

LONG QUESTIONS

1. Describe signs, symptoms, management and postmortem findings in case of chronic lead poisoning.
2. Discuss signs, symptoms, management and postmortem findings in case of chronic arsenic poisoning.

SHORT NOTES

1. Burtonian line.
2. Basophilic stippling/Punctate basophilia.
3. Acrodynia.
4. Hatter's shake.
5. Phossy jaw.
6. Erethism.

MULTIPLE CHOICE QUESTIONS

1. A Burtonian line over gums is suggestive of poisoning with:

(a) Lead (b) Mercury
(c) Copper (d) Iron

2. A pinch of which of the following poisons can kill 8 to 10 persons?

(a) Endrin (b) Thallium
(c) Arsenic trioxide (d) Arsenic disulphide

3. Acrodynia or pink disease is seen in case of poisoning:

(a) Cadmium (b) Mercury
(c) Iron (d) Copper

4. Fatal dose of copper sulphate is:

(a) 30 mg (b) 100 mg
(c) 10 gm (d) 30 gm

5. Hatter's shake is seen in poisoning by:

(a) Thallium (b) Arsenic
(c) Copper (d) Mercury

6. Minamata Bay Disaster happened due to poisoning by:

(a) Arsenic trioxide (b) Thallium
(c) Lead subacetate (d) Methylmercury

7. Hair and nails are preserved for chemical analysis in suspected poisoning due to:

(a) Cyanide
(b) Strychnine
(c) Barbiturates
(d) Arsenic

8. Gastroenteritis, alopecia, polyneuropathy are features of poisoning due to:

(a) Thallium (b) Mercury
(c) Arsenic (d) Lead

9. Bronze Diabetes is related to accumulation of following metal in the body:

(a) Copper (b) Manganese
(c) Zinc (d) Iron

10. Itai-itai (ouch-ouch) disease is caused by:

(a) Mercury (b) Cadmium
(c) Arsenic (d) Thallium

11. Accidental poisoning in children by burning Pharoah serpents could be due to:

(a) Lead tetroxide
(b) Mercury thiocyanate
(c) Cadmium phosphate
(d) Thallium acetate

12. "Milk and roses" appearance of skin is seen in poisoning with:

(a) Mercury (b) Copper
(c) Lead (d) Arsenic

13. Basophilic stippling seen in lead poisoning is due to inhibition of enzyme:

(a) Purine-5'-nucleotidase (b) DNA Polymerase-III
(c) RNA Polymerase (d) Pyrimidine-5'-nucleotidase

14. Retinal stippling is seen chronic poisoning of:

(a) Thallium (b) Cadmium
(c) Arsenic (d) Lead

15. Which poison is called the "King of poisons"?

(a) Organophosphorus
(b) Aluminium phosphide
(c) Arsenic
(d) Lead

ANSWER KEY

1. (a)	2. (c)	3. (b)	4. (d)	5. (d)	6. (d)	7. (d)	8. (a)	9. (d)	10. (b)
11. (b)	12. (d)	13. (d)	14. (d)	15. (c)					

Irritant Poisons

39 CHAPTER

ORGANIC IRRITANT POISONS

ABRUS PRECATORIUS (INDIAN LIQUORICE OR RATTI)

The plant grows throughout India and all parts of the plant are poisonous but the seeds are particularly used for the purpose of poisoning. The seeds of Ratti are 1/3 inches long and 1/4 inches broad and are of the size of small pea. Usually the seeds are red coloured, egg shaped having a black spot on one end but it may be of white, black, or yellow colour (Figure 39.1). Ratti seeds are used as decorative ornaments. The seeds are tasteless and odourless. The active principle is **Abrin** that is a **toxalbumin** similar to ricin and its action resembles the viperine snakebite. Besides this, it contains some poisonous proteins such as: (i) Abrussic acid (fat splitting enzyme) (ii) Abrin (nitrogenous compound) (iii) Ureases (iv) Haemagglutinin (v) Abraline (glucoside) (vi) Glycyrrhizin present in root, stems and leaves.

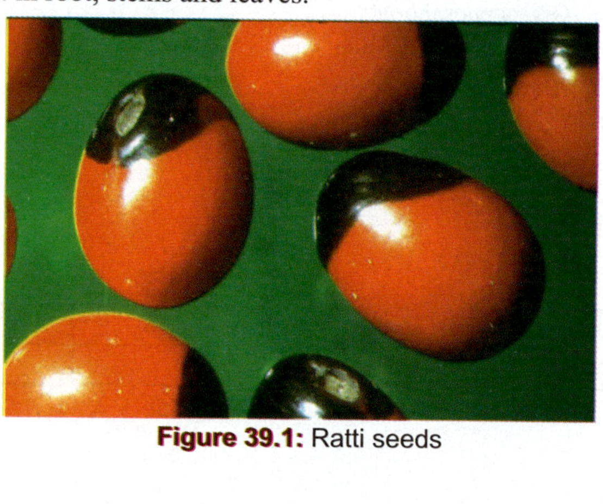

Figure 39.1: Ratti seeds

Preparation of 'Suis' or 'Sutari'

The seeds are first soaked in water, decorticated and made into a paste mixed with opium, onion, *dhatura*, little oil or water. The paste is then shaped in the form of small, sharp needles with pointed ends about 2.5 cm long and 90-120 mg by weight. The needles are then hardened by drying in the sun and then fitted to the holes of a bamboo pole. These needles are stabbed on the buttock of the animal, implanting the needles but detaching the handle. At the site of inoculation of **'sui'**, there will be inflammation, oedema or necrosis with oozing of haemorrhagic fluid from the puncture site similar to the viper bite. The animal stops eating food for 3-4 days, will be unable to move or stand. It will become apathetic and will develop convulsions before it gets comatosed. The collapse soon sets in and the animal dies by 48-96 hours later. The signs and symptoms simulate snakebite (viperine). The owner will not suspect homicidal cattle poisoning.

When the **'suis'** are stabbed in the human body, there will be painful swelling with ecchymosis at or about the site of injection. The inflammation sets up and necrosis begins soon. The patient suffers from headache, nausea, vomiting, vertigo, drowsiness and apathy. There is increasing prostration, dyspnoea, quick, weak, irregular and feeble pulse, and cold clammy skin. The blood pressure falls, oliguria, haemorrhagic manifestations and lately uremia may set in. Death occurs from 3-5 days from cardiac failure.

Signs and Symptoms

The ingestion of intact 'Ratti' seeds does not result in poisoning. Powdered seeds are boiled with milk and are used as a nerve toxin but when taken uncooked it acts as severe gastrointestinal irritant causing vomiting and diarrhoea. Abrin is slightly inactivated by gastric juice when crushed seeds are swallowed and it loses all its poisonous properties when boiled: (i) Extracts of seeds when injected under the skin of an animal cause inflammation, oedema and necrosis. (ii) In human beings, ingestion of crushed seeds results in: (a) Nausea and vomiting (b) Vertigo, tinnitus and giddiness (c) Cold clammy skin and fall of blood pressure (d) Irregular pulse and laboured breathing (e) Convulsions, haemolysis, oliguria (f) Death occurs from cardiac failure.

Fatal Dose: 90-120 mg (½ to 1 crushed seed).

Fatal Period: 3-5 days rarely even 24 hours.

Treatment

(i) Gastric lavage and emesis is carried out. (ii) Locally the part containing 'sui' should be excised in both humans and animals. (iii) Sodium bicarbonate 10 gm orally per day helps in maintaining alkalinity of urine and prevents agglutination of red cells and blocking of renal tubules with haemoglobin G. (iv) Antiabrin, an antiserum that is prepared by injecting abrin in rabbits, is to be administered. (v) A mixture of dilute hydrochloric acid and pepsin is to be given orally. (vi) Symptomatic treatment should be ensued.

Autopsy Findings

(i) Inflammatory oedema and necrosis at the site of injection (ii) Sometimes fragments of 'suis' are found at the site of injection (iii) Gastrointestinal tract is congested and haemorrhagic (iv) Petechial haemorrhages are seen in the skin, pleura, pericardium as well as peritoneum (v) The visceral organs are congested.

Medicolegal Aspects

(i) It is a mainly a cattle poison. (ii) 'Suis' are made by mixing with *Dhatura*, Opium, Onion and Spirit and used for poisoning the cattle and also for homicidal purposes. (iii) Seeds act as an abortifacient preventing conception. (iv) Application of powdered seeds on to the eye by malingerers to produce conjunctivitis. (v) Paste made from the powder of Ratti seeds is used as an arrow poison and also as an aphrodisiac.

SEMECARPUS ANACARDIUM (MARKING NUT, BHILAWAN)

The plant of marking nut is found all over India and the fruit of this plant is called marking nut (Bhilawan). The fruit is black, heart-shaped, having a rough projection at the base (Figure 39.2). It has a hard black rind, which contains a thick pericarp. This pericarp or fleshy pulp contains brownish oily acrid juice that turns black when mixed with the lime and exposed to air. It is used by washerman for marking cotton clothing and linen. That is why, it is known as **marking nut**. The juice mixed with the melted butter is used as a remedy for syphilis. The active principles are: (i) Semicarpol (0.1%) (ii) Bhilawanol (15-17%) (iii) Nonvolatile corrosive residue (18%) (iv) Fatty oils and tannic acids.

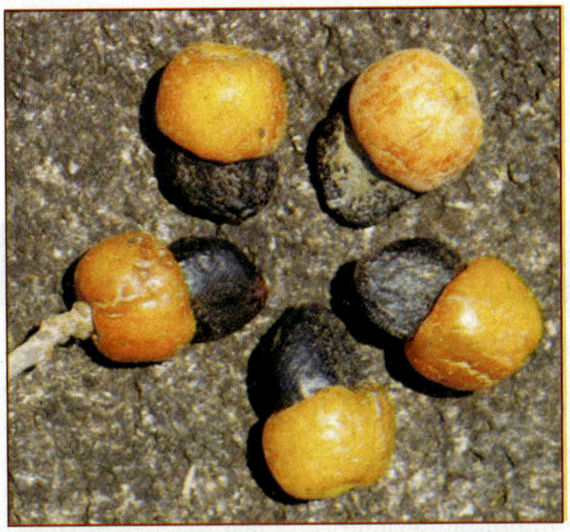

Figure 39.2: Fruits of semecarpus anacardium

Signs and Symptoms

On external application: (i) When applied externally, it causes irritation and itching (ii) When it is applied to the scrotum, it causes fever, haematuria and painful micturition (iii) Blisters are painful, black and raised containing acrid serum (iv) Acrid serum causes eczematous eruption of the contact area of skin (v) Blisters resemble bruises and may get infected and ulcerate (vi) Blisters are also associated with fever, dysuria, haematuria and painful defecation (vii) It is possible to detect poison from the serum and from the blisters.

When ingested: (i) Intense, painful irritation with blister formation locally in the mouth, tongue and throat (ii) Gastroenteritis with nausea and vomiting (iii) Tachycardia (iv) Quick weak pulse and hypotension (v) Pupils are dilated (vi) Cyanosis and dyspnoea (vii) Delirium and areflexia (viii) Collapse, coma and death occurs within 12-24 hours.

Fatal Dose: 5 gm.

Fatal Period: Uncertain, usually 12-24 hours.

Treatment

1. **External application:** Washing with lukewarm water with some antiseptic and application of antibiotic cream or ointment, if infected.
2. **When ingested:** Stomach wash with plain water; demulcent drinks; analgesics for pain and symptomatic measures to be employed.

Autopsy Findings

(i) Blisters in the mouth, throat and even stomach (ii) Fragments of seeds in stomach (iii) Fatty degeneration of the liver.

Medicolegal Aspects

(i) Accidental poisoning occurs when *Vaids* administer the juice of Semecarpus anacardium for the treatment of pain or for treating paralysis. (ii) Homicidal poisoning is rare. (iii) It is criminally introduced into the vagina as a punishment for infidelity. (iv) Juice of marking nut is applied on the skin to produce false bruise for levying charge against enemy. (v) It is applied on to the uterus for criminal abortion. (vi) It is sometimes applied on to the eyes by malingerers to produce ophthalmia.

RICINUS COMMUNIS (CASTOR OIL PLANT OR ARANDI)

History and background: Ricinus communis or the castor oil plant is cultivated in southern United States and also grows as a weed and ornamental plant (Figure 39.3). It is native to tropical Africa but has naturalised subtropical and temperate areas as well. The whole plant is poisonous, containing the heterodimeric ribosome inhibiting protein ricin that reaches the highest level in the seeds. It consists of a water-soluble glycoprotein, **Toxalbumin** that causes agglutination, cell destruction and haemolysis. Its residue contains the toxin, **ricin.** The seeds also contain purgative oil, the triglyceride of ricinoleic acid. The oil that is extracted does not contain any active principle. In the tropics, eating a single seed for the purgative effect is a widespread custom. The seeds have been used in folk medicine against many diseases for centuries. They appeared in classical Greek medicine and are described in the Sanskrit work on medicine, Sushruta Ayurveda from the 6th century BC. The oil is used for lubrication in the motor industry and is still being used as a laxative.

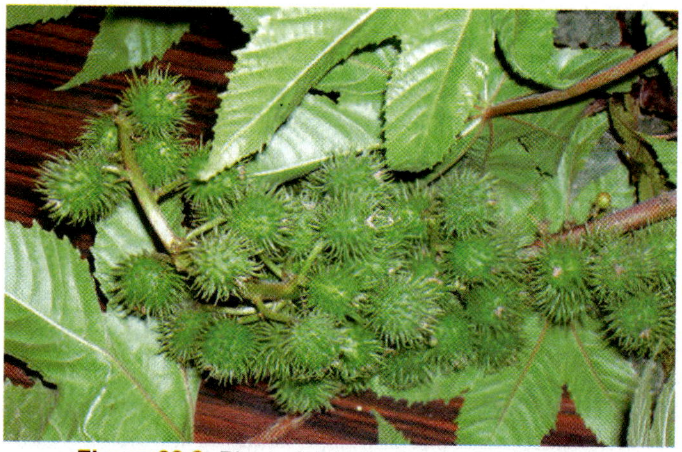

Figure 39.3: Plant of ricinus communis with fruits

The dust of this plant causes irritation of the eyes, nose and throat that causes asthma, allergy and dermatitis. Each fruit of Ricinus communis contains three mottled seeds, 5-15 mm long, that are red grey or polished brown in colour. The seeds exists in small and large forms. The poison is more effective when injected than when taken by mouth as it is destroyed by digestive enzymes. The plant also contains compounds which may elicit anaphylactic reactions. Because of this, ingestion of any dose of Ricinus communis can be fatal within minutes. Ricin has been known as a poison for years, usually through livestock deaths. The cattle may eat fruit or in our country, malicious neighbours are said to have administered extract of castor bean to their neighbour's cattle using a metal nail or 'Suis'. In Nigeria the beans are eaten as a food after careful preparation as heat inactivates the toxin, but in East Africa, unwanted children in the past have been murdered by adding castor beans to their food. The seeds of castor are commonly mistaken for that of croton but can be clearly distinguished on close inspection (Table 39.1, Figures 39.4 and 39.5).

Table 39.1: Differences between castor and croton seeds

Features	Castor seeds	Croton seeds
Appearance	Grayish with brown patches	Dark brown or brownish gray shell which on scrapping becomes black
Size	1.25 cm long and 0.85 cm broad	1.2 cm long and 0.82 cm broad
Transverse striae	Cells show ribbed appearance due to fine, transverse striae, polished	No transverse striae and no ribbed appearance, appear dull
Cross section	Lumen is circular	Lumen is slit like with radiating creases

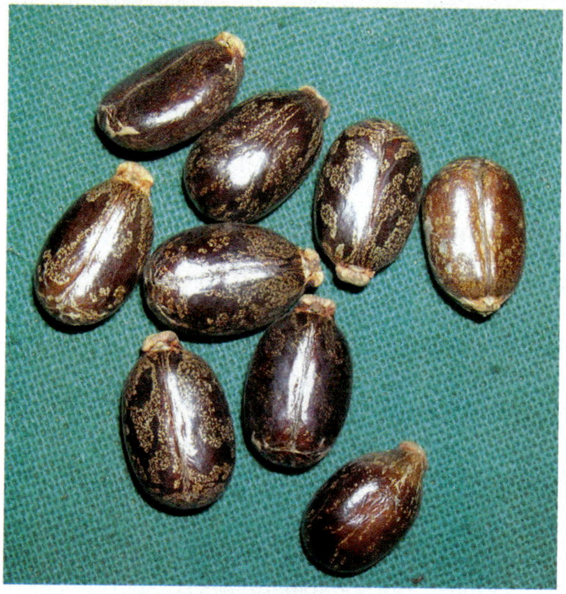

Figure 39.4: Castor seeds

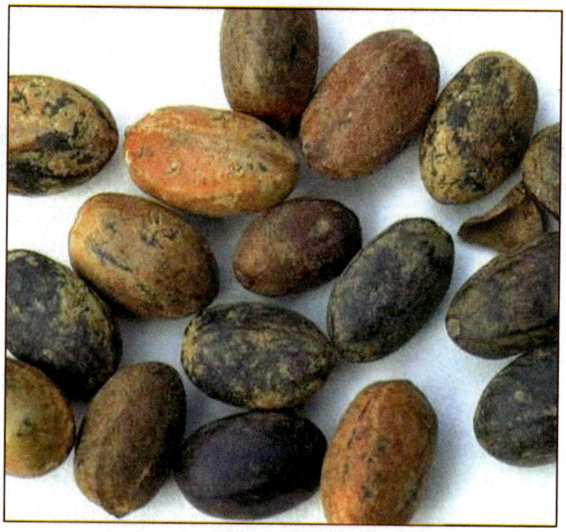

Figure 39.5: Seeds of croton tiglium

Fatal Dose: The fatal dose is 1 mg/kg or 8-10 crushed seeds in adults and 2-3 seeds in children. As lots of ricin is destroyed in the gastrointestinal tract, it is much more potent when administered parenterally. A dose of 2 millionths of the body weight may prove fatal.

Fatal Period: 2-24 hours.

Signs and Symptoms

Toxic effects of Ricin have a latent period and take 2-24 hours to develop.

After ingestion: The symptoms are: (i) Burning pain in the abdomen (ii) Vomiting and diarrhea often with blood (iii) Haemorrhages occur in intestines, mesenteries and omentum (iv) A diffuse nephritis and multiple necroses occur in liver and kidneys (v) Within several days there is severe dehydration, oliguria, thirst, burning throat, headache and patient may die of hypovolaemic shock (vi) Body temperature decreases before death and the patient often undergo a characteristic shivering (vii) Consciousness remains till the end (viii) Death occurs due to exhaustion or cramps.

When administered parenterally: Ricin is twice as toxic as cobra venom and is probably the most toxic parenteral substance in the plant kingdom. After parenteral administration, the patient may present with fever, leucocytosis and then hypotension and hypothermia. It primarily targets the liver and the kidneys.

Treatment

Measures should be undertaken to prevent absorption after ingestion of the poison as there is no specific antidote for Ricin: (i) Stomach wash using potassium permanganate should be carried out (ii) Syrup of ipecac and activated charcoal should be administered (iii) Stimulants should be given (iv) Intravenous glucose saline to be administered for dehydration (v) Sodium bicarbonate (vi) Supportive care including blood transfusion to combat blood loss (vii) Patient should be constantly monitored for hypoglycemia, haemolysis and hypovolaemia.

Medicolegal Aspects

(i) Poisoning is usually accidental when is taken by children by mistake (ii) It is also given mixed in food for criminal intent (iii) Powder when instilled into the eyes causes conjunctivitis (iv) Castor oil is non-poisonous and is used as purgative, for lighting purposes (v) Triglyceride of ricinoleic acid may act as an irritant poison (vi) It is used to make 'Suis' and injected into the buttock of the animal.

Autopsy Findings

(i) There is congestion of stomach, intestine and other visceral organs (ii) Inflammation and haemorrhages in the stomach, intestines, mesenteries and omentum are identifiable (iii) There is softening of the organs (iv) Fragments of seeds may be recovered from the stomach (v) There are findings of hepatic and renal necrosis.

CROTON TIGLIUM (JAMALGOTA OR NAEPALA)

The plant grows all over India and the seeds as well as oil expressed from the seed and the root of the plant are highly poisonous. The seeds are 0.65 × 0.85 cm in size, grayish white in colour with a white oily kernel having some longitudinal lines over the surface. Croton oil is vesicating agent, has brown colour and disagreeable odour and contains *crotonoleic acid*, *methyl crotonic acid*, *crotonol* and other fatty acid. The oil does not contain *crotin* that is left out in the croton seed cake on expression of the oil. When applied on the skin, it causes burning, redness, vesication and suppuration. When the seeds are swallowed, they cause irritation of the gastrointestinal tract. Croton seeds are poisonous to fish and a case is reported where croton oil was used to poison fishes at Midnapur, West Bengal.

Active principles: The active principles of seeds are: (i) Crotin a toxalbumin is less poisonous than ricin (ii) Crotonaside is a glycoside.

Signs and Symptoms

It is a gastrointestinal irritant and produces symptoms similar to Ricin poisoning (i) Severe hot burning pain in mouth, throat and abdomen. (ii) Salivation, nausea, copious vomiting. (iii) Frequent watery stools mixed with blood and mucus accompanied with gripping pain abdomen, anal irritation and tenesmus. (iv) Features of dehydration are prominent. (v) Quick weak pulse, shallow respiration and vertigo. (vi) Circulatory collapse and death. (vii) Being toxalbumin, it produces agglutination of red cells causing hemolysis, jaundice, pain in renal angles, haemoglobinuria. (viii) Blocking of renal tubules leads to oliguria, anuria and uremia and resulting renal failure accounts for delayed deaths. (ix) On application to skin, it produces burning, redness and vesication. The vesicles may suppurate resulting in scarring on healing. (x) On contact with eyes will produce conjunctivitis and corneal ulcer.

Fatal Dose: Four seeds; 1-2 ml of oil.

Fatal Period: 4-6 hours to 3 days.

Autopsy Findings

(i) Gastrointestinal tract mucosa shows erosion, inflammation and congestion (ii) Liver and spleen are congested (iii) Kidneys may show cloudy swelling and tubular necrosis (iv) In rare cases, there may not be any autopsy findings.

Medicolegal Aspects

(i) Poisoning results from eating seeds or inhaling dusts (ii) Accidental poisoning results from overdosage of croton oil that is used as purgative or administered after mixing with food (iii) It is rarely suicidal (iv) Used for homicidal purposes by boiling the root and adding to food (v) Root of the plant is commonly used as abortifacient (vi) It is used as an arrow poison.

CALOTROPIS PROCERA AND GIGANTEA (MADAR OR AKDO) (Figure 39.6)

The Calotropis plant is found all over India in two varieties; *Calotropis gigantea* and *Calotropis procera*. The dried root freed from its outer cortical layer is called *Madar*. Its constituents are Madaralbum, a crystalline colourless substance; Madarfluavil, an amber coloured viscid substance and Mudarine, gelatinizes on heating.

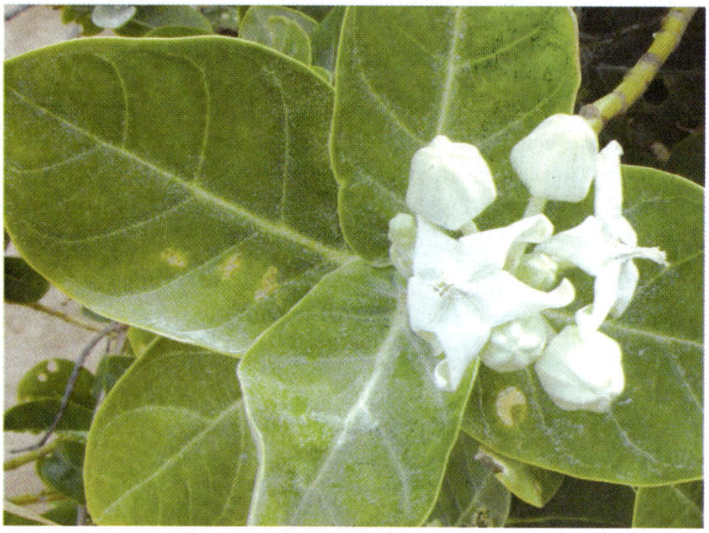

Figure 39.6: Calotropis procera

Active Principles: (i) Uscharin (ii) Calotoxin (iii) Calotropin (cardiac glycoside) (iv) Calactin.

Fatal Dose: Uncertain.

Fatal Period: 6-12 hours.

Uses: (i) Flowers are dried and powdered and used as digestive, carminative and tonic. (ii) Dried leaves are used as purgative in small doses; applied locally it relieves headache and in large doses act as an emetic. (iii) Tincture prepared from bark or root may be used in dysentery. (iv) Acrid milky juice may be used as an emetic, purgative, vesicant and also for treatment of chronic skin diseases. (v) Dried bark is used by vaids as an expectorant, emetic and purgative; bark may also be utilized for making madar or ushar fibres. (vi) Madar juice or the powdered bark or root of the plant may be used by tanners as a depilatory; this imparts yellow colouration to the skin and destroys offensive odour of fresh leather. (vii) Plant may also be used for treatment of impotence, asthma, syphilis, gonorrhoea and elephantiasis.

Medicolegal Aspects

(i) Madar juice is commonly used as an abortifacient either taken by the mouth or applied locally into the uterus by abortion stick, either alone or in the form of paste with lead oxide or arsenic preparation. (ii) Madar juice may be used for the purpose of homicide, suicide or infanticide; for infanticide, the madar juice may often be given by mouth mixing it with milk and water. (iii) Madar juice is commonly used as a cattle poison, when a cloth or rag smeared with the juice is either given with fodder or introduced into anal or vaginal canal of the animal. (iv) The root of calotropis procera is reputed to be strongly poisonous to cobras and other poisonous snakes, who cannot stand its smell. Hence, snake charmers may carry it to control freshly caught cobras. (v) When used with snuff, powdered madar root may cause death. (vi) The juice can often be used to produce artificial bruises. (vii) It may also be used as arrow poison.

CAPSICUM ANNUM (LAL MIRCH, CHILLIES) (Figure 39.7)

Capsicum fruits or seeds are extensively used in India as a condiment, in preparation of curries, *chutneys* etc. They have pungent acrid odour and taste, which lasts for a long time; may be used as stomachic and carminative.

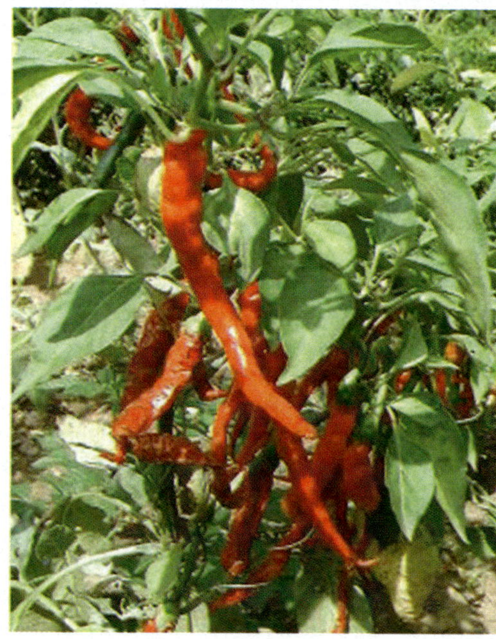

Figure 39.7: Capsicum annum plant

Chilli seed is approximately 0.30 cm (1/8″) long and 0.20 cm (1/10″) wide; they resemble very much *dhatura* seeds.

Active Principles: (i) Capsicin (ii) Capsaicin.

Signs and Symptoms

(i) Burning sensation in mouth (ii) Profuse salivation, thirst and difficulty in swallowing (iii) Pain in abdomen and constipation (iv) Burning sensation around the anus during passing stool (v) Nausea and vomiting (vi) Irritation and vesication on the skin, when applied locally (vii) Burning, lacrymation and chemosis, when applied to eyes (viii) Burning, lacrymation, coryza and cough, due to fumes of burned chillis (ix) **Hunan hand syndrome (Chilli burn):** It is a transient, painful, contact dermatitis usually developed on the hands of the cooks and chili pepper workers after prolonged exposure to chili peppers. The active ingredient capsaicin present in the peppers triggers the release of substance P which in contact with free nerve endings causes a sensation of intense burning pain. At the site of contact, usually there is no injury, no blister formation with an occasional finding of erythema. It is so named because it was observed commonly in the Hunan Province of China. Other terms used when different body parts involved are like "**Hunan nose**", "**Hunan eye**" and "**Chili Willie**".

Fatal Dose: Low toxicity.

Fatal Period: Fatality is unknown.

Treatment

(i) No specific treatment (ii) Stomach wash with plain water (iii) Cathartics should be given (iv) Irrigation of eyes with plenty of cold water or sterile normal saline and application of eye drops, in case of eye contamination (v) Skin contamination should be treated with plenty of water and an emollient cream locally.

Medicolegal Aspects

(i) Chilli powder may be thrown into the eyes to rob or steal valuables, money etc. from the persons by burglars and robbers specially from the bank counters. (ii) It can also be used to stupefy and disable a person to facilitate commission of crime. (iii) Chilli powder may be used for the purpose of torture to extract money or to extort confession of guilt, when it is introduced into the nostrils, eyes, vagina or urethra or rubbed over the breasts of females, burnt under the nose or when head is covered by nose-bags containing chilli powder. (iv) Burning of chilly seeds may at times be done by superstitious people to scare away devils and ghosts.

PLUMBAGO ROSEA, PLUMBAGO ZEYLANICA OR LAL CHITRA OR CHITRA

They grow as two types: *Plumbago rosea* (red flowers) and *Plumbago zeylanica* (white flowers) all over India (Figures 39.8 and 39.9).

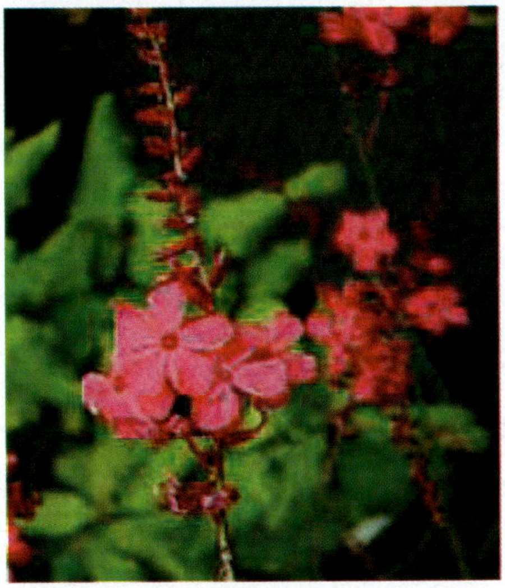

Figure 39.8: Plumbago rosea plant

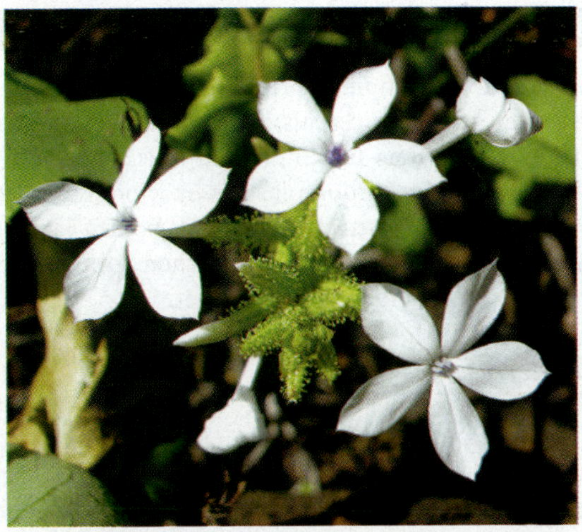

Figure 39.9: Plumbago zeylanica plant

Active Principles: The active principles is plumbagin contained in the roots and other parts of the plants. It is a highly acrid crystalline glycoside, the non-alkaloidal active principle. Plumbagin is powerful irritant and in small doses it stimulates contractions of heart, intestine and uterus. In large doses, it produces respiratory failure.

Fatal Dose and Fatal Period: Uncertain.

Signs and Symptoms

On external application of crushed roots and twigs of plants in the form of paste causes swelling, redness and inflammation and blister formation.

Ingestion of crushed roots in large doses causes: (i) Burning pain in mouth, throat and stomach with vomiting (ii) Intense thirst and diarrhea (iii) Convulsions (iv) Uterine contractions leading to abortion (v) Collapse and death from cardiorespiratory failure.

Treatment

(i) In case of local application of paste or abortion stick, it should be removed and vaginal douching with warm water and an antiseptic solution should be done. (ii) In case of ingestion, stomach wash with plain warm water, demulcents, stimulants, analeptics to combat shock and collapse.

Autopsy Findings

(i) Inflammation and injury in vagina, cervix and uterus when used as an abortifacient. (ii) Gastrointestinal irritation with congestion of all internal viscera.

Medicolegal Aspects

(i) Crushed roots of plumbago are used to procure abortion. The quacks used crushed roots as birth control pills. (ii) It is less commonly used for homicidal purposes. (iii) The paste or milky juice of crushed stems or leaves is applied to the skin to form reddish brown artificial bruise. (iv) Powdered leaves and roots may be used in the treatment of leprosy, scabies and influenza etc.

ERGOT

Ergot is dried sclerotium of the parasitic fungus *claviceps purpurea* that grows on cereals like wheat, rye, oat, barley and *bazra* etc. in wet seasons and ill-drained soils. The spores of ergot contaminate the grains through insects or wind. The spores then replace the grain and form dark purplish bodies larger than the original grain. These diseased grains when collected, dried and powdered constitutes ergot for the market.

Alkaloids of Ergot

These are grouped into:

1. Amino-acid alkaloids that comprises: (i) Ergotoxine (mixture of ergocrystine, ergocornine and ergocryptine) (ii) Ergotamine (iii) Ergosine.
2. Lysergic acid and amino-alkaloids that comprises: (i) Lysergic acid (ii) Lysergic and diethylamide (iii) Ergonovine (ergometrine) (iv) Methyl ergonovine (v) Methysergide.

Ergotoxine: It promotes contraction of pregnant uterus in last months of pregnancy but no or little effects are there on the uterus in other periods. It also produces gangrene by causing vasoconstriction.

Ergometrine: It is an active ecbolic and it causes prolonged uterine contraction especially on post-parturial uterus. It does not usually produce gangrene.

Lysergic acid and amino-alkaloids: They cause stimulation of central nervous system.

Ergot acts on smooth muscles of intestine, uterus and arterioles and it is commonly used in obstetrics for its ecbolic action. It is also used in the treatment of migraine, as abortifacient and in veterinary practice.

Fatal Dose: 1-2 grams.

Fatal Period: The death does not occur from single large dose but when small or medicinal doses are given for a long time. The fatal period is usually one day but death may be delayed for several days.

Signs and Symptoms

Acute Poisoning: The signs and symptoms of acute poisoning are: (i) Dryness and irritation of throat with intense thirst (ii) Nausea and vomiting (iii) Pain abdomen and diarrhoea (iv) Vertigo, giddiness and dizziness (v) Tightness and sense of constriction in chest (vi) Disturbance of speech and vision (vii) Tingling of hands and feet with feeling of numbness and coldness (viii) Muscular weakness and cramps in muscles (ix) Body temperature falls with hypoglycemia and suppressed urine (x) There may be abortion or bleeding from uterus (xi) Epistaxis, haemetemesis and haematuria may occur (xii) Convulsions and confusion leading to stupor and coma and finally death results from cardiorespiratory failure (xiii) In survivors, the extremities may develop gangrene.

Chronic Poisoning (Ergotism): Ergotism develops in those taking medicinal preparation of ergot or consumption of flour contaminated with ergot for a long time. The patients with focal sepsis and hepatic damage are more sensitive to ergot alkaloids. Signs and symptoms may present in convulsive or gangrenous form.

Convulsive Form: This form is presumed to occur with consumption of flour containing about 10% of ergot and is associated with vitamin A deficiency. The patient presents with (i) Tingling and itching (ii) Feeling of numbness in hands and feet and pain on walking (iii) Sensation of insects crawling under the skin (iv) Drowsiness and giddiness (v) Dimness of vision and fixed dilated pupil (vi) Loss of hearing and ataxia (vii) Loss of arterial pulsation and finally tonic or clonic convulsive seizures (viii) Paralysis of sensory nerves and maniac depressive psychosis (ix) Death results from asphyxia due to spasm of respiratory muscles.

Gangrenous Form: This form occurs with consumption of flour containing more than 10% of ergot. The following signs and symptoms are produced (i) There is swelling and pain in the limbs with feeling of intense heat, commonly known as **St. Anthony's fire or Holy fire** (ii) Tingling and numbness in fingers and toes resulting from vasospasm of arterioles (iii) Swelling of limbs and feet with red patches and blisters (iv) Loss of sensation of the part followed by gangrene formation from vasospasm and vasoconstriction with obliteration of the lumen of small blood vessels (v) The gangrene is of dry type affecting fingers, toes and limbs that become cold to touch and dark in colour. The gangrene may extend upto elbow or knee and may affect the nose, ears or even intestines with formation of ulcers.

Treatment

In Case of Acute Poisoning: (i) Stomach wash with plain warm water, tannic acid or activated charcoal (ii) Purgatives or enema can be given (iii) Vasodilators such as Nitroprusside or Nitroglycerine given parenterally (iv) Prazosin 1mg thrice daily orally and Captopril 50 mg thrice daily orally can be given for peripheral dilatation (v) The convulsion should be treated (vi) Heparin should be given I.M. for hypercoagulability of blood (vii) Hyperbaric oxygen to correct local tissue ischemia.

In Case of Chronic Poisoning: (i) The patient should be removed from the source of poisoning. (ii) Vasodilators as mentioned above. (iii) Gangrene to be treated by amputation.

Autopsy Findings

(i) Gastrointestinal tract will be congested with inflammatory changes (ii) All the visceral organs will be congested (iii) Gangrene of toes and fingers is evident (iv) Small blood vessels will show evidence of intimal degeneration.

Medicolegal Aspects

(i) Acute ergot poisoning may result from over dose of ergot preparations to cause abortion. (ii) Use of ergot preparations for a long time can result in ergotism.

CANTHARIDES (SPANISH FLY)

The dried beetle *Cantharis vesicatoria*, known as 'Spanish fly' contains a vesicant, **cantharidin.** Contact of either the live or the dried beetle with the skin results in immediate burning with vesication. Besides this, other beetles causing similar pictures include *Epicauta cinerea* (blister beetle) and members of genus *Paederus*. The compound is used as an aphrodisiac in both humans and cattle. It can cause **priapism** which is a persistent (more than 4 hours), usually painful erection unrelated to sexual activity.

Signs and Symptoms

A. **Ingestion results in:** (i) Burning sensation and vesication in mouth (ii) Nausea, vomiting and bloody diarrhoea (iii) Circulatory collapse (iv) Coma, convulsions and death.

B. **Local application on genitals results in:** (i) Intense haemorrhagic cystitis and urethritis with resulting priapism (ii) An intense pelvic congestion leading to abortion and priapism (iii) Onset of oliguria, haematuria and finally anuria heralds the appearance of several renal involvements.

Fatal Dose: 15-50 mg of cantharidine or 1½-3 g of powdered cantharides.

Treatment

(i) Gastric lavage to be carried (ii) Supportive and symptomatic treatment.

Autopsy Findings

(i) Forewings of the beetle may be found in the gastrointestinal tract (ii) Vesication of mouth and oesophagus may or may not be present (iii) Intense congestion and haemorrhage of the gastrointestinal tract (iv) Urinary bladder may be haemorrhagic (v) Haemorrhagic toxic nephritis in patient who survive longer.

SNAKES

Snakes belong to the class Reptilia, order squamata and suborder Serpentes. The snakes are found all over the world except New Zealand, Ireland and in Arctic lands. Of the 2500-3000 species of snakes distributed worldwide, about 500 are poisonous to humans. There are 238 species of snakes in India out of which only 52 are poisonous. Of these 52 poisonous species majority of bites and consequent mortality is attributable to 5 species viz. *Ophiophagus hannah* (king cobra), *Naja Naja* (common cobra), *Daboia rusellii* (Russell's viper), *Bungarus caeruleus* (krait) and *Echis carinatae* (saw-scaled viper).

In India, deaths as a result snake-biting are mainly accidental in nature. It has been reported that in most developing countries, up to 80% of individuals bitten by snakes first consult traditional practitioners before visiting a medical centre. In the year 1954, about 200,000 bites and 15,000 deaths were reported in India due to snake bite poisoning as far back as 1954. In Sri Lanka, the overall annual mortality from a single venomous species ranges from 5.6 per 100,000 to as high as 18 per 100,000 in some areas. Myanmar seems to have the highest mortality in Asia and 70% snakebites are by Russell's viper. However, this may only reflect a better reporting system prevalent in that country. Maharashtra, one of the states of India with the highest incidence, reported 70 bites per 100,000 population and mortality of 2.4 per 100,000 per year. The other states with a large number of snakebite cases include West Bengal, Tamil Nadu, Uttar Pradesh and Kerala.

General Characteristics of Snakes

A snake is a reptile without limbs and has a short tail. Vent is the opening in the rear part of the body for intestinal and genitourinary system. The part behind the vent is the tail that is flat in sea snakes and round in land snakes. The body of snakes is covered with scales. On the head, there are two eyes, two nostrils but no external ear. The eyes are covered with transparent scale bearing no eyelids and the pupils are round or vertical. All snakes are cold-blooded creatures with carnivorous habits. They use sharp teeth and strong muscles to catch the prey. The lower jaw comprises two bones, in front joined by an elastic ligament and it does not properly articulate with the upper jaw. The mouth of the snake is easily distensible allowing it to swallow even large animals as a whole. Their pointed and backwardly teeth are found on both jaws and palate. The upper marginal teeth get modified to form fangs. A new fang will appear in place of a broken one within 4-6 weeks. The fangs are solid in non-poisonous snakes but are grooved or channeled in poisonous ones for transport of venom from the poison glands to which they are connected through ducts. In poisonous snakes, parotid glands situated behind and below the eyes, one on each side secreting toxic saliva, and act as poison glands. The fangs of elapid snakes and sea snakes are short, fixed and grooved while those of vipers are long, movable and canalized. The tongue of the snake is forked at the tip and it acts as a sense organ for its search for food, other sex or enemy. Because of the shape of the body, the paired organs are laid one behind another. Poisonous snakes have only one right lung. The snake moults its skin several times a year throughout its life to keep oneself active. The snakes move by gliding motion.

Some snakes lay eggs, others give birth to young ones. Several species of egg layers such as pythons, cobras and water snakes have been found to stay with the eggs until hatching. The King Cobra is the only snake in the world that builds nest. In India the snakes range from the giant reticulated python (*Python reticulates*) that grows to 10 meters, to the tiny worm snake (*Typhina bramina*) which grows just 10 cm, and often mistaken for a worm. The King Cobra (*Ophiophagus Hannah*), the largest venomous snake in the world, which grows to 5 meters in India, is 'ophiphagus' that is they eat mostly snakes.

Differences between poisonous and nonpoisonous snakes (Table 39.2): There are certain physical characteristics that help to distinguish between the venomous and non-venomous snakes. Of these there are the belly scales that can be seen after turning the snake with belly upwards. The other distinguishable features are the size of head scales, fangs, appearance of tail, the teeth bite mark over the body of the victim and the habits of the snake whether they are nocturnal or diurnal.

Table 39.2: Differences between venomous and non-venomous snakes (Figures 39.10 to 39.12)

Features	Venomous snake	Non-venomous snake
Belly scales		
• Size	Large	Small
• Distribution	They cover the entire breadth of the belly. Some non-poisonous snakes may also possess such scales similar to those on the back or may be moderately large (Figure 39.13)	Never cover the entire breadth of the belly
Size of head scales	Usually small as in vipers except in pit vipers, Cobras or coral snakes and Kraits where they are large	Usually large
Fangs	Are hollow like hypodermic needles	Short and solid
Tail	Compressed	Not markedly compressed
Habits	Usually nocturnal	May be nocturnal or diurnal
Teeth-bite marks	Two fang marks are left at the site of bite usually with or without marks of other teeth. Usually they have two long teeth or fangs	Two fang marks are left at the site of bite and a number of several small teeth marks

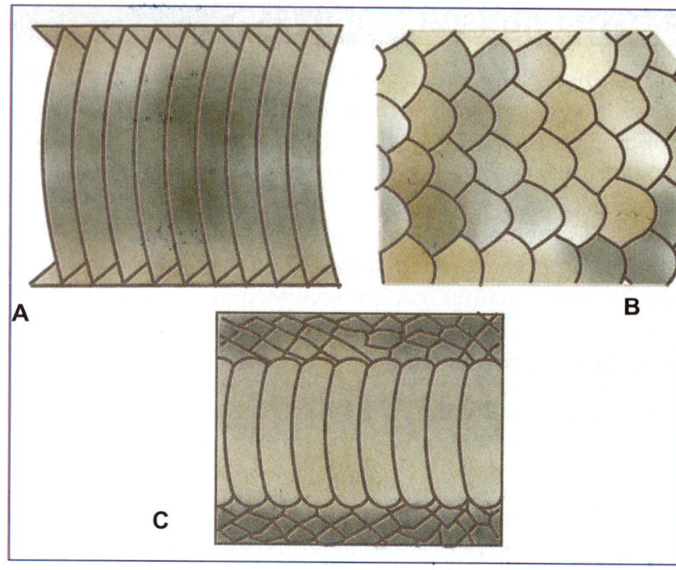

Figure 39.10: Large belly scales of venomous snakes with variations as in (A) Belly scales small like those on the back as in (B) or moderately large but not covering the entire breadth of belly as in (C)

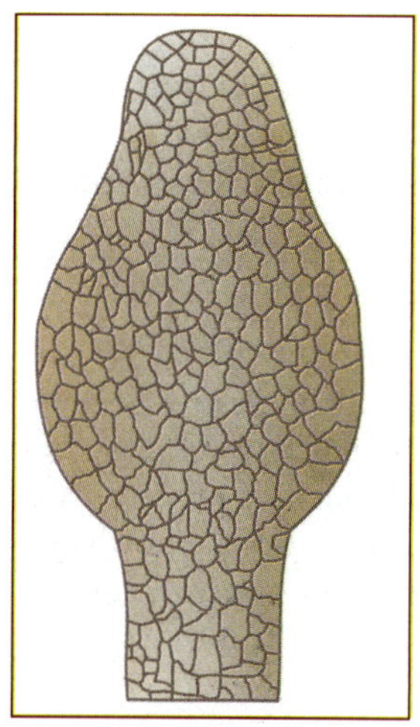

Figure 39.11: Small head scales of venomous snakes, e.g., Russel viper

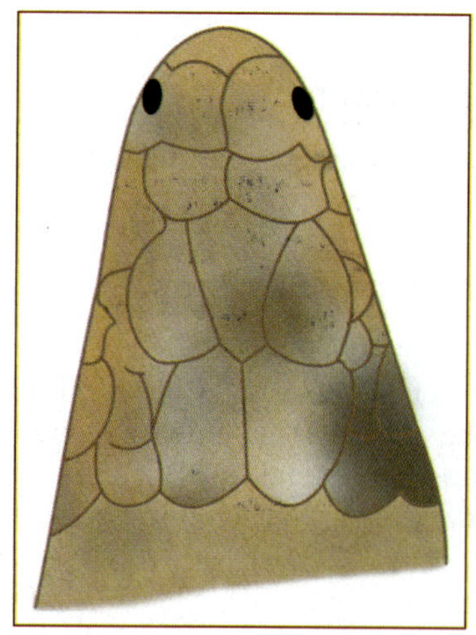

Figure 39.12: Large head scales of non-venomous snakes

Venomous Snakes

There are more than 52 species of venomous snakes in India of which there are four important types of snakes. These are King cobra, Krait (*Bungarus Russell*), Russell's viper (*Vipera Russell*) and the saw-scaled viper (*Echis carinatus*). Each of these snakes is easily distinguishable, though it is easy to confuse them with other harmless species. The venomous snakes are classified into three families based on the type of poison secreted.

I. **Elapidae or Colubridae that Secrete Neurotoxic Poisons**

Colubridae (Colubrid Snakes): The colubrine snakes lay eggs. Their oval heads covered by large scales are nearly of the same girth as of their neck that is indistinct and the pupils are circular. Their anteriorly situated fangs are short, fixed and grooved, thus they cannot effectively bite through the clothing and inject a complete lethal dose. The Colubrid snakes are sometimes referred to as "typical snakes". They comprise the largest family by far with over 2000 species worldwide. Most are medium sized snakes, and all lack a pelvic girdle and have no vestigial hind limbs and whose left lung is either absent or greatly reduced. Most species are considered members of two large subfamilies, Colubrine and Natricinae which are distinguished by the presence (Natricinae) or absence (Colubrinae) of spines on the lumbar vertebrae. The colubrines are subdivided into elapidae or land snakes, viperidae and hydrophidae or sea snakes.

Elapidae (Cobras and Coral Snakes): The cobra family is thought to have evolved from Colubrid snakes and many appear very similar in appearance with long, slender bodies and large scales (plates) on the head. They differ in having more advanced venom delivery systems than the venomous Colubrids. Elapids have fangs that are effectively tubular in that the fangs contain grooves that are enclosed by an infolding of the edges. The fangs are in the front of the mouth rather than the rear as is seen in venomous Colubrids. The Elapidae contains some of the world's most dangerous snakes including: (i) Common cobras (Naja Naja) (ii) King cobra (Naja hanna) (iii) Kraits: Kraits are bluish black in colour, shiny with transverse thin white cross bands, which may be very faint or sometimes even absent. They are subdivided into

(a) Common Krait (*Chitti*) and (b) Banded Krait (*Sankhini*) (iv) Mambas *(Dendroaspis)* (v) Sea snakes (Hydophinae and Laticaudinae) (vi) Coral snakes. In cobras and the coral snakes the third labial head scale touches the eye and nasal shields.

II. **Viperidae that Secrete Vasculotoxic Poisons**

The viperines are viviparous that is they give birth to young ones. The vipers are generally considered to be the most advanced family of snakes since they possess a very sophisticated venom delivery system. Large movable and tubular fangs are placed in the front of the mouth and they are hinged, allowing them to be folded back when not in use. The vipers can bite through the clothes and inject the venom. Their triangular heads are covered with numerous small scales and their eyes have vertically elliptical pupils. All the viperine species are poisonous. The viperine snakes have following subfamilies: (i) Saw scaled viper (ii) Pit viper (iii) Russell's vipers.

III. **Hydrophidae or Sea Snakes that Secrete Myotoxic Poisons**

There are about twenty types of sea snakes found in India and all are venomous. They have small heads, small eyes and a flat tail that helps in swimming. Their valved nostrils are situated on the top of the snout for free breathing. The belly plates are not broad and have dull trabeculated scales on their back. The poison glands are delicate with short fangs that are situated posteriorly. Their bodies are greenish black, dark black or bluish black in colour.

Common Cobra (Naja Naja, Nag, Gokhurra) (Figures 39.13 and 39.14): Common cobra is seen throughout India, Sri Lanka and Burma. These are 1.5-2 meters long. The cobra varies in colour from cream to black, though generally it is brown. The hood may have the typical spectacle or monocle marking on its underside, which are two dark round spots and at times only one spot surrounded by an ellipse. The characteristic hood of the cobra is visible only when it raises its head while in danger, enraged or about to strike. The underside of the hood also bears three dark bands on the central part and a white band in an area where hood touches the body. The divided tail shield helps in identifying a cobra when hood is not visible. The maxillary bone extends beyond the palate and the poison fangs are followed by one or two small teeth. In cobra, head scales are large and third labial touches the eye and nasal shields with round pupil (Figure 39.15).

King Cobra (Naja bangarus, Raj Nag or Daras): The King cobra is found in the hills and forests of South India, Orissa, Assam and the Himalayas. It is bigger in size compared to the common cobra and its length is usually 2.5-4.5 meters. The head is flat with a hood but no spectacle mark on it. It is usually jet black but can also be brownish to greenish and sometimes yellow. The tail scales are entirely present in their proximal ends but divided in the distal ends.

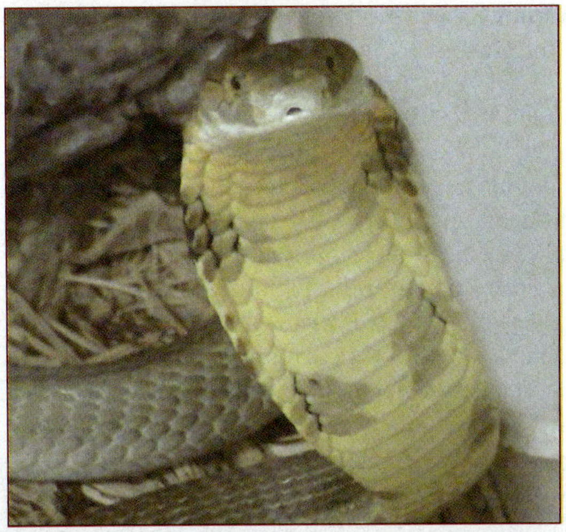

Figure 39.13: Cobra and its moderately large belly scales

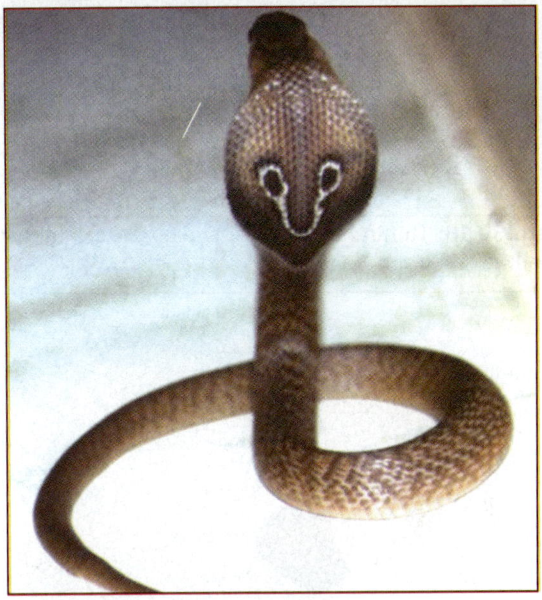

Figure 39.14: Hood of cobra showing spectacle mark

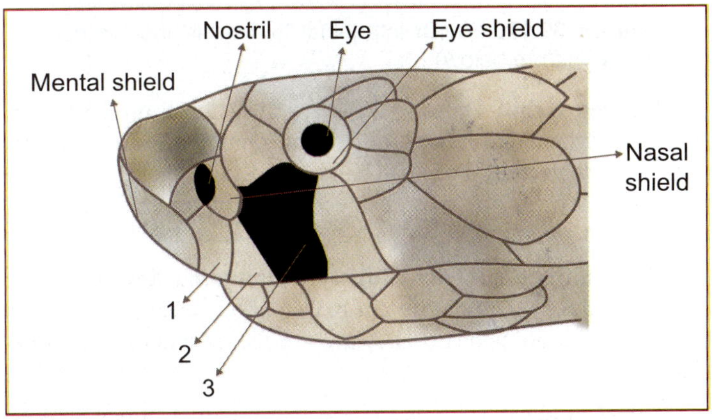

Figure 39.15: In cobra head scales are large and third labial touches the eye and nasal shields with round pupil

Common Krait (Bangarus Caeruleus): The common krait is found throughout India and is known by the names of *Chitti* (Calcutta), *Kawriya* (Punjab), *Maniyar* (Maharashtra). They are nocturnal and their habitat is near dwelling houses. The size may be 1.5 meters long and are usually steel black in colour. They bear single or double narrow bands across their back that extends from below the head up to the tip of tail. The belly is creamy white in colour. Their head are oval with one enlarged central row of hexagonal scales on the back (Figure 39.16). The undersurface of the mouth has only four infralabials–the fourth is the largest and there are bands or half rings across the back (Figure 39.17). The third labial scale does not touch the nose and eye. The tail is round with tail scales that are entirely placed and not divided.

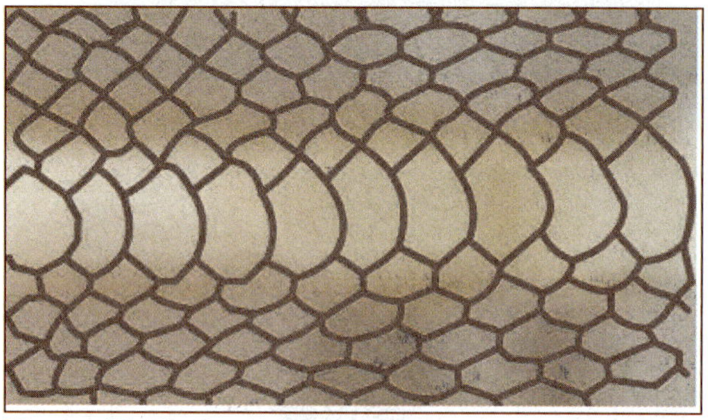

Figure 39.16: Central hexagonal scales on the middle of the back of krait

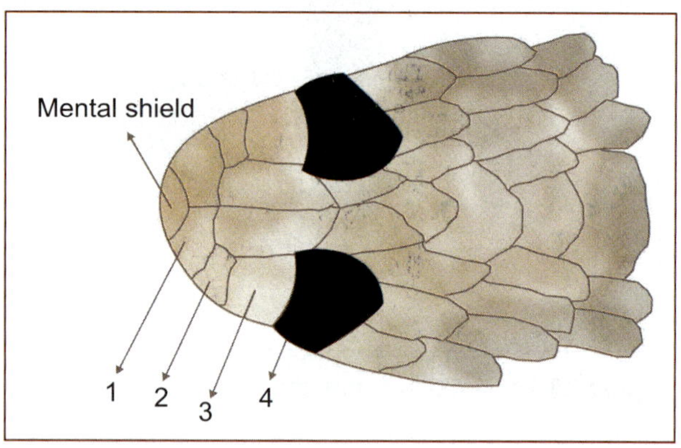

Figure 39.17: Fourth infralabial in krait is the largest (View is from below)

Banded Krait: These snakes vary in length from 2.5 to 3.5 meters, longer, bigger and stouter than common krait. It bears alternate jet black and yellow bands across its back, hence the name. It has a black mark on its neck spreading up to the eyes. It is deadly poisonous snake (Figures 39.16 and 39.18).

Rat Snake (Zamenis Mucosus, Dhamana Samp): They may look like a cobra but do not have a hood, spectacle mark or monocle mark on its head. They are 5-6 feet in length with large nostrils.

Coral Snakes: The coral snakes are relatively small snakes that spend most of their time underground and are found in hilly areas. Their size may be up to 1.5 meters (3 feet) and their primary food is other snakes. The bellies are pinkcoral coloured and the

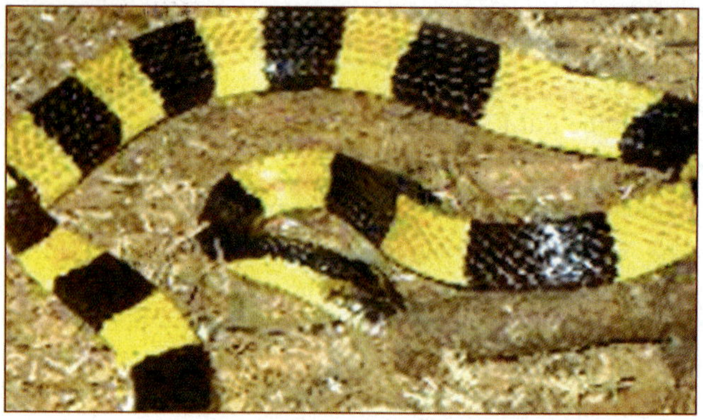

Figure 39.18: Banded krait

tail is round. Despite their small size and small fangs, their venom is extremely toxic.

Pit Vipers (Crotalidae): Pit vipers have a pair of heat sensing pits located on the head between each eye and nostril (Figure 39.19). The pit helps in detecting warm blooded prey in the dark. They are usually 2-4 feet (30-100 cm) in length and are found in the hills. These snakes are seldom fatal to humans. Their body is flat and broad with triangular head. They are found in hilly areas with their distinct green or sometimes yellow colour).

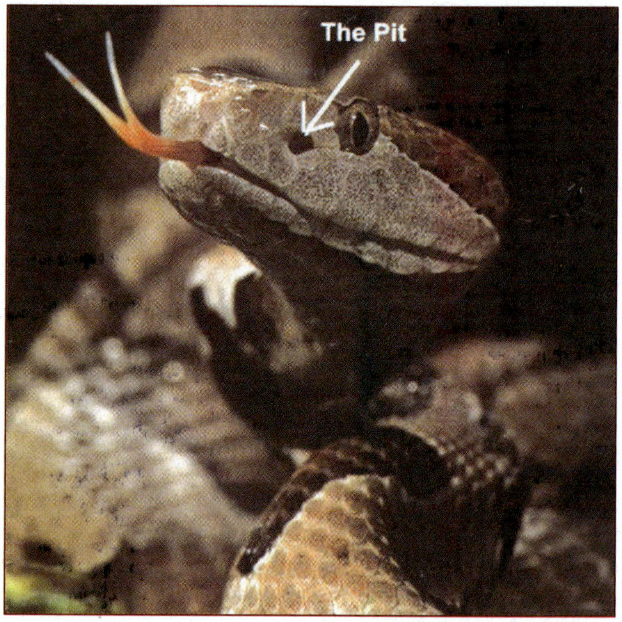

Figure 39.19: Pit viper

Russel's Viper (Chandra Bora or Daboia): Russel's vipers are heavy bodied snakes with narrow necks, triangular heads and three longitudinal regular chain-like pattern or rows on the back. The scales are quite rough and the overall colour is yellowish and brown. It is found throughout India in the plains. It is 1-1.5 meters long and is stouter than any other poisonous snake. Head scales are small and the nostrils are bigger than any other Indian snake. The tail is short with divided shields and the belly scales are broad. It makes a loud hissing sound before striking the enemy (Figure 39.20).

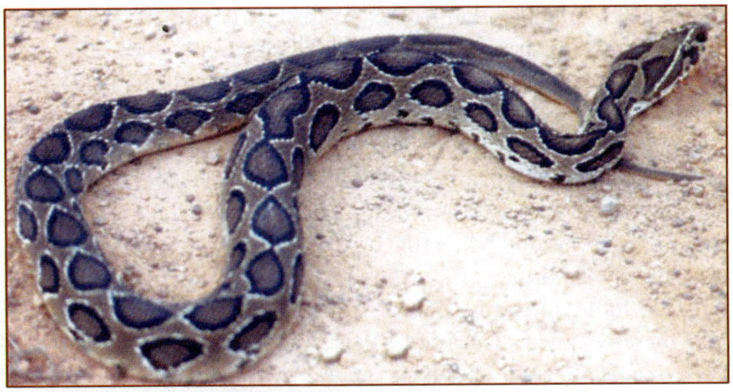

Figure 39.20: Russel's viper

Saw-Scaled Viper (Phoorsa or Echis Carinata): The saw-scaled viper is the smallest of these four types of snake, growing to just a foot. It is brownish with white marking and has a triangular head typical of the vipers (Figure 39.21).

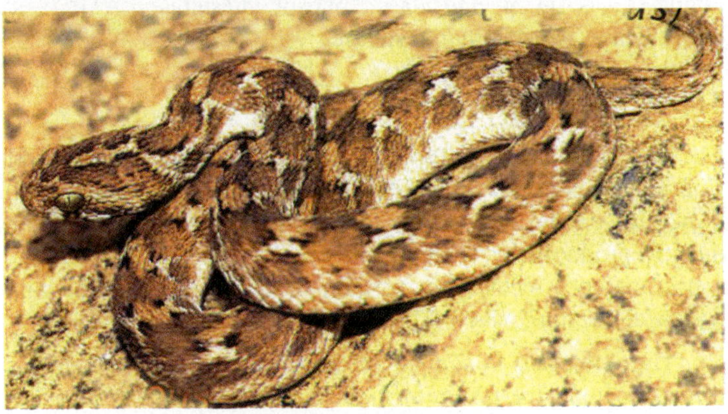

Figure 39.21: Saw-scaled viper

The scales on the head are small and that on the body are broad having serrated edges. It makes a peculiar rustling sound while moving because of its saw-like scales on the body.

The differences between cobra and viper are given in Table 39.3.

Table 39.3 Differences between cobras and vipers

Features	Cobras	Vipers
Body	Long and cylindrical	Short and stout
Head	Small and seldom broader than body, same width as neck, covered with large scales	Larger and broader than body, wider than neck, triangular and covered with small scales
Upper jaw	Has 2 poison fangs and other teeth	Only poison fangs
Eyes	Round pupil	Vertical pupil
Fangs	Grooved, short and fixed	Canalized, long and mobile
Tail	Round	Tapered
Venom	Neurotoxic	Haemotoxic
Eggs	Oviparous (lays eggs)	Viviparous (gives birth to young one)

SNAKE VENOM

The snake venom is the secretion of the racemose salivary glands that is a modification of the parotid salivary gland of other vertebrates, and is usually situated on each side of the head below and behind the eye, invested in a muscular sheath. It is provided with large alveoli in which the venom is stored before being conveyed by a duct to the base of the channelled or tubular fang through which it is ejected. Snake venom is poisonous only when it is injected but is not absorbed by the stomach mucosa when ingested. The blood of animal bitten by snakes will be poisonous and lethal when injected into the human body.

The Vipers furnish examples of the most highly developed poison apparatus, although inferior to some in its toxic effects, the poison gland is very large and in intimate relation with the masseter or temporal muscle, consisting of two bands, the superior arising from behind the eye, the inferior extending from the gland to the mandible. When the snake bites, the jaws close up, causing the gland to be powerfully wrung, and the poison pressed out into the duct. From the anterior extremity of the gland the duct passes, below the eye and above the maxillary bone, where it makes a bend, to the basal orifice of the poison fang, which is ensheathed in a thick fold of mucous membrane, the vagina dentis. By means of the movable maxillary bone hinged to the prefrontal, and connected with the transverse bone which is pushed forward by muscles set in action by the opening of the mouth, the tubular fang is erected and the poison discharged through the distal orifice in which it terminates.

Proteroglyphous Colubrids: The poison fangs are not tubular, but only channelled and open along the anterior surface. As the maxillary bone in these snakes is more or less elongate, and not or but slightly movable vertically, the poison duct runs above the latter, making a bend only at its anterior extremity, and the transverse bone has not the same action on the erection of the fangs. Otherwise the mechanism is the same.

Opisthoglyphous Colubrids: The grooved teeth are situated at the posterior extremity of the maxilla and a small posterior portion of the upper labial or salivary gland is converted into a poison-secreting organ. This is distinguished by a light yellow colour, provided with a duct larger than any of those of the labial gland, and proceeding inward and downward to the base of the grooved fang. The duct is not in direct connection with the groove, but the two communicate through the mediation of the cavity enclosed by the folds of mucous membrane surrounding the tooth, and united in front.

The reserve or successional teeth, which are always present just behind or on the side of the functional fang of all venomous snakes, are in no way connected with the duct until called upon to replace a fang that has been lost.

When biting, a Viperid snake merely strikes, discharging the venom the moment the fangs penetrate the skin, and then immediately leaves it. A Proteroglyph or Opisthoglyph Colubrid, on the contrary, closes its jaws like a dog on the part bitten, often holding on firmly for a considerable time.

The poison, which is mostly a clear limpid fluid of a pale straw or amber colour, more rarely greenish, sometimes with a certain amount of suspended matter, is exhausted after several bites, and the glands have to recuperate. The venom retains its poisonous properties for several years in dried state. The Cobra venom is slightly viscous and when exposed to sun it becomes a little turbid. The venom of Russel's viper is usually white or yellow.

It must be added that the poison can be ejected otherwise than by a bite, as in the so-called **Spitting snakes**, when irritated they are in the habit of shooting poison from the mouth, at a distance of 4 to 8 feet. In all probability, the poison escapes from the sheath of mucous membrane surrounding the base of the fangs, and is mixed with ordinary saliva, the membranes of the mouth perhaps acting as lips, in which case the term "spitting" would not be incorrect. The spitting, which may take place three or four times in succession, has been observed to be preceded by some chewing movements of the jaws. If reaching the eye, the poisonous fluid causes severe inflammation of the cornea and conjunctiva, but no more serious results if washed away at once.

Snakes emerging out from hibernation after winter usually give fatal bite. Nocturnal bites are more serious than those occurring during the day. Less venom will be injected if the fangs are broken or if the snake had bitten a prey previously. The vipers give a strong and complete bite whereas in cobra bite the transfer of venom is not complete. Bite on limbs and adipose tissue is less dangerous than those on the trunk, face or scalp.

It is noteworthy that the size of the poison fangs is in no relation to the virulence of the venom. The comparatively innocent Indo-Malay Lachesis alluded to above have enormous fangs, whilst the smallest fangs are found in the most justly dreaded of all snakes, the Hydrophids.

Venoms of different species of poisonous snakes varies in the toxicity, composition and antigenic structure. It is basically a mixture of one or more of the toxic substances, toxalbumins and enzymes in varying proportions such as: (i) *Proteolytic enzymes or proteolysins:* It causes liberation of histamine from the damaged muscular endothelium leading to dissolution of walls of blood vessels with extravasation of blood in the tissue space, also causes digestion of tissue proteins and peptides and produces marked tissue destruction. (ii) *Fibrin ferments or fibrinolysin thromboplastin* enhancing the coagulation process. (iii) *Neurotoxins* (mainly in elapidae venom) producing curare like effect causing paralysis especially of respiratory center. (iv) *Cholinestrase* (mainly in elapidae venom) causing hydrolysis of acetylcholine to choline and acetic acid thus causes impairment of neuromuscular transmission. (v) *Haemolysin* (mainly in viper venom) causing widespread hemolysis in presence of lecithinase. (vi) *Cytolysin* (mainly in viperine venom) causing lysis of cell structures of blood and tissues. (vii) *Agglutinins* causing agglutination of red blood cells. (viii) *Phosphatidases* produce haemolysis and toxic effects on heart and circulation with haemorrhage from lungs. (ix) *Proteinases* have trypsin like action, causing tissue damage. It produces anticoagulant effect from destruction of fibrinogen. It also catalyses the conversion of prothrombin to thrombin thus producing coagulant effect. (x) *Phospholipase* A, B, C, D acts as catalyst in hydrolysis of lipids. By destroying phospholipids in nervous tissues, it alters neuromuscular conduction. It also helps in penetration of neurotoxin into nervous tissue. (xi) *Hyaluronidase* helps in rapid spreading of the venom from the local site of bite and thereby quick absorption. It is present in all snake venoms. (xii) *Ribonuclease* and *deoxyribonulease* helps in rapid spreading of the venom from the local site of bite and thereby quick absorption. It is present in all venoms. (xiii) *Ophioxidase* helps in autolysis. (xiv) *Protease* causes dissolution of vascular wall and help in spreading of red blood cells and serum in the tissues. (xv) *Lecithinases* acts on the lipid layer of the cells causing increasing fragility and permeability leading to cell destruction. (xvi) It also contains enzymes such as: Acetylcholine, 5-Hydroxytryptamine, 5-nucleotidases, endonucleases, transaminases, NAD nucleosidase, phosphodiesterase, ATP, acid phosphatase, phosphomonoesterase.

The Colubrine Venom

The effect of the poison of Proteroglyphous Colubrids (Hydrophids, Cobras, Bungarus, Elapides, Pseudechis, Notechis, Acanthophis) is mainly on the nervous system. Respiratory paralysis being quickly produced by bringing the poison into contact with the central nervous mechanism which controls respiration; the pain and local swelling which follow a bite are not usually severe.

The colubrine venom is predominantly neurotoxic and is primarily toxic for respiratory and cardiac centres. It also has some toxic effects on the cardiovascular system. The cobra venom produces muscular paralysis involving firstly the muscles of the mouth, throat and lastly muscles of respiration, seat of action of venom being upon the motor nerve cells, the action resembling curare. It consists of: (i) Neurotoxin (ii) Cholinesterase (iii) Proteases (iv) Phosphotidases (v) Hyaluronidase (vi) Ribonuclease (vii) Thromboplastin (viii) Fibrinolysin (ix) Proteolysin (x) Cardiotoxin (xi) Phospholipase. Cobra venom produces convulsions and paralysis, while krait venom produces only muscular paralysis.

The Viperine Venom

The viperine venom is predominantly hemolytic and hemotoxic. It produces cytolysis of cells of vascular endothelium; causes lysis of red cells and other tissue cells and coagulation disorders. It consists of: (i) Proteases (ii) Hyaluronidase (iii) Haemorrhagin (iv) Haemolysin (v) Leucolysin (vi) Lecithinase (vii) Cytolysin (viii) Thromboplastin (ix) Phospholipase A (x) Proteinases.

Viper poison (Vipera, Echis, Lachesis, Crotalus) acts more on the vascular system, bringing about coagulation of the blood and clotting of the pulmonary arteries; its action on the nervous system is not great, no individual group of nerve-cells appears to be picked out, and the effect upon respiration is not so direct;

the influence upon the circulation explains the great depression which is a symptom of viperine poisoning. The pain of the wound is severe, and is speedily followed by swelling and discoloration.

There will be haemorrhage from the site of bite, associated with the necrosis of renal tubules, convulsions from intracerebral haemorrhage. Locally, there will be severe swelling of the bitten part, with oozing of blood and spreading cellulitis. Blood from such patients fails to clot even on addition of thrombin, because of the very low level of fibrinogen. The oozing of blood and serum is very much pronounced in case of viper bite than in cobra bite. Absence of oozing will indicate that the venom has not been injected into the wound.

A Cobra can inject about 40 times the fatal dose in a single bite. The amount of dried venom produced in a single bite is: (i) In Cobra bite (200-250 mg) (ii) In Viperine bite (150-200 mg) (iii) In Krait bite (20 mg) (iv) In Saw-scaled viper (4.5-5 mg).

Fatal Doses of various bites are: (i) Dried cobra venom—12- 15 mg (ii) Dried viper venom—15-20 mg (iii) Dried krait venom—5-6 mg (iv) Dried saw-scaled viper venom—8 mg.

Fatal Period: The death may occur instantaneously from neurogenic shock resulting from fright otherwise the fatal period is: (i) In colubrine bite—1/2-24 hours (ii) In viperine bite—2-4 days.

Signs and Symptoms of Ophitoxaemia

1. **Psychological trauma:** The most common and earliest symptom following snake bite (poisonous or nonpoisonous) is fright, particularly of rapid and unpleasant death. Owing to fright, a victim attempts 'flight' which unfortunately results in enhanced systemic absorption of venom. These emotional manifestations develop extremely rapidly (almost instantaneous) and may produce psychological shock and even death. Fear may cause also transient pallor, sweating and vomiting.
2. **Local manifestations:** With the possible exception of the psychological trauma of being bitten, local changes are the earliest manifestations of snake bites. Features are noted within 6-8 minutes but may have onset up to 30 minutes (i) Local burning pain with radiation and tenderness and the development of a small reddish wheal are the first to occur. (ii) This is followed by oedema, swelling and appearance of bullae all of which can progress quite rapidly and extensively even involving the trunk. (iii) Tingling and numbness over the tongue, mouth and scalp and paraesthesia around the wound occur mostly in viper bites. (iv) Local bleeding including petechial and/or purpuric rash is also seen most commonly with viperine bites. (v) Local area of bite may become devascularized with features of necrosis predisposing to onset of gangrenous changes. (vi) Secondary infection including tetanus and gas gangrene may also result.
3. **Systemic manifestations:** Regional lymphadenopathy has been reported as an early and reliable sign of systemic poisoning. The time onset of poisoning is similar in different species. Cobra produces symptoms as early as 5 minutes or as late as 10 hours after the bite. Vipers take slightly longer the mean duration of onset being 20 minutes. However, symptoms may be delayed for several hours. Sea snake bites almost always produce myotoxic features within 2 hours so that they are reliably excluded if no symptoms are evident within this period. Other systemic manifestations depend upon the pathophysiological changes induced by the venom of that particular species. As mentioned previously, based on the predominant constituents of venom of a particular species, snakes were loosely classified as neurotoxic (notably cobras and kraits), hemorrhagic (vipers) and myotoxic (sea snakes). However, it is now well recognized that such a strict categorization is not valid as each species can result in any kind of manifestations.

Features of neurotoxicity: Neurotoxic features are a result of selective d-tubocurarine like neuromuscular blockade which results in flaccid paralysis of muscles. Cobra venom is however 15-40 times more potent than tubocurarine (i) Ptosis is the earliest neuroparalytic manifestation followed closely by ophthalmoplegia. (ii) Paralysis then progresses to involve muscles of palate, jaw, tongue, larynx, neck and muscles of deglutition but not strictly in that order. (iii) Generally muscles innervated by cranial nerves are involved earlier. However, pupils are reactive to light till terminal stages. (iv) Muscles of chest are involved relatively late with diaphragm being the most resistant. This accounts for the respiratory paralysis, which is often terminal. (v) Reflex activity is generally not affected in ophitoxaemia and deep tendon jerks are preserved till late stages. (vi) Onset of coma is variable, however several cases of cobra bite progress to coma within 2 hours of bite. (vii) Symptoms that precede paralysis include repeated vomiting, blurred vision, paraesthesiae around the mouth, hyperacusis, headache, dizziness, vertigo and signs of autonomic hyperactivity.

Features of cardiotoxicity: Cardiotoxicity occurs in about 25% viperine bites (i) There are fluctuations in rate, rhythm and blood pressure in the form of tachycardia, hypotension and ECG changes. (ii) In addition, sudden cardiac standstill may also occur owing to hyperkalemic arrest. (iii) Non dyselectrolytemic acute myocardial infarction has also been reported.

Tetanic contraction of heart following a large dose of cobra venom has been documented. There is a single case report of nonbacterial thrombotic endocarditis following viper bite. Myalgic features are the most common presentation of bites by sea snakes. Muscle necrosis may also result in myoglobinuria.

Haemostatic defects: Snake venoms cause haemostatic defects by a number of different mechanisms. Some cause activation of intravascular coagulation and result in consumption coagulopathy. Notable in this group is Daboia russelli which has procoagulant activating factors V and X. Certain other venoms cause defibrinogenation by activating endogenous fibrinolytic system. Besides direct effects on the coagulation cascade, venoms also can cause qualitative and quantitative defects in platelet function. In India and Sri Lanka, Russell's viper envenomation is often associated with massive intravascular haemolysis. Haematological changes, both local as well as systemic are some of the most common features of snake bite poisoning (i) Bleeding may occur from multiple sites including gums, GIT (haematemesis and melaena), urinary tract, injection sites and even as multiple petechiae and purpura. (ii) Even subarachnoid haemorrhages, subdural haemorrhages and extradural hematoma have also been reported. (iii) Almost every species of snake can cause renal failure. It is fairly common following Russell's viper bite and is a major cause of death. In a series of 40 viper bites, renal failure was documented in about a third. The extent of renal abnormality in them correlated well with the degree of coagulation defect; however in a majority renal defects persisted for several days after the coagulation abnormalities normalised: suggesting that multiple factors are involved in venom induced ARF.

Rarer systemic manifestations: These include: (i) Hypo-pituitarism (ii) Bilateral thalamic hematoma (iii) Hysterical paralysis.

4. **Delayed manifestations of snake bite:** The delayed onset of signs and symptoms of snake bite is rare but definitely occurs in the form of bleeding manifestations including brain haemorrhages up to one week after the bite. Some patients develop compartment syndromes several weeks after the bite. The possible explanation for delayed bleeding is that local blebs constitute a venom depot, which is suddenly released into the blood stream, especially when the wound is handled surgically. Differences in clinical manifestations produced by cobra and viper are given in Table 39.4.

Table 39.4: Comparative features of clinical manifestations of colubrine and viperine bites

Features	Colubrine bite	Viperine bite
Onset of signs and symptoms	Within 10-20 minutes	Within second to 10 minutes
Development of gangrene	Early, wet type	Slower onset, dry type
Feeling of intoxication	Marked	Not marked
Gait	Staggering	Not so but features of general paralysis
Speech and power of deglutition	Lost	Not so
Involvement of tongue and larynx	Are paralysed with trickling of saliva from mouth	Not affected, salivation is absent
Pupils	Normal	Dilated, not reacting to light
Respiration	Slow, weak and laboured	Quick and laboured
Blood coagulability	Not affected	Completely dearranged
Haemorrhagic manifestations	Not present	Most important feature
Death	From respiratory paralysis	When rapid, due to pulmonary thrombosis; when slow, from toxic action of venom on heart and blood

Laboratory Diagnosis in Ophitoxaemia

The laboratory serves rather poorly in the diagnosis of snakebite but laboratory tests are useful for monitoring, prognosticating victims of Ophitoxaemia, as well as determining stages of intervention (i) *Enzyme linked immunoabsorbent assay (ELISA):* ELISA studies which are now available to identify the species involved, based on antigens in the venom. These tests are expensive and not freely available and hence of limited value except for epidemiological study. (ii) Blood changes include anaemia, leucocytosis and thrombocytopenia. (iii) Peripheral smear may show evidence of haemolysis, particularly in viperine bites. (iv) Deranged coagulant activity manifested by prolonged clotting time and prothrombin time may also be evident. The quality of clot formed may be a better indicator of coagulation capability than the actual time required for formation, since clot lysis has been observed in several patients who had normal clotting time. Hypofibrinogenemia may also be evident. (v) Among the metabolic changes, hyperkalaemia and hypoxemia with respiratory acidosis, especially with neuroparalysis may be present. (vi) Urine examination could reveal haematuria, proteinuria, haemoglobinuria or myoglobinuria. (vii) In cases of acute renal failure, all features of azotemia are also present. (viii) CSF haemorrhage has been documented in a minority. of victims. (ix) ECG changes are generally nonspecific and include alterations in rhythm (predominantly bradycardia) and atrioventricular block with ST segment elevation or depression. In addition, cases who develop hyperkalaemia manifest typical changes of this dyselectrolytaemia. (x) Serum cholesterol levels correlates negatively with severity of envenomation. (xi) Recently EEG changes have been noted in up to 96% of patients bitten by snakes; starting within hours of the bite. Interestingly none of them showed any clinical features suggestive of encephalopathy. These abnormal EEG patterns were picked up mainly in the temporal lobes.

20-Minute Whole Blood Clotting Test (20 WBCT): It is a simple, effective, affordable bed site test to determine venom-induced consumption coagulopathies (VICC) in snakebite patients. One ml of fresh whole blood is placed in a 5 ml clean dry glass tube and left undisturbed. 20 minutes later, the tube is inverted. Failure to clot is considered a positive test which gives clue for diagnose hemotoxic (viper bite) envenomation and rule out elapid bite.

Management of Venomous Snakebite (Ophitoxaemia)

A. **First Aid for Snakebite:**

(i) **Reassurance to the patient:** 70% of all snakebites are by nonvenomous snakes and 50% of bites by venomous species are dry bites. The victim should be explained that death is not imminent and medical care is available. (ii) Remove shoes, jewellery, watches, rings and tight clothing from the bitten area, as these can act as tourniquet, if swelling occurs. (iii) **Immobilization of the bitten limb:** The affected limb should be immobilized in the same way as a fractured limb. The principle is to minimize the movement of the venom around the body until the victim reaches hospital by using a splint (e.g., wooden stick) or sling. Use bandages or cloth just to hold the splints without applying any pressure, as it can block the blood supply which is dangerous. (iv) The victim should be shifted immediately to a hospital where optimal medical care with anti-snake venom (ASV) is available.

Practice of Pressure Immobilization Techniques: The use of this first aid technique in snakebite is controversial and currently, most toxicologists do not recommend. The bitten limb is wrapped with a compression bandage like crepe bandage or elastic bandage (if both not available cloth or other suitable material can be used), 10-15 cm wide, in overlapping turns, starting at the fingers or toes and continuing as far up the limb as possible to apply pressure of 50-70 mm Hg (for lower limb) or 40-70 mm Hg (for upper limb). It should be applied about as tight as that used for a sprained ankle. Enough space to allow one finger between the limb and bandage is most appropriate. The compression bandage should be tight enough to occlude the lymphatics, but not venous drainage. The limb is then immobilized by applying a splint or sling which again can be incorporated under the layers of the bandage. When applied properly, this method can trap the venom in the bitten area for many hours. The victim might not suffer any effects of the venom until the compression is released, which is done in hospital where antivenom can be administered, if required. This technique may be applied by a qualified medical professional when the victim is expected to reach the hospital in more than 30 minutes but less than 3 hours. The pressure immobilization technique (application of firm crepe bandage combined with splinting of bitten limb) was developed by Australian scientist **Struan Sutherland.** It can be helpful in neurotoxic elapid bites and should not be used for viper bites (can cause localized tissue necrosis). **Compression Pad and Ring:** A pad is placed over the bite wound site which is held in place with a nonelastic band with a pressure of at least 70 mm Hg, combined with a splint to immobilize the extremity **(Monash Technique).** When the bite is on torso (like thoracic or abdominal part), a circumferential compression device consisting of a ring with two hooks for attaching a band to apply pressure may be used as pressure immobilization bandages could not be used for these sites. Presently these techniques for first aid is no more recommended.

Status of Other Practices: (i) **Bite wound site should not be washed:** As traces of venom that are left on the skin can be used to identify the snake, and therefore the type of antivenom that should be used if required. (ii) **No incision and suction of the bite wound site:** Since the venom is injected deeply, so there is no benefit in cutting or sucking the bite site. It was formerly believed that incision over the bite drains out venom. However, it has now been established from animal experiments that systemic venom absorption starts almost instantly that is why incising and sucking is nowadays being questioned. However, some experts suggest that longitudinal incisions within fifteen minutes of the bite may be beneficial. (iii) **No tourniquets:** Use of tourniquets as a first aid technique is no more recommended in India. It can cause limb ischemia and necrosis. If tourniquet is already present in situ, precaution should be taken before removing tight tourniquets, as sudden release can lead to a massive surge of venom, leading to paralysis, hypotension, etc. The distal pulse should be checked first, if the tourniquet has occluded the distal pulse, then blood pressure cuff should be applied and pressure should be slowly reduced. In case of Viper bites, tourniquets are also a risk as the Viper's venom contains procoagulant enzymes which can cause the blood to clot in the small space below the tourniquet. When the tourniquet is released the clot will rapidly enter the body and can cause embolism and death. (iv) There is disagreement over the use of drugs as part of first-aid care. It has been suggested that NSAIDs particularly aspirin may be beneficial to relieve local pain. **Russell,** however, dissuades use of analgesic and in particular aspirin for fear of precipitating bleeding. In **Reid's** experience, pain relief with placebo was as effective as NSAID. Codeine may be useful in some cases. Similarly, there are proponents as well as opponents for use of sedatives. (v) **Nil by mouth:** No solid food or drinks should be given. (vi) No elevation of extremity and excessive physical activity. It should be avoided because they may hasten systemic absorption of venom. (vii) **No cryotherapy:** Ice should not be applied on the bitten area. (viii) **No electric shock:** Dangerous in experimental studies and is not recommended. (ix) **No to use of traditional first aid methods** like black stones, scarification etc. and alternative medical/herbal therapy as they have no role and do more harm than good by delaying treatment.

B. **Specific Therapy (Anti-Snake Venom):**

Anti-Snake Venom (ASV) is prepared by immunizing horses with venom from poisonous snakes and extracting the serum and purifying it. Antivenoms or antivenins may be species specific (monovalent) or effective against several species (polyvalent). The polyvalent ASV is only available in India which is effective against four common poisonous snakes (Cobra, Common Krait, Russel's Viper and Saw-scaled Viper). Monovalent antivenom is ideal, but the cost and non-availability, besides the difficulty of accurately identifying the offending species makes its use less common.

Indications for use: There are specific indications for use of antivenom. Not every bite, even if by poisonous species merits its use. This caution against the empirical use of antivenom is due to the risk of hypersensitivity reactions. Therefore, antivenin is indicated only if: (i) Serious manifestations of envenomation are evident viz coma, neurotoxicity, hypotension, shock, bleeding, DIC, acute renal failure, rhabdomyolysis and ECG changes. (ii) In the absence of these systemic manifestations, swelling involving more than half the affected limb, extensive bruising or blistering and progression of the local lesions within 30-60 minutes are other indications. (iii) There are no absolute contraindications to ASV.

Dose: The freeze-dried polyvalent ASV powder is reconstituted with 10 ml of distilled water/saline/dextrose. Despite widespread use of antivenom, there are virtually no clinical trials to determine the ideal dose. Conventionally: (i) 50 ml is infused for mild manifestations like local swelling with or without lymphadenopathy, purpura or ecchymosis. (ii) Moderate envenomation defined by presence of coagulation defects or bradycardia or mild systemic manifestations, merits the use of 100 ml. (iii) 150 ml is infused in severe cases, which includes rapid progression of systemic features, disseminated intravascular coagulation, encephalopathy and paralysis.

Administration: (i) *ASV hypersensitivity test:* Now-a-days, it is not recommended. It does not reliably predict early or late antivenom reactions as they are not mediated by IgE but by direct activation of complement system. The test also can pre-sensitize the patient and thereby cause more risk. (ii) *Prophylactic regimes for prevention of ASV reactions:* The role of prophylactic regimes for prevention of ASV reactions is not yet proved. Usually, two regimens are normally administered, i.e., hydrocortisone (100 mg) + antihistamine or 0.25–0.3 mg adrenaline subcutaneously. (iii) *Route of administration:* ASV is administered by intravenous route slowly and never to be given by intramuscular route. It should not be given at local bitten area as the systemic administration of antivenom has been shown to be effective at the local site as well. (iv) After administering ASV, the patient should be monitored for clinical features of anaphylaxis like urticaria, itching, fever, chills, nausea, vomiting, diarrhoea, abdominal cramps, tachycardia, hypotension, bronchospasm and angio-oedema. To manage anaphylaxis, adrenaline is given. ASV is to be temporarily discontinued.

Timing: There is no consensus as to the outer limit of time of administration of antivenom. Best effects are observed within four hours of bite. It has been noted to be effective in symptomatic patients even when administered up to 48 hours after bite. Reports suggest that antivenom is efficacious even 6-7 days after the bite. It is obvious that when indicated, antivenom must be administered as early as possible and data showing efficacy with delayed administration is based on use in settings where patients present late.

Response: Response to infusion of antivenom is often dramatic with comatose patients sitting up and talking coherently within minutes of administration. Normalization of blood pressure is another early response. Within 15 to 30 minutes, bleeding stops though coagulation disturbances may take up to 6 hours to normalize. Neurotoxicity improves from the first 30 minutes but may require 24 to 48 hours for full recovery. If response to antivenom is not satisfactory, use of additional doses is advocated. However, no studies establishing an upper limit are available. Infusion may be discontinued when satisfactory clinical improvement occurs even if recommended dose has not been completed. In experimental settings, normalization of clotting time has been taken as endpoint for therapy.

Side effects: Hypersensitivity reactions including the full range of anaphylactic reactions may occur in 3-4% of cases, usually within 10 to 180 minutes after starting infusion. These usually respond to conventional management including adrenaline, antihistamines and corticosteroids.

Availability: Several antivenom preparations are available internationally. In India, polyvalent antivenom prepared by C.R.I., Kasauli is effective against the 4 most common species. Antivenom produced at the Haffkine Corporation, Parel includes more species as well. This is about 10 times as expensive as the former. The WHO has designated the Liverpool School of Tropical Medicine as the international collaborating centre for antivenom production and/or testing.

C. **Supportive Therapy:**

(i) In cases of bleeding, replacement with fresh whole blood is ideal. Fresh frozen plasma and fibrinogen are not recommended. (ii) Volume expanders including plasma and blood are recommended in shock, but not crystalloids. (iii) Persistent shock may require inotrope support under C.V. P. monitoring. (iv) Early mechanical ventilation is advocated in respiratory failure though dramatic responses have also been observed with edrophonium followed by neostigmine. (v) Cases of acute renal failure generally respond to conservative management. (vi) Occasionally peritoneal dialysis may be necessary. (vii) In cases of Disseminated Intravascular Coagulation, use of heparin should be weighed against risk of bleeding hence caution is to be taken. (viii) Routine antibiotic therapy is not necessary though most Indian authors recommend use of broad-spectrum antibiotics. Chloramphenicol has been claimed to be useful as a post bite antibiotic even when used orally since it is active against most of the aerobic and anaerobic bacteria present in the mouths of snakes. Alternatives include cotrimoxazole, flouroquinolones with or without metronidazole or clindamycin for anaerobic cover. A study of the organisms isolated from the mouth of the Malayan pit vipers suggests that crystalline penicillin with gentamicin would also be appropriate antibiotic cover following snakebite. (ix) Recent studies have reported the beneficial effects of intravenous immunoglobulin in ophitoxaemia. There are suggestions that its administration may improve coagulopathy, though its effect on neurotoxicity is questionable. A pilot study indicates that IGg with antivenom eliminates the need to repeat antivenom for envenomation associated with coagulopathy. (x) A compound extracted from the Indian medicinal plant *Hemidesmus indicus* R (2-hydroxy-4 methoxy benzoic acid) has been noted to have potent anti-inflammatory, antipyretic and antioxidant properties, particularly against Russell's viper venom. These experiments suggest that chemical antagonists from herbs hold promise in the management of ophitoxaemia; particularly when used in the presence of antivenom. (xi) Injection of tetanus toxoid is necessary. (xii) Early surgical debridement is generally beneficial though fasciotomy is usually more harmful than useful. (xiii) There is no role for steroid therapy in acute snakebite. Although it delays the appearance of necrosis, it does not lessen the severity of outcome.

Autopsy Findings

Findings in a colubrine snakebite: (i) Puncture marks of fangs are usually 1.2 cm (½″) deep and are well visible by hand lens with oozing of serum, blisters and necrosis at the site of bite. (ii) Blood remains fluid showing features of hemolysis. (iii) Froth in mouth and nostrils. (iv) Features of asphyxia are prominently seen. (v) Microscopically, the nervous tissue will show changes in Nissl's granules, fragmentation of reticulum of the nerve cells, opacity, fragmentation and swelling of the nuclei. Cells of medulla shows acute granular degeneration.

Findings in a viperine snakebite: (i) Puncture marks are usually 2.5 cm (1″) deep with swelling, extravasation of blood, inflammation, cellulitis and discolouration in and around it. (ii) Blood-tinged serum oozes out of the punctured marks. (iii) Blood is fluid with purplish tinge. (iv) Evidence of haemorrhages from G.I.T., respiratory and urinary tract is there. (v) Petechial haemorrhages in pleura, pericardium and substance of kidney, liver, lungs and brain with congestion of these organs. (vi) Haemorrhage in the endocardium of left ventricle, interventricular septum and papillary muscles. (vii) Regional lymphadenopathy is there.

Medicolegal Aspects

(i) Always occurs accidentally. (ii) Suicide is unknown except by Cleopatra. (iii) Homicides, rarely where are allegations of snake being thrown into the enemy's place or the person is left in a room full of snakes but this cannot be proved without circumstantial evidences. (iv) Cattle poisoning does occur by placing snake and banana in an earthen pot and irritating snake by firing it. The cobra bites the banana injecting the venom into it. The fruit is taken out and smeared into a rag to be injected into rectum of the animal by bamboo stick.

SCORPIONS

Scorpions are poisonous insects that have a fleshy segment body with four pair of legs, a pair of claws and a tail. Scorpions lack fangs. The posterior segment is long and bulbous and contains the venom gland and a hollow sting at the end of the tail in its last joint. The sting communicates with the venom gland by means of a duct. The stings inject venom in the injury produced by it. The adult scorpion are 2-20 cm long and big, black coloured are more dangerous than the small, brown ones. The scorpion's bites are always accidental as they live in cracks and holes in the houses.

Scorpion venom: Scorpion venom is a clear and colourless toxalbumin that is more toxic than the snake venom. The small quantity of venom is injected. The scorpion venom consists of a neurotoxin (acts on the preganglionic and postganglionic nerve terminals and muscle endplates), haemolysins, agglutinins, haemorrhagins, proteinases, phospholipase A, leucocytolysin, coagulins, cholesterin and lecithin.

Signs and Symptoms

(i) Site of bite is having a red wheal with a hole in the centre and severe burning pain radiates from the site. The area is swollen, red and oedematous. (ii) Increased temperature with chills and headache. (iii) There is feeling of giddiness and fainting. (iv) Excessive sweating and salivation. (v) Muscular cramps and convulsions followed by unconsciousness. (vi) Paresis and muscular weakness persist for a week. (vii) Death occurs in children from pulmonary oedema and respiratory depression and it is rare in adults.

Treatment

(i) Immobilize the limb. (ii) Application of tourniquet or pressure bandage above the site of bite and incising and washing the bitten area with weak solution of potassium permanganate, borax or ammonia. The tourniquet should be loosened for 1-2 minutes after every 10-15 minutes. (iii) NSAIDS for pain relief. (iv) Local ice packs. (v) Local infiltration of 5% cocaine, or lignocaine solution in and around the bite relieves pain. (vi) Restoration of fluid volume by I.V. fluid. (vii) Calcium gluconate 10 ml of 10% solution should be given intravenously to combat muscular cramps. (viii) **Prazosin** is a α_1-adrenergic blocker, which can antagonize the hemodynamic, hormonal and metabolic effects of scorpion venom action. This is given as an immediate measure in all with evidence of autonomic storm. The dose recommended is 30 microgram/kg/dose. (ix) **Dobutamine** infusion alone has been reported to be able to improve the impaired heart function (left as well as right ventricular), helps in reducing pulmonary edema. The optimal dose of dobutamine to start with was between 5 and 10 μg/kg/min. (x) **Scorpion antivenom:** Early antivenom treatment is recommended. Its usefulness varies between countries and value remains controversial. Antivenom against the toxins of Indian scorpion (Buthus tamulus/red scorpion) is available for clinical use.

BEES, WASPS AND ANTS

(i) Produce a painful local reaction, which recedes with time. (ii) An allergic phenomenon produced by them may kill the patient because of prior sensitization. (iii) Number of stings may be so great or the patient is so young as to be killed with primary toxicity.

Signs and Symptoms

(i) Nausea and vomiting (ii) Thoracic oppression (iii) Cardiac irregularities (iv) Pulmonary oedema (v) Nephrosis (vi) Cyanosis, coma, convulsions and death.

The fatalities may result a short while after the infliction of stings.

Fire Ants: This insect *Solenopsis saevissima richteri* causes an immediate and very painful local reaction in the form of vesicles and swelling. The insect inserts its stinger number of times and as a result, number of sensitization occurs to its bite. The systemic reaction can also be produced in sensitized persons that can be febrile and allergic.

SPIDER

Spiders are arthropods fall into the subphylum chelicerata and class of arachnids. Except two small groups in the arachnid family, all spiders are poisonous. However, most spiders do not bite and not harmful to humans. Whenever spider bite occurs, there is a risk for life and should be taken seriously. Clinically significant spider species are Black widow spider (Latrodectus), Brown recluse spider (Loxosceles) and Funnel-web spider. Atrax robustus (a genera of funnel web spider) is considered as the deadliest spider in the world. In India, bite due to brown recluse spiders and poecilotheria spiders have been reported. Spiders have fangs and the bites are mostly accidental.

Spider Venom: It consists of different proteins, peptides, proteases and substances which affects sodium, calcium and potassium channels in neurons and also glutamate, dopamine, norepinephrine, epinephrine and acetylcholine receptors.

Signs and Symptoms

Fang marks may be present, pain, swelling and necrosis at the site of bite, muscle spasm pyrexia, pulmonary edema, respiratory distress, hypertension, kidney dysfunction and death.

Latrodectism is the severe symptoms caused by black widow spider bite. It is characterised by systemic toxicity with diffuse pain, muscle spasm and autonomic dysfunction.

Loxoscelism is clinical features caused by brown recluse spider bite. Local soft tissue destruction (necrotic arachnidism) at bite site is the main finding.

Funnel-web spider syndrome resulted from Funnel-web spider bite which is characterized by a painful bite with abrupt onset sweating, piloerection, fasciculations, cerebral and pulmonary edema and coma.

Treatment

(i) Supportive measures. (ii) Antivenom: For funnel web spider, antivenom FWSAV is used. No antivenom is available for brown recluse spider bite poisoning. (iii) Local wound management and tetanus prophylaxis. (iv) Opioids for pain. (v) Benzodiazepines to relieve muscle spasm.

INORGANIC IRRITANT POISONS

PHOSPHORUS

Phosphorus is a nonmetallic, hepatotoxic and protoplastic irritant type of poison. It exists in two forms: red phosphorus and white phosphorus. Of the two, red is not poisonous but white phosphorus is a deadly one.

White or Yellow Phosphorus: White phosphorus occurs in the form of white, waxy, translucent and pliably soft sticks. It is insoluble in water, somewhat soluble in alcohol and ether and readily soluble in carbon disulphide. On exposure to air, it slowly oxidizes or **'phosphorescences'**. Phosphorescence is the condition of white phosphorus, when it emits white fumes of phosphorus trioxide, which is luminous in the dark giving strong garlic odour. At 34°C, it ignites in the air emitting greenish-white flame, hence it is to be preserved under water or kerosene oil. It should not be handled even by wet finger as even the body heat can cause ignition.

Red Phosphorus: Red phosphorus is prepared by heating white phosphorus at 240°-250°C in an atmosphere with nitrogen or carbon dioxide gases. It occurs ordinarily as violet red solid mass that is odourless, tasteless, is insoluble in carbon disulphide, and does not luminescence in the dark (Table 39.5).

Table 39.5: Differences between red and yellow phosphorus

Properties	Red phosphorus	Yellow phosphorus
Colour	Violet-red or reddish brown	Originally white, turns to yellow on exposure
Appearance	Amorphous, solid mass	Waxy, translucent and soft pliable sticks
Taste and odour	Tasteless, odourless	Garlicky taste and odour

Contd.

Contd.

Luminosity in dark	Non-luminous	Luminous
Solubility in carbon disulphide	Soluble	Insoluble
Exposure to air	Does not phosphorescenses, non fuming	Phosphorescenses
Toxicity	Non-toxic	Highly toxic
Ignition in air	Not so	Possible

Uses of Yellow Phosphorus

(i) It is used in the preparation of vermin pastes that contain arsenic, fluor, oil, sugar, some colouring agents mixed with 1-4% conc. of yellow phosphorus. (ii) In manufacture of gunpowder, fireworks, and incendiary ammunitions and for creating smoke screens during warfare. (iii) In various chemical and fertilizer industries.

Medicolegal Aspects

(i) Phosphorus is not commonly used for homicidal purposes due to its characteristic garlicky odour, taste, luminosity in the dark makes for its easy detection. But it acts as a god homicidal poison as phosphorus containing rat poison mixed with strong tea is not easily detectable. Besides, there is delay in onset of clinical features and postmortem findings simulate that caused by hepatotoxic drugs and diseases. (ii) Vermin pastes, rat killers containing phosphorus are commonly used for suicidal purposes. (iii) Accidental poisoning can occur in children as they may ingest rat-poison. The poisoning can also occur from fragments of projectiles containing yellow phosphorus, inhaling hydrogen phosphide gas produced in ship holds from cargo and inhaling the gas evolved from ferrosilicon used in steel industry. (iv) Arson using phosphorus is done in villages when moist cow-dung and yellow phosphorus are mixed together and thrown over thatched cottage-roof that when dries in sun catches fire from phosphorescent phosphorus.

Fatal Dose: Adults—60-120 mg.
Children—10-25 mg.

Fatal Period: Upto 24 hours (4-10 hours).

Mechanism of Action

(i) Locally it acts as an irritant. (ii) On absorption, it remains in the blood in elemental form for a day or two, then gets oxidized into hypophosphorus and phosphorus acid when it acts as hepatotoxic, protoplasmic poison disturbing the normal cell metabolism by affecting cellular oxidation. (iii) It produces widespread fatty infiltration with degeneration of different organs especially the liver and cells of cerebral cortex. (iv) It also causes tissue destruction by interfering with carbohydrate, fat and protein metabolism especially by deposition of fat in the liver at the cost of glycogen. (v) Chronic absorption of phosphorus leads to bone formation in the epiphyseal cartilage and in the bone marrow and Haversian canal thus impairing blood circulation in bones. This leads to necrosis and sequestration of bones with or without spontaneous fractures.

Acute Phosphorus Poisoning

Signs and Symptoms

The signs and symptoms of acute phosphorus poisoning usually appear within a few minutes and sometimes may be delayed for up to 6 hours.

First Stage (General Symptoms): (i) Garlic like taste in mouth and smell in breath that is luminous in the dark. (ii) Sense of warmth with burning pain in mouth and throat radiating down to oesophagus, stomach and finally all over the abdomen. (iii) Intense uncontrollable and non-quenchable thirst with frequent gastric eructations and patient drinks lots of water trying to quench his thirst. (iv) Copious vomiting occurs that is frequent, profuse and persisting; has garlicky odour, luminous in the dark, bile stained and even blood tinged in later stages. (v) Painful throat as a result of repeated retching and vomiting. (vi) Diarrhoea though uncommon is in the form of dark, offensive and phosphorescent motions (**Smoking stool syndrome)** usually preceded by colicky pain. (vii) Abdomen is tender and distended with epigastric discomfort. (viii) Hypoglycemia may result. (ix) Cardiac and respiratory depression, cold clammy skin, hypothermia occurs. (x) Delirium is followed by convulsion, collapse, coma and death. occurring within 12-24 hours of ingestion of poison. (xi) Patient usually does not die in first stage but he enters second stage by 36-48 hours when signs and symptoms reduce in intensity and vitals improve.

Second Stage (Asymptomatic): This is a stage of apparent improvement of signs and symptoms that may last for 2-4 days. There may be little pain in the abdomen with occasional vomiting and purging, malaise and headache.

Third Stage (Advanced): (i) Vomiting and diarrhoea reappear and is more intense and distressing and contains mucous and blood. (ii) Abdomen distended with severe abdominal pain. (iii) Jaundice sets in and deepens quickly. (iv) Liver is enlarged, soft and tender. (v) Skin becomes cold, respiration laboured and pulse is feeble. (vi) Haemorrhages in the form of epistaxis, haematemesis, haematuria, malena and menorrhagia are commonly seen. (vii) Petechial haemorrhages over the mucous membranes. (viii) Blood urea is usually raised. (ix) Urine is scanty, high coloured, contains blood, ammonia, casts, albumen, free fat globules, excess of lactic acid, bile and some amino acids like leucine, tyrosine and cysteine. (x) Headache, restlessness, insomnia may be seen. (xi) Tinnitus and vertigo are usually present. (xii) Impaired vision, cramps, muscle twitchings and even paralysis, delirium and frequent priapism may also develop. (xiii) Features of increasing hepatic and renal insufficiency followed by hypoglycemia, quick weak and irregular pulse, fall of B.P., pulmonary oedema, dyspnoea, cyanosis, oliguria, even anuria, subnormal temperature progressing to death.

Yellow phosphorus produces usually second or third degree burns that are slowly healing and are surrounded by blisters on the skin.

Diagnosis

There is no specific diagnostic test for phosphorous poisoning. The blood phosphorous level is not useful for diagnosis. It is diagnosed by exclusion method after taking a detailed history and physical examination.

Treatment

(i) Stomach wash using 0.5% potassium permanganate solution that oxidizes phosphorus into harmless phosphoric acid and phosphates itself changing into manganese dioxide. (ii) Stomach wash using 0.1% copper sulphate solution or 250 mg of copper sulphate in a glass of water may be given by mouth every 5 minutes until free emesis starts. Copper sulphate also acts as an antidote as it is reduced by phosphorus and is precipitated as copper phosphide forming a coating over the phosphorus particles thus rendering them inert. However, its clinical utility has not been well demonstrated. There is no specific antidote for phosphorous poisoning. (iii) Hydrogen peroxide 2% solution can also be used as gastric lavage fluid. (iv) Activated charcoal also helps in adsorbing the poison. (v) Oils, fats, milk etc. should not be given to the patient as they help in dissolving phosphorus and promotes its absorption. (vi) Liquid paraffin retards absorption of phosphorus and hastens its elimination but castor oil should not be used. (vii) Whole bowel irrigation with polyethylene glycol. (viii) Glucose and alkaline drinks by mouth in plenty to protect liver. (ix) High carbohydrate and low protein and fat diet should be given. (x) To combat shock and dehydration plenty of glucose saline (500 ml of 5%) fluids and 10 ml of 10% calcium gluconate should be administered intravenously. (xi) Symptomatic treatment such as non-narcotic analgesics for pain, multivitamins especially injections of vitamin K should be given. (xii) N-acetylcysteine may helpful in early course of illness. (xiii) Liver transplantation for acute liver failure. (xiv) Locally, skin can be irrigated with 1% copper sulphate solution in water for at least 10 minutes.

Autopsy Findings

The postmortem findings will depend on the period of survival:

Death within first 24 hours: (i) Slight icteric tinge of the skin. (ii) Mucous membranes of pharynx, oesophagus, stomach and intestines show signs of inflammation, redness, ulceration and corrosion. (iii) Stomach is contracted and mucosa is inflamed, softened, yellowish green with garlicky odour that luminesce in dark.

Death after 24-48 hours: (i) Skin will look jaundiced. (ii) Petechial haemorrhages under the skin and over serous and submucous surfaces of the lungs, brain, leptomeninges, uterus and kidney. (iii) Garlicky odour from the body. (iv) Mucosa of stomach and intestine is yellow or yellowish green with evidence of inflammation, softening, corrosion and haemorrhagic. This is also luminous in the dark. (v) Liver is usually enlarged though it may be normal or contracted also. It is lemon yellow with doughy, soft and greasy consistency. A moderate pressure will allow the pressing finger to sink deep down into the liver substance, which will be easily friable. Small haemorrhagic spots are seen on the glisson's capsule and in liver substance. Evidence of fatty degeneration, cellular necrosis, fibrosis, cellular infiltration is there. Evidence of accumulation of fat in Kupffer's cell is the earliest manifestation of necrobiosis the liver undergoes in phosphorus poisoning the findings are distinguished from yellow atrophy of liver (Table 39.6). (vi) Heart is soft, flabby and dilated with evidence of fatty degeneration and subendocardial haemorrhages. (vii) Kidneys may be filled with cellular debris, fatty casts, albumen etc. and are enlarged, soft, greasy, yellow with petechial haemorrhages and fatty degeneration.

Table 39.6: Difference in liver in yellow phosphorus poisoning and yellow atrophy of liver

Morphology of liver	Yellow phosphorus poisoning	Yellow atrophy of liver
Size	Usually enlarged, normal or even contracted	Contracted with wrinkling of Glisson's capsule
Consistency	Doughy and soft	Leathery
Colour	Uniformly yellow	Dirty yellow
Greasiness	Greasy to touch and fingers dips easily	Soft and greasy to touch
Microscopic features of liver	Extensive fatty infiltration with degeneration, cellular necrosis and haemorrhages	Extensive cellular necrosis

Although phosphorus is readily oxidized in air, it may be detected in unoxidised form in dead body several days after death, even when the body is in an advanced state of decomposition. This may be explained by the fact that reducing gases that are formed during decomposition protects phosphorus from oxidation. Phosphorus occurs in combination with food articles, in tissue and body fluids mainly as phosphates. Hence, detection of phosphate has little medicolegal importance; but when detected in elementary form in the body, it is taken to be sufficient to have produced phosphorus poisoning as it does not occur in free form in nature.

Chronic Phosphorus Poisoning

Chronic phosphorus poisoning usually occurs due to inhalation of fumes of white phosphorus amongst those employed in manufacture of fireworks and some ammunitions where phosphorus is being used, inhalation of phosphorated hydrogen in preparation of acetylene gas from carbide and also from escape of the gas from ferrosilicon results in poisoning. It is also seen in workers in matchbox and sticks factory.

Signs and Symptoms

The symptoms and signs usually develop after working for weeks, months or even years in these factories: (i) Nausea, vomiting, garlicky smelling eructations and purging. (ii) Generalized wasting, weakness, lassitude, emaciation and joint pain. (iii) Abdominal discomfort and pain. (iv) Anaemia, jaundice, shallow complexion. (v) Tracheitis and bronchitis. (vi) ***Phossy jaw:*** It is osteomyelitis and periostitis of jaw due to chronic phosphorus poisoning associated with necrosis of the alveolar part of jawbone along with the sloughing of gums and loosening or falling of teeth. At first, there is history of toothache, swelling of jaw, loosening of teeth, sloughing of gums, necrosis and sequestration of mandible with multiple foul-smelling pus discharging sinuses. Phosphorus mainly attacks the lower jaw through carious or decayed teeth or through interspaced between the missing teeth adjoining the raw surface.

Bis-phossy jaw (bisphosphonate-induced osteonecrosis of the jaw): It is a modern equivalent of phossy jaw **(Phossy jaw of the 21st Century)** found in patients who have used bisphosphonates (chemical with two phosphonates (PO_3) groups) for prolonged period either as a preventive or as treatment for osteoporosis, bone metastasis, multiple myeloma, and Paget's disease. The patient presented with pathological fractures and other similar features like phossy jaw. The exact mechanism of this not known, however, it is speculated that bisphosphonates produces osteonecrosis by inhibiting bone remodelling and reducing endosteal blood flow.

Treatment

(i) Prophylactic measures such as cleanliness and ventilation of factories; oral hygiene of workers regularly that is washing mouths with soda bicarbonate solution and extraction or filling up of carious tooth should be followed. (ii) If necrosis of mandible occurs surgical intervention is undertaken.

IODINE

Iodine occurs in the form of bluish black, soft, scaly crystals that have a metallic sheen and unpleasant taste. It is freely soluble in water, the solubility increasing in presence of iodide. Idiosyncrasy is more common than bromide. It is very commonly used household antiseptic and potassium iodide is largely used as medicine.

Mechanism of Action

It acts as corrosive and coagulates cellular protein causing necrosis. The iodine vapours are irritant to respiratory passages. Iodine is converted to iodide in the body. The normal iodide content of the blood is 2-5 mg/100 ml. The prognosis is good if the patient survives for 48 hours after ingestion of the poison.

Fatal Dose: 2-4 gm (in solid form) and Two drachms of tincture iodine.

Fatal Period: 24 hours.

Signs and Symptoms

(i) Burning pain in mouth radiates to throat, oesophagus, stomach and abdomen. (ii) Increased thirst, nausea, vomiting, salivation and purging. (iii) The lips and angles of mouth are stained brown; the vomitus and faeces are stained dark brown or blue mixed with blood smelling of iodine. (iv) Urine is scanty or suppressed and reddish brown containing albumen; painful micturition. (v) Headache, muscle cramps, giddiness. (vi) Cold clammy skin and fall of B.P. (vii) Respiratory depression, quick weak pulse. (viii) Delirium and collapse. (ix) Consciousness is retained till the end. (x) Iodides may cause enlargement of salivary glands and lymph nodes. (xi) Application of iodine to skin causes weeping eruptions, with raised temperature in sensitive individuals. (xii) Injection of compound of iodine may cause sudden fatal collapse due to idiosyncrasy. (xiii) Inhalation of iodine vapours results in glottic oedema and death from asphyxia.

Chronic Iodine Poisoning (Iodism): It results from chronic use of potassium iodide in large doses as medicine. The clinical features are in the form of frontal headache, running nose, sneezing, watering from eyes, conjunctivitis, bronchitis, parotitis, excessive salivation, nausea, vomiting and diarrhoea associated with oedema of face and eyelids that clears up once the medication is discontinued.

Treatment

(i) Gastric lavage using 5% sodium thiosulphate solution or water containing soluble starch and albumen. (ii) Emetics should be given. (iii) Demulcents as barley water, egg albumen, milk, alkaline drinks and castor oils should be given. (iv) Shock and dehydration to be treated with 5% dextrose saline drip I.V. with mephenetin and other analeptics to maintain blood pressure. (v) Glucocorticoids and antihistaminics in repeated doses help in allaying oedema. Tracheostomy to be performed to relieve glottic oedema. (vi) 5% sodium thiosulphate 100-150 ml orally helps to reduce free iodine to nontoxic iodides. (vii) Fluid and electrolyte balance should be maintained. (viii) In chronic poisoning discontinue the drug and give large doses of sodium bicarbonate or sodium chloride with fluids to hasten recovery.

Autopsy Findings

(i) Face and eyes are swollen and there is evidence of glottic oedema. (ii) Mucosa of gastrointestinal tract is stained yellow or brown, is congested, inflamed and excoriated at places. Also the stomach contents are turned blue due to interaction of iodine with starchy food. (iii) Lungs are congested and oedematous. (iv) Heart and liver shows fatty change. (v) Kidneys may show glomerular and tubular necrosis. (vi) Brain is usually congested and oedematous.

Medicolegal Aspects

(i) Accidental poisoning is common in children from accidental drinking of tincture iodine, betadaine etc. or when an alcoholic solution is excessively used for external application. (ii) Suicidal and homicidal poisoning is rare.

CHLORINE

Chlorine is a greenish yellow gas having an unpleasant irritating odour even when diluted. It is largely used in industry as bleaching agent and disinfectant.

Fatal Dose: Exposure to air containing 1/1000 chlorine for 5 minutes is fatal by causing acute pulmonary oedema.

Fatal Period: Inhalation of pure chlorine gas results in death within 12-24 hours.

Signs and Symptoms

(i) Inhalation causes intense irritation of respiratory passages, throat and eyes causing dry harsh painful violent cough with yellowish expectoration, intense watering eyes and coryza. (ii) Headache, nausea, vomiting, and abdominal pain occur. (iii) Tachypnoea, extreme dyspnoea, palpitation and pyrexia results. (iv) In extreme cases, glottic oedema, asphyxia, intense cyanosis, tachycardia occurs. (v) Unconsciousness soon supervene and death results from acute respiratory or cardiac failure. (vi) Chronic exposure to chlorine vapours shows features of anemia, cachexia, dyspepsia, chronic bronchitis and emphysema.

Treatment

(i) Patient to be removed to fresh air immediately. (ii) Oxygen inhalation, artificial respiration and suction of frothy fluid from air passages. (iii) 5% dextrose saline drip with sodium bicarbonate to combat dehydration and shock. (iv) Treatment of pulmonary oedema, acidosis etc. should be ensued. (v) As a prophylactic measure the respirator masks soaked in sodium bicarbonate solution and sodium hyposulphite and goggles for eyes should be used.

Autopsy Findings

(i) Respiratory tract mucosa shows intense congestion. (ii) Lungs are congested, oedematous exuding frothy, tenacious bloodstained fluid and showing areas of patchy haemorrhages and collapse. (iii) Stomach and intestines are congested. (iv) Heart is also enlarged. (v) Odour of chlorine from the ventricles of brain that is congested. (vi) All organs are congested.

Medicolegal Aspects

Poisoning is usually accidental by chlorine and its compounds especially bleaching powder in industry. Use of chlorine gas in 1st World War caused numerous casualities.

BROMINE

Bromine is a dark reddish brown liquid that volatilizes at ordinary temperatures giving out irritating fumes of unpleasant odour. Compounds of bromine displace chlorides from the plasma and cells thereby causing depression of central nervous system hence are not commonly used in medicine as sedatives. They are also used as anticonvulsant agents. Children may get more readily affected from bromide poisoning than adults. The poison gets rapidly eliminated in the urine, saliva, sweat and milk.

Fatal Dose: Uncertain; 20-30 gms of sodium or potassium bromide can cause alarming symptoms.

Fatal Period: One ounce of undiluted bromine causes death in about 7 days.

Signs and Symptoms

(i) Intense burning sensation in mouth, throat, oesophagus and stomach. (ii) Intense thirst and excessive salivation. (iii) Nausea and vomiting, gaseous eructations, dysphagia and diarrhoea. (iv) Inhalation of bromine fumes causes acute bronchial catarrh, irritating cough, running nose and watering from eyes and intense chest constriction. (v) Oedema of glottis, pulmonary oedema develops with death from suffocation.

Chronic Poisoning (Bromism): Long continued use of bromides in large doses as medicines result in bromism, especially when the blood level reaches more than 50 mg%. Persons with low sodium level are more prone to bromism apart from those who are sensitive to these preparations.

Signs and Symptoms

(i) Bromide acne vulgaris with papular or pustular skin eruptions on the face, shoulders and upper part of chest. (ii) Headache, coryza, watering eyes. (iii) Swelling of face and eyelids. (iv) Indigestion with loss of appetite, constipation, furred tongue, foul breath. (v) Tremors, muscular weakness, staggering gait, loss of memory, slurred speech. (vi) Features of **bromide psychosis** such as confusion of ideas, delirium, delusions or hallucinations, loss of sexual ability with mental depression and drowsiness. (vii) Stupor and coma may result.

Treatment

(i) Patient to be removed to fresh air. (ii) Stomach wash with plain water containing starch or albumen. (iii) Emesis to be induced. (iv) Artificial respiration and oxygen inhalation. (v) Tracheostomy to relieve oedema of glottis. (vi) Sodium chloride 1-2 gm flavoured with fruit juice is given every 6 hours orally until bromide level falls below 50 mg%. (vii) 5% dextrose saline drip to be given I.V. that helps in excretion of bromides. (viii) Diuretics like furosemide or chlorthiazide help in excretion. (ix) Analeptics to treat shock and collapse.

Autopsy Findings

(i) Mucous membrane and skin bears dark brown parchment like stains. (ii) Gastrointestinal tract is congested with inflammation. (iii) There are features of pneumonia and pulmonary oedema. (iv) All organs are congested.

Medicolegal Aspects

(i) Accidental poisoning occur in those sensitive to bromides preparations. It was used in 1st World War when bromide vapours were used as asphyxiating and lacrymating agents. (ii) Used commonly for homicidal purposes.

MECHANICAL IRRITANT POISONS

The irritant mechanical poisons act mechanically to cause local irritation of the gastrointestinal tract when ingested. These are powdered glass, pins, needles, nails, diamond powder, and chopped human and animal hair.

POWDERED GLASS

The powdered glass and diamond dust does not act as poison as they are not absorbed in the blood but they do act mechanically causing irritation of the gastrointestinal tract. Their fatal periods as well as fatal doses are uncertain. The faint shadow of glass particles on X-ray due to presence of radiopaque silica helps in diagnosis.

Signs and Symptoms

(i) Burning pain in mouth, throat, stomach and intestines (ii) Nausea, vomiting and constipation (iii) Rarely diarrhoea with tenesmus and bloody stools occur (iv) Death may result from shock following perforation of stomach or intestines by sharp glass fragments.

Treatment

(i) Bulky foods such as rice, porridge should be given. (ii) Purgatives and cathartics should be given. (iii) Big pieces of banana when swallowed as a whole envelops the glass fragments within itself. (iv) Symptomatic treatment.

LONG QUESTION

1. Classify snakes, discuss clinical features and management in case of a snake bite.

SHORT QUESTIONS

1. Sui.
2. Phossy jaw.
3. First aid in snake bite.
4. Anti-snake venom therapy.

MULTIPLE CHOICE QUESTIONS

1. Toxalbumin is found in:

(a) Ricinus communis (b) Semicarpus anacardium
(c) Calotropis gigantea (d) Nerium odorum

2. "Human Hand syndrome" is observed in the following plant poisoning:

(a) Nerium odorum (b) Cannabis sativa
(c) Chilli peppers (d) Ricinus communis

3. Bulgarian dissident writer Georgi Markov was suspected to be poisoned by:

(a) Aconite (b) Cyanide
(c) Abrin (d) Ricin

4. "St. Antony's fire or Holy fire", a clinical feature seen in poisoning of:

(a) Aconite (b) Canthrides
(c) Ergot (d) Ricin

5. "Smoking Stool Syndrome" is seen in poisoning due to:

(a) THC (b) Nicotine
(c) Phosphorus (d) Mercury

6. Viper snake bite like clinical features are seen in poisoning by:

(a) Croton tiglium (b) Semecarpus anacardium
(c) Ergot (d) Abrus precatorious

7. Polyvalent antivenom available in India is effectively used in all snake bite cases *except:*

(a) Cobra (b) Russel's Viper
(c) Saw-scaled Viper (d) Banded Krait

8. Most characteristic feature of viperidae snake envenomation:

(a) Bleeding manifestations
(b) Neuro-paralytic symptoms
(c) Rhabdomyolysis
(d) Cardiotoxicity

9. Priapism is seen in poisoning due to:

(a) Ergot (b) Opium
(c) Cocaine (d) Canthrides

ANSWER KEY

1. (a)	2. (c)	3. (d)	4. (c)	5. (c)	6. (d)	7. (d)	8. (a)	9. (d)

40 CHAPTER

Deliriant Poisons

It is a class of compounds that cause delirium. The deliriant poisons are Dhatura, Belladonna, Cannabis and Cocaine.

DHATURA/DATURA

The term "datura" is derived from a Sanskrit word "dhatur". Datura is a deliriant poison, commonly known as Thorn Apple, Jimson Weed, Locoweed, Devil's Trumpet, Devil's apple, Moonflower, Metelnut and Solanum etc. It is a genus in the family Solanaceae that contains about 9 species. The more common species are **D. stramonium, D. fastuosa, D. atrox and D. metel** (Hindu datura). Dhatura stramonium is characterised by large white flowers which grows at high altitudes in the Himalayas. D. fastuosa exists in two varieties: (i) Datura Alba—'Safed' or white flowers (ii) Datura Niger—Kala datun with black or deep purple flowers. Both the varieties grow in waste places all over India. In India, the datura flowers and leaves are used to worship Lord Shiva and Ganesh.

Datura is a small shrub that attains a height up to 2 m. It has thick foliage of dark green ovate, pointed leaves. The flowers are trumpet-shaped and vary in length, some reaching 20–30 cm. The fruits are spherical with sharp spines—**Thorn apple** (Figure 40.1) and contains yellowish brown seeds. The seeds of Dhatura may be mistaken for capsicum seeds but the differences exist that are given in Table 40.1 and Figure 40.2. The entire plant is toxic; however, the seeds and roots are more poisonous.

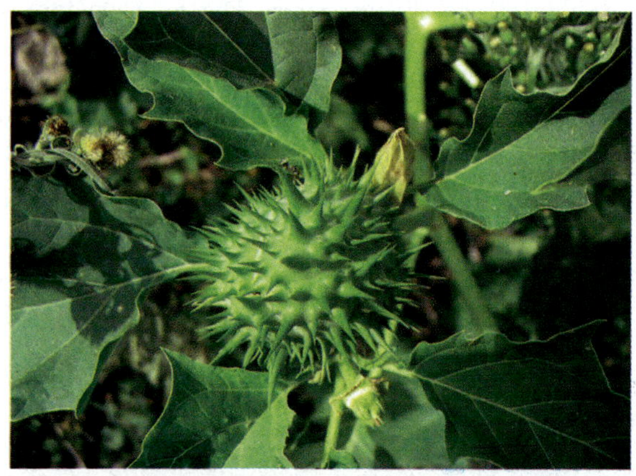

Figure 40.1: Dhatura plant with its fruit

Table 40.1: Differences between chilli and dhatura seeds

Features	Chilli Seeds	Dhatura Seeds
Size	Smaller in size	Larger in size
Shape	Round	Kidney shaped
Surface	Smooth	Finely pitted or reticulated
Colour	Yellowish	Brownish
Smell	Pungent	Odourless
Taste	Pungent	Bitter
Convex border	Single-edged	Double-edged
On section	The embryo lies embedded in the fleshy albumen and curved inwards	The embryo lies embedded in the white oily albumen and curved outwards

Active Principles

The plant contains belladonna alkaloids: (i) **Hyoscine (scopolamine)** (ii) **Hyoscyamine** (iii) Traces of **atropine**. It has been suggested that atropine does not exist as such but is a racemic form of Hyoscyamine that is converted to atropine during the process of extraction.

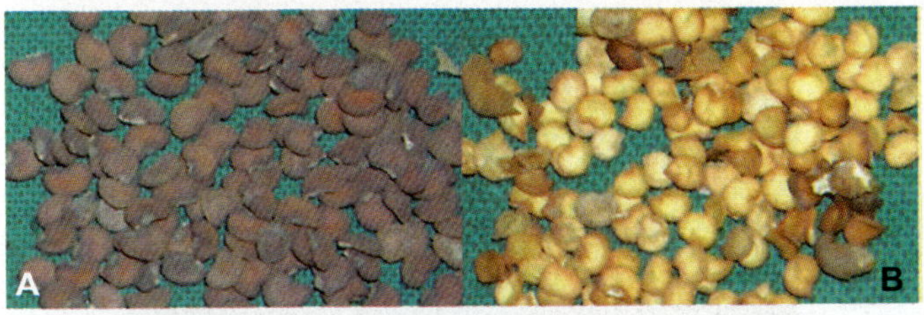

Figure 40.2: (A) Dhatura and (B) Chilli seeds

Mechanism of Action

They act as competitive antagonists to peripheral and central muscarinic acetylcholine receptors leading to a general paralysis of the parasympathetic innervated organs. Muscarinic acetylcholine receptors are located in smooth muscle, the ciliary body of the eye, salivary glands, sweat glands, and in the central nervous system (CNS). It also produces sympathomimetic action.

Signs and Symptoms

Dhatura poisoning can lead to all the classical features of anticholinergic syndrome.

(i) Contact with the leaves and flowers cause dermatitis in sensitive patients. (ii) Direct exposure of eyes of a person to sap or plant debris containing belladonna alkaloid while handling the plant in garden or cornfield produce mydriasis which is called **Gardeners eye** or **Cornpickers eye.** (iii) When the seeds are ingested, the symptoms appear within half an hour. (iv) At times vomiting occurs immediately after taking the seeds when crushed due to gastric irritation. (v) Bitter taste and dryness of mouth and throat. (vi) Burning pain in the stomach. (vii) Dysphagia and difficulty in talking. (viii) Headache followed by giddiness. (ix) Staggering gait and incoordination of muscles. (x) Flushing of face. (xi) Dry and hot skin with rise in body temperature to 107-108 ^{o}F. (xii) Pupils are dilated and there is photophobia. (xiii) There is loss of accommodation for near vision. (xiv) Conjunctiva is red and injected. (xv) There is inability to pass urine. (xvi) Drowsiness. (xvii) At times scarlentiniform rashes or exfoliation of skin are seen over most of the body. (xviii) Pulse is full and bounding, later on it is weak, irregular and intermittent. (xix) Respiration is increased. (xx) Muscle tone and deep reflexes are increased; muscular spasm is present at times. (xxi) Delirium is restless and purposeless. The person is silent or mutters indistinct or inaudible words, but usually he is noisy, tries to run up away from his bed, picks bed clothes, tries to pull imaginary threads from the tips of his fingers, threads imaginary needles (pin rolling movements). (xxii) Dreadful hallucinations of sight and hearing is present. (xxiii) Delusions are present.

The signs and symptoms of acute Dhatura poisoning can be summarized by **10 D's**: (i) Dysphagia (ii) Delusions (iii) Dermatitis (iv) Delirium (v) Drowsiness (vi) Dry skin and mucous membrane (vii) Dilated pupil (viii) Dreadful hallucinations (ix) Dysuria (x) Dysarthria.

The signs and symptoms can also be remembered as: (i) **Hot as a hare** (increased body temperature). (ii) **Blind as a bat** (disturbed vision due to mydriasis). (iii) **Dry as a bone** (Dryness of mouth and throat due to inhibition of salivation, intense thirst). (iv) **Mad as a hen** (mental symptoms—Delirium, hallucination, delusion, restlessness. (v) **Red as a beet** (flushing of the face due to dilatation of cutaneous blood vessels). (vi) **Full as flask** (distension of urinary bladder due to retention of urine).

As intoxication advances, this excitement phase passes off in 1-2 hours, deep coma or sleep ensues that may end in death from respiratory paralysis. Patient may stay ill for 2-3 days but definite improvement occurs in 24 hours. The cases that improve develop secondary delirium as stupor passes away. They remember nothing about the illness and are surprised to find themselves in the hospital.

Fatal Dose: 100 seeds or 0.5-1 gm.

Fatal Period: 24 hours.

Treatment

(i) Shift the patient to quiet and dark environment. (ii) Emetics can be used. (iii) Stomach wash using 5% tannic acid or a weak solution of potassium permanganate or activated charcoal. (iv) Enema should be given using sodium sulphate as purgative. (v) Physostigmine is an acetylcholinesterase inhibitor is the antidote of choice. The dose is 0.5- to 2-mg slow I.V. for adults and 0.02 mg/kg slow I.V. for pediatric patients with a maximum pediatric dose of 0.5 mg. The dose may be repeated after approximately 30 minutes if symptoms recur. It relieves both cerebral as well as peripheral clinical manifestations as it crosses the blood brain barrier. (vi) Morphine is contraindicated, though it is a physiological antidote. (vii) Short acting barbiturates like diazepam can be given for convulsions. (viii) Sponging to relieve high temperature. (ix) Dantrolene may be given where there is muscular hyperactivity (1 mg/kg IV to a maximum of 10 mg/kg). (x) Artificial respiration and oxygen inhalation should be given. (xi) Bladder catheterization.

Autopsy Findings

(i) Postmortem findings are not characteristic but signs of asphyxia are there. (ii) Seeds or their fragments may be found in the stomach or intestine. (iii) Stomach may show slight inflammation. (iv) Lungs are congested and oedematous. (v) All the organs are congested.

Medicolegal Aspects

(i) Dhatura is used mostly for criminal purposes. It is used to **stupefy travelers** for the purpose of robbery, rape and theft. It is also called **Road Poison** seeds that are mixed with rice, *dal*, coffee and sweets. Seeds and leaves are mixed with tobacco or *ganja* and smoked in *Chillum* (pipe). A decoction (boiling to extract the essence) of seeds is added to liquor to enhance its intoxicating property (the 'kick' effect). (ii) Accidental poisoning can result (a) When children and adults eat raw dhatura fruits (b) Seeds may be mistaken for capsicum seeds (c) Seeds have an aphrodisiac property (d) When dhatura is being used for medicinal purposes. (iii) Active principle is excreted unchanged in urine immediately after administration for 10-12 hours. Urine should be preserved for analysis. (iv) Dhatura seeds resist putrefaction for a long time but mydriatic principle contained in them is destroyed by putrefaction. It can be chemically detected even after a long time. (v) Dhatura is sometimes used for homicidal purposes. In 1921, the wife gave dhatura seeds to her husband in the food. (vi) It is used as an abortifacient. In a case report, a man administered *Dhatura* powder to a woman to produce abortion but she died 3 hours later. (vii) **Medicinal use of Dhatura:** (a) Dried leaves mixed with cannabis in the form of cigarettes are used for the treatment of asthma; the smoke is antispasmodic (b) Tinctures have been used for application on the wounds **(belladonna tinctures)** (c) Dhatura leaves are used to treat some types of fever (d) Juice of dhatura leaves is used to treat rheumatism and applied for pain and inflammation (e) *Vaids* and *hakims* use dhatura as medicine (f) Medicated ghee is prepared mixed with dhatura for local application (g) Used as an aphrodisiac (h) Used as a 'love potion'.

Differential Diagnosis of Dhatura Poisoning

(i) Poisoning by Hashish (ii) Opium poisoning; differentiated by pinpoint pupil and slow respiration (iii) Cerebral haemorrhage is differentiated by the presence of hypertension and CSF is diagnostic in such a case.

Test for Dhatura: (i) **Mydriatic test:** A drop of solution is instilled into the cat's eye. If dhatura is present, pupils will dilate within half an hour due to presence of atropine. (ii) **Vitali's test:** This is colour test for dhatura fastuosa. Add alcoholic KOH to the extracted residue. It produces a violet colour and then it changes to red and disappears. Again, add few drops of alcoholic KOH, if the colour reappears, then it is suggestive of dhatura fastuosa. (iii) **Microscopic test:** On a slide, dried residue of extract of vomit contents or viscera is taken. Presence of characteristics structure similar to eyelids under microscope suggestive of dhatura fastuosa.

ATROPA BELLADONNA (HYOSCYAMUS NIGER)

It is also known as belladonna or deadly night shade. The plant belongs to Solanaceae family. All parts of its plant are poisonous; mature being more poisonous (Figure 40.3).

Active Principles: (i) Hyoscyamine (ii) Atropine (iii) Scopolamine. They act by inhibiting muscarinic effects of acetylcholine. Root contains 82-97% hyoscyamine, 13-15% atropine and upto 2.5% scopolamine.

Fatal Dose: Atropine and hyoscyamine: 120 mg and hyoscine: 30 mg.

Fatal Period: Within 24 hours.

Absorption occurs through skin and parenteral route. Clinical features, treatment and autopsy findings are similar to Dhatura poisoning.

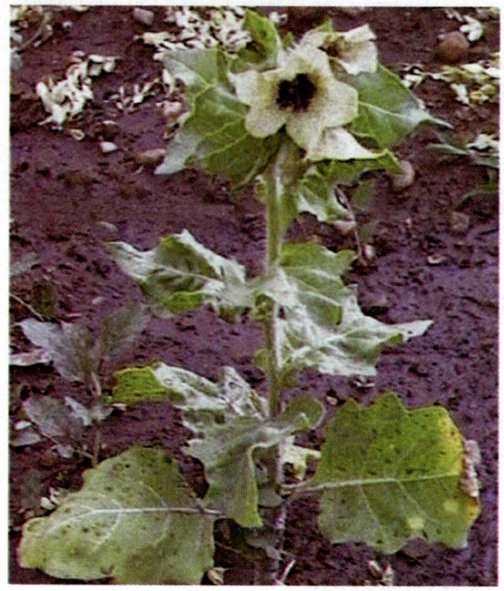

Figure 40.3: Hyoscyamus niger

CANNABIS INDICA OR MARIJUANA

Cannabis is one of the most commonly used illicit drug worldwide. It is a genus of flowering herb belonging to the Canabaceae family. There are three species of cannabis plant recognized namely Cannabis Sativa, Cannabis Indica and Cannabis Ruderalis. However, all three may be treated as subspecies of a single species C. sativa. Other names are **grass, pot, weed, tea, Mary Jane, dagga, sinsemilla, herb, reefer, dope, shunk, boom, gangster, kif, marihuana** etc. It is also called hemp plant and North American colonist used cannabis for making hemp ropes. The plant Cannabis indica and Canabis sativa grows all over India (Figure 40.4) but its cultivation is restricted due to the monopoly of the state government. Female plant is tall about 16-18 feet and has more dark and luxuriant leaf foliage than male plant. The all parts of the male and female plant contain active principles. The plant contains more than 60 cannabinoid compounds. The four major compounds are d-9-THC, Cannabidiol (CBD), d-8-THC and cannabinol. The chemical structures of these compounds are similar but their pharmacological effects are different. When cannabis is smoked, it characteristically smells like burnt rope.

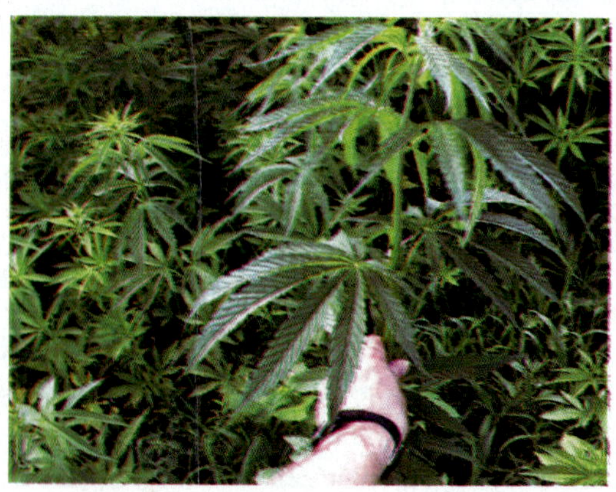

Figure 40.4: Cannabis sativa plant

Tetrahydrocannabinol (d-9-THC)

Tetrahydrocannabinol is the most important and main active principle of Cannabis. It is responsible for most of the intoxicating effects. It is absorbed into the blood stream through the walls of the lungs, when smoked and through the walls of stomach or intestine when ingested. It exerts quicker action through inhalation. The blood stream carries THC into the brain that produces the 'high' effects of the drug. The Tetrahydrocannabinols, are labile compounds that may change when exposed to U-V light or acid. THC acts through two type of cannabinoid receptor CB1 and CB2. CB1 found primarily in brain and mediate psychological effect and behavioural effect of THC. CB2 associated with immune system and modulate inflammatory responses. It has synergistic effects with other cannabinoids and cannabinols.

Medical Applications of the Drug

(i) THC appears to control nausea, vomiting, and lack of appetite in cancer patients receiving chemotherapy when other drugs such as antiemetics fail. (ii) Used as antidepressants for cancer patients. (iii) Marijuana dilates bronchioles but it is usually not given in asthma. (iv) THC in small doses acts as anticonvulsant but in large doses, it causes convulsions. (v) Workers have found that the topical application on the skin and mucous membrane has antibiotic activity. (vi) It dilates the vessels of iris that leads to increased intraocular pressure and glaucoma.

Effects of Cannabis

The effects of cannabis depend upon: (i) Amount of cannabis (ii) Route of intake, whether smoked or eaten (iii) Body size, weight and health of the person (iv) Tolerance and dependence (v) Individual's mood (vi) Circumstances under which it is taken whether to reduce stress or with others in a social setting.

Effects produced by the small doses: (i) Sense of wellbeing (Euphoria) (ii) Loss of inhibitions (iii) Tendency to talk and laugh (iv) Impairment of coordination and balance (v) Loss of concentration (vi) Munchies-increased hunger pains increased appetite (vii) Increased pulse and heart rate (viii) Reddened eyes (ix) Person passes to calm state of mind and sleepiness that lasts for 2-3 hours after smoking (x) There can be hangover, drowsiness and poor coordination for several hours.

Effects produced by large doses: (i) Confusion (ii) Restlessness (iii) Excitement (iv) Hallucination (v) Anxiety or panic. Sometimes inexperienced cannabis user can hallucinate in small doses. Cannabis also affects and impairs short-term memory, logical thinking, motor skills and ability to perform driving.

Various Preparations of Cannabis

Bhang (Siddhi, Patti or Sabji): Is formed of the dried leaves and flowering or fruiting shoots. It is used as an infusion in the form of beverage. It is prepared by rubbing on a stone and black pepper, dried leaves and sugar is added to form pill or bolus. Water is added and it is drunk after it is strained through the muslin cloth. People of Northern India consume this drink at festivals like Holi especially at some of the places like Varanasi. It is the least potent form containing about 15% of the active principle. Bhang is usually intoxicated to produce cheerful mood for dancing and singing. It acts as an appetizer so the individual consumes more food and also the person seeks sexual enjoyment. The intoxication lasts for 2-3 hours resulting in sleep. Fresh bhang is highly intoxicating and narcotic. Bhang that is kept for 2-3 years is mildly intoxicating and pleasure giving.

Majun: It is sweet meat confectionery prepared from bhang after treating with sugar, milk and butter. It has an agreeable odour and sweet taste and sold in the market in small lozenge shaped pieces. It increases appetite and sexual desire. The person feels happy and quite contented as if he belongs to Raja's family and he has all what he wants. Sometimes Dhatura is mixed with Majun.

Ganja: It is prepared from the flowering tops of female plant. Has rusty green colour and characteristic odour and its active principle is 15-25%. About 20-30 grains are rubbed with little water on palm till it becomes sticky and then mixed with tobacco and smoked in a pipe (*chillum*). The person on smoking feels heavy and lazy. Also conjunctiva gets suffused and tachycardia and hypotension is produced. The person indulges in pleasant reveries though he is able to discharge ordinary duties. *Sadhus*, *faqirs* and poor labourers, cut leaves and flowering tops of cannabis and roll them into cigarettes with their hands and then smoke them. These cigarettes are called **'reefers' or 'pot'.** A good quality cigarette contains 500 mg of marijuana that is effective after 15 minutes of smoking and produces benign ergosyntonic experience.

Marijuana: This term typically used for the tobacco-like preparations of the leaves and flowers of the plant cannabis sativa and Cannabis Indica. A typical marijuana cigarette **(a "joint")** generally contains 500-1000 mg of crude plant material and 15-30 mg of THC. When it is smoked in a modified pipe, it is called "**bongs**". It may be ingested as brownies, cookies, candy, and other food products. **Sinsemilla** is seedless marijuana with a fairly high THC content.

Charas or Hashish: Is of dark green or brown colour and commonly known as Hashish. It is a concentrated resin exuding from leaves and stem of the plant that grows in hilly areas, 6-8 thousand feet above the sea level. It has 25-40% active principle and is smoked with tobacco in a pipe or *hookah*. It is most potent of all the forms.

Hashish oil: It is an extract of cannabis and is thick, oily liquid spread on a tip of paper of cigarette. It is smoked and is strongest of all the preparations of Cannabis. Unlike alcohol it is always taken in a company. It produces the effects that are fleeting, brief and pass rapidly.

Signs and Symptoms

They appear soon after smoking ganja or charas and after half an hour after swallowing bhang. When taken in small doses, effects are slight and then patient becomes pleased with himself. He becomes talkative, cheerful though rarely violent or aggressive. With moderate doses, effects are intensified by impaired memory. There are two stages:

1. **Stage of Inebriation:** Person becomes dreamy or semiconscious. There are realistic visions of erotic nature. The person sees nude beautiful women dancing before him, playing music and singing amorphous songs. The higher faculties are depressed, the person may laugh, sing or make purposeless movements. Judgment in relation to time and space is lost and sensation of pain is lessened. It hampers the psychomotor activity (physical coordination, quick reaction time and visual perception) headed for driving and operating machinery. Interferes with immediate memory, arithmetic problem solving and thinking in general. Frightful hallucinations are there at 300-480 mg/kg oral and 200-250 µg/kg of THC. He is delirious, has homicidal tendency or a fear of death. Symptoms vary with the dose and personality of the user.
2. **Stage of Narcosis:** 0.5-1 mg/kg as single oral dose produces giddiness and ataxia. Speech may be confused and rambling. Tingling and numbness of skin occurs and in severe cases general anaesthesia and muscular weakness develops. The victim becomes drowsy and passes into deep sleep and wakes with lassitude and impaired mental function. Recovery occurs in about 6 hours. In extreme rare cases death is due to respiratory failure.

Fatal Dose: 1000-2000 mg or 30 mg/kg of THC
Charas 2 gm
Ganja 8 gm
Bhang 10 gm/kg body weight

Fatal Period: Cannabis is very rarely fatal and the period of fatality varies from 12 hours to several days.

Treatment

(i) Stomach wash to be done (ii) Purgatives should be administered (iii) Oxygen inhalation and artificial respiration to be given (iv) Symptomatic treatment should be administered.

Autopsy Findings

(i) Postmortem findings are not characteristic (ii) Only signs of asphyxia are present (iii) It's necessary to preserve urine (iv) On microscopic examination of the ingested material, the suspected material is placed on a slide and one drop of oil and potassium hydroxide is added, covered with cover slip and examined under the microscope. Morphological features of hair of the THC derivatives should be studied distinctly; ganja hairs are smooth and charas hairs are wavy or warty.

Chronic Poisoning

Regular users develop features of intoxication and may experience some physical, mental or social problems. There is an: (i) Increased risk of bronchitis, lung cancer and respiratory diseases associated with smoking. (ii) **Amotivational Syndrome:** There is loss of energy and will to work. The performance at the place of work suffers. When cannabis is stopped, the symptoms disappear. (iii) Decreased concentration, memory and learning abilities **(Toxic psychosis).** (iv) Interference with sexual and hormone production (Impotency, gynecomastia, low sperm count and irregular menstrual cycle). (v) THC is soluble in fatty tissue, can be deposited in fatty tissue including brain then gradually can be realized into blood stream. (vi) **Hashish Insanity/Hemp Insanity**: Hallucination, delusion of persecution develops. **Running Amok or Run Amok:** It is rare psychiatric condition caused by continued use or first time use of cannabis. Following a period of depression, the person suddenly run around and first kills a person or persons against whom they have entertained fancied or real enmity then kills anybody who comes in their way until homicidal tendency lasts. Later the person again become depressed and usually commit suicide or surrender before the police. (vii) Cannabis can produce short-term exacerbations of pre-existing psychotic diseases such as schizophrenia. (viii) **Cannabinoid hyperemesis syndrome (CHS):** It is a newly described adverse effect of chronic cannabis use. Actually, cannabis is used clinically to alleviate nausea, however in CHS the opposite effect is observed. The patient experiences cyclical nausea, vomiting and abdominal pain. There is intractable and excessive vomiting (sometimes 20 times per hour). The exact mechanism of CHS is not known. However, following mechanisms are suggested for development of CHS. (i) overstimulation of the CB1 receptor in the enteric nervous system could supersede the antiemetic effect of receptors in the CNS. (ii) Chronic consumption may desensitize or downregulate the CB1 receptors and remove the antiemetic effect of cannabinoids. (iii) Disruption of hypothalamic–pituitary–adrenal axis secondary to enhanced adrenocorticotropin (ACTH) secretion. It is variant of cyclical nausea and vomiting syndrome (abdominal migraine). The criteria used for diagnosis of CHS are (ROME IV criteria). (i)At least one discrete episode vomiting in the prior year and two episodes in the past 6 months, occurring at least 1 week apart. (ii) Presentation after prolonged excessive cannabis use (3–5 times daily for at least 2 years). (iii) Relief of vomiting episodes by sustained cessation of cannabis use. The diagnosis is supported by **pathologic bathing behaviour** (prolonged hot baths or showers). It has been associated with aspiration pneumonia, pneumonitis, acute kidney injury, severe electrolyte deficiency, Boerhaave's syndrome and even death.

Medicolegal Aspects

(i) Poisoning by bhang is mostly accidental. Majun and Charas are used as stupefying poisons. Cannabis can be used for homicidal purposes. (ii) To steady nerves before committing crime. (iii) ***Run amok***: There shall be no criminal responsibility of the person, since it is considered as a mental illness. (iv) ***Cannabis and other drugs***: Marijuana and alcohol when used together are more effective and dangerous than when it is used alone. There is no evidence as to the use of Cannabis automatically leading to the use of other drugs. (v) ***Cannabis and pregnancy:*** There is not much information about the effect of THC in an unborn child but experiments on animals do show some abnormal developments and behaviour in the offspring. (vi) ***Cannabis and the law:*** Cannabis is a banned drug and the punishment for cultivation of plant and ganja illegally is imprisonment of 5 years and fine of Rs 50,000. For other products the punishment can vary from 10-20 years with fine of 1-2 lakh. The small quantity for personal use of Hashish and *Charas* is 100 gms and for Ganja it is 1kg. Exceeding this quantity will be liable to punishment up to 1year or fine of Rs 10000 or both. (vii) ***Cannabis and driving:*** While driving intake of Cannabis affects motor and coordination skills along with the vision, perception of time and space. There are increased chances of vehicular accidents.

COCAINE

Cocaine is also commonly known by the names of **Coke**, **Snow**, **White lady** and **Cadillac** etc. It is an alkaloid derived from the leaves of the tropical shrub coca-tree (*Erythroxylon coca* and *E novogranatense*). These trees grow well in Central and South America, Mexico, Indonesia, East Indies and India. The leaves are traditionally chewed in many countries such as South America to allay fatigue. Purified cocaine first became commercially available in 1884. Cocaine acts as a good surface anaesthetic and it was introduced as first local anaesthetic for use as ocular anaesthetic. It was used in the original "Coca-Cola" beverage.

Cocaine along with heroin and its associated drugs forms the core of the hard-drug problem from which fatalities may result. In areas where cocaine use is common, a significant proportion of fetal deaths are associated with this narcotic. In a series reported in New York by Morild and Stajic, toxicology revealed cocaine in 64 out of 103 fetal deaths. The study also suggested that cocaine causes an increased incidence of fetal deaths, abortion and abruptio placentae. Many a times, the smugglers have died due to bursting of packets of cocaine in their gastrointestinal tract resulting in a massive overdosage.

The leaves of coca plant (Erythroxylon coca) contain about 0.5-1% cocaine. Cocaine, methylbenzoyl ecgonine may be synthetically prepared.

Routes of Administration

(i) Orally, it is rapidly destroyed. (ii) Injection. (iii) Snuffing via nasal (snorting) and oral mucous membranes when it is rapidly absorbed and causes cerebral stimulation followed by depression. (iv) Inhalation of freebase cocaine produces almost immediate absorption and a rapid onset of effects.

Various Forms Used for Abuse

1. **Cocaine hydrochloride:** It is water soluble and is typically used for injection or snorting but is not well suited for smoking as it is largely destroyed by heat of burning. The hydrochloride salt can be converted to the freebase form by treatment with alkali and extraction with organic solvents.
2. **Cocaine sulfate (coca paste, pasta basica, basuca)** is a crude intermediate product, usually contaminated with solvents is used for smoking.
3. **Crack:** Crude form of **freebase cocaine** may be obtained by heating the cocaine with sodium bicarbonate to yield 'crack', a hard white mass that is freebase plus impurities but without hydrochloride moiety. When smoked, this material gives off a cracking sound, hence the name.
4. **Speedball:** Sometimes cocaine abusers simultaneously inject intravenously a mixture of an opiate, such as heroin called speedball. This mixture is especially euphorigenic.

Mode of Action

Cocaine acts as a CNS stimulant and local anaesthetic with potent vasoconstrictor properties. It stimulates the vagal centre, vasomotor centre, vomiting centre and temperature regulating centre. It blocks uptake of noradrenaline and adrenaline into adrenergic nerve endings producing sympathomimetic effects. The reinforcing effects of cocaine are related to effects on dopaminergic neurons in the mesolimbic system.

Metabolism

The half life of a single dose of cocaine in the blood is only about 30-90 minutes. It is hydrolyzed by butyrylcholinesterase (plasma pseudocholinesterase) and the liver esterase into inactive metabolites, mostly benzoylecgonine and ecgonine methylester. With repeated high dosages, cocaine or its metabolites may accumulate in the body compartments such as fat and central nervous system from where it is then slowly released. Consequently, using sensitive techniques, cocaine may be detectable in the urine of heavy users for a couple of weeks. Metabolites can also be detected in blood, saliva, sweat and hair. Blood and saliva provide a better index of current concentrations, whereas urine provides a longer window of opportunity for detecting use over the previous few days.

Use in Conjunction with Other Drugs

Drugs such as cannabis, ethanol, sedatives and hypnotics are frequently taken with cocaine to reduce its unpleasant effects.

Use with alcohol: Alcohol is most commonly used along with cocaine as it modulates both the 'cocaine high' and 'dysphoria' associated with abrupt disappearance of cocaine's effects. The concurrent use of cocaine and alcohol may result in the accumulation of a distinct metabolite, cocaethylene.

Cocaethylene: Cocaethylene is an active metabolite and produces changes in the cardiovascular functions as that produced by cocaine alone. It produces long lasting effects than cocaine itself and also accounts for the enhancement of subjective effects as well as toxic symptoms when the two are used simultaneously.

Fatal Dose: As little as 20-50 mg when applied to nasal mucosa has caused deaths but even a gram when taken orally does not result in death. Chronic users of cocaine develop tolerance and habituation that is why it is difficult to estimate dangerous dose levels. Intravenous doses are of 100 mg and a lethal dose is ten times this dose, though there are chances that far larger doses can be tolerated by habitual users. Absorption through the nasal mucosa is less effective and larger doses are to be used to obtain the same effect as that produced by the intravenous route.

Fatal Period: Few minutes to few hours.

Acute Intoxication

Cocaine users develop the signs and symptoms of intoxication during the course of single binge and a hyperadrenergic state is produced.

Stage of euphoria: This stage is accompanied with (i) Increased suspiciousness and hypervigilance (ii) Anxiety, hyperactivity and talkativeness (iii) Grandiosity and excitement.

Signs and symptoms resulting from central stimulation: (i) Increased sense of well-being with increased power of endurance (ii) Tachycardia and ventricular arrhythmias (iii) Changes in blood pressure (iv) Pupillary dilatation (v) Perspiration and chills (vi) Hallucinations especially tactile (vii) Judgment is impaired but insight into drug induced nature of the hallucination is usually retained (viii) Dyspnea.

Stage of depression: (i) Loss of reflexes (ii) Paralysis of muscles (iii) Coma and tonic-clonic seizures (iv) Circulatory and respiratory failure (v) Sudden death may follow I.V. injection, smoking and snorting results in cardiac arrhythmias and cardiopulmonary arrest (vi) Complications such as pulmonary oedema after intravenous injection of freebase cocaine, pneumomediastinum and pneumothorax may occur after sniffing.

Crack lung is an acute pulmonary syndrome that occurs within 48 hours of smoking of crack cocaine. It is characterized by diffuse alveolar damage and haemorrhagic alveolitis. The common presenting symptoms are cough and dyspnoea.

Causes of death: (i) Cocaine overdose or hypersensitivity (ii) Sudden cardiac arrest in first time users.

Chronic Intoxication

It is also known as **Cocainism/cocainophagia/cocainomania.** Cocaine is usually abused by upper classes of society to enhance self-image or improve professional performance. There is a tendency for compulsive use of the drug though classical physical dependence is uncommon. Psychic dependence is common with chronic use of the drug and the euphoria following injection is short-lived, perhaps only for 15-20 minutes. Immediately upon intake there is: (i) Euphoria (*rush*) followed about an hour or so later by rebound depression (*crash*). To avoid unpleasant effects of rebound depression, the person feels compelled to take the drug again. (ii) It can also induce a toxic delirium and a more persistent toxic psychotic disorder characterized by: (a) Suspiciousness (b) Paranoia (c) Complex hallucinations—Tactile hallucination is the early hallucinatory phenomena observed in chronic cocaine users especially when used via IV route. There can be feeling of animals in the skin or bugs or insects under the skin or symptoms of itching (**formication**) which was described by Valentin Magnan (**Cocaine bugs or Magnan's sign**). It is felt primarily on hands and face but can also be felt on other parts of the body. The person does not believe the actual presence of the insects or objects, still scratch or rub the skin and probes under the skin to find the bugs. Visual hallucination is frequently observed which is characterized by shadows, flash lights (**snow lights**), objects moving and the bugs crawling on the arms. Olfactory, gustatory and auditory (hearing bugs) are observed. This condition is now considered under delusion of parasitosis**.** (d) Loss of insight. (iii) Chronic intake of cocaine in males causes impotence and gynaecomastia and in females menstrual disorders including amenorrhoea, galactorrhoea and infertility. (iv) In pregnant woman with cocaine abuse there is incidence of abortion, abruptio placentae and cerebrovascular diseases in mother. In the foetus also there is incidence of congenital malformations. The smoking of 'crack' results in production of **'crack babies'** (the baby shows congenital anomalies, low birth weight, undernourished and shows muscle twitchings. (v) On oral intake-black jet tongue is observed. (vi) Rarely, ulceration and perforation of the nasal septum occurs in chronic 'snorters'.

Delusion of Parasitosis (Ekbom's Disease or Morgellons): It is a psychodematologic condition in which a patient has firm and fixed belief that insects are living inside the skin despite absence of evidence. The patient brings specimen of alleged pathogens in a matchbox to the doctor in order to show the proof. It was first described by Perrin 1983 and is called **the matchbox sign**. The patients may try many methods to eradicate the parasites including using pesticides on themselves or hiring exterminators. A study by Freudenmann *et al.* observed, inanimate materials fibres and so-called Morgellons instead of living creatures for their infestation. They also recommended term "***delusional infestation***" rather than "delusional parasitosis".

Formication/Prickling is distinct form of Delusion of Parasitosis and the patient has tactile hallucination with similar symptoms of itching and a sensation of bugs crawling on the skin, but the patient is aware that there are no parasites involved. It can occur in delirium due to alcohol abstinence, following the intoxication by cocaine, methylphenidate, and amphetamines. It is also observed in various physiological and pathological conditions like in menopause, diabetic neuropathy, skin cancer, or herpes zoster etc.

Treatment

(i) To control seizures, intravenous diazepam 0.5 mg/kg may be given (ii) Propranolol 0.5-1 mg I.V. for ventricular arrhythmias

(iii) To treat psychosis, haloperidol should be given (iv) Treatment of chronic cocaine abuse requires combined efforts of primary care physicians, psychiatrists and psychosocial workers.

Autopsy Findings

(i) There are no specific autopsy features (ii) Findings of hypoxia are evident (iii) Oral ingestion results in findings of gastric ischemia (iv) Diluents such as quinine, mannitol and other bitter flavouring agents used to 'cut' the drug for illegal sale may be found at injection sites, the regional lymph nodes, in the lungs and in other organs (v) Particles of cocaine can be seen in the form of microemboli (vi) Adulterants used with cocaine are same as that in heroin such as talc, starch, quinine, lactose and dextrose. Quinine was used as diluent to treat falciparum malaria transmission was quite common amongst needle and syringe sharers (vii) Formation of foreign body granulomas in the lungs when cocaine mixed with talc or starch is used intravenously. This is due to filtering out of the undissolved components in the pulmonary capillary bed (viii) Evidence of cerebral haemorrhage is found at autopsy. These haemorrhages are the result of hypertension when blood pressure rises to over 300 mm Hg (ix) *Complication of the use of septic methods of injections:* (a) Infections HIV and Hepatitis (b) Endocarditis affecting the right heart valves (c) Phlebitis and distant embolic abscesses (x) Nasal swabs, one from each nostril should be taken and sent for analysis along with an unused cotton wool swab as control (xi) *Samples to be preserved:* (a) Swab from each nostril using a plain cotton swab along with another swab used as control (b) Routine viscera and blood sample for cocaine levels (c) Sample of urine as cocaine metabolites can be detected for varying lengths of time in urine depending on the dose of cocaine and sensitivity of the assay. The metabolite is generally detectable in the urine for 24-72 hours after brief periods of use (d) Injection prick site along with control sites (xii) According to **Baselt,** blood levels in fatal cases range from 1-21 mg/l with a mean of 5.2 mg/l.

Medicolegal Aspects

(i) Accidental cases occur from the addiction, hypodermic, urethral, vaginal or rectal injections. (ii) Drug is locally applied on penis as it is believed to be an aphrodisiac. Prostitutes sometimes inject cocaine solution into vagina to produce local constriction. Cocaine is also instilled in the urethra. (iii) Chronic users may develop metal derangements who may get involved in crimes, of which there are three categories: (a) Psychopharmacological effects (b) Economic compulsion (violent crimes committed to obtain money for drugs) (c) Systemic violence (associated with business methods and life-style of drug dealers). (iv) Cocaine induces states of paranoid and aggressive behaviour. (v) Protracted cocaine abuse may cause paranoid ideation and visual and auditory hallucinations, a state resembling alcoholic hallucinations.

MULTIPLE CHOICE QUESTIONS

1. Tactile hallucinations are seen with:

(a) Cocaine dependence (b) L.S.D. addiction
(c) Dhatura poisoning (d) Cannabis poisoning

2. Stupefying poisons are following *except:*

(a) Cannabis (b) Dhatura
(c) Belladonna (d) Aconite

3. Formication is a feature of:

(a) Chronic arsenic poisoning
(b) Opium addiction
(c) Atropine poisoning
(d) Chronic cocaine poisoning

4. The poison which can be detected in the viscera of a decomposed body:

(a) Phosphorous (b) Organophosphorus
(c) Acetic acid (d) Dhatura

5. An adult patient presented to medicine OPD with a black tongue, visual and tactile hallucination. The most likely poisoning is due to:

(a) Heroin (b) Cannabis
(c) Opium (d) Cocaine

6. Run-amok is observed in case of intoxication due to:

(a) Cocaine (b) Cannabis
(c) Barbiturates (d) Dhatura

7. Fatal dose of Ganja is:

(a) 4 gms (b) 8 gms
(c) 10 gms (d) 12 gms

8. Characteristic autopsy features of black tongue and teeth, nasal perforation and gangrene of nose tip is found in poisoning of:

(a) Chronic cadmium (b) Chronic mercury
(c) Chronic morphine (d) Chronic cocaine

9. Pathologic bathing behaviour supports the diagnosis of:

(a) Cannabis hyperemesis syndrome
(b) Atropine poisoning
(c) Chronic cocaine poisoning

10. Speed ball is a mixture of:

(a) Cocaine and Heroin (b) Cannabis and Cocaine
(c) Barbiturates and Cocaine (d) Dhatura and Heroin

11. Charas is the resin exuding from:

(a) Leaves and stem (b) Fruit
(c) Flower top and fruit (d) Root

12. A person with history of drug abuse by inhalation is brought for medical examination. X-ray reveals pneumomediastinum. He is likely to have used:

(a) Gajna smoke (b) Xylene
(c) Butane (d) Cocaine

13. Burnt rope like smell is found in which poisoning?

(a) Oleander
(b) Belladonna
(c) Cocaine
(d) Marijuana

14. Magnan's sign is found in:

(a) Cocaine addicts (b) Opium addicts
(c) Alcoholics (d) Cannabis addicts

15. Sinsemilla is a potent form of:

(a) Marijuana (b) Heroin
(c) Cocaine (d) Amphetamine

16. Amotivational syndrome is found in:

(a) Cannabis user (b) Heroin user
(c) Cocaine addict (d) Amphetamine addict

ANSWER KEY ☞

1. (a)	2. (d)	3. (d)	4. (d)	5. (d)	6. (b)	7. (b)	8. (d)	9. (c)	10. (a)
11. (a)	12. (d)	13. (d)	14. (a)	15. (a)	16. (a)				

41 CHAPTER

CNS Depressants

ALCOHOL

The term "alcohol" always means ethyl alcohol, which is one of the most widely used and abused substance in the world. Only human beings in the form of various alcoholic drinks consume ethyl alcohol (drinking alcohol). Alcohols are organic substances bearing 'OH' groups. The chemical formula for ethyl alcohol (ethanol) is C_2H_5OH. Its specific gravity is 0.79 that is 1 ml of alcohol weighs 0.79 gm. The term "toxic alcohols" is a collective term that includes methanol (wood alcohol), isopropyl alcohol (rubbing alcohol) and ethylene glycol (most commonly used in antifreeze).

Type of alcohol	Percentage of alcohol
Absolute alcohol	99.95%
Denatured alcohol	95% alcohol +
Or industrial spirit	5% wood naphtha
Rectified spirit	90%

Proof Spirit: It is a method to measure the alcohol content in an alcoholic beverage. It was originated in 16th century England, when spirits were being taxed according to their alcohol content. The British first developed the 'gunpowder method' to test the proof (something true or correct), by soaking a pellet of gunpowder in the spirit and attempting to light the wet pellet on fire. If the wet gunpowder could be lit, the alcohol was said to be a proof spirit and would therefore be taxed higher. Gunpowder soaked in spirit would not burn if it contained less than 57.15% alcohol by volume (ABV), meant it had 100 degrees proof. However, it was not an accurate method since the flammability of the liquor was dependent on its temperature, and the temperature wasn't kept consistent. It was modified in 1816 and again defined as "that mixture of alcohol and water, which at 10.5°C weighs exactly 12/13 part of an equal volume of distilled water". Proof spirit contains 57.07% alcohol by volume (ABV) or 49.24% by weight in the UK. In the USA it contains 50% alcohol by volume. A "proof spirit" has to be at least 100 proof. The weaker spirits are known as 'Under proof' and stronger spirits are called 'Over proof'. In India, alcohol content in bottles is 42.8% V/V or 75^0 Proof. Today, an alcohol by volume (ABV) percentage, which is the percentage of alcohol in the overall liquids, relatively easy to understand used internationally.

Alcoholic drinks contain ethyl alcohol with water and congeners (organic acids, acetones, butanol, aldehydes, tannins and esters). The congeners are produced during fermentation and distillation process. Wine and brandy have methyl alcohol as congeners. The % of alcohol in various drinks is given below:

Products of alcohol	Alcohol by volume
Rum	50-60%
Whisky	40-75%
Tequila	45-50.5%
Vodka	40-50%
Arrack (Liquor distilled from palm rice, sugar or jaggery)	40-50%
Gin, Brandy	40-45%
Port, Sherry	16-20%
Wine	10-15%
Beers	4-8%

Absorption: Alcohol is absorbed from the GI tract by simple passive diffusion along concentration gradients and does not involve an active transport system. **Alcohol is absorbed 20% through the empty stomach and 80% through the small intestine** to the blood because it provides larger absorption surface area by the villi and microvilli. From the blood, the alcohol goes to liver where it is damaged by a specific enzyme at a constant rate. Blood alcohol reaches the lungs through the venous circulation and through the arterial side of the heart into all the organs and tissues of the body mainly the brain. In brain, it interferes with the normal brain functions such as judgment and coordination of muscle movements. The blood concentration is influenced by many factors.

Only the concentration of alcohol in the blood influences the behavior. The amount in stomach and intestine indicates only the ingestion and has no effects as such. After death, alcohol in the stomach may diffuse into the blood and tissues. This results in higher blood level than actually existed during life, if the blood sample is taken from the part into which postmortem diffusion has taken place. In reference to absorption of alcohol when taken orally, gastric emptying seems to be the most important determinant of the rate of absorption, however, certain points need to be elaborated: (i) Absorption is slower in the stomach than intestine. (ii) Absorption is faster in empty stomach than when it contains food. (iii) Food affects the absorption by delaying the emptying time of the stomach: (a) Fatty foods, proteins and starch delay the absorption (b) Milk has similar effect, i.e., it delays absorption (c) Food prevents 10-20% of the ingested alcohol from being absorbed. (iv) Absorption of alcohol from GI tract is a first order kinetic process, i.e. the absorption rate is proportional to the concentration or amount of alcohol present in GI tract. Diluted form of alcohol like beer is absorbed slowly than the concentrated form. However, very high concentrated form of alcohol is also absorbed slowly, as it causes gastric irritation which leads to excessive mucous secretion, pyloric spasm and decreases gastric motility. Absorption is rapid when alcohol concentration in between 20 and 30%. (v) There is little difference in the rate of absorption of the same dose of alcohol administered in the form of different alcoholic beverages. (vi) It is a common belief that the use of a carbonated drinks increases the rate of alcohol absorption, however, there is little evidence to support it. (vii) Absorption of alcohol depends on habituation and tolerance of the individual as habituated heavy drinkers tend to absorb alcohol more rapidly. (viii) Emotional state of the person affects the contraction of the stomach resulting in rapid emptying time and the rate of absorption. (ix) Drugs like Benzedrine and atropine slows the absorption and retards the emptying time. Smoking delays gastric emptying time, thus, slows the absorption. Drugs like antihistamines, phenothiazines and metoclopramide enhances gastric emptying, thus accelerates absorption. (x) Age does not affect the rate of absorption of alcohol. (xi) Women have less active alcohol dehydrogenase enzyme (class IV) in the stomach mucosa to break down alcohol, i.e., reduced first pass metabolism, so more alcohol is available in GI tract for absorption. Women also absorb more alcohol during the premenstrual period than at other times. (xii) Individuals with gastrectomy, gastric ulcer and gastritis have an increased rate of absorption whereas, gastric malignancy and pyloric stenosis decreased rate of absorption. (xiii) *Inhalation:* Concentration in the blood is proportional to the concentration in the inspired air. (xiv) *Weight of the subject:* The same amount when taken by subjects of different weight has different blood levels depending upon the amount of bone, fat and muscles.

Distribution: (i) From GI tract, alcohol is absorbed into the blood from where it is distributed into the various organs and tissues in proportion to their water content. (ii) Women have a lower percentage of body water than men of comparable size, so there is less water to dilute the alcohol in women resulting in higher blood alcohol concentration. (iii) Alcohol can cross the placental barrier into the foetal circulatory system. (iv) It can easily cross the blood-brain barrier to cause impairment of brain functioning.

When equilibrium reached, the ratio of blood alcohol concentration (BAC) and other body fluid are as follows: (i) Blood: CSF:1:1.17 (ii) Blood: Vitreous:1:1.2 (iii) Blood: Urine: 1:1.3 (iv) Blood: Saliva: 1:12 (v) Blood: Breath Air: 1:2100.

Metabolism: The liver is the primary site for metabolism of alcohol. It is metabolized by both oxidative (mainly) and non-oxidative pathways. (i) **Oxidative Pathways** (Figure 41.1): About 90% of the alcohol metabolized through oxidative pathway. The enzymes alcohol dehydrogenase (ADH), cytochrome P450 2E1 (CYP2E1), and catalase all contribute to oxidative metabolism of alcohol. (a) *ADH enzyme:* Alcohol is oxidized to acetaldehyde primarily by enzyme alcohol dehydrogenase (ADH) and coenzyme nicotinamide-adenine dinucleotide (NAD) in the liver. This acetaldehyde is converted into free acetic acid (or acetyl coenzyme A). The acetate undergoes oxidation to carbon dioxide and water in the citric acid (Krebs cycle) (Figure 41.2). This acetate can form glycogen, proteins and also fats and cholesterol. The by-product acetaldehyde is toxic, responsible for tissue damage and, possibly the addictive process. There are five different isoenzymes of ADH (Class I-V) exist and each has a different affinity for alcohol. The class I ADH forms are mainly responsible for the oxidation of alcohol (b) *Cytochrome P450 2E1 (CYP2E1)/Microsomal alcohol oxidizing system*: This is a second oxidation pathway for alcohol metabolism which is present predominantly in the microsomes, or vesicles, of the endoplasmic reticulum in liver cell. It only accounts for ~10% of total alcohol clearance by the liver at low concentrations. (c) *Catalase:* This is a third oxidative pathway via the heme enzyme catalase, which is responsible for 0-2% of alcohol metabolism. (ii) **Nonoxidative Pathways:** The nonoxidative metabolism of alcohol is minimal, which produces ethyl glucuronide, ethyl sullfates, phosphatidyl ethanol and fatty acid ethyl esters. These metabolites used as biomarkers of ethanol intake and are mediators of ethanol toxicity.

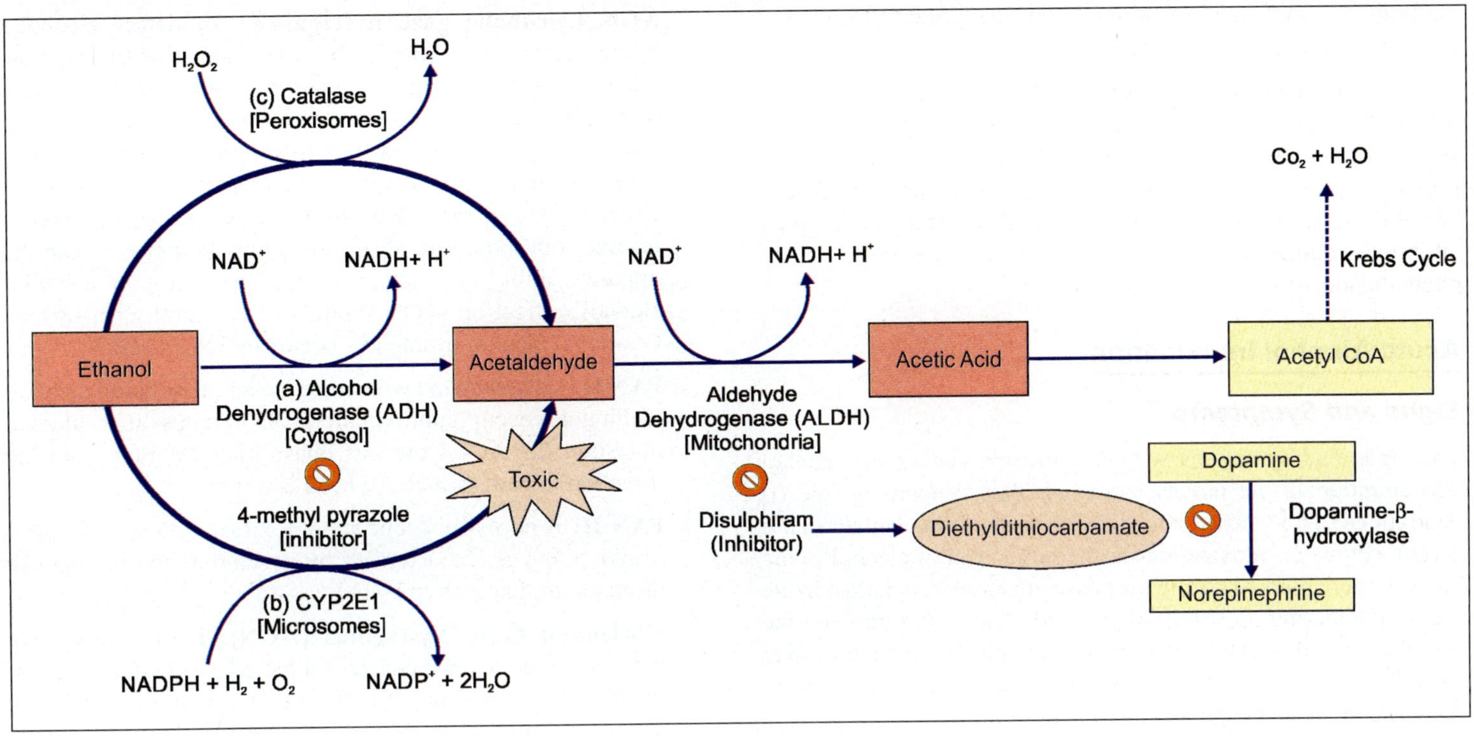

Figure 41.1: Ethanol oxidative metabolism pathway

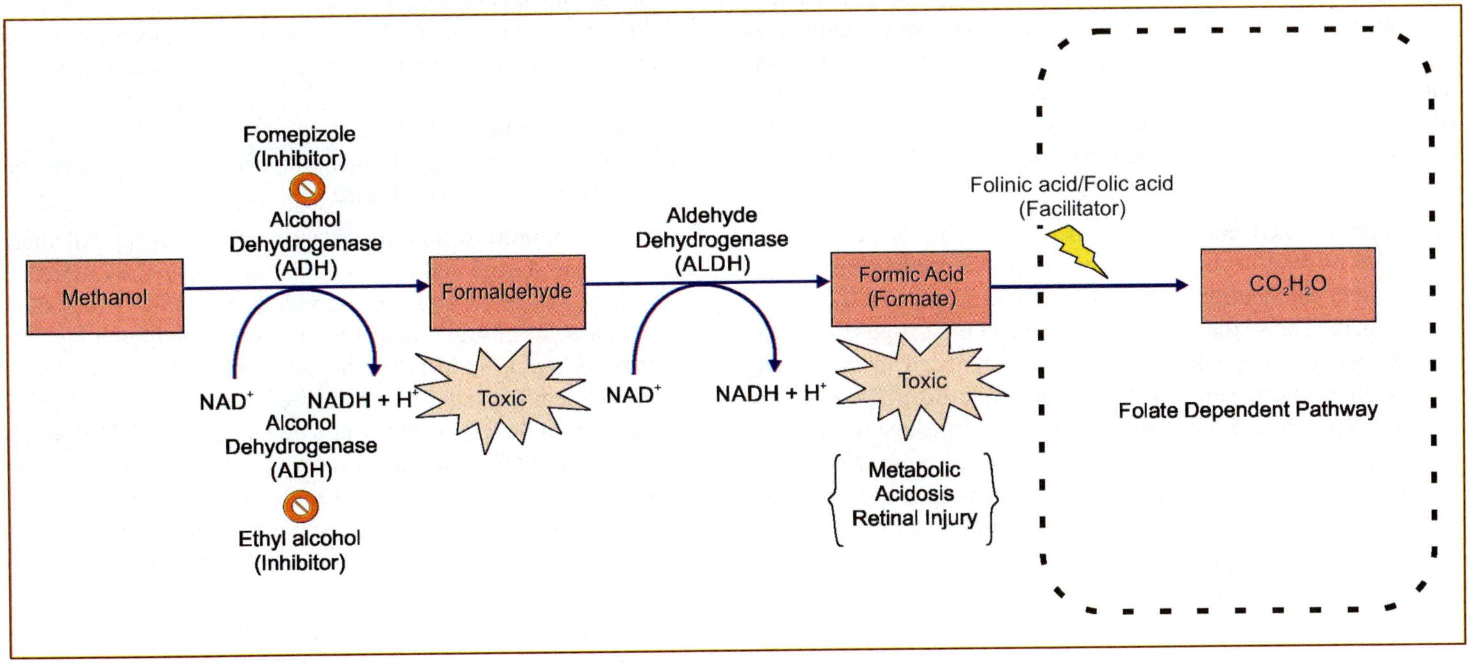

Figure 41.2: Methanol metabolism pathway

Elimination of the Alcohol

Majority of the ingested alcohol (95-98%) is metabolized and only small fraction is excreted unchanged via breath, urine or sweat. Due to an increase in liver enzymes, chronic alcoholic can metabolize alcohol faster at the rate of 40-50 mg%/hour. Alcohol from blood disappears at a rate of 10-15 ml/hour (15 mg%/hour) and is not stored in the tissues. Of the metabolized alcohol 10% get deposited in the tissues in the form of cholesterol and neutral fats. In hot climates, significant amount is lost through the sweat.

Pharmacological actions of alcohol: Alcohol being a central nervous system depressant causes an irregularly descending type of depression. Higher centres are depressed first followed by the midbrain and thalamus, spinal cord and finally the medulla. The recovery occurs in a reverse order.

Clinical consequences of alcohol: The disturbance of behaviour is due to the influence of alcohol on the central nervous system depending to what extent the brain function is affected. The initial symptoms such as feeling of well-being, self-confidence, garrulousness, exhilaration are due to the depression of the higher inhibitory control over the lower centres thereby causing a release phenomenon.

Acute Alcohol Intoxication

Signs and Symptoms

The signs and symptoms will be more marked as the alcohol concentration in the tissues increases. This depends on the (i) Amount (ii) Time lapsed and (iii) Tolerance. It is claimed that a certain degree of intoxication for the same level of alcohol in the blood is more marked during the phase of getting drunk than in the phase of sobering up (**Mellanby effect).** The departure from the normal is usually tested by a clinical examination of the subject to and the way in which the central nervous system is affected in response to acute mental and motor deterioration.

The normal discipline and controlled conduct are due to the control of higher centers of brain. When sufficient alcohol is taken the control of higher centers, normal inhibitions and restraints are removed. This is one of the earliest effects of alcoholic intoxication and may show in a variety of ways such as garrulity, impairment of judgment and recklessness. As the degree of intoxication advances, other CNS signs and symptoms manifest. There are three phases of intoxication:

1. **State of excitement:** This occurs at the blood alcohol level of 50-150 mg%, there is feeling of well-being, slight excitement, confidence is increased and a lack of self-control is there. The sexual desire is heightened but the performance is reduced. The visual acuity is also reduced in the blood alcohol concentration of 20 mg% in a nondrinker; 25-35 mg% in a moderate drinker and 40-70 mg% in a heavy drinker. The time and space orientation is altered with feeling of sleepiness. There is loss of critical judgment and the mental concentration is retarded. The memory is impaired.
2. **State of incoordination:** The symptoms of incoordination appear when the blood alcohol level is 150-250 mg/100 ml. The sense perception and skilled movements are affected. Inhibition of higher centers is lost resulting in change in the conduct of the individual. The person becomes irritable, gay, quarrelsome and sleepy. There is incoordination and clumsiness of fine and skilled movements. The speech is also altered. There are fine movements of fingers and tremors. Nausea and vomiting is common. Pulse is raised and face is flushed. The sense of touch, smell and hearing is diminished. Pupils are dilated and if light reflex is positive, it is a hopeful sign.

AGN (Alcoholic gaze nystagmus): To detect alcoholic intoxication, eyes should be examined for nystagmus. Alcoholic gaze nystagmus appears at blood alcohol levels of 50-100 mg%. Alcohol by acting on the vestibular system can cause **positional alcohol nystagmus (PAN)**. PAN is detected when the patient is lying supine with head turned to either the left or right. **Horizontal gaze nystagmus (HGN)** results from inhibition of the smooth pursuit system and the impaired ability to maintain eccentric gaze brought about by alcohol's effect on ocular moments via neural mechanisms. Positional alcohol nystagmus occurs in two stages:

PAN I: It is associated with acute elevation of blood alcohol, tending to occur approximately 30 minutes after alcohol ingestion. In PAN I the fast phase of nystagmus is in the direction towards which the head is turned.

PAN II: It normally occur at approximately 5-6 hours after drinking and is characterized by nystagmus in the opposite direction to that seen in PAN I.

Horizontal Gaze Nystagmus (HGN): It is a jerky eye moment noted when the gaze is directed to one side. The fast phase of HGN is in the direction of gaze, and it intensifies at a more eccentric gaze position. Although HGN can be seen in normal individuals at extreme gaze, when detected at lesser deviations, it is considered pathological. At angle of onset of 40° or less from the midline is a sensitive indicator of blood alcohol level in excess of 100 mg/dl. Blood alcohol levels of more than 80 mg% are consistently associated with HGN. Its presence should not be taken as proof of alcohol intoxication as HGN may be noted in pathological conditions, ingestion of sedatives and tranquilisers.

3. **Stage of coma:** Motor and sensory cells are deeply affected. Speech is slurred and the coordination is markedly affected. Gait is staggered and the individual may fall. The patient is in a state of coma and there is stertorous breathing. The pulse is rapid, temperature is subnormal and the pupils are constricted. On painful stimuli the pupils are dilated which then return slowly to the contracted stage called ***McEwan's sign.*** The patient may die or may recover in 8-10 hours with acute depression, nausea and headache. If coma is more than 5 hours, the death may occur resulting from asphyxia due to respiratory paralysis. In acute alcoholic intoxication even <400 mg% of blood alcohol concentration can cause death if the patient is suffering from heart or lung diseases.

Differential Diagnosis of Alcohol Poisoning: (i) Severe head injury (ii) Metabolic disorders such as diabetic or hypoglycemic coma (iii) Uraemic coma (iv) Intracranial tumours (v) Epilepsy (vi) Parkinsonism (vii) Disseminated sclerosis (ataxia, tremors and drowsiness simulating drunkenness is there) (viii) Cerebrovascular accidents (ix) Intake of drugs such as Insulin, barbiturates, atropine, antihistaminics, hallucinogens or morphine (x) Psychological disorders such as general paralysis of insane and hypomania (xi) High fever (xii) CO poisoning.

DRUNKENNESS

In 1927, the British Medical Council defined the word **Drunk** "The person concerned is so much under the influence of alcohol to have lost control of his faculties to such an extent as to render him unable to execute safely the occupation in which he is engaged at the material time".

In order to establish the diagnosis of drunkenness, the person should be carefully examined along with the collection of blood and urine samples for chemical analysis. Following points should be considered while examining a person for drunkenness: (i) The quantity of alcohol ingested is not related to the state of intoxication at the time of examination. (ii) The signs and symptoms, none of which is peculiar to this condition except the odour of the breath. (iii) An individual can react differently to different situations. Mentally unstable, epileptics and those with cerebral trauma may react even with small amount of alcohol. (iv) Even the smell of alcohol on the breath does not necessarily prove the person to be intoxicated because smell can persist for a longer time after the alcohol has been excreted from the body as it is due to the nonalcoholic constituents (congeners). (v) In many clinical conditions except for the smell of alcohol in breath, all or most of the symptoms and signs of alcoholic intoxication are found. These conditions are given under differential diagnosis. However, any of these clinical conditions can coexist with drunkenness or alcohol may modify the clinical features of these conditions specially the effects of drugs like barbiturates and tranquilisers are markedly potentiated by alcohol and many alcoholics develop the habit of taking alcohol and these drugs to experience 'kick'. (vi) A quite characteristic and aggressive odour of alcohol in the breath, loss of clearness of intellect and control of himself, unsteady gait, vacant look, dry and sticky lips, congested eyes, sluggish and dilated pupils, increased pulse rate, unsteady and thick voice, random talks and want of perception of the passage of time are the usual signs of drunkenness.

Model Performa for Examination of An Individual with Drunkenness

Special committee of British Medical Association has suggested the scheme of examination of an alleged case of drunkenness. In 1965 this committee has revised the original report of 1954 with a new title, "The drinking driver". The committee has defined **alcoholic intoxication** as "a condition produced in a person who has taken alcohol in a quantity sufficient to cause him to lose control of his faculties to such an extent that he is unable to execute the occupation on which he is engaged at the material time". The committee has proposed this proforma and protocol for such an examination. A written request should be obtained from the investigating officer.

1. Date, time and place of examination.
2. Preliminary details of the person being examined such as name of person with father's name, age, residential address etc.
3. Consent and name of the investigating police officer with name of police station.
4. Exclude injuries and pathological conditions, if any.
5. A brief history is to be recorded of (i) Amount of liquor taken (ii) Time of ingestion (iii) History of any disease (iv) Any treatment taken.
6. General behaviour (i) General appearance (ii) *State of clothing:* Whether soiled by vomiting or incontinence and the colour of the vomitus (iii) *Character of speech:* Whether it is thick, slurred with slight blurring of letters or over-precise. Memory of the recent things with mental alertness (iv) *Writing:* The following points should be noted: (a) Time taken to write (b) Repetition or omission of words or letters (c) Signatures can be compared (d) Ability to read his own handwriting.
7. **General examination should include:**

   (i) *Pulse*: Resting pulse at the beginning and at the end of the examination should be recorded; the pulse may be rapid. (ii) *Temperature* should be recorded; may be raised. (iii) *Skin: Is* dry or moist; flushed or pale. (iv) *Mouth:* Note the smell and whether the tongue is dry. (v) *Eyes*: Whether the lids are swollen (a) Is conjunctiva congested (b) Colour of the eyes (c) Visual acuity (d) Size of pupil (is dilated in early stages and constricted in late stages) (e) Reaction of eyes to light (f) Nystagmus. (vi) Smell of breath and any hiccups. (vii) *Ears:* Impairment of hearing. (viii) *Gait*: Manner of walking and turning (note any lurching or reeling) by asking the person to walk on a straight line and suddenly asked to turn back. He is then asked to stand with eyes closed and open and his ability to stand is noted **Romberg's sign.** (ix) *Muscular coordination*: This is assessed by finger nose test (asking him to touch nose with his index finger), picking up a pencil or coin from floor, lighting a cigarette, buttoning and unbuttoning clothes. (x) Knee and ankle reflexes are noted.
8. Systemic examination should be conducted.
9. **Opinion:** The opinion may be given as: I am of the opinion that the person examined (i) Did not consume alcohol; or (ii) Consumed alcohol but not under the influence; or (iii) consumed alcohol and under the influence (intoxicated).

Consumption of Alcohol

One unit = 10 grams of absolute alcohol.

60 grams = 66 ml of absolute alcohol.

In males: (i) Amount of absolute alcohol should not exceed 4 units/day (ii) 4-6 units/day is hazardous (iii) More than 6 units/day is harmful.

In females: (i) Amount of absolute alcohol should not exceed 2 units/day (ii) 2-4 units is hazardous (iii) More than 4 units is harmful.

Indications of Hazardous and Harmful Alcohol Consumption

Hazardous alcohol intake: (i) Regular intake of more than 60 gm/day in males and 40 gm/day in females (ii) Occurrence of episodes of intoxication twice monthly or more (iii) Drinking behaviour such as (a) Gulping the first drink (b) Difficulty in stopping drinking once started (c) Most of the leisure activities involve drinking (d) Most friends are heavy drinkers (e) Eating lightly or skipping meals while drinking (f) Attempts to cut down on drinking with limited success.

Harmful alcohol consumption: (i) *Psychological manifestations* in the form of: (a) Amnesic episodes while intoxicated and Blackouts (b) Insomnia and nightmares (c) Accidents where alcohol is involved (d) Charges of driving under influence (e) being late or absent from work (f) Concern or worry about driving by self or family. (ii) *Physical symptoms* such as (a) Dyspepsia (b) Morning nausea and vomiting (c) Recurrent diarrhoea. (iii) *General appearance* as (a) Bloated facies (b) Conjunctival injection (c) Coating of tongue and (d) Presence of scars and bruises especially of varying ages. (iv) *Demeanor:* Anxious and agitated. (v) *Cardiovascular system:* Tachycardia and hypertension. (vi) *Abdominal signs:* Soft hepatomegaly is there. (vii) Trauma; rib fractures may be there. The effects of alcohol, signs and symptoms and various medical terminologies are given in Table 41.1.

Other Effects of Alcohol

Delirium tremens: It is the unsoundness of mind resulting from long continued action of alcohol on the brain. It occurs in chronic alcoholics due to: (i) Temporary excess (ii) Sudden withdrawal of alcohol (iii) Shock after receiving injuries such as fracture of bone (iv) Acute infections.

The symptoms of delirium tremens are opposite to those of an intoxicated state and develop within 6 hours. Delirium tremens is a form of acute insanity in which the following signs and symptoms are present: (i) Coarse muscular tremors of the face, tongue and hands (ii) Hyperactivity of central nervous system (iii) Restlessness (iv) Loss of memory (v) Uncontrollable tears (vi) Sweating (vii) Agitation and anxiety (viii) Tendency to commit suicide, homicide, violent assault or to cause damage to the property (ix) Disorientation for time and place (x) Hallucination of hearing, sight and tactile when one feels that the insects are crawling under the skin (xi) Convulsions.

Medicolegal Aspects

It is an unsoundness of mind so the person is not responsible for his criminal acts.

Alcoholic polyneuritis: The signs and symptoms of alcoholic polyneuritis are: (i) Generalized weakness (ii) Pain in the extremities (iii) Wrist and foot drop (iv) Unsteady gait (v) Loss of deep reflexes (vi) Tenderness of muscles of arms and legs.

Wernicke's encephalopathy and Korsakoff's psychosis: Deficiency of vitamin B_1 occurs in heavy drinkers resulting in lesions of brain or spinal cord. This condition is rapidly fatal with death resulting within 24 hours. The patient becomes disoriented and forgetful of the recent past events. There is drowsiness, peripheral neuropathy, ophthalmoplegia, nystagmus, ataxia, delirium and stupor. This condition when untreated can progress to Korsakoff's psychosis in which there is impairment of short term memory, inability to learn new information and confabulation.

TREATMENT APPROACHES

The following treatment approaches are undertaken:

Detoxification

Detoxification is a process by which alcohol dependent persons recover from intoxication in a supervised manner so that the withdrawal symptoms are minimised. Delirium tremens is a medical emergency and its treatment is of two types, namely.

Table 41.1: Various medical terminologies and the effects of alcohol

Medical terminology	Blood alcohol concentration (mg%)	Effects	Symptoms and signs
Sober	<10	No effect	No features
Drinking	20-70	Impairment of cognitive function, motor coordination and sensory perception. Mild euphoria is produced	
Under the influence	80-100	Decreased inhibitions, increased self-confidence, alteration of judgment, euphoria	Flushing of face, dilatation of pupil, loss of inhibitions, speech is heavy, staggering gait, careless and in-coordinated
Drunk	150-300	Muscular incoordination, staggering gait, drowsiness, dizziness, disorientation, heaviness of speech and marked mental confusion	Face flushed, dilated and inactive pupil, rapid eyeball movement, loss of restraints, heaviness of speech, staggering gait and clouding of intellect
Coma and death	≥400	Respiratory failure, deep coma and death	The pupils are contracted, pulse is rapid, breathing stertorous and deep unconsciousness

Non-Medicated Detoxification

Home detoxification: When there is (i) No history of severe withdrawal, fits or acute organic brain syndrome (ii) No current signs of severe withdrawal (iii) No medical illness (iv) No evidence of psychiatric illness. In this treatment regimen, friends or relatives should stay with the patient and they should call the doctor if needed.

In patient detoxification: This treatment regimen is followed when the conditions at home atmosphere are not favourable. Here the withdrawal symptoms can be relieved by the provision of supportive counseling in a non-stimulating and nonthreatening environment. There are special techniques to relieve the anxiety and agitation.

Medicated Detoxification

In essence, one is substituting controlled drug intoxication for an uncontrolled one. Drugs that are used for medicated detoxification: (i) *Chloromethazole:* It is a short acting sedative and anticonvulsant (ii) *Diazepam:* It is a long acting drug given orally every two hours until sedation is achieved; maximum 120 mg can be given (iii) *Clonidine:* It is a major tranquilizer and antipsychotic drug that is given when the above drug fails (iv) Thiamine is administered intravenously (v) Electrolyte and acid base balance is corrected.

Pharmacological treatment: (i) *Disulfiram (Antabuse):* It was introduced about 40 years ago. It acts by inhibiting hepatic enzyme aldehyde dehydrogenase whenever alcohol is ingested. It produces symptoms such as flushing of face, upper trunk causes vomiting, dizziness and headache (Temposil 50 mg/day). (ii) *Serotonin uptake inhibitors:* They depend upon the neurochemical basis of alcohol uptake. These are Zimelidine, Viaqualine, they inhibit the uptake of Serotonin at nerve synapses. (iii) Alcohol antagonists is Imidazodiazepine: It antagonizes the effect of alcohol.

Behavioural treatment: Behavioural treatment is based on the theory that many important aspects of human learning takes place by imitating the behaviour of others by a much greater attention to cognitive process in specifically human learning. The behavioural therapy includes: (i) ***Aversion therapy***: Also known as counter conditioning is based on the work of **Pavlov** on conditioned reflex. The principle of aversion therapy is simply to attempt to create an aversive conditioned response to a drug by pairing a stimuli associated with drug taking (for example sight, taste, smell) with powerfully unpleasant unconditioned stimuli such as nausea and electric shock. Nausea induced by emetine has been used as the conditioned response from the 1940s. It has also been found that nausea based techniques are more effective than those based on electric shock. (ii) ***Cue exposure***: This method of treatment is based on the understanding of the nature of tolerance and withdrawal from addictive drugs with the idea that both tolerance and withdrawal are partly conditioned process. If tolerance, withdrawal and craving are conditioned phenomenon, it follows that they can, in principle, be extinguished. In other words if problem drinkers are exposed to cues for drinking but discouraged or prevented from drinking, the cues in question should loose their power to evoke a desire to consume alcohol and should also lead to lower tolerance in response to those cues. This hypothesis was tested by **Blakey and Baker**. The clients were encouraged to go into pubs where alcohol was placed in front of them but they were asked to resist from drinking. After some time the pubs which act as cues lost their influence over the alcohol drinkers. (iii) ***Alcoholic anonymous***: This is a voluntary organization with branches throughout the world. It comprises alcoholics that meet through group meetings, letters, media and e-mail. These alcoholics share their bad experiences related to alcohol with addicts who are desirous of giving up alcohol. This organization is self funding with contribution from its members. (iv) ***Psychotherapy and counselling:*** It involves the psychotherapeutic treatment and counselling of the alcoholics.

Medicolegal Aspects

S. 85 I.P.C.: Nothing is an offence which is done by a person who at the time of doing it, is by reason of intoxication incapable of knowing the nature of the act, or that he is doing what is either wrong or contrary to law; provided that the thing which intoxicated him was administered to him without his knowledge or against his will.

Scope S. 85 gives the same protection as S. 84 does to a person of unsound mind. Voluntary drunkenness is no excuse for commission of crime. As far as knowledge is concerned, the standard of test is same as in case of intention.

S. 86 I.P.C.: In cases where an act is done is not an offence unless done with a particular knowledge or intent, a person who does the act in a state of intoxication shall be liable to be dealt with as if he had the same knowledge as he would have had if he had not been intoxicated, unless the thing which intoxicated him was administered to him without his knowledge or against his will. Under S. 86 a person who gets into a state of intoxication voluntarily presumed to have the same knowledge as he would have had he not been intoxicated.

Principle: Since the criminal intention is the foundation of the criminal responsibility, it follows that a person who is drunk is in the same predicament as a person temporarily insane. However, since no man can be permitted to hear the clock of immunity by getting drunk, the rule justly accepts cases of voluntary drunkenness.

When drunkenness is a defence: Voluntary drunkenness as such is never a defence, still when habitual drunkenness produces frenzy that fact becomes material for showing how it was produced and when its existence is established, it will excuse a crime.

When drunkenness is relevant in considering intention: (i) Drunkenness caused without one's knowledge or against one's will excuses the crime. (ii) Voluntary drunkenness is an excuse only as regards 'intention' so that it is a complete excuse in crimes requiring the presence of an intention to complete a crime. (iii) However, voluntary drunkenness is no excuse for a crime, which requires the presence merely of knowledge as distinct from an intention. (iv) In any case, though voluntary drunkenness is no excuse for knowledge, it does not imply actual knowledge giving rise to the inference or presumed intention.

Scope of S. 86 I.P.C.: The law places insanity and involuntary drunkenness on the same footing by using the same criteria, that is incapability of knowing the nature of the act or that he is doing what is wrong or contrary to law.

A person who gets into a state of intoxication voluntarily is presumed to have the same knowledge as he would have if he had not been intoxicated. When the state of intoxication is such as to make him incapable of knowing the nature of the act or that he is doing wrong or contrary to law, he can only be punished based on knowledge and not of any particular intention.

Principle: Voluntary drunkenness does not afford the defence that the knowledge required to complete an offence was wanting, though it may be used to show that any intent if required was absent.

This section draws a distinction between presumption as to knowledge and presumption as to intention and though intention is to be inferred from knowledge.

Presumption of knowledge and intention: 'Knowledge' means knowing what is known, there is personal range of information whereas 'intention' means ultimate aim or purpose.

Even a drunken man is presumed to intend the natural consequences of his act, unless he proves incapacity in himself to form the intent necessary to constitute the crime. A distinction must be made between motive, intention and knowledge.

S. 510 I.P.C.: Misconduct by a drunken person in public is punishable with imprisonment upto 24 hours.

Alcohol and traffic accidents: There is deterioration in driving ability as blood alcohol level rises to 30-50% as it: (i) Increases reaction time (ii) Creates false confidence (iii) Impairs concentration (iv) Produces muscular incoordination (v) Decreases visual and auditory acuity.

At the blood alcohol concentration of 50 mg%, the drivers are able to carry out road safety rules properly. At the levels of 60 mg%, the chances of being involved in an accident increase two-fold. There is markedly increased risk at levels above 80 mg%; increases 12 times at 100 mg% and 25 times at over 150 mg%. At 150 mg%, there is a distinct impairment of driving whereas at 200 mg%, all drivers are intoxicated and again there is an increased risk of accidents. Drivers of motor vehicles often fail to realize that although after drinking, they may experience feeling of well being, their critical faculties are blunted and they are liable to take risks and make mistakes while driving. In some countries, such as Bulgaria, Russia, Romania, Hungary, Turkey and Belgium it is an offence to drive even with blood levels of 0 mg%. In other countries driving with certain blood alcohol levels is an offence such as:

• Poland and Sweden	20 mg%
• Czechoslovakia and India	30 mg%
• Australia, Netherlands, France, Finland and Greece	50 mg%
• France, Austria, Spain, Ireland, Canada, Germany and Italy	80 mg%
• USA	100-150 mg%

In India S. 185 Motor Vehicle Act 1988 (Amendment, 2019) states that statutory limit of blood alcohol is 30 mg% and for contravention the punishment involves fine up to Rs 10000- or 6-month imprisonment or both for the first offence. For a second or subsequent offence, the fine is up to Rs 15000 or imprisonment up to 2 years or both.

Alcohol and sudden death: (i) Alcohol predisposes to arrhythmia by its action on the myocardium. (ii) An intoxicated person would develop cardiorespiratory arrest and die during struggle. This results from release of catecholamines which on combination with alcohol produces cardiac arrhythmia and death. (iii) Conduction system lesions predisposes to arrhythmia that may be further aggravated by alcohol and release of catecholamines.

Laboratory Analysis of Alcohol

The concentration of alcohol in blood, urine, breath and saliva helps in estimating the degree of intoxication. Vitreous humour and urine are good for analysis as they are not effected by putrefaction for a longer period and also they do not contain much glucose. Blood is the best sample and gives the direct evidence of the concentration of alcohol in brain but it is difficult to collect the sample in an uncooperative patient. In addition the consent of the patient is necessary. If the patient is unconscious or unfit to give consent, examining doctor should not divulge the findings to the police but wait till patient regains consciousness or is in a fit condition to consent, then only doctor can divulge the findings. However, if the person is under arrest, no consent is required. Sometimes substances such as acetone, ether and paraldehyde may be estimated as alcohol.

1. **Breath analysis of alcohol:** 60-100 ml of breath is received into a dry balloon and analysed by drunkometer, intoximeter, alcometer or breath analyser. However, breath analyser is more reliable.

   Principle of breath analyser: The concentration of alcohol in deep lung air is directly proportional to the alcohol concentration in the arterial blood. This is based on the principle of **Henry's law**. Amount of alcohol in 2100 ml of alveolar air = amount of alcohol in 1 ml of blood. The converted breath tests are in close agreement with those obtained by direct blood analysis. The person is asked to blow into a plastic balloon through a glass tube containing a crystalline bichromate-sulphuric acid mixture. Blood alcohol >80 mg% is indicated by green colour in the spectrum.

Mechanism of operation: Alcohol absorbs radiations in the infrared region of spectrum and amount of infrared light absorbed by a vapour is proportional to the concentration of alcohol in that vapour.

Causes of false positive results: (i) Alcohol may remain in the mouth up to 20-30 minutes after a small peg. Therefore, the test is to be repeated after 20 minutes (ii) Hyperventilation (iii) Physical exercise (iv) Emesis (v) Regurgitation of stomach contents. Therefore, the plastic, aluminium and other flexible bags are made available so that the breath samples may be preserved for several hours.

2. **Blood analysis:** To clean the skin before withdrawing blood, spirit should not be used and syringe should not contain even a trace of alcohol in any form. The skin can be cleaned with a solution of 1:1000 mercuric chloride and can be washed with soap and water. 10 ml of blood is collected in a glass vial containing 10 mg of sodium fluoride or 30 mg of potassium oxalate as preservative. The bottle is tightly capped with screw and kept in a refrigerator but not frozen. The analysis should be performed within a week. **Whole blood alcohol concentration is 12-20% lesser than the serum or plasma concentration**. These tests are based on the presence of any volatile reducing agent. Basic principle being reduction of potassium bichromate by the test substance. The methods used are (i) **Kozelka and Hine test (macro test)** (ii) **Cavett test (micro test)**. Analytical methods such as chromatographs, spectrophotometric analysis and oxidation techniques are used. **Gas liquid chromatography** is more specific for medicolegal purposes.
3. **Saliva:** Before collecting saliva samples, mouth should be thoroughly rinsed with water. About 5 ml of sample should be collected in a test tube containing 10 mg of sodium fluoride.
4. **Urine analysis:** The concentration of alcohol in urine is 20% higher than blood when collected at the same time as urine has 25% more water compared to an equal volume of blood. **A ratio of 1.3:1 is acceptable** when urine and blood are in equilibrium. The concentration of alcohol in the second sample shows the blood level during the inter-specimen interval. When there is difference in alcohol concentration of the two urine samples, it indicates whether the patient was in absorptive phase, at peak or in elimination phase. An approximate value of blood alcohol level at the time when this sample was being secreted can be obtained by multiplying the alcohol concentration in second urine sample by 0.75. This calculation is based on a blood urine alcohol concentration ratio of 1:1.35. The extent of intoxication at the time of incidence can be detected by extrapolation from this blood level back to the time of incident. For urine analysis 2 samples should be obtained; first as soon as following the incident, completely emptying the bladder and second after a period of 25-30 minutes. The disadvantages of urine examination are (i) Maximum concentration in urine reaches 20-25 minutes later than the blood as a time lag before equilibrium is reached between blood and urine. (ii) After the maximum concentration of alcohol in blood has been reached, the urine alcohol concentration will be higher by 20-30% than in the blood at any given time as the sample of urine examined must have been secreted at some earlier period from the blood.
5. **Vitreous fluid analysis:** For every unit of alcohol in blood there are 1.2 units of alcohol in vitreous as it has a high-water content at equilibrium. Vitreous alcohol levels are analysed but these lag behind blood alcohol levels by 1-2 hours. These levels are lower than blood alcohol. **It is a good sample for alcohol estimation even in putrefied bodies.**

Widmark formula: This formula was created by Erik Widmark to determine (i) The amount of alcohol consumed by a person with known blood alcohol concentration (BAC). (ii) retrograde and anterograde calculations of BAC based on the amount of alcohol consumed by a person. This formula was devised taking into consideration the weight, sex of the person and type of alcoholic liquor consumed. The formula is applicable when there is complete absorption of alcohol and the equilibrium has been reached between blood and body tissue. The formula is:

a = cpr

where,

a = weight of alcohol ingested in gms

c = concentration of alcohol in blood (BAC) in mg/kg

p = body weight in kg

r = Widmark or distribution factor or 'r' factor (0.68 for males and 0.55 for females, it varies between 0.5-0.9)

For urine analysis, Widmark formula is: **a = 3/4 qpr**, where

a = weight of alcohol consumed (gms)

q = urine alcohol concentration (mg/kg)

p = body weight (kg)

r = Widmark or distribution factor or 'r' factor

This formula is however controversial.

Postmortem Alcohol

After death, alcohol diffuses through the stomach wall into surrounding blood, cavities (pleural, pericardial and peritoneal) and tissues. Therefore, it is important that for chemical analysis for alcohol, the blood sample should not be drawn from the areas in vicinity of the stomach. This would result in false high results due to gastric alcohol diffusion after death. If death has resulted from head injury due to trauma, **subdural hematoma should be preserved for analysis**, as it will contain the same concentration of alcohol as that in the blood at the time when incidence has occurred. After death, no appreciable loss of alcohol takes place by evaporation from body or blood. In conditions of advanced putrefaction as the entire contents of vascular compartment including the alcohol are destroyed, the brain should be preserved for analysis. Alcohols including **ethyl alcohol can be produced due to the action of enzymes, bacteria** such as E.coli, yeast or fungi on the carbohydrates and **proteins in putrefied bodies**. This production increases with the longer time interval after death and when the temperature of surroundings is raised. The concentration of alcohol in stages of advanced putrefaction could be as high as 0.2%. **When postmortem levels of alcohol are less than 0.2%, it could be attributed to the process of putrefaction**. There are circumstances when alcohol is found in blood and visceral organs but not in urine, this could be due to putrefaction. At autopsy, the blood samples should be collected from femoral vein, cubital vein or tibial vein. Postmortem blood alcohol concentrations are valid for a period of 36 hours after death. On analysis, if the person has consumed alcohol, concentration will be same in all these samples. The changes in concentration of alcohol cannot occur at exactly the same level in all the samples if it is due to bacterial and enzymatic putrefaction. The results could be erroneous due to hemolysis, diffusion from body fluids or tissues, collection of a wrong sample from the wrong site and also due to effect of putrefaction. Postmortem examination of urine sample is quite reliable qualitative index of antemortem intoxication than blood. If the urine alcohol concentration after death exceeds by more than 25% than that of blood it indicates a higher blood alcohol level during life. When the postmortem urine alcohol concentration is equal to or less than the blood alcohol level after death, it can be suggested that the individual was in absorptive phase at the time of death and about two hours could have passed after consumption of his last drink.

METHYL ALCOHOL

Methyl alcohol is prepared by destructive distillation of wood or molasses. When pure it is colourless, tasteless and odourless. It burns with pale blue non-luminous flame and its vapour produces explosive mixture in presence of oxygen or air.

Methanol, also known as methyl alcohol or wood alcohol, is a chemical compound with chemical formula CH_3OH. It is the simplest alcohol, and is a light, volatile, colourless, tasteless, flammable, poisonous liquid with a very faint odour. It is used as an antifreeze, solvent, fuel and as a denaturant for ethyl alcohol.

Methanol is produced naturally in the anaerobic metabolism of many varieties of bacteria. As a result, there is a small fraction of methanol vapour in the atmosphere. Over the course of several days, atmospheric methanol is oxidized by oxygen by the help of sunlight to carbon dioxide and water.

Methanol burns in air forming carbon dioxide and water:

$$2CH_3OH + 3\,O_2 \rightarrow 2CO_2 + 4H_2O$$

A methanol flame is almost colourless. Care should be exercised while burning methanol to avoid burning oneself on the almost invisible fire.

Because of its poisonous properties, methanol is also used as a denaturant for ethanol. Methanol is often called wood alcohol because it was once produced chiefly as a byproduct of the destructive distillation of wood. It is now produced synthetically by the direct combination of hydrogen and carbon monoxide gases, heated under pressure in the presence of a catalyst.

History: In their embalming process, the ancient Egyptians used a mixture of substances, including methanol, which they obtained from the pyrolysis of wood. Pure methanol, however, was first isolated in 1661 by Robert Boyle, who called it **spirit of box,** because he produced it via the distillation of boxwood. It was later came to known as **pyroxylic spirit.**

Uses of Methyl Alcohol

(i) It is used as a solvent for gums, fats and varnishes for cinematograph films and as an antifreeze. (ii) Methanol is used on a limited basis to fuel internal combustion engines, mainly by virtue of the fact that it is not nearly as flammable as gasoline. (iii) It is used for denaturation of ethyl alcohol. (iv) Industrial methylated spirit contains 95% by volume of ethyl alcohol, 5% by volume of wood naptha and 0.5% of crude pyridine. Methyl violet is added for colouring. It has disagreeable odour that is used for fouling rectified spirit, rendering it unfit for drinking. Nevertheless it is commonly consumed owing to its low cost and easy availability. (v) Surgical spirit contains industrial methylated spirit with methyl salicylate or mineral naptha and ethyl phthalate. (vi) Methanol is also used as a solvent and as an antifreeze in pipelines.

Toxicity: Methanol is toxic, as its metabolites formic acid and formaldehyde cause blindness and death. The toxicity results by: (i) Ingestion (ii) Inhalation (iii) Absorption through the skin. Foetal tissue will not tolerate methanol. Dangerous doses will build up if a person is regularly exposed to fumes or handles liquid without skin protection.

Mode of Action

Methyl alcohol is rapidly absorbed from the gastrointestinal tract and also through lungs and skin. It gets oxidized in liver into formaldehyde and formic acid by alcohol dehydrogenase (ADH) and aldehyde dehydrogenase (ALDH) respectively (Figure 42.2). The formic acid is not easily eliminated from body and mostly accumulates. Small amount of unprotonated form of formic i.e. formate, interacts with folic acid produce water (H_2O) and carbon dioxide (CO_2). The toxicity occurs as a result accumulation of toxic metabolites formate which causes high anion gap acidosis, widespread degenerative changes in the internal organs, CNS and retina. It concentrates in the vitreous body and optic nerve maximally.

Fatal Dose: 100–125 ml (4 fl. oz.); is quite variable as recovery has even occurred with large doses.

Fatal Period: 24-36 hours.

Signs and Symptoms

The effect of methyl alcohol on central nervous system is more intense and persistent than ethyl alcohol. The onset of clinical symptoms may be prolonged for 24-36 hours: (i) Headache, dizziness and vertigo (ii) Nausea, vomiting and severe epigastric pain (iii) Rise of serum amylase may result in acute abdominal pain due to pancreatitis (iv) Cardiac functions are depressed (v) Muscular weakness, dyspnoea and cyanosis (vi) Visual disturbances: (a) Concentric diminution of visual field for colour (b) Photophobia (c) Blurred (snow storm) vision (d) Retrobulbar optic neuritis or neuro-retinitis resulting in partial blindness. These are the most dangerous effect of methyl alcohol and are due to specific toxic effect of formaldehyde on retinal cells. The primary retinal damage is in the ganglion cells and optic atrophy is secondary (vii) Cold sweating and convulsions (viii) Subnormal temperature (ix) Delirium and coma may last for 2-3 days (x) Bradycardia and Kussmaul breathing (xi) Urine is strongly acid and contains albumen, acetone and formic acid (xii) Coma follows unconsciousness and coma induced is longer in onset and lasts longer compared to ethyl alcohol drunkenness (xii) Death occurs from cardiac failure.

Management

(i) The first step is to secure and maintain airway, breathing and circulation. (ii) The patient should be kept in a dark room to protect the eyes from light. (iii) **Correction of metabolic acidosis by Bicarbonate therapy** is the mainstay of treatment of methyl alcohol poisoning. It prevents retinal damage. (a) Gastric lavage using 4% soda bicarbonate solution in warm water and 500 ml of this solution is left in the stomach (b) Initial treatment with sodium bicarbonate 1-2 mg/kg via intravenously bolus is required for patient with pH below 7.3 followed by maintenance infusion till arterial pH is above 7.35. (iv) Potassium chloride (KCl) infusion is required only when hypokalemia occurs due to alkali therapy. (v) **Fomepizole** (Antizole, 4-Methylpyrazole or 4MP) is the antidote of choice which competitively inhibits alcohol dehydrogenase enzyme (ADH) that stops conversion of methanol to toxic metabolite formate. It has stronger affinity for ADH compared to ethanol, easy to administer and does not cause CNS depression. It is given IV with a loading dose of 15 mg/kg, and then maintenance dosing of 10 mg/kg every 12 hours for 4 doses or until the methanol concentration is less than 32 mg/dl with a normal acid-base status. (vi) **Ethyl alcohol:** It is used as an antidote in methanol poisoning. Both ethanol and methanol utilize same alcohol dehydrogenase (ADH) enzyme for their metabolism. However, ethanol has at least 10 times the affinity for ADH compared to methanol. When ethanol is given, it saturates ADH, there is limited availability of ADH for methanol metabolism resulting decreases the formation of toxic metabolites. Indications for ethanol administration include methanol levels > 20 mg/dl or an osmolol gap > 10 mosm/l. It can be given orally or intravenously. The therapeutic goal is to reach serum ethanol concentration in a range of 80 to 120 mg/dl. **Dose:** 50% (100 proof) oral ethanol may be administered with a loading dose of 2 ml/kg followed by 0.2 to 0.4 ml/kg per hour. 10% intravenous ethanol may be administered with a loading dose of 8 ml/kg over 30 to 60 minutes, followed by maintenance dosing of 1 to 2 ml/kg per hour. A close monitoring of serum ethanol concentration is required, since, it causes intoxication. It should only be given if fomepizole is unavailable. (vii) **Folate therapy**: Folinic acid or Folic acid is given in dose of 50 mg IV or orally 6 hourly for 24-48 hours as co-factor therapy as it accelerates the metabolism of the toxic metabolite, formate, to carbon dioxide and water. It has no significant role in treating already established methanol toxicity. (viii) **Haemodialysis:** It clears methanol as well as formate from the body and hastens recovery. Indications the procedure includes methanol ingestion (>30 ml), serum methanol level (> 20 mg/dl), visual complications, and no improvement in acidosis despite repeated sodium bicarbonate infusions. (ix) Stimulants and steroids are given. (x) Barbiturates are given to treat convulsions.

Autopsy Findings

(i) Stomach and intestines are hyperaemic, congested and inflamed with patchy submucous haemorrhages. (ii) Fat necrosis in the peritoneum. (iii) Brain and meninges are congested and oedematous. (iv) Lungs and kidneys are congested and oedematous. (v) Pancreas may show necrosis and haemorrhage. (vi) The eyes will show degenerative changes in the corneal epithelium, retina will show oedema of the optic disc and there may be optic nerve atrophy.

Medicolegal Aspects

(i) Poisoning is always accidental. (ii) Mass poisoning may result from consumption of liquor adulterated with methyl alcohol. (iii) It is also used inadvertently, when ethyl alcohol is not available. (iv) Consumption of **solox** (containing shellac, a paint solvent with ethyl alcohol and methyl alcohol) or **Khopadi**, a cheap liquor containing methyl alcohol and **French polish** or similar intoxicating products have given rise to methyl alcohol intoxication in various parts of the country.

ETHYLENE GLYCOL

Ethylene glycol (C2H6O2) is a toxic alcohol, colourless, nonvolatile, hygroscopic, water soluble, sweet-tasting liquid. It is commonly used as an antifreeze solvent, coolant, but used for other purposes, such as industrial solvents.

Mode of Action

It is poorly absorbed by dermal and pulmonary route. However, it is rapidly absorbed through the gastrointestinal tract after ingestion and the peak level reached approximately 2 hours after ingestion. The metabolism begins with gastric mucosal alcohol dehydrogenase, and occurs primarily in the liver. Ethylene glycol is first oxidized by alcohol dehydrogenase to glycoaldehyde, which is then oxidized by aldehyde dehydrogenase to glycolic acid, which is primarily responsible for the associated metabolic acidosis with increased anion gap and interstitial and tubular damage to the kidney. Glycolic acid finally oxidized to oxalic acid. The oxalic acid may precipitate as calcium oxalate crystals in the brain, kidney etc. and cause hypocalcemia. 80% of ethylene glycol metabolized in liver with the remainder renally excreted unchanged.

Signs and Symptoms

Early symptoms are similar to the feeling caused by drinking ethyl alcohol (euphoria etc.). However, after few hours, toxic effects become apparent. The features include nausea, vomiting, slurred speech, lethargy, nystagmus, convulsions, stupor, or even coma. A faint, sweet aromatic odor from breath.

Fatal Dose: Approx. 1.4 ml/kg of 100% Ethylene glycol.

Fatal Period: Upto 72 hours.

Diagnosis

It is established by measuring blood level of ethylene glycol and glycolic acids.

Treatment

(i) Supportive measures (ABC management). (ii) Gastric lavage and activated charcoal should be administered. (iii) Fomepizole or 4-methylpyrazole (15 mg/kg IV loading dose) is the antidote for toxic alcohols which acts by inhibiting alcohol dehydrogenase. (iv) Ethanol can be administered I.V. or oral route. (v) Hemodialysis indicated when the arterial pH is 7.3, or the osmolar gap exceeds 20 mOsm/kg. (vi) Seizure should be managed with benzodiazepines. (vii) Calcium for management of hypocalcemia.

OPIUM (PAPAVER SOMNIFERUM)

In Greek, Opium is the name for juice. The opium poppy originated in the Eastern Mediterranean and its use has been well documented by ancient civilizations. In particular, many famous Greeks espoused opium's therapeutic properties to elevated mood and work as a general tonic. Opium was originally used in its raw state. It was first prepared in the 15th century by **Paracelsus**, who mixed it with alcohol to produce laudanum tincture. Later in the 18th century, **Le Mort** combined opium with camphor to produce paregoric, which was used to treat diarrhoea. It wasn't until 1803 that the alkaloid morphine was isolated from opium by a German apothecary called **Serturner** who named the alkaloid morphine after *Morpheus*, the Greek God of dreams. By the 19th century, various derivatives of opium, such as codeine came into use. In 1874 diacetylmorphine, commonly known as heroin was discovered. Heroin a semisynthetic derivative of morphine was first made in London and was initially used to treat morphine addiction.

Papaver Sominferum (Figure 41.3A) grows throughout India but its cultivation is banned except on license obtained from the Central Government, for growing the plant strictly for the purpose of pharmaceutical industry. Government Opium factory is situated at Gazipur, U.P.

Various Forms of Opium

(i) Opium is the dried juice of Papaver somniferum, and dry capsule is used as a sedative fomentation and poultice. (ii) Opium when fresh is plastic and internally moist, coarsely granular or smooth. It is reddish brown to dark brown, hard and brittle (iii) *Post ka doda* contains 0.1-0.3% morphine. The morphine content of the opium varies from 9-14%, but when the morphine content is **10%** it is known as **standard opium.** (iv) *Poppy seeds (Khas khas)*: These are white, harmless demulcent, nutritive and used in various food preparation (Figure 41.3B). (v) *Poppy seeds oil:* It is used for lightening purposes and culinary.

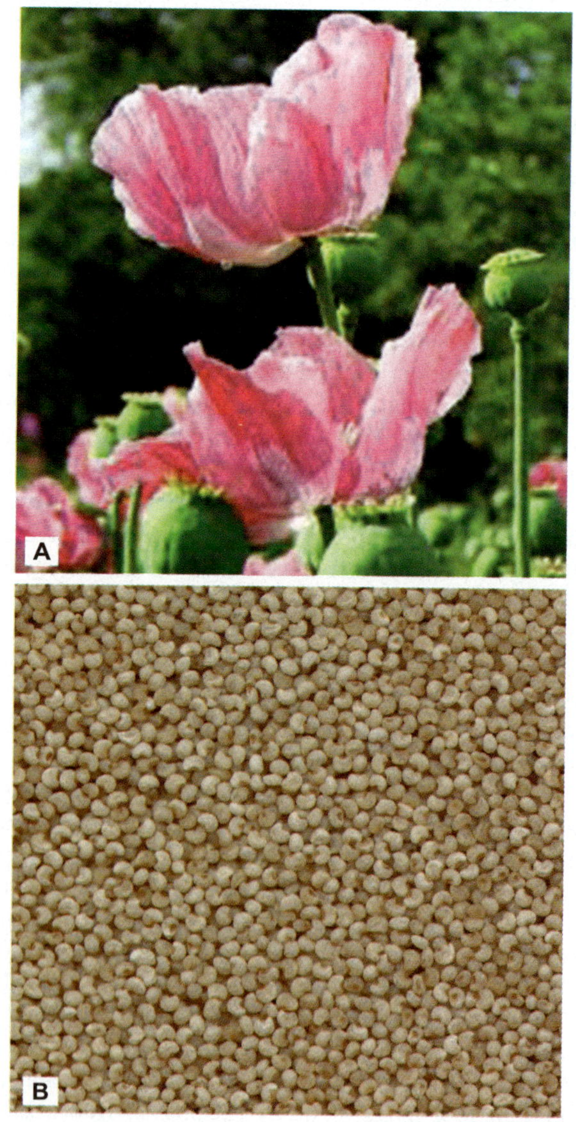

Figure 41.3A and B: (A) Opium plant with capsule (B) Poppy seeds

Opioid antagonists: Opiates may be classified as pure agonists and those with mixed agonistic and antagonistic actions. Opiates undergo oxidative metabolism, catalysed by cytochromes P-450 of which there are several hundred isoforms. Cytochromes P-450 requires the presence of molecular oxygen, NADPH cytochrome. The concept of antagonism of the actions of opioid is very complex. There are probably several subspecies of opioid receptor, each with its own self of affinities for exogenous drugs and endogenous ligands and each apparently mediating different effect, when activated. There is no theoretical reason to expect that any substance would have identical activity at those various binding sites. Naloxone comes closest being a relatively pure competitive antagonist.

Martin and Gilbert in 1976, 77 have postulated three subspecies of opioid receptors:

I. **μ receptors:** They are responsible for supraspinal analgesia and euphoric effects of opiates. They also cause respiratory depression, gastrointestinal dysmotility and miosis as well as physical dependence.

II. **κ- receptors:** These are responsible for supra spinal analgesia, miosis and dysphoria.

III. **α- receptors:** These are responsible for CNS stimulation.

Opium alkaloids: There are two groups of opium alkaloids: Phenanthrene and Isoquinoline. The *phenanthrene group* has following derivatives (i) Morphine (9-14%) (ii) Codeine (2-4%) (iii) Thebaine (0.5%). The derivatives of *isoquinoline group* are (i) Papaverine (1%) (ii) Narcotine (6%).

Fatal dose of various opiates	
Crude opium	2 g
Morphine	200 mg
Codeine	800 mg
Heroin	50 mg
Pethidine	1 gm
Methadone	100 mg
Pentazocine	300 mg
Propoxyphen	1 gm
Diphenoxylate	200 mg

Actions of Morphine

(i) Initially, morphine's analgesic effects were considered that they were the result of their ability to affect emotional responses to pain rather than to act directly on the transmission of pain. (ii) More recently, there is a belief that there are naturally occurring specific opiate receptors in CNS. (iii) The uptake of morphine in the spinal cord occurs only in substantia gelatinosa in the brainstem. This is a specific site of uptake, with opiate receptors found in solitary nuclei that receive afferent vagal fibres and in the area postrema, which contains chemoreceptor trigger zone (CTZ), the structure that is responsible for the mediation of respiration, cough, postural hypotension and nausea. (iv) It is the morphine's actions at CTZ that perhaps explains the common side effects of opiates, and indicates the main site where toxic levels of the drug will lead to death. (v) In the cortex, opiate receptors are most densely populated within the medial thalamic nuclei, the periaqueductal grey matter and most importantly the amygdaloid nuclei. It is at these sites within the cortex that addiction is thought to be mediated. (vi) Morphine is an agonist that: (a) Depresses the cortex, respiratory and cough center is stimulated (b) Relieves the pain by causing depression of cortex (c) Exerts euphoric effect (d) Vagal reflex and vomiting is stimulated (e) Spinal reflexes are also stimulated. Codeine is slightly less depressant to the cortex and medullary centers but stimulates the spinal cord.

Signs and Symptoms of Acute Morphine Poisoning

Stage of excitement: (i) There is sense of well being, restlessness, and hallucinations (ii) There is flushing of face, raised pulse when taken for a short period (iii) When large doses are taken, above symptoms may be absent (iv) In children, convulsions are seen and the adults are severely excited.

Stage of stupor: Nerve centers are depressed at this stage and the following symptoms are produced: (i) Headache, nausea and vomiting (ii) Giddiness and uncontrollable desire to sleep (iii) Patient cannot be aroused by external stimuli (iv) Pupils are contracted and conjunctiva are congested (v) Cyanosis (vi) Itching sensation (vii) Pulse and respiration are normal.

Stage of narcosis: (i) Patient is in deep coma (ii) Muscles are relaxed and reflexes are lost (iii) Secretions are suspected except of skin (iv) Face is pale and lips are livid (v) Lower jaw drops (vi) Pupils are contracted and not reacting to light (pinpoint pupil) and then dilated in terminal asphyxia (vii) Blood pressure is low (viii) Respiratory rate is 2-4/min leading to **cheyne stokes** breathing.

Triad of clinical features characteristic in opioid overdose (**Opioid overdose triad**) are pinpoint pupil, respiratory depression and decreased level of consciousness.

Unusual symptoms: (i) Vomiting (ii) Purging (iii) Convulsions (vi) Temperature is raised (v) Pupils are dilated (vi) Syncope occurs after subcutaneous injection.

Differential Diagnosis

(i) *Apoplexy:* The temperature is 103°F-104°F. (ii) *Uraemic coma*: In kidney diseases, presence of casts and proteins in the urine. (iii) *Epileptic coma:* The pupils are dilated and convulsions are seen. (iv) *Hysterical coma:* Is seen in the females, the tongue is not bitten and the reflexes remain unchanged. (v) *Acute alcoholic poisoning:* The face is congested, the pupils are dilated, and the smell of alcohol is there. The paralysis of muscles does not occur. (vi) *Carbolic acid poisoning:* (a) White patches are seen on the angles of mouth (b) Carboluria (Urine becomes dark or olive green on exposure to air due to the production of hydroquinone and pyrocatechol).

Treatment

(i) ABCDE protocol has to be followed. Maintenance of patent airways with assisted ventilation, Intravenous fluids to maintain fluid and electrolyte imbalance. (ii) Gastric lavage using potassium permanganate (I:5000). It useful even if opioids taken parentally because opiates (an alkaloid) undergo enterohepatic circulation. For the same reason, About 200-300 cc of $KmnO_4$ can be left in stomach after gastric lavage for oxidizing the alkaloid (iii) Activated charcoal should be administered. (iv) Whole bowel irrigation can be given in people who have ingested drug packets containing opiate (body packers). (v) Magnesium sulphate 15 gm for enema. (vi) Physostigmine salicylate can be given 0.04 mg/kg intravenously as it reverts symptoms of respiratory depression but is has an adverse effect of affecting the reticular system of the brain. (vii) Atropine is not to be given. (viii) **Naloxone hydrochloride** is antidote of choice for opiate poisoning. It can be administered via intravenous, intramuscular, subcutaneous, intranasal or via nebulization/endotracheal tube. The starting dose of 0.01-0.02 mg/kg I.V.; maximum up to 300 mg, may require repeat dose. **Side effects:** Acute opioid withdrawal symptoms. (ix) **Nalmefene and naltrexone:** These new agents on the market to reverse opiate toxicity, however not recommended because of the fear of precipitating a prolonged period of opiate withdrawal. (x) Symptomatic treatment.

Coma cocktail: In a comatose patient when the identity of the poison is not known, a combination of the therapy is given at emergency which includes dextrose (100 ml, 50%, I.V.), thiamine (100 mg I.V.) and naloxone (2 mg I.V.). The routine administration of coma cocktail is now discouraged.

Diagnosis

Marquis test: To a fragment of suspected residue of opium, a drop of mixture of 3 ml of concentrated sulphuric acid and 3 drops of formalin are added. The purple red colour is produced that changes to violet and finally blue.

Autopsy Findings

(i) Evidence of drug abuse in the form of injection prick marks, abscesses and old scars can be there (ii) Signs of asphyxia are present (iii) Froth comes out from the mouth and nostrils (vi) Blood is dark and fluid (v) In the stomach contents, lumps of opium may be present (vi) Lungs are congested (vii) Bladder is full of urine.

Medicolegal Aspects

(i) Opium is an ideal suicidal poison, because death is painless. When mixed with mustard oil, absorptive power increases. (ii) Opioid abuse is linked to the risk of unintentional overdose and suicide risk. Individuals who experience a nonfatal opioid overdose face a significantly greater risk of later dying by suicide. (iii) Due to its colour and smell, it is rarely used for homicidal poisoning. (vi) To poison the cattle it is mixed with *Gur*. (iv) It withstands putrefaction and can be detected after a long time. (v) Accidental poisoning can occur at times when the laborer given opium to their children while going for work. (vi) Morphine is one of the preferred drugs for euthanasia. (vii) **Brampton's cocktail:** It is a mixture of morphine/heroin, cocaine, ethyl alcohol and chlorpromazine, used as an effective method for controlling chronic pain in cancer patients. It was named after the Royal Brompton Hospital, London, where this mixture was standardized in the late 1920s. Later this cocktail was withdrawn.

Prolonged Use of the Opium (Morphinism or Morphinomania)

Opium is usually consumed by young people for a long time as it is probably an aphrodisiac and produces a sense of euphoria. The opium addicts can tolerate upto 3-6 gm per day. The prolonged use of the drug produces the following effects: (i) Emaciation (ii) Dry skin and hair (iii) Multiple scars of healed abscesses and tattooing of needles (iv) Pigmentation around the mouth and eyelids (v) Contracted pupils (vi) Dry and furred tongue (vii) Anorexia (viii) Nausea and marked constipation (ix) Disinterest and depression (x) Restlessness and irritability (xi) Disturbs sleep with insomnia (xii) Hallucinations (xiii) Impotence (xiv) Neurasthenia (xv) Dementia or mania (xvi) Sudden stoppage in pregnant woman addicts may be dangerous to foetus.

Withdrawal Symptoms

The following are the withdrawal symptoms when opium ingestion is stopped:

1st few hours :	Psychological effects due to fear, anxiety
8-16 hours:	Nervousness, restlessness, anxiety
14 hours :	Yawning, sweating and running of eyes and nose
24 hours :	Dilated pupils, goose skin and shivering
36 hours :	Severe twitching of muscles, painful cramps in legs and abdomen, vomiting, diarrhoea, insomnia
3-4 days :	Symptoms gradually subsides

Treatment of Withdrawal Symptoms

1. Opiates should be gradually withdrawn.
2. For opioid withdrawal, sometimes, different drug therapy (e.g., with an opioid agonist, opioid agonist-antagonist, opioid antagonist, or clonidine etc.) can be used.
   i. **Methadone:** It is a synthetic opioid, primarily acts on the mu-receptor (full opioid agonist). It alleviates opioid withdrawal symptoms and reduces cravings. Methadone was synthesized by a German scientist and was brought into clinical use at the end of World War II. It is sold under the trade names as 'Dolophine' and 'Westadone'. The starting dose is 10 mg oral or intravenous (IV), given every 4 to 6 hours, maximum 40 mg in 24 hours, if withdrawal persists. On the second day, the determined dose can be given once or twice a day. Titration is begun on the third day by decreasing 10% or 5 mg/daily of the total dosage. It is the preferred method of managing

opioid withdrawal for more seriously addicted patients because at appropriate doses, it has a long half-life and less profound sedation and euphoria. Methadone is an antidote of morphine but due to its own depressive action on respiration and other side effects has made it unsuitable for the purpose. It should be used with caution when the patient has respiratory deficiency, acute alcohol dependence, severe hepatic impairment, ulcerating or Crohn's disease and head injury.

ii. **Buprenorphine:** It is a synthetic opioid (analog of thebaine) and partial opioid agonist. It is used for the management of opioid-dependence (such as heroin, oxycodone, hydrocodone, morphine). It reduces cravings and improves the quality of life for patients undergoing addiction treatment. It is used when there is no availability of methadone, contraindications for methadone therapy, intolerance to methadone or failed methadone treatment. It is given sublingually, 4 to 12 mg initially and then tapered over a 5- to 10-day period. It can precipitate withdrawal symptoms in opiate dependence patients who don't have withdrawal signs. Thus, it must be started 12 to 18 hours after the last use of short-acting agonists like heroin or oxycodone and 24 to 48 hours after the last use of long-acting agonists such as methadone.

iii. **Clonidine:** A centrally acting α-adrenergic agonist can suppress the opioid withdrawal from low to moderate doses of methadone. It is a potent antihypertensive.

iv. **Nalorphine (Nalline/N-Allyl-normorphine):** It is a semisynthetic opiate. It causes analgesia, respiratory depression, dysphoria and hallucination. It was popularly used as antidote of morphine. However, its own depressive action on respiration and other side effects has made it unsuitable for the purpose. Nalorphine hydrochloride 5 mg I.V. is given for 15-30 minutes, then 10 mg I.V. to a total dose of 40 mg I.V.

v. **Naloxone Hydrochloride**: 0.4-0.8 mg I.M./ I.V. is given in adults and 0.01 mg/kg is given in children.

vi. **Newer Drugs:** (a) *Lofexidine hydrochloride*–the first non-opioid used for managing opioid withdrawal syndrome. It is an alpha-2 adrenergic agonist which acts which reduces and sympathetic tone and decreases norepinephrine release. It is an approved drug by FDA, can be used for up to 14 days.

vii. Symptomatic treatment in opioid withdrawal includes loperamide for diarrhea, promethazine for nausea/ vomiting and ibuprofen for myalgia.

viii. Psychological counselling of the patient has an important role.

HEROIN (BROWN SUGAR)

Heroin is diacetylmorphine and is a semisynthetic preparation of morphine. It is also known as **smack, dope or junk**. It was first prepared at St. Mary's Hospital, London by acetylation of morphine with acetic anhydride in 1898. Morphine was first used for the treatment of cough but soon it became the most potent drug used by drug addicts due to its habit forming properties. Manufacture of heroin and its use in Medicine is banned nowadays but it is being illegally manufactured and smuggled, as its cost is very high in international market (1 kg of morphine costs about one crore). This is quite profitable to India as it lies in the 'golden triangle' on eastern side and 'golden crescent' on the western side. India is one of the countries for transit of morphine and other drugs. Cultivation of opium and production of Heroin is done in 'golden quadrangle' namely Varanasi, Lucknow, Bareilly and Badauin district of U.P., and adjoining states of Rajasthan and Madhya Pradesh. About 10 kg of crude opium gives 1 kg of standard opium. This can be converted into Chinese Heroin (called No. 4 Heroin) and Brown sugar (called No. 3 Heroin, is 60% pure) that is available in India. Brown sugar is also called smack and its colour is brown due to presence of sugar of milk, starch, powdered coffee, tea and coco or brick powder. The smack of 'golden crescent' is grayish and that used of 'golden quadrangle' is blackish-brown in colour. Brown sugar is sold in small cellophane packets of 116 gms each. The amount of Heroin in each packet may be 1/16th, 1/18th, or ½ of a gram. These cellophane bags are kept in a matchbox to avoid suspicion. Heroin is used by diluting with quinine, lactose or mannitol to reduce cost.

Speed ball: It is a combination of heroin and cocaine.

Routes of Consumption

(i) Sniffing in the form of snuff (ii) Smoking in cigarettes or *bidis* after removal of some tobacco (iii) Chasing (a cigarette foil or Rs. 5 or 10 note is folded and instead of tobacco, the drug is put inside, this is then lighted using match stick, when thick smoke come out it is inhaled—called **Dragon chasing**) (iv) Injections by S.C. (***skin poppers***) and I.V. route (***main-liners***).

Signs and Symptoms

(i) Anorexia (ii) Nausea and vomiting (iii) Constipation (iv) Emaciation (v) Pigmentation around cheek (vi) Impotency.

Complications of Consumption

(i) Abscess formation along the routes of injection (ii) Formation of pigmented scars in cubital fossa described as **railroad track** (iii) Thrombosed veins (iv) Septicemia (v) AIDS and Hepatitis (vi) Chronic heroin smoking leads to impaired lung function and higher prevalence of dyspnea (vii) Heroin overdose leads to noncardiogenic pulmonary edema (**Heroin lung**).

Treatment

(i) Methadone 40 mg daily to prevent withdrawal symptoms should be increased to 80 mg in chronic addicts. The reduction of dose is to be achieved gradually by 20% daily. More than 20 mg methadone should not be given at one time. (ii) Narcotic antagonists such as naloxone, naltreoxone, clonidine, haloperidol and cyclazocine should be given. (iii) Detoxification techniques are useful.

Autopsy Findings

(i) Lungs are congested and rarely oedematous. Microscopically foreign body granulomas may be present (ii) Liver shows chronic inflammatory infiltrate with mononuclear cells.

PETHIDINE (MEPERIDINE, DEMEROL)

It is a colourless crystalline powder that is given I.M. or I.V. It is a synthetic opiate and is a narcotic. Some of its actions are in variation with morphine. It is a good analgesic and sedative. In contrast with the action of morphine it is mydriatic. It causes dryness of the skin. It has a direct inhibitory effect on the cardiac musculature. It liberates histamine from mast cells. Pethidine causes early loss of corneal reflex, due to its anaesthetic effect on the corneas. It is highly addictive agent and doctors and paramedical workers are the common victims. Pethidine is therapeutically contraindicated in cases of high intracranial pressure. It is also not given in toxemia of pregnancy.

Signs and Symptoms

(i) Addicts may have twitchings, tremors, mental confusion, hallucinations, convulsions and impairment of ability to work (ii) Abstinence syndrome similar to morphine withdrawal is present. Symptoms appear in 3-4 hours with maximum intensity after 8-12 hours.

Fatal Dose: 2 gms.

Fatal Period: 24 hours.

Treatment

Treatment is same as that of opium poisoning.

BARBITURATES

Since the synthesis of diethylbarbituric acid and its introduction into medicine as a sedative and hypnotic agent many other structural analogues have been prepared and investigated. Fisher and Von Mering introduced Diethyl Barbituric acid into medicine in 1904 under the name of *Venoral* (vera means true) that proved to be an effective hypnotic without serious side reactions.

The barbiturates were used as sleeping tablets and sedatives that led to their widespread abuse till 1960s when they were replaced by nonbarbiturate hypnotics, such as the benzodiazepines. Unfortunately, barbiturates are still available in the market either alone or in combination with other substances such as amphetamines.

Classification of Barbiturates

The classification of barbiturates into short, intermediate and long acting is arbitrary and may be misleading. The onset of action is about 15-30 minutes but the duration varies up to 8 hours or so for Phenobarbitone (Table 41.2).

Fatal Period: 1-2 days.

Table 41.2: Classification of barbiturates

Barbiturates	Duration of action	Fatal dose
Long acting	8-16 hours	3-4 gm
• Barbitone *(venoral)*, white tab		
• Barbitone sodium *(medinal)*, white tab		
• Phenobarbitone *(gardenal, luminal)*, white tab		
• Methyl Phenobarbitone *(prominal)*		
Intermediate acting	4-8 hours	2-3 gm
• Allobarbitone		
• Amylobarbitone		
• Butobarbitone *(Soneryl)*, pink tab		
• Pentobarbitone *(Nembutal)*, yellow tab		
Short acting	3-6 hours	1-2 gm
• Cyclobarbitone *(phanoderm)*, white tab		
• Hexobarbitone *(evipan)*, white tab		
• Quininalbarbitone *(seconal)*, red tab		
Ultra short acting	1-few min.	1.5-2 gm
• Thiopentone *(pentothal)*, white powders or ampoules		
• Metho- hexo- barbitone *(brevital)*		

Pharmacological Action of Barbiturates

Pharmacological action of barbiturates of all types is the same that is depression of central nervous system. However, the structural variations result in differences in rate of absorption and distribution. By altering the dose, the degree of depression can be altered. Phenobarbitone has a specific depressant action on cerebral motor cortex that makes it a valuable drug for epilepsy. In hypnotic doses, it has no analgesic action and if prescribed alone in painful conditions, there may be excitement, restlessness, mental confusion and delirium. Barbiturates act as synergists with analgesics and potentiate the action of alcohol.

As barbiturates are cumulative drugs, they are contraindicated in hepatic and renal disorders. After the oral ingestion, the peak concentration in blood and brain of:

1. Medium and short acting barbiturates is after: 1-2 hours.
2. Long acting is after: 4-8 hours after ingestion.
3. Ultra short acting is after: 30 seconds to a few minutes.

Barbiturates are rapidly absorbed from the gastrointestinal tract including rectum and from the subcutaneous tissues. They are concentrated in the liver for a short time and evenly distributed in the body fluids. Lipid solubility is the primary determinant of binding. Ultra short acting is 80% more bound to plasma proteins or stored in the body fat from which they are subsequently cleared and degraded in the liver. Long acting is only 5% bound to plasma proteins and mainly cleared by urinary excretion. Medium acting are bound more than the long acting and they are detoxified in liver and tissues and finally excreted quickly. Short acting barbiturates are also excreted quickly.

Highly lipid soluble barbiturates such as thiopental, methohexal reaches rapidly the vascular areas of brain and first to the gray matter. Maximum uptake occurs within 30 seconds and sleep may be induced within few minutes. Within 30 minutes, there is redistribution to the less vascular areas of the brain and other tissues. Other factors that affect the binding capacity are the dose absorbed and the patient's habit.

Excretion of Barbiturates: The barbiturates are removed from the body by two different mechanisms: (i) Long acting barbiturates are mainly excreted by the kidneys. As much as 85% of these compounds may be recovered from the urine. Excretion is slow and takes place in several days. (ii) Liver mainly metabolizes the short acting barbiturates. Other tissues may also participate in this process. These compounds are not recovered from the urine if taken in sedative doses.

Mechanism of Action

Barbiturates primarily act on the gamma-aminobutyric acid (GABA) chloride ion channels in the central nervous system (CNS) that suppress the activity of excitable tissue.

Mode of Action

Barbiturates are cellular, histotoxic agents. They (i) Produce histotoxic or tissue anoxia (ii) Partially inhibit the cytochrome enzyme system (iii) Toxic action may occur following a large single dose or repeated medication in slow excreting barbiturates.

Signs and Symptoms

The clinical staging of barbiturates has been classified into five stages by **'Sunshine and Hackett':** (i) Awake, competent and normally sedated (ii) Sedated: (a) Reflexes are positive (b) Prefers sleep (c) Answers question when aroused (d) Does not cerebrate properly (iii) Comatose with positive reflexes (iv) Comatose and areflexia (v) Comatose with difficulty in respiration and circulation and death is from respiratory failure. The various signs and symptoms are:

Central nervous system: (i) Drowsiness (ii) Transient period of confusion, excitement, delirium and hallucinations (iii) Ataxia, vertigo and slurring of sleep (iv) Headache (v) Consciousness is depressed in a variable degree; can be assessed by rubbing the clenched fist on patient's sternum. The response of the pupil and peripheral nerve reflexes are so erratic that it has a little help in assessing. (Pupils are constricted than dilated in terminal hypoxia) (vi) "Rising up" sign is there (vii) Babinski sign is positive (viii) The degree of consciousness can be expressed by the following classification:

Grade I : Response to vocal commands.

Grade II : Maximum response to minimal painful stimuli.

Grade III : Minimal pain to maximum stimuli.

Grade IV : Total unresponsiveness to maximal painful stimuli.

Respiratory system: They directly depress the medullary centers. The rate and depth of respiration is reduced and towards the end Cheyne-Stoke's type of breathing and then death occurs. If coma continues then infection, pneumonia and pulmonary oedema may develop.

Cardiovascular system: Barbiturates exert direct toxic effect on the myocardium and interfere with the myogenic tone of peripheral arterioles. There is (i) Fall in cardiac output (ii) Permeability of arterioles is increased leading to transudation and increase in extracellular fluid volume (iii) Cyanosis and hypotension (iv) Weak and rapid pulse (v) Cold and clammy skin.

Pupils: Pupils are little contracted and reacting to light; may be dilated and unequal in terminal asphyxia.

Body temperature: Barbiturates interfere with the control of body temperature; hypothermia is produced requiring the use of symptomatic measures. During recovery the patient may become febrile.

Gastrointestinal tract: Bowel sounds may be absent during severe poisoning and this is a bad sign. When bowel functions return further drug absorption may take place leading to fluctuating levels of consciousness. Incontinence of faeces may occur.

Renal symptoms: Renal functions may fail especially with hypotension and hypothermia. Incontinence of urine may occur and sugar and albumin may be present in the urine.

Dermatological symptoms: The skin lesions develop in about 6-10% of the cases of barbiturate poisoning; are diagnostic and very commonly present in poisoning with medium acting barbiturates. **Bullous lesions/Barbiturate blister** occur where the skin surface rubs the other part of the skin such as inner aspects of thigh and pressure bearing areas like hands and feet. Initially there are slightly raised areas of erythema and later on bullous eruptions are formed. The blister contains serous fluid, the rupture of which leaves a red raw surface that may be mistaken for burns. This rare entity is traditionally associated barbiturate poisoning but can also be seen in the setting of coma due to other etiologies. Hence, these lesions also referred as **coma blisters**. Blisters develop 48–72 hours after the onset of unconsciousness. The clinical course of the lesions is self-limiting and resolution occurred within 2 weeks. The exact mechanism of the bullous lesions remains unknown. It is suggested that bullous formation is either due to toxic effects of the drug or patient is unduly sensitive to the drug itself. Recent studies have proposed various immune mechanisms leading to bullae formation.

Differential diagnosis of bullous eruptions in barbiturate poisoning: (i) *CO poisoning*: The eruptions are present under the pressure areas, sacrum, spine, inner aspect of knee and ankle. They are produced due to impairment of circulation. (ii) *Thermal heat:* The blisters due to burns will show the effect of heat and the hair will be singed. (iii) *Pemphigus:* Pemphigus blisters are non-tense, larger and the bullous spreading test is positive. (iv) *Methaqualone (Mandrax) overdosage*: The following symptoms are present; hypoproteinemia, gastric bleeding and cardiac arrhythmias. (v) Glutethimide, meprobamate and tricyclic antidepressants overdosages. (vi) Prolonged contact with petrol and paraffin.

Clinical Diagnosis of Barbiturate Poisoning

1. In an unconscious patient, one has to rule out other causes of coma such as: (i) *Acute alcoholic poisoning:* (a) Odour of alcohol is present in the breathing (b) Eyes are congested and pupils dilated. (ii) *Carbolic acid poisoning:* (a) The odour is characteristic (b) White patches can be seen on lips and mouth (c) Carboluria is diagnostic. (iii) *Co poisoning:* (a) History of exposure to the carbon monoxide gas is there (b) Intermittent convulsions (c) Cherry red colour of the skin (d) Carboxyhaemoglobin is present in the blood. (iv) *Epileptic coma:* (a) There is history of fits (b) Pupils are fixed and dilated (c) Froth at mouth (d) Cyanosis. (v) *Diabetic coma*: (a) Gradual onset (b) Odour of acetone is present. (vi) Sugar and acetone is present in the urine. (vii) *Brain trauma*: (a) History is characteristic (b) Injuries and bleeding from the nose (c) Pulse is rapid (d) Paralysis may be present.
2. Clear history of ingestion of barbiturates.
3. Findings of general anaesthesia with low respiration and decreased respiratory function.
4. Presence or absence of bowel sounds.
5. Urine or first stomach wash is to be tested for barbiturates.
6. Blood levels by gas chromatography, calorimetric methods and spectrophotometry are: (a) For long acting (8-10 mg%) (b) For medium acting (4-7 mg%) (c) For short acting (2-4 mg%) (d) For ultra short acting (0.8-1 mg%).
7. ECG findings show inverted and flattened 'T' wave and depressed ST segment.
8. EEG findings in barbiturate poisoning:

   Mild intoxication: Normal activity is replaced by fast activity in the range of 20-30 Hz appearing first in the frontal regions and spreading to the parietal and occipital regions as intoxication worsens.

   More severe intoxication: The fast waves become less regular and interspersed with 3-4 Hz slow activity.

   Still more advanced cases: There are short periods of suppression of all activity, separated by bursts of slow (delta) waves of variable frequency.

   Extreme overdoses: All electrical activity ceases in extreme overdosages of the drug. This is one instance in which a flat EEG cannot be equated with brain death and the effects are fully reversible unless anoxic damage has supervened.

Treatment

Mild cases need no treatment but should be kept under observation. Before treatment in comatose patients, other causes of coma should be excluded. The treatment is mostly supportive.

(i) Maintenance of patient's airway, breathing and circulation (a) Clear the airway by tracheobronchial suction (b) Mechanical ventilation with oxygen (c) In comatose patient, intubation or tracheostomy may be considered (d) Intravenous saline drip for correction of shock and hypotension (e) Noradrenaline 2 mg with 500 ml of 5% glucose may be required. (ii) Gastric lavage: (a) These are more useful if it is done within 4 hours of the ingestion of the poison (b) Done with warm water mixed with potassium permanganate and suspension of activated charcoal and tannic acid. (iii) First sample is to be obtained in plain water. (iv) Magnesium sulphate is used for purgation as it minimizes. absorption. (v) Urine alkalization by administering I.V. sodium bicarbonate. Barbiturates are acidic drug and they become ionized in alkaline urine and eliminated. (vi) Hemodialysis and hemoperfusion: These methods are considered as more effective in phenobarbital poisoning because of its significant protein binding. (vii) **No specific antidote** is known. (viii) Supportive care for comatose patient.

Analeptics (Now-a-days not recommended): Analeptics stimulate the central nervous system especially respiratory center so they are used in the treatment of narcotic poisoning. The drugs used are caffeine, camphor and strychnine, picrotoxin, pentylenetetrazole and bemegride etc. Their use is opposed in barbiturate poisoning due to the following reasons: (a) Are generally ineffective in severe poisoning (b) Awakening effect is transient and followed by greater depression (c) Leads to cardiac arrhythmias and convulsions; cerebral ischemia and depression and then irreversible brain damage (d) Overall results without their use show a much-reduced mortality rate.

Scandinavian Method of Treatment: This is conservative method for treatment of barbiturate poisoning which was developed by **Scandinavian** physicians in mid-1940s. They have rejected the use of analeptics in barbiturate poisoning which was routinely practiced earlier. The method includes introduction of (a)

Effective anti-shock fluid therapy (b) Anaesthesiologic principles, including manual intermittent positive pressure ventilation into management (c) Centralisation of seriously poisoned patients in a dedicated unit.

Autopsy Findings

(i) External findings are not characteristic; signs of asphyxia are present and cyanosis of face and nails is seen. (ii) Traces of tablets and capsules of barbiturates may be found in the mouth, oesophagus and stomach. (iii) **Mucous membrane** of stomach is congested and eroded badly from the alkaline attack of drugs like sodium amytal which, being the sodium salt of a weak organic acid, hydrolyses in the stomach. The fundus may be thickened, granular and haemorrhagic. The cardia and lower oesophagus may be eroded from the reflux and if the victim regurgitates, then black, altered blood may appear at the nose and mouth. (iv) **Lungs** are congested, oedematous and findings suggestive of pneumonia may be present. The congested lungs in acute barbiturate poisoning are more intense than in any other condition. The lungs are almost black and the whole venous system is engorged with dark, deoxygenated blood. (v) **Petechial haemorrhages** are seen in the pleura, pericardium and meninges. (vi) Kidneys are congested and degenerative changes of the tubules are present. (vii) **Brain is oedematous**, softening of globus pallidus is seen and multiple petechial haemorrhages are seen in the white matter. (ix) All other organs are congested. (x) **Barbiturates blisters:** These blisters are found on the dependent parts of the skin surface, especially buttocks, backs of thigh, calves and forearms. (xi) For chemical analysis of viscera, besides the other organs, brain is to be preserved.

Medicolegal Aspects

(i) Barbiturates are commonly used for suicide as it is freely prescribed and easily available. (ii) ***Therapeutic uses:*** It is used for sleeplessness, anxiety states, epilepsy, strychnine, picrotoxin and cocaine poisoning. (iii) Rarely used for homicidal purposes. (iv) Repeated small doses cause addiction that leads to withdrawal symptoms, used for the relief of worries and anxiety of modern life. (v) ***Automatism:*** The accidental or suicidal overdose may lead to the poisoning. In ordinary doses, it induces natural sleep but occasionally instead of sleep, there is mental confusion. It is likely to happen in those cases where insomnia is due to pain and an analgesic is not taken for its relief. In these cases, the use of barbiturates may lead to mental confusion. As a result, to reduce pain patient takes more and more of the drug automatically and unknowingly that he has already taken a dose. This is known as **Barbiturate automatism**. In some cases, the patient continues to take the drug that leads to overdosage that is usually fatal.

However, some workers have a different concept; they feel that confusion and forgetfulness cannot account for overwhelming overdose that is found in these cases. It is possible that there are cases of intentional suicide or in alcoholics where confusion is more likely and the action of barbiturates is potentiated by alcohol. It is now over 40 years since 'automatism' was offered as a socially acceptable explanation of self-administered overdoses of barbiturates. The idea was often accepted without any real evidence that repeated therapeutic doses were taken by a patient who did not remember taking the drug and in some studies by Dorpat concluded that drug automatism is a myth.

LONG QUESTIONS

1. Clinical features, management and medicolegal aspect of acute ethyl alcohol poisoning.
2. Clinical features, management and medicolegal aspects of methyl alcohol poisoning.
3. Discuss signs, symptoms, management and postmortem findings in acute morphine/opium poisoning.

SHORT QUESTIONS

1. Proof of spirit.
2. Drunkenness.
3. Widmark's formula.
4. Delirium tremens.
5. Treatment of alcoholism.
6. Management of methyl alcohol poisoning.
7. Body packers.
8. Barbiturate automatism.
9. Medicolegal aspects of morphine poisoning.

MULTIPLE CHOICE QUESTIONS

1. MacEwan's sign is seen in:

(a) Organophosphorus poisoning
(b) Alcoholic intoxication
(c) Dhatura poisoning
(d) Opium poisoning

2. Widmark's formula is used for measurement of blood level of:

(a) Barbiturates (b) Organophosphorus
(c) Arsenic (d) Alcohol

3. All are given for treatment of methyl alcohol poisoning *except*:

(a) Ethanol (b) Sodium bicarbonate
(c) N-acetyl cysteine (d) Fomepizole

4. **Drug that inhibits aldehyde dehydrogenase:**

(a) Disulfiram (b) Fomepizole
(c) Pyridoxine (d) Folinic acid

5. **The ratio between the blood alcohol concentration and urine alcohol concentration at equilibrium is:**

(a) 1:1.3 (b) 1:3.1
(c) 1:13.1 (d) 1:131

6. **Pin point pupil seen in cases of poisoning by:**

(a) Dhatura (b) Opium
(c) Yellow oleander (d) Barbiturate

7. **Marquis' reagent test is done for presence of:**

(a) Morphine (b) Arsenic
(c) Phosphorous (d) Paraquat

8. **Following are the constituents of Brompton's cocktail:**

(a) Morphine (b) Ethyl alcohol
(c) Cocaine (d) Diazepam

9. **According to Motor Vehicles Act, 1988 (amendment, 2019), for first offence of drunken driving, the punishment shall be:**

(a) Up to 10000 fine or 6 months imprisonment or both
(b) Up to 2000 fine or 6 months imprisonment or both
(c) Up to 15000 fine or 2 years imprisonment or both
(d) Up to 2000 fine or 2 years imprisonment or both

10. **A person commits a crime under the influence of alcohol. He was given alcohol against his will by a friend. He will be not held responsible for his action is described in IPC section:**

(a) 82 (b) 83
(c) 84 (d) 85

11. **What is rectified spirit:**

(a) 99.5% ethyl alcohol by volume
(b) 99.9% ethyl alcohol by volume
(c) 95% ethyl alcohol by volume
(d) 90% ethyl alcohol by volume

12. **At postmortem, liquid blood sample for alcohol estimation is collected in vial containing:**

(a) Sodium Fluoride (b) Thymol Crystal
(c) Calcium Oxalate (d) EDTA

13. **If a person voluntarily consumes alcohol and commits a crime with an intent, he will be held responsible for his action is described in IPC section:**

(a) 83 (b) 84
(c) 85 (d) 86

14. **Kozelka and Hine method used for determination of:**

(a) Alcohol (b) Carbon monoxide
(c) Carbon dioxide (d) Phosphorous

15. **In alcohol poisoning, the viscera preserved in:**

(a) Rectified spirit
(b) Formalin
(c) Saturated common salt
(d) Glycerol

16. **For medicolegal purpose, blood alcohol estimation can be best determined by:**

(a) Cavett test
(b) Kozelka and Hine test
(c) Thin liquid chromatography
(d) Gas liquid chromatography

ANSWER KEY ☞

1. (b)	2. (d)	3. (c)	4. (a)	5. (a)	6. (b)	7. (a)	8. (d)	9. (a)	10. (d)
11. (d)	12. (a)	13. (d)	14. (a)	15. (c)	16. (d)				

42 CHAPTER

Spinal and Peripheral Poisons

SPINAL POISONS

This group of poisons mainly acts on the spinal cord, the cerebral symptoms being either slight or absent. The stimulation of spinal cord results in spasms and convulsions, while depression causes paralysis and loss of sensation. Nux vomica is a spinal stimulant whereas Gelsemium is spinal depressant.

STRYCHNOUS NUX VOMICA

Strychnous nux vomica, commonly known as *kuchla* is a spinal poison. It is called "slang nut" or "slang Thai nut" in Cambodia and Thailand. The plant grows wildly in all parts of India and its all parts are poisonous. The fruits of nux vomica are round, hard, slightly rough and glossy orange in colour (Figure 42.1). They contain 3-5 seeds and jelly like white pulp. The seeds are hard, flat circular discs with 2 cm diameter and 0.6 cm thickness being slightly convex on one side and concave on other. The seeds are ashy grey or light brown in colour and their shining surfaces are covered with fine, short, silky, yellowish grey hairs (Figure 42.2). The seeds are very hard and difficult to pulverize. The pulverized strychnine powder is extremely bitter.

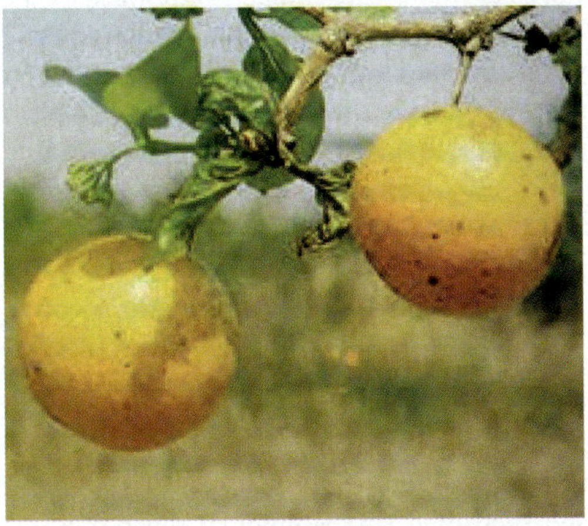

Figure 42.1: Nux vomica plant with fruits

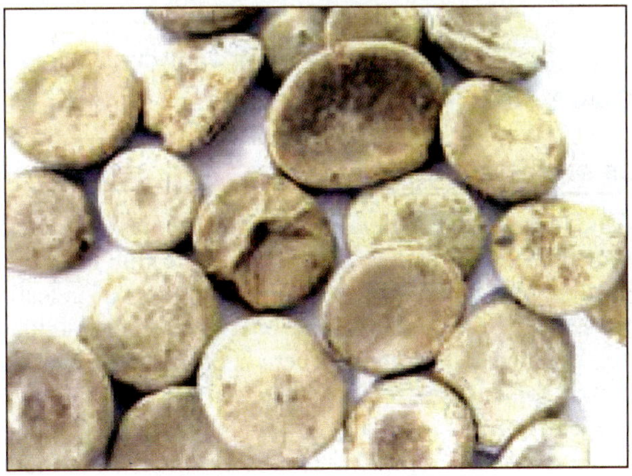

Figure 42.2: Nux vomica seeds

Alkaloids in the Seeds

The seeds contain two principal alkaloids: (i) **Strychnine** (1.3-1.5%) occurs as a powerful alkaloid in the dried ripe seeds of the plant *Strychnos nux vomica* and *Strychnos ignatii* (ii) **Brucine** (1.55%) (iii) It contains small amount of **loganin** which is a glycoside (iv)The pulp of the fruit has very low strychnine content whereas the bark, leaves and wood of the plant contains only Brucine. Brucine is similar in action to strychnine both chemically and physiologically but strychnine is 10-20 times more potent than brucine in its toxicity.

Absorption

The poison is absorbed from all the mucous membrane including the stomach and intestines and 20% of it gets eliminated slowly in the urine, some in bile, sweat, saliva and milk. Much of it is impounded either in liver or in the muscles. This release of the impounded strychnine in liver and muscles is either to be released again to the blood or to be destroyed. The release of strychnine results in producing convulsions on the second or third day.

Mechanism of Action

Strychnine is a competitive antagonist of the inhibitory neurotransmitter glycine at postsynaptic receptors. The loss inhibitory effect of glycine is resulted in release excitation. A slight stimulus can cause increased neuronal activity and excitability, leading to increased involuntary diffuse muscular contraction. It primarily affects anterior horn cells of the spinal cord. It has a little stimulant effect on the cerebral cortex as patient remains conscious till the end. The patient typically presents with severe muscle contractions that appear as if the patient having "awake seizures" or seizures with no postictal period. Death occurs from asphyxia due to spasm of muscles of respiration or from collapse occurring in the interval between spasms.

Fatal Dose: Strychnine: 30-120 mg.

One powdered nux vomica seed: 2 gms of alkaloid.

Extract of nux vomica powder: 200 mg.

Fatal Period: 1-2 hours.

Signs and Symptoms

Uncrushed seeds have no effect and they are passed intact with the faeces. The signs and symptoms appear within 5-10 minutes of ingestion of powdered seeds and half an hour of ingestion of crushed seeds. These are: (i) Intense bitter taste in the mouth when ingested in powdered form. (ii) There is difficulty in swallowing. (iii) Before convulsions, there is increased activity of perception, increased rigidity of muscles and twitching. (iv) Convulsions are due to the action on reflex centers of spinal cord and affect all the muscles at a time. They are clonic in nature to start with but become tonic very soon with paroxysms getting longer and interparoxysmal intervals becoming shorter. (v) Violent convulsive seizures occur involving all the muscles of the body all at a time. As a result, the antigravity muscles become markedly stiff and rigid, when the body is thrown into an arch, head bent backwards, arms being either flexed on the chest or stretched out extended and the hands tightly clenched; ultimately the body may assume the position of **Opisthotonos** (being arched on the back with the back of the head and heels touching the ground in a bow like position) the head hyperextended, feet arched and inverted legs extended and slightly thrown apart and abdominal muscles spasmodically fixed, resulting in serious interference with respiratory movements. (vi) **Emprosthotonus** that is forward bending of the body due to violent spasmodic contractions of abdominal muscles. The word *emprosthotonus* has been derived from the word emperor whom the people used to salute by bending forward. (vii) **Pleurosthotonus** is lateral bending of the body also occurs. (viii) Convulsions lasts for 1-2 minutes and occur after an interval of 10-15 minutes. Between convulsions the muscles are completely relaxed and the patient looks well though exhausted and looks cyanosed. (ix) Face is cyanosed and bears an anxious look. (x) Eyeballs are prominent with dilated pupil. (xi) **Risus sardonicus**: The corners of mouth drawback due to the contraction of jaws and facial muscles and the mouth is covered with froth that is frequently blood stained. Antigravity muscles are affected. (xii) Consciousness remains clear until the death. (xiii) Death usually occurs after 4-5 convulsions due to asphyxia and exhaustion. In nonfatal cases, convulsions become less severe and recovery occurs within 1-2 days.

Treatment

The treatment includes decontamination and supportive care. There is no specific antidote for strychnine poisoning. (i) To control the convulsions, the patient should be kept in bed in a dark room free from noise and disturbance (ii) Secure airway with endotracheal intubation, if necessary (iii) Stomach wash should be done using potassium permanganate (iv) Animal charcoal adsorbs the poison and tannic acid can be given (v) **Seizures Management:** It can be controlled by phenobarbital or diazepam. Diazepam is the anticonvulsant of choice but not effective in all cases. A combination with midazolam, fentanyl, and pancuronium is recommended (vi) Muscle relaxants such as dantrolene to combat muscle rigidity (vii) Intravenous fluid hydration.

Autopsy Findings

(i) Rigor mortis develops earlier and is prolonged (ii) Postmortem findings are not characteristic (iii) Signs of asphyxia are present (iv) Extravasation of blood is present in the muscles (v) Haemorrhages are seen in the peritoneal coat of the stomach (vi) Internal organs are congested.

Medicolegal Aspects

(i) Accidental poisoning results from (a) Ingestion of tablets by the children kept for use by the parents (b) When it is wrongly prescribed for quinine (c) Is prescribed as tonic (ii) Suicidal poisoning results when pharmacists or agricultural workers who have access to the drug may ingest it. In a case, a doctor injected himself of Strychnos hydrochloride, went upstairs, told his wife about it, and then died (iii) Homicidal poisoning occurs when the crushed seeds or tablets are mixed with the food to kill the person (iv) In Malaysia it is used as an arrow poison (v) Resists putrefaction, the poison can be detected in the viscera long time after death.

Diagnosis of Nux Vomica Poisoning

Physiological tests: Injection of aqueous solution of suspended material into the dorsal lymph sac of the Frog results in convulsions within few minutes. Stimulation of Frog will produce convulsions.

Differential Diagnosis of Nux Vomica Poisoning

(i) *Tetanus* (Differences between tetanus and nux vomica poisoning are given in Table 42.1). (ii) *Epilepsy*: This is differentiated by the history and the fits are clonic with loss of consciousness and the reflexes are normal (iii) *Meningitis*: Here fever and neck rigidity is present (iv) *Hysteria:* At times the two are difficult to distinguish so it's better to treat for the poisoning.

Table 42.1: Differences between the poisoning by strychnos nux vomica and tetanus

Features	Nux vomica poisoning	Tetanus
Onset	Sudden	Gradual
History	No history of injury	History of injury is there
Convulsions	All parts of the body involved at the same time	All parts of the body are not affected at the same time
Nature of paroxysms	Clonic	Tonic
Lower jaw	Does not start from the lower jaw	Usually starts from and specifically affects the lower jaw
Muscular condition between convulsions	Relaxed	Rigid
Fatal period	1-2 hours	>24 hours
Lab. Analysis	The poison can be detected from the food	No poison is found in the food
Microscopical and culture examination	Not helpful to diagnose the poison	Cl. tetani bacillus can be demonstrated

PERIPHERAL NERVE POISONS

CURARE

Curare, a generic term used for various alkaloid preparations obtained from different plants like Strychnos toxifera or S. guianensis (Family Loganiaceae) and of the Menispermaceae family, especially Chondrodendron tomentosum or Sciadotenia toxifera. It is not absorbed from GI tract, hence harmless if ingested. It can be absorbed through wounds or abrasions. At first, curare was known as South American arrow poison. It was also used as a muscle relaxant during an operation. Curare was used for the diagnosis of myasthenia gravis (curare test).

Active Principles: Alkaloids–Tubocurarine, curarine.

Mechanism of Action

It is a competitive antagonist of nicotinergic neuromuscular synaptic junctions.

Fatal Dose: 30-60 mg.

Fatal Period: 1-2 hours.

Signs and Symptoms

Headache, dilatation of pupil, blurred vision, gradual paralysis of voluntary muscles followed by respiratory muscles, death occurs due to asphyxia.

Treatment

(i) Artificial respiration (ii) A ligature can be applied proximal to the wound site/injection site in arrow poisoning (iii) Wash the wound site with solution of $KMnO_4$ (iv) Atropine 0.6-1.2 mg followed by physiostigmine1-2 mg or neostigmine 0.5-1 mg S.C., should be given.

Autopsy Findings

Features of asphyxia is present.

Medicolegal Aspects

(i) Arrow poisons (ii) Mostly accidental poisoning occurs (iii) Rarely used as a homicidal poison.

CONIUM MACULATUM (HEMLOCK)

Hemlock (Conium maculatum), is one of the most toxic poisonous plant belongs to Apiaceae family, has a worldwide distribution. It is also known as spotted hemlock, poison parsley, California fern or spotted cowbane. The plants have characteristic mousy smell when crushed, due to the presence of piperidine alkaloids. All parts of the plant are poisonous, the seeds are most toxic. The roots can easily be mistaken for wild parsnips, while the leaves can be mistaken for parsley.

Active Principles: Piperidine alkaloids–Coniine, N-methyl-coniine, conhydrine, pseudoconhydrine and gamma-coniceine (more toxic).

Mechanism of Action

It is a peripheral neurotoxin having curare-like effects in neuromuscular junctions and nicotinic effects in the autonomic ganglia.

Mode of Action

It affects the nervous system producing biphasic nicotinic effects (stimulation followed by paralysis of motor nerve endings and CNS stimulation and later depression). The neuromuscular blockage can stop the function of the respiratory muscles leads to respiratory paralysis and death.

Fatal Dose: 60 mg coniine.

Fatal Period: Few hours.

Signs and Symptoms

Nausea, vomiting, salivation, trembling, ataxia, slow and weak later rapid pulse, rapid respiration, urination, convulsions, dilated pupil coma and death. Skin exposure can cause contact dermatitis.

Treatment

(i) Gastric lavage with activated charcoal (ii) Supportive care along with I.V. fluids (iii) Mechanical ventilation, if necessary (iv) Treatment for seizures with benzodiazepines or barbiturates (v) Urine alkalization in case of rhabdomyolysis or myoglobinuria (vi) No specific is antidote available.

Autopsy Findings

Remains of the poison can be found in stomach contents. Features of asphyxia is present.

Medicolegal Aspects

(i) The poisoning is mostly accidental. Conium maculatum can be confused with edible vegetables of similar appearance. (ii) Toxicity from foraging is well-described in livestock. (iii) Homicidal poisoning by hemlock is rare. In 399 BC, Greek philosopher Socrates was sentenced to death by drinking a cocktail of extract from hemlock mixed with opium.

SHORT NOTES

1. Clinical features and management of Strychnine poisoning.
2. Differentiate poisoning by Strychnos nux vomica and tetanus.
3. Hemlock poisoning.

43 CHAPTER

Cardiac Poisons

Cardiac poisons have mainly actions on the heart, either directly on the musculature or through its nerve supply. Oleander, nicotine, digitalis and aconite belong to this group.

NICOTIANA TABACUM (TOBACCO)

Nicotine is a colourless, hygroscopic liquid alkaloid. It was first given to Columbus by Native Americans that subsequently spread to Europe. However, the use of cigarettes is a modern phenomenon throughout the world.

Uses: Preparations of nicotine are extensively used in agriculture and horticulture for fumigating and spraying, as insecticides, fumigants, vermin paste, worm-powder, sheep dip etc. The dried leaves of the plant Solanaceae comprise the tobacco used for smoking. These leaves of tobacco (*tambaku*) contain 1-8% of nicotine and are used in the form of smoking, snuff and for chewing. They are used for the preparation of cigars, cigarettes, *bidis* whereas powdered tobacco is used as a snuff. The tobacco is also consumed by mixing with lime alone (*khaini*) or with lime and betel.

Active Principles: All parts of the plant are poisonous except its ripe seeds. The leaves contain two active principles as toxic alkaloids; **Nicotine** and **Nicotianine.** Nicotine is very toxic and exists in all parts of the plant, in combination with malic acid and citric acid. The poisoning occurs in persons employed in tobacco extraction, processing or spraying of insecticides containing nicotine.

Absorption and Excretion: Concentrated liquid nicotine is exceedingly dangerous. However, tobacco is much less poisonous than would be expected from its nicotine content when smoked. Most of the nicotine is burned and when ingested in the form of tobacco, it is poorly absorbed from the stomach. Nicotine poisoning can occur from ingestion or application over skin and by inhalation. Nicotine in the cigarettes is rapidly absorbed through the arterial circulation to reach the central nervous system directly and the effect occurs within a few minutes. About 85-90% is metabolized in the liver, but some amount is metabolized in the kidneys and lungs. It has a half-life of about 2 hours.

Mechanism of Action

(i) Nicotine binds to nicotinic receptors, which are present mainly on the CNS, spinal cord and neuromuscular junctions. (ii) It also binds to autonomic nervous system and adrenal medulla. It first stimulates the vagus nerve, and then depresses the autonomic, central and spinal nervous system. (iii) In small doses, it contracts pupil but in larger doses, it causes dilatation.

Acute Poisoning: Following signs and symptoms are produced in acute poisoning: (i) Burning acid sensations in the stomach (ii) Salivation, nausea, vomiting and diarrhoea (iii) Headache, giddiness, numbness and faintness (iv) Muscular weakness and tremors (v) Cold and clammy skin (vi) Hearing and vision may be affected (vii) Cardiovascular manifestations include, slow pulse at first and then rapid, blood pressure is raised and arrhythmias also develop (viii) Pupils are first contracted then dilated (ix) Respiration is at first rapid then slow (x) Sometimes delirium and convulsions may occur (xi) Death occurs due to respiratory failure.

Chronic Poisoning: (i) Chronic poisoning is produced in heavy smokers and persons working in tobacco factories (ii)

Respiratory system is mainly affected; chronic cough, bronchitis and laryngitis are produced due to irritation of pyridine bases (iii) Pulmonary emphysema is quite common in smokers and smoking may lead to lung cancer.

The incidence of following diseases are more in smokers: (i) Coronary heart disease (ii) Oral cancer is directly related to smoking (iii) Hyperacidity and peptic ulcer are produced (iv) Dermatitis may be produced from dust and juice of tobacco leaves (v) Optic atrophy is also commonly observed in the smokers (vi) Hypertension, extrasystoles and ventricular fibrillation are frequent in the smokers (vii) Thromboangiitis obliterans may be present.

Fatal Dose: 60-100 mg of nicotine.

15-30 gm of crude tobacco.

Fatal Period: 5-15 minutes.

Treatment

(i) Gastric lavage with weak solution of potassium permanganate or warm water containing finely powdered charcoal or weak tannic acid solution (ii) Whole bowel irrigation (iii) Saline purgative to be given by mouth (iv) In mild to moderate cases, injection atropine sulphate 1-2 mg I.M. and hexamethonium chloride 25-50 ng S.C. to counteract peripheral autonomic disturbance and it also acts as a respiratory stimulant (v) Oxygen inhalation and artificial respiration (vi) Cardiac monitoring (vii) Seizures should be treated with anticonvulsant. (viii) Mecylamine (inversine) is the specific antidote. As it is the only antidote in tablet form, it is of little value, if the patient is vomiting.

Autopsy Findings

(i) Odour of tobacco and its leaves from the stomach contents (ii) Mucous membrane of stomach and intestines is congested and haemorrhagic due to caustic action of nicotine (iii) All the organs are congested and oedematous.

Medicolegal Aspects

(i) Accidental poisoning is quite common due to its extensive use and usually occurs under the following circumstances: (a) Tobacco is used in different ways like smoking, chewing, swallowing or by decoction. It is also widely used in agricultural and horticultural work (b) Accidental toxicity occurs when tobacco is applied as a poultice for ulcers or from mucous membranes when used as enema (c) Oral tobacco use can lead to gum diseases and oral cancer (d) Poisoning is usually accidental resulting from excessive smoking (e) Application of leaves or juice to the wound or abraded surface may lead to the absorption of the poison (f) Drinking hookah water and Cheroots in water are applied over the axilla. (ii) Suicidal and homicidal poisoning is rare. (iii) Malingering by soldiers to avoid duty, they soak the leaves in water and place in axilla with the bandage. (iv) Nicotine resists putrefaction so it can be recovered from the viscera for a long time after death. (v) As nicotine is completely excreted from the body within 16 hours thereafter, there is no danger to life.

DIGITALIS PURPUREA

The plant is cultivated in whole of Jammu and Kashmir of India and throughout the world (Figure 43.1). The entire plant of digitalis purpurea is toxic. Only leaves are used for medicinal purposes.

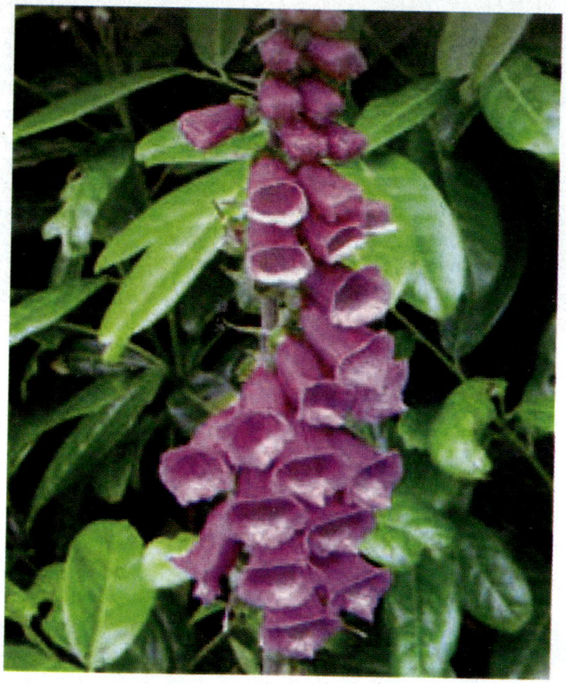

Figure 43.1: Digitalis purpurea plant

Active Principles: The active principles in the form of glycosides are present in the leaves, roots and seeds of the plant. There are about more than thirty glycosides out of which only four are important. Of this **digitalin**, **digitoxin** and **digitalein** are cardiac stimulants whereas **digitonin** is cardiac depressant. The poisoning by digitalis is mostly accidental as it is used in different types of cardiac diseases and overdoses do occur.

Mode of Action

The main action of the poison is on the heart due to its glycosides content. In the heart: (i) It prolongs the period of systole in cardiac cycle (ii) It regulates the rhythm of the heart by depressing both excitability and conductivity (iii) It shortens the period of diastole (iv) It causes rise of blood pressure (v) In toxic doses, there is increased excitability of the heart with development of extrasystole, ultimately toxic arrhythmia and bradycardia develops leading to heart failure.

Signs and Symptoms

The poison first acts on the gastrointestinal tract then the cardiovascular system. The signs and symptoms produced are: (i) *Gastrointestinal tract:* Anorexia, thirst, nausea, vomiting, abdominal pain, watery diarrhoea, vertigo and fatigue are produced. (ii) *Cardiovascular system*: Extrasystoles, pulsus bigeminus and heart block. (iii) *Respiration* is slow and sighing, pupils are dilated and visual derangements are there. (iv) *Central nervous system*: Headache, neuromuscular disorders, confusion, disorientation, drowsiness, delirium and hallucinations are present. (v) Death is due to ventricular fibrillation.

Tests for the glycosides: The glycosides can be extracted from the acidified organic matter. When these glycosides are treated with strong sulphuric acid, the reactions of all three are different: (i) Digitoxin will give green colour, which does not change with bromine (ii) Digitalin gives yellow colour that soon changes to brick red and to violet red on addition of bromine water (iii) Digitonin produces red colour and the colour intensifies with addition of bromine water.

Fatal Dose: Digitalis—2-3 gm.
Digoxin—5 mg.
Digitalin—15-20 mg.
Powdered leaves—2.5 gm.

Fatal Period: 24 hours.

Treatment

(i) Stomach wash using tannic acid and activated charcoal to be given (ii) Bowels should be evacuated (iii) Atropine 0.6 mg I.V. is given for bradycardia that can be repeated (iv) Quinidine sulphate 0.2 gm is given 4-6 hourly (v) Lignocaine 50 mg I.V. is given for ventricular tachycardia (vi) Digoxin specific antibody fragments (Fab) are given in the dose of 0.4-0.8 mg I.V. slowly (vii) Phenytoin 50 mg I.V./min, can be given up to 1 gm followed by 300 mg daily for ventricular fibrillation (viii) Lignocaine 100 mg I.V. to be given for arrythmias (ix) Potassium salts are administered to reduce extrasystoles (x) Electrolyte imbalance should be corrected using I.V. fluids.

Autopsy Findings

(i) Fragments of leaves of digitalis may be found in the stomach (ii) Mucous membrane of stomach is congested and inflamed (iii) All organs are congested.

Medicolegal Aspects

(i) Poisoning occurs due to intake of overdose of medicinal preparation accidentally (ii) It is also sometimes used for homicidal purposes (iii) Digitalis being a cumulative poison, accidental death may occur in **susceptible persons.**

ACONITE (MITHA BISH, MITHA ZAHER, BIKH)

The term aconite is derived either from Greek *akonitus* or from the Greek city *"acona"*. Few suggest that the word aconite has come from the hill of aconitus. The plant *Aconite* is grown in garden for its showy flowers in the Himalayan ranges in India (Figure 43.2).

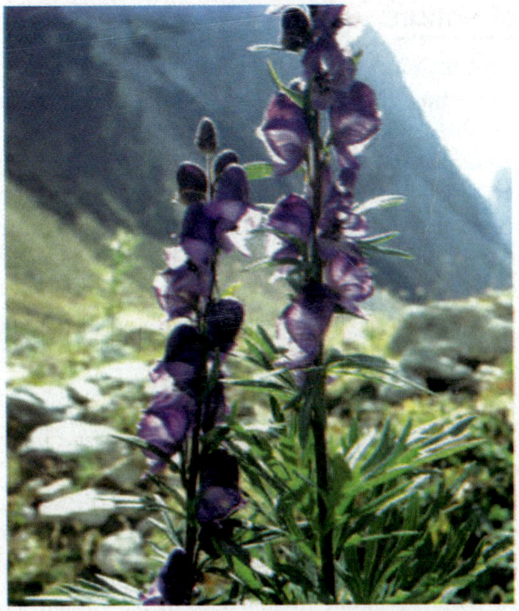

Figure 43.2: Aconite plant

Aconitum napellus belongs to the family Ranunculaciae. All parts of nearly all the varieties of the plant are poisonous but the root is chiefly used as poison. There are several species of aconite out of which *Aconitum ferox* and *Aconitum napellus* are commonly used as poison. They are also known as **Monk's hood, Blue Rocket, Bear's foot, Mitha zaher, Bish and Bikh etc.**

The dry root is conical and shows scars of broken rootlets. The upper end of it is usually about 2 cms thick and has a length of usually 8-10 cms. The root is dark brown in colour (Figure 43.3) that on cut section is whitish and starchy, which, on exposure to air, turns pink. It has to be differentiated from Horseradish root (Figure 43.4) that is long, cylindrical and yellowish white externally and whitish internally that does not change in colour on exposure to air and it has a pungent taste. Root of Aconite has no odour but is sweetish in taste hence the name **Mitha Bish**. On chewing tingling and numbness in the tongue, lips and mouth is felt.

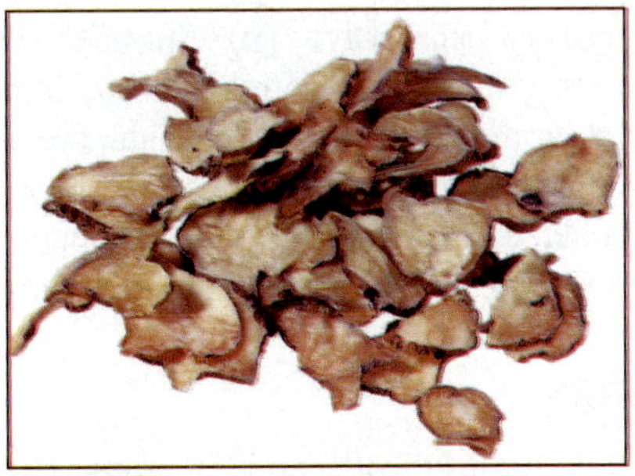

Figure 43.3: Roots of aconite

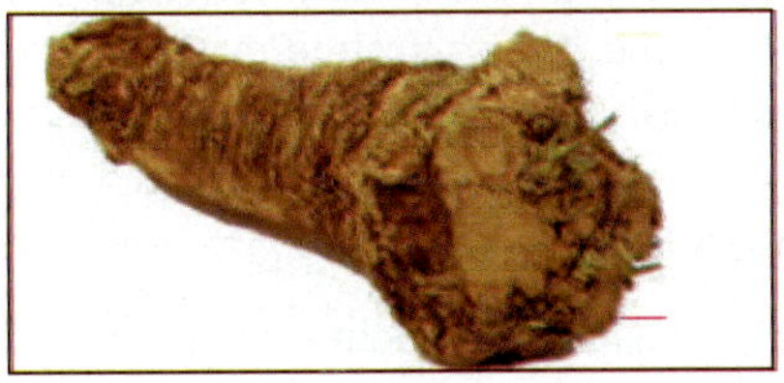

Figure 43.4: Horseradish root

Mode of Action

The poison first stimulates the sensory nerve endings, producing tingling sensation then paralyzing them causing numbness. It produces similar effect on the motor and secretory nerve endings, the centres of the medulla and cord, while the higher centres are always left out. The alkaloids depresses the myocardium, smooth muscles and skeletal muscles. Its depressant effect on motor ganglia and cardiac muscles produces heart block. Temperature falls gradually due to its action on thermogenic centre.

Elimination: Aconite is mainly excreted in urine, but traces are excreted in bile, saliva and sweat.

Active Principles: The alkaloids isolated from the different varieties of the Aconite are: (i) From *Aconite napellus* (a) *Aconitine* (Acetyl-benzoyl-aconine) (b) *Picraconitine* (Benzoyl-aconine) (c) *Aconine* (ii) From *Aconite ferox* (a) *Pseudoaconitine* (Veratroyl-aconine) (iii) From *Aconite charmanthum* (a) *Indaconitine* (iv) From *Aconite spicatum* (a) *Bikhaconitine.*

Of all these alkaloids obtained from the Indian varieties of the aconite plant, pseudoaconitine is the most toxic, Indaconitine and Bikhaconitine are less toxic than pseudoaconitine but a bit more poisonous than Aconitine.

Signs and Symptoms

The symptoms of aconite poisoning start immediately after its consumption: (i) Bitter taste in the mouth (ii) Burning pain in the abdomen (iii) Nausea, vomiting and salivation (iv) Diarrhoea is rare (v) Pupils alternately dilate and contract which is known as **hippus (pupillary athetosis)**, but at a later stage, they remain dilated. The diplopia is also present (vi) Pulse is slow and irregular (vii) Temperature is subnormal (viii) Consciousness usually remains clear till the end (ix) Death results from ventricular fibrillation.

Fatal Dose: 1-2 gm of root; 2-5 mg of aconitine.

Fatal Period: 1-5 hours.

Treatment

(i) Treatment is mostly supportive (ii) Stomach wash with tannic acid or milk (iii) No specific antidote is available (iv) For ventricular arrythmia-amiodarone and flecainide are reasonable first-line treatment (v) In refractory cases of ventricular arrhythmias and cardiogenic shock, early use of cardiopulmonary bypass is recommended (vi) Atropine should be used to treat bradycardia.

Autopsy Findings

(i) Bronchial tree contains froth and mucous (ii) Mucous membrane of stomach and small intestine may be congested (iii) All organs are congested.

Medicolegal Aspects

(i) As aconite is largely used as medicine, accidental poisoning is common (ii) It may be mistaken for Horse radish shoe (iii) It is given with betel leaf to mask its taste (iv) It is added with liquor to increase its intoxicating effect (v) It is used as arrow poison in hilly areas (vi) It is extremely unstable and is destroyed by putrefaction.

NERIUM ODORUM (WHITE OLEANDER, SWEET SCENTD OLEANDER OR KANER)

The plant grows wildly all over the country. It is also grown in gardens for its beautiful pink and white flowers (Figure 43.5A and B). The plant has lanceolate leaves and bears two folllicled fruit that contains numerous seed. All parts of the plant are poisonous.

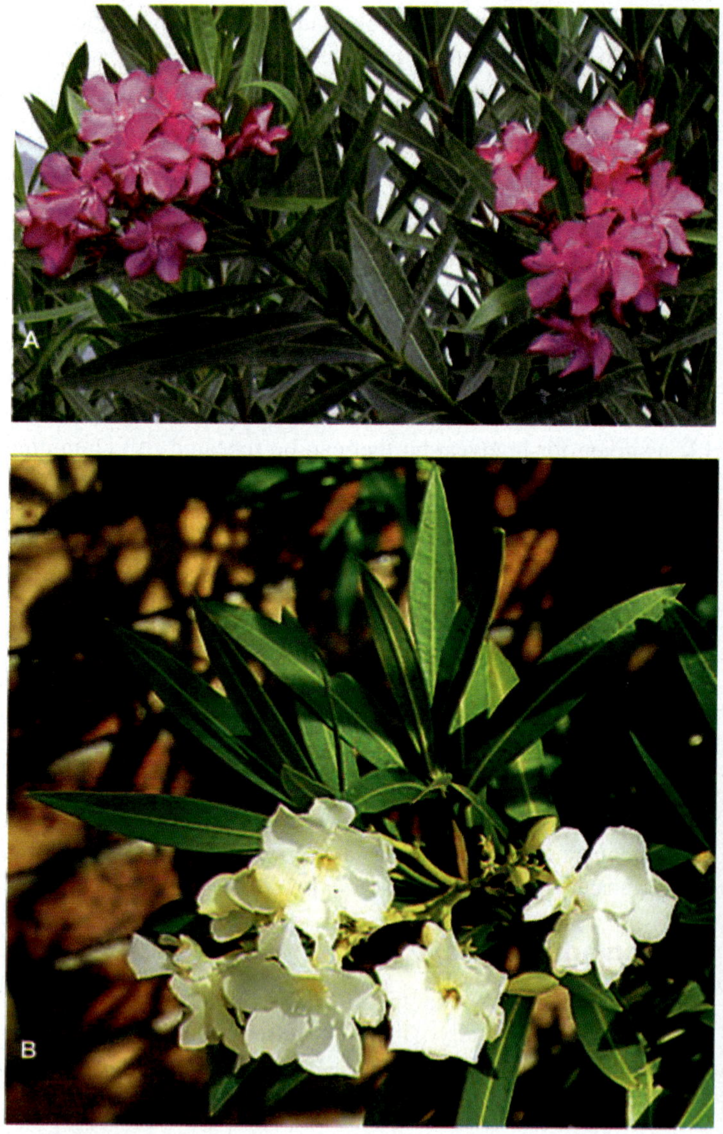

Figure 43.5A and B: Nerium odorum plants with flowers

Uses: (i) Powdered roots are used for the treatment of venereal diseases, epilepsy, malaria, skin diseases and menstrual disorders by the quacks (ii) The powdered roots are also applied as paste to treat ulcerations and cancerous growths (iii) Decoction of the leaves may be applied to reduce swelling of body.

Active Principles: The active principles are several cardiac glycosides known as (i) *Nerin* (ii) *Oleandrin* and (iii) *Karabin.*

Fatal Dose: Powdered root—15-20 gm.

Neriodorin and karabin—150 mg.

Signs and Symptoms

1. **On Ingestion:** (i) Peculiar taste in mouth (ii) Nausea, vomiting and profuse salivation (iii) Difficulty in deglutition and articulation (iv) Acute pain in epigastrium associated with diarrhoea (v) Fibrillary twitchings of muscles of upper limbs followed by tetanoid convulsion occurs. It affects nearly all muscles of the body, but may be unilateral. It is accompanied by lockjaw (vi) Pulse rate is slow, weak and feeble in late stages (vii) Fall of blood pressure and cardiac arrhythmias develop (viii) Respiration is hurried and stertorous with dilated pupil (ix) Exhaustion and drowsiness leading to insensibility, collapse and coma (x) Death occurs from heart failure.
2. **On Inhalation of the Smoke From Burning Plant:** (i) Cough, frothy salivation and dysphagia (ii) Fibrillary twitching of muscles (iii) Pulse is slow, weak and feeble (iv) Blood pressure is low and respiration is hurried and stertorous.

Treatment

(i) Stomach wash using weak solution of potassium permanganate or tannic acid (ii) Vomiting and diarrhoea should be controlled (iii) Morphine or pethidine 5 mg I.M. for sedation that will control spasm (iv) Absolute bed rest is a must (v) To treat cardiac arrhythmias, phenytoin 100-200 mg orally or 100 mg I.V. every 5 minutes until they are reverted (vi) Anti-digoxin ovine Fab fragments (vii) Symptomatic treatment for maintenance of circulatory collapse.

Autopsy Findings

(i) Stomach and intestinal mucosa are congested (ii) All the chambers of heart distended with blood (iii) All organs are congested (iv) Subendocardial haemorrhages are pathognomic.

Chemical Tests: Keller's test gives green colour appearing slowly in the acetic acid layer and crimson colour in the sulphuric acid layer when nerium extract obtained by Stass-Otto process is added. It is used to detect other alkaloids also.

Medicolegal Aspects

(i) Accidental poisoning can occur from ingestion of powdered root or decoction for treatment or when used as a love-potion (ii) The powdered roots, decoction of leaves or paste of the fruit may be ingested for committing suicide (iii) Cases are on record when it has been used for homicidal purposes (iv) It is commonly used as cattle poison; the paste of powdered root is smeared on a rag that is pushed into anal canal of the animal. It is also mixed with the cattle fodder (v) The paste is commonly smeared on the abortion stick to be used as an abortifacient (vi) The poison resists heat so it can even be detected in burnt human remains.

CERBERA THEVETIA (THEVETIA NERIFOLIA OR YELLOW OLEANDER)

The plant is also known by the names of *Bastard oleander, Pila kaner* etc. It belongs to N.O. Apocynaceae, alike Nerium odorum and is widely cultivated in gardens in India. The plant has linear lanceolate leaves and bears yellow coloured bell-shaped flowers (Figure 43.6). The fruit is globular in shape, green and contains a single pale-brown nut that is triangular in shape with a deep groove along the edge, having two cells (kernels), each enclosing a pale yellow cotyledon. All parts of the plant are highly poisonous.

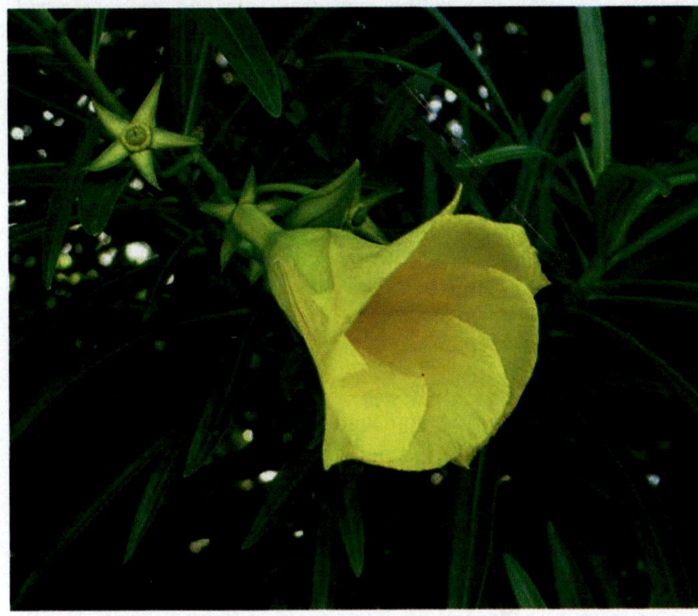

Figure 43.6: Yellow oleander

Uses: The powdered bark of the plant may be used as an antipyretic like Cinchona in the dose of 125 mg. In little bigger dose, it acts as an emetic and purgative and in further bigger dose, it is toxic.

Active Principles: The milky juice from nearly all parts of the plant gives out the active principle that are cardiac glycosides. Of these thevetin and thevetoxin can be recovered from the kernels of seeds: (i) *Cerberin* is a neurotoxic acts like strychnine (ii) *Thevetin* is a powerful cardiac toxin (iii) *Thevetoxin Action* is similar to digitalis (iv) *Nerifolin,* its action is similar to digitalis.

Fatal Dose: Uncertain but death can occur in adults by 8-10 seeds and children by 1-2 seeds.

Fatal Period: Uncertain but usually 2-3 hours.

Signs and Symptoms

(i) Burning sensation in the mouth with feeling of dryness (ii) Tingling and numbness of mouth, tongue and throat (iii) Headache, dizziness and faintness (iv) Dilated pupils with indistinct vision (v) Loss of muscular power and have fainting fits (vi) Nausea, vomiting and loose frequent motions due to the irritant action on bowel (vii) Depressant action on cardiac muscles causes slow and irregular pulse rate (viii) In late stages, pulse is weak, feeble, irregular with fall of blood pressure and heart block (ix) Respiration hurried and stertorous (x) Tetanic convulsions may occur (xi) Collapse, coma and death from peripheral circulatory failure.

Treatment

(i) Stomach wash using weak solution of potassium permanganate or tannic acid followed by animal charcoal suspended in water (ii) Barbiturates to control convulsions (iii) Stimulants, analeptics, digitalis, I.V. dextrose saline, noradrenaline and corticosteroids to counteracts cardiac failure (iv) To treat cardiac arrhythmias, phenytoin 100-200 mg orally or 100 mg I.V. every 5 minutes until they are reverted (v) Symptomatic treatment for maintenance of peripheral circulatory collapse.

Autopsy Findings

(i) Stomach and upper intestinal mucosa is congested (ii) Fragments of seeds may be recovered from the stomach contents (iii) All organs are congested (iv) Subendocardial haemorrhages are characteristic.

Chemical tests: As cerberine is easily destroyed by hydrolysis with dilute hydrochloric acid and gastrointestinal secretions, it is rarely detected in the viscera on chemical analysis. Thevetin is resistant to such destruction and is available for extraction in poisoning by yellow oleander. Thevetin contained in the acid ether extract obtained by subjecting the viscera of suspected yellow oleander poisoning to Stas-Otto procedure can be recognized by:

1. **Keller's test:** When the ether extract is dissolved in 1 ml of glacial acetic acid containing 5% ferric sulphate and this solution is put over a mixture of 100 parts of concentrated sulphuric acid and 1 part of ferric sulphate, blue colour appears on acetic acid layer and mauve colour on the sulphuric acid layer.
2. When portions of any part of yellow oleander is boiled with dilute hydrochloric acid, a blue colour develops and bluish colour also appears when alcoholic extract of the seed is warmed with dilute hydrochloric acid, this may disappear on adding potassium permanganate solution.

Medicolegal Aspects

(i) Accidental poisoning can occur from ingestion of powdered root or decoction for treatment and is common in children (ii) Powdered roots, decoction of leaves or paste of the fruit may be ingested for committing suicide (iii) It is not used for homicidal purpose (iv) It is commonly used as cattle poison that is given mixed with the cattle fodder (v) Paste is commonly smeared on the abortion stick to be used as an abortifacient. The powdered root or seeds are taken after mixing with food or drink to cause abortion.

CERBERA ODOLLAM (DABUR OR DAKUR)

This plant closely resembles that of cerbera thevetia that grows wild in the swams and the creeks of the seacoasts of India (Figure 43.7). The plant has a dark, fleshy lanceolate leaves similar to jasmine and the fruit resembles unripe mango that contains a single oval white seed that is flat and oval, has two cotyledons (kernels) that appears bluish when dry. Milky juice exudes out from all parts of the plant. The kernels yield a nonpoisonous oil that is used for burning.

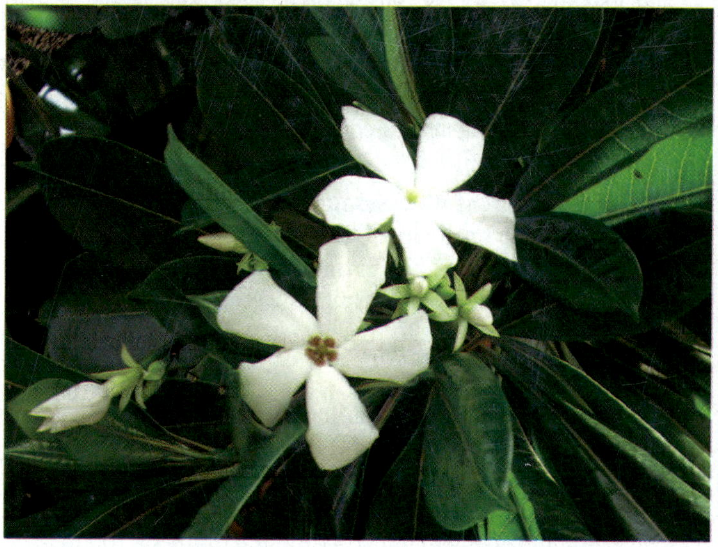

Figure 43.7: Cerbera odollam plant

Active Principles: The kernel contains a glycoside *cerberin* and alkaloid *Cerebroside* that has digitalis like action.

Fatal Dose: Kernel of one fruit.

Fatal Period: About 1-2 days.

Signs and Symptoms

They appear within one hour of ingestion. Initially gastrointestinal symptoms appear followed by cardiac toxicity: (i) Violent vomiting and diarrhoea (ii) Irregular respiration (iii) General paralysis and collapse (iv) Death results from heart failure (v) ECG changes (Sinus bradycardia, S.A. node block, atrial and ventricular fibrillation).

Treatment

(i) Mainly symptomatic treatment is given (ii) Stomach wash using weak solution of potassium permanganate or tannic acid followed by animal charcoal suspended in water (iii) Atropine sulphate 0.5 mg I.V. is to be given and repeated if needed (iv) Hyperkalemia should be corrected (v) Barbiturates to control convulsions (vi) Stimulants, analeptics, digitalis, I.V. dextrose saline, noradrenaline and corticosteroids for counteracting cardiac failure (vii) To treat cardiac arrhythmias, phenytoin 100-200 mg orally or 100 mg I.V. every 5 minutes until they are reverted.

Autopsy Findings

The autopsy findings are nonspecific.

Chemical test: The extract is treated with boiling dilute hydrochloric acid and cerberin will form a bluish or bluish green colour.

HYDROCYANIC ACID (CYANOGEN, PRUSSIC ACID)

Hydrocyanic acid is a vegetable acid that is widely distributed in nature in many fruits and leaves. Here it exists in the form of harmless glucoside known as **amygdalin**, which, coexist with the enzyme emulsion in the kernels of various fruits such as peaches, plums, apricots, bitter almonds, bamboo shoots, certain oil seeds and beans and leaves of cherry laurel. The emulsion can readily hydrolyse amygdalin in presence of water to form hydrocyanic acid, glucose and benzaldehyde. It is present in the leaves of Cherry laurel in the strength of 0.08-0.1% and 10% in oil of bitter almonds. Several people suffer from the effects of hydrocyanic acid poisoning after eating handful of bitter almonds.

Liquid hydrocyanic acid when pure, is a highly volatile colourless liquid having a peculiar odour of **bitter almonds or peach-kernels**. The hydrocyanic acid is usually obtained by distilling potassium cyanide or potassium ferrocyanide with dilute sulphuric acid.

Hydrocyanic acid is decomposed in neutral or alkaline solution with formation of ammonia. It rapidly decomposes when exposed to air and light.

The odour of hydrocyanic acid is that of bitter almonds and all persons cannot smell hydrocyanic acid gas as the ability to do so is a sex-linked trait and when a person is habituated to the smell for few minutes, it disappears and again he has to come to fresh air, then only he can smell it.

Uses of Cyanide

1. Potassium, sodium or silver cyanides are used in the industry for: (i) Metallurgy (ii) Photography (iii) Electroplating (iv) As spray to destroy blight (v) Fumigation of ships.
2. Sodium cyanide is extensively used in: (i) Metallurgy (ii) Electroplating (iii) Case hardening of steel and iron (iv) Tanning (v) Manufacturing of dyes.
3. Calcium cyanide is used for: (i) Mining industry (ii) As a source of hydrocyanic acid (iii) Fertilizer (iv) Preparation of basic chemicals for plastics.
4. Hydrocyanic acid is used for (i) Photography (ii) Electroplating (iii) Agriculture and horticulture for spraying citrus trees (iv) Fumigation of rooms, ship-holds to free them from bugs, lice and vermins (v) For metal cleaning, refining of ores and production of synthetic rubber.
5. *Flowering agent:* (i) Crude oil of bitter almond (2-10% HCN) (ii) Cherry laurel water (0.1 HCN) that looses strength on storing.
6. The hydrocyanic acid gas is capable of being absorbed by the skin, when it is moist with perspiration as the poison is readily soluble in water. It is too dangerous to remain too long in a high concentration of the gas in the atmosphere even when wearing a respirator. The hydrocyanic gas is used for fumigating premises and ship-holds.

Mode of Action

(i) Inhibits the action of cytochrome oxidase, carbonic anhydrase and other enzyme systems as a result the cells are unable to utilize oxygen by dissociating it from the oxyhaemoglobin of the red cells. Tissue anoxia or histotoxic anoxia results even with normal oxygen content in blood that accounts for bright red colour of the venous blood. (ii) There is an interference with the intracellular oxidative process in the tissues. (iii) Signs and symptoms appear at blood cyanide concentrations of approximately 40 mol/l. (iv) Death is due to histotoxic or cytotoxic anoxia although the blood may contain normal oxygen.

Absorption and Excretion

Cyanide gas is absorbed rapidly from the respiratory system whereas the acid and salts are absorbed from the stomach. The acid is also absorbed through the skin. Absorption is delayed when cyanide is taken on a full stomach or with much wine. Cyanide when ingested, in contact with hydrochloric acid of gastric juice leads to the formation of hydrocyanic acid and chloride. Therefore, it has been suggested that achlorhydric patients cannot be poisoned. It cannot be held true as the water in the gastric juice and tissues can cause hydrolysis and lead to liberation of hydrocyanic acid.

Signs and Symptoms

Signs and symptoms develop most rapidly when gas is inhaled and the action is instantaneous. Massive doses produce sudden loss of consciousness and the death due to respiratory failure. When large doses are inhaled, symptoms start immediately that is within 1-2 minutes. Voluntary acts are possible like walking and throwing some articles. On ingestion by mouth, the symptoms produced from cyanide poisoning may be delayed up to 15-20 minutes until the liberation of hydrocyanic acid by the action of gastric juice on salts of cyanide.

Double Cyanides: Potassium ferrocyanide and ferricyanide are practically nontoxic, but they give off hydrocyanic acid in certain conditions. They are toxic when they are taken with the acids. Potassium and sodium cyanide has a corrosive action on the mouth, throat and stomach. They produce: (i) Burning taste and feeling of constriction in the mouth and throat (ii) Nausea and vomiting (iii) Excessive salivation and blood-stained froth comes from the mouth (iv) Anxiety and confusion (v) Headache, vertigo and giddiness (vi) Initially hyperpnoea and dyspnea is present caused by stimulation of the chemoreceptors and the respiratory center. Then respiration becomes rapid, slow and irregular with short, inspiration and long expiration (vii) Smell of bitter almonds in breath and vomitus (viii) In early stages, blood pressure is increased and heart rate is decreased. Later on pulse is rapid, weak and irregular (ix) There is sense of constriction in the chest (x) Unconsciousness and violent convulsions; paralysis follows the convulsive state (xi) Opisthotonus and trismus may develop (xii) Involuntary micturition and defecation (xiii) Skin is covered with sweat and is pale appearance despite tissue hypoxia (xiv) Eyes are glassy and prominent; pupils are dilated and non-reactive to light (xv) Inhalation of gases produces: (a) Sense of constriction in throat and chest (b) Dizziness and vertigo (c) Insensibility and death from respiratory failure (d) Epigastric pain and vomiting (xvi) Death is due to respiratory failure.

Fatal Dose: HCN—50-60 mg.
KCN and NaCN—200-300 mg.
Air concentration 1:500 causes immediate death.

Fatal Period: HCN—2-3 minutes.
KCN and NaCN—Half an hour.

Treatment

(i) The person should be removed from the source poison. In case of dermal exposure, remove clothes and discard appropriately (ii) Stabilize the patient's airway, breathing and circulation (iii) No mouth to mouth resuscitation, because of risk of poisoning to the person who is doing resuscitation (iv) Artificial respiration to be given (v) In case of ingestion, gastric lavage by 3% hydrogen peroxide, sodium thiosulphate (5-10%) and potassium permanganate (1:5000) of which, 200 ml is left in the stomach. (vi) **Antidotes for cyanides:** Many efficient antidotes are available for cyanide poisoning. However, choice of antidotes in cyanide poisoning is still debated. FDA approved antidotes such as sodium thiosulfate and hydroxocobalamin for clinical use.

(1) **Hydroxycobalamin/Cyanokit (A Form of Vitamin B_{12}):** It is the ideal cyanide antidote because of rapid onset of action, easy to administer, tolerability, neutralization of cyanide without interfering with cellular oxygen use or oxygen transport, no harmful effects when administered to non-poisoned patients, safe to use especially if the patient has simultaneous carbon monoxide poisoning and conducive to use in the prehospital setting, as well as in the emergency department or intensive care unit. Hydroxycobalamin combines with cyanides to form the harmless vitamin B_{12} (cyanocobalamin) which is eliminated through the urine. The urine turned to reddish purple color (wine colored urine), because of cyanocobalamin, not due to myoglobinuria. It works both within the intravascular space and within the cells to combat cyanide intoxication. It is given in dose of 5 gms, IV over 15 minutes. It is the antidote of first choice for acute cyanide poisoning. However, it is relatively expensive and not universally available.

(2) **Cyanide Antidote Kit (CAK):** It is the most widely used antidote therapy. It may be used in place of hydroxocobalamin, if it is not available. It contains **amyl nitrite, sodium nitrite and sodium thiosulphate.** First step–Break 0.2 cc ampoule of amyl nitrite in a handkerchief and hold over the patient's nose for 15-30 minutes until sodium nitrite is given. Second step–Sodium nitrite 300 mg ampule or 10 mg/kg is given IV over 3-5 minutes in adults. The paediatric dose for sodium nitrite is 0.2 ml/kg, not to exceed 10 ml. Third step–12.5 gms of sodium thiosulphate in 50% solution is given I.V., over 30 minutes in adults. The paediatric dose for sodium thiosulfate is 7 g/m^2 and not to exceed 12.5 grams.

The exact mechanism of action of nitrites is not known. However, it is hypothesized that nitrites convert hemoglobin to methemoglobin, which then binds to cyanide producing cyanmethemoglobin (nontoxic). The cytochrome oxidase cyanide complex is revered which again allows cytochrome oxidase to reactivate the electron transport chain.

- Cytochrome oxidase + NaCN→cytochrome oxidase cyanide.
- Sodium Nitrite + Hb→Methemoglobin.
- Methemoglobin + NaCN→Cyanmethemoglobin (nontoxic).

Therapy with nitrites is not innocuous. The doses given to an adult can potentially cause a fatal methemoglobinemia in children or may cause profound hypotension. Treatment of children affected with cyanide intoxication must be individualized and is based upon their body weight and hemoglobin concentration. Amyl nitrite has rapid onset but short duration of action, weak and unpredictable methemoglobin-inducing effects. Hence, sodium nitrite is given subsequently which has a longer duration of action and more robust and predictable methemoglobin-inducing effects.

Sodium thiosulfate contains sulphane sulphur moiety, serves as a sulphur donor that increases the rate of rhodanese-catalyzed transformation of cyanide to less-toxic thiocyanates, which are renally excreted. It is efficient and safe, however, has a slow onset of action. It is given to confer additional antidotal efficacy in cyanide kit.

(3) **Other Antidotes:** (a) **4-Dimethylaminophenol (4-DMAP)** has been proposed in Germany as a more rapid antidote than nitrites and with reportedly lower toxicity. It is used currently by the German military and by the civilian population. In humans, intravenous injection of 3 mg/kg of 4-DMAP will produce 35% methemoglobin levels within 1-minute (b) **Cobalt salts** have also been demonstrated as effective

in binding cyanide. One current cobalt-based antidote available in Europe is dicobalt-EDTA, sold as *Kelocyanor*. This agent chelates cyanide as the cobalticyanide. This drug provides an antidote effect more quickly than formation of methemoglobin, but a clear superiority to methemoglobin formation has not been demonstrated. Cobalt complexes are quite toxic, and there have been accidents reported in the UK where patients have been given dicobalt-EDTA by mistake based on a false diagnosis of cyanide poisoning (c) **Methylene blue:** 50 ml of 1% aqueous solution is used. It converts hemoglobin to methemoglobin that combines with free cyanide, which is nontoxic and is removed from the circulation (d) In delayed cases, a mixture of ferric and ferrous sulphate with potassium carbonate is the chemical antidote that forms Prussian blue.

Autopsy Findings

(i) Rigor mortis starts early and lasts longer (ii) Eyes are bright, glistening, and prominent with dilated pupils (iii) Jaws are firmly closed (iv) Froth comes from the mouth (v) Postmortem staining is of cherry red colour due to the formation of cyanmethemoglobin, tissues cannot take up oxygen and oxygen remains in the cells as oxyhemoglobin; asphyxia occurs in the presence of oxygen (vi) On opening the body, the odour of cyanide can be felt from the stomach contents and other organs (vii) Brain is to be opened first as the odour is well marked here (viii) Trachea contains blood stained froth (ix) All the visceral organs are congested (x) Lungs are oedematous (xi) CNS shows degenerative changes (xii) Potassium and sodium cyanide cause corrosion of the mouth (xiii) Gastric mucosa is crimson red in colour that changes to rusty brown due to the formation of acid Haematin (xiv) Blood is cherry red coloured due to formation of cyanmethemoglobin.

Spectroscopic examination of blood: The spectroscopic examination of cyanides resembles that of reduced hemoglobin with a thick band between the lines D and E.

CHRONIC CYANIDE POISONING

Chronic poisoning may occur by continued inhalation of low concentration of cyanide gas for a long period; the symptoms are those of suboxia including cachexia, mental disturbance, visual defects, such as scotomata, optic atrophy and psychosis.

Judicial execution: The condemned or prisoner person is strapped to a chain in a closed room and several cyanide eggs are dropped into a pan of strong acid that leads to liberation of cyanide gas. Unconsciousness takes place very rapidly though heart continues to beat for 10-15 minutes then death occurs.

Medicolegal Aspects

(i) Commonly used for the purpose of suicide, as it is quick acting and only a small dose is fatal (ii) Oil of bitter almonds (2-10% HCN) and cherry laurel is used as flavouring agent (iii) Causes of accidental poisoning: (a) Inhalation of cyanide vapours used as fumigating agent (b) May be ingested in accidentally in lieu of some medicine (c) It may be accidental to the workers employed in the industry (iv) It is rarely used for homicidal purposes. During world war II, the Nazis used cyanide as an agent of genocide in gas chambers (v) Putrefaction produces 1/10th of the cyanide poison (vi) Cyanide is destroyed by embalming (vii) It is present in fire victims in very small amount (viii) Cattle poisoning results by eating *jawar, kadvi,* or *alsi* plants. Growing plants, flowers and seeds contain maximum hydrogen cyanide. One pound of flower is fatal to a bullock **(cyanogenic glucoside)** (ix) On keeping it for a long time harmless carbonate may be formed by the action of atmospheric carbon dioxide and moisture on potassium cyanide and potassium formate.

SHORT NOTES

1. Clinical features, management and medicolegal aspects of Aconite poisoning.
2. Management hydrocyanic acid poisoning.
3. Cyanide antidote kit.
4. Cardiac poisons.

MULTIPLE CHOICE QUESTIONS

1. **Smell of bitter almonds is observed in:**
   (a) Phosphorus (b) Nitric acid
   (c) Oxalic acid (d) Hydrocyanic acid
2. **4-DMAP (4-Dimethylaminophenol) is used for the treatment of poisoning due to:**
   (a) Barbiturate (b) Alcohol
   (c) Cyanide (d) Opioid
3. **Route of administration of Amyl nitrite given in cyanide poisoning is via:**
   (a) Intravenous (b) Intramuscular
   (c) Subcutaneous (d) Inhalational
4. **A 10-year-old boy is brought in casualty with history of accidental ingestion of something in wild. He is having perioral paraesthesia, irregular pulse and alternate contraction and dilatation of pupil. It is a case of poisoning by:**
   (a) Aconite (b) Abrus precatorious
   (c) Dhatura (d) Digitalis purpurea
5. **Cherry-red coloured postmortem observed in case of poisoning by:**
   (a) Nitrobenzene (b) Aniline
   (c) Potassium chlorate (d) Hydrocyanic acid

6. Cyanide antidote kit contains all *except*:

(a) Amyl nitrite (b) Sodium nitrite
(c) Sodium sulphate (d) Sodium thiosulfate

7. All are classified under cardiac poisons *except*:

(a) Nicotiana tabacum (b) Digitalis purpurea
(c) Cerbera thevetia (d) Dhatura

8. In white oleander plant, the glycosides present are all *except*:

(a) Oleandrin (b) Karabin
(c) Nerin (d) Cerberin

9. In yellow oleander plant, the glycosides present are all *except*:

(a) Karabin (b) Thevetin
(c) Thevotoxin (d) Cerberin

ANSWER KEY

1. (d)	2. (c)	3. (d)	4. (a)	5. (d)	6. (c)	7. (d)	8. (d)	9. (a)

44 CHAPTER

Drug Abuse

DRUG

In 1969, WHO Committee on Drug dependence defined drug as "A substance that when taken into a living organism, may modify one aspect of its function". As this definition included water and air also, certain modifications were made in the definition. These are: (i) Drug in the broadest sense is any chemical entity or mixture of entities other than those required for the maintenance of normal health, the administration of which alters the biological function and bodily structure (ii) Second level of definition could then specify the users to which these entities are put that is the drugs used for the treatment or alleviation of disease known as medications or therapeutic agents (iii) Third level of definition: One may differentiate chemical entities based on bodily system or function on which they exert their most marked or obvious affects, e.g., Diuretics, CNS Stimulants etc. (iv) Main concern is about the possible adverse effects on health or social function, e.g., Psychoactive drugs, Antihistaminics.

Use, Abuse and Misuse: Abuse and misuse are unsatisfactory concepts because these terms involve value judgment, they are impossible to define in such a way that they are appropriate for different drugs in different situations.

Drug Abuse

1969 WHO Expert Committee defined drug abuse as "Persistent or sporadic excessive drug use inconsistent with or unrelated to acceptable medical practice".

Further attempts to achieve a comprehensive definition of abuse have been considered depending on the medical need, individual and social harm and the degree of tolerance by the community.

Drug abuse refers to **the use usually by self-administration of any drug in a manner that deviates from the approved medical or social pattern within a given culture**. In some cultures, some drugs/substances are not considered against the society and so may not be against the legal system of the country. Use of medically prescribed drugs, e.g., barbiturates to induce sleep is permissible but if it is used to induce euphoria (when not medically indicated); it is called drug abuse, e.g., opiates can be taken when prescribed medically for the relief of pain but not solely for its euphoric effect. When people continue to take these drugs in the absence of disease, intensity of dependence varies from mild desire to the compulsion to use the drug is called drug abuse.

Clinicians and research workers can often manage without using the terms such as unsanctioned, hazardous, dysfunctional or harmful use as they are concerned more about the effects of drugs and their route of administration. Nevertheless, if such terms are to be used then following concepts may be useful (i) ***Unsanctioned use:*** Use of a drug, not approved by a society or a group within that society, it implies that we accept disapproval as a fact (ii) ***Hazardous use:*** Use of a drug that will probably lead too harmful consequences, for the users either to dysfunction or to harm, e.g., smoking 10-15 cigarettes per day may not be accompanied by any harm, but we know it to be hazardous (iii) ***Dysfunctional use:*** Use of a drug that is heading to impair psychological or social functioning such as loss of job, marital problems etc. (iv) ***Harmful use:*** Use of a drug that is known to have caused tissue damage on mental illness, in a particular person.

Drug addiction: Drug addiction is a state of periodic or chronic intoxication, produced by repeated consumption of a drug, which is harmful to the individual and to society such as Heroin, alcohol, cannabis, Hashish, barbiturates, opiates, cocaine, amphetamine, LSD, Mandrax and bromides. Of these, Heroin is the most dangerous.

Drug habituation: A condition resulting from the continued consumption of a drug, which does not cause much harm to the individual or to the society though there is psychological and emotional dependency on the drug. These are Caffeine, Nicotine etc.

Table 44.1: Differences between drug addiction and drug habituation

Features	Addiction	Habituation
Compulsion	Present	Desire
Dose	Increased tendency	No such
Dependence	Psychical and Psychological	Some degree of Psychological
Withdrawal symptoms	Characteristic	Mild or nil
Harm	Individual and society	Only to the individual

Causes of Drug Abuse

The drug abusers start with a smaller dose but gradually increase the dose and frequency of intake until they develop tolerance. The abusers use the drug due to many reasons such as: (i) To get respite temporarily from various physical or mental ailments (ii) For the purpose of recreation and relaxation (iii) For better performance and sports etc. (iv) For controlling feelings of anger or distress and to get relief from chronic tension (v) For performing spiritual exercises, e.g., LSD and Methaqulone (vi) For alleged aphrodisiac properties (vii) To get relief from frustration in life, love or sex (viii) Just out of curiosity.

Types of persons exposed: The persons likely to be exposed to drug abuse are: (i) Neurotic or mentally imbalanced subjects (ii) Persons in habit of taking risks and having rebellious nature (iii) Individuals with sexual promiscuity.

Classification of Drugs of Abuse

The abuse of narcotic as well as non-narcotic drugs is quite common and the non-narcotic drugs are commonly referred to as soft drugs to distinguish them from the narcotics or the hard drugs. The drugs of abuse are classified as: (i) ***Hypnotics*** such as barbiturates (called 'sleepers' or 'goof balls' by drug abusers) (ii) ***Stimulants*** are commonly used by drug addicts and the tolerance to these drugs develops slowly but can be acquired to the massive doses. These are Amphetamines (called 'Purple Hurts', 'Black bombers', 'pep pills' or 'desk), Benzedine and Ephedrine (iii) ***Antidepressants*** such as Tricyclic antidepressants and MAO inhibitors (iv) ***Hallucinogens*** drugs such as Cannabis, Mescaline, Cocaine, Lysergic, LSD, Phencyclidine, Methaquolone (Mandrax) and various hydrocarbon preparations (v) ***Sedatives*** *as well as hypnotic and tranquilizers* such as Benzodiazepines (vi) ***Narcotics*** such as opium and its derivative (pethidine and heroin) (vii) ***Alcohol*** and alcohol containing beverages (viii) ***Deliriants***.

The action of all these drugs overlap to a certain extent that is those substances acting as central nervous system stimulants can impair consciousness when taken in sufficient quantity whereas those that depress the CNS may arouse and cause loss of inhibitions before exerting their depressant action.

Routes of Administration

The route of administration depends predominantly on the nature of substance and the intensity of action desired. The possible routes are: (i) ***Orally*****:** This route is commonly employed but the absorption from the gastrointestinal tract is relatively slow and the impact of the drug on the brain is muted unless large quantities of the drug are taken (ii) ***Inhalation*****:** The method is also quite commonly employed as there is increase in the speed of absorption. This method is commonly employed for inhaling nicotine from tobacco and *charas* (iii) ***Snorting*****:** This route is not commonly employed except in cocaine. Cocaine is commonly dissolved and the solution sniffed up in the nostrils where a part of it is absorbed (iv) ***Injection:*** This method is the fastest method of getting the desired affect as high concentration of the drug is absorbed through the brain. Two methods are commonly employed; **Skin-popping** is injection via subcutaneous route and **mainlining** is injection via intravenous route. Besides this injection is also taken intramuscularly. Rapid I.V. injection of an opioids produces warm flushing of skin and sensation in the lower abdomen described by addicts similar in intensity to sexual orgasm that lasts for 45-50 seconds and is described as 'rush', 'thrill' or 'kick'.

Fatal Results of Drug Abuse

Overdosage of the drug: The overdosage of the drug commonly occurs accidentally, intravenous injection carries the highest risk of accidental overdosage, and when it occurs, the drug cannot be retrieved. When the supply of high quality drug is less, the drug pushers may *cut* (dilute) the drugs that are sold on the streets. In order to experience the 'kick' or 'rush', they tend to increase the dose.

Toxicity due to contaminants: The substances such as talc or quinine are commonly used to *cut* the drugs in order to reduce the cost. These are used by the drug addicts while preparing the drug for injection. The abuser may develop pulmonary granulomas due to these contaminants and other toxicity.

Infections: Infections such as Hepatitis B, HIV, bacterial abscesses, thrombophlebitis, endocarditis and moniliasis may result from the use of contaminated needles, sharing of needles following other unhygienic practices.

Gangrene: Gangrene may result from inadvertent intraarterial injections.

Anaphylactic reaction: The drugs of abuse are likely to cause hypersensitivity reactions.

Risks of body packing and body stuffing: A **'body packer'** or **'mule'** or **'courier'** is someone who voluntarily or through coercion swallow or insert drug-filled packets into his/her body cavity for the purpose of smuggling across secure borders. The drugs preparations that are financially lucrative such as cocaine (mainly), heroin, high-quality cannabis, and morphine are packed in small packets by using rubber, condom, plastic and aluminum foil etc. (Figure 44.1). The packets are swallowed by the individuals (*swallowers*) that can later on be recovered from the vomitus or excreted feces. The packets can be inserted into the body orifices like vagina, ear or rectum of the person. The drug abuser or dealer who ingest or insert drug packages into the body cavity when suddenly confronted by the authorities are called **body stuffers or quick swallowers.** There exists a risk of overdosage with these practices as the packets may burst and get absorbed through the gastrointestinal, vaginal or rectal mucosa which is called **Body packers syndrome**. The person may present with symptoms that vary from mild abdominal complaints to respiratory insufficiency and even death. There is also risk of acute intestinal obstruction as the drugs are commonly wrapped in aluminum foils, cellophane paper or condom etc. Abdominal radiograph usually helps in diagnosis of such packages and the sign seen on the X-ray is known as **'double-condom sign'** which is due to the trapped air in the individual layers of packing material. The CT scan help in revealing the physical characteristics of the wrapping material together with the nature of the drug contained therein. This helps the physician in deciding the protocol of management. The most common cause of the death among body packers is acute drug intoxication due to rupture of the package(s) within the gastrointestinal tract.

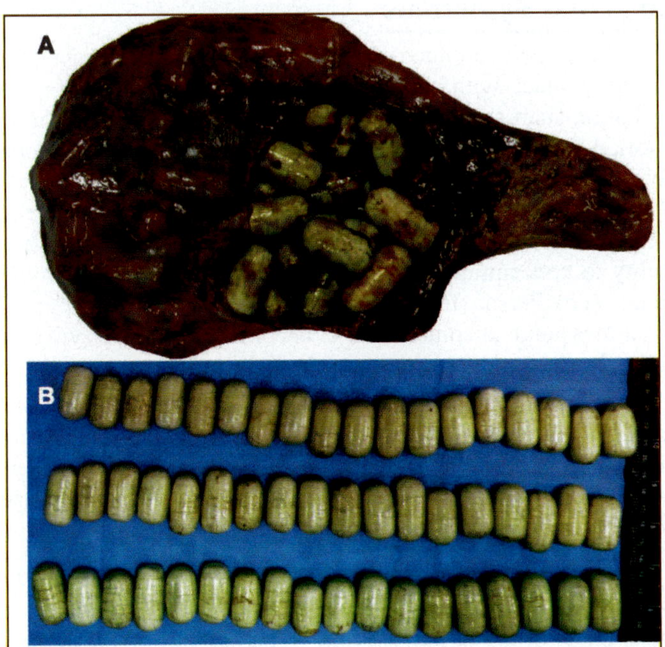

Figure 44.1: Body packaging (heroin) found in stomach at autopsy

Drug Dependence

According to WHO recommendations of 1964, drug addiction and drug habituation should be substituted by the term 'drug dependence' meaning deviation from normal social behaviour of the patient under the influence of drugs.

Types of Dependence

WHO has recognized five types of dependence. (i) ***Morphine type***: In this type of dependence there is an overpowering craving for the drug, which tends to increase with time. There is tendency to increase the drug. Tolerance and cross-tolerance is seen in this type of dependence. The drugs are usually taken by intramuscular, intravenous route or by sniffing. Withdrawal symptoms develop if the drug is withdrawn over a period of hours. Death may result from arrhythmias. (ii) ***Barbiturate type***: There is a strong desire to continue taking the drug. Tolerance develops to high doses of the drug. Cross-tolerance is seen in this type also and postural hypotension is also present in cases. There is development of withdrawal symptoms with maximum intensity within 2-3 days of withdrawal. (iii) ***Cocaine type***: In this type of dependence there is desire to continue taking the drug but there is no tolerance. Psychological dependence is present and there are no withdrawal symptoms. (iv) ***Cannabis type***: In this type also there is no tolerance and there are no withdrawal symptoms. There is no desire to increase the drug dose also. (v) ***Amphetamine type***: This type may be combined with barbiturates. There is increased desire to take the drug and there is a tendency to increase the dose. Tolerance and psychic dependence is present. No abstinence syndrome is seen and continuous use may lead to toxic psychosis.

Signs and Symptoms

(i) Loss of weight and appetite (ii) Unsteady gait (iii) Tremors (iv) Reddening of eyes (v) Puffiness of eyes (vi) Slurring of speech (vii) Impairment of memory and concentration.

Withdrawal symptoms: These are the symptoms, which are seen due to sudden stoppage of the regular supply of drugs. Usually the symptoms start within 6-8 hours following stoppage of drug but may be delayed depending on the type of drug. The intensity of withdrawal symptoms depend upon the dose and type of drug, duration of addiction and whether the drug has been withdrawn suddenly or gradually.

Early symptoms: (i) Sensation of cold and chills (ii) Uneasiness (iii) Rhinorrhoea (iv) Yawning.

Late symptoms: (i) Respiration: Rapid and laboured (ii) Loose skin (iii) Lachrymation (iv) Gross tremors (v) Dilated pupil (vi) Anorexia.

Third stage: Final stage of sleep lasting for 8-16 hours is seen and on awakening all the previous symptoms become intense. Other symptoms produced are: (i) Fever (ii) Tachypnoea (iii) Hypertension (iv) Pain and cramps in legs (v) Perspiration (vi) Diarrhoea and vomiting.

In newborns: Newborns of addicted mothers develop withdrawal symptoms within 5-6 hours of birth in the form of hyperactivity, convulsions and twitching.

Causes of Deaths in Drug Abuse

Most of the drug addicts die as result of complications of drug administration such as: (i) Infection and septicemia (ii) Endocarditis (iii) Hepatitis (iv) Tetanus (v) Pulmonary and cerebral abscess (vi) AIDS complications (vii) Suicidal tendency from overdose of drugs during withdrawal of certain drugs particularly amphetamine (viii) Person may die due to electrocution, fall resulting in head injury or fall in water (drowning) under the effect of drugs (ix) Accidental aspiration of food, vomitus or artificial dentures resulting in choking.

Autopsy Findings

External: (i) Person is emaciated with a shabby appearance with lots of tattoos and scars over the body (ii) Froth over mouth and nostrils is there (iii) The fingertips may be stained with different types of drugs used (iv) IV drug addicts show typical linear needle prick and scar marks usually over veins of cubital fossa, forearms, dorsum of hands, lower extremities, neck, and dorsal vein of penis known as ***mainliners*** (v) S.C. heroin drug users develop typical depressed, circular, atrophic scars and ulcers known as ***skin-poppers*** (vi) Superficial veins in hands and legs and rarely in scalp, penis and popliteal area may be thrombosed due to the injections (vii) Punctate areas of tattooing are seen along the needle tracks due to deposition of carbonaceous material along the needle track known as **turkey skin** (viii) Various recent and old injection sites may show zones of inflammation and perivenous fibrosis (ix) Multiple recent as well as scars of old healed abscesses may be seen (x) Habitual inhalation of cocaine or heroin by snorting and snuffing may lead to perforation of nasal septum.

Internal: (i) Gastrointestinal tract may still contain pills or capsules if they have been ingested recently. Active filler material like starch, talc or cellulose may be seen adherent to the gastric mucosa (ii) Microscopic examination of the various scars often shows foreign material like fibres of cloth, talc or dirt particles in the scar (iii) On repeated I.M. and I.V. injections, there is abscess formation in the muscle and at injections sites near the veins (iv) Hepatic lymphadenopathy is a very common finding. The lymph nodes in the porta hepatitis are enlarged and microscopically show nonspecific hyperplasia (v) There is nonspecific pulmonary edema, bronchopneumonia and aspiration of gastric contents. Froth is present in the upper respiratory tract (vi) Right ventricular hypertrophy may be present due to presence of extensive microcrystalline pulmonary emboli (vii) Lungs appear congested and edematous (viii) IgM and IgG concentration is increased in the spleen and lymph nodes indicating acute and chronic antigenic stimulation (ix) The skin, subcutaneous tissue, muscle and vein surrounding the area of recent injections along with the control from opposite side should be preserved in normal saline for chemical analysis.

Treatment

(i) Chlorpromazine/promethazine is given in 5% dextrose 8 hourly along with vitamin B complex (ii) For the treatment of pain proxyvan is given (iii) To treat insomnia, alprazolam or nitrazepam can be given (iv) After 3 days, Methadone, Naloxone, Naltrioxone can be given (v) By 2-3 weeks, the dose of Heroin is reduced gradually (vi) At the end of 3 weeks the drug is totally stopped and all other drugs tapered.

Treatment of addiction: (i) Steps to guide abuser to come back to a sober way of life (ii) Gradual withdrawal of drugs (iii) Use of other drugs (iv) Keep a careful watch to avoid obtaining secrete supply of drugs (v) Person should be removed to an institution (vi) Administration of drugs like sedative, benzedrine and hyoscine is beneficial (vii) Group and individual psychotherapy with counselling about bad effects of drugs on the patients and society (viii) Diverting the mind of the person by engaging physically/mentally in vocational courses (ix) Improving general health to the person with adequate nutrition and food (x) Symptomatic treatment should be undertaken.

HALLUCINOGENS (PSYCHEDELICS)

Hallucinogens are psychotomimetics, psychotogen, psychedelics or psychodysleptics. These are drugs that causes excitation of central nervous system characterized by: (i) Hallucination (ii) Mood changes (iii) Anxiety (iv) Sensory distortion (v) Delusion (vi) Depersonalization (vii) Increased pulse rate, temperature and blood pressure (viii) Dilatation of pupil (ix) Psychic dependence and (x) Depressive or suicidal psychosis. Since prehistoric times man has used many natural products having hallucinogenic property. However, a number of synthetic compounds have also been formed. These are: (i) LSD (Lysergic Acid Diethyl amide) (ii) Mescaline (iii) Psilocybin and (iv) Phencyclidine. There is individual variation in response to these drugs but autonomic and perceptual reactions are prominent.

Signs and Symptoms

(i) Hallucinogens produce a dream like state with disorientation, loss of contact with reality (ii) There is distortion of visual perception such as swaying of the field of vision, objects appear distorted similar to images in a curved mirror and face may appear grotesque (iii) There is an awareness of intense luminosity of colour and on closing eyes colourful images appear to surge (iv) There is alteration of time sense and music appears tangible (v) Ability to concentrate is impaired (vi) Ataxia is not a prominent feature (vii) Person feels relaxed and is extremely happy; may sometimes laugh uncontrollably or become sad or weep (viii) With higher doses, panic reactions and sinking sensations are common.

Tolerance and dependence: Tolerance is readily induced by hallucinogenic drugs and cross tolerance has also been demonstrated. Physical dependence does not occur but psychological dependence varying from mild (**occasional trips**) to marked (**compulsive abuse**) does occur.

Medicolegal Aspects

Few of the hallucinogenic drugs are primary causes of death but due to abnormal behaviour of the person who is under their influence there is increased incidence of homicidal deaths.

Lysergide

It is psychomimetic, semisynthetic derivative of Ergot that acts at multiple sites in the central nervous system from the cortex to spinal cord.

Signs and Symptoms

Small doses of 20-25 mg produces: (i) Pupillary dilatation (ii) Increased blood pressure (iii) Hypereflexia (iv) Tremors (v) Muscle weakness.

Large doses produce: (i) Dizziness (ii) Drowsiness (iii) Euphoria (iv) Colours may be heard (v) Sounds are visualized (vi) Time passes slowly (vii) Psychological dependence may develop (viii) Serious depression and (ix) Paranoid behaviour.

Treatment

(i) Antianxiety drugs should be given (ii) Barbiturates to be given (iii) It is better to talk to the patient.

LYSERGIC ACID DIETHYLAMIDE (LSD)

It is also known by the names of **Acid, microdot, purple haze, white lightning** etc. LSD has derived its name from the German '*lyserge saure diethlyamid*'. It is the most powerful hallucinogen known to man. It is one of the indole alkaloid derivative; others being psilocybin and psilocin that is contained in the Mexican mushroom (*Psilocybe mexicana).* LSD was synthesized by Hofmann in 1938 who was working on the chemistry of ergot alkaloids and himself experienced its hallucinogenic effects. The properties of LSD were known in 1943. The discovery of psychedelic effects of LSD in 1947 led to an epidemic of LSD abuse during the 1960s. It is the most potent psychedelic and doses as low as 25-50 μg may induce profound psychological and physiological effects. The action of LSD may persist for 12-18 hours even though the half life of the drug is only 3 hours. Abrupt abstinence following continued use does not produce withdrawal signs and symptoms. The use of LSD for therapeutic purposes should be undertaken only with great caution.

Signs and Symptoms

LSD causes alteration in consciousness; there is dream like state and sense of unreality. Easily induces laughter and crying. There are visual and tactile hallucinations (i) *Within minutes of oral administration of LSD, following symptoms are produced:* (a) Tachycardia (b) Hypertension (c) Pupillary dilatation (d) Tremors and (hypereflexia) (ii) *Within half an hour of oral intake, following symptoms are produced:* (a) Bizarre and conflicting perceptual and mood changes (b) Visual illusions (c) Synthesias (d) Extreme lability of mood (iii) Time seems to pass very slowly (iv) Behaviour becomes disturbed with paranoid delusions occur (v) **Flashbacks** in which effects of LSD may be reexperienced without further exposure to the drug for several years (vi) **Bad trip:** It is a medical emergency associated with use of LSD consisting of panic episode and that may persist for 24 hours.

Dose: (i) 1-3 mg/kg produces moderate effect and duration of action is 1-56 hours (ii) 20-100 mg produces the effect (iii) 14 mg is Fatal dose.

Treatment

(i) Supportive measures (ii) Anxiolytic drugs in small doses (iii) Chloropromazine counteracts the effects of LSD.

Medicolegal Aspects

Individual intoxicated with LSD rarely present for medical help. The drug was most popular with the hippies in the West in the 1960s. The deaths are commonly attributed to the bizarre behaviour induced by the drug that can result in accidental and suicidal deaths. Suicidal and homicidal tendency occurs. The persons explore their own feelings.

MESCALINE

Mescaline is a phenylalkyl amine that was isolated in 1896 from Mexican "Peyote cactus" *Lohophora Williamsi* growing in the deserts of Central America. Of the four alkaloids, mescaline is most important. The extracts are used as an intoxicating drink called **Mescal buttons**. 3-15 mg/kg produces the moderate effects and duration of action is 1-56 hours. 200 mg of Mescaline Sulphate produces intoxicating effects. This is the oldest known drug with a primary hallucinogenic action.

Signs and Symptoms

(i) Dilated pupil (ii) Static tremors (iii) Sweating (iv) Increased pulse rate (v) Visual hallucinations (vi) Disorientation of speech and time (vii) Other effects such as: (a) Insomnia (b) Vertigo and (c) Headache are also produced (viii) Large doses produce symptoms of poisoning such as: (a) Nausea (b) Vomiting (c) Bloody diarrhoea and shallow breathing (d) B.P. is low and death is due to respiratory failure.

PHENCYCLIDINE

Phencyclidine is also known by pseudonyms as **Angel dust, Peace pill, Hog, Goon, Rocket fuel, Cadillac, Super grass** etc. Phencyclidine (PCP) was developed for use as an anaesthetic in the late 1970s but was abandoned quickly because of an unacceptably high incidence of postoperative psychotic reactions. PCP (1-phenylcyclohexyl piperidine) is easily synthesized and several variants exist. It is usually smoked in combination with tobacco and less frequently with marijuana but it may also be ingested or injected. Phencyclidine binds to inotropic n-methyl-d-aspartate (NMDA) receptors in the nervous system, blocking ion current through these channels. The most common street preparation, angel dust, is a white granular powder that contains 50-100% of the drug.

Signs and Symptoms

1. **Pleasurable effects:** (i) Initial euphoria and a feeling of dissociation (ii) Numbness (iii) Perceptual distortion (iv) Visual hallucinations.
2. **Users may show:** (i) Horizontal or vertical nystagmus (ii) Flushing (iii) Diaphoresis (iv) Hyperacusis.
3. **Behavioural changes:** (i) Distortions of body images (ii) Disorganization of thinking (iii) Feelings of estrangement.
4. **Higher doses of PCP (5-10 mg) may be complicated by:** (i) Hypersalivation (ii) Profuse sweating (iii) Generalized seizures (iv) Prolonged psychotic reactions (v) Dystonias (vi) Hypoglycemia (vii) Rhabdomyolysis and acute renal failure.

Diagnosis

(i) Determination of phencyclidine levels in the urine as PCP is excreted in the urine for a long time after ingestion and autopsy samples may also be positive for up to a week (ii) The levels of PCP in the serum are also diagnostic but CSF concentrations may be three to four times higher than those in the serum and may take much longer time to clear.

Treatment

(i) Gastric lavage is helpful in achieving excretion of PCP from the body and gastric suction may be of some value by removing PCP secreted in gastric juice and preventing its reabsorption (ii) Oral diazepam is preferred but chlorpromazine can be given if hypertension is there (iii) Diaphenhydramine I.M. has been reported to abolish acute dystonic reactions (iv) Acidification of urine enhances renal elimination (v) Supportive measures including treatment of coma, convulsions and respiratory depression.

Medicolegal Aspects

(i) It is commonly smoked by sprinkling on parsley or marijuana leaves and the intoxication can result from this as cases have been reported in children who are in the same room with adult smokers (ii) It is sometimes used as an adulterant in expensive drugs of abuse such as cocaine (iii) Addiction may lead to violent behaviour, psychosis, suicidal and homicidal behaviour.

TRICYCLIC ANTIDEPRESSANTS

Tricyclic antidepressants and benzodiazepines, the ubiquitous sedatives and hypnotics are the major causes of clinical problems with drugs which depress the central nervous system. Imipramine was found during clinical trial in 1958 to selectively benefit depressed but not agitated psychotics. Tricyclics include: (i) Imipramine (ii) Amitriptyline (iii) Nortriptyline (iv) Trimipramine (v) Doxepin (vi) Dothiepin and (vii) Clomipramine.

Mode of Action

Tricyclic antidepressants have complex actions which account for the diverse nature of the features seen after overdosage. They inhibit the active uptake of biogenic amines noradrenaline (produces antidepressant action), 5-hydroxytryptamine (produces antidepressant and sedative action) and dopamine (produces stimulant action) into their respective neurons. They however differ markedly in their selectivity and potency for the different amines. They have potent anticholinergic and antiarrhythmic activity.

Signs and Symptoms

Features of poisoning usually appear within an hour or so after an overdose and usually reaches maximum intensity in 4-12 hours. The features are: (i) *Anticholinergic symptoms*: (a) Dry mouth (b) Constipation (c) Epigastric distress (d) Urinary retention (e) Dilated pupil and blurred vision (f) Palpitations are produced and (g) There is peculiar clumsy feeling (ii) Tiredness and light headedness (iii) Drowsiness and sleepiness (iv) Difficulty in concentrating (v) Unsteady gait (vi) Increased reflexes and extensor planter responses (vii) Tachycardia is due to anticholinergic and noradrenaline potentiating actions (viii) Postural hypotension is due to inhibition of cardiovascular reflexes (ix) *ECG changes*: T wave suppression or inversion is the most common consistent change (x) Arrhythmias occur due to interference with intraventricular conduction, combination of noradrenaline potentiating and acetylcholine blocking actions and direct myocardial depression that are major causes of death.

Tolerance and dependence: Tolerance to the anticholinergic and hypotensive effects develop gradually, though antidepressant action is sustained. Psychological dependence on these drugs is rare as their acute effects are not pleasant. There is some evidence of physical dependence occurring when high doses have been used for long periods.

Withdrawal symptoms: Withdrawal symptoms do occur on discontinuation of the drug that is why gradual withdrawal of these drugs should be done. The features such as malaise, chills, muscle pain may occur on discontinuation of the drug.

Treatment

(i) Gastric lavage with administration of activated charcoal (ii) Supportive measures such as adequate oxygen inhalation and control of convulsions (iii) Correction of acidosis by bicarbonate infusion intravenously (iv) Physostigmine 0.5-2 mg I.V. should be given to reverse the anticholinergic effects (v) To treat arrhythmias, propranolol or phenytoin should be used (vi) Diazepam may be injected intravenously to control delirium with auditory and visual hallucinations as well as convulsion that occur during recovery phase.

AMPHETAMINES

Amphetamines were first synthesized in 1887 but began to be therapeutically used only since 1930s. Amphetamines are drugs of abuse and are capable of producing but little or no physical dependence. Because of its abuse potential, its therapeutic administration is greatly restricted today. **Ecstasy** (methylenedioxymeth-amphetamine), was developed in 1914 and was used in as a conscious altering agent in psychotherapy.

Mode of Action

Amphetamines predominantly stimulate the central nervous system and maximum selectivity is exhibited by dextroamphetamine and methamphetamine, which in the usual doses produce few peripheral effects. They also cause stimulation of respiratory system especially when it is depressed. They inhibit hypothalamic feeding centre and also have a weak anticonvulsant, analgesic and antiemetics actions.

Derivative of amphetamines: The derivatives of amphetamine are: (i) Methamphetamine (ii) Dextroamphetamine (iii) Fenfluramine (iv) Phentermine (v) Mephentermine (vi) Methyl phenidate and (vii) Synthetic amphetamines (**'Designer drugs'**)—Methylenedioxymeth-amphetamine (MDA or **'Love drug'**) and Methylenedioxyeth-amphetamine (MDEA or **'Ecstasy'**).

Signs and Symptoms

(i) Alertness and increased concentration (ii) Initial euphoria and more extrovert behaviour (iii) Increased talkativeness with rapid speech (iv) Increased work capacity with allaying of fatigue (v) Improvement of athletic performance initially followed by further deterioration (vi) Stimulation of reticular activating system causing wakefulness and postponement of sleep deprivation induced physical stress (vii) Hunger is suppressed (viii) Tremors (ix) Pupils are dilated (x) Tachycardia and hypertension are not so significant (xi) High doses produces euphoria, marked excitement, that may progress to metal confusion, delirium, hallucinations and an acute psychotic state (xii) Peripheral component of toxicity include vasomotor effects, palpitation, arrhythmias, vomiting, abdominal cramps and vascular collapse (xiii) Death is uncommon and is usually preceded by convulsions and coma.

Autopsy Findings

(i) No specific findings (ii) Cerebral or subarachnoid haemorrhage from induced hypertension may be produced.

Treatment

(i) Chlorpromazine should be used for sedation (ii) β-adrenergic blockers are used to antagonize the peripheral sympathomimetic actions of amphetamines (iii) Acidification of urine helps in increased renal elimination of methamphetamine (iv) Supportive measures.

Medicolegal Aspects

(i) Acute overdosage is not so common (ii) Amphetamine abusers are generally teenagers seeking thrill or kick which is obtained on rapid I.V. injection and designer drugs are commonly abused by youngsters during parties (iii) Amphetamine abuse is also seen in athletes who use it to enhance their athletic ability and Amphetamine is one of the drugs included in the **'dope test'** for athletes.

BENZODIAZEPINES

The benzodiazepines are one of the most important groups of psychotropic drugs. They are widely used as tranquilizers, sedatives and hypnotics. They include the following compounds: (i) Chlordiazepoxide (ii) Diazepam (iii) Temazepam (iv) Lorazepam (v) Triazolam (vi) Bromazepam (vii) Clonazepam (viii) Desmethyldiazepam (ix) Medazepam (x) Prazepam.

Signs and Symptoms

Benzodiazepines are one of the safe drugs when their overdosage occurs alone. Cases have been reported when as many as 70 tablets of any of them are unlikely to produce any thing more than mild effect in most adults. Many benzodiazepines have active metabolites that account for their prolonged sedative effects. Benzodiazepines potentiate the effects of other CNS depressants, particularly alcohol, tricyclic antidepressants and barbiturates. Flurazepam is most likely to produce significant CNS depression. The signs and symptoms that are produced are: (i) Drowsiness (ii) Dizziness (iii) Ataxia and slurred speech (iv) Respiratory depression (v) Hypotension and coma.

Treatment

(i) Supportive measures started (ii) Gastric lavage is doubtful (iii) Flumazenil, specific benzodiazepine antagonist in the dose of 0.5 mg I.V. over 30 seconds and further 0.5 mg over next 30 seconds can be repeated, if necessary.

LONG QUESTION

1. Define drug abuse and what are the differences between drug abuse and drug dependence. How will you investigate a case of drug abuse?

SHORT NOTES

1. Body packer syndrome.
2. Body packer and body stuffer.
3. Flashbacks.
4. Ecstasy.
5. Designer drugs.

MULTIPLE CHOICE QUESTIONS

1. Flashback phenomenon is observed due to effect of:

(a) Dhatura (b) Alcohol
(c) LSD (d) Barbiturates

2. **"Turkey skin" is the punctate areas of tattooing characteristically seen in cases of:**
   (a) Close range firearm injuries of shotgun
   (b) Close range firearm injuries of pistol
   (c) Intravenous drug abusers
   (d) Grazed injuries caused in Road Traffic accidentally

3. **The following are true about body packer *except*:**
   (a) It is a method to smuggle drugs across border
   (b) The individual smuggles illicit drugs through parcels
   (c) X-ray examination can detect the packaging material
   (d) The person may die accidentally

4. **'Bad trip' is seen in drug abuse of:**
   (a) Cocaine (b) Alcohol
   (c) LSD (d) Morphine

5. **Following are the features suggestive of drug habituation except:**
   (a) Harm only to individual
   (b) Tendency to increase the dose
   (c) Withdrawal symptoms are mild
   (d) Some degree of psychological dependence

ANSWER KEY ☞

1. (c)	2. (c)	3. (b)	4. (c)	5. (b)

45 CHAPTER

Asphyxiants

CLASSIFICATION OF ASPHYXIANT GASES

Henderson and Haggard divided asphyxiant gases into five groups: (i) ***Irritants:*** The gases in this group infiltrates the air passages or lungs or both and produces inflammatory changes, such as smoke, ammonia, formaldehyde and chlorine. (ii) ***Chemical asphyxiants:*** These are gases that by combining with hemoglobin or by acting on some tissue constituents prevent oxygen from reaching the tissues, or from using it. These are hydrocyanic acid and carbon monoxide; produce histotoxic anoxia. (iii) ***Simple asphyxiants:*** These are inert gases which, when breathed in high concentration act mechanically by excluding oxygen. These are carbon dioxide and nitrous oxide. (iv) ***Volatile drugs:*** Have little or no irritant effect after absorption; they act as an anaesthetic agent or are toxic to the liver, kidney etc. (v) ***Systemic poison:*** These are insecticides, arsine gas etc.

CARBON MONOXIDE POISONING

Concentration of carbon monoxide in the air: In the atmosphere: (i) 0.01% the safe limit (ii) 0.02-0.05% produces toxic symptoms (iii) 0.25-3.0 or 3.33% is fatal to an adult within 4 hours.

Sources of Carbon Monoxide Gas

(i) Carbon monoxide is prepared by the decomposition of organic substances such as oxalic acids and formic acids by means of sulphuric acid. (ii) Where there is incomplete combustion of carbonaceous material on carbon, carbon monoxide is produced. (iii) It is found in the gaseous products from charcoal fires, salamanders, refineries, blast furnaces, limekilns, gas engines, water heaters, gas refrigerators and burning houses. (iv) It is also generated upto 8% in gunpowder, dynamite explosion and coalmine explosion. (v) In coal gas it is present in 4-10%. (vi) When blown into red-hot coal, it is 30-40%. (vii) In diesel engines, exhaust gas of motorcars and trucks, it is 7-13% that is represented as 1% of carboxyhaemoglobin. (viii) In city dwellers and smokers there is 3-5% of carboxyhaemoglobin. (ix) CO produced per minute by 20 horse power motor car is approximately 1 cubic foot that is enough to render the atmosphere of small closed garage (10 × 20 feet) poisonous in less than 10 minutes.

Properties

Carbon monoxide is colourless, tasteless, odourless and lighter than air. It is a highly poisonous gas that is absorbed into the lungs and combines with haemoglobin of the RBC in the blood and forms a stable compound carboxyhaemoglobin. The affinity of haemoglobin for carbon monoxide is **240 times** more than that of oxygen. The affinity of CO for myoglobin is **40 times greater** than oxygen. When combined with chlorine, it produces a dangerous poisonous respiratory irritant gas known as carbonyl chloride or phosgene gas.

Mechanism of Action

Since carbon monoxide has 200-300 times greater affinity for haemoglobin than oxygen, it displaces oxygen for haemoglobin and forms a stable compound known as **carboxyhaemoglobin.** It reduces oxygen content of blood and then of tissues. Since carboxyhaemoglobin does not take part in oxygen transport, symptoms of oxygen deprivation will follow inhalation of the carbon monoxide gas. Carbon monoxide acts as a chemical asphyxiant and it has a direct toxic effect on the myocardium. Since the main action of carbon monoxide is oxygen deprivation and not a toxic manifestation due to the carbon monoxide alone, the important factor is not the level of carboxyhaemoglobin in the blood but the percentage of haemoglobin that is prevented from carrying oxygen. Normally after somatic death, cells near the capillaries continue to function by extracting oxygen from oxyhaemoglobin and cause blue staining. Nevertheless, in CO poisoning this cannot occur because the cells cannot break carboxyhaemoglobin compound. In potent cellular poisons such as cyanide, fluroacetate and freezing break the metabolism of cells so fast that they cannot extract oxygen from oxyhaemoglobin. In these cases, blood under the skin and tissues will remain cherry red due to oxyhaemoglobin. Some people are in a metabolic state in which they can withstand the oxygen lack better than the others are. This is the reason why some persons may recover and live with a level of carbon monoxide that would be lethal to others. It must be taken into consideration also that patients with anemia, coronary artery sclerosis and pulmonary disease are much less able to tolerate oxygen lack.

Types of Poisoning

1. **Acute poisoning:** The acute poisoning is further divided depending on the percentage of carboxyhaemoglobin in the blood. The percentage of CoHb is 10-30% (mild poisoning), 30-40% (moderate poisoning) and severe (more than 40%).
2. **Chronic poisoning:** The toxicity depends upon (i) Concentration (ii) Duration of exposure (iii) General health of the person.

Signs and Symptoms

The signs and symptoms run parallel to the percentage of saturation of CO in the blood. The effects produced are those of suboxia. The symptoms are not noticeable until 20% saturation of haemoglobin occurs. The central nervous system is the first to be affected. (1) ***When the gas is inhaled in concentrated form:*** (i) Sudden weakness and dizziness is followed by coma and death due to respiratory failure (ii) Pale or cyanosed appearance (iii) Colour of the skin is cherry red due to carboxyhaemoglobin; the colour is characteristic of the poisoning but its absence by no means excludes it (iv) Coma may last for 3-5 days, sometimes even longer so bronchopneumonia and oedema of the lungs occur. (2) ***When the gas is inhaled in dilute form:*** (i) Tightness of the forehead (ii) Dizziness (iii) Agitation (iv) Muscular weakness (v) Emotional instability and confusion (vi) Lethargy (vii) Slurred speech (viii) Dilated and fixed pupil (ix) Coma (x) Sudden apnea and death (xi) In some cases rapid and feeble pulse, low B.P. and tremors are seen (xii) Myocardial ischemia, infarction and arrhythmias have also been reported. ECG findings are suggestive of prolonged PR interval, A-V block, bundle branch block, prolonged QT interval and ST depression (xiii) Liver is enlarged (xiv) There is tendency to bleed resulting in retinal haemorrhages and papilloedema (xv) Increased sweating (xvi) Glycosuria and albuminuria. (3) ***When recovered after prolonged illness:*** Due to hypoxic changes in the brain, nervous and mental symptoms are produced, that are: (i) Cerebral haemorrhage (ii) Encephalitis (iii) Optic neuritis (iv) Retrograde amnesia (v) Mental confusion. (4) **There is formation of bulla in CO poisoning,** these are discrete and isolated, contains thick and cellular fluid with an inflammatory ring around them. The bullous eruptions can be localized by external pressure and are produced due to sudden hypoxia. (5) Presence of other diseases like respiratory diseases or severe anaemia with barbiturate etc. reduces the lethal concentration of Carbon monoxide. (6) Physical activity during the exposure increases the rate of saturation. Children saturate their blood more rapidly due to increased rate of respiration. (7) Depending on the concentration of carboxyhaemoglobin in the blood, following signs and symptoms are produced (Table 45.1).

Diagnosis of Carbon Monoxide Poisoning

(i) Presence of smell of utility gas on the victim's clothing (ii) Exposure is fairly sudden (iii) Face is livid or sweaty (iv) Cherry red colouration of skin (v) Blood is highly saturated with CO (vi) There is anaemia (vii) Cyanosis is present (viii) Cheyne-stroke breathing in comatose patients (ix) In mild cases, little involvement of the cardiovascular system with raised pulse and blood pressure (x) In severe cases, low B.P.; thready and irregular pulse with extrasystoles are produced (xi) Heart dilates rapidly after exposure and death is due to acute circulatory failure (xii) Pupils are dilated, loss of light reflex occurs late, and other

Table 45.1: Signs and symptoms produced depending on % saturation of *Carboxyhaemoglobin*

CoHb level in % *saturation*	Signs and symptoms
<10%	No appreciable symptoms
10-20%	Breathlessness on moderate exertion, mild headache and tightness across forehead
20-30%	Throbbing headache, irritability, emotional instability, defective memory, rapid fatigue and lethargy
30-40%	Severe headache, nausea, vomiting, dizziness and confusion and dimness of vision
40-50%	Increasing confusion, hallucinations, severe ataxia like a drunk and rapid respiratory collapse
50-60%	Syncope and coma with convulsions, tachycardia and tachypnoea
60-70%	Coma is increased with incontinence of urine and feces
70-80%	Prolonged coma, weak thready pulse, absent reflexes and convulsions
>80%	Rapid death from respiratory arrest

reflexes are decreased (xiii) In deep coma extensor planter response is there but limb reflexes and muscle tone are lost (xiv) There is hyperpyrexia and neurological involvement (xv) In the urine glycosuria and albuminuria occurs (xvi) **Bullous eruptions** on the skin are seen on the pressure areas (xvii) **Laboratory Tests**: (a) ***Hoppe-Seyler's test***: Blood is added to twice volume of a solution of sodium hydroxide (NaOH) with specific gravity 1.3. Normal blood turns brownish-green, but if CO is present, the colour will remain bright-red (b) ***Kunkel's test***: Few drops of 3% tannic acid is added to blood diluted 1:10 with distilled water; the appearance of a crimson red coagulum indicates the presence of Carboxyhaemoglobin (c) Other colour tests used for detection of CO are ***Katayama's test*** and ***Potassium Ferrocyanide test (d) Spectrophotometric method:*** On spectroscopic examination of blood, the line that is nearer to 'D' is half of the other and is unchanged after the addition of ammonium sulphate. It is the most reliable method for detection of carboxyhaemoglobin level in blood.

CHRONIC CARBON MONOXIDE POISONING

This results from intermittent exposure to the gas in the workers of automobile workshops, gas houses, and steel plant blast furnaces and in those staying in ill ventilated rooms for a long time. The following signs and symptoms are produced: (i) Dull frontal headache (ii) Nausea and vomiting (iii) Digestive disturbances (iv) Palpitations (v) Dyspnea (vi) Loss of memory (vii) Anaemia (viii) Visual disturbances (ix) Ataxia (x) Tachycardia (xi) Hepatomegaly (xii) Skin lesions (xiii) Angina (xiv) Mental symptoms (xv) Polycythemia.

Treatment

1. **Prophylactic:** The industry and domestic plants should be properly installed and well maintained. Adequate ventilation should be maintained and special masks should be used,
2. **Therapeutic:** (i) Removal of the patient to fresh air (ii) Clearing of the airway by suction (iii) Mouth to mouth respiration should be given (iv) 100% Oxygen inhalation can be employed through the mask for greater dissociation of carboxyhaemoglobin. Some advocate the use of 5% CO_2 and 95% O_2 (v) In serious cases, 0.5-1% adrenaline sulphate and 5 ml of 25% solution should be given intravenously for half to one hour and repeated (vi) Antibiotics should be given to combat infection (vii) Dehydration should be corrected (viii) In cases of acute heart failure, I.V. digoxin to be given (ix) CSF pressure taken by lumbar puncture, if elevated then 500 ml of 10% mannitol I.V. and furosemide to be given to relieve cerebral oedema (x) Body should be kept warm by hot water bottles and blankets (xi) *In cases of severe collapse:* (a) Normal saline should be administered subcutaneously (b) Hypothermia or exchange transfusion may be helpful (c) If cerebral oedema is there, 500 ml of 20% mannitol and corticosteroids should be administered (d) Procaine hydrochloride 500 mg in 500 ml of 5% dextrose I.V. once a day should be given for 7 days (e) Cytochrome C should be administered intravenously (f) Patient should be kept in a chamber filled with **hyperbaric oxygen** at two atmospheric pressure; the oxygen dissolved in the plasma is raised from 0.25 to 3.8-vol % and rate of dissociation of CO for haemoglobin is greatly increased. The disadvantages of hyperbaric oxygen are oxygen poisoning, pulmonary oedema and haemorrhages (g) After the breathing is established, tea and coffee is given and antibiotics to counteract infection.

A man when brought to normal oxygen atmosphere, the carboxyhaemoglobin level reduces to half in 4 hours and with 100% oxygen inhalation, the carboxyhaemoglobin concentration reduces to half in just 40 minutes.

Prognosis

(i) A close watch should be kept on the complications like renal failure, gangrene, pulmonary oedema and progressive paralysis due to hypoxia and local pressure (ii) Neurological sequel is well known but may leave residual disability after 20-30 days (iii) If the degree and duration of hypoxia has damaged vital centers, the period of coma may be prolonged but may be followed by complete or partial recovery (iv) Muscle rigidity and increased tone of limbs in severe poisoning (v) Persons more than 60 years of age and coma for 24 hours usually succumb to its effects (vi) Repeated exposure may lead to polycythemia.

Autopsy Findings

External Findings: (i) Bright red colour of the lips and fingertips (ii) Postmortem staining is cherry red in colour; to be differentiated from cold exposure and cyanide poisoning (iii) Fine froth is present at mouth and nostrils (iv) Muscle necrosis and skin blebs are present.

Internal Findings: (i) Blood is cherry red and fluid (ii) Mucous membrane is red in colour (iii) Hyperemia is general and serous effusions are common (iv) Lungs are congested and oedematous and consolidations may be present (v) Heart shows haemorrhages and necrotic changes (vi) Brain is oedematous and has serous effusions in the ventricles, punctiform haemorrhages in the white matter and softening in the cerebral cortex, globus pallidus and corpus striatum. The bilateral symmetrical necrosis of ventricular nuclei is present (vii) Renal failure is the pathological evidence.

Medicolegal Aspects

(i) Carbon monoxide poisoning is mostly **accidental**. It is the most common form of unintentional poisoning. The diseased, drugged and drunk persons are involved more in the poisoning. The poisoning usually occurs in ill ventilated rooms where incomplete combustion of wood or coal occurs and the persons' sense of smell and hearing are impaired. It can also occur in dwellings with faulty fittings with leaky gas pipes and taps. In small garages people die from the gas from the motor exhausts. The poisoning can also result in narrow streets where there is dense traffic. Some sexual deviants may also be poisoned when they inhale coal gas. In suspected cases of poisoning air samples should be taken for analyses of carbon monoxide. In deaths due to fire more than 50% concentration is of carboxyhaemoglobin. In some victims with blood carboxyhaemoglobin concentration of 15-20%, the symptoms similar to drunkenness are produced. (ii) Sometimes Carbon monoxide poisoning may be confused with vehicular accidents. (iii) Presence of occasional bullous lesions similar to the 3rd degree burns on the body is diagnostic of CO poisoning. (iv) Tendency of the dying person to become wild may cause an impression of violent quarrel, can cause an erroneous suspicion of murder. (v) Carbon monoxide poisoning is suicidal mostly in western countries when the room is closed after placing the fire. (vi) In the garage the exhaust fumes are inhaled through a pipe or sometimes the gas is inhaled through the gas taps. It is sometimes associated with suicidal pacts, e.g., the mother ends life along with her children. (vii) The poisoning is very rarely homicidal unless drink, drugs or disease incapacitates the person when a gas tap is opened when the person is sleeping in the bedroom. (viii) Carbon monoxide with chlorine leads to the formation of carbonyl chloride (**phosphene**) that is war gas. (ix) Putrefaction has a little effect on the carboxyhaemoglobin as it is extremely stable, may be detected in the blood after several days even up to seven months after death.

CARBON DIOXIDE POISONING

The carbon dioxide intoxication usually results from the physiological disturbances. The gas may disperse slowly if ventilation is poor. The carbon dioxide gas may also be: (i) Formed during fermentation reactions (ii) Found also in grain bins, caves, ships' holds and in fires (iii) Released from water in wells by changes in atmospheric pressure (iv) Released from some fire extinguishers (v) Released from dry ice. Features of hypoxia are prominent in carbon dioxide poisoning.

LONG QUESTION

1. Describe the clinical features, diagnosis, management, autopsy findings and medicolegal aspects in a case of carbon monoxide poisoning.

MULTIPLE CHOICE QUESTIONS

1. Hope-Seyler's test used for detection of:

(a) Cyanide (b) Carbon monoxide
(c) Hydrogen sulphide (d) Carbon dioxide

2. The most reliable method for detection of carboxyhaemoglobin level in blood is:

(a) Spectrophotometric method
(b) HPLC method
(c) Gas chromatography method
(d) TLC method

3. The signs and symptoms in carbon monoxide poisoning usually begin when the Carboxyhemoglobin concentration rises above:

(a) 5% (b) 10%
(c) 15% (d) 25%

4. Bullous eruptions on the skin found in poisoning due to:

(a) Cyanide (b) Carbon monoxide
(c) Hydrogen sulphide (d) Carbon dioxide

ANSWER KEY

1. (b)	2. (a)	3. (b)	4. (b)

46 CHAPTER

Biological and Chemical Warfare Agents

CHEMICAL WARFARE

Chemical warfare is warfare (and associated military operations) using the toxic properties of chemical substances to kill, injure or incapacitate an enemy. They are also used in civilian conditions to disperse unruly mobs. Chemical warfare is different from the use of conventional weapons or nuclear weapons because the destructive effects of chemical weapons are not primarily due to any explosive force.

The use of nonliving toxic products produced by living organisms (e.g., toxins such as botulinum toxin, ricin or saxitoxin) is considered chemical warfare under the provisions of the Chemical Weapons Convention. Under this Convention, any toxic chemical, regardless of its origin, is considered as a chemical weapon unless it is used for purposes that are not prohibited.

Biological warfare: The offensive use of living organisms (such as anthrax) is considered to be biological warfare rather than chemical warfare.

Chemical weapon agents: A chemical used in warfare is called a chemical weapon agent (CWA). About 70 different chemicals have been used or stockpiled as chemical weapon agents during the 20th century. These agents may be in liquid, gas or solid form. Liquid agents are generally designed to evaporate quickly; such liquids are said to be volatile or have a high vapour pressure. Many chemical agents are made volatile so they can be dispersed over a large region quickly.

Chemical weapons are classified as weapons of mass destruction by the United Nations, and their production and stockpiling was outlawed by the **Chemical Weapons Convention of 1993.** Under the Convention, chemicals that are toxic enough to be used as chemical weapons, or may be used to manufacture such chemicals, are divided into three groups according to their purpose and treatment:

Schedule 1: Have few, if any, legitimate uses. These may only be produced or used for research, medical, pharmaceutical or protective purposes (mustard gas, lewisite).

Schedule 2: Have no large-scale industrial uses, but may have legitimate small-scale uses (dimethyl methylphosphonate, a precursor to sarin).

Schedule 3: Have legitimate industrial uses (phosgene, chloropicrin).

The earliest target of chemical weapon agent research was not toxicity, but development of agents that can affect a target through the skin and clothing, rendering protective gas masks useless. In July 1917, the Germans first employed mustard gas, the first agent that circumvented gas masks. Mustard gas easily penetrates leather and fabric to inflict painful burns on the skin.

Chemical weapon agents are also divided into lethal and incapacitating categories. A substance is classified as incapacitating if less than 1/100 of the lethal dose causes incapacitation, e.g., through nausea or visual problems. The distinction between lethal and incapacitating substances is not fixed, but relies on a statistical average called the LD_{50}.

Classes of chemical weapon agents: Chemical weapon agents are organized into several categories according to the manner in which they affect the human body. There are other chemicals used militarily that are not technically considered to be chemical weapon agents, such as:

1. *Defoliants* that destroy vegetation, but are not immediately toxic to human beings. (Agent Orange, for instance, used by the United States in Vietnam, contained dioxins and is known for its long-term cancer effects and for causing genetic damage leading to serious birth deformities).
2. *Incendiary or explosive chemicals* (such as napalm, extensively used by the United States in Vietnam, or dynamite) because their destructive effects are primarily due to fire or explosive force, and not direct chemical action.
3. *Biological warfare agents* that includes the viruses, bacteria, or other organisms, e.g., Bacillus anthracis, Clostridium botulinum, Brucella, Yersinia pestis, Ebola virus etc.

Use of Poison Gas in World War I: The French were the first to use chemical weapons during the First World War, using teargas. The first full-scale deployment of chemical weapon agents was during World War I, originating in the Second Battle of Ypres, when the Germans attacked French, Canadian and Algerian troops with chlorine gas.

Although crude chemical warfare has been employed in many parts of the world for thousands of years, modern chemical warfare began during World War I. Initially, only well-known commercially available chemicals and their variants were used. These included chlorine and phosgene gas. The methods of dispersing these agents during battle were relatively unrefined and inefficient.

Chemical Warfare in World War II: During World War II, chemical warfare was revolutionized by Nazi Germany's accidental discovery of the nerve agents tabun, sarin and soman. The Japanese used mustard gas and the recently-developed blister agent Lewisite against Chinese troops. During these attacks, the Japanese also employed biological warfare by intentionally spreading cholera, dysentery, typhoid, bubonic plague and anthrax.

Developments by the Western Governments: In 1952 the U.S. Army patented a process for the "Preparation of Toxic Ricin", publishing a method of producing this powerful toxin. Also in 1952, researchers in Porton Down, England, invented the VX nerve agent but soon abandoned the project. In 1958 the British government traded their VX technology with the United States in exchange for information on thermonuclear weapons; by 1961 the U.S. was producing large amounts of VX and performing its own nerve agent research. This research produced at least three more agents; the four agents (VE, VG, VM, VX) are collectively known as the "V-Series" class of nerve agents.

Classification of the Warfare Agents

Poisons used as war gases can be classified according to their primary physiological actions as:

Lung irritants (Asphyxiants or choking gases): (i) Chlorine (ii) Phosgene (iii) Chloropicrin (iv) Diphosgene.

Lacrimators (Tear gases): (i) Chloroacetophenone (C.A.P.) (ii) Bromobenzyl cyanide (B.B.C.) (iii) Ethyl-iodo-acetate (K.S.K.).

Vesicants (Blister gases): (i) Mustard gas (ii) Lewisite.

Sternutators (Nasal irritants or vomiting gases): (i) Diphenylchlorarsine (D.A.) (ii) Diphenyl-amine-chlorarsine (D.M.) (iii) Diphenyl-cyan-arsine (D.C.).

Paralysants (Nerve poisons): (i) Carbon monoxide (ii) Hydrocyanic acid (iii) Hydrogen sulphide.

Nerve gases: These are toxic chemicals having acetylcholine like action. These are (i) Tabun (GA) (ii) Sarin (GB) (iii) Soman (GD) and (iv) VX.

LUNG IRRITANTS

These are irritant gases that exert their main action on the pulmonary alveoli through the upper respiratory passage. Of these, chlorine and phosgene are the gases that are kept liquid under pressure. Chlorine has bleaching powder like smell whereas phosgene has musty odour. These can be released from tanks, gas shells and canisters.

Chloropicrin is a yellowish oily liquid having flypaper like odour and Diphosgene is also an oily liquid with smell of phosgene. Both phosgene and diphosgene are known as **Green cross**. Phosgene is 21/2 times more toxic than chloropicrin. Their effects are insidious that is why the victims can carry on work for a few hours after exposure.

Signs and Symptoms

Signs and symptoms develop within 2-4 hours of inhalation: (i) Lachrymation with conjunctivitis (ii) Coughing, dyspnoea with intense air hunger (iii) Feeling of pain and constriction in throat (iv) Headache, retching and vomiting (v) Restlessness, rapid and stertorous breathing (vi) Cyanosis and collapse (vii) Death from respiratory failure with acute pulmonary oedema within 24-48 hours.

Treatment

(i) The victim is removed into fresh air (ii) Artificial respiration and oxygen inhalation (iii) Cardiac and respiratory stimulants may be given (iv) Antibiotics should be given to combat infection (v) Atropine sulphate to relieve pulmonary oedema.

Autopsy Findings

(i) Lungs are congested and oedematous (ii) On dissection, frothy fluid mixed with blood oozes out of the lungs (iii) Petechial haemorrhages are seen markedly on pleura, pericardium and peritoneum (iv) There may be serous effusion in pleural cavities (v) All the organs are congested.

LACHRYMATORS (TEARGASES)

These are usually fired in artillery shells for the control of riots and are ordinarily harmless to life in concentrations obtained under such conditions. These are:

1. **Chloroacetphenone (C.A.P.):** It occurs in the form of finely divided powder that is colourless and odour of 'locust flowers' soluble in organic solvents.
2. **Bromobenzyl cyanide (B.B.C.):** It is a heavy dark brown oily liquid having the odour of 'sour' fruit.
3. **Ethyl-iodo-acetate (K.S.K.):** It is also a brown coloured liquid with odour of 'pear drops'.

Signs and Symptoms

Exposure to vapours of any of these compounds will produce: (i) Intense irritation of the eyes with severe lacrimation along with spasm of eyes and temporary blindness (ii) Irritating cough, burning sensation in throat with tracheitis and bronchitis (iii) Chest discomfort (iv) Nausea and vomiting (v) Pneumonitis, keratitis and corneal ulceration in rare cases (vi) B.B.C. and K.S.K. before volatilization may cause blistering and ulceration of skin and conjunctiva due to splashing.

Treatment

(i) Victim should be removed to fresh air (ii) Eyes should be thoroughly washed with fresh water or normal saline (iii) Respirators should be used to protect eyes and lungs from tear gases.

VESICANTS (BLISTERING) GASES

Both the mustard gas (dichlorethyl sulphide) and lewisite (chlorvinyl dichlorarsine) are volatile irritant liquids. The mustard gas is a heavy, dark and oily liquid that gives out vapours at ordinary temperatures. It has a garlicky odour whereas Lewisite has smell of geraniums. These are harmful in both gaseous and liquid form. They vapourise slowly and persist long after discharge. Mustard gas is more persistent than lewisite. The terrain occupied by mustard gas remains poisonous to human beings for 2-5 days. Mustard gas is also known as **'yellow cross'** was largely used during the Great wars.

Signs and Symptoms

Mustard gas acts insidiously and the effects usually appear after 2-4 hours: (i) Coryza and laryngitis (ii) Irritation of eyes, nose, throat and respiratory passages (iii) Lachrymation, conjunctivitis and photophobia (iv) Nausea, vomiting and pain abdomen (v) Intense itching, redness, vesication and ulceration of the skin of the moist areas such as axilla, groin and perineum as mustard gas passes through the clothes (vi) In severe cases, suppuration of eyelids, destruction of eyeball, fever, intractable cough and respiratory difficulties may occur (vii) The patients of mustard gas poisoning may die of bronchopneumonia and chronic bronchitis and bronchiectasis that are common complications.

Lewisite rapidly blisters the skin and causes inflammation of mucous membrane of larynx, trachea and bronchi. It also causes hemolysis, leucopenia and features similar to arsenic poisoning.

Treatment

(i) Patient should be immediately removed to fresh air (ii) All the clothing should be removed and body should be thoroughly washed with soap and water (iii) Eyes should be irrigated with cold water or 2% soda bicarbonate solution (iv) Nostrils to be irrigated with 5% soda bicarbonate solution (v) Burns should be treated with sodium bicarbonate dressing or tannic acid jelly (vi) B.A.L. can be given for Lewisite poisoning.

STERNUTATORS (NASAL IRRITANTS)

The sternutators or nasal irritants are diphenyl chlorarsine (D.A.), diphenylamine chlorarsine (D.M.), diphenyl cyanarsine (D.C.) which are fired by artillery shells. They are solid organic compounds of arsenic and get dispersed by heat on detonation in the form of fine particulates hanging in the air like cloud or smoke.

Signs and Symptoms

The persons inhaling the air or drinking the water contaminated by these chemicals suffer from: (i) Irritation of nostrils and sinuses (ii) Sneezing and coryza (iii) Generalised malaise and headache (iv) Excessive salivation (v) Nausea and vomiting (vi) Pain and oppression in the chest and prostration.

Sometimes features of arsenic toxicity result but fatality is unknown. The nasal irritants destroy the morale of the victim in losing confidence in the respirators.

Treatment

(i) Removal of the victim to fresh air (ii) Sodium bicarbonate is used as mouth wash (iii) Nasal irrigation with 5% sodium bicarbonate solution is advocated.

PARALYSANTS (NERVE AND BLOOD POISONS)

These include carbon monoxide, hydrocyanic acid and hydrogen sulphide gases. These are not very useful in chemical warfare as it is difficult to obtain them in lethal concentrations.

NERVE GASES

The nerve gases were developed in World War II but facts about them have been kept a secret. These are colourless and odourless liquids related to phosphate esters which produce poisonous vapours on evaporation. These are: (i) Tabun (GA) (ii) Sarin (GB) (iii) Soman (GD) and (iv) VX. They are absorbed from the lungs, G.I.T., skin and conjunctivae. They cause inactivation of cholinesterase and produce features of acetylcholine poisoning with constriction of pupil, coryza, choking, bronchial constriction and photophobia. Absorption of large amount causes severe bronchospasm, hypotension, unconsciousness and bradycardia resulting in cardiac arrest.

Efforts to Eradicate Chemical Weapons

1. **August 27, 1874: The Brussels Declaration** Concerning the Laws and Customs of War is signed, specifically forbidding the "employment of poison or poisoned weapons".
2. **September 4, 1900: The Hague Conference**, which includes a declaration banning the "use of projectiles the object of which is the diffusion of asphyxiating or deleterious gases", enters into force.
3. **February 6, 1922:** After World War I, the **Washington Arms Conference Treaty** prohibited the use of asphyxiating, poisonous or other gases. It was signed by the United States, Britain, Japan, France and Italy, but France objected to other provisions in the treaty and it never went into effect.
4. **September 7, 1929: The Geneva Protocol** enters into force, prohibiting the use of poison gas and bacteriological methods of warfare. As of 2004, there are 132 signatory nations.
5. **May 1991:** President George H.W. Bush unilaterally commits the United States to destroying all chemical weapons and to renounce the right to chemical weapon retaliation.
6. The U.S. Congress has since passed legislation requiring the destruction of the entire stockpile by December 31, 2004. Official U.S. policy is to support the Chemical Weapons Convention as a means to achieve a global ban on this class of weapons and to halt their proliferation.
7. **April 29, 1997:** The **Chemical Weapons Convention** enters into force, augmenting the Geneva Protocol of 1925 by outlawing the production, stockpiling and use of chemical weapons.

SHORT NOTE

1. War gases.

MULTIPLE CHOICE QUESTIONS

1. Which of the following is not a teargas?

(a) Chloroacetophenone (b) Ethyl iodoacetate
(c) Bromobenzyl cyanide (d) Diphenyl chlorarsine

2. Mustard gas is also known as:

(a) Yellow cross (b) Orange cross
(c) Golden cross (d) Silver cross

3. Both phosgene and diphosgene are known as:

(a) Yellow cross (b) Orange cross
(c) Green cross (d) Silver cross

4. Which of the following is not a nerve gas?

(a) Tabun (b) Sarin
(c) Soman (d) Chloropicrin

ANSWER KEY ☞

1. (d)	2. (a)	3. (c)	4. (d)

47 CHAPTER

Agrochemical Poisons

Pesticides are chemical compounds that are used to kill pests, including insects, rodents, fungi, unwanted plants and other organisms. The Food and Agriculture Organization (FAO) has **defined pesticide as**:

"*Any substance or mixture of substances intended for preventing, destroying or controlling any pest, including vectors of human or animal disease, unwanted species of plants or animals, causing harm during or otherwise interfering with the production, processing, storage, transport, or marketing of food, agricultural commodities, wood and wood products or animal feedstuffs, or substances that may be administered to animals for the control of insects, arachnids, or other pests in or on their bodies.*"

Pesticides enable the farmers to control their crops, from being destroyed by these agents. As a result, though the yields of food crops have reached new high levels but their extensive use by the agriculturists has resulted in poisoning of human beings and domestic animals.

Classification of Pesticides

I. Based on the Pests Which They Kill

A. **Insecticides:** Insecticides are the compounds that are employed for killing insects. They can be classified based on the origin and chemical composition.

1. *Chemical insecticides:* (A) *Inorganic* (i) Phosphorus (ii) Compounds of arsenic, antimony, mercury, barium, zinc, thallium (B) *Organic* (i) Organophosphorus compounds (a) Alkyl phosphates (b) Aryl phosphates (ii) Carbamates (iii) Chlorinated hydrocarbons (a) Indane derivatives (chlordane, heptachlor, aldrin, dieldrin, endrin, diendrin) (b) Chlorobenzene derivatives (DDT, chlorophenothane) (c) Benzene hexachloride (lindane, gammexane) (d) Chlorinated camphenes (toxaphene, strobane).
2. *Insecticides of vegetable origin:* (i) Nicotine (ii) Pyrethrins (iii) Rotenone.

B. **Rodenticides:** These are compounds that are employed to rats or other rodent pests. They are (i) *Inorganic compounds* (a) Aluminium phosphide (b) Zinc phosphide (c) Thallium (d) Phosphorus (ii) *Organic compounds* (a) Fluoroacetate (iii) Convulsants (a) Strychnine (iv) Anticoagulant (a) Warfarin.

C. **Fungicides:** These are chemicals that destroys fungus. These are mainly mercurial compounds.

D. **Herbicides:** Since the growth of undesirable herbs and weeds in the field yields low production, the herbicides or weed killers are used to protect the field. These are: (i) Sulphuric acid (1%); is a corrosive acid (ii) Sodium chlorate; is irritant (iii) Potassium cyanide; causes tissue anoxia (iv) Paraquat.

E. **Others:** (a) *Bactericides:* Kill bacteria, e.g., Oxytetracycline (b) *Avicides:* Kill birds, e.g., Strychnine (c) *Algicide:* Kill or inhibit algae, e.g., Copper sulphate (d) *Molluscicides:* Kill slugs and snails, e.g., Metaldehyde (e) *Acaricides:* Kill mites and ticks, e.g., DDT, permethrin (f) *Piscicides:* Act against fishes, e.g., Rotenone (g) Silvicides: Act against woody vegetations, e.g., Tebuthiuron.

II. Classification of Pesticides Based on Toxicity Levels

WHO classification has been aligned with the Acute Toxicity Hazard Categories from *The Globally Harmonized System of Classification and Labelling of Chemicals* (GHS). It is based primarily on the acute oral and dermal toxicity to the rat since these determinations are standard procedures in toxicology. The LD_{50} value is a statistical estimate of the number of mg of toxicant per kg of body weight required to kill 50% of a large population of test animals: the rat is used unless otherwise stated.

III. Based on Mode of Entry into the Body of Insects

1. ***Contact poisons***: E.g., Paraquat 2. ***Stomach poisons***: Calcium and lead arsenate 3. ***Fumigants***: It acts by producing vapor, e.g., Aluminum phosphide 4. ***Systemic insecticides***: Methyl demeton 5. ***Repellents***: Keep pests away, e.g., Methiocarb.

IV. Miscellaneous Classifications

The pesticides can also be classified based on the (i) Chemical composition (ii) Mode of action (iii) Stage specificity.

ORGANOPHOSPHORUS COMPOUNDS

Historical considerations: The first organophosphate insecticide was tetraethyl pyrophosphate (TEPP) and it was developed in Germany as a substitute for nicotine, which was in short supply in the country during World War II and in 1944, Parathion was synthesized. They are extensively used as agricultural insecticides being effective against a wide range of insects and pests. Nevertheless, a number of these compounds have proved to be more toxic to human beings, than to the insects and rodents. It is the most common agrochemical poisons.

Mode of Action

Organophosphates cause some degree of irritation to mucous membrane. They are primarily nerve poisons affecting both autonomic and central nervous system. On autonomic nervous system, it exerts parasympathomimetic action by inactivating cholinesterase. Therefore, both muscarinic and nicotinic action of acetylcholine is increased. It causes depression of central nervous system.

Acetylcholine is recognized as mediator of impulses of autonomic ganglia. It is present in an inactive form that bounds loosely with a protein or lipoprotein. Acetylcholine as chemical transmitter plays a vital role to propagate nerve impulse across the synapses of peripheral and central nervous system. Traces of acetylcholine are produced at the myoneural junctions and synapses of the ganglions. On stimulation of the nerve, acetylcholine is set free and diffuses down the nerve fibers. These same nerve fibers contain an enzyme cholineacetylase that is capable of synthesizing acetylcholine with great rapidity. Free acetylcholine is unstable and gets spontaneously hydrolysed to choline and acetic acid, the hydrolysis getting accelerated by the enzyme, acetylcholinesterase present in the plasma, cell membrane or cytoplasm of many cells of the body. In blood and nerve tissue, cholinesterase inactivates acetylcholine after its liberation as shown below:

$$\text{Acetylcholine} \xrightarrow[\text{ACh esterase}]{} \text{Acetic acid + Choline}$$

Cholinesterases are of two types namely **true cholinesterase** that is present in blood cells and central nervous system whereas plasma and white matter of brain contains **pseudocholinesterase.** Usually true cholinesterase inactivates acetylcholine but when excess of acetylcholine escapes in the blood, plasma or

Table 47.1: WHO classification of pesticides

Class		LD_{50} for the rat (mg/kg body weight)		Examples
		Oral	Dermal	
Ia	Extremely hazardous	< 5	< 50	Parathion, Dieldrin, Phorate
Ib	Highly hazardous	5–50	50–200	Aldrin, Dichlorvos
II	Moderately hazardous	50–2000	200–2000	DDT, Chlordane
III	Slightly hazardous	Over 2000	Over 2000	Malathion
U	Unlikely to present acute hazard	5000 or higher		Carbetamide, Cycloprothrin

Table 47.2: GHS classification of pesticides

GHS Category	Criteria for Classification			
	Oral		Dermal	
	LD_{50} for the rat (mg/kg bw)	Hazard statement	LD_{50} for the rat (mg/kg bw)	Hazard statement
Category 1	< 5	Fatal if swallowed	< 50	Fatal in contact with skin
Category 2	5-50	Fatal if swallowed	5-50	Fatal in contact with skin
Category 3	50-300	Toxic if swallowed	50-300	Toxic in contact with skin
Category 4	300-2000	Harmful if swallowed	300-2000	Harmful in contact with skin
Category 5	2000-5000	May be harmful	2000-5000	May be harmful

pseudocholinestrase also plays a role. Cholinesterases are most effective in the presence of small amount of acetylcholine.

Organophosphorus compounds inactivate acetylcholine-sterase by the process of phosphorylation to facilitate the action of acetylcholine. This occurs first at the plasma level then at the cellular level of brain. As a result, there is accumulation of acetylcholine at the nerve endings resulting in interference at the passage of nerve impulses across the myoneural junctions and synapses of autonomic ganglions. As such, these compounds are known as Cholinesterase inhibitors. Hence, the action of organophosphorus will simulate actions of physostigmine, acetylcholine, pilocarpine and muscarine. A drop in the activity of cholinesterase to 25-30% of the normal value will be characterized by signs and symptoms compounded as: (i) Muscarinic like effect on the parasympathetic system affecting the postganglionic cholinergic nerve fibres (ii) Nicotinic like actions followed by paralysis of preganglionic sympathetic fibres and somatic motor nerves (iii) Effect on central nervous system with stimulation followed by depression (iv) Porphyrinuria leading to shedding of red tears **(Chromolachyrorrhoea)** due to accumulation of porphyrin in the lachrymal gland.

The Organophosphorus Compounds May Cause:

1. **Irreversible inhibition of cholinesterase due to:** (i) Direct action (TEPP) (ii) Delayed action (Parathion and Malathion).
2. **Reversible inhibition of cholinesterase:** (i) Carbamates (a) Carbaryl (b) Mactacil.

Organophosphorus compounds are divided mainly in two groups:

i. **Alkyl phosphate:** (a) TEPP (Tetraethyl-pyrophosphate) (b) HETP (Hexa-ethyl-pyrophosphate) (c) Dimefox (d) Malathion (e) Sulfotepp (f) Systox.

ii. **Aryl phosphates:** (a) Parathion (b) Paraoxon (c) Chlorothion (d) Methyl parathion (e) Diazinon (Diazion, TIK 20) (f) Methyl umbeliferone.

Routes of Absorption

(i) Absorption through intact skin (ii) Respiratory system by inhalation (iii) Gastrointestinal tract by ingestion (iv) Circulatory system by intramuscular and intravenous route.

Signs and Symptoms

1. **Muscarinic like effects:** Muscarinic receptors for acetylcholine are found primarily in the smooth muscles, the heart and exocrine glands. The muscarinic like effects produced by the organophosphorus compounds are: (i) Tightness in the chest (ii) Wheezing respiration (expiration due to bronchoconstriction) (iii) Increased bronchial secretion (iv) Increased salivation (v) Increased sweating (vi) Tone and peristalsis is increased (vii) Nausea, vomiting and abdominal cramps (viii) Diarrhoea (ix) Tenesmus and involuntary defecation (x) Bradycardia and heart block (xi) Frequent and involuntary urination due to constriction of smooth muscles of bladder (xii) Constriction of pupil causing miosis. The muscarinic effects can be remembered by the acronym **SLUDGE**: **S**alivation, **L**acrimation, **U**rination, **D**efecation/Diarrhoea, **G**astrointestinal distress and **E**mesis.
2. **Nicotinic like symptoms:** Nicotinic signs and symptoms result from the accumulation of acetylcholine at the endings of motor nerves to skeletal muscle and autonomic ganglia. The effects include: (i) Easy fatigability and mild weakness followed by involuntary twitching, fasciculation and cramps (ii) Muscles of respiration are affected leading to dyspnea and cyanosis. Nicotinic action at autonomic ganglia masks the muscarinic effects. Thus: (iii) Tachycardia is produced instead of bradycardia (iv) Pallor (v) Blood pressure is raised (vi) Hyperglycemia (vii) Cardiac arrhythmias (viii) Pulmonary edema.
3. **Accumulation of acetylcholine in central nervous system** (i) Anxiety, tension and confusion (ii) Restlessness, insomnia and headache (iii) Irritability and neurosis (iv) Excessive dreaming and nightmares (v) Slurred speech and tremors (vi) Ataxia and convulsion (vii) Depression of respiratory and circulatory centers (viii) Coma leading to death.

Intermediate syndrome is a distinct clinical entity characterized by prominent weakness of neck flexors, muscles of respiration and proximal limb muscles. It usually occurs 24 to 96 hours after the ingestion of an OP compound after an initial cholinergic crisis, but before organophosphate-induced delayed polyneuropathy. The exact pathogenesis of intermediate syndrome is not known; however, the proposed mechanisms include persistent inhibition of AChE leading to functional paralysis of neuromuscular transmission, muscle necrosis, and oxidative free radical damage to the receptors.

Fatal Dose: TEPP is most toxic whereas HETP is the least toxic comparatively as 5 mg I.M. or 25 mg taken orally of TEPP produces toxic symptoms. The fatal dose of various organophosphorus compounds are:

- *TEPP:* 50 mg I.M. or 100 mg oral.
- *Parathion:* 80 mg I.M. or 100-175 mg oral.
- *HETP:* 160 mg I.M. or 350 mg oral.
- *OMPA:* 80 mg I.M. or 175 mg oral.
- *Malathion and Diazinon (Tik 20):* 1 gm oral.

Fatal Period: In fatal doses symptoms start within half an hour and death occurs within three hours. In nonfatal cases, effects last for 36 hours and fade off in 48-72 hours to 3 weeks. Blood cholinesterase level drops to 22-28% that is up to 50% of the normal value. Normal value is 77-142 units in red blood cells that is more appropriate than the plasma levels of 41-140 units. About 3% of the population suffers from congenital cholinesterase deficiency and the level decreases in patients with severe liver disease.

Diagnosis

1. **Cholinesterase level in blood:** As organophosphates inhibit cholinesterase activity, level of cholinesterase should be estimated in the blood. The normal level of cholinesterase is about 77-142 in red cells and 41-140 in the plasma. In organophosphorus poisoning, the cholinesterase activity of blood and plasma falls by 25-85% of its normal value. Periodic measurements of blood cholinesterase level helps in detection of poisoning because marked depression of cholinesterase activity of blood occurs, before the symptoms become evident. Normally the symptoms may not appear until the level of cholinesterase falls by 20% or less. Five ml of heparinized blood should be collected for estimating level of cholinesterase in blood.
2. **Cholinesterase level in the motor end plates:** The cholinesterase level can be demonstrated histochemically in muscles kept at room temperature for 1-2 days and up to several months when kept at 4° C. The cholinesterase activity at the myoneural junction is not affected by embalming the body or if the tissue is fixed by formalin or acetone up to 24 hours.
3. **Test by atropine:** When 2 mg of atropine is given intravenously, there are signs of atropinisation in a normal individual, while in a case of organophosphorus poisoning it will have no effect.

Treatment

(i) Remove the patient from the source of exposure (ii) Strip off contaminated clothing (iii) Wash all parts with soap and water under the shower bath (iv) Give life supporting measures such as oxygen inhalation (v) Gastric lavage with 2% potassium permanganate (vi) Purgatives like sodium or magnesium sulphate 30 gm orally (vii) Dehydration and shock must be treated (viii) Diazepam intravenously should be given to control convulsions (ix) Morphine and aminophylline are not to be given (x) ***Exchange transfusion:*** It takes 2-3 months for complete recovery after exchange transfusion. Blood cholesterol level should be checked every 15 days (xi) ***Atropine sulphate*** is the readily available best-known antidote against all organophosphorus compounds. It inactivates acetylcholine, arrests muscarinic and other effects but not the nicotinic action. Atropine sulphate, 2-4 mg is given I.V. or I.M. in adults and 0.05 mg/kg in children. The dose is to be repeated as 2-4 mg I.M. every 20-30 minutes until full **atropinization** is achieved. Then the dose has to be decreased and given less frequently. The repetition of dose of atropine depends upon severity of case:

- In mild cases, 2-4 mg I.M./I.V. initially that is to be repeated after 20 minutes as 2 mg and then repeated again.
- In moderate cases, 2-4 mg I.M./I.V. that is to be repeated after 10 minutes interval.
- In severe cases, 4-6 mg I.M./I.V. that is to be repeated after 3-10 minutes interval. Then total 50 mg is administered in 24 hours.
- Usually 40-50 mg may be required during first 24 hours and 12 mg may be given safely in the first 6 hours.

Signs of atropinization: (i) Flushing of face (ii) Dry mouth and dry, warm skin (iii) Blurring of vision (iv) Dilatation of pupil (v) Rapid and irregular pulse (vi) Loss of neuromuscular coordination.

Precautions while atropinization: (i) Adequate oxygen therapy should be given simultaneously to prevent myocardial infarction (ii) Drug should be withdrawn judiciously as there may be rapid development of pulmonary oedema and respiratory depression (iii) Atropine is ineffective against autonomic ganglionic actions of acetylcholine and peripheral neuromuscular paralysis occurs (iv) To combat overdosage of atropine, physostigmine salicylate should be administered in the dose as given below:

- In adults, 1-2 mg I.M./I.V.; to be repeated up to a total of 6 mg.
- In children, 0.5 mg I.M./I.V.; to be repeated up to a total of 2 mg.

The dose of atropine should be reduced when oximes are given together.

(xii) ***Specific Reactivator Oximes***: Relief of muscle weakness in particular respiratory paralysis can be achieved with certain Oximes (pralidoxime, obidoxime, HLö 7 and HI-6), which can reactivate the cholinesterase by reversing the phosphate ester bond formed at the enzyme active site (Cholinesterases and organic phosphates are bound by phosphate bond). However, the choline esterase enzyme does not remain susceptible to reactivation by the oximes forever because of the phenomenon of ageing. Ageing refers to a process whereby phosphorylated acetylcholinesterase may lose an alkyl side chain non-enzymatically, leaving a hydroxyl group in its place. Oximes should be used within 48 hours. Pralidoxime (2-PAM) remains the most widely used amongst oximes and it has four salts namely: Pralidoxime chloride (2-PAM Cl), methiodide, metilsulfate and mesylate (P2S).

- **PAM (Pralidoxime chloride):** Protopam chloride is to be given 1 gm I.V. over a period of 2 minutes or in 250 ml of normal saline infusion for 20-30 minutes that is to be repeated after 8-12 hours. In children 25-50 mg I.M. or I.V./kg body weight is to be given within 2 minutes or as an infusion for 20-30 minutes.
- **P_2AM (Pyridine-2-aldoxime methiodide)** can be given as 50 mg/kg in one litre of normal saline slowly to be followed by another litre of same infusion over a period of 12 hours.
- **DAM (Diacetyl monoxime)** can be given as 2 gm in one litre of normal saline slowly.

- **P_2S (Pyridine-2-aldoxime methane sulfonate)** is given in the dose of 1-2 gm in adults and 25-50 mg/kg in children. The dose is to be repeated every 12 hours.

  Atropine works on muscarinic and other effects but not on the nicotinic action and oxime works on nicotinic effects. Hence, atropine must be given before 2-PAM to avoid worsening of muscarinic-mediated symptoms.

  Adverse reactions of Specific Reactivator Oximes: (i) When given intravenously, it produces tachycardia and muscular rigidity (ii) When given intramuscularly, conjunctival hyperemia is produced (iii) When given orally nausea, vomiting and diarrhoea may result.

(xiii) ***Newer modalities of treatment:*** Various studies have been conducted regarding these modalities of therapy but results are inconclusive. These new therapies can be used as adjuvant to standard therapy.

(a) **Magnesium sulphate:** It blocks ligand-gated calcium channels which inhibits acetylcholine release in the central nervous system and at peripheral sympathetic and parasympathetic synapses. It also reduces CNS overstimulation mediated via NDMA activation. Few studies reported use of intravenous MgSO4 decreases mortality compared to usual care (b) **Clonidine:** It is a centrally acting alpha-2 receptor agonist which inhibits presynaptic release of acetylcholine, thereby decreasing the cholinergic symptoms caused by organophosphate poisoning. It has synergistic action with atropine (c) **Sodium bicarbonate:** It is used to treat metabolic acidosis. IV infusion of sodium bicarbonate may even be more beneficial in nerve agents poisoning (d) **Fresh frozen plasma (FFP) or albumin:** Useful therapy through clearing of free organophosphates (e) **Antioxidant:** Vitamin E reduces oxidative stress in OP poisoning (f) **Haemodialysis, hemoperfusion or hemofiltration:** Its role still not clear (g) **Recombinant bacterial phosphotriesterases and hydrolases that are able to transfer organophosphorus:** Degrading enzymes are very promising in delayed treatment of OP poisoning.

Prophylaxis from organophosphorus poisoning: (i) Body should be properly protected while spraying in the fields with aprons, gloves and masks. (ii) Agriculturist should not spray for more than 2-4 hours a day and should not work for more than 6-7 successive days. (iii) He should not eat, drink, chew or smoke while spraying. (iv) After the operation, the face, hands, feet, eyes should be washed thoroughly with soap and water. (v) Even the spraying machines, tanks or containers and hoses should be washed after each operation. (vi) When the worker is suffering from upper respiratory tract infection, he should restrain from spraying.

Autopsy Findings

(i) Findings of asphyxia such as congestion of face and cyanosis of lips, nails and mucous membranes is present. (ii) At times blood-tinged froth is found over the nostrils and mouth. (iii) Smell of kerosene may be present on opening the oesophagus and stomach. (iv) The mucosa of stomach is congested and submucosal petechial hemorrhages are present. (v) Frothy fluid at times tinged with blood may be found in the trachea and bron[illegible] (vi) Lungs show congestion and gross edema and submucosal hemorrhages. (vii) Brain shows petechial hemorrhages, is congested and oedematous and the meninges are dilated.

Medicolegal Aspects

(i) Accidental poisoning occurs usually during manufacturing, spraying or dusting in the field and when mixed with other foodstuffs. In the Kerala food poisoning tragedy in 1958, about 100 people died due to inadvertent stocking of foodstuffs and parathion. (ii) It is less frequently used as homicidal poison. (iii) Most commonly used for suicidal purposes next to barbiturates due to their easy availability, quick action, are cheap and can be easily purchased for domestic use.

CARBAMATES POISONING

Carbamates are derivatives of carbonic acid. They are marketed in the form of dusts or solutions. These are of two types depending on their toxicity such as: (i) *Highly toxic:* Carbaryl (Sevin), Carbofuran (Furaxdan), Propoxur (Baygon), Methomyl. (ii) *Moderately toxic:* Aminocarb (Matacil), Aprocarb (Baygon), Aldicard (Temik), Carbendezin, Triallate.

Signs and Symptoms

Signs and symptoms are similar to those of organophosphorous poisoning except: (i) Symptoms begin within 15 min-2 hours. (ii) Carbamates hydrolyse spontaneously from sites of cholinesterase enzyme within 24-48 hours. (iii) Carbamates do not penetrate effectively central nervous system thus their toxicity is limited.

Treatment

(i) Atropine is specific. (ii) Pralidoxime (2-PAM) is helpful in diminishing severity of symptoms and preventing morbidity. Besides this it improves respiratory functions as well as patient's well-being. (iii) Benzodiazepines are used for the treatment of seizures and agitation for intubated patients.

PARAQUAT POISONING

Uses: Paraquat is a herbicide that is sprayed on unwanted weeds and other vegetation before planting crops. It is absorbed by the foliage and rapidly kills the plant, but is inactivated when in contact with the soil, so cannot harm the seeds or young plants that are placed in the same ground a short time later.

Properties: Paraquat and the Diquat are both dipyridyl compounds and paraquat is 1 : 1 dimethyl 4 : 4 bipyridium. It is produced commercially as a brownish concentrated liquid of the dichloride salt at 10-30% strength. Both are water soluble herbicides supplied in 20-25% concentration in bulk to the farmers and horticulturists. It is marketed under the trade name Gamaxone or Weedol.

Toxicity: (i) Ingestion most commonly (ii) Inhalation through spraying of liquid stored in soft drink bottles (iii) Skin contamination during spraying.

Fatal Dose: 4 mg/kg body weight.

Fatal Period: 3-5 days.

Signs and Symptoms

(i) Paraquat is irritant to epithelial tissues in concentrated form and causes erosion of the mucous membrane of the lips, tongue (paraquat tongue) mouth, pharynx and esophagus. The presence of prominent pharyngeal membrane can lead to an erroneous diagnosis of tonsillar diphtheria. (ii) Burning sensation of mouth and throat, nausea, vomiting and diarrhea observed. (iii) At times esophageal perforation occurs resulting in mediastinitis. (iv) Lungs are usually affected because of aspiration of irritating liquid while regurgitation or swallowing. The lungs become markedly edematous and at times weigh upto 2000 gm. The outer surface may be indented by the ribs. On cut section frothy fluid comes out. (v) Paraquat produces lung damage in two phases, initially from destructive alveolitis over 1-3 days followed by proliferative phase leading to fibrosis. This type of lung is known as **Paraquat lung.** (vi) Renal failure may develop within 2-3 days. (vii) Death is due to failure of vital organs like liver and kidney.

Laboratory Findings

(i) Elevation of blood urea, serum alkaline phosphatases and bilirubin are characteristic of kidney and liver damage (ii) Serum trypsin inhibitor gets depressed indicating extent of damage to lungs.

Treatment

(i) Stomach wash using 4-7% bentonite-magma solution and repeated with caution and some of it is left in the stomach (ii) Activated charcoal should be given orally (iii) There is no known antidote (iv) Forced diuresis is started as early as possible to prevent renal damage (v) Hemodialysis to remove any poison left after forced diuresis (vi) Glucocorticoids for progressive lung proliferative lesions (vii) Supportive therapy (viii) Fullers earth or 7% bentonite should be given.

Autopsy Findings

(i) Ulceration of mouth and lips may be present (ii) Centrilobular necrosis of the liver with giant mitochondria and crystalline inclusion bodies are seen on electron microscopy (iii) Diffuse tubular damage of the kidneys (iv) Proliferative damage to the lungs is characteristic lesion of paraquat poisoning. When paraquat reaches the distal air spaces, diffuse pulmonary oedema and haemorrhages occur.

Medicolegal Aspects

(i) Suicidal poisoning by deliberate self ingestion of the liquid (ii) Accidental poisoning resulting from ingestion.

CHLORINATED HYDROCARBON INSECTICIDES

D.D.T. (Chlorophenothane) is the most commonly used chlorinated hydrocarbon insecticide in agriculture and public health. The commonly used agents are Endrin, Aldrin, Chlordane, Dieldrin, Lindane (Gammexene), Methoxychlor, Toxaphene and D.D.D. (Dichloro-diphenyl-dichloroethane). Even though some of the compounds individually exhibit differences in chemical configuration and physiological actions, from chemical standpoint, their effects on human beings are essentially the same and hence can be described in a group. Poisoning by Endrin is more common than D.D.T. in rural India.

D.D.T. (DICHLORODIPHENYLTRICHLOROETHANE)

Properties: D.D.T. is white crystalline powder with faint aromatic odour. It is insoluble in water but soluble in kerosene, vegetable oil and other organic solvents. While dusting as powder, it is to be diluted to 10% with powdered chalk or kaolin. It can be used as spray in 5% solution diluted with suitable solvents.

Uses: D.D.T. acts as both insecticide and pesticide to kill mosquitoes, flies, bedbugs, lice, arthropods and other insects. They usually become resistant to D.D.T. later on.

Routes of Absorption

In pure solid form, it does not get absorbed through skin but when it is dissolved in kerosene oil or other solvents, it gets easily absorbed through the gastrointestinal tract, skin and lungs. A 2% solution of D.D.T. acts as poison to human beings and its solution in fatty acids increases the toxicity. D.D.T. powder is safe for dusting animals.

Mode of Action

(i) It first stimulates then depresses the cerebellum and motor cortex. (ii) It sensitizes the myocardium to the action of catecholamines, so that injection of epinephrine may induce ventricular fibrillation. (iii) It depresses adrenal cortex causing irritation and sensitization of the skin. (iv) Locally it acts as an irritant, when swallowed. (v) Chronic exposure causes liver necrosis, degeneration of renal tubules, myocardium and voluntary muscles.

Fatal Dose:

- *D.D.T.:* 30 gm or 0.5 gm/kg.
- *Lindane:* 15 gm.
- *Chlordane:* 30 gm.
- *Methoxychlor:* 350 gm.

Acute Poisoning

The signs and symptoms develop within half an hour of ingestion of the poison: (i) Salivation, nausea, vomiting and abdominal pain (ii) Apprehension, hyperexcitability, restlessness, nervousness (iii) Tinnitus and vertigo (iv) Blurred vision with twitching of eyelids that is followed by muscular tremors, first affecting the head and neck, then involving the extremities (v) Tonic clonic convulsions are characteristic of D.D.T., Aldrin, dieldrin and lindane poisoning (vi) Generalised epileptiform convulsions occur in toxaphene poisoning (vii) Rarely muscular weakness, ataxia, incoordination, numbness and paralysis may occur (viii) Pulmonary oedema, respiratory distress, fall of B.P., delirium and unconsciousness, coma and collapse occurs (ix) Death occurs from respiratory failure.

Chronic Poisoning

After absorption, these insecticides gets accumulated in body fat and concentration gradually falls over several months. The workers with history of many months of exposure having more than 648 ppm of D.D.T. in their fat suffer from chronic poisoning. The signs and symptoms are: (i) Anorexia, nausea and vomiting (ii) Cachexia, loss of weight, anaemia (iii) Anxiety, headache, hyperirritability (iv) Blurred vision (v) Tremors, convulsions and coma (vi) Liver is moderately enlarged.

Treatment

(i) Immediate gastric lavage with 0.2% potassium permanganate (ii) Emetics should be given (iii) There is no known antidote of D.D.T. (iv) Cathartics, fats or oils should be avoided as they promote absorption (v) Atropine sulphate should be administered (vi) Oxygen inhalation and artificial respiration is given (vii) To control muscular twitching, tremors and convulsion, Thiopentone sodium 100-250 mg I.V. followed by I.M. injection of 100 mg of Phenobarbital sodium (viii) Calcium gluconate 10 ml of 10% with glucose I.V. and calcium lactate orally are beneficial (ix) Adrenaline, epinephrine should not be used as they induce ventricular fibrillation. Morphine is also avoided (x) For skin contamination, thorough washing with soap and water (xi) In chronic poisonings, the patient should be removed from the site of exposure and given low fat, high protein and carbohydrate diet. The treatment is symptomatic.

Autopsy Findings

(i) Stomach contents may smell of kerosene and are bloodstained (ii) Mucosa of stomach and intestines is congested and haemorrhagic (iii) Liver is enlarged with fatty degeneration (iv) Lungs are congested and oedematous (v) Spleen, brain and kidneys are congested.

ENDRIN

Properties: Endrin is the most toxic of all the chlorinated hydrocarbons. It is 12-15 times more toxic than D.D.T. and 3 times more toxic than Aldrin and dieldrin. It is insoluble in water, sparingly soluble in alcohol and freely soluble in aromatic hydrocarbons and fats. It remains stable for months or years.

Uses: Several preparations containing endrin are sold in the market in 20-25% concentration mixed with petroleum hydrocarbon. They all smell like kerosene. Endrin is also known as **plant penicillin** as it is a popular pesticide against insect pests of cotton, paddy, sugarcane and tobacco. It is used as spray in solutions, or as dust mixed with some other inert powders. It is marketed under the trade name Endox DR-50 Trafdrine and Endrex.

Absorption: Endrin is not absorbed through intact skin in dry powder state and poorly absorbed from the gastrointestinal tract mucosa but when it is dissolved in oil it gets freely absorbed from skin as well as mucous membrane.

Fatal Dose: 5-6 gms.

Fatal Period: Usually 1-2 hours (1-2 days rarely).

Mode of Action

(i) Has no effect on cholinesterases (ii) It is neurotoxic primarily acting on central nervous system, causing respiratory failure.

Signs and Symptoms

(i) Salivation, nausea, vomiting and abdominal discomfort (ii) Apprehension, hyperexcitability, restlessness, nervousness, incoordination and ataxia followed by mental confusion and delirium (iii) Profuse frothing at mouth and nostrils (iv) Tonic clonic convulsions (v) Unconsciousness, coma and collapse and death from respiratory failure.

Diagnosis

To diagnose, chemical examination of blood and subcutaneous fat is undertaken.

Treatment

(i) Immediate gastric lavage with 0.2% potassium permanganate (ii) Emetics should be given (iii) There is no known antidote of endrin (iv) Cathartics, fats or oils should be avoided as they promote absorption (v) Atropine sulphate should be administered (vi) Oxygen inhalation and artificial respiration (vii) To control convulsions, Thiopentone sodium 100-250 mg I.V. followed by I.M. injection of 100 mg of Phenobarbital sodium should be given (viii) Calcium gluconate 10 ml of 10% with glucose I.V. and calcium lactate orally are beneficial (ix) Adrenaline, epinephrine should not be used as they induce ventricular fibrillation. Morphine is also avoided (x) For skin contamination, thorough washing with soap and water is recommended (xi) In chronic poisonings, the patient should be removed from the site of exposure and given low fat, high protein and carbohydrate diet. The treatment is entirely symptomatic.

Autopsy Findings

(i) Congestion of face. (ii) Cyanosis of lips and fingertips. (iii) Conjunctiva is congested and pupils are dilated. (iv) Blood stained frothy fluid discharge smelling of kerosene comes out of mouth and nostrils. (v) Gastrointestinal tract is congested and stomach contents are bloodstained and smell of kerosene is present. (vi) Respiratory tract mucosa is congested, oedematous containing bloodstained frothy fluid mixed with mucus. (vii) Lungs are congested and oedematous with subpleural ecchymotic patches. (viii) Evidence of hepatic and renal tubular degeneration. (ix) Blood remains fluid and dark for long. (x) Subpericardial and subendocardial haemorrhages are seen.

Medicolegal Aspects

(i) For homicidal purposes, it may be given mixed with sweets, food and alcohol to mask its smell. (ii) Suicidal use is quite common in spite of its unpleasant smell and painful death. (iii) Accidental poisoning occurs commonly from skin contamination while spraying. (iv) Endrin resists putrefaction for a long time that is why it can be detected in the viscera for long after death.

PYRETHROIDS

Pyrethroids are insecticides (according to the WHO classification belongs to fourth group of insecticides) widely used in agriculture, household forestry and horticulture. They are synthetic derivatives of natural pyrethrins extracted from *Chrysanthemum cinerariaefolium*. Pyrethroids are divided into two groups: Type I and Type II, depending on the structure of the compound, and their action and undesirable symptoms they cause. Common Pyrethroids used are permethrin (Type I), deltamethrin (Type II), and cypermethrin (Type II). They primarily enter the body through skin contact but also through inhalation or food/water ingestion. They are highly toxic to insects (2250 times more toxic to insects than mammals) because insects have increased sodium channel sensitivity, smaller body size, and lower body temperature.

Mechanism of Action

Type I pyrethroids are ion channel toxins (mainly on sodium) prolonging neuronal excitation, but are not directly cytotoxic. Type II pyrethroids act on chloride channels, including GABA-dependent ones in addition to their effects on sodium channels.

Signs and Symptoms

Type I pyrethroids cause *Band or tremor type syndrome* which is characterized by tremors of the whole body, aggressive behaviour, hypersensitivity and ataxia.

Type II pyrethroids produce salivation, hyperexcitability, choreoathetosis and seizures. Both produce potent sympathetic activation. Skin contamination produces paresthesia. Ingestion causes sore throat, nausea, vomiting, mouth ulceration, convulsions and coma.

Treatment

(i) Management is mainly supportive care and symptomatic (ii) Gastric lavage (iii) Atropine (0.5-10 mg) is given to decrease salivation and pulmonary edema (iv) Seizures should be controlled (ii) No specific antidote is available.

Medicolegal Aspects

(i) Toxicity is mostly accidental (ii) Suicide and homicide due to pyrethroids are rare.

NAPHTHALENE (TAR, CAMPHOR, $C_{10}H_8$)

Properties: It occurs as large white crystalline plaques from coal tar distillation having a characteristic odour. It is insoluble in water but freely soluble in ether, chloroform, alcohol and oils. It sublimes at ordinary temperatures.

Uses: (i) It is used commercially as **moth repellant**, wool preservative and as deodorant in lavatories. (ii) It is also used in the manufacture of indigo and azo dyes. (iii) Chlorinated naphthalene is used for giving insulated coating on electrical wires and other electrical equipments.

Mode of Action

It produces haemolysis, causing blockade of renal tubules by precipitated haemoglobin and may cause hepatic necrosis. Only the patients with deficiency of glucose-6-phosphate-dehydrogenase in the red cells result in low level of reduced glutathione and increased susceptibility to hemolysis by the metabolites of naphthalene. In children below 6 years absorption occurs quickly.

Fatal Dose: 2 gm.

Fatal Period: Few hours to 2-3 days.

Signs and Symptoms

On ingestion of naphthalene: (i) Nausea, vomiting, diarrhoea, abdominal pain and hepatomegaly (ii) Headache, excitement, delirium, muscular twitchings and staggering gait (iii) Cyanosis, tachycardia and drowsiness resulting in coma, collapse and death (iv) Profuse sweating (v) Burning micturition, pain in loin and hypogastrium, oliguria and haematuria (vi) Urine is dark brown containing albumin, casts and haemoglobin (vii) Acute nephritis, haemolytic anemia, jaundice and optic atrophy are characteristic features (viii) Anemia and leucocytosis on hematological examination.

On inhalation of naphthalene vapours: (i) Headache, malaise and tinnitus (ii) Photophobia, conjunctivitis, retina and choroid plexus are affected (iii) Nausea and vomiting (iv) Anemia and jaundice (v) Severe hyperthermia due to the formation of **naphthylamine**.

Contamination of skin: (i) Dermatitis with scaling-weeping-crusting of skin and pruritis (ii) Conjunctivitis (iii) Headache (iv) Anemia, jaundice and hematuria.

Treatment

(i) Stomach wash with warm water to be followed by one ounce of saturated solution of magnesium sulphate. (ii) Oily and fatty preparations should be avoided as they dissolve the poison. (iii) Whole blood transfusion followed by sodium bicarbonate 15 gm orally every 4 hours or exchange transfusion will be helpful in nervous complications. (iv) 5% Dextrose saline is given I.V. for anuria. (v) Glucocorticoids should be administered as they prevent naphthalene hemolysis. (vi) Diet rich in proteins, carbohydrates and vitamins but poor in fat to be given.

Autopsy Findings

(i) Skin is pale and yellow due to anemia and jaundiced (ii) Gastrointestinal tract mucosa is inflamed, congested and tinged yellow (iii) Larynx and trachea contains blood stained froth (iv) Kidneys are congested (v) Liver is enlarged and congested and showing features of fatty degeneration.

Medicolegal Aspects

(i) Accidental poisoning is common in children as they ingest naphthalene balls and in adults resulting from inhalation of naphthalene vapours due to heavy dusting of bed clothes. (ii) Very few cases of suicide using naphthalene balls have been reported. (iii) Homicidal poisoning is also quite rare.

ALUMINIUM PHOSPHIDE

Aluminium phosphide (AlP) is a metal phosphide (other examples Zinc phosphide, potassium phosphide, sodium phosphide, etc.), solid, cheap, effective, commonly used fumigant. It can be formulated in the form of tablets, pellets, granules or as a dust. Aluminium phosphide (AlP) tablets are dark grey in colour, marketed under the names of 'Celphos', 'Alphos' or 'Quickphos' etc. It is known as the **Agent of sure death.** A single grayish green tablet weighs 3 gm mixed with urea and ammonium carbonate. Each tablet releases 1 gm of phosphine gas (PH_3) that on contact with water or acids is poisonous not only to rodents and insects but also to human beings.

Fatal Dose: 150-500 mg (1 tablet).

Fatal Period: 12-36 hours.

Mechanism of Action

On exposure to air and moisture or gastric acid the aluminium phosphide tablets releases phosphine gas. The reaction is:

$$ALP + 3H_2O \rightarrow Al(OH)_3 + PH_3 \text{ (Phosphene)}$$

$$ALP + 3HCl \rightarrow AlCl_3 + PH_3 \text{ (Phosphene)}$$

The phosphene inhibits cytochrome c oxidase in mitochondria that blocks cellular respiration. Pure phosphene gas is colourless and odourless, however, due to the presence of substituted phosphines and diphosphines, it has a foul odour resembling **decaying fish or garlic.** Phosphene gas is inflammable and may spontaneously ignite in air.

Uses: Aluminium phosphide is widely used in grains and fruit preservatives. It is also used as fumigant to destroy grain insects and rodents. The tablets are removed from airtight containers and mixed with grains that on contact with moisture and air, liberates phosphine and thus fumigates the grains.

Signs and Symptoms

Phosphene when inhaled by human beings results in severe pulmonary oedema. Due to the release of phosphine gas in contact with moisture, symptoms of severe gastrointestinal tract irritation are produced that cause cardiovascular collapse and death. The aluminium phosphide poisoning has a high mortality.

The signs and symptoms produced because of aluminium phosphide poisoning are: Nausea, vomiting and burning pain in the epigastrium: (i) **Garlicky (fishy) odour from breath** (ii) Intense thirst and diarrhoea (iii) Tightness in the chest and dyspnoea (iv) Excitement and agitation (v) Oliguria (vi) Arrhythmias (vii) Hypocalcemia tetany, convulsions and coma (viii) Shock (ix) Hypotension (x) Myocardial damage (xi) Cold clammy skin with respiratory distress in terminal stages (xii) Rarely muscular wasting, bleeding diathesis, cardiac complications like pericarditis, congestive cardiac failure (xiii) Death occurs due to cardiac failure.

Laboratory Diagnosis

(i) ECG abnormalities such as (a) P waves and PR interval is normal (b) Elevation of ST segments in V_1-V_5. Later depression of ST segment (c) T-inversion in all leads (d) Sinus tachycardia, bradycardia and heart block (ii) Increased SGOT level suggestive of myocardial necrosis (iii) Chest X-ray shows pulmonary oedema.

Tests for aluminum phosphide: Silver nitrate impregnated paper test is a simple, reliable, sensitive bedside method to detect phosphine (PH_3) of aluminum phosphide ingestion. The patient is asked to breathe on a piece of filter paper in the form of mass impregnated with 0.1 N silver nitrate solution for a period of 5-10 minutes. If the paper is blackened, it indicates presence of phosphine in breath as silver nitrate is reduced to silver on exposure to phosphine. The gastric fluid also can be tested for presence of phosphene.

Management

(i) There is no specific antidote of aluminium phosphide. (ii) Early stomach wash using 3-5% sodium bicarbonate, 1% copper sulphate, 1% potassium permanganate (1:5000 solution) or mineral oil should be carried. All these compounds convert it to phosphate within half an hour and thus reduces the available toxic dose of phosphene. Recent studies advocate not to carry out stomach wash because in contact of moisture, the remaining aluminium phosphide in the stomach is converted into phosphine. (iii) *Magnesium sulphate (25%)* is given I.M. or I.V. to correct arrhythmias as 3 gm bolus followed by an infusion of 6 gm for 24 hours for a period of 5-7 days. (iv) Digoxine 0.5 mg I.V. is given followed orally by1 tablet. Aluminium phosphide depresses cardiac functions due to toxic myocarditis that can be reversed by rapid digitalization. (v) Steroids are given to control pulmonary oedema. (vi) Calcium salt is given intravenously. (vii) Low dose dopamine infusion to be given. (viii) Antibiotics are given to treat infection. (ix) To combat metabolic acidosis, sodium bicarbonate 50 meq is given every 15 minutes until arterial bicarbonate level increases above 15 mmol/l. (x) Oxygen inhalation and artificial respiration to maintain respiratory distress.

Role and distribution of magnesium in the body: In adults, 2000 meq of magnesium is present in the body, of which 60% is concentrated in the bones and 40% in the soft tissue. The plasma concentration of magnesium is 1.5-2.2 meq/l and 4-8 meq/day is excreted through the kidney into urine, milk, saliva and gastrointestinal tract. In cardiovascular system high concentration of magnesium of about 10-15 meq/litre produces symptoms similar to hyperalkalinity in where conduction time is increased and PR interval and QRS complex is lengthened. More than 15 meq/litre of magnesium causes cardiac arrest. Hypermagnesemia due to renal insufficiency results from the decreased excretion of magnesium. The manifestation starts at 12-15 meq/litre level resulting in respiratory paralysis. The above concentrations can vary independently and deficit in one compartment may not be accompanied by a significant change in the other.

Magnesium sulphate has membrane stabilizing effect. The exact mechanism is not known. It is used in patients with acute myocardial infarction and for treatment of tachycardia. Plasma concentration and muscle biopsy is required to diagnose magnesium deficiency, but exchange of magnesium does not occur between bone, plasma and intracellular components. In patients with renal failure the administration of magnesium is of little value as there is risk of hypermagnesemia.

Autopsy Findings

(i) Cyanosis is present (ii) In few cases, froth over the mouth and nostrils are present (iii) On opening the body, fishy or garlicky smell of phosphine gas is present (iv) All the internal organs are congested with petechial haemorrhages (v) Lungs are congested and oedematous with rupture of alveoli. In a study, pulmonary oedema is well established was 30 cases resulting from irritation from the phosphene gas (vi) Liver shows fatty degeneration and necrosis (vii) Heart shows myocardial necrosis.

Medicolegal Aspects

(i) Poisoning is most commonly suicidal and there is a drastic increase in mortality due to this poisoning in Haryana, Rajasthan and U.P. since the last 20-25 years. (ii) Accidental poisoning may occur rarely in farmers. (iii) Homicidal poisoning is uncommon owing to its taste and odour.

ZINC PHOSPHIDE

Zinc phosphide (Zn_2P_3) is a metal phosphide, dark grey, crystalline compound. It is commercially available in powder or pellet form. The trade names are 'Ratol', 'Ridal', 'Arrex', 'Commando' etc. It is commonly used as a rodenticide because of its low cost and high availability. It enters the body via skin, respiratory and gastrointestinal tracts.

Mechanism of Action

This is same as aluminum phosphide (phosphide on contact with moisture converted to phosphene which affects cellular respiration by inhibiting cytochrome c oxidase).

Signs and Symptoms

The features are non-specific like aluminum phosphide poisoning.

Treatment

Same as aluminum phosphide poisoning.

Medicolegal Aspects

(i) Mostly used as a rodenticide (ii) Commonly used for suicidal purpose (iii) Can be consumed accidentally.

LONG QUESTIONS

1. Describe the clinical features, diagnosis, management, autopsy findings and medicolegal aspects in a case of organophosphorus poisoning.
2. Classify pesticides. Describe in details signs and symptoms, management and autopsy findings in aluminium phosphide poisoning.

SHORT NOTES

1. Atropinisation.
2. Paraquat lung.
3. Pralidoxime.
4. Chromolachyrorrhoea.

MULTIPLE CHOICE QUESTIONS

1. **All of the following are the features of organophosphorus poisoning *except:***
   (a) Sweating
   (b) Miosis
   (c) Respiratory Depression
   (d) Tachycardia

2. **Pralidoxime is not useful in poisoning with:**
   (a) Malathion (b) Parathion
   (c) Endrin (d) DFP

3. **Estimation of blood cholinesterase level helps in the diagnosis of poisoning due to:**
   (a) Endrin (b) Opium
   (c) DDT (d) Parathion

4. **Atropine is not used as antidote in poisoning by:**
   (a) TIK-20 (b) Parathion
   (c) Malathion (d) Endrin

5. **Gastric lavage sample of which poisoning turns black on exposure to silver nitrate:**
   (a) Mercury (b) Malathion
   (c) Aluminium phosphide (d) Barbiturates

6. **Which is known as plant penicillin?**
   (a) Malathion (b) DDT
   (c) GBH (d) Endrin

7. **Following clinical features are the nicotinic effects of organo-phosphorous poisoning *except:***
   (a) Hypertension (b) Fasciculation
   (c) Tachycardia (d) Miosis

8. **A pharyngeal membrane, which closely resembles that of diphtheria, is found in the poisoning of:**
   (a) Paraquat (b) Endrin
   (c) Manganese (d) Selenium

9. **Chromolachryorrhoea is seen in case of poisoning due to:**
   (a) Aluminium phosphide
   (b) Organophosphorus
   (c) Dhatura
   (d) Belladonna

10. **Which poison is known as agent of sure death?**
    (a) Aluminium phosphide
    (b) Paraquat
    (c) Organophosphorus
    (d) Carbamates

ANSWER KEY ☞

1. (d)	2. (c)	3. (d)	4. (d)	5. (c)	6. (d)	7. (d)	8. (a)	9. (b)	10. (a)

48 CHAPTER

Organic Solvents

Organic compounds used in industry or at home may result in death from their careless use for improper purposes. Environmental exposure occurs from improper disposal and leakage from toxic dump sites resulting in contamination of drinking water. The various compounds are: (i) Gasoline (ii) Lighter fluids (iii) Aerosol sprays (iv) Spot removers (v) Paint removers (vi) Floor/tile cleaners.

The compounds such as anaesthetic agents, solvents and fluorohydrocarbons are used as propellants in aerosol products.

SOLVENT ABUSE

Solvent abuse is deliberately inhaling a variety of substances especially organic solvents that results in symptoms similar to alcoholic intoxication.

The distortion of consciousness, euphoria (sometimes of erotic nature), distortion of perception and actual hallucinations are produced.

Predominantly males of 14-22 years to beyond the either end or solitary users are commonly involved. Most common substance inhaled was toluene-based adhesive that is why it is also called **'Glue sniffing'**.

Common Method of Solvent Abuse

1. A solvent or chemical is taken in a plastic bag; the open end is placed against the nose and mouth and air re-breathed. The warm air results in vaporization of solvent, enters tidal air stream and absorbed through pulmonary membranes into blood.
2. The inhalant is placed on the hanky and inhaled directly as pad over nose and mouth. Gaseous substances (butane or propane) are taken from either a large cylinder used for camping, heating or cooking or from small ampoule cylinders sold for refilling gas cigarette lighters are introduced into mouth or nose.
3. They may be used directly from pressurized aerosol cans or pain relieving sprays. They can be derived from tins, jerry cans and petrol filters of motor vehicles. Fire extinguishers contain an organic bromine derivatives that when inhaled sensitizes the myocardium to catecholamines.

Various Compounds Used For Solvent Abuse

Aliphatic Hydrocarbons

C1-C4 Aliphatic hydrocarbons: Straight chain hydrocarbons with ≤ 4 carbon atoms are present in:

- *Natural gas (Methane and ethane):* Are simple Asphyxiants, act by high concentration in air and decreased oxygen concentration.
- *Bottled gas (Propane and butane):* Are used directly from pressurized containers, are light hydrocarbons from upper fractions of oil distillation.

C5-C8 Aliphatic hydrocarbons: Like most organic solvents it depresses CNS causing dizziness and incoordination:

- n-hexane is a widely used solvent contained in glue and polyneuropathy is primary toxic reaction.

- 2-hexane (methyl n-butyl ketone) is metabolized to 2, 5 hexanenedione binds to amino groups of neurofilaments, aggregates and axonal swelling is produced.

Clinical Symptoms

There is symmetrical sensory dysfunction of distal portion of extremities, muscle weakness in toes and fingers and loss of deep sensory reflexes.

Mechanism

Peripheral neuropathy associated with exposure to these solvents is due to cytochrome P450-mediated biotransformation of n-hexane and 2-hexane to 2, 5 hexanedione.

GASOLINE AND KEROSENE

Gasoline and kerosene are petroleum distillates prepared by fractionation of crude petroleum oil. They contain aromatic, aliphatic and variety of branched and unsaturated hydrocarbons. They are used as illuminating fuels, heating fuels, motor fuels and vehicles for many pesticides and cleaning agents. Accidental poisoning occurs due to being preserved in containers for beverages and is common in children. Chronic exposure to gasoline (2% benzene) results in leukemia.

Signs and Symptoms

Signs and symptoms are similar to that of ethyl alcohol poisoning such as: (i) Incoordination. (ii) Restlessness. (iii) Excitement. (iv) Confusion. (v) Disorientation. (vi) Ataxia. (vii) Delirium and coma. (viii) Severe irritation of skin with resulting chronic eczemoid dermatitis and causes second degree burns of skin if left in contact for some time. (ix) Gasoline and kerosene may sometimes be inhaled or 'sniffed' resulting in elation and hypoxia. (x) When inhaled, the toxic effects are produced on the tracheobronchial tree resulting in chemical tracheobronchitis and pneumonitis.

Inhalation of high concentration of gasoline vapours by workman cleaning storage tanks leads to immediate death as a result of: (i) Sensitive myocardium such that small amounts of circulating epinephrine precipitate ventricular fibrillation. (ii) Rapid depression of central nervous system and death from respiratory failure. (iii) Inhalation of high concentration for hours results in pneumonitis.

Cause of Death

(i) Sudden cardiac arrest following arrythmia (ii) Persistent rebreathing in toxic environment results in hypoxia or hypercapnia (iii) **Plastic bag asphyxia** (iv) Aspiration of vomitus.

Poisoning results from inhalation of vapours and ingestion of liquid. Ingestion of liquid is more hazardous due to low surfaces tension of liquid. The liquid is aspirated into respiratory tract by vomiting or eructation with resulting chemical peritonitis, secondary bacterial pneumonia and pulmonary oedema. The last two are the most serious sequel to aspiration. Death occurs with in 16-18 hours.

Autopsy Findings

1. Lungs are heavy, oedematous, haemorrhagic and congested.
2. Alveoli are filled with an exudate that is rich in proteins, cells and fibrin.
3. Alveolar walls are weakened thus rupture occurs with resulting emphysema and pneumothorax.
4. Inflammation and enlargement of pulmonary lymph nodes is present.

Radiological Findings

On X-ray examination many small areas of pneumonitis similar to virus pneumonitis, except in the areas of infiltration; nimbus-like clouds in the chest may give the impression of consolidation.

Treatment

Treatment mainly consists of symptomatic and supportive care.

Medicolegal Aspects

1. Accidental poisoning due to being preserved in containers for beverages.
2. Chronic exposure to gasoline (has 2% benzene) results in leukemia.
3. It is commonly used for glue sniffing.

49 CHAPTER

Miscellaneous Poisons

ANALGESICS AND ANTIPYRETICS

ACETYLSALICYLIC ACID (ASPIRIN)

It is white powder commonly used as an antipyretic and analgesic.

Signs and Symptoms

(i) Burning pain (ii) Vomiting, occasional diarrhoea (iii) Sweating (iv) Rise of temperature (v) Dyspnea (vi) Vertigo (vii) Ringing in the ears and deafness (viii) Impairment of vision (ix) Headache (x) Restlessness (xi) Confusion (xii) Delirium and hallucinations (xiii) Pupils are dilated.

Blood level of 50 mg% are toxic whereas of 100 mg% are fatal to life.

Fatal Dose: 15-30 gm.

Fatal Period: Few minutes to several hours.

Causes of Death

(i) Uraemia leading to circulatory failure (ii) Respiratory failure.

Treatment

(i) Stomach wash with sodium bicarbonate (ii) Dialysis should be given (iii) Exchange transfusion should be undertaken (iv) Symptomatic treatment should be administered.

Autopsy Findings

(i) Pupils are dilated (ii) Skin rashes may be present (iii) Gastric mucosa is congested (iv) Subpleural haemorrhages (v) Lungs are congested and oedematous (vi) Hepatitis (vii) Myocardium, liver and kidney are soft and greasy to touch, if the survival rate is for few days.

Medicolegal Aspects

(i) Poisoning is almost always suicidal (ii) It is not accidental due to its bitter taste.

PARACETAMOL

Paracetamol is also known as acetaminophen, N-acetyl-p-aminophenol or 4'-hydroxyacetanilide. It is an analgesic and antipyretic, without the anti-inflammatory properties of aspirin, for which it is often used as an alternative because of the lack of gastric irritation.

In combination with other drugs such as codeine and dextropropoxyphen, Paracetamol is one of the most common agents used in self-induced poisoning by medicinal products. Acetaminophen toxicity is the second most common cause of liver transplantation worldwide. It is used alone in therapeutic doses of upto 500 mg. Overdoses of 20 g or more are potentially lethal, but much less is needed in combination with other drugs, such as propoxyphen.

Paracetamol poisoning is more common in children who have low hepatic glucuronide conjugating ability. When a large dose (more than 150 mg/kg or more than 10 g in an adult) is taken, it causes serious toxicity. Fatality is common with doses more than 250 mg/kg. Paracetamol is a potent liver poison, as a small portion is converted by the liver enzyme 'P450' (microsomal mixed function oxidase) into a toxic compound, probably N-acetyl-p-benzoquinone. Normally glutathione and other sulphydryl compounds detoxify this substance, but in overdose, these are exhausted and the toxic agent causes a profound centrilobular necrosis. The plasma half-life is a guide to hepatotoxicity; it is dangerous to have a half-life of more than two hours at a level of 300 mg/l at four hours after ingestion. Typical blood levels in overdoses when at least 10-15 gm has been taken are 100-400 mg/l with an average around 250 mg/land the urine may contain 150-800 mg/l. All the levels depend on dose and survival time.

Mechanism of Toxicity

N-acetyl-benzoquinone-imine is a highly reactive arylating minor metabolite of Paracetamol, which is detoxified by conjugation with glutathione. When a very large dose is taken, hepatic glutathione is depleted and this metabolite binds covalently to proteins in liver cells and renal tubules causing necrosis. Toxicity thus shows a threshold phenomenon, manifesting only when the glutathione is depleted to a critical point. In chronic alcoholics, even 5-6 gm/day taken for a few days can cause hepatotoxicity. Paracetamol is not recommended in premature infants that are of less than 2 kg for fear of hepatotoxicity.

Fatal Dose: 10-20 gm.

Fatal Period: 2-4 days.

Signs and Symptoms

Early manifestations: (i) Nausea, vomiting and abdominal pain (ii) Tenderness of liver (iii) No impairment of consciousness.

After 12-18 hours: (i) Centrilobular hepatic necrosis (ii) Renal tubular necrosis (iii) Hypoglycemia progressing to coma (iv) Fulminating hepatic failure and death may occur when plasma levels are above the level of 200 μg/ml at 4 hours and 30 μg/ml at 15 hours.

O-Cresol test: It is a rapid color test for determination of acetaminophen especially in urine sample. Acetaminophen and its metabolites are hydrolyzed in acid solution to p-aminophenol, which is then coupled with o-cresol to give a distinctive indophenol blue.

Treatment

Treatment should be started as early as possible as it is practically ineffective if started 16 hours or more after paracetamol ingestion. This includes: (i) Gastric lavage and induction of vomiting (ii) Activated charcoal given orally or through the tube (iii) **N-acetylcysteine** 150 mg/kg should be infused intravenously over 15 minutes followed by the same dose over the next 20 hours. Alternatively, 75 mg/kg may be given orally every 4-6 hours for 2-3 days. It replenishes the glutathione stores of liver and prevents binding of the toxic metabolite to other cellular constituents.

Autopsy Findings

(i) There are no specific findings in the gastrointestinal tract (ii) In massive overdoses, death may result from depression of central nervous system (iii) Most deaths are delayed for 2-4 days when liver failure develops; the liver may be enlarged but is often less than 1500 gms. It is pale yellow to tan coloured and centrilobular necrosis is visible microscopically (iv) Renal tubular necrosis may be seen (v) Myocardial fibril damage may be visible histologically.

INSULIN POISONING

Insulin is a peptide hormone secreted in the body by beta cells of islets of Langerhans of the pancreas and regulates blood glucose levels. It is primarily used for glycaemic control in patients with diabetes mellitus type-1 and sometimes diabetes mellitus type-2. On the basis of duration of action, Insulin is categorized as rapid acting (lispro and aspart), short-acting (regular insulin), intermediate-acting (neutral protamine hagedorn and lente insulin), and long-acting (glargine and determir).

Signs and Symptoms

Insulin is regarded as a 'high alert medication' since misuse of it leads to development of hypoglycaemia which can be life threatening. There can be signs and symptoms of neuroglycopenia like dizziness, weakness, headache, confusion, drowsiness, seizures and coma. Autonomic features include nausea, sweating or clammy skin, trembling hands, arrhythmias and hypotension. Electrolyte abnormalities include hypokalemia and hypomagnesemia.

Treatment

(i) Infusion of bolus dose dextrose (0.5 to 1 g /kg) followed by various concentration of intravenous dextrose for correction of hypoglycemia (ii) Correction of hypokalemia and hypomagnesemia (iii) Benzodiazepines for control of seizures. (iv) Alert patient should be fed.

Medicolegal Aspects

Death from parenteral administration of insulin is quite common. Fatal insulin toxicity can be accidental, suicidal and even homicidal. Accidental fatalities are mostly medical errors resulting from misreading the label on the box or ampoule. Suicide by insulin is also quite common in non-diabetics, especially medical and paramedical personnel and relatives of diabetic patient. As insulin is inactive orally and has to be given parenterally for its hypoglycemic action.

Autopsy Findings

(i) Peripheral blood samples, skin, and underlying tissue from the injection as well as control site should be preserved. The needle marks are usually not evident at autopsy unless a small vessel has been damaged. The samples should be either frozen or kept in refrigerator (ii) Frozen serum separated from red cells should be sent for analysis (iii) Porcine or bovine insulin can be detected as such but immunoassay of the insulin itself, measuring C-peptide, produced on a one-to-one basis by the pancreas assists in distinguishing endogenous from exogenous insulin (iv) Attempting to prove insulin-induced hypoglycemia by measuring glucose levels in human postmortem fluids is impracticable, due to the unreliability of such estimations after death (v) Very low vitreous humour glucose levels suggest hypoglycemia but is not well acceptable.

ANTI-INFECTIVES/ANTIBIOTICS

Anti-infectives is a general term used to describe any medicine which is used to treat or to prevent infections. It includes antibacterial, antifungal, antiviral and antiparasitic medications.

Antibiotics are the group of medicines that are used to inhibit the growth or kill various bacteria and other microorganisms. Misuse of antibiotics sometimes called antibiotic abuse or antibiotic overuse which may produce serious health effects. It can lead to multidrug resistant bacteria, informally called 'super bugs'.

Many researchers have treated antibiotics as potential poisons. The adverse events tend to occur only after prolonged antibiotic therapy or with high doses. Antibiotics are the second most common cause of drug related adverse events and important cause of mortality in the health care context. Use of antibiotics is commonly associated with medical malpractice claims.

The most common adverse events associated with the use of antibiotics are diarrhoea, allergic reactions, hepatotoxicity, nephrotoxicity, ototoxicity, neurotoxicity and phototoxicity. β lactam antibiotics (penicillin, cephalosporin, carbapenems etc.) are most commonly associated with hypersensitivity reaction. Aminoglycosides commonly cause ototoxicity. Quinolones is known for neurotoxicity.

Treatment

(i) Early diagnosis is required for minimizing adverse effects. (ii) Stop taking the medication immediately. (iii) Specific treatment as per the nature of adverse events.

LITHIUM

Lithium (Li) is a soft, white, lustrous, alkali metal and lightest of the solid elements. It is used in batteries, nuclear fusion reactions and thermonuclear weapons.

Salts of lithium, especially lithium carbonate is used to treatment of major depression and bipolar disorder. Its mechanism of action is still incompletely understood. Lithium has narrow therapeutic index, hence, continuous monitoring of plasma lithium level is required to avoid toxicity in patient. Toxicity due to lithium is due to excessive intake and impaired renal excretion. There are 3 types of lithium intoxication namely acute, chronic, and acute-on-chronic.

Signs and Symptoms

Acute and Acute on chronic intoxication is most often associated with GI symptoms such as nausea, vomiting, and diarrhoea, at times with significant volume loss. Cardiotoxic effects like arrhythmias, prolonged QTc interval, bradycardia is observed. Late developing neurological signs are also observed.

Chronic intoxication primarily manifested as neurological symptoms, including confusion, myoclonus and seizures. Renal toxicity which includes nephrogenic diabetes insipidus (most common cause of drug induced diabetes insipidus), impaired urinary concentrating ability and nephrotic syndrome are commonly observed.

Treatment

(i) *In acute intoxication:* In unconscious patient-Airway management. (ii) Gastric lavage by using a nasogastric tube may be considered, if the patient presenting early to the emergency. (iii) Oral activated charcoal has no effect as it cannot bind lithium ions. (iv) Whole bowel irrigation with polyethylene glycol in case of poisoning with sustained released drugs. (v) Haemodialysis is the most appropriate method lithium for elimination of lithium. (vi) Peritoneal dialysis can be done, if haemodialysis is not available.

Medicolegal Aspects

(i) Though lithium has anti-suicidal effect, suicide attempt and suicide cases have been reported by ingestion of lithium. (ii) Lithium toxicity due to accidental overdose is common.

PHENYTOIN

Phenytoin (earlier known as diphenylhydantoin or DPH) is a hydantoin derivative, odourless, tasteless, fine white or almost white crystalline powder drug. It commonly used for management of epilepsy, generalized tonic-clonic seizures, complex partial seizures and status epilepticus.

It acts by blocking voltage-gated sodium channel that is responsible for increasing the action potential. Through this mode of action, it obstructs the positive feedback that sustains high-frequency repetitive firing, thus preventing the spread of the seizure focal point.

It is metabolized by cytochrome P450 enzyme. It has narrow therapeutic index, hence pose a high risk of poisoning in clinical practice.

Signs and Symptoms

Acute toxicity results in nausea, nystagmus, ophthalmoplegia, ataxia, dysarthria, confusion, depressed conscious state and coma. Allergic reactions and mental health issue can be observed. It can lead to paradoxical seizures.

Chronic toxicity leads to phenytoin encephalopathy and peripheral neuropathy. Phenytoin causes Gingival hyperplasia as it affects the gingival connective which is constantly inflamed and subjected to microtrauma leading to hypertrophy.

Purple glove syndrome: Intravenous phenytoin administration results in microvascular thrombosis and subclinical extravasation which is manifested as progressive distal limb edema, discoloration and pain.

Fetal hydantoin syndrome: Phenytoin easily crosses placentae. Children born to epileptic mother who took phenytoin may have significant malformations such as orofacial clefts and cardiac defects), dysmorphic skull and facial features, nail and digit hypoplasia, growth abnormalities and cognitive deficits.

Management

(i) Basic life support (ii) Gastric lavage with charcoal, if the patient presents early (iii) Use cathartics (iv) No antidote is available.

Medicolegal Aspects

(i) Death is a rare complication of phenytoin intoxication. (ii) Phenytoin toxicity may result from intentional overdose, dosage adjustments, drug interactions, or alterations in physiology.

NEUROLEPTICS/ANTIPSYCHOTIC DRUGS

These are the drugs primarily used to manage symptoms of psychosis such as delusions, hallucination, psychomotor agitation etc. They are classified as: first-generation or "typical" antipsychotics and second-generation or "atypical" antipsychotics.

The first-generation antipsychotic acts through strongly blocking the dopamine receptor (mainly D2), in the CNS. It also blocks cholinergic or histaminergic receptors. The second-generation antipsychotics differ from first-generation by transiently occupying D2 receptors, followed by rapidly dissociating, allowing normal dopamine neurotransmission. They also have fast D2 dissociation, antagonistic properties on 5HT2A receptor, and 5HT1A agonism. Second-generation antipsychotics have less side effects comparison to first generation and generally considered safe in adult and older populations.

The first-generation antipsychotics include fluphenazine, trifluoperazine, haloperidol (butyrophenones), loxapine, pimozide, perphenazine, and thiothixene etc. The second-generation antipsychotics include risperidone, olanzapine, quetiapine, ziprasidone, aripiprazole, paliperidone, asenapine, lurasidone, iloperidone, cariprazine, brexpiprazole and clozapine etc.

HALOPERIDOL

Haloperidol is a first-generation neuroleptic drug having antipsychotic and antianxiety effects. It is used for treatment of schizophrenia, acute psychosis, Tourette syndrome, and other severe behavioural disorder in children.

Signs and Symptoms

The most prominent feature of haloperidol overdose is severe extrapyramidal reactions such as tremor, rigidity and an intense feeling of physical restlessness (akathisia).

Anticholinergic side effects include dry mouth, constipation, difficulty urinating, blurred vision and paralytic ileus.

Other common symptoms of overdose are drowsiness, hypotension or hypertension, tremors, hypothermia, ventricular arrhythmias and in severe cases, coma.

Neuroleptic malignant syndrome is a rare, but life-threatening neurological condition associated with the use of antipsychotic (neuroleptic) agents and is characterized by a distinctive clinical syndrome of mental status change, rigidity, fever and dysautonomia.

Treatment

(i) Supportive therapy is the mainstay of treatment (ii) Maintenance of ABC (iii) Oxygen supplement via nasal prongs or facemask (iv) Cardiac monitoring (v) If an oral overdose is identified early, induction of emesis and gastric lavage can be tried to eliminate the drug from the stomach (vi) No antidote is available.

Medicolegal Aspects

(i) Accidental haloperidol poisonings have been reported. (ii) Suicidal poisoning is uncommon.

GENERAL ANAESTHETICS

General anaesthesia renders a patient reversibly unconscious order to allow surgeons to operate on that patient. There are 5 main classes of anaesthetic agents: intravenous (IV) anaesthetics, inhalational anaesthetics, IV sedatives, synthetic opioids, and neuromuscular blocking drugs. Commonly used general anaesthetics are propofol, ketamine, thiopental etc.

Propofol

Propofol is a phenol derivative, highly lipid soluble, short acting drug. It is the most commonly used IV general anaesthetic agent. It is often utilized as an induction agent for general anaesthesia. It has sedative property in addition to anxiolytics and analgesics. The exact mechanism action of propofol is not known, however, it primarily potentiates GABA receptors in the brain. Propofol is rapidly metabolized in liver.

Signs and Symptoms

Propofol Infusion Syndrome (PRIS): This is a rare but serious side effect of prolonged infusion of propofol at high doses (4 mg/kg/hr for more than 48 hours). The features include metabolic acidosis, hyperkalemia, hyperlipidemia, and rhabdomyolysis and the patient may proceed to renal and cardiac failure and ultimately death can happen. The exact mechanisms of PRIS is not known.

Treatment

Treatment of PRIS (i) Discontinuation of propofol infusion and supportive treatment (ii) In severe case, advanced cardiorespiratory support such as extracorporeal membranous oxygenation (ECMO) may be required (iv) Electrolyte imbalance should be corrected (v) Continuous renal replacement therapy (CRRT), therapeutic plasma exchange, haemodialysis, and hemofiltration may help in reducing serum levels of propofol, propofol metabolites and elevated electrolytes.

Medicolegal Aspects

(i) Cases of accidental overdose due to propofol are reported (ii) Suicide cases are reported in health workers (iii) Homicide by using propofol is rarely reported.

LOCAL ANAESTHETICS

Local anaesthetics are used in many medical and dental procedures. Administration of local anaesthesia is usually safe, however, toxic reactions to local anaesthetics may occur due to overdose, accidental intravascular injection, idiosyncratic response, allergic reaction, or interactive effects with other agents like sedatives. The toxicity due to local anaesthetics can be local or systemic (LAST-local anaesthetic systemic toxicity).

LIDOCAINE

It is a tertiary amine derived from xylidine. Because of the superior safety profile, it is the most common local anaesthetic used for various superficial and invasive procedures. It is also used as an antiarrhythmic drug (class IB) to depress ventricular arrhythmia. The route of administration of lidocaine is by injection, inhalation and can be applied a topically. Infusion of lidocaine is also done to supplement general anaesthetic techniques. For local application, it is given in combination with epinephrine which acts as a vasopressor and extends its duration of action at a site by opposing the local vasodilatory effects of lidocaine. It blocks the voltage gated sodium channel, so that the neurons of local tissues incapable of signalling the brain regarding sensations.

Signs and Symptoms

Early symptoms include circumoral numbness, slurred speech, tongue paraesthesia and dizziness. Later, there may be muscle twitches, seizures, unconsciousness and coma.

Treatment

(i) ABC management (ii) For local anaesthetic systemic toxicity– the treatment is symptomatic (iii) Seizures should be controlled with benzodiazepines and or barbiturates or propofol (iv) Administration of lipid emulsions which will bind free circulating local anaesthetics and lower the plasma levels.

Medicolegal Aspects

(i) Lidocaine toxicity is mostly due to accidental overdose.

MUSCLE RELAXANTS

Muscle relaxants are group of drugs that act as central nervous system depressants and have sedative and musculoskeletal relaxant properties. They are beneficial for short term use for acute, painful musculoskeletal conditions. It includes baclofen, chlorzoxazone, cyclobenzaprine, chlorphenesin dantrolene, methocarbamol and orphenadrine etc. They are primarily metabolized in liver.

Signs and Symptoms

Nausea, vomiting, headache, dizziness, nystagmus, hypotonia and CNS depression are observed in chlorzoxazone, chlorphenesin, carisoprodol and methocarbamol toxicity. Baclofen causes CNS depression, muscle weakness, seizures etc.

Treatment

(i) Gastric lavage by single dose activated charcoal (ii) In baclofen poisoning, repetitive charcoal administration may be used (iii) Whole bowel irrigation may be considered after ingestion of sustained released preparation (iv) Physiostigmine1-2 mg, IV over 2-3 minutes will reverse the anticholinergic effects of cyclobenzaprine and orphenadrine. (v) IV lipid emulsion may be beneficial.

Medicolegal Aspects

Both intentional poisoning and accidental overdose cases have been reported.

MULTIPLE CHOICE QUESTIONS

1. O-Cresol test is used for:

(a) Paracetamol (b) Benzene
(c) Alcohol (d) Toxic mushrooms

2. Antidote used for paracetamol poisoning is:

(a) N-acetylcysteine (b) Physostigmine
(c) Neostigmine (d) Pralidoxime

ANSWER KEY ☞

1. (a)	2. (a)

50 CHAPTER

Food Poisoning

Food poisoning or the food borne illness includes all the illnesses resulting from ingestion of food containing bacterial products, toxins, viruses, prions or parasites or acute gastroenteritis due to bacterial infection of food or drink. The contamination may result from improper handling, preparation or storage of food. Food borne illness can also result by adding pesticides or medicines to food or by accidentally consuming naturally poisonous substances like poisonous mushrooms or fish. Contact between food and pests, especially rodents, flies and cockroaches are further cause of contamination of food.

WHO defines food poisoning as "diseases, usually either infectious or toxic in nature, caused by agents that enter the body through the ingestion of food".

Ptomaines: An early theory on the causes of food poisoning involved the ptomaines that are alkaloidal bodies formed as a result of bacterial decomposition of protein in decaying animal or vegetable protein. These alkaloidal bodies when formed in the dead tissues are called **'cadaveric alkaloids'**. These are not bacterial poisons and do not cause food poisoning but are formed only when food becomes too disagreeable to eat. The ptomaines are usually nonpoisonous except for neurine and mydalein that are produced in traces 5-7 days after death. The signs and symptoms produced resemble that of atropine poisoning.

Leucomaines: These are alkaloids that are secreted by living cells during metabolism and are toxic when injected but harmless when they are ingested. While some poisonous alkaloids are the cause of poisoning, the discovery of bacteria left the ptomaine theory obsolete.

Causes and Incidence of Food Poisoning

(1) *Poisoning due to bacteria and toxins* (2) *Poisoning of vegetable origin (natural food poisons):* (i) Lathyrus sativus (ii) Poisonous mushrooms (iii) Ryes, Oats, Barley etc. (iv) Poisonous berry such as Atropa belladonna (v) Argemone mexicana (vi) Cotton seeds (vii) Groundnuts (viii) Cabbage (ix) Soyabeans (x) Sweet clover (3) *Poisons of animal origin:* (i) Poisonous fish (ii) Mussel (4) *Chemicals that are added intentionally:* (i) Flavouring agents in processed form (ii) Colouring agents (iii) Preservatives (iv) Extraction of fat by solvents like hydrocarbons (v) Accidentally added such as pesticides and insecticides (vi) Products of food processing such as smoking of fleshy food (vii) Radionuclides.

Incidence: (i) Chemical (28.4%) (ii) Staphylococcal (21.4%) (iii) Salmonella (17.4%) (iv) C. botulinum (10.4%) (v) Parasitic (8%) (vi) C. perfrigens (7.5%) (vii) Other bacterial (4%) (viii) Viral (3%).

Infectious dose: The infectious dose is the amount of agent that must be consumed to give rise to symptoms of food poisoning. The infective dose varies according to the causative agent and the victim's age and generalized health. In Salmonella food poisoning, as few as 15-20 cells may suffice.

BACTERIAL FOOD POISONING

Bacterial infection is the most common cause of food poisoning. The symptoms are delayed for 12-36 hours after consumption of contaminated food. Bacterial food poisoning is divided into two groups: (i) *Infection type:* The pathogenic organisms in food

Table 50.1: Difference between infection and toxin types of bacterial food poisoning		
Features	**Infection type**	**Toxin type**
Causative organisms	1. *Salmonella group* (i) S.enteritidis (ii) S.typhimurium (iii) S.cholerasuis (iv) S.paratyphi 2. Shigella sonnei 3. Proteus, E.coli, Streptococci, Shigella flexneri are also involved	1. Staphylococcus toxin 2. Botulinum toxin 3. Bacillus cereus
Type of food ingested	Ingestion of contaminated, uncooked or imperfectly cooked food	Ingestion of: (i) Preformed toxin in prepared (canned and preserved) food (ii) Imperfectly or undercooked food such as cheese, meat, fish and eggs

multiplies in the body (ii) *Toxin type:* Ingestion of poisonous substances that are formed in the food due to bacterial proliferation (Table 50.1).

The common bacterial foodborne pathogens are Aeromonas, Bacillus, Brucella, Campylobacter, Corynebacterium, Coxiella burnetii, E. coli, Listeria, Salmonella, Shigella, Streptococcus, Vibrio cholera, Vibrio parahaemolyticus and Yersinia enterocolitica. The incubation period of various food poisonings is given under Table 50.2.

Table 50.2: Incubation periods of food poisoning caused by various organisms	
Causative organism	**Incubation period**
C. botulinum	2 hours-several days (12-36 hours)
C. perfrigens	8-20 hours
Salmonella except S.typhi	12-48 hours
S.typhi causing typhoid fever	10 days or less to 14 days or more
Staphylococcus aureus	1-6 hours (24-48 hours)

Some foodborne illnesses are caused by exotoxins that are secreted by the cell as the bacterium grows. Exotoxins can produce illness even when the microbes that produced them have been killed. Symptoms typically appear after 1-6 hours depending on the amount of toxin ingested. These are caused by Clostridium botulinum, Clostridium perfringens and Staphylococcus aureus.

CLOSTRIDIAL FOOD POISONING

Clostridium is gram positive, anaerobic, spore forming bacilli that are responsible for three major diseases namely tetanus (Cl tetani), gas gangrene (Cl perfringes, Cl septicum, Cl novyi, Cl histolyticus and Cl fallax), food poisoning (Cl botulinum and Cl perfringens type A and C) and acute colitis (Cl difficile). Infant botulism is produced by ingestion of contaminated honey.

Clostridium perfringens food poisoning: The organism is a square ended gram positive, nonmotile rod that is fastidious anaerobe. It is an important cause of gas gangrene. The incidence is more often reported at restaurants and public gatherings. The organism is found in soil and is a normal inhabitant of intestinal tract of man and animals. It has been isolated from meat, poultry and fish purchased from the market. The organism is heat resistant and if the meat is left unrefrigerated the level rises to hazardous concentrations. The organism grows in a food that is improperly refrigerated after initial cooking.

Clostridium botulinum toxin: Cl botulinum elaborates powerful exotoxin that is produced intracellularly and released only on the death and autolysis of the organism. This is the most powerful toxin known to humans. The lethal dose for humans is just 1-2 mg or 1 picogram/kg. It is basically a neurotoxin that acts slowly taking several hours to kill. The food contaminated by the toxin can be rendered safe by pressure cooking or boiling for 20 minutes. The spores resist boiling at 100°C even for several hours.

Mode of Action

Botulinum toxin enters preganglionic nerve terminals by endocytosis and binds rapidly and irreversibly to the cell membrane. It inhibits calcium dependent exocytosis preventing the release of acetylcholine that results in presynaptic blockade and interference with cholinergic transmission at all acetylcholine dependent synapses in peripheral nervous system. The toxin has no effect on the central nervous system or on axonal conduction system.

Foodborne botulism: This type of botulism occurs when Cl. botulinum multiplies in food such as Sausages, tinned meat, fish, fruits and vegetables infected with soil contamination, as Cl. botulinum is normally present in the soil. The incidence of food borne botulism in: (i) Canned food is 2% (ii) Restaurant food is 4% (iii) Family home canning is more than 90%.

It produces a powerful exotoxin and is caused in humans by its distinct strains type A, B, E and rarely F. The food contaminated by type A, B and E strains looks and smells abnormal due to the action of proteolytic enzymes and that contaminated by type E strain is normal in appearance and odour. The initial phase is so subtle as to go unnoticed or misdiagnosed. The clinical features are: (i) Vomiting, thirst and abdominal pain (ii) There may be constipation (iii) Ptosis, difficulty in visual accommodation, mydriasis and diplopia (due to ocular paresis) (iv) Dysphonia and dysphagia (v) Bilaterally symmetrical descending motor paralysis beginning with abducens or oculomotor nerve palsy and progressing to respiratory insufficiency (vi) Urinary retention (vii) Mental status, sensorium, reflexes, body temperature and pulse are usually normal.

Wound botulism: It is a rare life threatening complication of trauma. It occurs after spores of Cl. botulinum have germinated in a wound and the produced botulinum toxin results in flaccid paralysis. It may also result from fatal intravenous drug abuse. Cocaine and Heroin when injected subcutaneously result in wound botulism. Deep wounds, crush injury and compound fracture treated with open reduction predisposes to wound botulism. The incubation period is 4-18 hours and the clinical features are: (i) Fever associated with sinusitis, abscess and tissue infection acts as a focus of infection (ii) There is absence of gastrointestinal manifestations (iii) Cranial nerve palsies result in ptosis, diplopia, poor accommodation, ophthalmoplegia, dysphagia, dysphonia and dysarthria (iv) Flaccid paralysis (v) Shortness of breath (vi) Respiratory failure.

Infant botulism: This type of botulism results from the ingestion of Cl. botulinum organism with subsequent in vivo production of the toxin followed by absorption from the gastrointestinal tract. Bacterial growth associated with breast-feeding may favour Bifibobacterium development instead of bacteria known to inhibit Cl botulinum, i.e., Coliforms, Enterococcus and Bacteroides species. Honey is the most common food source contaminated with Cl botulinum spores. The clinical features produced are: (i) Feeding difficulties (ii) Constipation (iii) Feeble crying (iv) **Floppy infant syndrome** sometimes referred as **rag-doll syndrome** characterized by decreased muscle tone particularly of neck and limbs (v) Loss of facial grimacing (vi) Ophthalmoplegia (vii) Diminished gag reflex (viii) Dysphagia (ix) Poor anal sphincter tone (x) Respiratory failure.

Diagnosis

The diagnosis is made from: (i) History of ingestion of canned food, vegetables, fruits and honey is there (ii) Clinical features suggestive of clostridial food poisoning (iii) Laboratory analysis of sample of blood, stool, vomitus, gastric contents and suspected food item, which are tested for Cl botulinum and botulinum toxin (iv) **Tensilon test:** Tensilon (edrophonium) is a rapid acting anticholinestrase used to differentiate botulism from myasthenia gravis. 10 mg of the drug is injected slowly intravenously, 1-2 mg at first followed by rest of it by next 5 minutes. The muscle strength in myasthenia will improve within ½-1 minute and lasts for about 5 minutes whereas there will be no or little improvement in botulism (v) *Electromyography:* In all forms of botulism, EMG pattern is characterized by brief, small, abundant motor unit action potential. The motor nerve conduction velocity is normal.

Treatment

(i) All patients should be hospitalized (ii) Respiratory status should be monitored for vital capacity, peak expiratory flow rate, negative inspiratory force, pulse oximetry and gas reflex. The moment signs of bulbar palsy occur; intubation or tracheotomy should be done (iii) Evacuate GIT of spores and toxins with the help of activated charcoal, emetics, gastric lavage and catharsis-Sorbitol (iv) *Botulinum antitoxin:* Trivalent botulinum antitoxin is available in 10 ml vial containing: (a) 7500 I.U. of type A (b) 5500 I.U. of type B (c) 8500 I.U. of type E produced by horses immunized against botulinum toxin and then defibrinated, digested and dialyzed and prepared as a 20% protein antitoxin. Equine globulin preparation is available in the west since 1960s but not yet produced in India. One vial is administered by slow I.V. as a 1:10 vol/vol dilution in 0.9% saline, and intramuscular dose of single vial and then after 2-4 hours again I.V. dose is administered. The antitoxin is not administered in infant botulism. It has got serious side effects such as anaphylaxis and serum sickness. It has a lack of effect on toxin producing organisms in the gut (v) *Guanidine:* Its use is controversial as its efficacy is low and there is high incidence of adverse effects. If found appropriate, the dose is 15-40 mg/kg/day orally until EMG improvement occurs at least in ocular muscles (vi) *Human derived Botulism Immunoglobulin (BIG):* It is used to treat infant botulism. It is a pentavalent (types A, B, C, D and E) immunoglobulins harvested by plasmapheresis from donors who received multiple immunizations with pentavalent botulinum toxoid. It avoids the use of foreign equine protein, thereby eliminating the risk of hypersensitivity reactions (vii) *Supportive measures:* These include the nutritional supplementations as oral feeds are contraindicated unless there is intact gag reflex and respiratory supportive measures.

Prevention of Botulism

(i) Improperly preserved home canned food should be avoided especially the green beans, Asparagus and peppers. (ii) Food should be pressure cooked at temperatures above 100°C for 10 minutes that kills spores. (iii) Jams and jellies can be consumed, as they do not contain Cl. botulinum due to their high sugar content. (iv) Cooked food should not be kept at temperatures of 4°-6°C for more than four hours. (v) Boiling the food before eating destroys the toxin. (vi) Food pH should be maintained to less than 0.5; NaCl should be more than 3.5% and nitrites level should also be sufficiently high. (vii) Acidifying agents like citric and phosphoric acids are used while canning low acid food like mushrooms, beets, beans, corns and olives etc.

Medicolegal Aspects

The poisoning is commonly accidental and in literature, there is no incidence of use of botulinum toxin as homicide. Its incidence is more common in western countries and recently in Iran, Russia and Japan. It is quite rare in developing countries like India due to non-popularity of preserved and canned food.

Autopsy Findings

(i) Visceral organs and meninges are congested (ii) Mucosa of gastrointestinal tract is congested, swollen and haemorrhagic (iii) Microscopically fatty degeneration of the liver can be seen.

Viruses

Viral infections make up perhaps one third of cases of food

poisoning in developed countries. They are usually of intermediate (1-3 days) incubation period, cause illnesses which are self-limited in otherwise healthy individuals, and are similar to the bacterial forms described above. The viruses that commonly cause food poisoning are: (i) Norovirus (formerly Norwalk virus) (ii) Rotavirus (iii) Hepatitis A is distinguished from other viral causes by its prolonged (2-6 weeks) incubation period and its ability to spread beyond the stomach and intestines, into the liver. It often induces jaundice, or yellowing of the skin, and rarely leads to chronic liver dysfunction (iv) Hepatitis E.

Parasites

Most foodborne parasites are zoonoses and are caused by: (i) Platyhelminthes (*Taenia saginata* and *Taenia solium*) (ii) Fasciola hepatica (iii) Nematode (*Ascaris lumbricoides*, *Trichinella spiralis* and *Trichuris trichiura*) (iv) Protozoa (*Acanthamoeba* and other free-living amoebae, *Cryptosporidium parvum*, *Entamoeba histolytica*, *Giardia lamblia*, *Sarcocystis hominis*, *Sarcocystis suihominis*) (v) Toxoplasma gondii.

Prevention of Food Poisoning

(i) In a final product, it must be important to know the origin of the ingredients (originating farm, identification of the harvesting or of the animal) and where and when it was processed (ii) Respect of hygiene procedures with maintenance of "cold chain" (iii) There should be power of control and law enforcement of the veterinarians (iv) At home, the prevention mainly consists of: (a) Separating foods while preparing and storing to prevent cross contamination (i.e., clean cutting boards, utensils, and hands after handling meat and before cutting vegetables, etc.) (b) Wash hands and/or gloves before handling ready-to-eat foods (c) Respect of the food storage (that is hot foods hot and cold foods cold) and food preservation methods (especially refrigeration), and checking the expiration date (d) Washing the hands before preparing the meal and before eating (e) Washing the fresh fruits and vegetables with clear water, especially when not cooked (e.g., fruits, salads). Scrub firm fruits and vegetables with a brush to clean (f) Washing the dishes after use (g) Keeping the kitchen and cooking utensils clean (h) Bacteria need warmth, moisture, food and time to grow. The presence, or absence of oxygen, salt, sugar and acidity are also important factors for growth. In the right conditions, one bacterium can multiply using binary fission to become four million in eight hours. Since bacteria can be neither smelled nor seen, the best way to ensure that food is safe is to follow principles of good food hygiene. This includes not allowing raw or partially cooked food to touch dishes, utensils, hands or work surfaces previously used to handle even properly cooked or ready to eat food (v) High salt, high sugar or high acid levels keep bacteria from growing, which is why salted meats, jam, and pickled vegetables are traditional preserved foods (vi) Most frequent causes of bacterial foodborne illnesses are cross-contamination and inadequate temperature control. Therefore control of these two matters is especially important (vii) Thoroughly cooking food until it is piping hot, i.e., above 70°C (158°F) will quickly kill virtually all bacteria, parasites or viruses, except for *Clostridium botulinum* and *Clostridium perfringens*, which produces a heat-resistant spore that survives temperatures up to 100°C (212°F). Once cooked, hot foods should be kept at temperatures out of the danger zone. Temperatures above 63°C (145°F) stop microbial growth (viii) Cold foods should also be kept colder than the danger zone, below 5°C (41°F). However, *Listeria monocytogens* and *Yersinia enterocolitica* can both grow at refrigerator temperatures.

POISONOUS FOODS

POISONOUS MUSHROOMS (Figure 50.1)

The *Amanita* genus of mushroom that is *Amanita phalloides*, *Amanita muscaria* and *Amanita pantherina* are responsible for most cases of mushroom poisoning. These are:

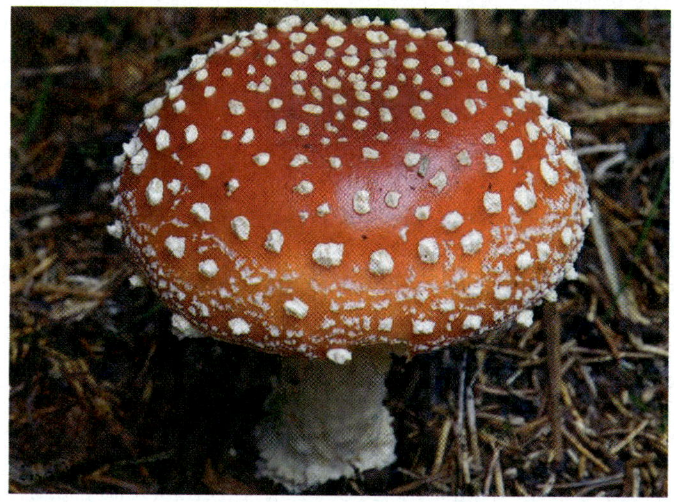

Figure 50.1: Amanita mushroom

Amanita Phalloides Poisoning

Amanita phalloides, also known as **'death cap'**, is responsible for majority of deaths in cases of mushroom poisoning worldwide. This specie of mushroom is very toxic even after cooking. It contains three main group of toxins: amatoxins, phallotoxins and virotoxins. α-amanitin is mainly responsible for the toxic effects in humans. It inhibits RNA polymerase II, causing protein deficit and ultimately cell death. The main target organs involved are liver and kidneys. The onset of symptoms is slow and the prognosis grave.

Signs and Symptoms

The signs and symptoms vary with the passage of time after ingestion of mushroom: (i) *After 8-12 hours of ingestion* (a) Nausea (b) Vomiting (c) Diarrhoea and dysentery (d) intense thirst occurs (ii) *Within 24 hours of onset:* (a) Circulatory collapse (b) Restlessness (c) Twitching (d) Delirium proceeding to coma (iii)

After 3-4 days (a) Hepatic damage (b) Renal damage (c) Death results after 2-4 days.

Meixner test: It is color test for detection of α-amanitin in cases of Amanita mushrooms poisoning.

Treatment

(i) Gastric lavage (ii) Saline cathartics and (iii) Symptomatic treatment is the mainstay.

Medicolegal Aspects

(i) Mainly accidental poisoning (ii) Mushrooms have been rarely used for homicidal purposes.

Autopsy Findings

(i) Extensive fatty infiltration of the liver (ii) Renal tubular necrosis (iii) Haemorrhages in gastrointestinal tract (iv) Renal and hepatic haemorrhages (v) Basal ganglia necrosis.

Amanita Muscaria and Amanita Pantherina Poisoning

Both these mushrooms contain muscarine and give rise to a syndrome resembling that seen in pilocarpine poisoning.

Signs and Symptoms

They appear within a short time of ingestion of the mushroom: (i) Profuse salivation (ii) Perspiration (iii) Severe nausea, vomiting (iv) Watery diarrhoea (v) Pupil is miotic with no reaction to light (vi) Muscular twitching may be present (vii) Sensorium is usually clear (viii) Maniac excitement or hallucinations may be present occasionally more common with *A. pantheria* than *A.muscaria* (ix) In fatal cases death may occur within a few hours.

Autopsy Findings

(i) Congestion of all visceral organs (ii) Findings suggestive of effects of hypoxia.

TOXIC HONEY

The Bees have little selection in the type of nectar, which they transport back to the hive to make honey, as it requires about 17,000 bee-loads to make 1 kg of honey, the stand of poisonous plants must be rather great for enough of the toxic material to get into the honey. The most common type of toxic honey is that from the **laurels or rhododendrons** plants which contain diterpene grayanotoxins. Grayanotoxin containing honey is called "**mad honey**". The following plants have been thought to be present in large enough planting to cause production of toxic honey: (i) The laurels: Sheep laurel (*Kalmia angustifolia*), Mountain laurel (*K. latifolia*), Swamp laurel (*K. polifolia*), Great laurel (*Rhododendron maximum*), Black laurel (*Leucothoe davisiae*), Dog laurel (*L.catesbaei*) (ii) Rhododendron *(Rhododendron species)*: California rose bay (*R. californicum*) and Rose bay (*R. catawbiense*) (iii) Bog rosemary (*Andromeda glaucophylla*) (iv) Jasmine (*Gelsemium sempervirens*) (v) Soapberry (*Sapindus drumondii*) (vi) Indian hemp (*Cannabis indica*) (vii) Oleander (*Nerium odorum*) (viii) Black locust (*A androsaemifolium*) and Clammy locust (*R.viscosa*) (ix) Lily of the valley (*Convallaria majalis*) (x) Death campus (*Zygadenus*) (xi) California buckeye (*Aesculus californican*) and Horse chestnut (*A. hippocastanum*) (xii) Dogbane (*Apocyanum cannabinum*).

Signs and Symptoms

These are of the toxic material in the honey. In addition there is: (i) Tingling of fingers (ii) Vomiting and diarrhoea (iii) Inability to stand (iv) Features of mania.

Other toxic compounds in honey: A compound not naturally present in honey, named 5-hydroxymethylfurfural (HMF), may be formed by the Maillard reaction during the heating or preservation processes of honey. Several types of heavy metals such as lead (Pb), arsenic (As) and mercury (Hg) may also be present.

FISH POISONING

Poisoning by ingestion of fish may result from bacterial growth in partially decomposed fish or by the presence in certain fishes of a neurotoxin. The neurotoxin is present in the whole fish but is concentrated in the ovaries, testes and liver. This is particularly marked during spawning. The syndrome is called **'ichthyotoxicosis' or 'ciguatera'.**

Signs and Symptoms

The signs and symptoms begin within 10-30 minutes following ingestion of the fish: (i) Burning of the throat (ii) Nausea, vomiting and pain abdomen (iii) Ascending motor and sensory paralysis (iv) Mydriasis (v) Hypotension and bradycardia (vi) Respiratory difficulties (vii) Conduction disturbances (viii) Syncope and death resulting from respiratory failure.

Treatment

(i) Gastric lavage (ii) Symptomatic treatment (iii) Cerebral depressants should be avoided.

Venomous Fish (Figure 50.2)

(i) Some fishes cause poisonous wounds with their spines either while trying to get the fish off a hook or out of net. These fishes are commonly *Plutosus* and *Paraplutosus*. They cause painful wound with swelling and redness. The patient is treated with morphine and prevention of secondary infection. (ii) One genus of fish, the *Muraena* (eel) inflicts poisonous bite producing local symptoms of pain to general symptoms of coma, respiratory failure and death. (iii) Stingrays' fishes are most important, the

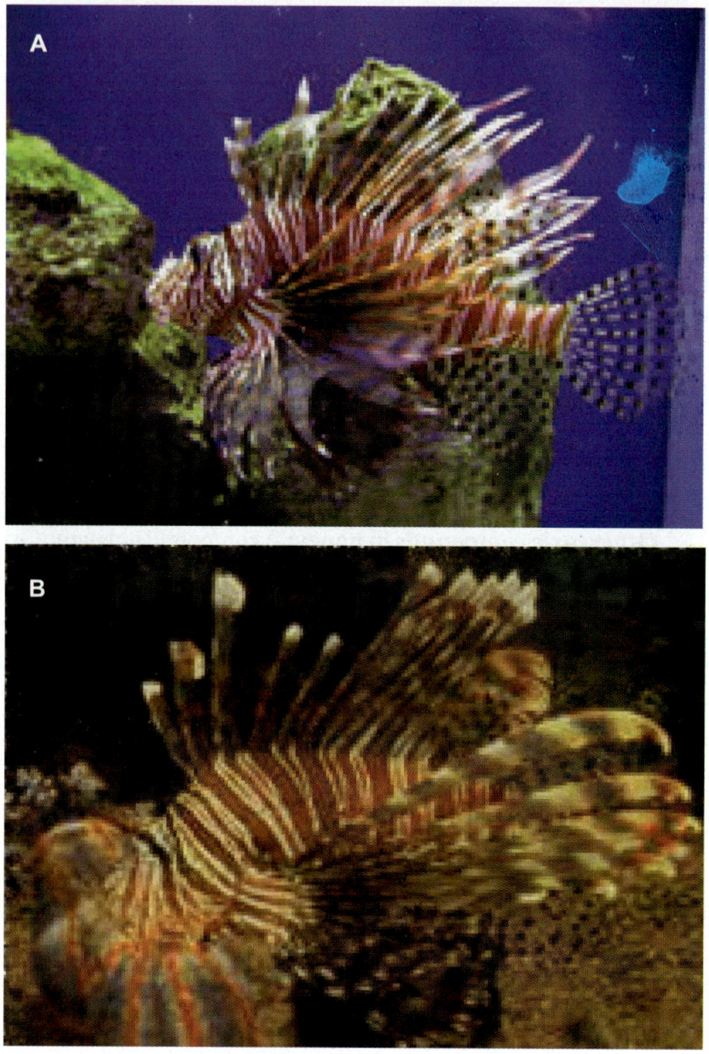

Figure 50.2: Venomous fishes

tail has a series of barbs which close down for the thrust into the victim, flesh and then swing open to make the exit very painful. These fishes lie in the sand and mud at the bottom of water and attack with the poison tail or string when disturbed or frightened. The tail is cut out to remove it from the victim's body. Intense pain is produced and paralysis and other systemic manifestations may develop. Marked abdominal pain with cramps is produced. Respiratory difficulty, delirium and circulatory collapse progress until death ensues. In cases that recover, the necrosis of sting site occur and sloughing and healing may be delayed.

Coelenterate Urtication

This group of invertebrates includes jellyfish, corals, Portuguese man of war and medusae and is present in waters in great numbers. Especially dangerous is the Rhizostoma sp. that causes severe fatigue and depression along with others symptoms. This group of fish's causes release of an urticating fluid that contains several toxic fraction, a neurotoxin, a primary irritant, a haemotoxin and an anaphylactic principle. It causes intense burning pain and irritation, severe abdominal pain, muscular cramps, convulsions and respiratory depression. The treatment is symptomatic.

Shellfish Poisoning

Both mussels and clams contain neurotoxins during certain months. These are heat stable and not destroyed by cooking. The shellfish contains poisonous plankton ingested as food. Intoxication has been reported with two species of *Gonyaulax catanella*, these dinoflagellates in larger numbers impart a reddish tinge to the water and luminosity at night.

Signs and Symptoms

The signs and symptoms appear within 10-20 minutes after ingestion of shellfish. These are: (i) Nausea and vomiting (ii) Burning paraesthesiae of the hands and feet (iii) Numbness of lips and tongue (iv) Ataxia (v) Extreme mydriasis (vi) Convulsive seizures (v) Death from respiratory failure 2-12 hours later.

Treatment

Gastric lavage and symptomatic treatment to be undertaken.

LATHYRUS SATIVUS (KESHARI DAL)

Keshari dal grows under extreme conditions of drought in several parts of India. It is a staple diet of people from low socioeconomic strata. Continuous consumption of this pulse in quantities more than 30% of the total diet for more than six months results in a condition called Lathyrism. When mixed with three times its weight of wheat, the grain becomes apparently harmless but when cooked alone, it acts as a poison. The pulse loses 90% of its toxic amino acid when it is steeped in hot water or parboiled.

Lathyrism

Lathyrism is a condition characterized by features of paralytic manifestations due to the presence of a neurotoxin 1% BOAA [B (N) Oxalyl amino-L-Alanine], a free water-soluble amino acid in the seed cotyledons. This neurotoxin has predilection for pyramidal tract.

Signs and Symptoms

(i) Patient suffers from severe agonizing pain in the calf muscles and limbs that are paralyzed (ii) There is weakness in the legs with difficulty in sitting and getting up (iii) Patient later on finds difficult to walk with spastic gait characterized by walk on tiptoes (iv) Complete spastic paraplegia of lower limbs occurs in late stages and patient can just crawl (v) Motor nerves of the muscles of trunk, upper limbs and sphincters are spared (vi) There will be no atrophy or loss of muscle tone and no reaction of degeneration (vii) Knee jerks will be increased, ankle clonus well marked and there is extensor planter reflex (viii) There are no sensory changes and no loss of consciousness (ix) There is usually no involvement of bladder and rectum unless the lumbar segment gets affected.

Treatment

(i) No specific treatment (ii) Pulse should be excluded from the diet and if it is necessary to consume, it should never exceed 25% of the total amount of cereals and pulses consumed per day (iii) Diet rich in vitamin A, carotene and other vitamins should be given (iv) Physiotherapy for muscular and neurological involvement is quite beneficial.

ARGEMONE MEXICANA

The plant *Argemone Mexicana (Mexican prickly Poppy Pila dhatura/Phirangi Dhatura/Satyanasi)*, grows widely all over India in winters at the same time when mustard plants are growing. The seeds are commonly confused with the mustard seeds and are deliberately or accidentally mixed with mustard seeds. Mustard oil is widely used for cooking purposes in Bengal, Assam, Maharashtra, Odisha and Bihar and is often adulterated with the oil of Argemone mexicana. The plant has thistle like, sessile and spiny leaves and yellow flowers (Figure 50.3). The seeds of argemone are dark brown, globular, smaller than the mustard seeds and are covered by regular minute projections and depressions. The seeds on pressing burst with a sound giving out argemone oil whereas mustard seeds on pressing burst without any sound and give out mustard oil.

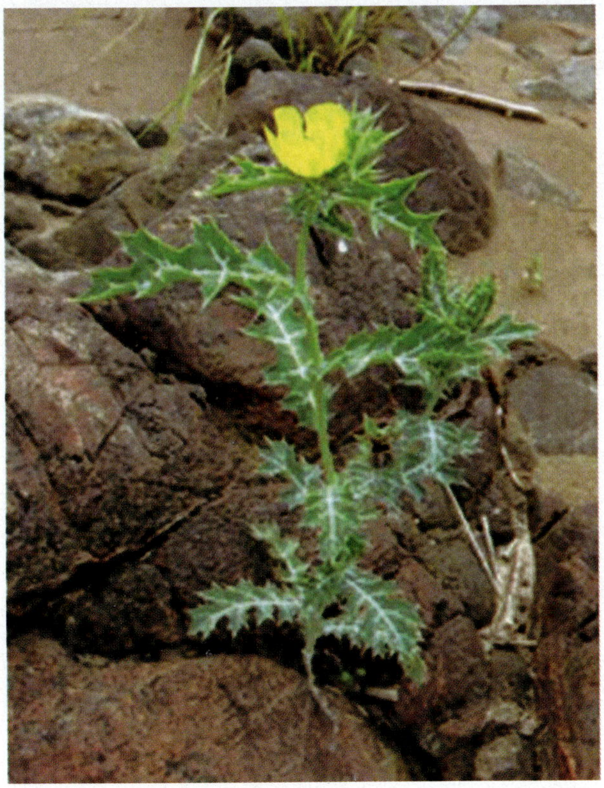

Figure 50.3: Agremone mexicana plant with its flower

All parts of this plant are poisonous and seeds being more poisonous. The plant contains two alkaloids *berberine* and *protopine,* whereas oil extracted from the seeds contains *sanguinarine* and *dihydrosanguinarine,* the former being more toxic. The adulteration of mustard oil with the oil of Argemone mexicana causes **Epidemic dropsy and glaucoma.** The symptoms usually break out in an epidemic form amongst the consumers of adulterated oil. More than 1% concentration of argemone oil in edible oil is enough to produce symptoms.

Signs and Symptoms

The symptoms appear gradually on consumption of the adulterated oil: (i) Loss of appetite, nausea, vomiting, dyspepsia and diarrhoea (ii) Oedema of legs and generalized anasarca (iii) Fall of blood pressure, quick weak pulse, dyspnoea with features of myocardial damage (iv) Breathlessness on slight exertion (v) Enlarged, tender liver (vi) Subcutaneous telangiectasis or hemangiomas due to peripheral vasodilatation (vii) Small fleshy dark red growths may be noticeable on various body parts and also on the mucosa of cheek, gums, tongue and nose (viii) Tingling and hyperaesthesia with diminished or even absent jerks (ix) About 1/10th of the cases develop glaucoma with dimness of vision and raised intraocular pressure (x) Application of adulterated oil on scalp causes burning and fall of hairs (xi) Death results from heart failure.

Tests for Argemone

To the edible oil mix equal volumes of nitric acid, the development of crimson colour indicates presence of argemone oil.

Treatment

(i) Adulterated oil should be discarded and sent for analysis (ii) Mainly symptomatic treatment should be undertaken (iii) Supportive treatment to combat heart damage in the form of digitalis, diuretics and prednisolone (iv) Good nutritious diet with multiminerals and multivitamins especially B complex group should be administered.

SHORT NOTES

1. Toxic honey.
2. Lathyrism.
3. Epidemic dropsy.

MULTIPLE CHOICE QUESTIONS

1. **Ichthyotoxicosis or Ciguatera is a toxicity due to poisonous substance derived from:**
   (a) Fish
   (b) Honey
   (c) Amanita Muscaria
   (d) Amanita Phalloides

2. "Pila Dhatura" is the common name of:

(a) Argemone Mexicana
(b) Dhatura Fastuosa
(c) Dhatura Stromonium
(d) Yellow oleander

3. The active principle of argemone mexicana is:

(a) B(N) oxalyl-amino-alanine
(b) Ptomaine
(c) Ergotamine
(d) Sanguinarine

4. Which of the following is known as death cap?

(a) Tricholoma pardinum
(b) Amanita pantherina
(c) Amanita muscaria
(d) Amanita phalloides

5. Meixner Test used for detection of:

(a) Amatoxins in stool
(b) Botulinum toxin in stool
(c) Arsenic in blood
(d) Mercury in blood

6. Active principle in lathyrus sativus:

(a) Berberine
(b) Protopine
(c) Sanguinarine
(d) B(N) Oxalyl amino-alanine

7. 'Floppy infant syndrome' is seen in case of:

(a) Botulism
(b) Epidemic dropsy
(c) Tetanus
(d) Lathyrism

ANSWER KEY

1. (a)	2. (a)	3. (d)	4. (d)	5. (a)	6. (d)	7. (a)

Brief Index of Various Poisonings

Poison (properties)	Mechanism of action (cause of death)	Fatal dose	Fatal period	Antidote
Organophosphorus compounds	Inhibitors of acetylcholinesterase and pseudocholinesterase	1. TEPP: 50 mg I.M./100 mg oral 2. HETP: 60 mg I.M./350 mg oral 3. OMPA and parathion: 80 mg I.M./175 mg oral 4. Malathion and diazinon: 1 gm oral	24 hours with proper treatment upto 10 days in an untreated patient	1. Atropine sulphate 2-4 mg I.V. and 0.05 mg/kg in children 2. Specific cholinesterase reactivators
Aluminium phosphide	**Inhibitor of:** 1. Respiratory chain enzymes 2. Electron transport resulting from preferential inhibition of cytochrome oxidase	One tablet is fatal (150-500 mg)	Varies from 1 hour-4 days, but 24 hours in majority	No specific antidote
Sulphuric acid • Odourless • Colourless • Heavy • Non-fuming • Hygroscopic • Oily brown or Dark in colour	• Circulatory collapse • Oedema glottis • Perforation of stomach→ collapse • Toxaemia Delayed deaths may result from hypostatic pneumonia, secondary infection, renal failure and starvation due to oesophageal stricture	5-10 ml	12-24 hours	—
Nitric acid • Colourless • Fuming • Heavy • Choking odour	-do-	10-15 ml	12-24 hours	—
Hydrochloric acid • Colourless • Fuming • Pungent	-do-	15-20 ml	12-24 hours	—

Contd.

Contd.

Oxalic acid • Colourless • Transparent • Prismatic crystals	• Shock • Hypocalcemia • Renal damage	15 - 20 gms	1-1/2 hours	–
Carbolic acid • Colourless • Prismatic needle like crystals • Burning, sweetish taste • Turns pink on exposure to air • Carbolic or phenolic smell dark brown liquid (commercial)	• Nervous system depressant especially of the respiratory centre • Syncope • Respiratory failure • Oedema glottis • Brochopneumonia	1-2 gms	3-4 hours	–
Caustic alkalis • Ammonia • KOH • NaOH • $Ca(OH)_2$ • NH_4CO_2 • KCO_3 • $NaCO_3$	• Absorbs water from the tissues • Precipitates proteins • Liquefaction necrosis • Saponification of fat	NaOH/KOH-5 gm KCO-8 gm $NaCO_3$ and ammonia-30 gm		–
Arsenic compounds 1. Arsenic oxides • Arsenious oxide or Arsenious trioxide (Sankhya) • Arsenious acid (white arsenic) 2. Sulphides of arsenic • Arsenic trisulphide (yellow orpiment–*Hartal*) • Arsenic disulphide (Red realgar–*Manseel*) 3. Copper compounds of arsenic • Copper arsenite (Paris green or emerald green–*Hirwa*) 4. Others • Lead arsenate Sodium arsenites Potassium arsenite 5. Arseniuretted hydrogen (Arsine)—colourless garlicky, non-irritating odour	Interferes with cellular respiration by combining with SH group of mitochondrial enzymes especially pyruvate oxidase and certain phosphatases	120-200 mgs	24 hours	Freshly prepared ferric oxide

Contd.

Contd.

Mercury compounds • $HgCl_2$ • HgO_2 • HgI_2 • $HgCN_2$ • $HgNO_3$ • $HgSO_4$ • Ammonia mercuric dichloride • Organic compounds		0.5 to 1 gm	3-5 days	Chelating agent–BAL, DMSA/Succimer
Lead compounds • Lead acetate • Lead carbonate • Lead monoxide • Lead tetraoxide (*Sindur*) • Lead chromate	Interacts with SH groups and interferes with action of enzymes necessary for haem synthesis, for Hb and cytochrome production	Lead acetate—20 gm Lead carbonate—40 gms	2-3 days	Chelating agents–BAL, BAL analogues, Ca Na 2 EDTA
Copper compounds • Copper sulphate (blue vitriol) • Copper subacetate (verdegris) • Cupric carbonate		15-30 gms	1-3 days	Freshly prepared 1% solution of potassium ferrocyanide
Potassium permanganate		10-20 gm	Few hours	10% sodium thiosulphate
Phosphorus • Red (amorphous) • White (crystalline)		60-120 mg	Upto 24 hours	No specific antidote
Ricinus communis	Blocks synthesis of protein by inhibiting RNA polymerase	Ricin—6 mg (1 mg/kg body wt.) Seeds—8-10	2-24 hours	No specific antidote
Croton tiglium • Crotin (Toxalbumin) • Crotonoside (glycoside)		Seeds—4 Oil—1-2 ml	6 hours-3 days	No specific antidote
Abrus precatorius		90-120 mg 1/2-1 crushed seed	3-5 days	Antiabrin
Semecarpus anacardium (Bhilawa) • Semicarpol • Bhilawanol		5 gm	12-24 hours	No specific antidote
Ergot		1-2 gm	1 to several days	No specific antidote
Calotropis		Uncertain	6-12 hours	No specific antidote
Opium	1. Phenanthrene gp. • Morphine (10%) (narcotic) • Codeine (1-2%) (narcotic) • Thebaine (0.3%) (convulsant) 2. Isoquinoline gp • Papaverine (1%) • Narcotine (6%) both analgesic and non-narcotic	Opium—2 gm Morphine—200 mg Codeine—800 mg	6-12 hours	Naloxone HCL

Contd.

Contd.

Barbiturates	• Short acting • Medium acting • Long acting	1-2 gm 2-3 gm 3-5 gm	1-2 days	No specific antidote
Datura fastuosa	• Hyoscine • Scopolamine • Hyocyamine • Traces of atropine	0.5-1 gm (100-125 seeds)	24 hours	Physostigmine
Cocaine		1-11/2 gm	Few min-few hours	No specific antidote
Hydrocyanic acid	Inhibits respiratory enzyme cytochrome oxidase	60 mg of anhydrous acid and 20 mg of cyanides	10 min for HCN and 30 min for Cyanides	Cyanide antidote kit Hydroxycobalamin, cobalt salt

Appendices

Confidential

Medicolegal Examination Report of Survivors/Victims of Sexual Violence

(Proforma Issued by MOHFW, Govt of India)

1. **Name of the Hospital** .... **OPD No.**.................... **Inpatient No.**....................

2. **Name** .... **D/o or S/o (where known)** ....

3. **Address**..

4. **Age (as reported)** .... **Date of Birth (if known)**..............................

5. **Sex (M/F/Others)**..

6. **Date and Time of arrival in the hospital** ....

7. **Date and Time of commencement of examination**..

8. **Brought by**.. **(Name and signatures)**

9. **MLC No.** .... **Police Station** ....

10. **Whether conscious, oriented in time and place and person**...

11. **Any physical / intellectual / psychosocial disability** ....

    (Interpreters or special educators will be needed where the survivor has special needs suchas hearing/speech disability, language barriers, intellectual or psychosocial disability.)

12. **Informed Consent/refusal**

    I .... D/o or S/o ....

    hereby give my consent for:

(a) Medical examination for treatment	Yes	☐	No	☐
(b) Medicolegal examination	Yes	☐	No	☐
(c) Sample collection for clinical and forensic examination	Yes	☐	No	☐

    I also understand that as per law the hospital is required to inform police and this has been explained to me.

    I want the information to be revealed to the police Yes ☐ No ☐

I have understood the purpose and the procedure of the examination including the risk and benefit, explained to me by the examining doctor. My right to refuse the examination at anystage and the consequence of such refusal, including that my medical treatment will not be affected by my refusal, has also been explained and may be recorded. Contents of the above have been explained to me in............................... language with the help of a special educator/interpreter/support person (circle as appropriate) ....

If special educator/interpreter/support person has helped, then his/her name and signature..

Name and signature of survivor or parent/Guardian/person in whom the child reposes trust in case of child (<12 years) ....
With date, time and place...

Name and signature/thumb impression of Witness ....

With Date, time and place...

13. **Marks of identification** (Any scar/mole etc.)

(1) ....

(2) ....

Left Thumb Impression

14. **Relevant Medical/Surgical history**

(i) Onset of menarche (in case of girls) Yes/No, Age of onset ....

(ii) Menstrual history: Cycle length and duration .... Last menstrual period ....

(iii) Menstruation at the time of incident - Yes/No

(iv) Menstruation at the time of examination - Yes/No

(v) Was the survivor pregnant at time of incident - Yes/No, If yes duration of pregnancy .... weeks

(vi) Contraception use: Yes/No .... If yes – method used: ....

(vii) Vaccination status – Tetanus (vaccinated/not vaccinated), Hepatitis B (vaccinated/not vaccinated)

15. **A. History of Sexual Violence**

(i) Date of incident/s being reported

(ii) Time of incident/s

(iii) Location/s

(iv) Estimated duration: 1-7 days .... 1 week to 2 months .... 2-6 months .... > 6 months ....

Episode: One .... Multiple .... Chronic (>6 months) .... Unknown ....

(v) Number of Assailant(s) and name/s..

(vi) Sex of assailant(s)..Approx. Age of assailant(s)................................... If known to the survivor – relationship with the survivor..............................

(vii) Description of incident in the words of the narrator:
Narrator of the incident: survivor/informant (specify name and relation to survivor)

B. Type of physical violence used if any (Describe):

Hit with (Hand, fist, blunt object, sharp object) /Burned with .... Biting/Kicking/Pinching/Pulling Hair

Violent shaking/Banging head/Dragging/Any other:

C.

(i) Emotional abuse or violence if any (insulting, cursing, belittling, terrorizing) ....

(ii) Use of restraints if any ....

(iii) Used or threatened the use of weapon(s) or objects if any ....

(iv) Verbal threats (for example, threats of killing or hurting survivor or any other person in whom the survivor is interested; use of photographs for blackmailing, etc.) if any: ....

(v) Luring (sweets, chocolates, money, job) if any: ....

(vi) Any other ....

D.

(i) Any H/O drug/alcohol intoxication:

(ii) Whether sleeping or unconscious at the time of the incident: ....

E. If survivor has left any marks of injury on assailant/s, enter details: ....

F. Details regarding sexual violence:

Was penetration by penis, fingers or object or other body parts (Write Y=Yes, N=No, DNK=Don't know)
Mention and describe body part/s and/or object/s used for penetration.

	Penetration			Emission of Semen		
Orifice of Victim	By Penis	By body part of self or assailant or third party (finger, tongue or any other)	By Object	Yes	No	Don't know
Genitalia (Vagina and/or urethra)						
Anus						
Mouth						

Oral sex performed by assailant on survivor	Y	N	DNK
Forced Masturbation of self by survivor	Y	N	DNK
Masturbation of Assailant by Survivor, Forced Manipulation of genitals of assailant by survivor	Y	N	DNK
Exhibitionism (perpetrator displaying genitals)	Y	N	DNK
Did ejaculation occur outside body orifice (vagina/anus/mouth/urethra)?	Y	N	DNK

If yes, describe where on the body			
Kissing, licking or sucking any part of survivor's body	Y	N	If Yes, describe
Touching/Fondling	Y	N	If Yes, describe
Condom used*	Y	N	DNK
If yes status of condom	Y	N	DNK
Lubricant used*	Y	N	DNK
If yes, describe kind of lubricant used			
If object used, describe object:			
Any other forms of sexual violence			

*Explain what condom and lubricant is to the survivor

Post incident has the survivor	Yes/No/Do Not know	Remarks
Changed clothes		
Changed undergarments		
Cleaned/washed clothes		
Cleaned/washed undergarments		
Bathed		
Douched		
Passed urine		
Passed stools		
Rinsing of mouth/Brushing/ Vomiting (Circle any or all as appropriate)		

Time since incident .... H/o vaginal/anal/oral bleeding/discharge prior to the incident of sexual violence...............

H/o vaginal/anal/oral bleeding/discharge since the incident of sexual violence ....

H/o painful urination/painful defecation/fissures/abdominal pain/pain in genitals or any other part since the incident of sexual violence.

16. **General Physical Examination:**

(i) Is this the first examination..

(ii) Pulse.......... .... BP..

(iii) Temp... Resp. Rate..

(iv) Pupils ....

(v) Any observation in terms of general physical wellbeing of the survivor...

17. **Examination for injuries on the body if any**

The pattern of injuries sustained during an incident of sexual violence may show considerable variation. This may range from complete absence of injuries (more frequently) to grievous injuries (very rare).

(Look for bruises, physical torture injuries, nail abrasions, teeth bite marks, cuts, lacerations, fracture, tenderness, any other injury, boils, lesions, discharge specially on the scalp, face, neck, shoulders, breast, wrists, forearms, medial aspect of upper arms, thighs and buttocks). Note the injury type, site, size, shape, colour, swelling signs of healing simple/grievous, dimensions.)

Scalp examination for areas of tenderness (if hair pulled out/dragged by hair)	
Facial bone injury: orbital blackening, tenderness	
Petechial hemorrhage in eyes and other places	
Lips and buccal mucosa / Gums	
Behind the ears	
Ear drum	
Neck, shoulders and breast	
Upper limb	
Inner aspect of upper arms	
Inner aspect of thighs	
Lower limb buttocks	
Other, please specify	

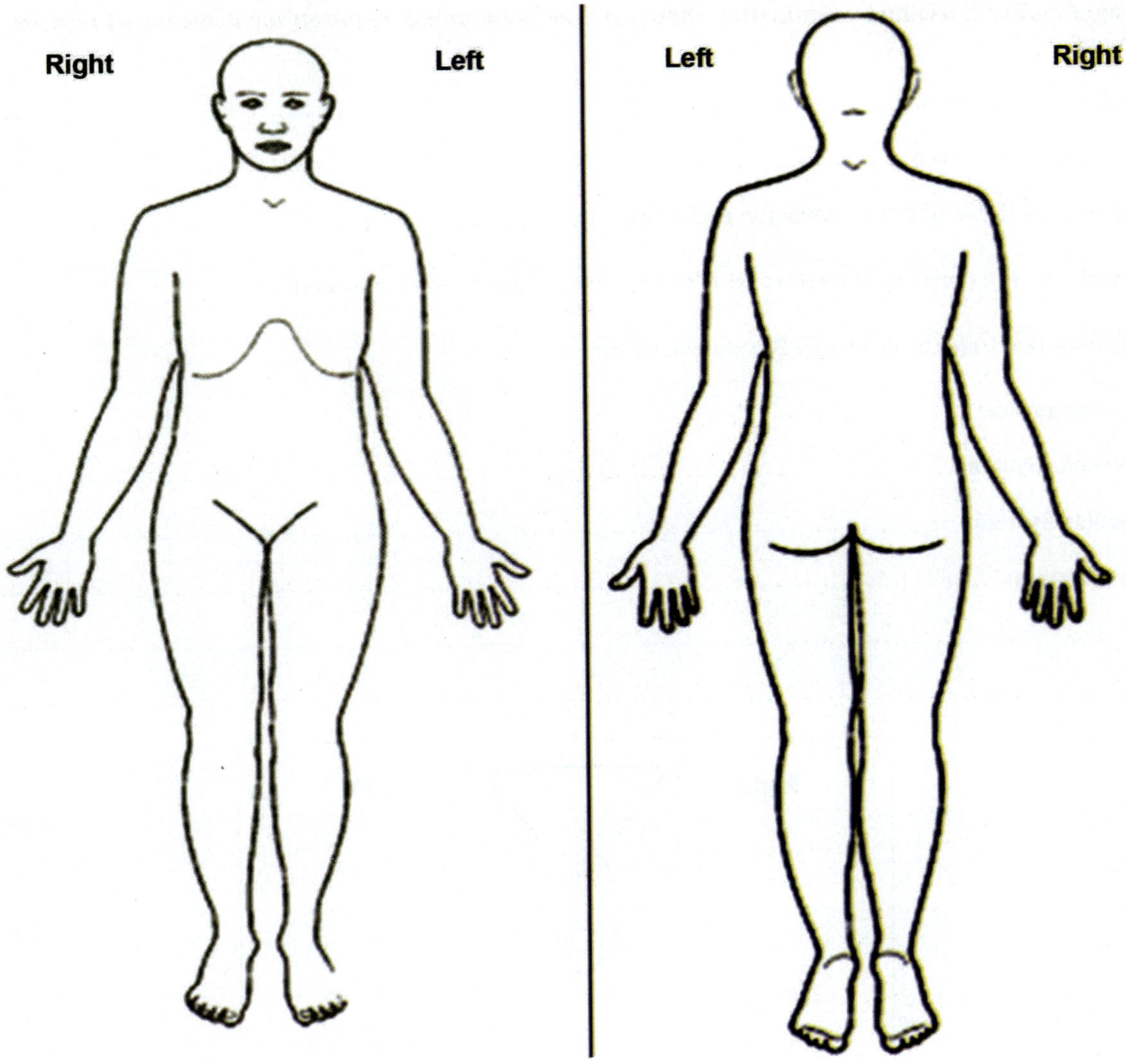

18. **Local examination of genital parts/other orifices*:**

A. External Genitalia: Record findings and state NA where not applicable.

Body parts to be examined	Findings
Urethral meatus and vestibule	
Labia majora	
Labia minora	
Fourchette and Introitus	
Hymen Perineum	
External Urethral Meatus	
Penis	
Scrotum	
Testes	
Clitoropenis	
Labioscrotum	
Any Other	

B. **Per Vaginum/Per Speculum examination should not be done unless required for detection of injuries or for medical treatment.**

P/S findings if performed ....

P/V findings if performed ....

Record reasons if P/V of P/S examination performed ....

C. **Anus and Rectum (encircle the relevant)** Bleeding/tear/discharge/oedema/tenderness

D. **Oral Cavity (encircle the relevant)** Bleeding/discharge

19. **Systemic examination:**

Central Nervous System: ....

Cardiovascular System: ....

Respiratory System: ....

Chest: ....

Abdomen: ....

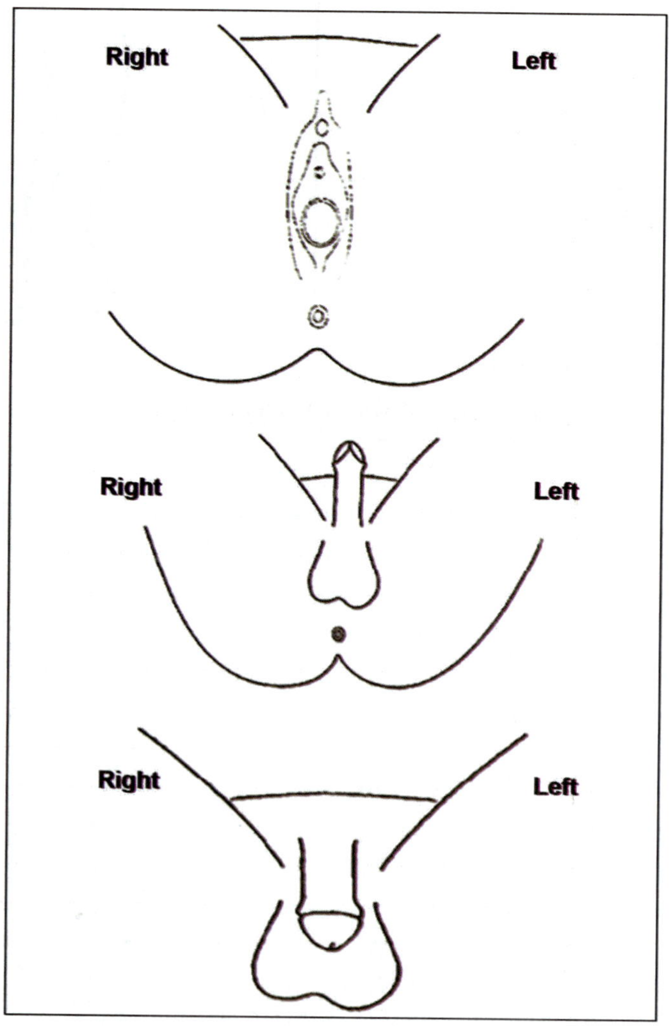

20. **Sample collection/investigations for hospital laboratory/Clinical laboratory**

(1) Blood for HIV, VDRL, HbsAg

(2) Urine test for pregnancy

(3) Ultrasound for pregnancy/internal injury

(4) X-ray for injury

21. **Samples Collection for Central/State Forensic Science Laboratory**

(1) Debris collection paper

(2) Clothing evidence where available (to be packed in separate paper bags after air drying)

List and Details of clothing worn by the survivor at time of sexual violence ....

(3) Body evidence samples as appropriate (duly labelled and packed separately)

	Collected/Not Collected	Collected/Not Collected
Swabs from Stains on the body (blood, semen, foreign material, others)		
Scalp hair (10-15 strands)		
Head hair combing		
Nail scrapings (both hands separately)		
Nail clippings (both hands separately)		
Oral swab		
Blood for grouping, testing		

(4) **Genital and Anal evidence** (Each sample to be packed, sealed and labelled separately–to be placed in a bag)

* Swab sticks for collecting samples should be moistened with distilled water provided.

	Collected/Not Collected	Collected/Not Collected
Matted pubic hair		
Pubic hair combing (mention if shaved)		
Cutting of pubic hair (mention if shaved)		
Two Vulval swabs (for semen examination and DNA testing)		
Two Vaginal swabs (for semen examination and DNA testing)		
Two Anal swabs (for semen examination and DNA testing)		

*Samples to be preserved as directed till handed over to police along with duly attested sample seal.

22. **Provisional medical opinion**

I have examined (name of survivor) ....M/F/Other.................aged.............reporting (type of sexual violence and circumstances) ...., XYZ days/hours after the incident, after having (bathed/douched etc) .... My findings are as follows:

- Samples collected (for FSL), awaiting reports
- Samples collected (for hospital laboratory)
- Clinical findings
- Additional observations (if any)

23. **Treatment prescribed:**

Treatment	Yes	No	Type and comments
STI prevention treatment			
Emergency contraception			
Wound treatment			
Tetanus prophylaxis			
Hepatitis B vaccination			
Post exposure prophylaxis for HIV			
Counselling			
Other			

24. **Date and time of completion of examination** ....

This report contains .... number of sheets and .... number of envelopes.

Signature of Examining Doctor

Name of Examining Doctor

Place: Seal

25. **Final Opinion** (After receiving Lab reports)

Findings in support of the above opinion, taking into account the history, clinical examination findings and Laboratory reports of .... bearing identification marks described above, ... hours/days after the incident of sexual violence, I am of the opinion that:

Signature of Examining Doctor

Name of Examining Doctor

Place: Seal

COPY OF THE ENTIRE MEDICAL REPORT MUST BE GIVEN TO THE SURVIVOR/VICTIM FREE OF COST IMMEDIATELY

PROFORMA FOR EXAMINATION OF AN ACCUSED OF SEXUAL OFFENCES

MLC No.. Ref. No..

Date.. time.................................. and place of Examination..

Name.. Age.................. Marital status..............................

Address..

S/o...Occupation................................Religion..

Brought by Constable...................................... Belt No/ID. .... Police Station..

Identification Marks: 1.

2.

Informed Consent: I give my full, free and voluntary consent for my medical examination and sample collection. The nature and consequences of such an examination has been explained to me by Dr.____.

Signature/Thumb impression..

Witness (Name, Signature with Date) ....

Short History:

Examination of clothing:

G.P.E.: Built .... Ht.................................... Wt.................................. Dentition......................................

Injuries on the body..

Local Examination:

(a) Development of genitals

(b) Pubic hair

(c) Penis: I. Condition:

II. Injuries to frenum:

III. Presence of smegma:

IV. Presence of stains:

(d) Testis and epididymis

(e) Signs of venereal disease

(f) Material collected for investigation

Opinion:

Signature of M.O.

Date

PROFORMA FOR INJURY REPORTING

MLR.No.. Date....................... Time..................... Place of Examination..

Name.. Age......... Sex.......... S/o, D/o, W/o.......................................Occupation..........................

Address...

Brought by Constable... Belt No/ID. .... Police Station...

Brief History:

Consent: I give my full, free and voluntary consent for my medical examination for the purpose of preparation of injury report. The nature and consequences of such an examination has been explained to me by Dr.________________________________.

Witness (Signature and Date) ....

Signature/Thumb impression

Marks of identification: 1.

2.

General physical examination:

Examination of injuries

S. No	Type of injury	Dimensions of injury	Site of injury	Age of injury	Nature of injury	Type of weapon used	Remarks

Material sent for chemical analysis...Investigations advised...

Signature of M.O. with Date

PROFORMA FOR EXAMINATION OF A CASE OF DRUNKENNESS

MLC. No...C.R. No...................................

Name...S/D/W of...Age............ Sex....................

Address..

Referred by P.S.. Brought by..

Informed Consent: I .... give my full, free and voluntary consent for my medical examination, collection of specimens for laboratory analysis for the purpose of preparation of drunkenness report. The nature and consequences of such an examination has been explained to me by Dr.______________________________________.

Signature/Thumb impression ....

Witness (Signature and Date) ....

Identification Marks: 1 ....

2 ....

Place of Examination... Date...............Time.........

Short History:

Examination:

1. General behavior:
2. Clothing:
3. Speech:
4. Self-control:
5. Memory and mental alertness:
6. Writing:
7. Pulse:
8. Temp.:
9. Skin:
10. Mouth:
11. Teeth:
12. Eyes: a. Conjunctiva
    b. Pupil
    c. Muscle coordination
        i. McEvan's Sign:
        ii. Lateral nystagmus:

13. Ears:
14. Gait:
15. Stance:
16. Reflexes:
17. Muscle Coordination:
18. C.V.S.
19. Respiratory system:
20. Abdominal examination:

Blood alcohol level estimation by using Breath Analyzer: .... mg%

Collection and preservation of samples for estimation of alcohol in Forensic Science Laboratory:

(i) Blood (in sodium fluoride or potassium oxalate)

(ii) Urine (in sodium fluoride)

Opinion: Based on clinical and laboratory (chemical) examination, I am of the opinion that the person has:

(a) Not consumed alcohol.

(b) Consumed alcohol, but not under its influence.

(c) Consumed alcohol and under influence of it.

Signature of M.O. with Date

PROFORMA FOR AGE ESTIMATION

Age Report No: .... Dated .... Time ....

Requisition from .... of P.S./Court of ....

vide letter no.. Dated ....

Name .... S/o, W/o, D/o .... Sex ....

Residence ....

Occupation .... Marital status ....

Brief History:

MLC No .... Casualty/CR No ....

Age as alleged by (a) Individual to be examined ....

(b) Police or person accompanying .... Relation ....

Informed Consent: I am willing to undergo my/my ward's medical examination for the purpose of estimation of my age. The nature and consequences of such an examination has been explained to me. ....

(Signature or thumb impression of the individual/guardian)

(Signature of witness) ....

Identification Marks: 1.

2.

Name of the female attendant present ....

General Physical Examination:

Height .... cms Weight .... kgs

General built ....

Hair: Beard .... Moustache.................................... Axillary .... Chest ....

Pubic — P_1 / P_2 / P_3 / P_4 / P_5

Breast development — B_1 / B_2 / B_3 / B_4 / B_5

Acne .... Genitals .... Date of menarche ....

Voice ....

Dental Examination:

Dental Formula

1 8	1 7	1 6	1 5	1 4	1 3	1 2	1 1	2 1	2 2	2 3	2 4	2 5	2 6	2 7	2 8
4 8	4 7	4 6	4 5	4 4	4 3	4 2	4 1	3 1	3 2	3 3	3 4	3 5	3 6	3 7	8 8

5 5	5 4	5 3	5 2	5 1	6 1	6 2	6 3	6 4	6 5
8 5	8 4	8 3	8 2	8 1	7 1	7 2	7 3	7 4	7 5

Radiological Examination:

X-ray Registration Nos .... Total X-ray films.

Ossifications:

OPINION: From general physical examination, dental examination and radiological examination taken together. I am of the opinion that the age of the person examined is between .... and .... years.

(Signature of the M.O. with Date)

Annexure

Comparative tables showing relevant sections of Indian Penal Code (IPC), 1860/Criminal Procedure Code (Cr. Pc), 1973/ Indian Evidence Act (IEA), 1872 WITH Bharatiya Nyay Sanhita (BNS)/ Bharatiya Nagarik Suraksha Sanhita (BNSS)/Bharatiya Sakshya Adhiniyam Sanhita (BSA), 2023

Table 1: Comparative table showing relevant sections of Indian Penal Code(IPC), 1860 and Bharatiya Nyay Sanhita (BNS), 2023

Section of IPC,1860	Description	Clause of BNS, 2023	Description	Change in BNS
-	-	2(3)	**Definition of 'child'- any person below the age of 18 years**	**This is a new addition**
29 & 29A	Document	2(8)	Document	The word **"electronic and digital record" are added.** BNS Section 2(8) incorporates both the sections 29 and 29A of IPC.
44	Injury	2(14)	Injury	-
46	Death	2(6)	Death	-
51	Oath	2(23)	Oath	-
52	Good faith	2(11)	Good faith	-
53	Punishments	4	Punishments	**'Community service' is added** to punishments
54	Commutation of sentence of death	5	Commutation of sentence	-
55	Commutation of sentence of imprisonment for life	5	Commutation of sentence	-
80	Act in doing a lawful act	18	Act in doing a lawful act	-
81	Act likely to cause harm, but not done without criminal intent, and to prevent other harm	19	Act likely to cause harm, but not done without criminal intent, and to prevent other harm	-
82	Act of child under 7 years of age	20	Act of child under 7 years of age	-
83	Act of child above 7 and under 12 of immature understanding	21	Act of child above 7 and under 12 of immature understanding	-
84	Act of a person of unsound mind	22	Act of a person of unsound mind	-
85	Act of a person incapable of judgment by reason of intoxication caused against his will.	23	Act of a person incapable of judgment by reason of intoxication caused against his will.	-

Contd.

Contd.

86	Offence requiring a particular intent or knowledge committed by one who is intoxicated.	24	Offence requiring a particular intent or knowledge committed by one who is intoxicated.	-
87	Act not intended and not known to be likely to cause death or grievous hurt, done by consent.	25	Act not intended and not known to be likely to cause death or grievous hurt, done by consent.	-
88	Act not intended to cause death, done by consent in good faith for person's benefit.	26	Act not intended to cause death, done by consent in good faith for person's benefit.	-
89	Act done in good faith for benefit of child or insane person, by or by consent of guardian.	27	Act done in good faith for benefit of child or **person of unsound mind**, by or by consent of guardian.	Words "insane person" are replaced with **"person of unsound mind"**.
90	Consent known to be given under fear or misconception.	28	Consent known to be given under fear or misconception.	-
91	Exclusion of acts which are offences independently of harm caused.	29	Exclusion of acts which are offences independently of harm caused.	-
92	Act done in good faith for benefit of a person without consent.	30	Act done in good faith for benefit of a person without consent.	-
93	Communication made in good faith.	31	Communication made in good faith.	-
166B	Punishment for non-treatment of victim.	200	Punishment for non-treatment of victim	-
171E	Punishment for bribery	174	Punishment for bribery	-
172	Absconding to avoid service of summons or other proceeding.	206	Absconding to avoid service of summons or other proceeding.	The upper limit of the **fine is increased** from five hundred to five thousand rupees and one thousand to ten thousand rupees; 'Court of justice' is replaced by 'Court' etc.
173	Preventing service of summons or other proceeding, or preventing publication thereof.	207	Preventing service of summons or other proceeding, or preventing publication thereof.	-
174	Non-attendance in obedience to an order from public servant	208	Non-attendance in obedience to an order from public servant	-
177	Furnishing false information	212	Furnishing false information	-
178	Refusing oath or affirmation when duly required by public servant to make it.	213	Refusing oath or affirmation when duly required by public servant to make it.	-
181	False statement on oath or affirmation to public servant or person authorized to administer an oath or affirmation	216	False statement on oath or affirmation to public servant or person authorized to administer an oath or affirmation	-
191	Giving false evidence	227	Giving false evidence	-
192	Fabricating false evidence	228	Fabricating false evidence	-

Contd.

Contd.

193	Punishment for false evidence	229	Punishment for false evidence	**Fine is defined** in sub-section (1) as up to ten thousand rupees and in sub-section (2) as up to five thousand rupees
197	Issuing or signing false certificate	234	Issuing or signing false certificate	-
201	Causing disappearance of evidence, or giving false information to screen offender.	238	Causing disappearance of evidence, or giving false information to screen offender.	-
202	Intentional omission to give information of offence by person bound to inform	239	Intentional omission to give information of offence by person bound to inform	-
299	Definition of culpable homicide	100	Definition of culpable homicide	-
300	Definition of murder	101	Definition of murder	Formal changes, but essence is the same, Secondly, thirdly, and fourthly, are replaced by clauses (a), (b), (c), and (d). The word "it" is replaced by the words "the act by which death is caused".
301	Culpable homicide by causing death of person other than person whose death was intended.	102	Culpable homicide by causing death of person other than person whose death was intended.	-
302	**Punishment for murder.-** Whoever commits murder shall be punished with death or imprisonment for life, and shall also be liable to fine.	103(1)	**Punishment for murder. -** Whoever commits murder shall be punished with death or imprisonment for life, and shall also be liable to fine.	**No change,** except IPC section is included as subsection in BNS.
		103(2)	**Punishment for murder. -** "When a group of five or more persons acting in concert commits murder on the ground of race, caste or community, sex, place of birth, language, personal belief or any other similar ground each member of such group shall be punished with death or with imprisonment for life, and shall also be liable to fine".	**This is a new addition**
303	Punishment for murder by life-convict.	104	Punishment for murder by life- convict.	**BNS gives an alternate punishment for the life-convict murderer** as death 'or with imprisonment for life, which shall mean the remainder of that person's natural life', whereas in IPC, only punishment is a death sentence for murder by a life convict.

Contd.

Contd.

304	Punishment for culpable homicide not amounting to murder	105	Punishment for culpable homicide not amounting to murder	**Minimum imprisonment for 5 years is added** and **fine is made mandatory**.
304A	**Causing death by negligence. -** Whoever causes the death of any person by doing any rash or negligent act not amounting to culpable homicide shall be punished with imprisonment of either description for a term which may extend to **two years,** or with fine, or with both. (Cognizable, Bailable offence, Trial by First class Judicial Magistrate)	106 (1)	**Causing death by negligence. -** Whoever causes death of any person by doing any rash or negligent act not amounting to culpable homicide, shall be punished with imprisonment of either description for a term which may extend to **five years**, and shall also be liable to fine; and if such act is done by a registered **medical practitioner while performing medical procedure,** he shall be punished with imprisonment of either description for a term which may extend to **two years,** and shall also be liable to fine. **Explanation:** For the purposes of this sub-section, "registered medical practitioner" means a medical practitioner who possesses any medical qualification recognized under the National Medical Commission Act, 2019 and whose name has been entered in the National Medical Register or a State Medical Register under that Act. (Cognizable, Bailable offence, Trial by First class Judicial Magistrate)	**Imprisonment is increased and offence by registered medical practitioner and its explanation are added.**
		106(2)	**Causing death by negligence. -** Whoever causes death of **any person by rash and negligent driving of vehicle not amounting to culpable homicide, and escapes without reporting it to a police officer or a Magistrate soon after the incident**, shall be punished with imprisonment of either description of a term which may extend to ten years, and shall also be liable to fine.	**This is a new addition.**
304B	Dowry death	80	Dowry death	-
305	Abetment of suicide of child or insane person	107	Abetment of suicide of child or person of unsound mind.	Formal changes but essence is same- 'insane person' is replaced by **'person of unsound mind'**.
306	Abetment of suicide	108	Abetment of suicide	-

Contd.

Contd.

307	Attempt to murder	109	Attempt to murder	**Under IPC, Section 307 Clause 2** prescribes the **death penalty only for an attempt to murder by a life-convict**, but alternate punishment is given **in Section 109(2) of the BNS, which states that "be punished with death or with imprisonment for life, which shall mean the remainder of that person's natural life"**.
308	Attempt to culpable homicide	110	Attempt to culpable homicide	-
309	Attempt to commit suicide	**No equivalent section in BNS, 2023.**	-	**It has been removed from the text of BNS**, since **attempt to commit suicide is decriminalized** as per "The Mental Healthcare Act, 2017".
-	-	**226**	Attempt to commit suicide to compel or restraint exercise of lawful power. - **Whoever attempts to commit suicide with the intent to compel or restrain any public servant from discharging his official duty shall be punished** with simple imprisonment for a term which may extend to one year or with fine or with both or with community service.	**This is New Addition.** Though attempt to suicide is decriminalized, **attempt to commit suicide with the intent to compel or restrain any public servant from discharging his official duty remains a punishable offence**.
312	Causing miscarriage	88	Causing miscarriage	-
313	Causing miscarriage without woman's consent.	89	Causing miscarriage without woman's consent.	-
314	Death caused by act done with intent to cause miscarriage	90	Death caused by act done with intent to cause miscarriage	Heading of para-2 **"if act done without woman's consent" is excluded**. The words "Where the act referred to in sub-section (1)" are added.
315	Act done with intent to prevent child being born alive or to cause it to die after birth.	91	Act done with intent to prevent child being born alive or to cause it to die after birth.	-

Contd.

Contd.

316	Causing death of quick unborn child by act amounting to culpable homicide.	92	Causing death of quick unborn child by act amounting to culpable homicide.	-
317	Exposure and abandonment of child under twelve years, by parent or person having care of it.	93	Exposure and abandonment of child under twelve years, by parent or person having care of it.	-
318	Concealment of birth by secret disposal of dead body.	94	Concealment of birth by secret disposal of dead body.	-
319	Hurt	114	Hurt	-
320	Definition of Grievous Hurt	116	Definition of Grievous Hurt	Suffering threshold period for grievous hurt is **reduced from 20 (twenty) days to 15 (fifteen) days.**
321	Voluntarily causing hurt.	115(1)	Voluntarily causing hurt.	-
322	Voluntarily causing grievous hurt	117(1)	Voluntarily causing grievous hurt	-
-	-	117(3)	**Voluntarily causing grievous hurt. -** "Whoever commits an offence under sub-section (1) and in the course of such commission causes any hurt to a person which causes that person to be in permanent disability or in persistent vegetative state, shall be punished with rigorous imprisonment for a term which shall not be less than ten years but which may extend to imprisonment for life, which shall mean imprisonment for the remainder of that person's natural life".	**New addition in BNS, 2023**
-	-	117(4)	**Voluntarily causing grievous hurt. -** When grievous hurt of a person is caused by a group of five or more persons on the ground of his, race, caste, sex, place of birth, language, personal belief or any other ground, each member of such group shall be guilty of the offence of causing grievous hurt, and shall be punished with imprisonment of either description for a term which may extend to seven years, and shall also be liable to fine.	**New addition in BNS, 2023**
323	Punishment for voluntarily causing hurt	115(2)	Punishment for voluntarily causing hurt	Section is included as sub-section in BNS sans heading. **Fine is increased** which may extend to ten thousand rupees.
324	Voluntarily causing **hurt** by dangerous weapons or means	118(1)	Voluntarily causing **hurt or grievous hurt** by dangerous weapons or means	IPC section is included as a sub-section in BNS. **Fine is increased** which may extend to twenty thousand rupees and **words "grievous hurt" are added in heading.**

Contd.

Contd.

325	Punishment for voluntarily causing grievous hurt.	117(2)	Punishment for voluntarily causing grievous hurt	-
326	Voluntarily causing **grievous hurt** by dangerous weapons or means	118(2)	Voluntarily causing **hurt or grievous hurt** by dangerous weapons or means	IPC section is included as a sub-section in BNS sans heading. **Mandatory minimum imprisonment for one year is added**.
326A	Voluntarily causing grievous hurt by use of acid etc.	124(1)	Voluntarily causing grievous hurt by use of acid etc.	The IPC section is included as a subsection in BNS. Words "causes a person to be in a **permanent vegetative state**" are added in Section 124(1) of the BNS.
326B	Voluntarily causing grievous hurt by throwing or attempting to throw acid.	124(2)	Voluntarily causing grievous hurt by throwing or attempting to throw acid.	IPC section is included as a sub-section in BNS, sans heading. Words **"permanent vegetative state" are added.**
328	Causing harm by means of poison etc. with intent to commit an offence.	123	Causing harm by means of poison etc. with intent to commit an offence.	-
350	Criminal force	129	Criminal force	-
351	Assault	130	Assault	-
354	Assault or use of criminal force to woman with intent to outrage her modesty.	74	Assault or use of criminal force to woman with intent to outrage her modesty.	-
354A	Sexual harassment	75	Sexual harassment	-
354B	Assault or use of criminal force to woman with intent disrobe.	76	Assault or use of criminal force to woman with intent disrobe.	Words "Any man who" is replaced by "Whoever".
354C	Voyeurism	77	Voyeurism	-
354D	Stalking	78	Stalking	-
359	Kidnapping	137(1)	Kidnapping	-
360	Kidnapping from India.	137(1)(a)	Kidnapping from India.	-
361	Kidnapping from lawful guardianship	137(1)(b)	Kidnapping from lawful guardianship	The IPC section is included as a clause in the BNS. Words "minor under the age of 16 years of male or under 18 years of age if a female" are **replaced by "child"** thus making it **gender neutral**.

Contd.

Contd.

362	Abduction	138	Abduction	-
363	Punishment for kidnapping.	137(2)	Punishment for kidnapping	-
370	Trafficking of person.	143	Trafficking of person.	Word "minor" is replaced by "child".
375	Rape definition	63	Rape definition	**Age of Consent: 15 years is replaced by 18 years in BNS. Exception 2 of Section 63 states that "sexual intercourse or acts by a man with his wife, the wife not being under 18 years of age, is not rape".**
376(1) & 376(2)	Punishment for rape.	64	Punishment for rape.	Word "military" is replaced with "army".
376(3)	Punishment for rape in certain cases-rape on a woman under sixteen years	65(1)	Punishment for rape in certain cases-rape on a woman under 16 years	Section is included as sub-section in BNS sans heading
376AB	Punishment for rape in certain cases-rape on a woman under twelve years	65(2)	Punishment for rape in certain cases-rape on a woman under 12 years	Section is included as sub-section in BNS sans heading
376A	Punishment for causing death or resulting in persistent vegetative state of victim.	66	Punishment for causing death or resulting in persistent vegetative state of victim.	-
376B	Sexual intercourse by husband upon his wife during separation.	67	Sexual intercourse by husband upon his wife during separation.	-
376C	Sexual intercourse by a person in authority.	68	Sexual intercourse by a person in authority.	-
-	-	69	**Sexual intercourse by employing deceitful means etc**. "Whoever, by deceitful means or by making promise to marry to a woman without any intention of fulfilling the same, has sexual intercourse with her, such sexual intercourse not amounting to the offence of rape, shall be punished with imprisonment of either description for a term which may extend to ten years and shall also be liable to fine. **Explanation:** "deceitful means" shall include inducement for, or false promise of employment or promotion, or marrying by suppressing identity."	**It is a New section in BNS, 2023**
376D	Gang rape	70(1)	Gang rape	No Change except IPC section is included as subsection in BNS.
376DA	Punishment for gang rape **under 16 years** of age	70(2)	**Punishment for gang rape** on women **under the age of 18 years.**	This Section is included as a sub-section in BNS, sans heading

Contd.

Contd.

376DB	Punishment for gang rape **under 12 years** of age		**Punishment:** Imprisonment for life, which shall mean imprisonment for the remainder of that person's natural life, and with fine, or with **death**.	-
376E	Punishment for repeat offenders of rape and related sexual offences	71	Punishment for repeat offenders of rape and related sexual offences	-
377	Unnatural offences	-	-	**The BNS repealed S. 377 IPC. No Section in BNS.** In *Navtej Vs Johar* case, the supreme court decriminalized consensual sexual relations between adults regardless of their gender, thereby partially striking down Section 377 of the IPC.
390	Robbery definition	309(1),(2),(3)	Robbery definition	-
391	Dacoity definition	310(1)	Dacoity definition	-
392	Robbery-Punishment	309(4)	Robbery-Punishment	-
395	Dacoity Punishment	310(2)	Dacoity Punishment	
497	Adultery	-	-	Adultery is not criminal offence. **There is no section in BNS.**

Table 2: Comparative table showing relevant sections of Criminal Procedure Code (Cr. Pc), 1973 and Bharatiya Nagarik Suraksha Sanhita (BNSS), 2023

Section of Cr. Pc,1973	**Description**	**Clause of BNSS, 2023**	**Description**	**Change in BNSS, 2023**
2	Definitions	2(1)&(2)	Definitions	Several new subsections, such as 2(1)(a), 2(1)(b), 2(1)(d), and 2(1)(e), are added, while others, namely 2(f), 2(k), 2(q), and 2(t) of CrPC, are excluded. Furthermore, certain subsections are modified.
6	Classes of Criminal Courts	6	Classes of Criminal Courts	Words **"in any Metropolitan area, Metropolitan Magistrates" are excluded.**
9	Court of Session.	8	Court of Session.	Under the BNSS, **the positions of Judicial Magistrate of the third class, Metropolitan Magistrate, and Assistant Session Judges have been abolished**.
11	Courts of Judicial Magistrates	9	Courts of Judicial Magistrates	The words "not being a Metropolitan area" are excluded.

Contd.

Contd.

12	Chief Judicial Magistrate and Additional Chief Judicial Magistrate, etc.	10	Chief Judicial Magistrate and Additional Chief Judicial Magistrate, etc.	-
21	Special Executive Magistrates.	15	Special Executive Magistrates.	**New addition in BNSS** -State Government may **appoint police officers of the rank Superintendent of Police or equivalent, as Special Executive Magistrates**
27	Jurisdiction in the case of juveniles	-	-	**No equivalent section in BNSS.** Addressed under Juvenile Justice (Care and Protection of Children) Act
28	Sentences which High Courts and Sessions Judges may pass	22	Sentences which High Courts and Sessions Judges may pass	-
29	Sentences which Magistrates may pass.	23	Sentences which Magistrates may pass.	**Change in amount of fine:** ten thousand is replaced by fifty thousand, and five thousand is replaced by ten thousand. The explanation of Section 23 **defines "community service"**
39	Public to give information of certain offences	33	Public to give information of certain offences	-
40	Duty of officers employed in connection with the affairs of a village to make certain report	34	Duty of officers employed in connection with the affairs of a village to make certain report	-
53	Examination of accused by medical practitioner at the request of police officer.	51	Examination of accused by medical practitioner at the request of police officer	In BNSS, sub-section (1), **"not below the rank of sub-inspector" is excluded**.
53A	Examination of person accused of rape by medical practitioner.	52	Examination of person accused of rape by medical practitioner.	The words **"police officer not below the rank of Sub-Inspector" are replaced by "any police officer"**.
54	Examination of arrested person by medical officer	53	Examination of arrested person by medical officer	**A new provision added to subsection (1) regarding one more examination can be done if it is necessary, in the opinion of the medical practitioner**
61	Form of summons	63	Form of summons	**A new clause** (ii) "in an encrypted or any other form of electronic communication and shall bear the image of the seal of the Court or digital signature" is **added**.
62	Summons how served	64	Summons how served	**Two new provisos regarding electronic communication, under subsections (1) and (2), are added.** The word "personally" is added in sub-section (3).

Contd.

Contd.

63	Service of summons on corporate bodies and societies	65	Service of summons on corporate bodies, firms, and societies	In subsection (1), Director and Manager is added. New subsection (2) regarding service of summons on any partner of a firm or other association of individuals
64	Service when persons summoned cannot be found	66	Service when persons summoned cannot be found	The word **"male" is excluded** to make the provision **gender neutral.**
65	Procedure when service cannot be effected as before provided	67	Procedure when service cannot be effected as before provided	-
66	Service on government servant	68	Service on government servant	-
67	Service of summons outside local limits	69	Service of summons outside local limits	-
68	Proof of service in such cases and when serving officer not present	70	Proof of service in such cases and when serving officer not present	**A new subsection (3) is added**, mentioning that service of summons through electronic communication shall be considered duly served, and a copy of such summons shall be attested and kept as proof of service of summons
69	Service of summons on witness by post	71	Service of summons on witness by post	**The words "by electronic communication or" are added** in subsection (1). In subsection (2) words "or on the proof of delivery of summons under sub-section (3) of section 70 by electronic communication to the satisfaction of the Court," are added.
87	Issue of warrant in lieu of, or in addition to, summons	90	Issue of warrant in lieu of, or in addition to, summons	-
160	Police officer's power to require attendance of witnesses	179	Police officer's power to require attendance of witnesses	-
164A	Medical examination of the victim of rape	184	Medical examination of the victim of rape	**In BNSS, "without delay" is replaced by "Within a period of seven days"** for medical practitioner to forward the report to Investigating officer.

Contd.

Contd.

173	Report of police officer on completion of investigation	193	Report of police officer on completion of investigation	Section 193(2) **extends** this requirement to **complete the investigation within two months,** offences U/S 4, 6, 8, 10, and 12 of **POCSO Act, 2012 in addition to offences of rape and gang rape.** Section193(3)(i) of the BNSS provides that **reports to Magistrate can also be forwarded through electronic communication**. **The newly inserted clause (i) of sub-section 193(3) (i)** of BNSS provides that the report shall also contain 'the sequence of custody in the case of electronic devices'. **Clause 193(3)(ii) of BNSS provides that the police officer shall, within 90 days, inform the progress of investigation** by any means including electronic communication to informant or the victim. **Subsection (8) is newly inserted**, which mandates the police officer investigating the case to submit such number of copies of police report for supply to the accused. Proviso to the same authorizes electronic communication for this purpose. **The new proviso to subsection (6) provides for further investigation during the trial with the permission of the Court.**
174	Police to enquire and report on suicide, etc.	194	Police to enquire and report on suicide, etc.	In subsection (2) "forthwith" is replaced by **"within 24 hours"** for sending the report to DM and SDM. The word "man" is replaced by "person".
175	Power to summon persons	195	Power to summon persons	Proviso to Subsection (1) of 195 provides **immunity to male persons under the age of 15 years** or **above the age of 60 years**, or a **woman** or a **mentally or physically disabled persons** or a **person with acute illness shall not be required to attend at place other than the place where such person resides.** However, they can attend at police station willingly

Contd.

Contd.

176	Inquiry by Magistrate into cause of death	196	Inquiry by Magistrate into cause of death	The words "Judicial Magistrate" are replaced by "Magistrate", and Metropolitan Magistrate is excluded.
231	Evidence for prosecution	254	Evidence for prosecution	**Newly added proviso to section 254 of BNSS** provides that **evidence of a witness may be recorded by audio-video electronic means**. Newly added subsection (2) provides that the deposition of evidence of any police officer or public servant may be taken through audio-video electronic means.
242	Evidence for prosecution	265	Evidence for prosecution	The new proviso to subsection 265(3) of the BNSS states that **evidence of a witness may be recorded by audio-video electronic means** at the designated place to be notified by the State Government
311	Power to summon material witness, or examine person present	348	Power to summon material witness, or examine person present	-
312	Expenses of complainants and witnesses	350	Expenses of complainants and witnesses	-
344	Summary procedure for trial for giving false evidence.	383	Summary procedure for trial for giving false evidence.	**The fine increased** to "one thousand rupees" from "five hundred rupees".
293	Reports of certain Government scientific experts	329	Reports of certain Government scientific experts	-
350	Summary procedure for punishment for non-attendance by a witness in obedience to summons	389	Summary procedure for punishment for non-attendance by a witness in obedience to summons	**The fine increased** to "five hundred rupees" from "One hundred rupees"
357A	Victim compensation scheme	396	Victim compensation scheme	-
357B	Compensation to be in addition to fine under section 326A or 376D	396	Victim compensation scheme	-
357C	Treatment of victims	397	Treatment of victims	-
-	-	530	**Trial and proceedings to be held in electronic mode**	**New Addition in BNSS**

Table 3: Comparative table showing relevant sections of Indian Evidence Act, 1872 and Bharatiya Sakshya Adhiniyam Sanhita (BSA), 2023

Section of IEA,1872	Description	Clause of BSA, 2023	Description	Change in BSA
3	Interpretation clause	2(1)	Definitions	Definitions, where each word and expression is given individual alphabetical clauses **BSA excludes the interpretation of "India".**
		2(2)	**"Words and expressions used herein and not defined but defined in the Information Technology Act, 2000 (21 of 2000), the Bharatiya Nagarik Suraksha Sanhita, 2023, and the Bharatiya Nyaya Sanhita, 2023, shall have the same meanings as assigned to them in the said Act and Sanhitas."**	**New Addition**
32	Cases in which statement of relevant fact by person who is dead or cannot be found, etc., is relevant.	26	Cases in which statement of relevant fact by person who is dead or cannot be found, etc., is relevant.	-
45	Opinions of experts.	39(1)	Opinions of experts.	Words **"or any other field" are added.** Thus, scope is expanded greatly
45A	Opinion of Examiner of Electronic Evidence.	39(2)	Opinion of Examiner of Electronic Evidence.	Heading is dropped as section is added as a subsection
47	Evidence of character or previous sexual experience not relevant in certain cases	53A	Evidence of character or previous sexual experience not relevant in certain cases	-
60	Oral evidence to be direct	55	Oral evidence to be direct	-
61	Proof of contents of documents	56	Proof of contents of documents	-
62	Primary evidence.	57	Primary evidence.	-
63	Secondary evidence	58	Secondary evidence	-
64	Proof of documents by primary evidence	59	Proof of documents by primary evidence	-
65	Cases in which secondary evidence relating to documents may be given.	60	Cases in which secondary evidence relating to documents may be given.	

Contd.

Contd.

-	-	61	**Electronic or digital record. -** Nothing in this Adhiniyam shall apply to deny the admissibility of an electronic or digital record in the evidence on the ground that it is an electronic or digital record and such record shall, subject to section 63, have the same legal effect, validity and enforceability as other document.	**New Addition in BSA**
65B	Admissibility of electronic records.	63	Admissibility of electronic records.	-
101	Burden of proof	104	Burden of proof	-
118	Who may testify.	124	Who may testify.	The word **"Lunatic" is replaced by "A person of unsound mind"**.
137	Examination of witnesses.	142	Examination of witnesses.	-
138	Order of examinations	143	Order of examinations	-
139	Cross- examination of person called to produce a document.	144	Cross- examination of person called to produce a document.	-
141	Leading questions	146(1)	Leading questions	-
142	When they (leading) must not be asked.	146(2)&(3)	When they (leading) must not be asked.	-
143	When they (leading) may be asked.	146(4)	When they (leading) may be asked.	-
147	When witness to be compelled to answer.	150	When witness to be compelled to answer.	-
157	Former statements of witness may be proved to corroborate later testimony as to same fact	160	Former statements of witness may be proved to corroborate later testimony as to same fact	-
159	Refreshing memory.	162	Refreshing memory.	-
165	Judge's power to put questions or order production.	168	Judge's power to put questions or order production.	-

Index

D

E

T